PATIENT CARE STANDARDS

Nursing Process, Diagnosis, and Outcome

WITHDRAWN

PATIENT CARE STANDARDS

Nursing Process, Diagnosis, and Outcome

SUSAN MARTIN TUCKER, R.N., M.S.N., P.H.N.

Director of Nursing
Kaiser Permanente Medical Center
Panorama City, California

MARY M. CANOBBIO, R.N., M.N.

Cardiovascular Clinical Specialist
Assistant Clinical Professor, School of Nursing
University of California, Los Angeles
Los Angeles, California

ELEANOR VARGO PAQUETTE, R.N., B.S., P.H.N.

Assistant Director of Education and Training
Department of Education and Training
Kaiser Foundation Health Plan of North Carolina
Raleigh, North Carolina

MARJORIE FYFE WELLS, R.N., B.S., P.H.N.

Director of Illness Prevention Clinic
Senior Citizen's Guild
Ann Arbor, Michigan

FIFTH EDITION

with 315 illustrations

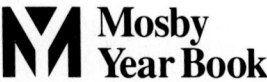
Mosby Year Book

St. Louis Baltimore Boston Chicago London Philadelphia Sydney Toronto

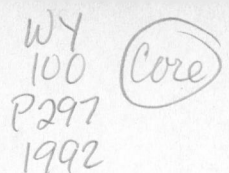 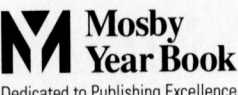

Mosby
Year Book
Dedicated to Publishing Excellence

Editor: Terry Van Schaik
Developmental Editor: Janet R. Livingston
Project Manager: John Rogers
Senior Production Editor: Helen Hudlin
Production Editor: Shauna Burnett Sticht
Manuscript Editors: Joseph Lawler, Roger McWilliams
Book and Cover Design: Gail Morey Hudson

FIFTH EDITION

Mosby–Year Book, Inc.
11830 Westline Industrial Drive, St. Louis, Missouri 63146

Library of Congress Cataloging in Publication Data
Patient care standards : nursing process, diagnosis, and outcome /
Susan Martin Tucker . . . [et al.].—5th ed.
    p.cm.
    Includes bibliographical references and index.
    ISBN 0-8016-6268-0
    1. Nursing—Standards. I. Tucker, Susan Martin, 1943—
    [DNLM: 1. Nursing Care—standards. 2. Patient Care Planning
    —standards. WY 100 P297]
    RT85.5.P38 1991
    610.73'0218—dc20
    DNLM/DLC
    for Library of Congress
                                                                    91-36073
                                                                    CIP

92 93 94 95 96 GW/MV 9 8 7 6 5 4 3 2 1

TO THE FIFTH EDITION

S. LORRAINE DASKAL, R.N., M.S.N.

Clinical Nurse Specialist
Department of Education and Training
Kaiser Permanente Medical Center
Los Angeles, California

EZELIA R. GOODE, R.N., M.S.N.

Clinical Nurse Specialist
Department of Education and Training
Kaiser Permanente Medical Center
West Los Angeles, California

TO THE FOURTH EDITION

DIANE COOPER, R.N., M.N.

Lecturer, School of Nursing
University of California
Los Angeles, California

DIANE R. DANMEYER, R.N., F.N.P., M.N.

Parent-Child Clinical Nurse Specialist
Pediatric Supervisor, Kaiser Permanente Medical Center
Anaheim, California

S. LORRAINE DASKAL, R.N., M.S.N.

Clinical Nurse Specialist
Department of Education and Training
Kaiser Permanente Medical Center
Los Angeles, California

EZELIA R. GOODE, R.N., M.S.N.

Clinical Nurse Specialist
Department of Education and Training
Kaiser Permanente Medical Center
West Los Angeles, California

CHRISTINE F. RODEMICH, R.N., B.S.N., M.S.N

Assistant Professor of Allied Health
Glendale Community College
Glendale, California

RENATA A. SZLAKIEWICZ-JONES, R.N., M.N.

Clinical Educator
Department of Education and Training
Kaiser Permanente Medical Center
Bellflower, California

SARAH MOTTRAM VAUGHAN, B.S.N., M.S.N.

Pediatric Clinical Specialist
Southern Connecticut State University
New Haven, Connecticut

MICKIE D. WELSH, R.N., M.S.N.

Former Lecturer, School of Nursing
University of California
Los Angeles, California

ELLEN R. WHALEN, R.N., M.S.N.

Director, Medical Nursing Services
USC University Hospital
Los Angeles, California

MARY E. WILLMANN, R.N.

Pediatric Clinician
Utilization Review Coordinator
Kaiser Permanente Medical Center
Los Angeles, California

KATHRYN ADAMS, R.N.

Ophthalmology Nurse
Ann Arbor, Michigan

JAN TRESTON AURAND, R.N., M.S.N.

Infection Control Practitioner
Catherine McAuley Health Center
Ann Arbor, Michigan

JANET T. BARRETT, R.N., Ph.D.

Director, B.S.N. Program
Deaconess College of Nursing
St. Louis, Missouri

CORAZON G. BARRIOS, R.N., M.S.N

Department Administrator
Education and Training
Kaiser Permanente Medical Center
Los Angeles, California

BARBARA BOYLAN-LEWIS, R.N., B.S.N., M.A.

Enterostomal Therapist
Catherine McAuley Health Center
Ann Arbor, Michigan

BARBARA J. BOSS, R.N., Ph.D.

Professor of Nursing
University of Mississippi Medical Center
Jackson, Mississippi

TONI CASCIO, R.N., C.C.R.N., M.N.

Clinical Educator—Critical Care
Ochsner Foundation Hospital
New Orleans, Louisiana

FRANCIS CHUNG, Pharm.D.

Pharmacist Specialist—Oncology
Kaiser Permanente Medical Center
Los Angeles, California

JACQUELINE J. CLIBOURN, R.N.

Product Manager, Blood Bank Marketing
Haemonetics Corporation
Braintree, Massachusetts

DIANE COOPER, R.N., M.N.

Lecturer, School of Nursing
University of California, Los Angeles
Los Angeles, California

EMIGDIA DUARTE, R.N., B.S.N.

Member Health Educator
Certified Diabetic Practitioner
Kaiser Permanente Medical Center
Los Angeles, California

WANDA CLEVELAND DUBUISSON, B.S., M.N.

Assistant Professor of Nursing
University of Southern Mississippi
Hattiesburg, Mississippi

FRANCES R. EASON, R.N.C., Ed.D.

Professor
School of Nursing
East Carolina University
Greenville, North Carolina

MIKEL GRAY, C.U.R.N., Ph.D.

Clinical Urodynamics
Egelston Children's Hospital
Scottish Rite Children's Hospital
Shepherd Spinal Center
Atlanta, Georgia

BARBARA N. GRIMM, R.N., B.S.

Assistant Director of Nursing
Labor and Delivery/Pediatrics
Kaiser Permanente Medical Center
Panorama City, California

DEBRA HAIRE-JOSHU, R.N., Ph.D.

Director, Diabetes Education Center
Washington University School of Medicine
St. Louis, Missouri

MARCIA J. HILL, R.N., M.S.N.

Manager, Nursing
Methodist Hospital
Clinical Assistant Professor
Department of Dermatology
Baylor College of Medicine
Houston, Texas

CHRISTINA BERGH JACKSON, C.R.N.P., M.S.N.

Faculty, Eastern College
St. Davids, Pennsylvania
Pediatric Nurse Practitioner
Chestnut Grove Pediatrics
Coatesville, Pennsylvania

MERTIE JONES, C.U.R.N., B.S.N., M.Ed.

Staff Nurse, PACU
Cox Medical Center
Springfield, Missouri

CHARMAINE KLEIBER, R.N., C.P.N.P., M.S.

Clinical Nurse Specialist II
Pediatric Nursing
University of Iowa Hospitals and Clinics
Iowa City, Iowa

GAIL L. KONGABLE, C.C.R.N., C.N.R.N., B.S.N.

Assistant Professor
University of Virginia Health Sciences Center
Charlottesville, Virginia

EDWINA A. McCONNELL, R.N., Ph.D.

Independent Nurse Consultant
Madison, Wisconsin

NOELLA McCRAY, R.N., O.C.N., M.N.

Director, Oncology Program
Independence Regional Health Center
Independence, Missouri

ROYANNE A. MOORE, R.N.C.C., M.S.N.

OB/GYN Nurse Practitioner in Private Practice
Adjunct Faculty
Vanderbilt University School of Nursing
Nashville, Tennessee

JUDITH L. MYERS, R.N., M.S.N.

Assistant Professor
St. Louis University
St. Louis, Missouri

MARIE NEATON, R.N., C.S., M.S.

Clinical Nurse Specialist
Catherine McAuley Health Center
Ann Arbor, Michigan

JOYCE POWERS, R.N., C.S., M.S.N.

Clinical Nurse Specialist
Cardiology Consultants
Albuquerque, New Mexico

CATHERINE R. RATLIFF, R.N., C.S., C.E.T.N., M.S.

Clinical Nurse Specialist
University of Texas M.D. Anderson Cancer Center
Houston, Texas

EUGENE RODRIQUEZ, R. Ph.

Kaiser Permanente Medical Center
Panorama City, California

LEONARD SADOFF, M.D.

Internal Medicine
Oncology Specialist
Kaiser Permanente Medical Group
Los Angeles, California

CARRALEE SUEPPEL, R.N., C.U.R.N., B.L.S.

Clinical Nursing Specialist
Urology Nursing
University of Iowa Hospitals and Clinics
Iowa City, Iowa

LYNNE ANN THELAN, R.N., M.N.

Critical Care Consultant
La Jolla, California

SARAH JANE TOBIASON, R.N., M.A.

Assistant Professor
Arizona State University College of Nursing
Tempe, Arizona

MARY WALLACE, R.N.C., M.S.N.

Associate Professor
Department of Nursing
Northern Michigan University
Marquette, Michigan

SUSAN M. WEINER, R.N.C., M.S.N.

Perinatal Clinical Nurse Specialist
Thomas Jefferson University Family Center
Philadelphia, Pennsylvania

PREFACE

Welcome to the fifth edition of *Patient Care Standards*. We are pleased to offer this revised volume to help you continue promoting consistency, continuity, and quality care. Many of you have used this book as your primary source of patient care plans and now that the Nursing Care Standards of The Joint Commission on Accreditation of Healthcare Organizations (JCAHO) have been revised, this book may serve more of you as your single source of patient care guidelines. The JCAHO standards require that each patient's nursing care be based on a nursing diagnosis or patient's need/problem that is identified as the end result of the assessment process. This is achieved when objective and subjective data that is collected by competent nursing staff members is assessed by the registered nurse through a process of cognitive synthesis of the information. The end result of this assessment process is the identification of the nursing diagnosis or patient's need/problem. The care that is planned and subsequently provided based on the assessment should be consistent with the therapies of other disciplines.

Policies and procedures can describe the role and use of patient care standards in implementing interdisciplinary treatment plans and describe how nursing diagnoses and standards of care will guide the nurse in providing care to patients. According to the JCAHO, protocols and guidelines such as *Patient Care Standards* can be used to achieve this purpose for specific patient populations. Although JCAHO does not require a written plan of care, licensing agencies or other regulatory bodies may require them. In that event *Patient Care Standards* can be used as the source to create individualized, goal-directed written plans of care for patients.

The initial edition of *Patient Care Standards* was the first major book on standards of patient care when it was published in the mid 1970s. Over the years we have significantly changed the format and updated the content to ensure usable, readily retrievable guidelines for patient care. We are proud that this book has become the foundation for many others who have emulated its format for more limited patient populations because such texts also serve to assist the nurse in providing quality patient care. As inpatient length of stays decrease and acuity increases, and as nursing care time becomes more valuable, *Patient Care Standards* can contribute to efficient operations by providing the nurse with instant information.

Some of the changes you will find in this edition include an Expected Outcome/Evaluation section for each nursing diagnosis. Essentially this is stated in a manner to effect goal-directed patient care in achieving the identified expected outcome. Other new information includes standards on cardiac transplantation, biliary lithotripsy, thrombolytic therapy, use of leech therapy for digital transplantation, and a broadened Neoplasia chapter with care designated for oncologic emergencies and biological response modifiers. A new chapter is provided on immune diseases, and each of the other chapters has been updated to reflect the dynamic changes in medical and nursing practice.

The first chapter includes specific North American Nursing Diagnosis Association (NANDA) nursing diagnoses and care for physiologic and psychobehavioral patterns, as well as some general care standards that relate to patients with special needs and special equipment. The subsequent chapters are divided into body systems, and the related standards are preceded by an extensive assessment tool.

To assist the nurse in the nursing process, each standard has been divided into sections. The following describes the components of most of the standards.

Title. The medical condition, surgical intervention, procedure, or pharmacologic agent that is the basis for the standard is identified.

Definition. A brief description of the condition, surgical procedure, disease, or condition is given.

Assessment

Observations/findings. Defining characteristics, as well as objective and subjective signs and symptoms, are presented. Generally for medical conditions the observations/findings listed are what one would most expect to see. In contrast those listed for surgical procedures are provided as a patient-monitoring guide to prevent complications and promote a positive outcome.

Laboratory/diagnostic studies. Condition-appropriate studies are identified, as well as some laboratory values and trends.

Potential complications. Potential condition/procedure-related complications are identified. Nursing interventions are directed toward preventing these complications.

Medical management. Major therapeutic interventions are listed, as well as those functions requiring a physician's orders.

Nursing diagnoses/interventions/evaluation

Nursing diagnoses. Nursing diagnoses are listed in a priority sequence and are those most commonly associated with the condition. They are related to the etiologies or other factors from the assessment data to assist the nurse in understanding the reason or rationale for performing the intervention. NANDA–approved nursing diagnoses are used except on rare occasions, and these exceptions are clearly identified in a footnote.

Interventions. Nursing care activities are prioritized under the specific nursing diagnosis. They describe actions to perform in order to achieve the specific identified outcome and to prevent complications. Some rationales are linked with the intervention when it is of utmost importance.

Patient teaching relating to cognitive, affective, and psychomotor skills based on patient education are identified under the nursing diagnosis "knowledge deficit."

Expected outcome/evaluation. Summary statements reflect goal attainment and provide an indicator of the quality and appropriateness of care resulting in a positive patient outcome.

Patient Care Standards can be used by the bedside nurse for reference when caring for the hospitalized patient; the primary nurse, case manager, team leader, or clinical specialist can use them as a guide to patient care planning and patient/family education; the nursing administrator, nurse manager and quality assurance staff should find them invaluable in assuring the quality and appropriateness of care. They should prove to be an important study aid for the student nurse, giving a concise overview of standards of care related to a specific patient condition. They should also be useful to nurses who come in contact with clients outside the acute care hospital, including skilled nursing and extended care facilities, as well as public health nurses, home health nurses, and those engaged in discharge planning, utilization review, quality assurance, patient teaching, and administration of ambulatory outpatient care facilities. Staff development educators should find the standards helpful in the identification of nursing performance problems that are resolved by planned educational experiences.

Patient Care Standards is presented to promote continuity, consistency, and quality care and to promote the delivery of safe, effective, and appropriate care by guiding nurses in implementing the nursing process using nursing diagnoses and providing a tool to evaluate the outcome of patient care.

Susan Martin Tucker
Mary M. Canobbio
Eleanor Vargo Paquette
Marjorie Fyfe Wells

CONTENTS

1 GENERAL CARE AND NURSING DIAGNOSES, 1

Standards of Care Related to Nursing Diagnoses, 1
Functional Health Pattern I: Health Perception/
  Management, 1
  Potential for infection, 1
  Potential for injury, 2
Functional Health Pattern II: Nutritional/Metabolic, 3
  Altered nutrition: more than body requirements, 3
  Altered nutrition: less than body requirements, 3
  Altered oral mucous membrane, 4
  Potential impaired skin integrity, 5
  Potential altered body temperature, 6
Functional Health Pattern III: Elimination, 6
  Constipation, 6
  Diarrhea, 7
  Altered patterns of urinary elimination, 7
Functional Health Pattern IV: Activity/Exercise, 8
  Potential activity intolerance, 8
  Impaired physical mobility, 8
Functional Health Pattern V: Sleep/Rest, 9
  Sleep pattern disturbance, 9
Functional Health Pattern VI: Cognitive/Perceptual, 10
  Pain, 10
  Knowledge deficit (specify), 10
  Altered thought processes, 11
  Decisional conflict, 12
Functional Health Pattern VII: Self-Perception/Self-
  Concept, 13
  Anxiety, 13
  Hopelessness, 15
  Body image disturbance, 16
  Self-esteem disturbance, 17
  Personal identity disturbance, 18
Functional Health Pattern VIII: Role/Relationship, 18
  Dysfunctional grieving, 18
  Altered role performance, 19
  Potential for violence: self-directed or directed at others, 19
  Impaired social interaction, 22
Functional Health Patterns X: Coping/Stress
  Tolerance, 25
  Ineffective individual coping, 25
Functional Health Patterns XI: Value/Belief, 26
  Spiritual distress (distress of the human spirit), 26
Care of Patient with Special Needs, 27
  General preoperative care/teaching, 27
  Recovery room care, 28
  Care of the aging patient, 29
  Care of the dying patient, 30
  Enteral nutrition, 32
  Total parenteral nutrition (TPN), 36
Care of Patient with Special Equipment, 53
  Central lines, 53
  Intravenous continuous drip narcotics, 58
  Patient-controlled analgesia (PCA), 59

Permanent epidural catheter, 59
Transcutaneous electrical nerve stimulation (TENS), 60

2 CARDIOVASCULAR SYSTEM, 63

Cardiovascular assessment, 63
Peripheral vascular assessment, 68
Venous thrombosis, 70
Vein ligation and stripping, 72
Chronic arterial insufficiency, 73
Carotid endarterectomy, 75
Aortofemoral bypass graft, 77
Hypertensive crisis, 78
Angina pectoris, 81
Acute myocardial infarction (AMI), 85
Vasodilator drugs, 88
  Sodium nitroprusside (Nipride), 88
  Nitrates, 89
  Hydralazine, 90
  Prazosin, 90
  Nifedipine, 91
  Captopril, 91
Infective endocarditis, 91
Valvular heart disease, 95
Pericarditis, 98
Pericardiocentesis, 100
Cardiac tamponade, 100
Heart failure, 101
Shock, 105
Cardiac surgery (open-heart procedure), 108
Cardiac transplantation, 115
Postcardiac injury syndrome, 116
Cardiac rehabilitation, 116
ECG rhythms, 120
Pacemaker insertion, 134
Automatic implantable cardioverter-defibrillator
  (AICD), 138
Cardiac catheterization, 139
Percutaneous transluminal coronary angioplasty
  (PTCA), 140
Thrombolytic therapy, 142
Hemodynamic monitoring, 143
Anticoagulant therapy, 148

3 HEMATOLOGICAL SYSTEM, 152

Hematological assessment, 152
Pernicious anemia (Hyperchromic macrocytic anemia), 155
Iron deficiency anemia (Hypochromic, microcytic
  anemia), 158
Hemolytic anemia, 160
Sickle cell anemia and crisis, 162
Aplastic anemia, 164
Polycythemia, 169
Thrombocytopenia, 171
Disseminated intravascular coagulation (DIC), 173

Splenectomy, 175
Apheresis therapy, 177
Blood transfusions, 179

4 RESPIRATORY SYSTEM, 186

Respiratory assessment, 186
Therapeutic bronchoscopy, 191
Thoracentesis, 192
Aspiration of secretions, 193
Oxygen therapy, 194
Humidity and aerosol therapy, 196
Chronic obstructive pulmonary disease (COPD), Chronic
    obstructive lung disease (COLD), 196
Asthma, 202
Pulmonary rehabilitation, 204
Pneumonia/pneumonilis, 205
Pulmonary edema, 209
Pulmonary embolism, 211
Pulmonary hypertension, 212
Pulmonary tuberculosis, 214
Pneumothorax, 216
    Tension pneumothorax, 216
    Hemothorax, 217
Thoracic empyema, 219
Atelectasis, 220
Pleural effusion, 221
Flail chest, 222
Respiratory failure, 223
Adult respiratory distress syndrome (ARDS), 225
Thoracotomy, lobectomy, pneumonectomy, 227
Chest tubes, 229
Artificial airways, 230
    Oral (oropharyngeal) airway, 230
    Nasal, 230
    Nasopharyngeal airway, 230
Endotracheal tube, 231
Tracheostomy, 232
Continuous mechanical ventilation, 235
    Care of patient on continuous mechanical
        ventilation, 235
    Pressure-limited positive-pressure ventilator, 236
    Volume-cycled positive-pressure ventilator, 236
Intermittent positive pressure breathing (IPPB), 237
Incentive spirometer, 238

5 DIGESTIVE SYSTEM, 240

Gastrointestinal assessment, 240
Esophagus, 243
Esophageal stricture, esophagitis, achalasia,
    diverticulosis, 243
Bleeding esophageal varices, 244
Esophageal surgery, 246
Endoscopy: esophageal, gastric, duodenal, 247
Segstaken-Blakemore tube or Linton tube, 248
Stomach, 249
Anorexia nervosa/bulemia nervosa, 249
Peptic ulcer disease (gastric and duodenal), 252
Gastric bleeding, 253
Gastric surgery, 254

Dumping syndrome, 256
Surgical intervention for obesity, 257
Nasogastric tubes, 262
Esophagostomy, gastrostomy, duodenostomy-jejunostomy
    management, 263
Intestine, 265
Inflammatory bowel disease: regional enteritis (Crohn's
    disease) and ulcerative colitis, 265
Peritonitis, 267
Short bowel syndrome, 268
Intestinal obstruction, 269
Paralytic ileus, 271
Diverticular disease of colon, 272
Intestinal surgery, 273
Continent ileostomy (Knock's pouch), 275
Ileoanal reservoir, 279
Care of naso-oral intestinal tube (Cantor or Miller-Abbott
    tube), 282
Ileostomy, colostomy management, 283
Colostomy irrigation, 285
Rectal surgery, 286
Gallbladder, 287
Biliary obstruction (stones, infection), 287
Biliary surgery, 288
Biliary lithotripsy, 290
Laproscopic, endoscopic laser cholecystectomy, 291
T tube management, 292
Transhepatic, bilary decompression catheter
    management, 292
Liver, 293
Cirrhosis: portal, postnecrotic, biliary, 293
Viral hepatitis, 295
Hepatic surgery, 298
Portacaval-splenorenal shunts for portal hypertension, 299
Liver biopsy, 302
Pancreas, 302
Acute and chronic pancreatitis, 302
Pancreatic surgery, 304

6 ENDOCRINE SYSTEM, 308

Endocrine assessment, 308
Hypothyroidism: myxedema, 312
Hyperthyroidism: thyroid crisis (storm, thyrotoxic
    crisis), 315
Hypoparathyroidism, 318
Hyperparathyroidism, 320
Adrenocortical insufficiency, 322
Cushing's syndrome and Cushing's disease, 324
Primary aldosteronism, 326
Pheochromocytoma, 328
Hypopituitarism, 329
Central diabetes insipidus, 330
Diabetes mellitus, 332
Diabetic ketoacidosis (DKA), 340
Hyperosmolar hyperglycemic nonketotic coma
    (HHNC), 343
Hypoglycemia, 343
Surgical Interventions, 345
Thyroidectomy, 345

Parathyroidectomy, 347
Adrenalectomy, 347
Hypophysectomy, 349

7 MUSCULOSKELETAL SYSTEM, 353

Musculoskeletal assessment, 353
Orthopedic sepsis: acute pyogenic arthritis, acute osteomyelitis, 355
Progressive systemic sclerosis (scleroderma), 356
Gouty arthritis, 358
Fractures, 359
Maxillomandibular fixation, 361
Spinal surgery, 362
Fracture or dislocation of cervical spine, 365
Ankylosing spondylitis, 367
Hip surgery, 368
Total joint arthroplasty: hip, knee, ankle, shoulder, elbow, wrist, finger, 370
Amputation of leg: above or below knee, 374
Arthroscopic surgery of knee, 376
External fixation for complicated fractures, 377
Digital replantation, 379
Compartment syndrome, 382
Tissue pressure monitoring, 384
Bunionectomy (Keller or Mayo arthroplasty), 384
Traction management, 385
Cast management, 385
Continuous passive motion device, 389

8 NEUROLOGICAL SYSTEM, 391

Neurological assessment, 391
Diagnostic procedures, 396
Care of patient with altered consciousness, 396
Seizure disorder (convulsions, epilepsy), 399
Cerebrovascular disruptions, 402
Cerebrovascular accident (CVA) (stroke), 404
Brain tumors, 408
Craniocerebral trauma, 411
Spinal cord injuries, 413
Surgical intervention of central nervous system, 416
Alzheimer's disease, 418
Parkinson's disease, 419
Multiple sclerosis (disseminated sclerosis), 422
Myasthenia gravis, 424
Myasthenia gravis crisis, cholinergic crisis, 426
Amyotrophic lateral sclerosis (ALS), 427
Guillain-Barré Syndrome (acute infectious polyneuritis; polyradiculitis), 429
Neurological infections, 432
Substance abuse (drug abuse and intoxication), 434
Lumbar puncture (spinal tap), 437
Hypothermia: care of patient, 438
Increased intracranial pressure (ICP), 439
Intracranial pressure (ICP) monitoring, 440
Bowel training, 441
Skull tongs and halo traction, 441
Care of patient on a circle bed, 442
Stryker frame, 442
General rehabilitative care of neurological patient, 442

Paraplegia, 444
Quadriplegia, 445

9 GENITOURINARY SYSTEM, 447

Genitourinary assessment, 447
Urinary tract infection (UTI), 451
Urinary incontinence, 453
    Functional incontinence, 453
    Stress incontinence, 455
    Reflex incontinence, 457
    Urge incontinence, 459
    Total incontinence, 460
Acute urinary retention, 462
Surgery for female urinary incontinence, 464
Artificial urinary sphincter (AUS), 466
Indwelling urethral catheter management, 469
Urinary diversion, 470
Polycystic kidney disease, 475
Glomerulonephritis, 477
Urinary calculi (urolithiasis), 479
Renal failure, 482
Peritoneal dialysis, 486
Care of patient after hemodialysis, 490
Nephrectomy: total/partial, 493
Renal transplant: care of recipient, 497
Prostatic hypertrophy, 501
Prostatectomy, 502
Penile implant, 506

10 FEMALE REPRODUCTIVE SYSTEM, 510

Female reproductive system assessment, 510
Pelvic inflammatory disease (PID), 513
Toxic shock syndrome (TSS), 514
Hydatidiform mole, 515
Dilation and curettage (D & C), 515
Tubal pregnancy and salpingectomy, 516
Total abdominal hysterectomy and bilateral salpino-oophorectomy (TAH-BSO), 518

11 INTEGUMENTARY SYSTEM, 521

Integumentary system assessment, 521
Pressure ulcer, 523
Cellulitis, 525
Burn management, 525

12 OPTIC AND AUDITORY SYSTEMS, 532

Optic system assessment, 532
Visually impaired patient, 533
Acute glaucoma: adult onset, 535
Eye surgery, 536
Contact lens removal, 538
Instillation of eye drops/ointments, 539
Auditory system assessment, 539
Auditory-impaired patient, 540
Ear surgeries, 541

13 IMMUNE SYSTEM, 544

Immune system assessment, 544
Acquired immune deficiency syndrome (AIDS), 546
Rheumatoid arthritis, 558
Systemic lupus erythematosus (SLE), 560
Sarcoidosis, 563
Bone marrow transplantation (BMT), 565

14 NEOPLASIA, 581

Cancer detection and prevention, 581
  General, 581
  Skin cancer, 581
  Cancer of head and neck, 582
  Lung cancer, 582
  Cancer of esophagus and stomach, 583
  Colorectal cancer, 584
  Renal, pelvis, and bladder cancer and cancer of ureter and urethra, 585
  Testicular cancer, 586
  Prostate cancer, 587
  Breast cancer, 587
  Vaginal cancer, 590
  Ovarian cancer, 590
  Cervical cancer, 591
  Uterine cancer (endometrial), 591
  Leukemia, 592
  Hodgkin's disease, 593
Oncology assessment, 593
  Laryngectomy: radical neck dissection, 600
  Esophageal carcinoma, 603
  Gastric carcinoma, 605
  Intestinal carcinoma, 606
  Hepatic carcinoma, 607
  Pancreatic carcinoma, 610
  Osteosarcoma, 611
  Orchiectomy for testicular tumor, 613
  Modified radical mastectomy, 614
  Radical hysterectomy, 616
  Vulvectomy, 617
  Pelvic exenteration, 619
  Choriocarcinoma, 621
  Acute leukemia, 621
  Multiple myeloma, 625
  Hodgkin's disease, 628
  Malignant lymphoma, 632
Oncologic Emergencies, 634
  Hematological emergencies, 634
  Cardiovascular emergencies, 635
  Metabolic emergencies, 636
  Neurological emergency, 638
  Pulmonary emergencies, 638
Renal emergency, 639
Cancer therapy, 641
  Surgery, 641
  Radiotherapy, 642
  Care of patient receiving radium (Cesium) therapy sealed in a mould, afterloader, colpostat, or Ernst applicator, 644
  Unsealed radioactive therapy, 648
  Antineoplastic chemotherapy, 649

Safety in handling cancer chemotherapy agents, 667
Extravasation, 669
Symptomatic care in chemotherapy, 670
  Hematological, 670
    Leukopenia, 670
    Thrombocytopenia, 672
    Anemia, 674
  Gastrointestinal, 675
    Nausea, vomiting, and anorexia, 675
    Stomatitis/mucositis, 677
    Diarrhea, 678
    Constipation, 679
  Integumentary, 680
    Dermatological, 680
    Alopecia, 681
  Cardiotoxicity, 682
  Pulmonary toxicity, 683
  Renal, 683
    Nephrotoxicity, 683
    Hemorrhagic cystitis, 684
  Neurotoxicity, 685
  Hepatotoxicity, 686
  Gonadal dysfunction, 687
Biological response modifiers, 687

15 PERINATAL/NEONATAL STANDARDS, 695

Mother, 695
Antepartum assessment, 695
Pregnancy-induced hypertension (PIH; preeclampsia), 697
Eclampsia, 701
Hyperemesis gravidarum, 702
Amniocentesis, 703
Care of diabetic mother during last trimester of pregnancy, 704
Care of diabetic mother during labor and delivery, 705
Premature rupture of membranes (PROM), 706
Placenta previa, 707
Abruptio placentae, 708
Prolapsed umbilical cord, 709
Preterm labor, 711
Care of mother in first stage of labor, 714
Procedural care of mother during delivery: second stage of labor, 717
Oxytocin infusion: augmentation or induction of labor, 718
Fetal distress, 720
Care of mother on fetal monitor, 722
Nonstress test (NST), 722
Contraction stress test (CST), 723
Postpartum care, 724
Cesarean delivery, 728
Breast-feeding, 731
Postpartum hemorrhage, 734
Newborn, 735
Care of newborn, 735
Care of premature infant, 740
Small for gestational age (small for date, low birth weight, intrauterine growth retardation, dysmaturity), 742
Large for gestational age (dysmaturity, high birth weight), 742

Postterm infant (postmaturity), 743
Infant of diabetic mother (IDM), 744
Care of infant with hyperbilirubinemia, 745
Exchange transfusion, 747
Umbilical catheterization, 748
Neonatal sepsis, 749
Neonatal drug withdrawal, 750
Necrotizing enterocolitis (NEC), 752
TORCH infections, 753
Respiratory distress syndrome (hyaline membrane disease), 755
Meconium aspiration syndrome, 756
Care of newborn with endotracheal tube, 757
Care of newborn on a ventilator, 758
Bronchopulmonary dysplasia, 758
Intermittent gavage feeding, 760
Family-centered care of high-risk infant, 761

16   PEDIATRICS, 763

Basic standards of care, 763
Infant age-group care, 763
Toddler age-group care, 766
Preschool-age child care, 766
School-age child care, 767
Adolescent age-group care, 770
Respiratory system, 770
Croup: laryngotracheobronchitis, 770
Epiglottitis, 776
Pertussis: whooping cough, 777
Pneumonia, 779
Asthma, 780
Bronchiolitis, 782
Cystic fibrosis, 783
Gastrointestinal system, 776
Cleft lip repair, 786
Cleft palate repair, 788
Tracheoesophageal fistula, 789
Tracheoesophageal fistula repair, 791
Pyloric stenosis, 793

Ruptured (perforated) appendix, 794
Hirschsprung's disease: aganglionic megacolon, 796
Abdominoperineal pull-through procedure, 798
Gastroenteritis, 800
Diet for control of diarrhea, 801
Oral rehydration therapy, 802
Incarcerated inguinal hernia, 802
Intussusception, 802
Central nervous system, 803
Hydrocephalus, 803
Ventricular shunt insertion, 805
Myelomeningocele, 806
Meningitis, 810
Genitourinary system, 811
Acute glomerulonephritis, 811
Nephrosis (nephrotic syndrome), 813
Hematology, 815
Acute leukemia, 815
Failure to thrive (FTT), 818
Cardiovascular system, 821
Congenital heart defects, 821
Congenital heart surgery, 828
Preoperative preparation, 828
Palliative procedures, 829
Corrective surgery, 830
Open-heart surgery, 832
Congestive heart failure (CHF), 835
Pediatric digitalis therapy, 836
Temporary artificial pacemaker, 837
Other aspects of pediatrics, 838
Child abuse, 838
Vital signs, 840
Nutrition, 841
Drugs, 843

APPENDIXES

A Medical-surgical care, 845
B Guidelines for patient care planning and nursing care, 847

1

CHAPTER

General Care and Nursing Diagnoses

Standards of Care Related to Nursing Diagnoses

The standards of care in this section are the basic nursing functions required for all patients regardless of medical diagnosis. They are included to assist the nurse in selecting appropriate interventions for the following nursing diagnoses, on which the nurse may act independently. To list by priority and to combine related diagnoses, they are divided into Functional Health Patterns.* The interventions under each diagnosis are not meant to be inclusive, and the nurse must select those that are appropriate based on the related/risk factors and the defining characteristics. The nursing diagnoses included here were accepted in 1989 by the North American Nursing Diagnosis Association (NANDA). This is a partial list of NANDA-approved nursing diagnoses.

Functional Health Pattern I: Health Perception/Management

POTENTIAL FOR INFECTION

Definition† *The state in which an individual is at increased risk for being invaded by pathogenic organisms*

Risk Factors

Inadequate primary defenses (broken skin, traumatized tissue, decrease in ciliary action, stasis of body fluids, change in pH secretions, altered peristalsis)
Inadequate secondary defenses (e.g., decreased hemoglobin, leukopenia, suppressed inflammatory response, immunosuppression)
Inadequate acquired immunity
Tissue destruction and increased environmental exposure
Chronic disease
Invasive procedures
Malnutrition
Pharmaceutical agents and trauma
Rupture of amniotic membranes
Insufficient knowledge to avoid exposure to pathogens

---

*From Thompson JM et al: *Mosby's manual of clinical nursing*, ed 2, St Louis, 1989, CV Mosby.
†Definitions, risk factors/related factors, and defining characteristics in this section for NANDA nursing diagnoses are from Kim MJ et al: *Pocket guide to nursing diagnoses*, ed 4, St Louis, 1991, Mosby-Year Book.

Interventions

Assess body systems for type, location, and cause of infections
  Wear gloves, gown, mask, goggles appropriate to procedure
  Wash hands after each patient contact
Monitor vital signs
Monitor laboratory values; elevated WBC, UTI, positive blood culture
Initiate cooling measures as needed
Administer antipyretics, antibiotics as indicated; assess for effectiveness and side effects
Discuss with and teach patient about adequate nutrition and fluid intake
Provide and review immunization requirements to maintain health
Integumentary
  Maintain aseptic technique during dressing changes and change prn
  Promote and provide skin care and oral hygiene daily and prn
  Assess pressure points prn and apply lotion, protective covering as needed; massage skin only if it is not reddened
  Monitor insertion sites of intravenous and central lines daily
  Maintain sites and dressings according to policy
  Discuss with and teach patient about principles of autocontamination and cross-contamination
Respiratory
  Assess respiration for dyspnea, shortness of breath, rales
  Assess frequency of expectorating; color, consistency of sputum; culture as indicated
  Encourage coughing and deep breathing at least q1hr to 2hr
  Assist with respiratory aids; incentive spirometer, oxygen therapy
  Encourage ambulation or frequent position changes
  Elevate head of bed to promote more comfortable breathing
  Encourage fluid intake to liquefy sputum
Genitourinary
  Maintain closed drainage system for urethral catheters as indicated
  Monitor intake and output
  Provide daily catheter care as indicated
  Culture urine as indicated

1

Expected Outcome/Evaluation

Patient

Understands cause of infection

Expresses knowledge of methods of preventing further or recurring infections

Demonstrates ability to promote own wellness

POTENTIAL FOR INJURY

***Definition** The state in which an individual is at risk of injury as a result of environmental conditions interacting with the individual's adaptive and defensive resources*

Risk Factors

Interactive conditions between individual and environment that impose a risk to defensive and adaptive resources of individual

Internal

Biochemical

Regulatory function

Sensory dysfunction

Integrative dysfunction

Effector dysfunction

Tissue hypoxia

Malnutrition

Immune-autoimmune

Abnormal blood profile

Leukocytosis or leukopenia

Altered clotting factors

Thrombocytopenia

Sickle cell

Thalassemia

Decreased hemoglobin

Physical

Broken skin

Altered mobility

Developmental

Age

Physiological

Psychosocial

Psychological

Affective

Orientation

External

Biological

Immunization level of community

Microorganism

Chemical

Pollutants

Poisons

Drugs

Pharmaceutical agents

Alcohol

Caffeine

Nicotine

Preservatives

Cosmetics and dyes

Nutrients (vitamins, food types)

Physical

Design, structure, and arrangement of community, building, and/or equipment

Mode of transport/transportation

Nosocomial agents

People/provider

Nosocomial agents

Staffing patterns

Cognitive, affective, and psychomotor factors

Interventions

Assess patient's mental, visual, and auditory acuity

Monitor neuromuscular status, age, medication history, and nutritional status

Assess ability to perform activities of daily living (ADLs), exercises, and to ambulate

Maintain safe environment

Orient patient to surroundings

Provide needed equipment and maintain within easy reach; avoid clutter

Maintain side rail, bed position, and use of restraints per policy as written

Remind patient that there is no smoking in room

Assist patient with ADLs and teach use of safety rules of mobilizing devices as needed

Explain all treatments, procedures, and care

Provide adequate lighting

Instruct patient on safety precautions to observe at home

Maintain electrical and hospital equipment in good repair

Maintain safe medication administration

Monitor laboratory profiles for signs of impending problems

Administer medications according to policy

Understand and monitor side effects

Instruct patient to take medications as prescribed on discharge and explain side effects to report to physician

Advise patient to avoid over-the-counter (OTC) medications unless prescribed by physician

Provide safety teaching according to maturational age

Home hazards

Fire, flammable items

Floor, stairs, ramps

Tubs, showers, pools

Lighting

Chemicals, medications

Expected Outcome/Evaluation

Patient

Demonstrates understanding of potential health hazards

Practices injury prevention measures for self

Remains injury free

Functional Health Pattern II: Nutritional/Metabolic

ALTERED NUTRITION: MORE THAN BODY REQUIREMENTS

Definition The state in which an individual is experiencing an intake of nutrients that exceeds metabolic needs

Related Factor

Excessive intake in relation to metabolic need

Defining Characteristics

Weight 10% over ideal for height and frame
Weight 20% over ideal for height and frame
Triceps skinfold greater than 15 mm in men and 25 mm in women
Sedentary activity level
Reported or observed dysfunctional eating patterns
  Pairing food with other activities
  Concentrating food intake at end of day
  Eating in response to external cues (e.g., time of day, social situation)
  Eating in response to internal cues other than hunger (e.g., anxiety)

Interventions

Assess patient for signs of fluid retention
Weigh patient daily; same clothes, time, and scale
Assess patient's desire for weight loss
Determine triceps fold measurements
Determine ideal body weight (Table 1-1)
Collaborate with dietitian, patient; set realistic goals for weight loss; reward goals attempted and attained
Encourage patient to keep a diary of intake; what, when, and where food is eaten; feelings at time of eating
Emphasize importance of a regular exercise program
Provide information on a weight loss program

Expected Outcome/Evaluation

Patient
  Expresses understanding of factors causing weight gain
  Demonstrates desire to maintain normal weight for age and height

ALTERED NUTRITION: LESS THAN BODY REQUIREMENTS

Definition The state in which an individual experiences an intake of nutrients insufficient to meet metabolic needs

Related Factor

Inability to ingest or digest food or absorb nutrients because of biological, psychological, or economic factors

Defining characteristics

Loss of weight with adequate food intake (Table 1-2)
Body weight 20% or more under ideal for height and frame
Reported inadequate food intake, less than Recommended Daily Allowance
Weakness of muscles required for swallowing or mastication
Reported or evidence of lack of food

TABLE 1-1. Height and Weight Tables with Desirable Weights for Persons Age 25 and Over

Men					Women				
Height		Small frame (lb)	Medium frame (lb)	Large frame (lb)	Height		Small frame (lb)	Medium frame (lb)	Large frame (lb)
Feet	Inches				Feet	Inches			
5	2	128-134	131-141	138-150	4	10	102-111	109-121	118-131
5	3	130-136	133-143	140-153	4	11	103-113	111-123	120-134
5	4	132-138	135-145	142-156	5	0	104-115	113-126	122-137
5	5	134-140	137-148	144-160	5	1	106-118	115-129	125-140
5	6	136-142	139-151	146-164	5	2	108-121	118-132	128-143
5	7	138-145	142-154	149-168	5	3	111-124	121-135	131-147
5	8	140-148	145-157	152-172	5	4	114-127	124-138	134-151
5	9	142-151	148-160	155-176	5	5	117-130	127-141	137-155
5	10	144-154	151-163	158-180	5	6	120-133	130-144	140-159
5	11	146-157	154-166	161-184	5	7	123-136	133-147	143-163
6	0	149-160	157-170	164-188	5	8	126-139	136-150	146-167
6	1	152-164	160-174	168-192	5	9	129-142	139-153	149-170
6	2	155-168	164-178	172-197	5	10	132-145	142-156	152-173
6	3	158-172	167-182	176-202	5	11	135-148	145-159	155-176
6	4	162-176	171-187	181-207	6	0	138-151	148-162	158-179

Weights at ages 25-59 based on lowest mortality.
Weight in pounds according to frame (in indoor clothing weighing 5 pounds, shoes with 1-inch heels).

Weights at ages 25-59 based on lowest mortality.
Weight in pounds according to frame (in indoor clothing weighing 3 pounds, shoes with 1-inch heels).

Metropolitan Life Insurance Co, New York, 1983.

TABLE 1-2. Effect of Some Drugs on Nutritional Status

Drug	Effect
Aspirin	Malabsorption of folate
	Excretion of vitamin C
Barbiturates	Malabsorption of thiamin, vitamin B_{12}
	Excretion of vitamin C
Corticosteroids	Malabsorption of calcium, zinc, phosphorus
Hydralazine	Excretion of pyridoxine
Methotrexate	Malabsorption of vitamin B_{12}, folate, fat
Mineral oil	Malabsorption of fat-soluble vitamins, calcium, phosphorus
Neomycin	Malabsorption of major nutrients
Oral contraceptives	Possible decreased absorption of vitamin C, B complex vitamins, magnesium, zinc
Penicillin	Loss of potassium
Tetracycline	Malabsorption of calcium, iron, magnesium, pyridoxine
	Excretion of vitamin C, riboflavin, niacin, folic acid
Thiazides	Excretion of potassium, magnesium, zinc, riboflavin

Modified from Long BC, Phipps WJ: *Medical-surgical nursing: a nursing process approach*, ed 2, St Louis, 1989, CV Mosby.

Lack of interest in food
Perceived inability to ingest food
Aversion to eating
Reported altered taste sensation
Satiety immediately after ingesting food
Abdominal pain with or without pathological conditions
Sore, inflamed buccal cavity

Interventions

Assess nutritional status, past eating patterns, and medications (see box)
Assess causative factors; anorexia, dysphagia, altered taste, age, unavailability of food
Assess food preferences; likes and dislikes
Monitor intake and weigh daily
Monitor laboratory values; CBC, electrolytes
Assess oral cavity and ability to chew and swallow
Provide meals in quiet environment and encourage patient to eat slowly and chew well
Maintain position of comfort during meals
Encourage family, significant other involvement with meals, eating with patient, bringing food from home
Maintain clean environment to prevent nausea, anorexia
Collaborate with dietitian about special food preparation
Discuss and teach patient/significant other nutritional guidelines, importance of regular meals, and foods to include

---

MEDICATIONS TO BE TAKEN WITH FOOD	
Aminophylline	Nitrofurantoin (Macrodantin)
Chlorothiazide (Diuril)	Phenylbutazone (Butazolidin)
Ferrous sulfate	
Indomethacin (Indocin)	Phenytoin (Dilantin)
	Prednisolone
Metronidazole (Flagyl)	Reserpine (Serpasil)
	Triamterene (Dyrenium)

From Long BC, Phipps WJ: *Medical-surgical nursing: a nursing process approach*, ed 2, St Louis, 1989, CV Mosby.

Expected Outcome/Evaluation

Patient
Expresses understanding of nutritional deficit
Demonstrates knowledge of adequate nutritional intake
Gains weight as needed to meet body needs

ALTERED ORAL MUCOUS MEMBRANE

***Definition** The state in which an individual experiences disruptions in the tissue layers of the oral cavity*

Related Factors

Pathologic conditions: oral cavity (radiation to head and/or neck)
Dehydration
Trauma
Chemical (e.g., acidic foods, drugs, noxious agents, alcohol)
Mechanical (e.g., ill-fitting dentures; braces; tubes: endotracheal, nasogastric; surgery in oral cavity)
NPO instructions for more than 24 hours
Ineffective oral hygiene
Mouth breathing
Malnutrition
Infection
Lack of or decreased salivation
Medication

Defining Characteristics

Coated tongue
Xerostomia (dry mouth)
Stomatitis
Oral lesions or ulcers
Lack of or decreased salivation
Leukoplakia
Edema
Hyperemia
Oral plaque
Oral pain or discomfort

Desquamation
Vesicles
Hemorrhagic gingivitis
Carious teeth
Halitosis

Interventions

Assess mucous membrane, tongue, and gums daily
Observe for moisture, cleanliness, integrity, edema, color, bleeding, and odor
Assess teeth for cleanliness, integrity, sensitivity to heat or cold, presence of dentures, and sordes
Brush teeth bid and prn with toothpaste, powder, baking soda, or mouthwash
Promote regular flossing
Advise to avoid foods that cause discomfort
Encourage adequate fluid intake
Advise to rinse with water or mouthwash
Apply petroleum jelly, lip balm, or glycerin-lemon mixture to lips for dryness
Remove dentures and cleanse bid with toothpaste or powder and running water; protect from breakage and place in marked denture cup when not in use
Cleanse mouth with equal parts of hydrogen peroxide and water prn for sordes
Encourage routine dental checkups

Expected Outcome/Evaluation

Patient
    Demonstrates correct technique to promote proper oral care
    Has oral cavity that is clean, moist, and odor free

POTENTIAL IMPAIRED SKIN INTEGRITY

Definition The state in which an individual's skin is at risk of being adversely altered

Risk Factors

External (environmental)
    Hypothermia or hyperthermia
    Chemical substance
    Mechanical factors
        Shearing forces
        Pressure
        Restraint
    Radiation
    Physical immobilization
    Excretions and secretions
    Humidity
Internal (somatic)
    Medication
    Alterations in nutritional state (obesity, emaciation)
    Altered metabolic state

Altered circulation
Altered sensation
Altered pigmentation
Skeletal prominence
Developmental factors
Alterations in skin turgor (change in elasticity)
Psychogenic
Immunological

Interventions

Assess patient for causative factors
Assess bathing needs; complete or partial bed bath, tub, or shower using warm water and mild superfatted soap
    Provide privacy and avoid chilling
    Massage skin with mild lanolin-based lotions to increase circulation and maintain integrity
    Dry skin thoroughly
Assess skin for redness, lesions, blisters, swelling, or drainage
Monitor for incontinence
Encourage ambulation; limit chair sitting to 1 hour
Assist with and/or teach range-of-motion (ROM) exercises
Provide nutritious diet and adequate fluid intake
Assess perineal and perianal areas as needed; observe for excoriation, vaginal discharge, and pain; apply lotions or cornstarch to area as needed
Assess feet and hands; observe nail beds and observe for signs of rash, dryness, or skin breaks
    Soak in warm soap and water, dry well, and apply lotion prn
    Cleanse and trim nails prn
Assess condition of hair; observe for matting, tangles, signs of alopecia, lice, cradle cap scales, and dryness
    Comb hair daily and shampoo as needed
    Apply baby oil and massage into scalp; leave on 1 hr for scales, then gently shampoo and comb
    Apply alcohol to release tangles
    Style for attractiveness, comfort, and easy care
Assess male patient for shaving needs
    Apply warm towels to face before shaving
    Rinse skin well and apply lotion after shaving
Maintain physical comfort
Change bed linen daily and prn; keep linen neat, dry, wrinkle-free, and clean
Provide adequate warmth
Change position frequently: small changes of body parts prevent pressure and fatigue

Expected Outcome/Evaluation

Patient's
    Skin integrity is maintained
    Impairment is minimal if present
    Maximal circulation is maintained
    Optimal nutrition is demonstrated

POTENTIAL ALTERED BODY TEMPERATURE

Definition The state in which an individual is at risk for failure to maintain body temperature within normal range

Risk Factors

Extremes of age
Extremes of weight
Exposure to cold/cool or warm/hot environments
Dehydration
Inactivity or vigorous activity
Medications causing vasoconstriction/vasodilation, altered metabolic rate, sedation
Inappropriate clothing for environmental temperature
Illness or trauma affecting temperature regulation

Interventions

Hyperthermia
  Assess for causative factors
  Monitor vital signs q1hr
  Monitor intake and output; report output less than 30 ml/hr to physician
  Monitor electrolytes, CBC, glucose
  Monitor for tachycardia, tachypnea
  Maintain parenteral fluids as indicated
  Initiate cooling measures as indicated; cool slowly; handle body gently
    Monitor mental acuity
    Monitor temperature q10min during procedure and q1hr after
    Discontinue cooling measures when temperature is 1° F above normal
    Dry skin thoroughly (avoid friction) and provide clean, dry linen
  Reduce physical activity and urge fluids as tolerated
  Administer prescribed antibiotics and antipyretics
  Reinstitute cooling measures as needed
  Maintain cool room temperature
Hypothermia
  Monitor vital signs q1hr
  Monitor mental acuity
  Initiate warming measures as prescribed—warm slowly; handle body gently
  Monitor for bradycardia, hypotension
  Monitor blood gases, electrolytes, glucose; report abnormal results to physician
  Monitor intake and output q1hr; if less than 30 ml/hr notify physician
  Maintain warm, comfortable environment

Expected Outcome/Evaluation

Patient's
  Temperature is normal
  Vital signs are normal
  Skin is warm and dry

Functional Health Pattern III: Elimination

CONSTIPATION

Definition The state in which an individual experiences a change in normal bowel habits characterized by a decrease in frequency and/or passage of hard, dry stools

Related Factors

Less than adequate intake
Less than adequate dietary intake and bulk
Less than adequate physical activity or immobility
Personal habits
Medications
Chronic use of medication and enemas
Gastrointestinal obstructive lesions
Neuromuscular impairment
Musculoskeletal impairment
Pain on defecation
Diagnostic procedures
Lack of privacy
Weak abdominal musculature
Pregnancy
Emotional status

Defining Characteristics

Frequency less than usual pattern
Hard-formed stool
Palpable mass
Reported feeling of rectal fullness
Straining at stool
Decreased bowel sounds
Reported feeling of abdominal or rectal fullness or pressure
Less than usual amount of stool
Nausea

Other Possible Defining Characteristics

Abdominal pain
Back pain
Headache
Intereference with daily living
Use of laxatives
Decreased appetite
Appetite impairment

Interventions

Assess cause(s) of constipation
Determine normal elimination pattern
Assess daily defecation routine and maintain pattern as much as possible
Provide natural stimulants (coffee, prune juice) as allowed
Maintain privacy
Monitor and record daily bowel movements; monitor for melena as needed
Initiate diet changes to maintain normal consistency; high-fiber foods (fruits, vegetables, whole grains)

Avoid excessive use of bran

Increase activity, exercise, and fluid intake

Provide natural laxatives initially, before administering laxative or enema

Instruct patient to avoid routine use of laxatives

Explain that medications often cause constipation

Explain importance of defecating as soon as urge occurs

Instruct patient to set schedule for defecating daily, such as after a meal

Initiate relaxing techniques to assist in defecation

Reduce rectal pain/discomfort from hemorrhoids through use of lubricants, cool compresses, stool softeners, suppositories

Administer perianal care after each defecation

Expected Outcome/Evaluation

Patient

Expresses understanding of causative factors of constipation

Demonstrates knowledge of importance of diet, fiber, fluids, and exercise

Verbalizes need to avoid straining and using laxatives to defecate

DIARRHEA

Definition The state in which an individual experiences a change in normal bowel habits characterized by the frequent passage of loose, fluid, unformed stools

Related Factors

Stress and anxiety

Dietary intake

Medications

Inflammation, irritation, or malabsorption of bowel

Toxins

Contaminants

Radiation

Defining Characteristics

Abdominal pain

Cramping

Increased frequency

Increased frequency of bowel sounds

Loose, liquid stools

Urgency

Changes in color

Interventions

Assess for causative factors including impaction

Maintain NPO and parenteral fluids as ordered

Collaborate with physician, initiate fluids, and progress to soft, bland diet as tolerated

Avoid irritating foods; milk, caffeine, raw fruits and vegetables

Weigh daily; same time, clothes, and scale

Monitor serum electrolytes

Monitor bowel sounds

Encourage patient to verbalize situations that cause stress

Assist and teach stress management techniques

Assess perineal area for excoriation, irritation

Provide perineal skin care after each bowel movement; apply soothing ointments as indicated

Provide bedpan/commode and keep within easy reach

Maintain uncluttered room for easy access to bathroom; provide a night light

Expected Outcome/Evaluation

Patient

Verbalizes causative factors of diarrhea

Reports improved frequency and consistency of stools

Presents normal electrolytes and fluid intake

ALTERED PATTERNS OF URINARY ELIMINATION

Definition The state in which an individual experiences a disturbance in urine elimination

Related Factors

Sensory motor impairment

Neuromuscular impairment

Mechanical trauma

Defining Characteristics

Dysuria

Frequency

Hesitancy

Incontinence

Nocturia

Retention

Urgency

Interventions

Assess for causative factors

Determine usual urinary pattern

Measure intake and output

Monitor urine for color, frequency, amount, and consistency

Monitor for sugar, acetone, blood, and pH

Monitor for residual urine

Monitor for frequency, urgency, dysuria, and distension

Administer and teach female perineal care after urination; explain correct wiping procedure

Provide privacy

Maintain uncluttered room for easy access to bathroom

Provide a night light

Increase fluid intake, if allowed, to maintain hydration

Institute voiding measures as needed: running water, leaning forward; peppermint in bedpan

Maintain bedpan within easy reach

Monitor indwelling urethral catheters for patency, correct

position of collection unit, and infection; teach self-catheterization as needed

Provide daily meatal care according to hospital policy

Monitor for incontinence

Initiate voiding schedule of q2hr-4hr

Provide protective padding as needed

Expected Outcome/Evaluation

Patient

Expresses understanding of causative factors of altered urinary pattern

Verbalizes and demonstrates correct post-urinating hygiene

Reports urination returning to a normal pattern

Functional Health Pattern IV: Activity/Exercise

POTENTIAL ACTIVITY INTOLERANCE

Definition *The state in which an individual has insufficient physiological or psychological energy to endure or complete requried or desired daily activities*

Related Factors

Generalized weakness

Sedentary lifestyle

Imbalance between oxygen supply and demand

Bed rest or immobility

Defining Characteristics

Verbal report of fatigue or weakness

Abnormal heart rate or blood pressure response to activity

Exertional discomfort or dyspnea

Electrocardiographic changes reflecting dysrhythmias or ischemia

Interventions

Physical

Assess body systems for possible cause of inactivity

Disturbance in oxygen maintenance

Fluid or electrolyte imbalance

Deficiencies in nutrition

Neuromuscular disorders

Observe patient for pain and insufficient rest/sleep

Monitor side effects of all medications and diagnostic studies

Assess patient's tolerance of activity

Assess past activity pattern

Explain procedure, activity, or treatment

Monitor resting vital signs

Have patient perform activity at own rate

Monitor vital signs immediately and again in 3 min

Discontinue activity if any of the following occur

Chest pain, dyspnea, cyanosis, vertigo, confusion, hypotension, failure of systolic pressure increase, increased diastolic pressure, decreased respiratory rate, continuing tachycardia

Reduce energy expenditure where possible

Increase activity slowly to increase patient's tolerance; assist as needed

Coordinate care to allow for rest periods

Maintain and increase strength with active or passive range-of-motion (ROM) exercises

Encourage self-care activities as soon as patient is able

Provide adaptive devices to assist in activities of daily living (ADLs) as needed, such as padded eating utensils, long-handled tongs

Psychological

Assess patient for presence of depression or lack of incentive; assess for maladaptive behaviors

Explain importance of activity to tolerance

Involve patient in care plan and short-term goal setting

Acknowledge and praise attempted or completed tasks

Discuss and assist patient with identifying possible incentives to increase activity

Assist patient in identifying successful past coping behaviors

Involve family/significant other in supporting/participating with patient in daily activities

Expected Outcome/Evaluation

Patient

Participates in activities that increase ability to perform ADLs, other activities

Expresses understanding of a balanced rest/activity program

Seeks support of others to maintain optimal level of activity

IMPAIRED PHYSICAL MOBILITY

Definition *The state in which an individual experiences a limitation of ability for independent physical movement*

Related Factors

Intolerance of activity; decreased strength and endurance

Pain and discomfort

Perceptual or cognitive impairment

Neuromuscular impairment

Musculoskeletal impairment

Depression, severe anxiety

Defining Characteristics

Inability to purposefully move within physical environment, including bed mobility, transfer, and ambulation

Reluctance to attempt movement

Limited range of motion (ROM)

Decreased muscle strength, control, and/or mass

Imposed restrictions of movement, including mechanical, medical protocol

Impaired coordination

Interventions

Assess patient's mobility tolerance and motivation

Maintain circulatory function

Encourage and teach leg exercises q1hr

Apply antiembolic hose

Monitor for thrombophlebitis; pain, warmth, edema of extremity

Assist and teach turning techniques

Monitor vital signs after activity at 3 min and 15 min

Observe for hypertension or hypotension, tachycardia or bradycardia

Maintain respiratory function

Encourage and teach deep breathing q1hr

Assist and teach incentive spirometer

Maintain patent airway

Monitor respirations q1hr-2hr

Increase fluid intake to liquefy secretions

After activity monitor vital signs

Observe for dyspnea, cyanosis, shortness of breath, tachypnea, bradypnea

Maintain normal elimination

Provide increased fluid intake

Encourage exercise activity

Provide diet to promote elimination

Bowel: high fiber, roughage, prunes

Bladder: meat, fish, cereals

Provide privacy

Assist and teach perianal, perineal hygiene

Provide bedpan within easy reach

Maintain musculoskeletal function

Perform active or assist with and teach passive ROM exercises q4h; note tolerance and motivation

Maintain body alignment while in bed

Provide bed cradle as needed

Prevent footdrop with foot board

Support dependent limbs as needed with pillows or immobilizing devices; avoid pillow under knee

Avoid long periods in any one position: frequent small changes prevent pressure, discomfort, and fatigue

Maintain casts, braces, traction, or prosthetic devices in correct position to avoid discomfort or pressure

Help patient progress in mobility slowly as tolerated

Assist patient as needed with sitting up, dangling, standing, and ambulation

Initiate and teach use of mobilizing devices as needed: crutches, walker, wheelchair, sling

Maintain skin integrity

Assess pressure points for signs of breakdown

Administer gentle massage to pressure areas; apply lotion as needed

Encourage activity as tolerated

Prevent shearing force with use of turn sheet

Provide nutritious diet of protein, carbohydrate

Increase fluid intake; monitor intake and output

Maintain psychological integrity

Encourage patient to express fears/anxieties

Promote support of significant others

Provide diversional activities

Encourage self-care involvement

Maintain positive communication

Reinforce positive coping patterns

Expected Outcome/Evaluation

Patient's

Ability to interact with others, make own decisions, and use positive coping behaviors is increasing

Vital signs are normal

Elimination is normal

Activity is at optimal level

Skin integrity is maintained

Functional Health Pattern V: Sleep/Rest

SLEEP PATTERN DISTURBANCE

Definition Disruption of sleep time causes discomfort or interferes with desired lifestyle

Related Factors

Sensory alterations

Internal factors

Illness

Psychological stress

External factors

Environmental changes

Social cues

Defining Characteristics

Verbal complaints of difficulty in falling asleep

Awakening earlier or later than desired

Interrupted sleep

Verbal complaints of not feeling well rested

Changes in behavior and performance

Increasing irritability

Restlessness

Disorientation

Lethargy

Listlessness

Physical signs

Mild, fleeting nystagmus

Slight hand tremor

Ptosis of eyelid

Expressionless face

Thick speech with mispronunciation and incorrect words

Dark circles under eyes

Frequent yawning

Changes in posture

Interventions

Assess and identify risk factors

Assess patient's normal rest/sleep pattern

Control environmental disturbances, noise, and lighting

Maintain quiet environment; close doors, pull drapes and dividers; decrease incoming stimuli

Provide night lights, soft music

Coordinate nursing functions to allow for rest periods and fewer interruptions during night

Limit visitors during rest periods and limit fluid intake where possible after 6 PM

Maintain balance of daytime activity and rest

Increase activity to point of tolerance to promote tiredness

Limit sleep during daytime and stimulate wakefulness as required

Involve in unit and diversional activities

Provide comfort measures

Maintain warm, clean, comfortable bed

Provide needed equipment within easy reach

Encourage usual sleeping aids

Administer hs care as close to bedtime as possible

Monitor sleep medication for effectiveness

Encourage patient to express fears/anxieties that may prevent or disrupt sleep

Monitor for pain, discomfort; administer analgesics

Teach patient alternative pain/stress management techniques

Expected Outcome/Evaluation

Patient

Expresses understanding of causative factors of sleep disturbance

Demonstrates optimal balance of rest and activity

Expresses increased ability to sleep

Functional Health Pattern VI: Cognitive/Perceptual

PAIN

Definition The state in which an individual experiences and reports the presence of severe discomfort or an uncomfortable sensation

Related Factors

Injuring agents
Biological
Chemical
Physical
Psychological

Defining Characteristics

Subjective
Communication (verbal or coded) of pain descriptors
Objective
Guarding behavior; protective
Self-focusing
Narrowed focus (altered time perception, withdrawal from social contact, impaired thought process)
Distraction behavior (moaning, crying, pacing, seeking out other people and/or activities, restlessness)

Facial mask of pain (eyes lack luster, "beaten look," fixed or scattered movement, grimace)

Alteration in muscle tone (may span from listless to rigid)

Autonomic responses not seen in chronic, stable pain (diaphoresis, blood pressure and pulse rate change, pupillary dilation, increased or decreased respiratory rate)

Interventions

Assess location, type, duration, and frequency of pain

Assess intensity of pain using scale 0-5; 0 meaning absence of pain and 5 being intense pain

Assess risk factors

Discuss past effective/ineffective pain relief measures

Assess effect of pain on patient
Altered sleep/activity pattern
Decreased energy, sexual activity
Reduced feelings of self worth

Assess effectiveness of pain-relief measures

Develop trusting relationship
Encourage patient to talk about self
Be a good listener
Avoid judgmental statements
Be truthful and consistent
Accept pain as patient sees it
Set realistic goals
Assist patient with understanding pain
Explain relationship of pain to disease process
Estimate duration of pain when possible
Explain painful procedures realistically

Involve patient in care; allow some control over daily activities where possible

Encourage pain reduction techniques as appropriate:
Rocking movements, external warmth, visual focal point with breathing patterns, imagery, relaxation techniques, touch

Discuss alternate interventions such as biofeedback, TENS unit, hypnosis, self-controlled pain procedure

Encourage support of family/significant others

Expected Outcome/Evaluation

Patient
Expresses understanding of causative factors of pain
Demonstrates ability to reduce or control pain using learned skills

KNOWLEDGE DEFICIT (SPECIFY)

Definition The state in which specific information is lacking

Related Factors

Lack of exposure
Lack of recall

Misinterpretation of information
Cognitive limitation
Lack of interest in learning
Unfamiliarity with information resources
Patient's request for no information

Defining Characteristics

Verbalization of the problem
Inaccurate follow-through of instruction
Inadequate performance of test
Inappropriate or exaggerated behaviors (e.g., hysterical, hostile, agitated, apathetic)
Statement of misconception
Request for information

Interventions

Establish expected outcomes for learning
Use information obtained in assessment
Set expected outcomes according to priority, patient's needs, and readiness to learn
Set small, specific, and realistic expected outcomes to provide patient with a sense of accomplishment
Reward goals attempted/completed
Write expected outcomes in nursing care plan
Incorporate principles of learning/teaching
　Desire to learn must be present before learning can take place
　Each individual learns at own pace
　Environment must be free from stress, discomfort, pain, or distractions
　Information is best learned if it is meaningful, organized, and relevant
　Individual will learn only if he sees value of information
Present information in small segments
Use language that is easily understood
Teach from a well-organized plan
Allow time for questions
Obtain feedback after each segment is presented
Continue with plan only when understanding is ensured
Maintain eye contact during presentation
Present information step by step and obtain a return demonstration when teaching a procedure
Present information using different techniques based on patient's learning preference
Use as many audiovisual aids as possible
　Films
　Slides
　Booklets
　Diagrams
　Procedure pictures
　Procedure equipment
Offer praise when learning takes place
Initiate teaching plan as soon after admission as possible, predicated on patient's condition and readiness to learn

Expected Outcome/Evaluation

Patient
　Verbalizes understanding of given instructions/information
　Demonstrates learned procedure(s) correctly

ALTERED THOUGHT PROCESSES

***Definition** The state in which an individual experiences a disruption in cognitive operations and activities*

Related Factors

Physiological changes
Psychological conflicts
Loss of memory
Impaired judgment
Sleep deprivation

Defining Characteristics

Inaccurate interpretation of environment
　Cognitive dissonance
　Distractibility
　Memory deficit or problems
　Egocentricity
　Hypervigilance/hypovigilance
　Decreased ability to grasp ideas
　Impaired ability to make decisions
　Impaired ability to solve problems
　Impaired ability to reason
　Impaired ability to abstract or conceptualize
　Impaired ability to calculate
　Altered attention span—distractibility
　Obsessions
　Inability to follow commands
　Disorientation to time, place, person, circumstances, and events
　Changes in remote, recent, immediate memory
　Delusions
　Ideas of reference
　Hallucinations
　Confabulation
　Inappropriate social behavior
　Altered sleep patterns
　Inappropriate affect

Other Possible Defining Characteristic

Inappropriate/nonreality-based thinking

Disorientation
Description*

Disorientation is the inability to correctly identify self in relation to time, place, or person.

---

*Descriptions and their related characteristics in this chapter on nursing diagnoses are not NANDA approved.

Defining Characteristics of Disorientation

Chronic dementia

Acute delirium

Psychomotor agitation

Insomnia

Excessive fear

Visual hallucinations

Aggressive behavior

Purposeless activity

Reversible causes such as the following: alcohol intoxication, altered cerebral blood flow, dehydration, electrolyte imbalance, high fever, infection, metabolic disturbance, sleep pattern disturbance, toxic reactions, head trauma, malnutrition, sensory deprivation or overload, overmedication

Irreversible causes such as the following: senile dementia (Alzheimer's disease), chronic progressive neurologic conditions, neoplasms that present with the following behaviors: psychomotor agitation or retardation, disinterest in personal care, confabulation, "sundowner's" syndrome, short-term memory loss, inability to concentrate, loss of intellectual abilities, delusions, lability of affect and concrete thinking

Interventions

Assess causative factors and possible etiology of disorientation (acute and reversible delirium versus chronic and irreversible dementia)

Treat acute delirium as a medical emergency

Protect patient from self-injury with attention to equipment at bedside

Provide soft restraints or restraint jacket to prevent unescorted wandering

Cover adequately to avoid unintentional physical exposure

Wear clearly visible name tag

Introduce self to patient before giving care

Relate date, time of day, and recent activities

Speak in kind tone using short, simple sentences

Give one direction at a time

Adjust lighting to prevent shadows and distortions

Leave a night light on

Assist patient in self-care activities

Maintain a therapeutic environment; orient patient to room, display familiar items, place personal items in accessible place, display clock and calendar, keep equipment and possessions in same place

Post list of daily activities in clear view

Label bathroom and other areas with large-lettered signs or use a color code to help patient identify personal items and room

Encourage ambulation when possible

Encourage socialization

Provide radio, television, newspapers

Address patient by name

Tell patient when you do not understand his statements

Do not point out deficits of behavior

Do not laugh at misinformation or misperceptions

Provide repetitive schedules

Encourage independence

Encourage visits from family and significant others

    Assess patient's response to visitors

    Assist family with their emotional reactions

    Help family in goal setting that is realistic

Provide tasks that do not require new learning

Give positive reinforcement for participation in activities

Provide same staff when possible

Expected Outcome/Evaluation

Patient

    Maintains orientation to time, place, and person

    Demonstrates increased cognitive functioning

    Remains in reality

    Maintains safety consciousness

DECISIONAL CONFLICT

Definition *A state of uncertainty about the course of action to be taken when choice among competing actions involves risk, loss, or challenge to personal life values; (specify focus of conflict, e.g., choices regarding health, family relationships, career, finances, or other life events)*

Related Factors

Unclear personal values/beliefs

Perceived threat to value system

Lack of experience or interference with decision making

Lack of relevant information

Support system deficit

Defining Characteristics

Verbalized feeling of distress related to uncertainty about choices

Verbalization of undesired consequences of alternative actions being considered

Vacillation between alternative choices

Delayed decision making

Self-focusing

Physical signs of distress or tension (increased heart rate, increased muscle tension, restlessness, etc.)

Questioning personal values and beliefs while attempting to make a decision

Interventions

Assess any physical condition that may affect decision-making or cognition

Assist patient with clearly identifying a problem

Provide accurate data; be consistent to avoid misconceptions

Decrease anxiety (see Anxiety care plan, p. 15)

Assist patient with identifying potential alternatives

Encourage patient to write down pros and cons of each alternative

Assist patient with identifying previous successful decisions

Encourage verbalization and recognition of factors that hinder decision making

Reassure patient that it is acceptable to make mistakes

Remind patient that any decision will have negative aspects

Encourage patient to make simple choices first
Choice of activity
Selection on menu
Time of procedures

Explain importance of not making decisions based on preference of others

Reinforce patient's verbalization of independent opinions, thoughts, and decisions

Assist and reinforce progression to more complex decision making

Point out resources that are available for decision to be made

Teach assertive communication techniques

Assist with appropriate action once decision has been made

Expected Outcome/Evaluation

Patient
Makes contribution to treatment plan
Seeks increasing responsibility for own activity and behavior
Verbalizes alternative solutions to problems

Functional Health Pattern VII: Self-Perception/Self-Concept

ANXIETY

Definition A vague, uneasy feeling, the source of which is often nonspecific or unknown to the individual

Related Factors

Unconscious conflict about essential values and goals of life
Threat to self-concept
Threat of death
Threat to or change in health status
Threat to or change in socioeconomic status
Threat to or change in role functioning
Threat to or change in environment
Threat to or change in interaction patterns
Situational and maturational crises
Interpersonal transmission and contagion
Unmet needs

Defining Characteristics

Subjective
Increased tension
Apprehension
Increased helplessness
Uncertainty
Fearful
Scared
Feelings of inadequacy
Shakiness
Fear of unspecific consequences
Regretful
Overexcited
Rattled
Distressed
Jittery
Objective
Sympathetic stimulation: cardiovascular excitation, superficial vasoconstriction, pupil dilation
Restlessness
Insomnia
Glancing about
Poor eye contact
Trembling; hand tremors
Extraneous movements: foot shuffling; hand, arm movements
Expressed concern regarding changes in life events
Worried
Anxious
Facial tension
Voice quivering
Focus on self
Increased wariness
Increased perspiration

Mild Anxiety
Description

Mild anxiety is normal anxiety that motivates an individual on a daily basis wherein the ability to perform and problem solve is enhanced.

Defining Characteristics of Mild Anxiety

Slight discomfort
Restlessness
Mild insomnia
Mild change in appetite
Irritability
Repetitive questions
Attention-seeking behaviors
Increased alertness
Increased perception and problem solving
Easily angered
Focus on future problems
Fidgety movements
All of the NANDA nursing diagnoses may be associated with anxiety in one of its levels

Interventions

Watch for signs of increasing anxiety

Help client channel energy constructively
Use prn medication sparingly
Encourage problem solving
Provide accurate and factual information
Be aware of defense mechanisms used
Assist in identifying successful coping skills
Maintain a calm, unhurried manner
Teach client that mild anxiety is a normal part of living
Teach relaxation exercises and techniques

Expected Outcome/Evaluation

Patient
  Uses capabilities of effective coping to solve potential
    or actual threat
  Increases knowledge of self and/or situation
  Reports an enhancement of self-esteem

Moderate Anxiety
Description

Moderate anxiety is anxiety that interferes with new learning by narrowing the perceptual field so that the individual grasps less but is able to attend with direction by others.

Defining Characteristics of Moderate Anxiety

Progression of mild anxiety
Selective attention to environment
Concentration on individual tasks only
Moderate subjective discomfort
Increase in amount of time spent on problem situation
Voice tremors
Change in voice pitch
Tachypnea
Tachycardia
Tremulousness
Increased muscle tension
Nail biting, finger drumming, toe tapping, or foot
  swinging

Interventions

Maintain calm, unhurried manner when dealing with pa-
  tient
Speak in calm, firm, reassuring manner
Use short, simple sentences
Avoid becoming anxious, angry, or defensive
Listen to patient with respect and interest
Offer some physical contact with patient; touch patient's
  hand or arm
Administer tranquilizers and sedatives as ordered
Assist patient with labeling and recognizing anxiety
Assist patient with identifying and describing feelings and
  the source of distress
  Do not probe
  Allow patient to cry
  Allow for verbal expression of anger

Assist patient with correcting events that precipitated
  anxiety
Encourage participation in diversional activities
  Reading
  Watching television
  Listening to the radio
  Writing letters
  Physical activity; walking
  Visiting with relatives or friends
Assist patient with identifying coping mechanisms that
  will reduce anxiety and with using those that have been
  successful in the past
Teach patient to use relaxation techniques with assistance
Encourage patient to engage in activities using large mus-
  cle groups
Establish and maintain familiar routines
Teach patient the importance of establishing daily exer-
  cise to control stress level
Continue with mild anxiety care

Expected Outcome/Evaluation

Patient
  Perceives threat realistically
  Expresses diminished anxiety level

Severe Anxiety
Description

During an episode of severe anxiety the perceptual field is narrowed to the point that the individual is unable to problem solve or learn. The focus is on small or scattered details, and communication patterns are disrupted. The patient may exhibit many aborted attempts to reduce anxiety and usually verbalizes great subjective distress.

Defining Characteristics of Severe Anxiety

Sense of impending doom
Excessive muscle tension (headache, muscle spasms)
Diaphoresis
Respiratory changes
  Sighing
  Hyperventilation
  Dyspnea
  Dizziness
GI changes
  Nausea, vomiting
  Heartburn
  Belching
  Anorexia
  Diarrhea or constipation
Cardiovascular changes
  Tachycardia
  Palpitations
  Precordial discomfort
  Greatly reduced range of perception
  Inability to learn

Inability to concentrate
Sense of isolation
Difficult or inappropriate verbalization
Purposeless activity
Hostility

Interventions

Isolate patient in quiet and safe environment
Provide frequent-to-constant contact and care
Administer medications as ordered
Assist and/or make decisions for patient; do not ask patient to do this entirely for self
Observe for signs of increasing agitation
Do not touch patient without permission
Assure patient that he will be safe
Assess for safety in the immediate environment

Expected Outcome/Evaluation

Patient
  Verbalizes decreased behavioral, affective, physiologic symptoms of anxiety
  Demonstrates ability to concentrate and attends with assistance to immediate environment
  Uses coping strategies to reduce anxiety
  Identifies thoughts, perceptions that preceded anxiety

Panic
Description

Anxiety has escalated to the level that the individual is now a danger to self and/or others and may become immobilized or strike out in a random fashion.

Defining Characteristics of Panic

Severe hyperactivity or immobility
Extreme sense of isolation
Loss of identity; personality disintegration
Severe shakiness and muscular tension
Inability to communicate in complete sentences
Distortion of perception and unrealistic appraisal of environment and/or threat
Disorganized behavior in attempting to escape
Assaultive

Interventions

Remain with patient; call for assistance
Remove as many physical and psychologic stressors from environment as possible
Speak in a calm, reassuring manner using low voice tones
Tell patient that you (staff) will not allow him to harm self or others
Isolate patient in quiet, safe area
Continue with severe anxiety care

Expected Outcome/Evaluation

Patient
  Does not harm self or others

Expresses a decreased feeling of anxiety
Begins to make decisions for self

HOPELESSNESS

***Definition** The subjective state in which an individual sees limited or no alternatives or personal choices available and is unable to mobilize energy on own behalf*

Related Factors

Prolonged activity restriction creating isolation
Failing or deteriorating physiological condition
Long-term stress
Abandonment
Loss of belief in transcendent values/God

Defining Characteristics

Passivity, decreased verbalization
Decreased affect
Verbal cues (indicating despondency, "I can't," sighing)
Lack of initiative
Decreased response to stimuli
Turning away from speaker
Closing eyes
Shrugging in response to speaker
Decreased appetite, increased/decreased sleep
Lack of involvement in care; passively allowing care

Interventions

Maintain a kind but firm attitude in all patient care activities
Maintain adequate hydration and nutrition
Measure intake and output as ordered or if indicated
Allow patient to wear own clothes when possible
Involve patient in decision-making process when formulating care plan
Help patient set small, realistic goals
Give positive reinforcement for independent functioning
Assess patient with identifying areas over which he has control
If appetite is poor and patient is eating insufficiently, offer soft, nutritious foods that are easily chewed; include high-protein between-meal snacks and a variety of liquids such as milk shakes, custards, and eggnog
Maintain liquids and foods within easy reach
Offer frequent small amounts
Discourage intake of nonnutritive items such as coffee and foods high in refined sugar
Encourage intake of water
Serve food attractively and at proper temperature
Provide foods that patient prefers; assit with menu selection
Do not give patient choice of not eating by asking, "Do you feel like eating?" Offer foods, saying, "I have something for you to eat"

Administer stool softeners or laxatives as ordered

Encourage intake of foods rich in fiber

Reinforce and assist grooming efforts and personal hygiene; encourage male patient to shave and female patient to apply makeup and style hair

Encourage patient to do things for self in order to feel better rather than waiting to feel better first before doing things for self

Assist with positioning in bed, sitting, and ambulation

Offer positive recognition for increased activity level

Provide noncompetitive activities (handicrafts, sewing, simple puzzles) before progressing to competitive activities such as board games

Promote planned rest periods during the day based on physical condition

Discourage sleeping all day or remaining in bed

Decrease environmental and other stimuli at night to promote sleep

Promote bedtime rituals

Avoid stressful conversation

Discourage caffeine-containing substances

Discourage exercise before bedtime

Offer back rub and warm milk

Do not encourage dependence on hypnotics, especially those that suppress REM (rapid eye movement) sleep

Continually assess for suicide potential

If patient expresses plan for suicide, ask for details of plan

Support all verbalization of feelings, especially anger

Report suicidal ideation to attending physician

Observe closely for any self-destructive behavior as mood-elevating medications take effect or if patient demonstrates a sudden change in affect or behavior

Plan time to sit with patient; do not act rushed and remain comfortable during silent periods; do not require patient to always talk

Do not discourage patient from crying; remain with and support patient unless patient requests privacy

Do not belittle patient's statements or offer inappropriately cheerful remarks or platitudes such as "Everything's going to be all right"

Be sure reassurances are realistic and are meant for patient, not nurse

Assess your own feelings of powerlessness and helplessness

Avoid agreement with self-deprecating statements and cast doubt on their validity, but do not argue with patient

Reinforce positive statements about self and others; do not be overcomplimentary

If patient expresses feelings of guilt, assist him with exploring their origin and with exploring associated feelings of anger and resentment

Respect denial of illness if patient is unable to accept it; do not force reality on patient

Assist and support gradually increasing amounts of independent self-care

Provide for physical exercise at patient's level of tolerance

Maintain a clean orderly environment

Ask if visit by religious or spiritual support person is desired

Administer antidepressants as ordered

Be aware of lag time of up to 2 weeks before they take effect

Familiarize yourself with side effects; most common are anticholinergic

Be aware of possible "cheeking" of medication or hoarding at bedside: antidepressants are lethal

Expected Outcome/Evaluation

Patient

Demonstrates relief of symptoms of moderate and severe depression

Reaches acceptance stage of death and dying if terminal illness is present

Uses problem solving to increase individual capabilities

Verbalizes source of hope

Participates fully in own treatment

Verbalizes no self-destructive thoughts

Establishes social network for support

BODY IMAGE DISTURBANCE

Definition Disruption in the way one perceives one's body image

Related Factors

Biophysical

Cognitive perceptual

Psychosocial

Cultural or spiritual

Defining Characteristics

Either the following A or B must be present to justify the diagnosis of body image disturbance:

A. Verbal response to actual or perceived change in structure and/or function

B. Nonverbal response to actual or perceived change in structure and/or function

The following clinical manifestations may be used to validate the presence of A or B:

Objective

Missing body part

Actual change in structure and/or function

Not looking at body part

Not touching body part

Hiding or overexposing body part (intentional or unintentional)

Trauma to nonfunctioning part

Change in social involvement

Negative feelings about body

Feelings of helplessness, hopelessness, or powerlessness

Preoccupation with change or loss

Emphasis on remaining strengths, heightened achievement

Extension of body boundary to incorporate environmental objects

Personalization of part or loss by name

Depersonalization of part or loss by impersonal pronouns

Refusal to verify actual change

It may be possible to identify high-risk populations such as those with the following conditions:

Missing parts

Dependence on machine

Significance of body part or functioning with regard to age, sex, developmental level, or basic human needs

Physical change caused by biochemical agents (drugs)

Physical trauma or mutilation

Pregnancy and/or maturational changes

Interventions

Determine patient's perception of change in body image and subsequent threat to self

Encourage verbalization of emotions such as anger, fear, frustration, and anxiety about altered functioning or lost body part

Encourage patient to look at and touch changed or lost body part

Assist family in adapting to change through providing resources, encouraging verbalization, and including in care of family member

Encourage discussion of physical changes in simple, direct, and factual manner

Assess own attitudes and values related to wholeness and physical appearance

Give realistic feedback about loss or change

Discuss sexual concerns openly and honestly

Encourage patient to participate in all therapeutic modalities offered in treatment

Give positive feedback for attempts to enhance and integrate new body image

Allow patient to progress at own rate; do not force independent functioning or allow too much dependency

Help patient discriminate between internal stimuli and those that come from environment

Use active listening for nonverbal clues as well as verbal statements

Assess previous adaptive and maladaptive responses to stressors and illness

Assess for self-destructive behavior

Display empathy rather than sympathy

Provide patient and family with hospital and community resources

Discuss options available, such as cosmetic procedures, mechanical devices, and rehabilitative services

Teach patient and family the stages of grief and importance of grief work

Expected Outcome/Evaluation

Patient

Progresses toward completion of grief work

Verbalizes an acceptance of altered body functioning or loss

Plans realistically for future role functioning

Incorporates prosthesis, stoma, or device into changed body image

Verbalizes an interest and willingness to rejoin and resume social interactions and activities

Uses hospital and community support systems

SELF-ESTEEM DISTURBANCE

Definition *Negative self-evaluation/feelings about self or self-capabilities, which may be directly or indirectly expressed*

Defining Characteristics

Self-negating verbalization

Expressions of shame/guilt

Evaluation of self as unable to deal with events

Rationalizing away/rejecting positive feedback and exaggerating negative feedback about self

Hesitancy to try new things/situations

Denial of problems obvious to others

Projection of blame/responsibility for problems

Rationalizing personal failures

Hypersensitivity to criticism

Grandiosity

Interventions

Provide for success experiences by introducing tasks at patient's level of functioning

Assess for possible alcohol or drug dependency

Communicate acceptance of patient and show genuine concern by spending unstructured, undemanding time

Explore patient's feelings and give validation for their expression

Provide for positive feedback on accomplishments

Explore alternative approach or coping strategies

By giving observations, comment on positive attributes; avoid false praise

Explore with patient his current strengths

Encourage group interaction and explore possible support groups for aftercare

Assist with grooming and hygiene when necessary; promote attractiveness

Help patient list past success experiences

Teach assertive techniques: use of "I" statements, ability to say "no," body posture, eye contact, tone of voice, personal space, tactics for negotiation

Teach difference between assertion and nonassertion; aggressive and passive behaviors

Practice role playing

Discuss activities that might increase self-esteem

Expected Outcome/Evaluation

Patient

Verbalizes realistic appreciation of self, including attributes and limitations

Presents a positive personal appearance that reflects good grooming and hygiene

Initiates approach strategies to potentially threatening events or changes in environment

Demonstrates appropriate assertive behavior in social interactions

Reports a minimal level of interpersonal anxiety

Displays no overt self-destructive behaviors

Communicates needs effectively

PERSONAL IDENTITY DISTURBANCE

Description

Personal identity is the coherent sense of self as a unique and separate identity that develops through successful resolution of developmental issues. Identity rests on the ability to distinguish self from others and the environment.

Defining Characteristics

Disturbance in body image

Sex role disturbance

Gender identity confusion

Pathologic symbiotic relationships

Undifferentiated or fused family

Dissociative states

Developmental crisis such as adolescence

Delirium or dementia

Functional psychotic states: schizophrenia, bipolar disorder

Severe anxiety and/or panic

Hypnagogic states

Interventions

Assist patient with identifying actual threats to self from misinterpretation of perceived threat

Provide accurate information about threat

Provide calm, structured environment

Encourage self-care activities and taking responsibility for self

Direct activities that support reality issues: simple and concrete

Use simple, direct, and concise statements

Assess for altered homeostasis caused by physiologic disequilibrium

Assess developmental issues: age, crisis, regression

Encourage verbalization of anxiety concerning sexual identity and sexual preference; be nonjudgmental

Assess for loss of contact with reality: hallucinations and/or delusions

Do not argue with delusions; do not reinforce; look for

needs they might satisfy and find more appropriate manner of meeting them

Objectively point out your reality when hallucinations are present; help patient focus on here and now; decrease stimuli and help reduce level of anxiety

Use anxiety-reducing interventions

Teach principles of normal growth and development

Refer to psychiatric unit or psychotherapy as necessary

Expected Outcome/Evaluation

Patient

States ability to define and identify self

Maintains contact with reality

Verbalizes realistic plan to meet actual threats to self

Acknowledges and accepts developmental changes into new personal identity

Functional Health Pattern VIII: Role/Relationship

DYSFUNCTIONAL GRIEVING

Definition *The state in which actual or perceived object loss (object loss is used in the broadest sense) exists; objects include people, possessions, a job, status, home, ideals, parts and processes of the body, etc*

Related Factors

Actual or perceived object loss

Thwarted grieving response to a loss

Absence of anticipatory grieving

Chronic fatal illness

Lack of resolution of previous grieving response

Loss of significant others

Loss of physiopsychosocial well-being

Loss of personal possessions

Defining Characteristics

Verbal expression of distress at loss

Denial of loss

Expression of guilt

Expression of unresolved issues

Anger

Sadness

Crying

Difficulty in expressing loss

Alterations in

Eating habits

Sleep patterns

Dream patterns

Activity level

Libido

Idealization of lost object

Reliving of past experiences

Interference with life functioning

Developmental regression

Labile effect
Alterations in concentration and/or pursuits of tasks

Interventions

Identify significance of loss or multiple losses
Discuss ambivalence
Assess stage of grief and support patient's expression of grief
Use active listening and permit verbalization of anger
Observe for suicidal ideation
Facilitate discussion of positive and negative aspects of loss
Facilitate exploration of support groups
Provide opportunities for social interaction, especially with those who have coped successfully with similar loss
Teach patient and significant other about grief process
If individual attempts to consistently deny grief, plan to spend time each shift talking about loss but avoid confrontation during discussion if patient changes subject and shifts reference; take cues from patient; be available to reopen subject when patient initiates conversation; use times of silence to convey support by offering your presence nonverbally
Assure individual that all feelings are normal, including anger, hatred, and feelings of desertion, guilt, or betrayal
Expect individual to meet reponsibilities and give positive reinforcement for resuming role responsibilities
Withdraw attention (negative reinforcement) if individual does not fulfill responsibilities for own care, which he is capable of doing
Assist individual with identifying ways of adapting lifestyle to accommodate the loss
Explore ways to assist patient to make new emotional investments
Be aware that it is acceptable to share your feelings with individual as long as these activities serve to support patient through his grief and are not expressions of unresolved loss on your part
If you become uncomfortable with your own unresolved feelings of loss, have another nurse who is comfortable talk with individual

Expected Outcome/Evaluation

Patient
  Relates realistically to both the pleasures and the disappointments of the lost relationship
  Establishes new and meaningful relationships and interests
  Displays no exaggerated or distorted emotional reactions to the deceased or loss
  Engages in constructive, meaningful lifestyle (pre-crisis level of functioning)
  For anticipatory grief: maintains a constructive and meaningful relationship with the dying significant other without displaying characteristics of dysfunctional grief

ALTERED ROLE PERFORMANCE

Definition Disruption in the way one perceives one's role performance

Defining Characteristics

Change in self-perception of role
Denial of role
Change in others' perception of role
Conflict in roles
Change in physical capacity to resume role
Lack of knowledge of role
Change in usual patterns of responsibility

Interventions

Assess nature and degree of disturbance in role performance
Assess patient's and significant other's perceptions of role disturbance
Assess cultural and economic factors
Determine number and types of roles within family structure
Assist patient and family with clarifying expected roles and those that must be relinquished or altered
Assist patient with verbalizing realistic expectations of role and concrete behaviors necessary to implement performance
Support grief work if role has been lost
Allow time for expression of fears/anxieties
Be nonjudgmental
Determine if patient is in role that is compatible with sexual orientation, sexual functioning, and self-concept
Provide role model for patient or reference to groups that supply new models
Assist in role rehearsal through role playing

Expected Outcome/Evaluation

Patient
  Verbalizes realistic perception and acceptance of new, lost, or altered role
  Demonstrates role mastery
  Develops with family or significant other specific behavioral strategies for assimilating role-specific changes in existing system

POTENTIAL FOR VIOLENCE: SELF-DIRECTED OR DIRECTED AT OTHERS

Definition The state in which an individual experiences behaviors that can be physically harmful either to the self or others

Risk Factors

Antisocial character
Battered women
Catatonic excitement

Child abuse
Manic excitement
Organic brain syndrome
Panic states
Rage reactions
Suicidal behavior
Temporal lobe epilepsy
Toxic reactions to medication

Potential for Violence: Self-Directed—Suicide

Description

Self-directed violence is characterized by any activity that has negative consequences for the individual's physical or mental well-being.

Defining Characteristics of Suicidal Behavior

Low self-esteem
Major loss
Terminal illness or major disability
Lack of future orientation
Lack of impulse control; history of substance abuse
Severe depression
Agitation and increased restlessness
Excessive guilt
Hopelessness; person feels like a failure
Moderate or greater levels of anxiety
Powerlessness
Verbal statements concerning thoughts of death
    "I just can't cope with life anymore"
    "My family would be better off without me"
Decreased verbal communication with family and/or significant others
Giving needed things away
Making a will
Checking on life insurance
Refusing to spend money for new possessions
Diminished ability to care for self
Writing letters saying "goodbye" or asking for forgiveness

Interventions

Maintain a safe environment to protect patient from injury
    Attempt to place in room with shatterproof windows
    Do not leave patient alone until full assessment of intent is made
    Remove patient's personal belongings that might prove to be harmful—drugs, razors, glass objects, cords, belts, panty hose, neckties—and explain to patient that you are doing this to remove potential danger from area
    Assure adequate staffing on unit, especially during intershift report and meal breaks; understand that most hospital suicides occur at this time
    Check site of incision, drains, and drainage tube insertion sites and document

    Consider reducing amounts of drugs (e.g., morphine, heparin) piggybacked to main IV lines
    Face IV pump or controller-regulating mechanism away from patient and out of reach
    Note IV rate of flow and level in bottle each time you enter room
    Give medication in liquid form rather than tablets, as tablets may be saved or concealed
Remember that no one can prevent a person intent on suicide from harming self
Understand that relationship building is more essential than removing hazards from immediate environment
Observe for sudden changes in patient's mood
Have same nurse each shift if possible
Ask patient for details of suicide plan
Do not withhold patient's thoughts of suicide from staff
Notify physician of patient's intent to commit suicide
Be aware that as depression lessens, patient may acquire energy needed to carry out a suicide plan
Be aware that previous attempts at suicide increase the risk for a repeated attempt
Remember that the more violent the plan, the more likely it is that the patient will commit suicide
Encourage patient to talk about feelings
Encourage communication with significant others who are viewed as supportive or as a potential means of support by patient
Avoid overly cheerful remarks
Do not change subject if patient begins to discuss his self-destructive thoughts
Assist patient with identifying alternatives to problem (see care plans for coping and anxiety)
Be aware of your own anxiety when caring for patient; understand that everyone has some fantasy of suicide at some time
Be aware that patient's dependency as well as your responsibility for preventing self-destructive behaviors in patient can be frustrating and burdensome; use support of peers to talk out own feelings
Encourage diversional activities that will promote outlet for angry feelings
Assist family with identifying and sharing their feelings with staff
Write down and give patient, family, and significant others phone numbers to contact (physician, suicide prevention center, hot lines, etc.)
Be certain that family and significant others can identify patient's cries for help and know to stay with patient at these times while calling for assistance

Expected Outcome/Evaluation

Patient
    Demonstrates ability to manage stressors without resorting to violence against self
    Develops discharge plans with staff

Expresses satisfaction with current life situation
Demonstrates increased self-esteem

Potential for Violence: Directed at Others—Excessive Hostility or Assaultive Behavior

Description

A potential for violence directed at others is characterized by the acting out of anger, hostility, or resentment in such a manner that it brings threat or harm to others in a socially unacceptable context. Hostility may be considered different from anger in that it is viewed as destructive, whereas anger can be seen as constructive. Anger is often justified and can be a healthy response to threatening, fearful, or frustrating situations. Expressing anger may enhance self-esteem and give an individual a sense of power in a situation. Expressing anger appropriately involves the creative use of energy. Unexpressed anger tends to pile up and create a negative and resentful individual who often vents anger inappropriately or not at the original source. Aggressive behavior is hostility acted out and may involve significant danger to others. There are important ethical and legal issues involved in managing aggressive behavior. It is the responsibility of the nurse to become familiar with those issues within the institution. Aggression indicates that behavior is out of control, and it is the responsibility of the staff to protect the patient and others from harm, not to punish.

Defining Characteristics of Actual or Potential Acting Out of Violence or Assaultive Behavior

Verbal abuse
Rising agitation, pacing
Low self-esteem
Lack of impulse control, history of substance abuse
Panic
Resistance to hospitalization or treatment
Psychosis: loss of contact with reality (delusions and/or hallucinations)
Intoxication by drugs or alcohol
Increased voice volume: shouting, swearing
Destruction of property

Interventions

Call patient by name; speak in calm, firm, and reassuring manner
Do not approach an openly hostile, aggressive patient by yourself; obtain assistance from another staff member
Act interested in what patient has to say
Do not invade personal space
Do not touch patient
Direct patient to calm and control self
Remove others from immediate area
Do not threaten, argue, or respond with hostility
Move around room while speaking with patient

Watch patient's eyes: body part that will be attacked will be observed by patient
State that you cannot allow patient to harm self or anyone in environment
Do not leave patient alone
Be aware of your own feelings and behavior
   Maintain and communicate control to patient
   Do not become personally insulted or demonstrate anger at patient's behavior
   Do not give in to patient's inappropriate demands
   Have another nurse remain with patient if you become upset or defensive
Decrease environmental stimulation
Give patient as much control over his own area as is safely possible
Focus on patient's feelings
Avoid pat reassurances and overgeneralizations
Use the same terms patient uses: "upset," "frustrated," "ticked off"
Avoid use of physical restraint unless patient is also using physical violence
Make every attempt to talk patient out of intended assaultive behavior
Apply mechanical restraints only if absolutely necessary and according to policy of institution
Offer medication
Administer chemical restraint (medications) according to institutional policy
When incident has passed
   Assist patient with identifying and discussing feelings
   Assist patient with identifying what triggered loss of control
   Assist patient with identifying alternative ways of expressing emotion and relieving tension
Be aware of importance of staff continuing with routine patient care activities
Manage emotional reactions of other patients to the incident
Involve patient in activities to promote release of energy and feelings: large muscle movement
Understand that rejection of patient by staff can increase patient's anxiety and perpetuate anger
Teach difference between assertive and aggressive behavior

Expected Outcome/Evaluation

Patient
   Verbalizes alternative ways of dealing with aggressive feelings in conflict situations
   Uses energy of anger constructively
   Remains in reality
   Demonstrates nondestructive ways of interacting with others and environment
   Displays effective coping strategies in reducing anxiety and in assessing potentially threatening situations

Develops increased self-awareness and increased self-esteem

IMPAIRED SOCIAL INTERACTION

Definition *The state in which an individual participates in an insufficient or excessive quantity or ineffective quality of social exchange*

Related Factors

Knowledge/skill deficit about ways to enhance mutuality
Communication barriers
Self-concept disturbance
Absence of available significant others or peers
Limited physical mobility
Therapeutic isolation
Sociocultural dissonance
Environmental barriers
Altered thought processes

Defining Characteristics

Verbalized or observed discomfort in social situations
Verbalized or observed inability to receive or communicate a satisfying sense of belonging, caring, interest, or shared history
Observed use of unsuccessful social interaction behaviors
Dysfunctional interaction with peers, family, and/or others
Family report of change in style or pattern of interaction

Manipulative Behavior
Description

Manipulative behavior involves two ways of controlling the behavior of others to achieve one's goals: passive behavior gets needs met indirectly through others; aggressive behavior is directed against or toward others in an attempt to get one's own needs met. These two ways of interacting are used when an individual feels powerless to meet his own needs through assertive interaction.

Defining Characteristics of Manipulative Behavior

Lack of insight toward problems and/or denial of problems
Inabilty to express anger openly
Changing subject of conversation or activity of group
Crying or acting helpless when confronted
Attention-seeking behavior such as monopolizing conversations in both social and therapeutic interactions
Constantly seeking approval and recognition
Being overly solicitious and ingratiating
Attempting to gain special attention or privileges
Demonstrating anger and feeling hurt, deserted, and unworthy when above attempts are denied
Reporting confidential information to others
Attempting to use others' weaknesses against them; playing one person against the other
Consistently breaking rules and routines and disrupting procedures

Intellectualizing and rationalizing problems away
Projecting blame onto others
Viewing self as uniquely special and deserving
Attempting to get others to rescue him by being helpless and boosting others' self-esteem by relying on them to fix the problem

Interventions

Assess needs that patient is trying to meet through manipulation
Decrease patient's manipulation of staff
 Avoid discussing yourself and other staff members with patient
 Assign consistent staff when possible
 Develop plan of care with other staff members and communicate to all involved with patient's care
 Communicate frequently with other staff members to ensure continuity and consistency of approach
Point out manipulative behavior to patient if patient states
 "You're the only one who understands . . ."
 "You're the only one who cares about me"
 "You're the only one I can talk to"
Caution staff to not attempt to be liked or to be patient's favorite nurse
Do not accept favors as gifts, which foster a personal relationship
Be matter of fact in interactions with patient
Avoid angry, negative, and punitive responses to patient when patient is being manipulative
Offer limited choices (e.g., "Would you like to ambulate now or at 9 o'clock?")
Be direct in interactions; do not bargain or rationalize
Assist patient in recognizing his own patterns of manipulative behavior by providing nonthreatening similar examples
Point out relationship between need to control and inability to achieve self-control
Encourage identification of alternate and appropriate behaviors for meeting needs; use role playing
Give verbal and nonverbal positive reinforcement when patient functions without being manipulative
Encourage and support verbalization about feelings, medical conditions, and/or surgery and current treatment; listen nonjudgmentally
Build trust through consistency and keeping promises
Assure patient that if limits are set, it is because you care and that caring and limit setting are neither mutually exclusive nor opposites
Involve patient in his own plan of care without allowing patient to dictate aspects of care

Expected Outcome/Evaluation

Patient
 Verbalizes satisfaction with improved social interaction
 Demonstrates ability to define and meet needs without manipulative behavior
 Participates actively in planning own care

Demanding Behavior
Description

Demanding behavior occurs in syndromes involving anxiety, fear, helplessnes, inadequacy, inferiority, hostility, manipulation, and dependent behavior. The individual believes he is incapable of fulfilling his own needs or having his needs met by making requests in a direct, matter-of-fact manner. Attempts are then made to coerce others to meet these needs by making requests with forceful and manipulative behavior with implied threat.

Defining Characteristics of Demanding Behavior*

Making frequent requests
Constant attention seeking
Attempting to coerce others to meet needs
Asking others to do what he is capable of doing
Displaying helplessness when making requests
Displaying anger when requests are not met immediately
Detaining staff with subsequent requests after inital request has been met
Acting domineering, sarcastic, or ridiculing
Using threats if requests are not met
Not using proper channels of communication: goes over nurses' authority by talking to supervisors, etc.

Interventions

Be aware that dynamics between staff and patient can create and maintain the problem situation
Be aware that staff's responses to patient will influence whether or not patient continues to be demanding; avoid displaying annoyance or anger with patient's request; understand that such a display perpetuates patient's demands
Be aware that depersonalization caused by hospitalization promotes anxiety and contributes to patient's perception of lack of control and self-esteem
Assess unfilled needs of patient
Involve patient in deciding how needs will be met
Assist patient with identifying demanding behaviors
Relate to patient your own responses to demanding behavior in nonemotional tone of voice
Assist patient with developing alternative behavior by
  Asking directly for what is wanted
  Taking responsibility for behavior by using the personal pronoun "I" before a request
  Becoming more aware of responses and associated feelings when requests are not met immediately
  Reinforcing independently made direct questions
Do not refuse or ignore request
Give reasons why requests cannot be met
Anticipate realistic requests and meet them rapidly
Allow patient as much control as possible in own care
Spend time with patient when he is not demanding; set up a regular schedule of checking in with patient that is independent of his using the call light
Give full attention to patient during verbal interactions

and recognize positive qualities to promote self-esteem
Demonstrate interest and be attentive to patient as a person
Allow opportunity for appropriate ventilation of feelings regarding annoyances and restrictions; feeling of powerlessness
If you tell patient that you will be back in 20 minutes, be sure that you are
Avoid withdrawing from patient by insensitive mechanistic actions

Expected Outcome/Evaluation

Patient
  Displays a positive regard for assertive social interactions
  Makes realistic requests of staff in situations that patient is unable to meet by self or without help

Withdrawn Behavior
Description

Withdrawn behavior is an attempt to avoid interaction with others and thus avoid relatedness; it is a defense against anxiety that is related to a stressor or threat. The range of behavior can be from disinterest in others to severe withdrawal with an accompanying increase in primary process thinking. This may ultimately lead to autistic behavior or delusions and hallucinations as the individual withdraws more from the environment and attends to internal thoughts and stimuli.

Defining Characteristics of Withdrawn Behavior

Dull, flat, or inappropriate affect/mood
Apathy
Depression
Absence of spontaneity
Inappropriate response to environmental stimuli
Excessive fear and increasing levels of anxiety
Decreased or absent verbalization
Decreased motor activity or agitation
Lack of awareness of surroundings
Inattention to grooming and personal habits
Inappropriate social behavior, including open masturbation, obscene language, handling of excreta
Regression: may assume fetal position
Disturbance in thought content, such as delusions
Disturbance in perception, such as hallucinations

Interventions

Communicate with patient in a positive, accepting manner
Plan time to sit with patient
Consider touching patient's hand if a negative response is not anticipated
Avoid attempts to oververbalize with patient
Remain comfortable during silent periods
Avoid asking questions that require "yes" or "no" answers
Expect patient to respond to conversation
Provide reality-oriented conversation focusing on the here

and now; avoid generalizations and abstract concepts

Allow sufficient time for patient to respond

Avoid placing patient in private room

Administer phenothiazines and antidepressants as ordered

Measure intake and output if indicated

Assist with meeting basic needs: eating, drinking, elimination, bathing, and ambulation

Assist and teach ROM exercises and turn q2h if bedridden

Maintain skin integrity

Use television and/or radio in room

Provide newspapers and magazines

Involve patient in plan of care

Assist patient with identifying alternate and appropriate behaviors

Orient patient to time, place, and person; use clock and calendar in room

Provide positive reinforcement for self-care activities

Be aware that logical arguments only increase delusional thought content

Encourage and support verbalization of feelings about concrete issues: medical condition, menu, etc.

Decrease anxiety level (see anxiety care plan)

Provide a regular schedule of activities (routines)

Ask patient to look at you when you are speaking to him

Share with patient that you do not see or hear hallucinatory material

Use empathy: "That must be frightening"

Gradually introduce patient to more people in environment

Expected Outcome/Evaluation

Patient

Reports a satisfying social interaction with nurse

Identifies increased self-esteem

Responds with positive and appropriate affect to social interaction

Remains in reality

Initiates and completes self-care activities

Dependent Behavior
Description

Dependent behavior includes impaired decision making; a tendency to lean on others for guidance, direction, support, protection, and advice; and a compelling need to relate to a stronger person in coping with stressors.

Defining Characteristics of Dependent Behavior

Constant attention seeking

Whining

Helplessness when making a request

Refusing to make decisions

Asking others to do what he could do himself

Feeling no responsibility for

Decisions

Behaviors

Feelings

Thoughts

Lack of initiative

Low self-esteem

Procrastination

Passiveness

Low frustration tolerance

Lack of social skills

Few adaptive coping skills

Lack of problem-solving skills

Moderate interpersonal anxiety

Moderate-to-severe depression

Covert expressions of anger

Repeated hospitalizations; many physical complaints

Substance abuse and/or dependency

Inability to define or express needs appropriately

Interventions

Assess for suicidal thoughts and behaviors

Assess patient's dependence on drugs and/or alcohol

Maintain consistent approach

Set limits for unrealistic and inappropriate requests

Use calm, firm tone of voice when speaking

Do not display anger or frustration toward patient

Do not reward attention-seeking behavior

Meet dependency needs at first while gradually assisting patient in becoming more independent in stages: (1) do for patient; (2) do with patient; (3) allow patient to take lead while you provide support; (4) provide positive reinforcement for independent behaviors

Avoid making simple decisions for patient

Offer alternative choices

Investigate physical symptoms reported by patient but do not encourage "sick role" behavior

Assist patient with verbalizing and identifying strengths

Do not be the only one with whom the patient can talk; involve other staff with patient

Avoid feelings of sympathy; do not give phone number to patient or allow patient to call you at work or home

Assist patient with identifying consequences of behavior, including indecisiveness

Assist patient with expressing anger in open and direct manner when his demands or requests are not met

Positively reinforce expression of genuine feelings

Refer to self-help groups when appropriate

Teach about physical and/or psychologic dependency that occurs with continued use of tranquilizers and/or alcohol

Expected Outcome/Evaluation

Patient

Assumes responsibility for major areas of life

Resumes appropriate role functioning

Reports satisfying social interactions

Makes decisions independently

Copes with stressors without using tranquilizers and/or alcohol

Functional Health Pattern X: Coping/ Stress Tolerance

INEFFECTIVE INDIVIDUAL COPING

Definition Impairment of adaptive behaviors and problem-solving abilities of a person in meeting life's demands and roles

Related Factors

Situational crises
Maturational crises
Personal vulnerability
Multiple life changes
No vacations
Inadequate relaxation
Inadequate support systems
Little or no exercise
Poor nutrition
Unmet expectations
Work overload
Too many deadlines
Unrealistic perceptions
Inadequate coping methods

Defining Characteristics

Verbalization of inability to cope or inability to ask for
   help
Inability to meet role expectations
Inability to meet basic needs
Inability to problem solve
Alteration in societal participation
Destructive behavior toward self or others
Inappropriate use of defense mechanisms
Change in visual communication patterns
Verbal manipulation
High illness rate
High rate of accidents
Overeating
Lack of appetite
Excessive smoking
Excessive drinking
Overuse of prescribed tranquilizers
Alcohol proneness
High blood pressure
Chronic fatigue
Insomnia
Muscular tension
Ulcers
Frequent headaches
Frequent neckaches
Irritable bowel
Chronic worry
General irritability
Poor self-esteem
Chronic anxiety

Emotional tension
Chronic depression

Interventions

Understand that patient may not know what the problem is
Assist patient with clearly identifying precipitating event
Explore major changes that have occurred in previous 2 weeks
Ask patient how he feels and help patient to put a label on the emotion
Assist patient with identifying
   How problem affects his life and future
   How problem is affecting family or significant other
   If other factors could be influencing the way he sees problem
Assist patient with identifying strengths and coping skills
   Ask whether anything like this has happened to him before
   Ask how past crises were handled
   Inquire as to how patient usually decreases tension and anxiety
   Ascertain whether patient has tried to use any of the same anxiety-reducing methods this time
   If not, attempt to explore possible reasons or blocks to using prior coping skills
   If anxiety-reducing methods were tried and were unsuccessful, ask what kept them from working
   Assist patient with exploring and identifying what else he thinks might work
Assist patient with identifying nature and strength of situational supports; collect data about current and potential sources of support
   Persons with whom patient lives
   Persons with whom patient is close
   Friends or best friend
   Persons available to help
   Persons whom patient trusts and feels are understanding
   Community services
Assist patient with planning alternative solutions using patient's own coping skills and situational and environmental supports
Offer suggestions of other adaptive coping strategies
Confront self-defeating and destructive behavior in a factual and nonjudgmental manner; make observations about amount of alcohol intake, use of tranquilizers, or overindulgence in food or cigarette smoking
Acknowledge patient's feelings about crisis
Assist patient with sorting out feelings and validating them as acceptable and normal
Assist patient with exploring alternative coping skills
Assist patient with testing role playing or rehearsing new approaches to problem
Present self as role model for open and direct communication, innovative thinking, flexibility, and self-awareness

Provide positive reinforcement for all adaptive coping skills used in situation

Teach relaxation techniques

Teach psychological and physiological effects of chronic stress

Expected Outcome/Evaluation

Patient

Returns to precrisis level of functioning

Develops an adequate response repertoire

Displays no symptoms of excessive anxiety or lasting physiological responses to stress

Increases self-esteem

Acknowledges increased confidence to solve future problems effectively

Functional Health Pattern XI: Value/Belief

SPIRITUAL DISTRESS (DISTRESS OF THE HUMAN SPIRIT)

Definition Disruption in the life principle that pervades a person's entire being and that integrates and transcends one's biological and psychosocial nature

Related Factors

Separation from religious and cultural ties

Challenged belief and value system (e.g., result of moral or ethical implications of therapy or result of intense suffering)

Defining Characteristics

Concern expressed regarding the meaning of life and death and/or belief systems

Anger toward God (as defined by the person)

Questioning the meaning of suffering

Verbalizing inner conflict about beliefs

Verbalizing concern about relationship with deity

Questioning meaning of own existence

Inability to choose or choosing not to participate in usual religious practices

Seeking spiritual assistance

Questioning moral and ethical implications of therapeutic regimen

Displacement of anger toward religious representatives

Description of nightmares or sleep disturbances

Alteration in behavior or mood evidenced by anger, crying, withdrawal, preoccupation, anxiety, hostility, apathy, etc.

Regarding illness as punishment

Not experiencing that God is forgiving

Inability to accept self

Engaging in self-blame

Denying responsibility for problems

Describing somatic complaints

Interventions

Assess cause(s) of spiritual distress

Patient's belief in divide power, its existence, and credibility

Meaning of religion; description or relationship of divine power

Means of communicating with divine power

Effect of beliefs on personal life

Sense of identity, worth, and purpose

Relationship with others: value, need, changes caused by illness

Meaning of illness or suffering in relation to belief

Important features of religious faith

Assistance with fear, pain

Source of strength, hope, love

Religious practices, symbols, medals, garments

Provide a quiet, private atmosphere for expressions of faith, self, and meaning of life

Listen with attention, understanding, and compassion

Be available and sensitive to patient's needs to express feelings

Talk with, not at, patient

Be cognizant of your nonverbal behavior, biases, preconceptions, and judgments

Do not impose your beliefs on patient

Accurately interpret and clarify meanings expressed and behavior observed

Assist patient with facing reality; explore experience of illness and meaning of suffering

Encourage self-awareness and mobilization of internal strengths and resources

Assist patient through uncompleted developmental stages to attain trust, hope, love, forgiveness, and purpose in life

Assist patient with exploring life situations and discovering practical solutions to problems

Allow and encourage free choice and decision making

Praise successes: physical, emotional, and spiritual

Convey to patient that he is important and what he does with his life matters

Use touch therapeutically when providing daily care: stroking, holding hands, and grooming

Provide pleasant view and special pictures

Control odors and smoking as necessary

Provide articles necessary for religious practice: special clothing, rosary, books, etc.

Arrange religious symbols for easy viewing

Arrange for favorite music: recordings and tapes

Read favorite, comforting passages from Bible, Koran, Torah, Book of Mormon, poetry, other meaningful works

Share in prayers or special practices when appropriate

Provide uninterrupted time for meditation, silence, and prayer

Arrange for communion, anointment, and other practices

Arrange easy access for communication with loved ones, chaplain, priest, rabbi, or minister

Provide special foods, meals, and periods of fasting as needed

Consider needs in special situations

Birth: baptism or circumcision
Medical procedures: amputation, burial, transfusions
Note schedule for holy days
Religious observances
Anointment
Laying-on of hands
Healing services
Confession
Communion
Holy days
Restrictions or needs in diet or appearance
Not cutting or shaving of hair
Use of special clothing
Death
   Rite for anointing the sick
   Bathing and placement of body
   Positioning of extremities

Expected Outcome/Evaluation

Patient
   Expresses increased sense of hope and well being
   Demonstrates desire to interact with others in a meaningful manner
   Uses available religious resources

Care of Patient with Special Needs

GENERAL PREOPERATIVE CARE/TEACHING

Assessment
Observations/findings
EMOTIONAL STATUS

Understanding of operative, preoperative, and postoperative procedures
Ability to verbalize fears and anxieties
Relationship, response, and behavior of patient and family
Family's knowledge of operative procedure

PHYSICAL STATUS

Nutritional and hygienic state
Elimination habits
Medications being taken
Medical background
   Diseases
   Surgery
Socioeconomic background
Allergies
Physical handicaps, limitations
Signs of infection
Mental, visual, auditory acuity

LEGAL STATUS

Informed consent signed for operation
Physician's preoperative orders complete
Identification bands on and correct
Patient's willingness to receive blood noted
Environmental understanding

Use of equipment in room
Use of call bell
Purpose and use of side rails

Interventions

Maintain NPO after midnight or as ordered
Take a record BP, T, P, R, and weight; report abnormalities to physician
Check and record allergies
Monitor laboratory work; report abnormalities to physician
Assess surgical preparations for completeness
Administer enemas as ordered; avoid giving too many, too fast as they may tire or dehydrate patient
Complete bowel preparation if ordered
Monitor for electrocardiogram (ECG) and chest x-ray examinations
Assess history and physical for completeness
Assess blood type and cross match results; note number of units available
Administer preoperative medications; make sure side rails are up after injection
Insert nasogastric tube and/or indwelling bladder catheter if ordered
Initiate parenteral fluids if ordered
Encourage patient to void before leaving for operating room
Remove dentures, contact lenses, nail polish, makeup, prosthesis, and/or valuables before leaving for operating room; religious medals may be pinned to gown

Preoperative Teaching
EMOTIONAL

Reinforce physician's explanation of surgical procedure
Answer questions as honestly as possible
Allow time for and encourage verbalization of fears and anxieties
Avoid standard clichés such as "Don't worry," "Everything is just fine," "I know how you feel"
Listen to and *hear* patient
Avoid rushing through explanations
Accept patient's behavior unless it is unsafe; avoid judging it or trying to change it
Involve family or significant other in care and instructions when possible

PHYSICAL

Explain all procedures, the reason for them, and their importance
Preoperative
   Enema
   Skin preparation
   NPO
   Laboratory work
Postoperative

Parenteral fluids
Vital signs
Dressings
Pain and availability of medications
Nasogastric and other tubes
Indwelling urethral catheter
Incentive spirometer, oxygen therapy
Not touching the incision
Teach patient, using return demonstration, how to
Turn, cough, and deep breathe, depending on surgical procedure
Support incision during coughing
Deep breathe hourly postoperatively
Exercise lower extremities actively
Sit up, get up, and ambulate; chair sitting should be avoided
Explain importance of progressive care
Early ambulation
Self-care encouraged as soon as patient is able
Discuss with patient and family purpose of recovery room
Visiting policies
Type of care
Length of stay if applicable
Possibility of placement in intensive care unit (ICU) if indicated
Explain other hospital policies as indicated
Visiting hours
Number of visitors
Location of waiting rooms
How physician will contact them after operation

RECOVERY ROOM CARE

Assessment
Observations/findings
GENERAL ANESTHESIA

Level of consciousness
Unconscious
Absence of cough or gag reflex
Presence of endotracheal tube or airway
Semiconscious
Absence of endotracheal tube
Presence of oral or nasal airway
Partial return of all reflexes
Conscious
Return of all reflexes
Respiration
Rate
Rhythm
Depth
Quality
Laryngospasm
Endotracheal tube or airway present
Position
Adequate ventilation
Pulse

Rate
Rhythm
Quality
Blood pressure
Hypotension
Hypertension
Normal
Parenteral infusion
Flow rate
Type of solution
Site
Patent vein
Medications
Pain
Location
Amount, severity, type
Tolerance of
Skin
Color
Normal
Flushed
Cyanotic
Pallid
Condition
Dry
Moist
Hot
Cold
Nail beds: color
Normal
Cyanotic
Return of reflexes
Type of surgery performed
Site of incision
Dry
Bleeding
Drainage
Drains
Dressing
Dry
Intact
Drainage tubes: patency and connections
Past and current medical problems

SPINAL ANESTHESIA

Monitor each item under general anesthesia section and check legs for the following
Mobility
Color
Temperature, pedal pulses
Return of sensation

Interventions

Maintain patent airway
Endotracheal tubes, nasal and oral airways
Suction prn

Inadequate airway
  Hyperextend neck
  Bring chin forward
  Turn head to one side
  Insert oral or nasal airway
  Notify anesthesiologist of respiratory impairment
Take initial BP, P, and R and report to anesthesiologist
Monitor q15min and prn until stable
  BP, R, and apical pulse
  Level of consciousness
  Return of reflexes
  IV site
  Site of incision
  Drainage tubes and equipment
  Movement of extremities
Monitor rectal or axillary temperature q1h to 4h
Auscultate chest for breath sounds q30min
Maintain NPO
Maintain parenteral fluids as ordered
Measure intake and output; report <30 ml/hr output to
  physician
Administer oxygen, incentive spirometer
Reinforce dressing prn; notify physician if drainage is ex-
  cessive
Administer blood and blood components as ordered
Administer all medications as ordered
Encourage patient to move legs and feet if not contrain-
  dicated
Position to maintain optimal ventilation and comfort
Maintain pain management; administer narcotics in one-
  fourth, one-third, or one-half doses until patient has
  reacted fully
Monitor patient-controlled analgesia (PCA) or continu-
  ous epidural anesthesia (CEA) as warranted
Keep patient warm and dry; cover with warm blankets if
  necessary
Remain with patient if restless
  Turn patient's head to one side at first sign of vomiting
  Suction as needed
Administer oral hygiene q1h to 2h; keep patient's mouth
  and tongue moist
Assist patient to turn, cough, and deep breathe q1h to
  2h when reactive: support incision as needed
Monitor traction equipment for accurate placement and
  weights
Monitor casts for position and body alignment
Maintain quiet environment; avoid discussions over pa-
  tient's bed
Discharge to room when
  Patient is fully reactive
  Patient is moving extremities well
  Vital signs have been stable for 1 hr
  Patient is medicated for pain and vital signs are stable
  Dressings have been checked and no bleeding or ex-
    cessive drainage is noted

All drainage tubes are functioning
Patient has been cleared by anesthesiologist

CARE OF THE AGING PATIENT

***Aging** Part of the continuum of life; effects vary widely from one individual to the next; does not progress at a uniform rate, and at any given time patient may exhibit only a few of the characteristics (disease should not necessarily be equated with aging; however when one health problem is identified, others must be suspected since multiple disease conditions are a primary characteristic of advancing years); classification of aging has changed in recent years because of increasing longevity. 65 to 75 yrs: older adult, over 75 yrs: elder-older adult*

Normal Variations During the Aging Process
Assessment
Observations/findings

General
  Height 1/2 inch or more below height during youth
  Steady weight loss in men over 65 years old (weight
    gain in women)
  Ears and nose appear large in relation to size of face
  Wrinkling and sagging of skin
  Loss of hair pigmentation and thinning of hair
Eyes
  Dry and lusterless
  Discoloration of sclera
  Arcus senilis (opaque ring near edge of cornea)
  Diminished pupil size
  Pale brown discoloration in iris
  Diminished peripheral vision
Ears
  Hearing loss
  Initial loss of high-frequency tones
  Suspiciousness and irritability may or may not be
    present
Mouth
  Loss of taste perception
  Recession of gums if not edentulous
Breasts: pendulous, elongated, and/or flaccid
Respiratory system
  Decreased tidal volume
  Decreased peripheral perfusion
  Tracheal deviation if upper dorsal scoliosis present
Cardiovascular system
  Decreased resting heart rate and cardiac output
  Easily palpable arterial pulse
Gastrointestinal system
  Diminished salivation and gastric acid secretion
  Constipation
Genitourinary system
  Nocturnal micturition frequent
  Incontinence

Difficulty in initiating and ending the stream in male (caused by prostatic hypertrophy)
Female reproductive system
  Narrowing and shortening of vagina
  Diminished vaginal lubrication
  Dyspareunia
  Long-term estrogen therapy effects
    Uterine bleeding
    Mastalgia
    Weight gain
    Fluid retention
    Hypertension
  Uterine contractions with orgasm may be uncomfortable
Male reproductive system
  Decrease in size and firmness of testes
  Enlarged prostate gland
  Decrease in amount and viscosity of seminal fluid
  Increased diameter of penis
  Longer duration of excitement and plateau or orgasmic phases; resolution phase may last 12 to 24 hr
  Libido and sense of satisfaction usually do not change
Musculoskeletal system
  Decrease in quick voluntary movements
  Decrease in muscle mass; not necessarily associated with loss of strength
  Osteoarthritic changes in joints
    Heberden's nodes at distal finger joints
    Bouchard's nodes at proximal finger joints
  Dupuytren's contracture of lateral fingers, preventing full extension
  Osteoporosis: kyphosis may be an early indication
  Broad-based stance
Skin
  Thinning of skin over back of hands
  Decreased activity of sebaceous and sweat glands; may result in "dry skin"
Thinning and/or loss of scalp, pubic, and axillary hair
Small, scattered scarlet growths (senile telangiectasis)
Paler skin with increased pigment deposition (freckles)
Local or general skin areas lacking pigmentation (vitiligo); increases with age
Hyperkeratosis, or warts with raised pale, brown, or black epidermal overgrowth usually located over long axis of skin creases
Cutaneous skin tags (acrochordons) around lower neck, axillary area; usually soft and flesh colored and on pedicles
Neurologic system
  Decrease in conduction velocity of some nerves
  Diminished sense of smell
  Diminished sense of position
  Decreased tactile sense
  Deep tendon reflexes may be decreased
  Diminished sensitivity to hot and cold extremes in temperature

Interventions

Assess support systems and recent changes in life that may have bearing on ability to meet needs
Monitor fluid/nutrition intake
  Observe for retention/dehydration/malnutrition
  Assess skin turgor
  Provide fluids/diet within parameters of disease process
  Assess ability to chew, swallow, presence of dentures
Monitor elimination patterns
  Observe for incontinence
  Constipation, diarrhea
  Provide bedpan, urinal within easy reach
Monitor activity/rest
  Observe ability to perform ADLs
  Provide balance between activity and rest
Monitor communication/social skills
  Provide alternate means of communicating as needed
  Involve in care plan
  Promote self-care as tolerated
  Encourage family/significant other support
Monitor medications
  Administer medications judiciously
  Absorption, detoxification, and excretion of drugs is diminished; lower dosage levels and decreased frequency of administration may be indicated
  Assess need for analgesia carefully since sensitivity to pain is usually decreased
Monitor side effects carefully

CARE OF THE DYING PATIENT

Death *An unavoidable part of life and the part most difficult to accept. Each person dies uniquely and therefore must be cared for uniquely; that is, the nurse must develop and maintain a positive needs-perceptive relationship with the patient and family that will allow the patient to die in comfort and with dignity*

Nurse Self-Assessment/Interventions

To care for the dying patient, the nurse must
  Learn about self and own feelings concerning dying
  Look at own cultural background
  Examine own exposure to death
    Family and friends
    Reactions to these experiences
  Be honest about own feelings: anxiety, depression, avoidance, coping mechanisms
  Examine how nurse sees own death
  Share feelings about death with others; initiate open discussion to better understand behavior
  Learn to listen; realize that all of a patient's questions do not require answers—often patient will answer own questions if nurse does not provide "pat" answers
  Explore feelings about life: respect, discontent, etc.
  Recognize own power in controlling patient and his responses to care

Avoid using this power as threat to patient
Use it to give respectful, humane care
Consider effect patient has on nurse; examine how nurse sees him as an individual human being
Consider the following in caring for the dying patient
Be aware of what physician has told patient; avoid conflicting statements
Realize that decision to tell patient of outcome of disease lies with physician and family
Be honest in dealing with patient who has not been told of impending death (ask patient what he thinks or feels about his question "Am I going to die?")
Communicate situations and conversations with patient to others on the staff; provide continuity and avoid discrepancies in emotional care

Family Assessment/Interventions

Realize that family or significant other will need support during patient's illness
Assess and evaluate patient and family feelings about death and work within the framework of those feelings
Do not judge actions or behavior of family
Realize that family members may have gone through a lot with a long illness and are no longer able to cope
Understand that a change in family structure is occurring
Emotional: loss of a loved member
Financial: long illnesses become a burden
Be aware that preillness relationships and/or problems will continue
Encourage family involvement with patient
Frequent visits and telephone calls
Staying with patient
Bringing valued objects to patient
Providing home-cooked meals
Bringing children and pets for visits
Assist family in grieving process
Understand that they, too, will go through the stages of dying
Be aware that timing of stages is very often not the same as the patient's
Understand that family very often may not reach stage of acceptance
Work with famiy past denial stage so that they can let patient know the truth, thus permitting open and frank communication with patient
Assist family in making plans, both intermediate and long-term
Help family see patient's need to live as normally as possible for as long as possible
Assist family in making arrangements for home care when it is possible and desirable for patient
Teach methods of care that will be required
Arrange help through social service department and community resources
Explore possibility of hospice care

Patient Assessment/Interventions

Realize patient needs compassionate, consistent, and realistic care during terminal illness
Be aware that he is sensitive to feelings of others
Understand that patient will avoid discussion of his death and feelings if he senses others are unable to talk of dying
Be aware that he will very often discuss feelings with nursing staff rather than with the physician
Provide needed hope, human contact, and caring
Understand that hope must be realistic; patient needs treatment for alleviation of pain rather than getting well
Do not avoid patient during any of the stages of dying
Realize that patient needs continuous caring by all members of staff
Be aware that patient has many fears
Encourage expression of feelings
Provide an accepting environment
Demonstrate warmth and friendliness
Encourage use of spiritual resources
Explore past coping strengths
Explain all procedures and nursing functions
Discuss fears with patient
Fear of the unknown
Loss of control of body and behavior
Pain: Patient needs explanation of availability of different drugs and therapies, such as radiation or surgery
Helplessness: Patient needs general nutrition, some activity, and deep breathing every day, which usually help initially
Understand that patient needs to have each day be as comfortable, positive, and productive as possible
Promote self-care and diversional activities
Maintain a normal lifestyle for as long as possible

Care During the Stages of Dying

DENIAL AND SHOCK
Assessment
Observations/findings

Ignoring or distorting reasons given for illness
Refusal to participate in care
Refusal to follow directions of physician or staff

Interventions

Recognize that denial and shock will be used by the patient after he is told of impending death
Do not interfere with this mechanism unless it becomes destructive (patient refuses further treatment and care)
Spend time with patient to show that he will not be left alone
Do not support denial; conversations should include reality
Continue to teach and encourage self-care and activities

ANGER

Assessment

Observations/findings

Abusive language
Refusal of care
Refusal of nutrition and self-care
Negative criticism of staff
Striking out
   Not permitting others to be close to him
   Throwing objects
   Removing IV needle, leads, etc.
   Calling for nurse and then asking why nurse is there

Interventions

Recognize that patient is not angry with nurse personally
Do not allow physically harmful behavior to continue
   Spend time with patient and discuss his anger
   Encourage verbalization of anger; be empathetic
Plan care with patient and encourage mutual problem solving
Question how patient evaluates care being given
Continue to question and discuss patient's anger

BARGAINING

Assessment

Observations/findings

Statements such as "I hope I live until. . .," "If only I could . . ."

Interventions

Realize patient needs time to accept death and needs this mechanism
Spend time with patient
Discuss importance of valued objects and people
Set small, realistic, attainable goals
Provide praise for goals reached or attempted

DEPRESSION

Assessment

Observations/findings

Apathy
Decreased ability to concentrate
Insomnia
Inability to wake up
Crying
Constant fatigue
Poor appetite
Lack of interest in people or environment

Interventions

Recognize that patient is beginning to separate himself from life
Do not attempt to cheer patient
Be available to sit quietly and if appropriate hold patient's hand

Accept crying and do not interrupt
Realize that patient may only want most beloved person to be with him
Promote positive relationships to maintain patient's dignity

ACCEPTANCE

Assessment

Observations/findings

Devoid of feelings
Absence of emotional affect
Peacefulness
Less pain and discomfort, usually

Interventions

Plan care to allow person with whom patient is comfortable to care for him
Realize that patient may not want to be alone

ENTERAL NUTRITION

Provision of nutritional support to meet nutritional requirements via a nasogastric tube, orogastric tube, esophagostomy, gastrostomy, duodenostomy, or jejunostomy; preferred for the patient who has a functional GI tract but is unable to consume an adequate nutritional intake, or when oral intake is contraindicated; may be indicated in the following clinical conditions: physical impairments (e.g., obstructive lesions of the esophagus or pharynx, following radical head and neck surgery, following fracture of facial bones); neurologic conditions associated with impaired swallowing and oropharyngeal trauma; increased metabolic needs caused by trauma, burns, or sepsis, or the presence of an endotracheal tube

Assessment

Observations/findings

Dietary history
   Lactose intolerance
   Food allergies, dietary restrictions
Medical history
   Chronic renal disease
   Liver disorders
   Diabetes mellitus
   Heart disease
Cerebrovascular accident (CVA)
   Coma
Respiratory
   Respiratory distress
   Aspiration
   Coughing
   Choking
   Cyanosis
   Increased respiratory rate
   Decreased breath sounds
   Rales at lung bases

Skin and mucous membranes
  Skin irritation and/or breakdown, nares, ostomy tube
  Poor skin turgor
  Dry mucous membranes
  Diaphoresis
Level of consciousness
  Coma
  Change in mental status
Gastrointestinal
  Nausea
  Vomiting
  Diarrhea
  Abdominal distention/delayed gastric emptying
  Decreased or absent bowel sounds
  Abdominal cramping
  Constipation
  Esophageal reflux
  Gastric residual
  Tube placement: stomach, duodenum, jejunum, esophagus

Laboratory/diagnostic studies

Serum electrolytes
Serum osmolality
Serum glucose
Urine glucose
Urine specific gravity
BUN
Serum creatinine
Serum albumin
Serum transferrin

Potential complications

Hypernatremia (p. 44)
Hyperchloremia
Azotemia
Dehydration
Tube feeding syndrome
Hyperglycemia
Nausea
Vomiting
Pulmonary injury during insertion
Aspiration/pneumonia
Diarrhea
Constipation
Gastric retention
Fluid overload (p. 50)
Gastric rupture
Dumping syndrome
  Weakness
  Diaphoresis
  Lightheadedness
  Tachycardia
  Cramping
Tube displacement

Tube obstruction
Intraperitoneal leakage and leakage of fluid around catheter (associated with gastrostomy and jejunostomy tubes)

Medical Management

Treatment of underlying disease process
Desired route
Tube selection, small bore tubes generally used
Type of formula (concentration and rate)
Intermittent or continuous feeding
Antidiarrheal agents
Laxatives
Insulin
Intake and output
Daily weights
Daily laboratory studies

Nursing diagnoses/interventions/evaluation

■ **NDX:** Diarrhea related to altered dietary intake, malabsorption, concomitant drug therapy, type of formula, bacterial contamination, stress/anxiety

Record color, odor, amount, and frequency of stool qday
Monitor intake and output q8h
Test stool for occult blood
Weigh patient daily at same time with same clothing and scale
Assess for signs and symptoms of dehydration
  Poor skin turgor
  Decreased urine output
  Increased urine specific gravity
  Dry mucous membranes
Monitor laboratory results; report abnormalities to physician
Review current medications, antibiotics, cimetidine, other H_2 blockers, electrolyte elixirs, antacids for possible side effects, such as diarrhea
Assess for intolerance to feeding solution q4h
Report untoward reactions to physician immediately
  Abdominal distention, delayed gastric emptying
  Nausea
  Vomiting
  Cramping
Auscultate bowel sounds q4h
Report hyperactive or hypoactive bowel sounds to physician
Assess for gastric residual q4h
If residual is greater than 100 ml, hold feeding and notify physician (replace residual)
Avoid rapid rate of infusion
  Initiate tube feeding slowly at half-strength concentration or as ordered by physician
  Increase rate according to patient tolerance

Regulate flow rate using enteral pump (some IV infusion pumps can be adapted to delivery enteral feedings)

Place time tape on formula bag or bottle; monitor rate q1h

Give formula at room temperature

Administer antidiarrheal agents as ordered

Avoid formula with high osmolality and high fat content

Contact physician regarding change in formula

Administer enteral feedings at approximate serum osmolality

Administer dilute strength and/or decrease volume per physician order

Intervene for lactose intolerance

Contact physician regarding change to lactose-free formula

Delete all milk products from diet

Avoid bacterial contamination

Wash hands thoroughly before preparation and handling of formula

Use ready-mix formula whenever possible

Allow formula to hang for no longer than 8-12 hrs

Refrigerate unused formula

Rinse feeding container and gavage set between feedings

Flush tube with water when feeding is disconnected

Change feeding container and gavage set daily

Expected outcome/evaluation

Patient

Tolerates tube feeding volume, concentration, and formula type

Evacuates soft-formed stool qod

Remains hydrated

■ **NDX:** Potential for aspiration related to reduced level of consciousness, diminished or absent cough and gag reflexes, incompetent esophageal sphincter, delayed gastric emptying, displaced feeding tube

Use small-bore feeding tubes: less likely to disrupt the esophageal sphincter and cause reflux

Ensure correct placement of tube in stomach q4h (with small-bore tube, x-ray examination may be necessary to confirm placement)

Confirm by radiograph placement of all intestinal tubes

Keep head of bed elevated 30 to 45 degrees during feeding periods and 1 hour after

Clamp tube feeding when patient must be placed flat

Check for residual q4h for continuous feeding and before each intermittent or bolus feeding

Report to physician if residual is 100 ml or more and hold feeding

Replace aspirate: prevents loss of gastric juices and electrolytes

Assess patient for cramping, bloating, nausea, and abdominal distension

Auscultate bowel sounds q4h

Monitor vital signs T, P, R, and BP q4h

Inflate cuff for cuffed tracheostomy tube or endotracheal tube and keep inflated for 1 hr after feeding

Assess for signs and symptoms of aspiration; report findings to physician

Shortness of breath

Fever

Cough

Discolored tracheal aspirate

Increased respiratory rate

Cyanosis

Diminished breath sounds

Rales/rhonchi

Before removal of orogastric or nasogastric tube, irrigate and clamp or pinch tube to minimize risk of aspiration as tube is being withdrawn

Expected outcome/evaluation

Patient's

Breath sounds are normal as evidenced by

No rales or rhonchi

No cough

Temperature is within normal limits

■ **NDX:** Fluid volume deficit related to insufficient fluid intake and abnormal fluid loss associated with high osmolality of enteral feeding

Assess q8h for signs and symptoms of fluid volume deficit

Report the following to physician

Poor skin turgor

Decreased urine output

Dry mucous membranes

Weight loss greater than 0.5 kg/day

Decreased blood pressure

Increased urine specific gravity

Measure intake and output q8h

Weigh patient daily at same time with same clothing and scale

Increase free water via feeding tube as prescribed

Thereafter, flush feeding tube with 30 to 50 ml of water q4h to 6h

Monitor urine specific gravity q8h

Administer hypertonic formulas using half-strength concentration

Change hypertonic formula to isotonic formula

Document baseline mental status

Assess mental status q4h; report changes to physician

Monitor continuous feedings q1h

Use enteral pump to regulate rate of feedings

Monitor urine or serum glucose q6h as ordered

Expected outcome/evaluation

Patient

Maintains good skin turgor, color

Presents moist mucous membranes

Maintains weight

Maintains urine specific gravity within normal limits

■ **NDX:**   Constipation related to formula composition, inadequate water intake, and immobility

Ensure administration of high-residue formula
Increase free water via feeding tube as prescribed
Flush feeding tube with 30 to 50 ml of water q4h to 6h
Administer stool softener as prescribed
Administer 4 to 6 oz of prune juice daily through tube, if allowed
Monitor medications (e.g., narcotics) for possible side effects
Encourage physical activity within limits
    Assist with ambulation
    Assist patient to chair twice a day
    Change position q2h
Monitor for fecal impaction
Allow for adequate time in bathroom or with commode/ bedpan
Provide privacy for patient
Monitor bowel elimination pattern

Expected outcome/evaluation

Patient
    Tolerates tube feeding
    Evacuates soft, formed stool qod

■ **NDX:**   Impaired tissue integrity: related to pressure from feeding tube and/or drainage from ostomy tube insertion site

Use small-bore feeding tube when possible
Position tube to prevent undue pressure on nares
Cleanse and lubricate nares q4h and prn
Provide oral care q4h and prn
Provide skin care at insertion site of ostomy tube
Assess tube insertion site q8h for tenderness, redness, and drainage
Report abnormalities to physician
Change ostomy site dressing q2d and prn
Cleanse site with soap and water
Apply stoma adhesive around tube at insertion site
Cover site with transparent or similar dressing
Secure ostomy tube
Report continuous leakage around tube to physician

Expected outcome/evaluation

Patient's skin around the tube insertion site is clean and dry

■ **NDX:**   Body image disturbance related to change in appearance resulting from nasal or ostomy tube

Assess level of anxiety and understanding of need for tube feedings; if feasible, select and/or change to a feeding tube that patient tolerates physically and psychologically
Encourage patient to express feelings about the way he feels and looks

Reassure patient that feelings are appropriate
Continue to be sensitive to patient's needs and feelings
Assess for readiness to begin self-care
Instruct patient and/or significant other regarding feeding procedure
Provide emotional support and positive feedback for participation in self-feeding
Provide opportunity for questions and reinforce instructions as necessary
Continue to support coping efforts
Provide referrals as necessary (social service, dietitian, support groups, clergy)
Encourage ambulation if not contraindicated
Provide small amounts of favorite foods orally, if allowed

Expected outcome/evaluation

Patient
    Expresses understanding of need for tube feeding
    Copes with imposed restrictions
    Participates in own care
    Shares feelings about how he views himself

■ **NDX:**   Knowledge deficit related to lack of information about purpose and administration of tube feedings, complications, nasal tube and enterostomy care, and/or activity

Purpose and administration of tube feedings

Explain that all necessary nutrients—protein, fats, carbohydrates, vitamins, and minerals—will be supplied by tube feeding
Discuss formula selection and reason for same
Instruct patient and/or significant other in formula preparation, storage, and feeding schedule
Instruct patient and/or significant other in administration of formula and medications via feeding tube

Complications

Discuss signs and symptoms of feeding intolerance
    Nausea, vomiting, diarrhea, cramping, bloating; discuss importance of reporting signs and symptoms to physician
Explain reasons for administration of feeding with patient upright
Demonstrate procedure for checking placement of feeding tube
Discuss signs and symptoms of possible aspiration
    Coughing, choking, difficulty in breathing, elevated temperature; discuss importance of reporting signs and symptoms to physician
Discuss importance of flushing tube with water after each feeding and after administration of medications
Demonstrate urine and/or serum glucose checking procedure; discuss importance of reporting abnormalities to physician
Discuss measures to prevent constipation

Contact home health nurse if tube is clogged, broken, or dislodged

Nasal tube and enterostomy care

Demonstrate taping of tube to prevent slipping

Demonstrate cleansing and lubrication of nares; explain that this should be done q4h and prn

Teach importance of maintaining good oral hygiene

Demonstrate ostomy care

Discuss importance of reporting redness, drainage, foul odor, or tenderness around stoma to physician

Teach patient how to remove and insert ostomy feeding tube per physician order (esophagotomy and gastrostomy tubes may be removed after several weeks and inserted only for feedings)

Activity

Instruct patient to increase activity/exercise as desired and tolerated

Discuss benefits of exercise

Promotes feeling of well-being

Increases gastric motility

Expected outcome/evaluation

Patient

Demonstrates administration of tube feeding, serum/glucose testing, ostomy care with application of skin barrier and appliance

Acknowledges understanding of purpose of tube feeding, complications with intervention, and need for follow-up care

TOTAL PARENTERAL NUTRITION (TPN)

Infusion of necessary nutrients—amino acids, fat, trace elements, carbohydrates, vitamins, and electrolytes— through a peripheral or central vein; peripheral or central venous nutrition may be chosen when the enteral route is not available because of mechanical or functional abnormalities of the GI tract; clinical conditions that may indicate the need for parenteral nutrition are short bowel syndrome, ileus, malabsorption, pancreatitis, hypermetabolic states (trauma, sepsis), and altered metabolic states (acute renal failure, hepatic insufficiency)

Assessment
Observations/findings

Insertion site

Pain

Warmth

Redness

Edema

Drainage at insertion site

Leakage at insertion site

Fever

Leukocytosis

Glucose intolerance

Laboratory/diagnostic studies

Potassium

Phosphorus

Magnesium

Blood glucose

Calcium

Sodium

Chloride

Blood urea nitrogen (BUN)

Prothrombin time (PT)

White blood cell count (WBC)

Liver enzymes

Bilirubin

Serum albumin

Transferrin

Potential complications

Mechanical

Pneumothorax (with subclavian vein catheterization)

Air embolism

Catheter and venous thrombosis

Septic

Catheter sepsis (bacterial or fungal)

Metabolic

Hyperglycemia

Hyperosmolar nonketotic coma

Hypoglycemia

Fatty acid deficiency

Electrolyte abnormalities

Liver dysfunction

Mineral and trace elements deficiency

Medical Management

Route of administration

X-ray examination to determine placement of central line

Keeping vein open with isotonic solution until catheter placement is confirmed

Rate of flow

Increase or decrease in rate of solution

Fat emulsion

Daily weights

Urine glucose

Blood glucose monitoring

Administration of insulin

Intake and output

Daily laboratory studies

Nursing diagnoses/interventions/evaluation

■ **NDX:** Potential for infection related to risk of invasive procedure and delivery of high concentrations of glucose parenterally

Peripheral venous nutrition

Wash hands thoroughly before insertion of IV needle or catheter

Wear gloves as per universal precautions

Select distal veins in upper extremities

Clip or shave hair at site according to hospital policy

Prepare site with povidone-iodine swab and allow to air dry

Cover site with occlusive dressing

Monitor for signs and symptoms of phlebitis and/or infiltration

Remove catheter or needle if phlebitis or infiltration is present

Rotate catheter site q72h or according to hospital policy

Tape IV tubing securely

Monitor catheter site every hour

Change IV tubing q24h or according to hospital policy

Use strict aseptic technique when assembling and changing administration set

Monitor vital signs T, P, and R q4h; report elevation of temperature to physician

Monitor blood glucose as ordered

Monitor urine for glucose as ordered, usually q6h (glucosuria may indicate impending sepsis)

Ensure that final amino acid concentration does not exceed 10% dextrose

Ensure continuous infusion of fat emulsion when 10% dextrose is infused peripherally

Refrigerate TPN solution until ready to use

Allow solution to hang no longer than 24 hr

Never piggyback medications other than fat emulsion via TPN line

Securely tape needle used for piggybacking fat emulsion

Central venous nutrition

Assist physician with insertion of central line catheter

Ensure catheter insertion under sterile conditions

Ensure proper site preparation

Change central line dressing using sterile technique

Prepare site with povidone-iodine and allow to air dry

Apply povidone-iodine ointment to catheter site

Cover site with sterile occlusive dressing

Observe site for signs of sepsis: erythema, swelling, tenderness, drainage at insertion site

Monitor vital signs T, P, and R q4h; report temperature elevation to physician

Monitor blood glucose as ordered

Monitor urine for glucose as ordered, usually q6h (glucosuria may indicate impending sepsis)

Monitor catheter site q1h

Tape tubing securely

Do not use stopcocks on TPN line

Change IV tubing q24h or according to hospital policy

Use strict aseptic technique when assembling and changing administration set

Allow solution to hang no longer than 24 hr

Never use line for piggybacking medications, taking central venous pressure (CVP) readings, or aspirating blood for laboratory studies

Expected outcome/evaluation

Patient's

Temperature is within normal limits;

Catheter insertion site is clean, dry, and intact with no sign of redness, edema, or drainage

■ **NDX:** Potential complications of total parenteral nutrition (TPN), metabolic abnormalities, pneumothorax, air embolism, adverse reactions to amino acid and/or fat emulsion therapy[*]

Metabolic abnormalities

Monitor for signs and symptoms of hyperglycemia

Polyuria

Glycosuria: elevated blood sugar

Polydipsia, polyphagia

Dimmed, blurred vision

Monitor for signs and symptoms of hypoglycemia

Tachycardia

Cold sweat

Posterior occipital headache

Irritability, jitteriness

Lethargy

Blood glucose level <60 mg/dl

Perform urine and/or serum testing q6h

Monitor vital signs and electrolytes (Table 1-3) q4h

Assess neurologic status q8h

Monitor intake and output q8h

Weigh patient daily at same time with same clothing and scale

Initiate TPN solution slowly

Increase rate per patient tolerance and physician order

Do not increase rate to catch up

Monitor flow rate of solution using infusion control device

Do not interrupt infusion for more than 1 hr q8h

Ensure patency of line

For hyperglycemia, administer insulin as ordered

For hypoglycemia, administer IV 50% dextrose as ordered

---

[*]Not a NANDA-approved nursing diagnosis.

TABLE 1-3. Observation of Fluid and Electrolyte Imbalances

Imbalances	Causes	Neuromuscular system	GI system
ELECTROLYTE IMBALANCES			
Hyperkalemia (potassium excess)	Excessive administration of potassium chloride Decreased renal excretion, as in renal failure, hypovolemia, potassium-sparing diuretics Trauma to tissues such as burns and crash injuries (will release intercellular potassium and result in hyperkalemia) Aldosterone insufficiency Respiratory or metabolic acidosis Banked blood	Weakness, flaccid paralysis, twitching, hyperreflexia, paresthesia or numbness and tingling sensations, (usually affect the face, tongue, hands, and feet), apathy, confusion	Diarrhea, intestinal colic, nausea
Hypokalemia (potassium deficit)	Increased renal loss (diuretics; diuresis phase after burns; diabetic acidosis, Cushing's syndrome; nephritis) Hypomagnesium Inadequate intake of potassium Acid base imbalance: alkalosis; loss from vomiting, diarrhea, excess use of laxatives, GI suction or fistulas, steroid administration	Muscular cramps, paresthesias, muscular weakness to flaccid paralysis, fatigue, mental confusion, hyporeflexia, drowsiness, apathy, irritability, tetany, coma	Anorexia, nausea and vomiting, abdominal distension, paralytic ileus

Respiratory system	Cardiovascular system	Renal system	Skin and mucous membranes	Blood gas values	Interventions
Respiratory paralysis and involvement of muscles of phonation	Bradycardia, lethal dysrhythmias, and cardiac arrest ECG changes: tall peaked T waves, shortened QT interval, disappearance of P waves, widening of QRS complex, flat-to-absent P wave and asystole				Observe patient for changes in heart rate, rhythm, and ECG pattern Be aware cardiac arrest can occur Restrict potassium-containing foods, fluids, and salt substitutes Monitor serum potassium levels Do not give calcium if patient is on digitalis since calcium potentiates the effect of digitalis Avoid potassium-containing medications such as potassium penicillin Administer IV glucose, insulin, and sodium bicarbonate as ordered (helps shift potassium into the cells) Administer cation-exchange resins as ordered (helps to remove potassium by way of GI tract) Peritoneal or hemodialysis may be ordered if other therapy fails
Respiratory muscle weakness, paralysis of the diaphragm, shallow respirations, apnea, and death may result	Irregular rhythm, ECG: flat or inverted T wave, appearance of U wave, short and depressed ST segment, peaking of P waves, QT interval prolonged, circulatory failure, hypotension and systolic arrest Effectiveness of digitalis enhanced (to the point of toxicity)				Monitor serum potassium and report significant changes Observe for signs and symptoms of metabolic alkalosis Watch for signs of toxicity in patients receiving digitalis (blurred vision, nausea, and vomiting) Monitor rate of IV administration of potassium Monitor intake and output (report changes)

Continued.

TABLE 1-3. Observation of Fluid and Electrolyte Imbalances—cont'd

Imbalances	Causes	Neuromuscular system	GI system
Hypokalemia (potassium deficit)—cont'd			
Hypercalcemia (calcium excess)	Hyperparathyroidism Prolonged immobilization (causes calcium displacement from bone to blood) Hypophosphatemia Metastatic carcinoma Alkalosis Thyrotoxicosis Vitamin D overdose Addison's disease Multiple myeloma Skeletal muscle paralysis Cardiac failure Prolonged thiazide diuretic therapy Excessive calcium intake Parathyroid tumor Sarcoidosis	Generalized muscle weakness Depressed or absent deep tendon reflexes (DTRs) Drowsiness Lethargy Headaches Loss of muscle tone Ataxia Mental confusion Impairment of memory Slurred speech Personality or behavior changes Stupor or coma Pathologic fractures may occur Flank or deep bone pain	Anorexia Nausea Vomiting Constipation Epigastric pain Polydipsia

Respiratory system	Cardiovascular system	Renal system	Skin and mucous membranes	Blood gas values	Interventions
	Bradycardia Hypertension ECG: QT interval shortened, T waves inverted Ventricular arrhythmias Enhanced effectiveness of digitalis	Development of renal calculi, kidney stones Polyuria			Encourage intake of food and fluids rich in potassium (orange juice, bananas, bouillon, meat broths, colas, tea, leafy vegetables) Observe for changes in heart rate, rhythm, and ECG pattern Determine source of potassium losses Assess for causes Administer loop diuretics to increase excretion of calcium Administer corticosteroids and mithramycin as ordered (lowers serum calcium concentration) Administer antacids cautiously: some contain calcium Position and move patient carefully to prevent pathologic fractures Administer isotonic fluids as ordered Encourage fluid intake of 2000 to 3000 ml a day Monitor intake and output Avoid dietary intake of calcium (dairy products and green leafy vegetables) Monitor serum calcium levels Observe for changes in heart rate, rhythm, and ECG pattern Observe for digitalis toxicity

Continued.

TABLE 1-3. Observation of Fluid and Electrolyte Imbalances—cont'd

Imbalances	Causes	Neuromuscular system	GI system
Hypocalcemia (calcium deficit)	Inadequate intake of calcium Decreased absorption from intestine Hypoparathyroidism Vitamin D deficiency Rapid dilution of the plasma by intravenous calcium-free solutions Chronic renal failure Chronic malabsorption syndrome Neoplastic diseases Hypomagnesemia Cushing's syndrome Acute pancreatitis Hyperphosphatemia Extreme stress situations Excessive citrated blood, alkalosis	Muscle tremors, paresthesias, especially numbness or tingling, skeletal muscle cramps, abdominal spasms and cramps Hyperactive reflexes Convulsions Positive Trousseau's sign Positive Chvostek's sign Emotional depression or confusion	Paralytic ileus GI bleeding
Hypernatremia (sodium excess)	Primary aldosteronism: excessive steroids (Cushing's disease) Excessive IV administration of large amounts of sodium chloride solution without water replacement Renal failure (with sodium retention) Neurohypophyseal dysfunction (as in diabetes insipidus) High-protein diets with minimal fluid intake Diabetes mellitus Excessive ingestion of sodium chloride Decreased water intake, severe vomiting or diarrhea Inadequate circulation of blood to the kidneys (congestive heart failure; CHF) Cirrhosis of the liver	Sodium ↑, water ↓ CNS depression (lethargy to coma), muscle weakness, muscle rigidity, muscle tremors	

Respiratory system	Cardiovascular system	Renal system	Skin and mucous membranes	Blood gas values	Interventions
	Dysrhythmias Hypotension Prolonged QT interval with normal T wave on ECG				Monitor rate, rhythm, and ECG pattern Administer calcium gluconate or calcium chloride 10% as ordered Monitor serum calcium levels every 12 to 24 hr Report calcium deficit to physician Monitor PT and platelet levels Observe for signs and symptoms of tetany Provide dietary calcium (i.e., cheese, cream, milk, yogurt) Administer vitamin D as ordered Monitor prothrombin and platelet levels Check for bleeding from any source (calcium aids in blood clotting) Monitor use of laxatives and antacids (those containing phosphate affect calcium metabolism)
Sodium ↑, water ↑ (increase in extracellular fluid volume) may cause pulmonary edema: shortness of breath, coughing, cyanosis, increased respiratory rate	Sodium ↑, water ↑: postural hypotension Sodium ↑, water ↑: elevated blood pressure; pitting edema		Increased sodium with decrease in fluid intake: observe for signs and symptoms of dehydration (dry mucous membranes, flushed skin, elevated temperature		Sodium ↑, water ↓: Increase po fluid intake Administer IV fluids as ordered Instill water with or between tube feedings Sodium ↑, water ↑: Administer diuretics as ordered Restrict NA intake Restrict fluid intake Monitor intake and output q8h Weigh daily Monitor vital signs q8h Check urine for specific gravity

Continued.

TABLE 1-3. Observation of Fluid and Electrolyte Imbalances—cont'd

Imbalances	Causes	Neuromuscular system	GI system
Hyponatremia (sodium deficit)	Inappropriate ADH syndrome Excessive intake of hypotonic fluids Severe malnutrition Vomiting Diarrhea GI drainage from suction or fistulas Severe diaphoresis Trauma such as surgery or burns Small bowel obstruction and peritonitis Renal disease Administration of sodium-removing diuretics Water intoxication (IV therapy, tap water enemas)	Headache Vertigo Anxiety Muscle weakness and cramps Lassitude, apathy, confusion Hyperreflexia	Anorexia, nausea, vomiting, diarrhea, cramping
Hypermagnesemia (magnesium excess)	Renal failure Adrenal insufficiency Excessive ingestion of magnesium-containing medications Diabetic ketoacidosis (with severe water loss) Hyperparathyroidism	Drowsiness, lethargy, loss of deep tendon reflexes Respiratory depression, coma, and cardiac arrest	Nausea
Hypomagnesemia (magnesium deficit)	Acute pancreatitis Malabsorption syndrome (non-tropical sprue or steatorrhea) Diarrhea, vomiting Excessive calcium intake Primary hyperparathyroidism and other hypercalcemic states Alcoholism Bowel resection, small bowel bypass, or inherited intestinal defects Gastrointestinal fistulas Excessive renal secretion Nasogastric suctioning Diabetic ketoacidosis Toxemia of pregnancy	Neuromuscular irritability Tremors, tetany, increased reflexes, clonus Convulsions Disorientation Agitation, depression Hallucinations Athetoid or choreiform movements, convulsions, clonus, positive Babinski's sign, positive Chvostek's sign, and positive Trousseau's sign Paresthesias of feet and legs	Anorexia Nausea

Respiratory system	Cardiovascular system	Renal system	Skin and mucous membranes	Blood gas values	Interventions
Hyperpnea	Hypotension Orthostatic hypotension Tachycardia Thready peripheral pulse or loss of peripheral pulse, collapsed neck veins	Decreased urine output Oliguria to anuria	Flushed, dry, hot skin Fever Loss of skin turgor		Administer IV normal saline solution as ordered (monitor rate carefully) Monitor serum sodium and potassium levels Administer sodium orally as ordered Maintain intake and output q8h Weigh daily Encourage foods and fluids high in sodium (milk, meat, eggs, fruit juices, bouillon) Use normal saline for all irrigations
Depressed respirations	Hypotension Bradycardia, weak pulse, prolonged QT interval on ECG Heart block				Avoid use of all magnesium-containing medications (Maalox, Mylanta, and Milk of Magnesia) Monitor vital signs and level of consciousness qlh Encourage fluid intake Administer IV calcium gluconate as ordered Monitor serum magnesium levels q6h Observe for flushing of skin and diaphoresis
	Tachycardia Hypotension Atrial or ventricular premature contractions Nonspecific T wave changes				Administer magnesium sulfate as ordered When administering IV magnesium sulfate, observe patient carefully Monitor for signs and symptoms of high serum magnesium Check for loss of patellar reflex q5 min Monitor respiratory rate q5 min

TABLE 1-3. Observation of Fluid and Electrolyte Imbalances—cont'd

Imbalances	Causes	Neuromuscular system	GI system
Hypomagnesemia (magnesium deficit)—cont'd			

ACID-BASE IMBALANCES

Imbalances	Causes	Neuromuscular system	GI system
Respiratory alkalosis (deficit of H_2CO_3 Decreased P_{CO_2})	Fever, bacteremia, shock Hyperthyroidism Severe pain Hyperventilation caused by hysteria, intentional overbreathing, brain trauma, or ventilators Overdose of epinephrine or salicylates CNS disturbances (meningitis, encephalitis, brainstem injury) Pulmonary embolism Interstitial lung diseases, CHF Hypoxia due to high altitude or severe anemia	Syncope, vertigo, headache, muscle spasm, and weakness Tingling in fingers and face Tetany, convulsions, or coma may develop	
Respiratory acidosis (excess H_2CO_3, elevated P_{CO_2})	Hypoventilation Emphysema Chronic obstructive pulmonary disease (COPD) Pneumonia Asthma Pickwickian syndrome Barbiturate poisoning Brain trauma with pressure on medulla	Anxiety, weakness, headache Depression of CNS Disorientation and coma	Nausea and vomiting may occur

Respiratory system	Cardiovascular system	Renal system	Skin and mucous membranes	Blood gas values	Interventions
					Observe for increased thirst, flushing of skin, diaphoresis, anxiety, or drowsiness
					Notify physician immediately if patient develops loss of patellar reflex, hypotension, or flushing of face
					Take precautions against seizures
					Monitor blood pressure, pulse, and neurological signs q4h
					Watch for signs and symptoms of digitalis toxicity (a deficit in magnesium may precipitate or aggravate digitalis toxicity)
					Monitor serum magnesium levels q6h
					Observe for diarrhea
Rapid respirations	Dysrhythmias may occur			pH: increased P_{CO_2}: decreased HCO_3: normal	Implement measures to treat underlying problem
					If alkalosis is caused by anxiety, attempt to calm and reassure patient
					Encourage breathing into a paper bag and/or other breathing techniques
					Administer sedatives as ordered
Distressed respirations Cyanosis	Rapid pulse Ventricular fibrillation may occur			pH: decreased P_{CO_2}: increased HCO_3: increased	Maintain patent airway
					Place patient in semi-Fowler's position
					Suction nasal and/or pharyngeal airways and trachea as necessary

Continued.

TABLE 1-3. Observation of Fluid and Electrolyte Imbalances—cont'd

Imbalances	Causes	Neuromuscular system	GI system
Respiratory acidosis (excess H_2CO_3, elevated PCO_2)—cont'd	Neuromuscular disorder (Guillain-Barré, myasthenia gravis) Spinal cord trauma Airway occlusion Pneumothorax Atelectasis Postanesthesia Inadequate mechanical ventilation		
Metabolic alkalosis (base bicarbonate excess)	Ingestion of large amounts of sodium bicarbonate (e.g., baking soda or antacids) Vomiting Prolonged gastric suction Diarrhea Potassium-free IV solutions Transfusion Alkalosis Adrenocortical hormone use Excess infusion of parenteral bicarbonate	Hypertonicity, tetany, tremors, convulsions, sensorium changes, irritability, disorientation	
Metabolic acidosis (base bicarbonate deficit)	Diabetic ketoacidosis Prolonged starvation Alcohol abuse Renal failure Vomiting of GI contents Systemic infections Salicylate intoxication Severe diarrhea Abnormal intake of exogenous acids (e.g., ammonium chloride and ferrous sulfate)	Muscle weakness Headache CNS depression, disorientation, stupor, coma	Nausea, vomiting, diarrhea

Respiratory system	Cardiovascular system	Renal system	Skin and mucous membranes	Blood gas values	Interventions
					Avoid sedation
					Monitor heart rate and rhythm
					Administer oxygen at flow rate ordered
					Monitor fluid and electrolyte levels
					Monitor arterial blood gases
					Assess for signs and symptoms of respiratory distress
					Administer sodium bicarbonate as ordered
					Maintain mechanical ventilation as ordered
					Perform chest physiotherapy and postural drainage as ordered
Shallow, slow respirations	Sinus tachycardia Dysrhythmias			pH: increased P_{CO_2}: normal or slightly increased HCO_3: increased	Monitor accurate intake and output
					Monitor vital signs q8h
					Perform neurological check q8h
					Take seizure precautions
					Irrigate gastric suction with isotonic solutions
					Avoid excessive amounts of $NaHCO_3$
					Avoid sedatives or hypnotics
					Administer medications, treatments, and fluids as ordered by physician
Kussmaul's respirations (rapid, deep breathing) Shortness of breath on exertion	Cardiac dysrhythmias Bounding pulse Increased blood pressure			pH: decreased P_{CO_2}: normal HCO_3: decreased	Monitor accurate intake and output
					Monitor serum electrolyte levels
					Monitor blood gas levels
					Observe for signs of hyperkalemia
					Monitor vital signs q4h
					Perform neurological checks q4h

Continued.

TABLE 1-3. Observation of Fluid and Electrolyte Imbalances—cont'd

Imbalances	Causes	Neuromuscular system	GI system
Metabolic acidosis (base bicarbonate deficit)—cont'd			
FLUID IMBALANCES			
Hypervolemia (extracellular fluid volume excess)	Excess sodium intake Malnutrition Excessive ADH secretion Oliguria phase of renal disease Excessive administration of IV fluids CHF Chronic liver disease with portal hypertension	Behavior change, loss of attention, confusion and aphasia; convulsions, coma, and death may follow	Anorexia Nausea and vomiting Constipation Thirst
Hypovolemia (extracellular fluid volume deficit)	Decreased fluid intake Anorexia Excessive output: vomiting, diarrhea, wounds, burns, excessive diaphoresis Uncontrolled diabetes leading to osmotic diuresis Antidiuretic hormone (ADH) insufficiency Diuretic phase of renal disease Excessive use of diuretics	Behavior change, apathy, restlessness, disorientation, lethargy, muscle weakness, tingling of extremities	Anorexia Nausea and vomiting Diarrhea Constipation Abdominal cramps and distention Thirst

Respiratory system	Cardiovascular system	Renal system	Skin and mucous membranes	Blood gas values	Interventions
					Take seizure precautions Administer medications, treatments, and fluids as ordered by physician
Dyspnea, orthopnea, rales, productive cough	Observe for symptoms of pulmonary edema: dyspnea, orthopnea, coughing, cyanosis Increased respiratory rate Edema Distended neck veins Increased CVP readings Auscultation of S_3	Oliguria	Skin warm, moist, and flushed		Monitor accurate intake and output Weigh daily Monitor vital signs q4h Monitor IV fluid rate carefully Explain reason for restricted fluid intake Observe for signs and symptoms of CHF Restrict sodium intake Administer diuretics as ordered
	Hypotension (postural systolic hypotension) Rapid heart rate Collapsed neck veins Decreased CVP readings	Oliguria Concentrated urine	Poor skin turgor, flushed skin, dry mucous membranes, furrows on tongue		Monitor intake and output Monitor vital signs q8h Administer IV fluids as ordered Encourage po intake, if allowed Set up 24-hr schedule for fluid intake Administer plasma or albumin as ordered Assist patient when moving from lying to sitting or standing position

Taper solution before discontinuing

Review medications that may affect glucose metabolism

Assess for possible sepsis

Monitor for signs and symptoms of fluid overload

Pedal or sacral edema

Rapid weight gain: 1 lb (0.45 kg) or more a day

Pitting edema

Increased blood pressure

Bounding pulse

Monitor for signs and symptoms of fluid deficit

Provide patient and/or significant other with instructions regarding

Reasons for TPN

Importance of therapy

Expected outcome

Need for protection of IV site

Need for prevention of tension on central venous catheter

Importance of intake and output measurement

Signs and symptoms to report to nurse and/or physician

Excessive urination

Chills

Elevated temperature

Feeling of warmth

Shortness of breath

Excessive thirst

Leakage of fluid at catheter site

Pain or tenderness at catheter site

Swelling at catheter site

Home total parenteral nutrition: provide patient and/or significant other with the following instructions regarding

Type of solution

Schedule of infusion

Obtaining the solution

Storage of solution

Inspection of solution

Procedure for changing central line dressing

Frequency of dressing change

Supplies needed

Where to obtain supplies

Cleansing of site

Observation of site

Procedure for flushing catheter

Purpose of flushing

Frequency of flushing

Solution used for flushing

Changing injection site cap

Frequency of change

Clamping of catheter before cap change

Signs and symptoms to report to physician

Elevated temperature

Rapid weight loss

Rapid weight gain

Increased fatigue

Shortness of breath

Tightness in chest

Redness, swelling, or drainage at insertion site

Glucose present in urine

Instruct patient regarding

Amount of physical activity allowed

Need to keep follow-up appointments

Poor skin turgor

Dry mucous membranes

Tachycardia

Hypotension

Weight loss

Review all routine laboratory tests for abnormalities

Assess for signs and symptoms of fatty acid deficiency, alopecia, brittle nails, desquamating dermatitis, decreased immunity, thrombocytopenia, and delayed wound healing

Report abnormalities to physician

Pneumothorax

Auscultate chest for breath sounds q1h

Assess respiratory status q1h and report signs and symptoms to physician

Sudden onset of sharp chest pain

Coughing secondary to pleural irritation

Dyspnea, cyanosis, hypotension

Obtain baseline BP, apical pulse, T, and R

Keep vein open with isotonic solution until chest x-ray examination confirms correct placement of central line

Air embolism

Assess for signs and symptoms of air embolism, dyspnea, tachycardia, cyanosis, and hypotension

Place patient in head-down position during subclavian or jugular vein insertion

Use Luer-Lok connections on all central line tubing

Securely tape all tubing connections

Use air-eliminating filters when possible

Clamp catheter or assist and teach patient to perform valsalva maneuver during tubing changes

Reaction to TPN

Assess patient for dyspnea, chest, abdominal, or back pain; fever, flushing, chills, headache, decreased blood pressure, cyanosis, diaphoresis, and/or urticaria

Stop infusion and report untoward reactions to physician

Monitor and report elevated triglyceride levels and/or elevated liver function tests

Expected outcome/evaluation

Patient's

Central line is patent

Laboratory results are within normal limits

Weight is stabilized and/or progressing toward patient's ideal

Skin turgor is good

Cardiopulmonary status is within normal limits

■ NDX: Knowledge deficit related to lack of information about purpose of TPN, complications associated with therapy, and/or expected outcome

Ensure patient/significant other understands
    Resources for assistance as needed
    Importance of avoiding crowds and persons with infections
    How to recognize and handle possible complications: air embolism, blood backup, catheter injury
Ensure that patient and/or significant other demonstrates
    Handwashing technique
    Preparation and infusion of TPN solution
    Use of infusion pump
    Clamping catheter
    Flushing catheter
    Changing injection site cap
    Central line dressing change
    Care of catheter insertion site
    Measuring and recording intake and output
    Testing urine for sugar and acetone
    Taking and recording temperature

Expected outcome/evaluation

Patient
    Verbalizes understanding of purpose of TPN, complications, and action to take
    Demonstrates handwashing technique, tubing change, use of infusion pump flushing and cap change, and dressing change

Care of Patient with Special Equipment

CENTRAL LINES

central line A venous catheter inserted into the superior vena cava through the subclavian, internal, or external jugular vein; can be used for monitoring of venous pressure, infusion of medications and TPN, rapid infusion of fluid and blood products, and blood withdrawal

Insertion of Catheter

Auscultate chest for breath sounds
Obtain baseline BP, apical pulse, T, and R
Provide emotional support
    Explain procedure to patient
    Reinforce physician's explanation of procedure
Prepare to assist physician with insertion of central venous catheter
    Maintain sterile technique
    Shave hair from insertion site
    Prepare skin around insertion site with povidone-iodine solution
    Establish and maintain a sterile field throughout insertion
Place patient in supine or Trendelenburg position if sub-

TABLE 1-4. Regulation of IV Drip Rates

Amount/ hr (ml)	Amount/8 hr (ml)	Amount/24 hr (ml)	Drops/ min
PEDIATRIC MICRODRIP (60 DROPS/ML)			
4	30	90	4
5	40	120	5
6	50	150	6
8	60	180	8
9	70	210	9
10	80	240	10
12	100	300	12
14	110	330	14
18	150	450	18
22	180	540	22
25	200	600	25
30	250	750	30
37	300	900	37
ADULT IV SET (10 DROPS/ML)			
125	1000	3000	21
100	800	2400	16
90	720	2160	15
80	640	1920	13
70	560	1680	11
60	480	1440	10
50	400	1200	8
40	320	960	6
30	240	720	5
ADULT IV SET (15 DROPS/ML)			
125	1000	3000	30
100	800	2400	25
90	720	2160	22
80	640	1920	20
70	560	1680	17
60	480	1440	15
50	400	1200	12
40	320	960	10
30	240	720	7

clavian or jugular vein is used as insertion site
Administer isotonic IV solution at a keep-open rate until position of catheter is verified by chest x-ray examination (Table 1-4)
Apply sterile occlusive dressing to catheter insertion site; label with date and time of insertion
Obtain chest x-ray film

Postinsertion Assessment
Observations/findings

Chest, shoulder, or neck pain
Edema in catheterized arm
Neck vein distention
Redness, swelling, or drainage at insertion site
Temperature elevation
Elevated WBC
Occlusion of central line
Rejection of catheter
Air embolization
Accumulation of serous fluid around site

Potential complications

Infection at site
Venous thrombosis
Catheter migration
Catheter embolus
Occlusion of catheter
Extravasation
Septicemia
Pneumothorax
Hemothorax
Hematoma
Cardiac tamponade
Cardiac dysrhythmias

Postinsertion Care
Immediate care

Observe patient for signs of pneumothorax until chest x-ray film is read
  Auscultate chest for breath sounds q30 min for two times and then qh; report diminished or absent breath sounds to physician
  Report respiratory distress and presence of chest pain to physician
Prepare for insertion of chest tubes if pneumothorax is present

Ongoing care

Check BP, T, P, and R q4h
Auscultate chest for breath sounds q8h
Monitor parenteral fluids
  Maintain a closed system
  Keep system free of air
  Have a rubber-tipped hemostat available to clamp catheter if necessary
  Maintain a continuous drip of parenteral solutions at all times unless obtaining a CVP reading or aspirating a blood specimen
Change dressing daily
  Inspect catheter insertion site for signs of infection, redness, tenderness, drainage, and edema
  Cleanse skin around insertion site with povidone-iodine solution
  Apply bacteriostatic ointment to catheter insertion site; avoid antibiotic ointment
  Apply sterile occlusive dressing
  Secure tubing to skin to prevent tension on catheter
Measure intake and output q8h
Send tip of catheter to laboratory for culture when catheter is removed

Patient Teaching/Discharge Outcome

Ensure that patient and/or significant other knows and understands
  Purpose of central catheter
  Importance of not touching catheter and tubing

Importance of reporting any difficulty in breathing, sudden chest pain at insertion site, or fever to nurse
  When to flush catheter
  When to change dressing
  Type and amount of parenteral solutions to be infused daily
  Need to keep solution refrigerated (bring to room temperature before administration)
  Where to purchase solution and supplies needed
  Name of medication, dosage, time of administration, and side effects
  Need to avoid crowds and persons with infections
Ensure that patient and/or significant other demonstrates
  Handwashing technique
  Dressing change
    Inspect catheter insertion site for redness, tenderness, drainage, or swelling
    Clean skin around insertion site with povidone-iodine solution
    Apply bacteriostatic ointment to insertion site
    Apply sterile occlusive dressing
  Flushing catheter
  Administration of parenteral solutions and/or medications as ordered by physician
  Use of infusion pump if necessary

Multilumen Subclavian Catheters

Three separate subclavian catheters contained in one sheath; allows infusion of incompatible drugs simultaneously—the solutions do not mix but exit via separate lumens; the catheters vary in length, gauge, and volume (Figure 1-1)

Postinsertion Assessment
Observations/findings

See Central Lines (p. 53)

Potential complications

See Central Lines (p. 53)

Postinsertion Care

Use larger gauge lumen for administration of blood products or blood withdrawal (i.e., 16-gauge CVP readings can be taken from distal lumen only)
Reserve one lumen for TPN use only
Keep occlusive clamp available at bedside

Site care

Observe site q1h
Inspect site for redness, drainage, swelling, leakage of fluid, or loose sutures
Notify physician if any of the preceding occur
Change dressing qd for gauze dressing, q5d for transparent dressing or when nonocclusive
Cleanse site with povidone-iodine solution

Apply povidone-iodine ointment to catheter insertion site

Apply occlusive gauze or transparent dressing

Maintaining patency of lumens

Flush each catheter lumen with heparin q12h if catheter lumen not in use

Flush after each intermittent medication infusion or blood sampling

Change catheter tip syringe intermittent injection site cap q3d or according to hospital policy

Cap change should coincide with heparin flush

Blood withdrawal

Collect blood specimen for laboratory studies as ordered

Stop infusion through other lumens

Perform procedure using sterile technique

Aspirate and discard the first 3 ml

Withdraw amount of blood needed for laboratory studies

Flush with normal saline, then heparin solution 3 ml

Resume infusion through other lumens

Patient Teaching/Discharge Outcome

See Central Lines (p. 53)

Silastic Atrial Catheter

A central line catheter (single or double lumen) tunneled subcutaneously and inserted by cutdown into the central venous system by way of the cephalic or internal jugular vein; procedure is performed under fluoroscopy using sterile technique; a Dacron cuff anchors catheter subcutaneously

Postinsertion Assessment
Observations/findings

See Central Lines (p. 53)

Potential complications

See Central Lines (p. 53)

Postinsertion Care

Clamp catheters with occlusive clamp only

Administer TPN as ordered by physician

Administer prescribed parenteral fluid

Administer antibiotics as ordered by physician

Administer blood and blood products as ordered by physician

Blood withdrawal

Collect blood specimen for laboratory studies as ordered

Stop infusion through both lumens

Perform procedure using sterile technique

Aspirate and discard first sample

  Adult: 5 ml

  Child: 3 ml

Aspirate amount of blood needed for laboratory studies

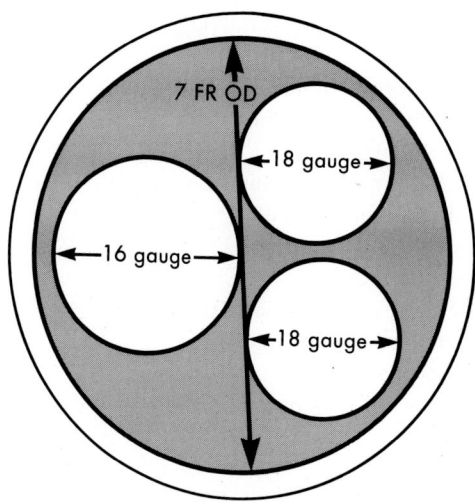

FIGURE 1-1. Multilumen catheter. French polyurethane catheter featuring three internal lumens: 18-gauge proximal, 18-guage middle, and 16-gauge distal. (Redrawn from Recker DH, Metzler DJ: *Crit Care Nurse* 4[3]:92, 1984)

Flush with normal saline, then heparin solution 5 ml

Resume infusion through other lumen

Site care

Change transparent dressing q5d or when nonocclusive

Inspect catheter insertion site for redness, drainage, or edema

Cleanse insertion site with povidone-iodine solution

Apply povidone-iodine ointment to catheter insertion site

Apply sterile transparent dressing

Secure IV tubing to prevent tension on catheter

Obtain order to remove site sutures within 7 days

Maintaining patency of catheter lumens

Flush each catheter lumen with heparin q12h if lumen is not in use

Flush after each intermittent medication infusion or blood sampling

Change injection site caps q3d or according to hospital policy

Use small-gauge (25-gauge or 22-gauge 1-inch) needle when entering injection site caps for flushing, etc.

Patient Teaching/Discharge Outcome

See Central Lines (p. 53)

Ensure that patient and/or significant other demonstrates

  Handwashing technique

  Method of changing dressing

  Technique for heparinizing the catheter

  Method of changing injection site caps

  Administration of prescribed medications and parenteral solution

  Use of infusion pump

Ensure that patient and/or significant other knows and understands
  Need to notify physician if any of the following occur
    Inability to flush catheter
    Broken catheter
    Swelling, redness, drainage at insertion site
    Dislodged catheter
    Burning sensation during flushing
    Fever of 100° F (37.8° C) or above
  Instructions regarding activity
    Resume activity as tolerated
    Shower daily
    Change transparent dressing after shower if wet
    May swim, if allowed

Implanted Port

Implantation of an infusion port under the skin to provide vascular access for patients requiring repeated infusion of drugs, TPN, blood products, and other fluids; the system consists of an implantable silicone catheter and an implantable stainless steel portal with a self-sealing septum; the IV system is inserted into the superior vena cava or right atrium via the subclavian or internal jugular vein with the portal placed over the third or fourth rib (Figures 1-2 and 1-3)

Postinsertion Assessment
Observations/findings

Accumulation of serous fluid around implant site
Aching discomfort to acute pain in shoulder, neck, or arm on ipsilateral or contralateral side
Supraclavicular or neck swelling
Venous dilation
Redness, swelling, tenderness, and drainage at site
Device rotation
  Palpate skin over device and check for possible rotation or migration of portal
Device extrusion

Potential complications

See Central Lines (p. 53)

Postinsertion Care
Site care

Always access the device, portal septum area, using sterile technique
Cleanse skin over portal septum area with providone-iodine solution

Accessing the system

Use special noncore needles to access the device (regular needle cannot be used)
Do not leave needle open to air while it is in the portal, as it may cause air embolus
Attach extension tubing or stopcock to needle; allows patient movement without dislodging needle and facilitates changing of syringe or connections

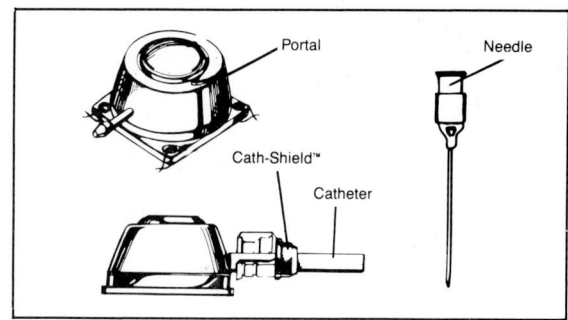

FIGURE 1-2. Parts of Port-A-Cath implantable drug delivery system. (Courtesy Pharmacia Deltec, Inc, St Paul, Minn.)

Prime needle and extension tube with normal saline before use

Maintaining patency of the device

Flush system with 5 ml of normal saline before administration of any drugs, then flush the heparin
Always leave system filled with heparinized saline after each use
For intermittent use, flush catheter q4 weeks
Avoid reflux when withdrawing needle from septum; press down on portal while maintaining positive injection pressure

Dressing/tubing/needle change

Change dressing and tubing q48h or according to hospital policy
Provide site care
Apply povidone-iodine ointment to needle site
Place sterile rolled gauze between skin and needle for support
Apply sterile transparent dressing over needle, gauze, and extension tube
Tape needle securely to skin
Administer prescribed parenteral fluids; TPN, antibiotics, blood/blood components
Follow hospital protocol for administration of chemotherapeutic agents

Blood sampling

Flush system with 5 ml of normal saline to ensure patency of line
Withdraw 3 ml of blood and discard
Aspirate amount of blood needed for laboratory studies
Flush with normal saline 20 ml, then heparinized saline 5 ml or according to hospital policy

Patient Teaching/Discharge Outcome

Ensure that patient and/or significant other demonstrates
  Handwashing technique
    Technique for accessing the system, always cleansing skin around site with povidone-iodine solution

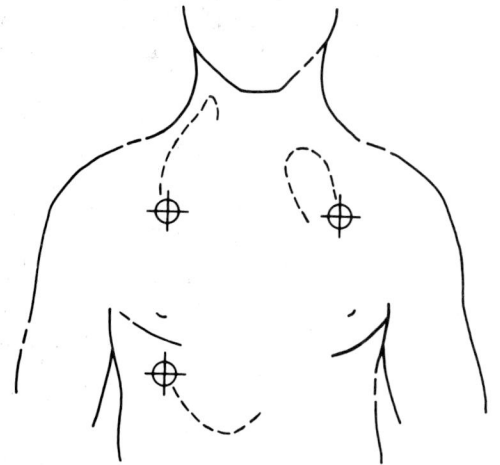

FIGURE 1-3. Some commonly used locations for placement of Port-A-Cath portal and catheter. (Redrawn from Patient information Port-A-Cath [booklet], Pharmacia Deltec, Inc, St Paul, Minn.)

 Technique for expelling all air from syringe, tubing, and needle (bandage or dressing on the site is not required)
 Technique for flushing the system
 Administration of parenteral solution as ordered
 Administration of medications as ordered; use of infusion pump
Ensure that patient and/or significant other knows and understands
 Instructions regarding activity
  Resume activity as tolerated
  Shower daily
  May swim, if allowed
  Carry special identification card
 Need to notify physician if any of the following occur:
  Inability to flush system
  Movement of portal; appearance of bruising, swelling, redness, or tenderness at portal site
  Fever of 100° F (37.8° C) or above

Peripherally Inserted Central Catheter

A peripherally inserted central catheter (PICC) is a radioopaque central catheter that is inserted peripherally, usually into a vein in the antecubita fossa through an introducer; the tip of the catheter is placed into the superior vena cava; it can be used for infusion of medications, TPN, fluids, or blood products

Indications

Venous access for intermediate-length infusion therapy
Eliminates the complications of neck and chest insertion

Insertion

Obtain and record baseline vital signs
Measure and record upper-arm circumference midway between shoulder and elbow of the arm to be used for insertion

Assist physician with insertion, providing a sterile field
Apply a sterile gauze dressing over insertion site
Obtain chest x-ray film

Postinsertion
Observations/findings

Shoulder, neck, or ear pain
Edema in catheterized arm
Neck vein distention
Redness, swelling, or drainage at insertion site
Occlusion of central line
Temperature elevation
Elevated WBC

Potential Complications

Infection at site
Venous thrombosis
Catheter migration
Catheter embolus
Occlusion of catheter
Extravasation
Septicemia

Interventions

Assess and record vital signs q4-8h
Administer fluids, blood products, or medications as ordered
Maintain scrupulous aseptic technique when manipulating catheter and fluid connections
Avoid use of multiple stopcocks to prevent contamination of IV system, potential blood loss, or air embolism
Use catheter tip syringe connections and tape all connections to prevent accidental opening of system
Administer one infusion at a time
 Flush catheter between IV treatments to prevent particulate formation and/or clotting
Assess insertion site, arm, and neck daily for pain, redness, warmth, swelling, or leakage; notify physician if present
Measure circumference of upper arm weekly
 Compare with baseline measurement
 Notify physician if increase is 2 cm or more
 Change dressing
 Remove gauze dressing 24 hours after insertion
 Handle carefully to prevent pulling on catheter
 Clean skin at insertion site with povidone-iodine solution
 Allow skin to dry at least 2 min to maximize action
 Apply transparent dressing; note date and initials
 Change dressing and cleanse site every 5 days or when dressing is moist or loose
Flush catheter and change cap
 Flush catheter after each infusion with normal saline
 Flush with an intermittent motion (stop briefly after each millimeter of normal saline instilled) to ensure that blood or other substances clear valve

Flush with 20 ml normal saline using intermittent motion after blood administration

Use a 1-inch or shorter needle for flushing to prevent puncturing the catheter

Never use force when flushing the catheter

Notify physician immediately if catheter ruptures and breaks

Seal catheter with a catheter tip syringe cap when not in use

Never use a clamp or hemostat: catheter is very soft and thin-walled and can be easily cut

Change catheter tip syringe cap

When infusion is restarted

Every 5 days when catheter is not in use

Blood collection

Do not use catheter to obtain routine blood samples as lumen is of small size

A single blood culture may be withdrawn if catheter-related sepsis is suspected

Teaching

Ensure that patient and/or significant other knows, understands, and demonstrates when appropriate

Purpose of central catheter

Importance of not touching catheter and tubing with hands

Need to report any pain in arm, neck, or ear; difficulty breathing; or fever

Need to avoid crowds and persons with infections

Handwashing technique, care of catheter, flushing method, dressing change, how to obtain supplies and solutions

Names of medications/solutions, purpose, dosage, side effects, and time and length of administration

INTRAVENOUS CONTINUOUS DRIP NARCOTICS

Indications

Inability to provide pain relief by other routes

Bleeding, pain, or tissue damage from intramuscular or subcutaneous routes

Rectal and oral routes contraindicated

Assessment

Observations/findings

Dosage necessary for maximum pain relief and minimum side effects

Side effects

Drowsiness

Mood changes

Mental cloudiness

Respiratory depression

Increased PA_{CO_2}

Decreased GI motility

Nausea

Vomiting

ELECTRONIC INFUSION DEVICES

Nonvolumetric devices	Deliver solution in drops/min	Drop rate–calibrated infusion pumps	Are designed to count drops and are set in terms of gtt/min; move solution through the line by application of positive pressure
Volumetric devices	Deliver a specific volume in a given time as shown in ml/hr		
Drop rate–calibrated infusion controllers	Regulate infusion rate via gravity by electronically counting or measuring drops (controllers that set the rate in drops/min are now considered obsolete)	Volumetric infusion pumps	Have rate setting adjustment calibrated in ml/hr rather than drops/min; pump output pressure limits are established by manufacturer and can range as high as 25 psi
Volumetric infusion controllers	Count the volume in each drop; permit flow rate to be set in ml/hr rather than gtt/min (controllers *do not* add pressure to the line to overcome resistance to flow)		
Infusion pumps	Apply positive pressure to the line to overcome flow; most deliver solution to a vein at an average pressure of psi (pounds per square inch) (*pressure can increase if a line is occluded partially or totally*)	Variable pressure limit volumetric infusion pumps	Are designed to provide only the pressure needed for specific clinical situations; allow nurse to set pressure limit based on clinical considerations

Alterations of endocrine and autonomic nervous systems

Desired effects
  Analgesia
  Alertness
  Increased coherence
  Decreased anxiety
  Improved coping ability
  Improved relationships with others
  Improved cardiac function
    Decreased tachycardia
    Modulation of BP
  Regular respiratory rhythm

Interventions

Choose narcotic based on minimum toxicity

Dilute solution based on dosage required for analgesia and amount of fluid per hour that is therapeutic for patient

Titrate hourly drip rate to level of analgesia desired without untoward effects

Regulate drip carefully with controller or pump as indicated (see box)

Involve patient in plans; encourage communication about how patient feels

Monitor BP, P, R, and level of consciousness qh while dosage is being adjusted

Monitor BP, P, R, and level of consciousness q2h when optimum dosage is achieved

Check arterial blood gases as ordered

Initiate flow sheet with vital signs and dosage per hour as indicated

PATIENT-CONTROLLED ANALGESIA (PCA)

Patient-controlled analgesia (PCA) enables the patient to self-administer a physician-prescribed dose of analgesia on demand; with PCA acute as well as chronic pain can be managed; more severe pain such as that encountered by a patient with terminal cancer can be controlled through use of the continuous infusion feature; the continuous infusion rate may also be used in conjunction with PCA to control severe chronic pain.

Indications

Acute postoperative pain
  Laminectomy
  Chest surgery
  Major abdominal surgery
  Orthopedic surgery
Acute pain in disease, such as sickle cell crisis
Chronic severe pain

Assessment
Observations/findings

Ability of patient, mentally and physically, to operate the device

Dosage adjustment for maximal pain relief with minimal side effects
Ability of patient to participate in his care
Side effects
  Respiratory depression
  Drowsiness
  Nausea
  Vomiting
  Mental cloudiness
  Increased $PaCO_2$
  Anxiety
  Decreased GI motility
  Constipation

Interventions

Ensure completeness of physician's order
  Name of drug
  Concentration of drug
  Loading dose
  Lock-out interval

Program prescribed information into PCA unit

Verify accurate program entry with another RN

Monitor baseline vital signs and level of consciousness

Instruct patient regarding purpose of PCA and operation of unit

Stay with patient as first dose is being administered

Be prepared to place the unit in stop mode if respiratory distress or change in sensorium is noted at any time during the infusion

Have naloxone hydrochloride (Narcan) available at all times

Monitor BP, P, R, and level of consciousness 30 min after the first dose and q4h thereafter

Monitor BP, P, R, and level of consciousness whenever there is change in the PCA dose, administration of a loading dose, or a change in the lock-out interval

Monitor patient for adequate pain relief; use flow sheet and pain rating scale

Collaborate with physician to determine dosage needed if pain relief is not obtained

Monitor for side effects of the narcotic drug

PERMANENT EPIDURAL CATHETER

The placement of a radioopaque silicone catheter into the epidural space for the administration of a narcotic drug can be used as a method of pain control; the catheter has two segments; the one with the smaller lumen is inserted at L1, and the proximal end is placed between T11 and C3 at the appropriate level to obtain pain relief; the segment with the larger lumen is inserted in the abdomen, tunneled to the lumbar site, and joined to that segment; a Dacron filter cuff is attached to the catheter 2 in from the abdominal incision; subcutaneous tissue adheres to the cuff, preventing bacterial entry

Indications

Chronic pain such as that in
  Cancer
  Degenerative joint disease
  Spinal trauma
Pain not controlled by conventional therapy
Restriction of activity by usual pain therapy

Assessment
Observations/findings

Severity of pain (rating scale)
Amount of pain relief (rating scale)
Dosage of narcotic that will control pain with minimal
  side effects
Side effects
  Respiratory depression
  Drowsiness
  Nausea
  Vomiting
  Mental cloudiness
  Increased $PaCO_2$
  Anxiety
  Decreased GI motility
  Constipation

Potential Complications

Infection
Displacement of catheter
Catheter malfunction

Interventions

Immediate postoperative care
  Epiduragram to confirm placement and determine the
    spread of fluid in the epidural space
  Maintain dressings at both incision sites, lumbar and
    abdominal, for the first 24 hours after operation
  Assess for bleeding at sites
  Reinforce dressings prn
  If bleeding is noted, apply ice packs or apply pressure,
    using sand bags, to the subcutaneous tunnel
Catheter care
  Change dressings at both incision sites daily until su-
    tures are removed from lumbar site
  Continue changing dressings at abdominal site daily
    Cleanse site with hydrogen peroxide followed by io-
      dine solution
    Cover with sterile occlusive dressing
Administration of drug
  Dilute prescribed drug with *preservative-free* normal sa-
    line solution to a volume of 5 to 10 ml as epidural
    space can safely handle only 15 ml/hour
  Cleanse injection site of the catheter cap with iodine
  Inject the drug into the catheter as rapidly as is com-
    fortable
  Change catheter filter daily for continuous infusion and

  q4d for intermittent infusion
Assess for signs and symptoms of infection at exit site q8h
  and report presence to physician
  Redness and edema
  Pain
  Seepage of fluid around catheter
  Fever of unknown origin
Assess severity/pain relief q4h; use rating scale
Monitor for medication side effects/toxicities q4-8h
  Assess BP, P, R, and level of consciousness
If unable to inject medication into catheter
  Change the filter
  Change patient position while trying to inject medi-
    cation
  NOTE: If label on catheter indicates it is not for IV
    access, and if IV accidently infused, remove filter,
    aspirate as much drug or solution as possible, attach
    a new filter, and notify physician *before* injecting any
    other drugs or solutions
If above interventions fail, report problem to physician

Teaching

Ensure that patient and/or significant other knows, un-
  derstands, and demonstrates
  Purpose of epidural catheter
  Handwashing technique
  Method of dressing change
  Name, purpose, dosage, and frequency of medication
  Side/toxic effects of medication to report
  Need to notify physician if pain relief is not obtained
  Preparation of medication
  Administration of medication
  Method of changing filter and injection cap
  Symptoms of infection to report as well as inability to
    inject medication

TRANSCUTANEOUS ELECTRICAL NERVE STIMULATION (TENS)

*Transmission of an electrical impulse to the body from a
battery-powered device through electrodes attached to
the skin; pain is relieved by production of a pleasant
tingling, tapping, or massaging sensation.*

Indications

Postoperative use
During labor and delivery
Acute injuries
Chronic conditions

Contraindications

Cardiac pacemaker
Significant dysrhythmias
Myocardial infarction (MI)
Cardiac monitoring (creates artifact)

First trimester of pregnancy

Placement over carotid sinus nerve, eyes, laryngeal/pharyngeal muscles

Assessment

Observations/findings

Muscle spasm

Increased pain

Nausea

Headache

Skin irritation

Sensations produced

    Tingling

    Pleasure

    Itching

    Burning

    Pricking

Unit function

    No stimulation

    Cuts in and out

Unit settings

    Rate: 2 to 200 pulses/min (hertz [Hz])

    Pulse width: 0 to 500 μsec

    Amplitude

Interventions

Assist patient in placing electrodes according to recommendations of manufacturer

Maintain electrodes in total contact with skin

Change electrode poistions prn to prevent skin irritation

Monitor patient for appropriate pain relief

Adjust rate and pulse width settings to prevent unpleasant sensations

Maintain electrodes in place

Activate unit in response to pain

For skin irritation

    Remove electrodes

    Expose to air

    Apply skin cream

    Reposition electrodes away from irritation

    Change type of electrode if necessary

For nausea

    Reposition electrodes

    Vary rate, pulse width, and amplitude

For headache

    Turn down pulse width dial

    Turn down amplitude

    Use shorter stimulation period

    Place electrodes farther apart

    Vary rate

If problems are not resolved

    Try different TENS device

    Discontinue using TENS

Refer patient for assistance by TENS specialist if available

Refer patient to pain clinic for assistance

Teaching

Ensure that patient and/or significant other knows and understands

    Mechanisms of rate, pulse width, and amplitude adjustments

    Appropriate sensations to be achieved

    How to adjust settings to

        Achieve maximum pain relief

        Avoid unpleasant sensations

        Avoid muscle spasm and pain exacerbation

    Need to

        Change electrode placement prn

        Maintain skin integrity

        Wear TENS all day: on 2 hr, off 1 hr—total stimulation of 6 to 8 hr

        Wear TENS all night if sleep is interrupted (turn unit on if awakened by pain)

        Maintain a record of settings that work

BIBLIOGRAPHY

Anderson KR et al: Bacterial contamination of tube-feeding formulas, J Parent Enter Nutr, 8(6):673, 1984.

Anderson KR, Norris DJ, Godfrey LB et al: Bacterial contamination of tube-feeding formulas, J Parent Enteral Nutr 8(6): 673, 1984.

Carpentino LJ: Handbood of nursing diagnosis, Philadelphia, 1990, JB Lippincott.

Colburn L: Preventing pressure ulcers: how to recognize and care for patients at risk, Nursing 90 20(12):50, 1990.

Doenges ME et al: Nursing care plans: guidelines for planning patient care, ed 2, Philadelphia, 1989, FA Davis.

Ehrhardt BS, Graham M: Pulse oximetry, an easy way to check oxygen saturation, Nursing 90 20(3):50, 1990.

Eisenberg P: Enteral nutrition: indications, formulas, and delivery techniques, Nurs Clin North Am 24(2):315, 1989.

Gallagher MT, Kahn C: Lasers: scalpels of light, RN 53(5):46, 1990.

Gulanick M et al: Nursing care plans, ed 2, St Louis, 1990, Mosby–Year Book.

Guzzetta CE et al: Clinical assessment tools for use with nursing diagnoses, St Louis, 1989, CV Mosby.

Heitkemper MM, Williams S: Prevent problems caused by enteral feeding: know about complications before they arise, J Gerontol Nurs 11(7):25, 1985.

Henrietta G: Lab tests you can't overlook, part II, Nursing 87 17(3):48, 1987.

Jones L, Brooks J: The ABCs of PCA, RN 53(5):54, 1990.

Kim MJ et al: Pocket guide to nursing diagnoses, ed 4, St Louis, 1991, Mosby–Year Book.

Kohn CL, Keithley JK: Enteral nutrition: potential complications and patient monitoring, Nurs Clin North Am 24(2):339, 1989.

McCaffery M: Patient-controlled analgesia, more than a machine, Nursing 87 17(11):63, 1987.

McFarland GK, McFarlane EA: Nursing diagnosis and intervention, St Louis, 1989, CV Mosby.

Petrosino BM, Christian BJ, Wolf J et al: Implications of selected problems with nasoenteral tube feedings, Crit Care Quart 12(3):1, 1989.

Petrosino BM et al: Implications of selected problems with nasoenteral tube feedings, CCQ 12(3):1, 1989.

Petrosino BM, Meraviglia M, and Becker H: Mechanical problems with small-diameter enteral feeding tubes, J Neurosci Nurs 19(5):276, 1987.

Santo-Novak DA: Seven keys to assessing the elderly, Nursing 88 18(8):60, 1988.

Smith CE et al: Diarrhea associated with tube feeding in mechanically ventilated critically ill patients, Nurs Res 39(3):148, 1990.

Smith CE, Marien L, Brogdon C et al: Diarrhea associated with tube feeding in mechanically ventilated critically ill patients, *Nurs Res* 39(3):148, 1990.

Spyr J, Preach MA: Pulse oximetry—understanding the concept, knowing the limits, *RN* 53(5):38, 1990.

Thelan LA et al: *Textbook of critical care nursing,* St Louis, 1990, Mosby–Year Book.

Thompson JM et al: *Mosby's manual of clinical practice,* ed 2, St Louis, 1989, CV Mosby.

Tribulski JA: Nursing diagnosis: waste of time or valued tool? *RN* 51(12):30, 1988.

Wilson MF, Haynes-Johnson: Cranberry juice or water? A comparison of feeding-tube irrigants, *Nutr Support Serv* 7(7):23, 1987.

2
CHAPTER

Cardiovascular System

CARDIOVASCULAR ASSESSMENT

Subjective Data

Pain
  Onset
  Duration
  Location
  Radiation
  Description
Indigestion
Weakness
Fatigue
Fainting
Dizzy spells, lightheadedness
Shortness of breath with or without activity or on waking
  at night
Palpitations
Sudden awakening at night with shortness of breath
Fever
Cough, wheezing, hemoptysis
Edema of extremities
Blue discoloration of lips, fingers
Nausea
Numb, cold extremities
Changes in vision
Headaches

Objective Data

Age
General appearance
  Color
  Assumed position
  Respirations
Vital signs
  Arterial pulses
    Rate
    Rhythm
    Equality
    Presence
    Absence
  Respirations
    Rate
    Character
    Type

Temperature
Neck veins
  Distension
  Venous pressure
  Pulsation
BP
  Position and extremity
  Pulse pressure
Pulsus paradoxus
Pulsus alternans
Urinary output
  Amount
  Character
  Color
Precordium (Figure 2-3)
  Point of maximal impulse (PMl)
  Lifts
  Bulges
  Pulsations
  Thrills
  Symmetry
  Cardiac border
Heart sounds (Figure 2-4)
  Intensity
  Pitch
  Duration
  Timbre
  Origin
  S_1, S_2
  Presence of S_3, S_4
  Murmurs
  Pericardial friction rub
Breath sounds
  Location
  Description
    Normal
    Decreased
    Pleural friction rub
    Adventitious
    Rhonchi
    Crackles
Skin
  Color
  Temperature

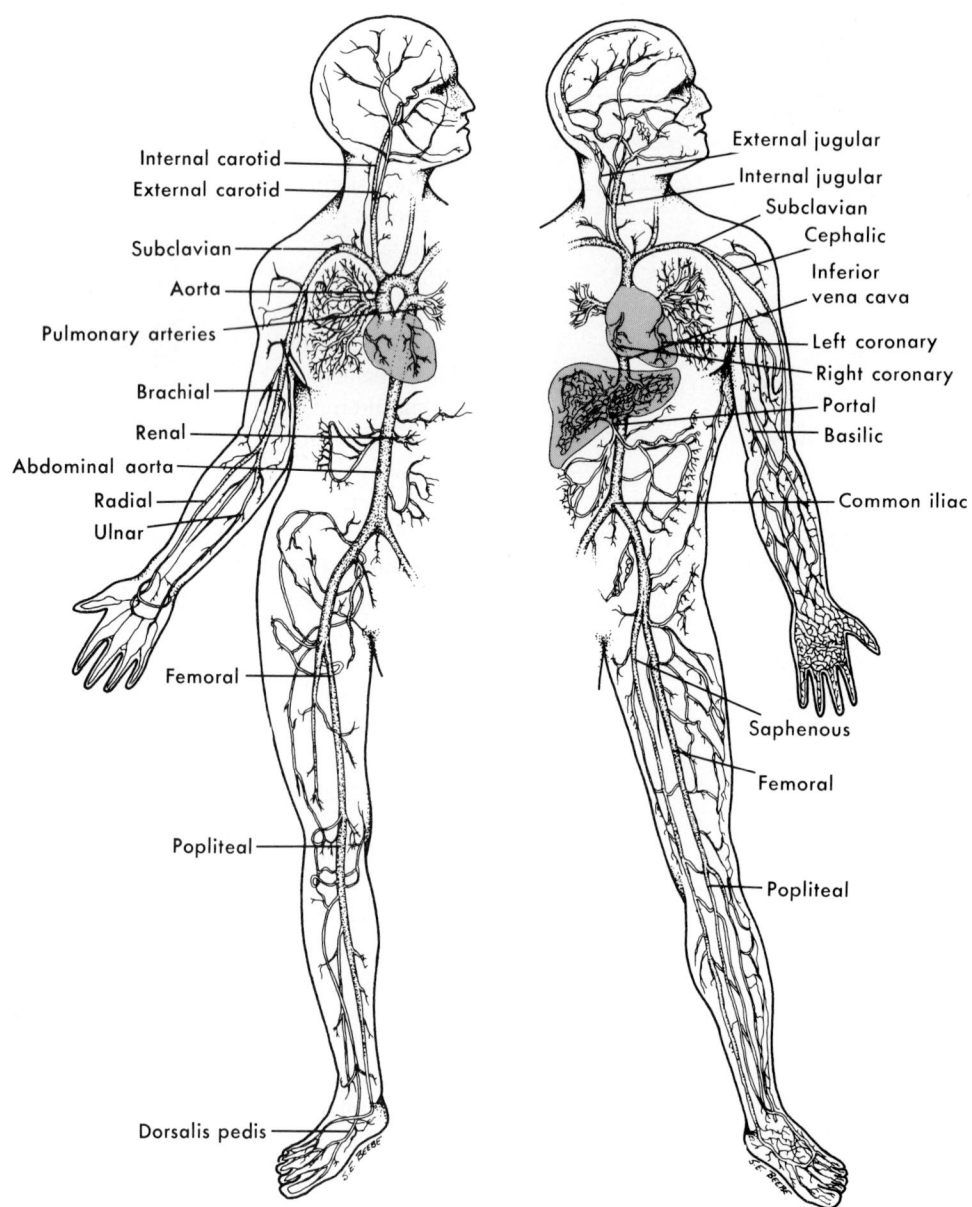

FIGURE 2-1. Arterial system *(left)* and venous system *(right)*.

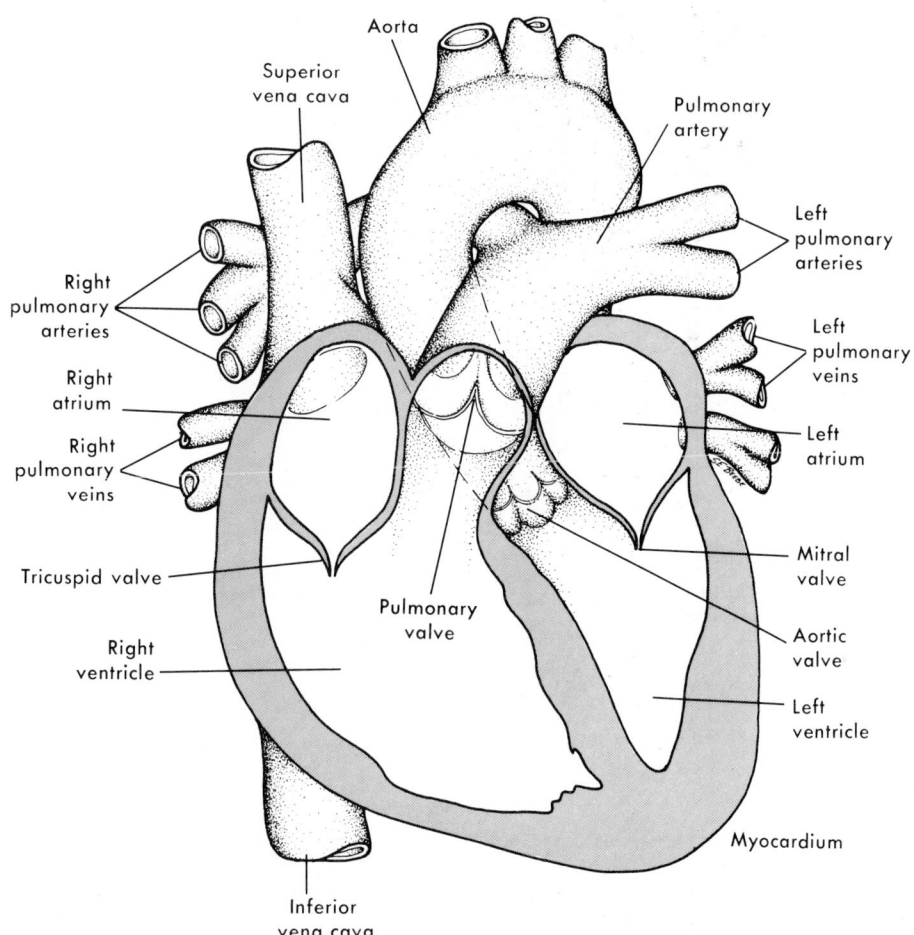

FIGURE 2-2. Circulatory system (heart).

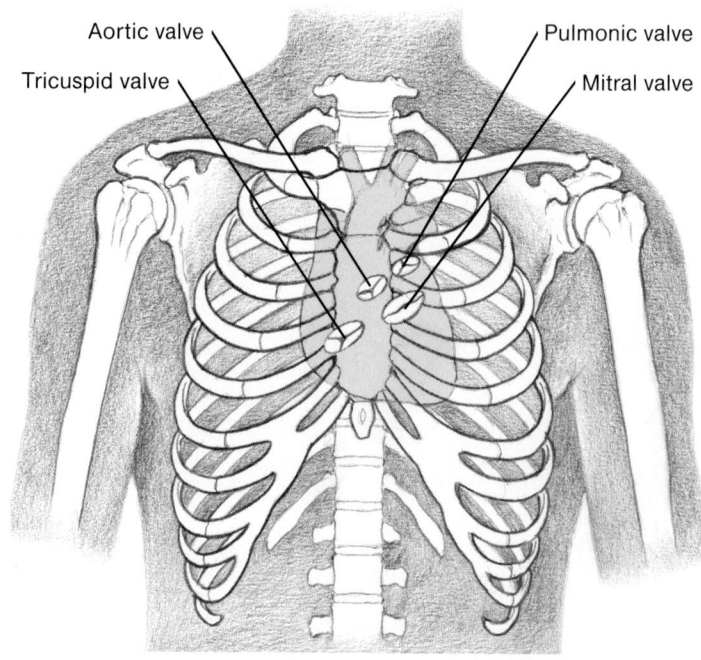

FIGURE 2-3. Chest wall landmarks. (From Malasanos L et al: *Health assessment,* ed 4, St Louis, 1990, Mosby–Year Book.)

Suprasternal notch

Angle of Louis

Midsternal line

Midclavicular line

Anterior | Posterior

Midaxillary lines

W.R. SCHWARZ.

Aortic valve

Tricuspid valve

Pulmonic valve

Mitral valve

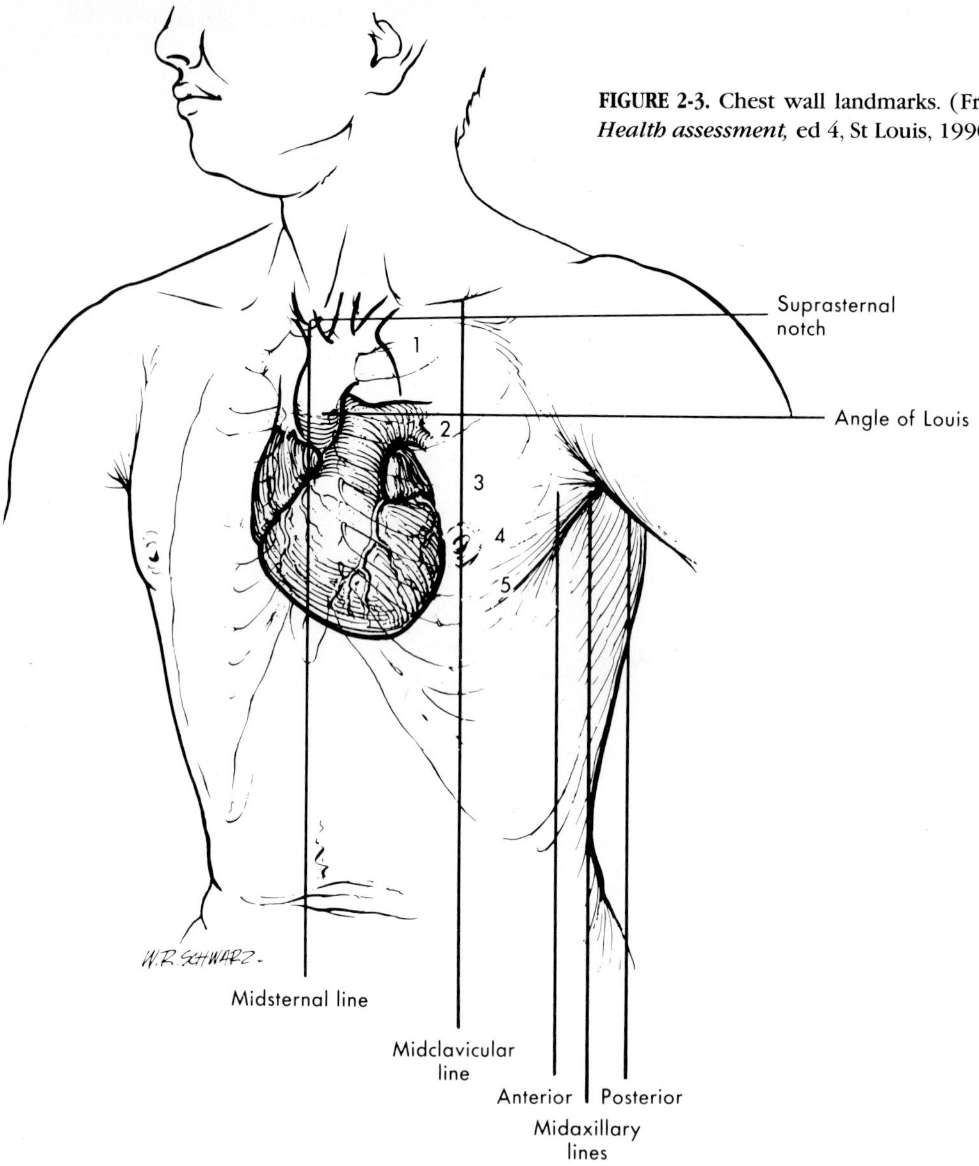

FIGURE 2-4. Anatomic location of cardiac valves. (From Canobbio MM, *Cardiovascular disorders: Mosby's clinical nursing series,* St Louis, 1990, Mosby–Year Book.

Turgor
Diaphoresis
Dryness
Extremities
　Appearance
　Color
　Temperature
　Edema
　Capillary filling time
　"Clubbing"
　Nail shape
　Description of lesions
Central nervous system (CNS)
　Level of consciousness (Figure 2-5)
　Neurological signs
　Reflexes
　Response to pain
Gastrointestinal system
　Ascites
　Hepatomegaly

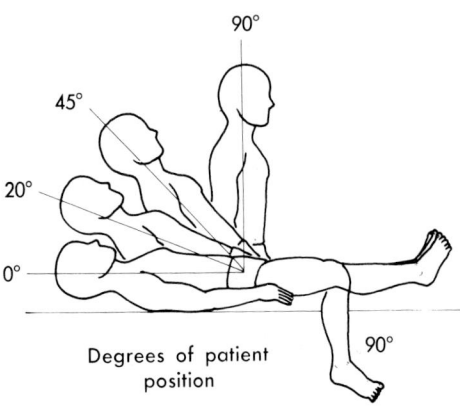

FIGURE 2-5. Degrees of patient position.

Pertinent Background Information

CONCURRENT DISEASES OR CONDITIONS

Atherosclerosis
Hyperlipoproteinemia
Hypertension
Obesity
Diabetes
Pulmonary conditions
　Pneumonia
　Emphysema
　Cor pulmonale
Renal conditions

BEHAVIORAL RESPONSES

Response to stress
Methods of coping
Response to pain
Relationships with others
Recent stressful life events

PREVIOUS MEDICAL HISTORY

Infancy and childhood
　Cyanosis at birth
　Murmurs
Systemic infection
　Rheumatic fever
　Endocarditis
　Kawasaki disease
Coronary artery disease
　Myocardial infarction (MI)
　Angina
　Heart failure
Heart murmur

Congenital heart disease
Cardiovascular surgery
Thromboembolism
Occlusive vascular disease
Pulmonary conditions
Renal conditions

FAMILY HISTORY

Heart disease
Hypertension
Diabetes
Obesity
Arterial and venous diseases
Cerebrovascular accident (CVA)
Kidney disease

SOCIAL/CULTURAL HISTORY

Cultural orientation
Educational level
Smoking
Alcohol use
Exercise and activity levels
Nutritional status
　Height
　Weight
　Less or more than body requirements
Occupation (sedentary or active)
Sleep patterns
Leisure activities
Environmental factors
Economic resources
Insurability status
Social support resources
　Marital status
　Number of siblings, children

MEDICATION HISTORY

Prescription medications
- Digitalis preparations
- Antihypertensives
- Anticoagulants
- Beta blockers
- ACE inhibitors
- Calcium channel blockers
- Vasodilators
- Diuretics
- Birth control pills
- Other

Over-the-counter medications
- Aspirin
- Cold and flu remedies
- Sleeping pills

Street or "illicit" drugs
- Cocaine
- IV drug use

Diagnostic Aids

LABORATORY STUDIES

Enzyme profile
- Serum glutamic oxaloacetic transaminase (SGOT)
- Creatine phosphokinase (CPK-MB)
- Lactic acid dehydrogenase (LDH)

Lipid profile

Electrolyte profile

Cholesterol value

Lipid levels; HDL:LDL ratio

Triglyceride value

Complete blood cell count (CBC)

Erythrocyte sedimentation rate (ESR)

Hemoglobin (Hgb)

Hematocrit (Hct)

Clotting profile

Prothrombin time (PT)

Partial thromboplastin time (PTT)

Heparin time

BUN, creatinine

Glucose level

Urinalysis

ELECTROCARDIOGRAM (ECG)

P wave

PR interval

QRS complex

QT interval

ST segment

T wave

U wave

Axis calculation

Rhythm identification

Chamber enlargement

OTHER PROCEDURES

Noninvasive

Radiologic studies
- Chest x-ray examination
- Fluoroscopy

Echocardiography
- M-mode
- Two-dimensional
- Doppler ultrasound

Transesophageal echocardiogram (TEE)

Treadmill (stress test)

Holter monitor

Signal averaging (SA) ECG

Atrial electrogram (AEG)

Nuclear studies
- Thallium uptake
- Computed tomography (CT) scan
- Multigated cardiac blood pool imaging (MUGA)
- Magnetic resonance imaging (MRI)

Invasive

Arterial pressure

Digital subtraction angiography (DSA)

Digital vascular imaging (DVI)

Cardiac catheterization

Coronary angiography

Ventriculography

Electrophysiologic (EP) studies
- His bundle recordings
- Programmed electrical stimulation (PES)
- Mapping (endocardial, epicardial)

PERIPHERAL VASCULAR ASSESSMENT

Subjective Data

Limb pain
- Initiating factors: onset
  - Continuous exercise
  - Rest
  - Amount of exercise tolerated
- Provoking factor: change in environmental temperature, exercise
- Alleviating factors
  - Rest
  - Exercise
  - Effect of prescribed medication
- Location
  - Calf
  - Foot

Swelling of extremity(ies)

Skin discoloration: pale, red, blue tinged

Numb, cold extremities

Transient ischemic attack (TIA)

Abdominal or back pain

Objective Data

General appearance
  Color
  Assumed position
Age
Vital signs: BP, T, P, and R
Pulses
  Rate
  Equality
  Rhythm
  Amplitude
  4+: strong, bounding (normal)
  3+: easily palpable
  2+: difficult to palpate
  1+: weak, thready
  0: absent
  Bruits
    Carotid
    Subclavian
    Femoral
Skin
  Temperature
  Tissue loss
    Ulceration
    Gangrene
  Lesions
Color
  Pale; increased pallor of lower extremities with walking,
    with elevation
  Mottled
  Cyanosis
  Redness (rubor); increased in dependent position
Hair loss
Opacification of nails
Lower extremities
  Cold feet
  Intermittent claudication
    Pain: calves, thighs, buttocks
    Onset with continuous exercise
    Localized or radiates from calf to thigh
    Relieved by rest or stopping activity
  Pain with rest
  Tissue loss
Upper extremities
  Digital ischemia
  Fingertip ulcerations
  Gangrene
  Allen test (positive)
Abdomen
  Pulsatile abdominal mass
  Bruits
Capillary filling time
  Normal: <3 sec
  Abnormal: >3 sec

Pertinent Background Information

CONCURRENT DISEASES OR CONDITIONS

Atherosclerosis
Hyperlipoproteinemia
Hypertension
Diabetes
Obesity
Heart failure
Renal conditions

PREVIOUS MEDICAL HISTORY

Thrombophlebitis
Cerebrovascular disease
Coronary artery disease
Aneurysm

FAMILY HISTORY

Premature deaths
Cerebrovascular diseases
Atherosclerosis

MEDICATION HISTORY

Over-the-counter: aspirin
Prescribed medications
  Antihypertensives
  Anticoagulants
  Antiinflammatories
  Steroids
  Birth control pills
  Fibrinolytics
  Vasodilators

SOCIAL HISTORY

Smoking, tobacco use
Alcohol and caffeine use
Occupation (sedentary or active)
Environmental factors
Exercise and activity levels
  Recent changes caused by increased symptoms
Leisure activities

Diagnostic Aids

NONINVASIVE

Segmental limb systolic pressure (SLPs)
  Normal
    Lower extremities
      Midthigh: 16 mm Hg
      Upper third of leg: 3 to 12 mm Hg
      Above ankle: 1 to 18 mm Hg
      Foot: 0.2 to 1 mm Hg
    Upper extremities
      Upper arm: 4 to 16 mm Hg
      Elbow: 3 to 12 mm Hg
      Wrist: 1 to 10 mm Hg
      Hand: 0.2 to 2 mm Hg

Phlebography (venography)
Intermittent claudication determination
Doppler flow velocity tracings
Plethysmography
Radioactive fibrinogen uptake
Infrared thermography (IRT)
Carotid phonoangiogram (CPG)
Stress testing
Allen test
    Radial
    Ulnar

INVASIVE

Radionuclide studies
Digital subtraction angiography (DSA)
Angiography

VENOUS THROMBOSIS

An abnormal vascular condition associated with thrombus formation within a blood vessel, which develops as a result of stasis, hypercoagulability, or damage to the internal lining of the vein; can occur in superficial or deep veins (Figure 2-6); the following are terms used to describe venous disorders that reflect thrombus (clot) formation

phlebitis *Inflammation of a vein*
phlebothrombosis (venous thrombosis) *Intraluminal thrombus with minimal or no inflammatory component; these have a greater tendency to embolize*
thromboembolism *Phenomenon of thrombus dislodgment and migration*
thrombophlebitis *An acute condition characterized by thrombus and inflammation in deep or superficial veins.*

Assessment
Observations/findings

Lower extremity (deep veins)
    Calf pains with dorsiflexion of foot (Homan's sign)
    Heavy feeling
    Pain and tenderness over involved extremity
    Cramping
    Redness
    Taut, shiny skin
    Swelling and edema
    Ulcerations
    Increased size compared with nonaffected extremity
    Increased skin temperature
    Peripheral pulses: present, absent
Upper extremity (superficial veins)
    Redness
    Warmth
    Tenderness
Elevated temperature

Laboratory/diagnostic studies

Phlebography (venography)
Doppler ultrasound
Phlethysmography
125 I fibrinogen uptake test

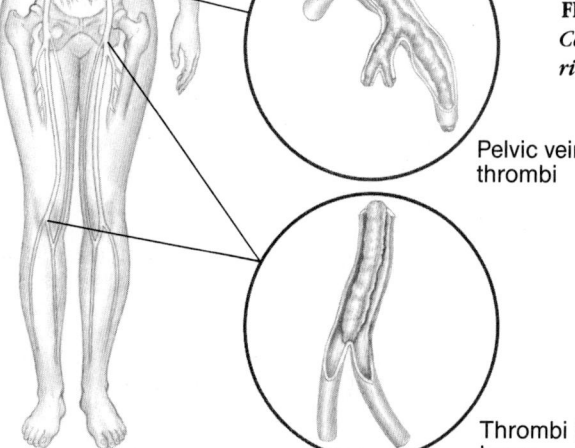

Embolism of
pulmonary
trunk

Pelvic vein
thrombi

Thrombi in
lower
extremity

FIGURE 2-6. Venous thrombosis. (From Canobbio MM: *Cardiovascular disorders: Mosby's clinical nursing series,* St Louis, 1990, Mosby—Year Book.)

Potential complications

Venous ulcers
Pulmonary embolism
Chronic venous insufficiency
CVA

Medical Management

Medications
    Anticoagulant therapy: heparin, warfarin (p. 148)
    Fibrinolytic agents: streptokinase
    Antiplatelet agents
        Dipridamole (Persantine)
    Analgesics
Surgical management
    Iliofemoral thrombectomy
    Procedures to prevent distal embolization
        Extravascular vena cava interruption
        Intracaval filter (Mobin-Udden umbrella, Kimray-Greenfield filter)

Nursing diagnoses/interventions/evaluation

■ **NDX:** Pain: peripheral related to inflammatory process

Assess quality and location of pain
Maintain bed rest, limit self-care activities
Elevate affected limb above level of right atrium
Apply warm, moist compresses as ordered; avoid burning edematous skin
Use bed cradle over affected extremity
Provide support or antiembolic stockings
Administer analgesics as ordered

Expected outcome/evaluation

Patient verbalizes relief from pain and absence of swelling and redness

■ **NDX:** Alteration in tissue perfusion: peripheral related to interruption of venous flow

Assess circulation of affected extremity q4h
Assess pulses in all extremities q4h; use Doppler sensor if pulse seems absent
Maintain complete bed rest during acute phase (4 to 7 days)
Position patient comfortably; avoid position that restricts venous return
Elevate affected limb above the level of right atrium
    Avoid use of pillows
    Never gatch knees without raising foot of bed
Measure and record size of affected limb qd
Do not wash or massage affected extremity
Provide support or antiembolic stockings
Administer anticoagulation and fibrinolytic therapy as ordered

Assess laboratory values as indicated
    PTT q4h to 12h to maintain 1½ to 2½ times control
    PT qd to maintain level 1½ to 2½ times control
Teach patient to avoid smoking
Implement progressive exercise program as ordered
    Ambulate as ordered
    Alternate with bed rest
    Never dangle
    Ambulate 10 min qh while awake or as ordered
    Apply stockings before ambulating
    Avoid having patient stand for long periods; have patient alternate position by standing on toes, then on heels
    Exercise toes and change weight distribution q10min to 15min
Elevate legs 10 min qh when sitting
    Do not constrict circulation in groin area
    Flex calf muscles and perform quadriceps contractions 10 min qh
    Avoid having patient cross legs at the knees
Advise patient to build exercise tolerance by increasing walking distance each day; continue after discharge, increasing distance 1 to 2 miles
Refer to cardiac rehabilitation program for monitored exercise program

Expected outcome/evaluation

Patient demonstrates adequate tissue perfusion as evidenced by palpable pulses and warm extremities

■ **NDX:** Potential for impaired gas exchange related to embolization of thrombus

Assess for signs of pulmonary embolism: chest pain, dyspnea, tachypnea, tachycardia, hemoptysis, pallor, anxiety
Auscultate chest for breath sounds q4h
Maintain bed rest during acute phase
Avoid exercising and massaging affected extremity during acute phase
Administer anticoagulant therapy as ordered
Encourage patient to turn, cough, and deep breathe q2h to 4h
Obtain and monitor PO_2 and PCO_2
Apply elastic support stockings when patient is ambulating or sitting for prolonged periods

Expected outcome/evaluation

Patient demonstrates effortless breathing and performs self-care activities without becoming short of breath

■ **NDX:** Potential alteration in skin integrity related to venous stasis and fragility of small blood vessels

Assess skin for redness, breakdown, or ulcerations

Administer daily hygiene measures
  Use small amount of mild soap
  Rinse well
  Dry gently but thoroughly; avoid vigorous rubbing
  Do not allow skin to remain wet
Use bed cradle for affected extremity
Do not wash or massage affected extremity
Assist and teach patient as appropriate to make small changes in position
Perform active or passive range-of-motion (ROM) exercises with unaffected extremities

Expected outcome/evaluation

Patient demonstrates no signs of skin breaks or ulceration and demonstrates management of home care

■ **NDX:** Knowledge deficit related to lack of information about disease process

Assess level of understanding
Plan exercise program that includes aerobic activities, such as swimming
Discuss importance of not smoking
Discuss skin care
  Avoid use of harsh soaps
  Do not rub or massage extremity
  Keep extremity warm and avoid exposure to extremes in temperature
Discuss need to avoid use of constrictive clothing such as garters, girdles, underwear with elastic groin bands, and knee-high or ankle stockings with elastic tops
Discuss symptoms of recurrence to report to physician (see Observations/findings p. 70)
Review medications: name, dosage, time of administration, purpose, and side effects
Explain need to avoid taking over-the-counter medications without checking with physician
Discuss anticoagulant precautions if appropriate (p. 148)
Discuss symptoms of complications to report to physician
  Pulmonary emboli
  MI
  CVA
  Renal problems
Explain importance of ongoing outpatient care
Teach application of support or antiembolic stockings
Teach deep-breathing exercises

Expected outcome/evaluation

Patient verbalizes an understanding of disease process and self-care management

VEIN LIGATION AND STRIPPING

Ligation of the saphenous vein and stripping (removal) from the groin to the ankle

Assessment
Observations/findings

Color, warmth, and sensation of affected extremity
Edema or heaviness of affected extremity
Dilation of leg veins
Leg cramps when standing

Potential complications

Thrombophlebitis
Phlebitis
Leg ulcers
Hemorrhage

Medical Management

Diet
Medications: analgesics

Nursing diagnoses/interventions/evaluation

■ **NDX:** Alteration in tissue perfusion: peripheral related to inadequate venous return and/or immobility

Assess color, warmth, and sensation of affected extremity qh for 6 hr; report any change to physician
Maintain bed rest
  Elevate legs as ordered
  Do not gatch knee
  Avoid dangling
Apply elastic bandages from toes to groin; leave in place for 24 hr
Remove elastic bandages or stockings as indicated
  Reapply q8h and prn
  Avoid constriction
  Keep snug and wrinkle free
  Assess frequently for slippage, especially after ambulation
Assist patient with ambulation within 24 hr as ordered
Have patient increase activity as ordered
  Ambulate with assistance
Do not allow chair sitting (patient must be either walking or in bed)
Perform active and/or passive ROM exercises to unaffected extremities q4h and dorsiflexion of foot of affected extremity

Expected outcome/evaluation

Demonstrates improved tissue perfusion
  Peripheral pulses are palpable
  Extremities are warm with normal color

■ **NDX:** Pain of lower extremities related to surgical incision

Assess quality and degree of pain; determine source of pain

Incision
Constrictive dressings
Bleeding
Local site infection
Assess bandages for bleeding qh; report excessive bleeding to physician
Assess dressings for signs of wound infection; report to physician
Low-grade temperature
Swelling, redness, pain, purulent drainage
Reinforce and/or change dressings
Assess BP, T, P, and R q4h as indicated
Administer analgesics as indicated

Expected outcome/evaluation

Patient verbalizes absence of pain

■ **NDX:** Knowledge deficit related to lack of information about home management

Assess level of understanding
Discuss possibility of varicosities recurring
Explain importance of avoiding constriction of venous blood return in extremities
Do not wear tight garters or girdles
Avoid crossing legs
Walk rather than sit or stand
Wear full-length support hose, elastic stockings, or bandages as ordered
Elevate legs while sitting
Sleep with legs elevated
Explain importance of skin care
Keep legs and feet warm and dry
Avoid chilling
Do not massage affected area
Discuss need to maintain normal weight for age and height and reduce if overweight
Explain need to check with physician before taking oral contraceptives
Discuss signs and symptoms of wound infection and bleeding to report to physician
Redness   Drainage
Pain   Edema
Explain importance of ongoing outpatient care

Expected outcome/evaluation

Patient verbalizes understanding of disease process and knowledge regarding self-care so recurrence of varicosities is minimized

CHRONIC ARTERIAL INSUFFICIENCY

Inadequate blood flow in arteries caused by occlusive atherosclerotic plaques or emboli, damaged or diseased vessels, aneurysms, hypercoagulability states, or heavy use of tobacco

Assessment
Observations/findings

Pain
Foot, calf, thigh, or buttocks
Sharp and viselike
Cramping
Tired feeling in legs
Usually occurs during exercise; decreases when exercise stops (intermittent claudication)
May occur at rest, especially at night, accompanied by very hot or cold feeling
Increases with elevation of legs
Diminished-to-absent pedal and popliteal pulses
Extremities
Numbness
Hair loss
Skin glossy, thin, smooth, cold, discolored, atrophied
Ulcerations, poor wound healing
Nails thickened: accumulation of cornified material
Pigmentation, rashes
Pallor
Increased with elevation of extremity
Decreased with extremity below heart level
Rubor
Edema
Delayed venous filling in dependent position

Laboratory/diagnostic studies

Doppler ultrasonography
Angiography
Arteriography

Potential complications

Peripheral ischemia, necrosis
Cellulitis
Gangrene

Medical Management

Medications
Thrombolytic enzymes: urokinase, streptokinase
Antiplatelets: aspirin, dipyridamole
Pentoxifylline (Trental)
Regular walking program
Diet therapy
Weight reduction
Low–saturated-fat, low-cholesterol diet
Percutaneous or peripheral transluminal angioplasty (PTA)
Laser thermal angioplasty (LTA)
Surgical management
Arterial reconstruction and/or revascularization
Endarterectomy
Bypass graft surgery
Femoropopliteal reconstruction: femoropopliteal bypass (Figure 2-7), profundoplasty

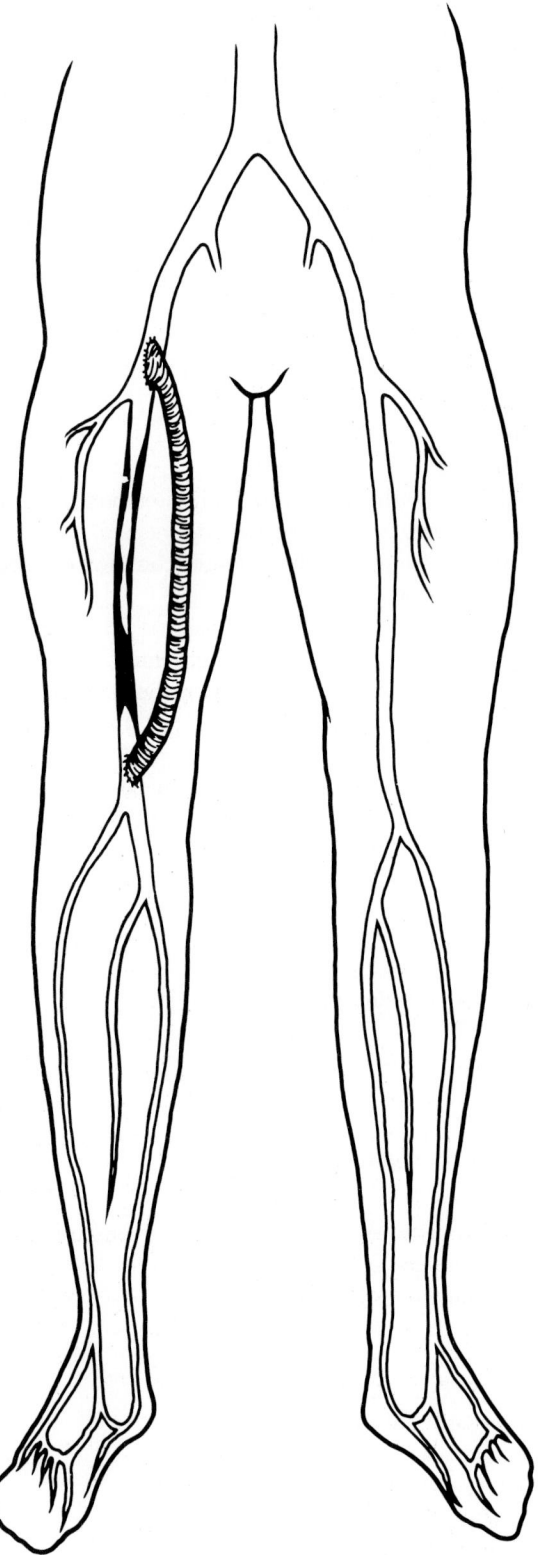

FIGURE 2-7. Femoropopliteal bypass graft to revascularize right lower limb. (From Guzzetta C, Dossey B: *Cardiovascular nursing: bodymind tapestry,* St Louis, 1985, CV Mosby.)

Lumbar sympathectomy
Amputation of limb

Nursing diagnoses/interventions/evaluation

■ **NDX:**   Alteration in tissue perfusion related to interruption of arterial flow

Assess arterial pulses; determine pulse volume qid
Auscultate for bruits before and after exercise
Elevate head of bed; use 4-inch to 6-inch block as ordered
Position patient confortably; avoid use of knee gatch
Protect affected extremity
   Place bed cradle over affected area
   Use heel guards (sheepskin) or white cotton socks
   Avoid use of heating devices on lower extremities
Keep patient warm
   Have patient wear socks when in bed or walking
   Use cotton blankets next to patient
   Use flannel or cotton bedclothes
   Use extra blankets if required
Assist patient with getting out of bed as ordered; avoid one position, sitting or standing, for long periods of time
Initiate scheduled walking exercise program; with increased pain, stand until pain eases, then continue walking
Have patient sit with feet dependent
Perform active or passive ROM exercises to all extremities q4h to 6h
Turn patient q2h while on bed rest
Change patient's position slightly q20 to 30 min
Avoid raising lower extremity above heart level
Instruct patient to avoid use of nicotine
Administer medications as ordered

Expected outcome/evaluation

Patient reports relief of pain (no claudication)
   Peripheral pulses are present, equal, and bilateral
   Skin is warm with normal color

■ **NDX:**   Pain related to peripheral ischemia

Assess quality and degree of pain
Assist patient with identifying activities that precipitate or aggravate pain, and to understand nature of pain
Instruct patient to stand or dangle at side of bed to obtain relief from ischemic pain
Encourage regular exercise program but instruct patient to stop and rest before claudication occurs
Administer analgesics as indicated
Initiate alternative pain relief measures
   Relaxation techniques: meditation, deep breathing
   Guided imagery
   Biofeedback

Involve patient in decision-making regarding measures to reduce pain

Assess effectiveness of pain relief measure(s)

Expected outcome/evaluation

Patient reports relief or control of pain

Verbalizes and demonstrates a variety of strategies to reduce pain level

■ **NDX:** Impairment of skin integrity, actual or potential, related to impaired circulation

Assess skin daily for signs of scaling, breaks, or cuts

Administer daily hygiene measures

Use small amount of mild soap

Rinse well

Dry gently but thoroughly; avoid vigorous rubbing

Apply lanolin-based lotions; do not allow skin to remain wet

Assess skin color and temperature in both legs qid

Treat ulcerated areas as they occur

Administer soak, topical, and/or systemic antibiotics and dressings as ordered

Avoid use of adhesive tapes directly on skin

Avoid use of tight, constrictive socks or hose; use cotton socks; avoid use of knee gatch; reposition extremities frequently

Expected outcome/evaluation

Patient shows no signs of skin breakdown

Demonstrates progressive healing of ulcerations

■ **NDX:** Knowledge deficit related to lack of information about disease process

Provide information regarding disease process and associated risk factors (see Risk Factor Profile p. 79)

Explain importance of care of legs and feet

Inspect legs, feet, and toes daily for blisters, skin breaks, and discolored areas

Wash daily with mild soap, dry well, and apply lanolin-based lotion but do not leave skin wet

Clean small cuts or abrasions with soap and water; protect from further injury

Report to physician cuts or skin breaks that do not begin healing in 2 to 3 days

Trim toenails straight across

Do not cut, file, or use over-the-counter medications on corns or calluses

Avoid exposing legs to extremes in temperature; wear warm coverings in cold weather and avoid exposure to sunshine

Do not apply indirect heat to legs, such as hot water bottles or electric pads; wear cotton or woolen socks to warm feet

Explain need to avoid injury to legs and feet

Always wear well-fitting shoes or slippers; never go barefoot

Wear well-fitting, correct size stockings

Avoid tight-fitting or constrictive clothing such as garters, girdles, underwear with elastic legs, and knee-high or ankle stockings with elastic tops

Avoid crossing legs

Avoid scratching legs or feet

Turn on lights when getting up at night to avoid bumps

Sleep with bed level or with head elevated

Avoid tight fitting covers over legs and feet

Instruct patient in daily progressive walking program

Walk to tolerance; increase time each week until able to walk without pain for 30 to 60 min; may initially experience decreased ability

Walk until pain increases, stop and stand still to decrease pain, then continue to walk

Do not sit or raise legs above heart level to decrease pain

Remember that same distance walked in one direction must also be walked on return

Explain need to avoid smoking or using other tobacco products

Discuss symptoms of recurrence to report to physician (see Observations/findings p. 73)

Explain importance of maintaining diet as ordered: low-calorie, low-cholesterol, low-fat

Discuss medications: name, dosage, time of administration, purpose, and side effects

Explain need to avoid taking over-the-counter medications without checking with physician

Explain importance of ongoing outpatient care

Expected outcome/evaluation

Patient verbalizes increased knowledge regarding disease process, risk factors, and home care management

CAROTID ENDARTERECTOMY

Surgical removal of atherosclerotic plaques or thrombus from the carotid artery to increase blood flow

Assessment

Observations/findings (Postoperative)

Respiratory distress

Bradypnea

Tachypnea

Cyanosis

Tracheal deviation to opposite side

Laryngeal edema

Stridor

Neurological deficit

Cerebral ischemia, TIAs

Decreasing BP, increasing P and R
Dizziness
Altered level of consciousness
Confusion
Disorientation
Memory loss
Unequal reaction of pupils to light
Unequal handgrips
Inability to protrude tongue
Muscle weakness of mouth on operative side
Dysphagia
Altered speech
Slurred
Indistinct
Dysrhythmias

Potential complications

Seizure activity
Hemorrhage
Shock
Embolism
Infection
CVA (p. 404)
Neurological deficit
Hematoma

Medical Management

Parenteral fluids
Medications
Antihypertensive
Vasopressor

Nursing diagnoses/interventions/evaluation

■ **NDX:** Altered cerebral tissue perfusion related to interruption of arterial flow

See Care of Patient in Recovery Room (p. 28)
Assess for changes in mental status
Assess and compare temporal pulses q15 min for four times, then q2h to 4h
Mark pulse site on skin: Note rate and volume
Assess neurological signs qh
Assess BP, R, and apical pulse q1h to 2h for 24 hr; report increase or decrease to physician immediately
Maintain bed rest in quiet environment; position with head elevated 30 to 45 degrees
Check rectal temperature q2h to 4h for 24 hr
Administer medications as ordered
Inspect incision qh for bleeding and edema
Report excessive bleeding or edema to physician
Reinforce dressing prn
Control pain as ordered; apply ice collar to neck as ordered
Provide emotional support
Gentle reassurance
Means of communicating; phrase questions for "yes" or "no" answers

Continue with immediate postoperative care and decrease frequency of nursing functions as patient's condition improves
Ambulate as ordered; check and report any altered gait
Change dressing prn
Continue assessing neurological signs q8h

Expected outcome/evaluation

Patient demonstrates adequate cerebral blood flow as evidenced by
Mental alertness and orientation
Absence of dizziness
Equal and reactive pupils
Normal motor-sensory function

■ **NDX:** Potential for injury: respiratory distress

Maintain patent airway
Perform oropharyngeal suctioning only if ordered
Assist and teach patient to turn and deep breathe q1h to 2h
Avoid having patient cough
Auscultate chest for breath sounds q1h to 2h
Report complaints of severe hoarseness, sore throat, or dysphagia to physician
Monitor oxygen saturation via arterial blood gases or peripheral O_2 saturation as indicated

Expected outcome/evaluation

Patient demonstrates effortless breathing

■ **NDX:** Knowledge deficit related to lack of information about postoperative self-care management

Assess level of understanding regarding disease process
Discuss risks associated with activities
Exercise to tolerance
Avoid bending from waist
Plan rest periods
Avoid lifting or straining
Explain importance of reporting sudden changes in vision, gait, speech, or the experience of muscle weakness
Report changes to physician immediately
Demonstrate care of incision
Discuss signs of wound infection
Redness
Pain
Drainage
Edema
Discuss diet
Explain importance of ongoing outpatient care

Expected outcome/evaluation

Patient verbalizes knowledge and skills in self-care management

AORTOFEMORAL BYPASS GRAFT

Surgical resection of an aortic aneurysm and insertion of a graft conduit to deliver blood to the femoral vessels, bypassing diseased segments

Assessment
Observations/findings (Postoperative)

Marked increase or decrease in BP, P, and R
Decreased arterial pressure or central venous pressure (CVP)
Signs of arterial graft occlusion of lower extremities (lower limb ischemia)
  Mottled or pale skin
  Skin cool to touch
  Absence of pulses
Site of incision
  Redness
  Pain
  Swelling

Potential complications

Embolism to extremities, cerebrum, or heart
Cardiac
  Congestive heart failure (CHF)
  Dysrhythmias
  Acute myocardial infarction (AMI)
Hemorrhage
Shock
Renal failure
  Decreased urine output
  Specific gravity <1.030
Bowel ischemia
  Diarrhea with or without blood
  Abdominal tenderness
  Leukocytosis
  Metabolic acidosis
Prosthetic graft infection
  Purulent wound drainage
  Low-grade fever without chills
  Sepsis
  Graft occlusion
  Local hemorrhage
  Septic embolization: cellutitis
  Sinus tract infection
Spinal cord ischemia
  Paraplegia
  Paraparesis

Laboratory/diagnostic studies

Doppler: systolic ankle pressure
White blood cell count (WBC), chemistries, electrolytes

Medical Management

Hemodynamic monitoring: pulmonary artery pressure (PAP), arterial pressure
Cardiac monitor
Medications
  Anticoagulation therapy
  Antibiotic therapy
  Vasodilators
Ankle-to-brachial systolic pressure index (0.95 mm Hg or more)

Nursing diagnoses/interventions/evaluation

■ **NDX:** Potential alteration in tissue perfusion related to interruption of arterial flow

Assess and compare pedal pulses q15 min for four times, then q4h; mark pulse site on skin
Assess lower extremities for color, warmth, and sensation q15 min for 4 hr, then q14h
Assess and compare ankle-to-brachial systolic pressure index (ratio) as ordered; report if less than 1 mm Hg
Maintain bed rest; elevate head 30 to 45 degrees
  Do not gatch knees
  Avoid sharp hip flexion
Provide antiembolic stockings or elastic bandages as ordered; remove, reapply, or rewrap q8h
Do not massage or apply heat to lower extremities
Ambulate as ordered; no chair sitting
Administer daily skin care
  Observe for signs of breaks or drainage
  Avoid use of adhesive tapes on sensitive skin of distal lower extremity
Protect affected extremity
  Place bed cradle over affected area
  Use sheepskins

Expected outcome/evaluation

Patient demonstrates improved tissue perfusion
  Graft is patent
  Peripheral pulses are palpable
  Extremities are warm with normal color
  Ankle-to-brachial pressure index is normal or improved

■ **NDX:** Potential for infection related to arterial prosthetic graft procedure

Observe for signs of infection of incision (see Observations/findings p. 77)
Check T q4h
Inspect dressing q1h to 2h
  Observe for healing process
  Reinforce dressing prn
  Report excessive drainage to physician
Administer prophylactic antibiotic as ordered
Avoid prolonged use of urinary catheters, nasogastric tubes, or pressure catheter that may cause transient bacteremia
Use strict aseptic technique in dressing change, venipressure, or suctioning procedures
If graft infection occurs

Administer antibiotic therapy as ordered
Perform irrigation of graft and wound as ordered
Prepare for surgical intervention as ordered
  Graft removal
  Revascularization
  Amputation

Expected outcome/evaluation

Patient demonstrates absence of graft infection
  Temperature is normal
  Graft is patent
  Skin integrity is maintained

■ **NDX:** Potential for complications: cardiac, bowel ischemia, renal failure, and hemorrhage*

Cardiac complications

Dysrhythmias
Acute myocardial infarction (AMI)
Heart failure
Monitor ECG, arterial pressures, PAP, CVP, qh
Assess BP, R, and apical pulse q4h for 48 hr
Auscultate heart and lung sounds q4h to 6h or as indicated
Record description of chest pain; report increase or significant change to physician
Administer antihypertensive, antiarrhythmic drugs as indicated
Obtain ECG rhythm strip during episodes of chest pain
Obtain isoenzymes (CPK-MB) as indicated
Monitor potassium levels

Bowel ischemia

Maintain NPO, usually for first 12 hr or until bowel sounds are present
Progress diet as tolerated and ordered after nasogastric tube removal
Connect nasogastric tube to intermittent suction as ordered
Auscultate abdomen q2h to 4h
Measure abdominal girth for distension q8h
Assess for and report increased distension to physician

Renal failure

Administer parenteral fluids with electrolytes as ordered
Measure intake and output
  Use indwelling urethral catheter as ordered
  Measure output qh
  Report output of less than 30 to 50 ml/hr

Hemorrhage

Assess for signs of bleeding q4h to 8h
  Hematoma in groin area
  Bleeding of skin incision

---

*Not a NANDA-approved nursing diagnosis.

Retroperitoneal bleeding: signs of hypovolemia—low CVP and pulmonary capillary wedge pressure (PCWP), decreased urine output, severe back pain
Evaluate laboratory studies q4h to 8h

Expected outcome/evaluation

Patient demonstrates no signs and symptoms of complication

■ **NDX:** Knowledge deficit related to lack of information about home care management

Assess for level of understanding
Explain importance of exercise and activity
  Avoid sitting or standing without moving for long periods
  Do not cross legs
  Exercise slightly beyond tolerance
Discuss importance of maintaining planned rest periods
Demonstrate correct application of antiembolic stockings or elastic bandages
Discuss care of legs and feet
  Do not wear constrictive clothing: girdles, garters, etc.
  Avoid extreme heat and cold
  Keep feet warm
  Exercise feet and legs as ordered
Demonstrate care of incision
Discuss signs of wound infection
  Redness
  Pain
  Swelling
  Drainage
Explain importance of not smoking
Discuss symptoms of recurrence to report to physician
Explain importance of ongoing outpatient care

Expected outcome/evaluation

Patient verbalizes increased knowledge level regarding home care management

---

HYPERTENSIVE CRISIS

Sudden severe elevation of BP (systolic greater than 200 mm Hg, diastolic greater than 140 mm Hg) with mean arterial pressure greater than 150 mm Hg

Assessment
Observations/findings

Severe suboccipital headache radiating frontally
  Neck stiffness, soreness
  Palpitations
  Pallor
  Diaphoresis
Hypertensive encephalopathy
  See Neurologic Assessment (p. 391)

```
┌─────────────────────────────────────────────────┐
│         CARDIOVASCULAR RISK FACTOR PROFILE        │
│                                                   │
│  Family history of heart    Elevated serum level  │
│    disease                    of lipids and       │
│  Sex: Males (35-55)           cholesterol         │
│       Females (>50 or       Diabetes mellitus     │
│         after menopause)    Physical inactivity;  │
│  Hypertension                 sedentary lifestyle │
│  Smoking                    Stress                │
│  Overweight/obesity         For women <40 years:  │
│                               use of estrogen     │
│                               (i.e., birth        │
│                               control pills)      │
│                               and smoking         │
└─────────────────────────────────────────────────┘
```

Confusion
Irritability
Stupor
Somnolence
Coma
Pulse
  Tachycardia
  Bounding
  Femoral delays
Vertigo
Nausea, vomiting
Anxiety
Eye signs and symptoms
  Diplopia
  Visual loss
  Optic fundi
    Hemorrhage
    Cotton exudates
    Arterial-venous nicking
    Papilledema
Cardiac symptoms
  Angina
  Dyspnea on exertion (DOE)
  Paroxysmal nocturnal dyspnea (PND)
  Orthopnea
  S_4 gallop
  Pulsus alternans
Renal symptoms
  Hematuria
  Nocturia
  Azotemia

Laboratory/diagnostic studies

Serum
  Electrolytes, chemistries
  Aldosterone
  Cholesterol, triglycerides
Urine
  Steroids, catecholamines; renin

Urinalysis: BUN, uric acid
24 hr VMA
Aldosterone
Electrocardiogram (ECG)
  Left ventricular hypertrophy (LVH)
  Ischemia
Echocardiogram
  LVH with/without dilation
Chest x-ray examination
  Increased cardiothoracic ratio
CT scan
  Cerebral ischemia, infarct
  Encephalopathy

Potential complications

Cardiac dysrhythmia
MI
Renal failure
Heart failure
CVA

Medical Management

Admission to intensive care unit (ICU)
Cardiac monitor
Hemodynamic monitoring: arterial pressure
Medications
  Antihypertensives
  Vasodilators: Nitroprusside, diazoxide
  Diuretics
  Beta blockers
  Anticonvulsants
  Sedatives

Nursing diagnoses/interventions/evaluation

■ **NDX:** Pain (headache) related to increased cerebral vascular pressure

Maintain bed rest; quiet, low-lighted environment
Minimize environmental distractions and stimulation
Limit activities
Avoid smoking or use of nicotine products
Administer analgesia and sedation as ordered
Administer comfort measures as indicated
  Ice packs
  Reassurance and frequent simple explanation
  Position of comfort; assist with turning gently, using pull sheet as indicated
  Relaxation techniques
  Guided imagery
  Avoidance of Valsalva maneuver
  Avoidance of constipation

Expected outcome/evaluation

Patient verbalizes absence of headache
  Appears comfortable

■ NDX: Potential alteration in tissue perfusion: cerebral, renal, cardiac related to impaired circulation

Immediate

Maintain bed rest; elevate head of bed; shock blocks may be ordered

Assess BP on admission in both arms: lying, sitting, and with arterial pressure monitor if available

Assess BP, R, apical pulse, and neurological signs q5min to 10min

Use same arm for BP each time

Use Doppler sensor if indicated

Monitor arterial pressure as ordered

Maintain parenteral fluids with medications as ordered

Administer medications as ordered

Antihypertensives: IV, IM

Observe for side effects or toxic effects of each medication

Monitor IV medications continuously

Titrate according to prescribed BP parameters as ordered

Observe for sudden hypotension

Place on cardiac monitor; record ECG rhythm strip q4h to 6h and prn

Measure intake and output

Output qh; note amount and color of urine

Report output of less than 30 ml/hr

Monitor electrolytes, BUN, creatinine as ordered

Check specific gravity and perform urinalysis as ordered

Keep NPO if nausea and/or vomiting is present

Restrict fluids as ordered

Do not allow smoking or use of nicotine products

Ongoing

Continue with immediate care and decrease frequency of nursing functions as patient's condition improves

Maintain progressive ambulation, observing at all times for orthostatic hypotension

Elevate head of bed slowly in beginning, then take BP

Progress to dangling for 10 min as ordered if BP is stable

Take BP while patient is sitting up

Take BP while patient is standing at bedside; then have patient take small steps when ordered

Ambulate to tolerance; avoid fatigue

Initiate Stepped Care Approach for the Treatment of High Blood Pressure as ordered (see box below)

Expected outcome/evaluation

Patient demonstrates improved tissue perfusion as evidenced by

BP within acceptable limits

No complaints of headache, dizziness

Laboratory values within normal limits

Urine output ≥30 ml/min

Vital signs stable

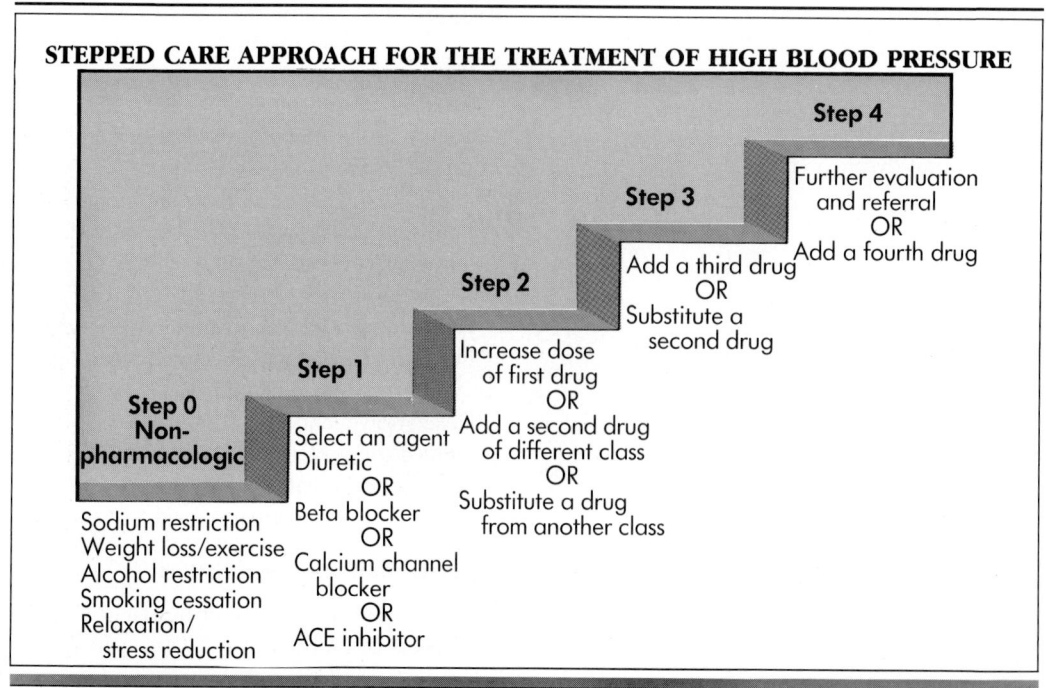

STEPPED CARE APPROACH FOR THE TREATMENT OF HIGH BLOOD PRESSURE

Step 0 Non-pharmacologic
Sodium restriction
Weight loss/exercise
Alcohol restriction
Smoking cessation
Relaxation/stress reduction

Step 1 Select an agent
Diuretic
OR
Beta blocker
OR
Calcium channel blocker
OR
ACE inhibitor

Step 2 Increase dose of first drug
OR
Add a second drug of different class
OR
Substitute a drug from another class

Step 3 Add a third drug
OR
Substitute a second drug

Step 4 Further evaluation and referral
OR
Add a fourth drug

From Canobbio MM: *Cardiovascular disorders: Mosby's clinical nursing series*, St Louis, 1990, Mosby–Year Book.

■ NDX: Knowledge deficit related to lack of information about disease process and self-care

Explain nature of disease and purpose of treatment and procedures

Explain importance of quiet, nonstressful environment

Discuss medications: name, dosage, time of administration, purpose, and side effects or toxic effects

Explain need to avoid taking over-the-counter medications without checking with physician

Discuss symptoms of recurrence or progression of disease to report to physician

Headache

Dizziness

Faintness

Nausea, vomiting

Discuss importance of decreasing weight or maintaining stable weight

Explain importance of not smoking

Discuss need to avoid fatigue and heavy lifting

Discuss importance of planned daily exercise program and rest periods

Explain need for low-calorie, low-sodium diet as ordered

Explain importance of maintaining proper fluid intake; amount allowed, limitations such as caffeinated coffee and tea, and alcohol

Explain need to avoid constipation and straining

Demonstrate taking and recording of BP and P if indicated

Expected outcome/evaluation

Patient verbalizes knowledge and skills in self-care management

Reports taking medication as ordered

ANGINA PECTORIS

Chest pain or discomfort caused by myocardial ischemia, which is the result of an imbalance between myocardial oxygen supply and demand (although angina pectoris most commonly occurs in the setting of coronary atherosclerosis, it may occur in patients with normal coronary arteries) (Table 2-1)

TABLE 2-1. Different Patterns of Angina

Observations	Stable angina pectoris	Variant (Prinzmetal's) angina	Unstable angina pectoris
CHEST PAIN			
Quality	Aching, sharp, tingling, or burning sensation or pressure	Similar to stable angina pectoris	Similar to stable angina pectoris but may be more severe
Location and radiation	Substernal with radiation to left shoulder, down inner aspect of left arm or both arms; neck, jaw, and scapula may be additional sites of radiation	Similar to stable angina pectoris	Similar to stable angina pectoris
Precipitating factors	Onset classically associated with exercise or activities that increase myocardial oxygen demand, e.g., physical exercise, heavy lifting, emotional stress, cold temperatures	Onset at rest; pain is cyclic, often occurring during sleep (most common in early morning hours)	Pain may be brought on with less than usual exertion; may occur at rest
Duration and alleviating factors	3-15 min; relieved by rest, stopping pain-inducing activities; taking sublingual nitroglycerin (NTG) tablet	Characteristically, pain intensifies quickly, tends to last longer than angina, and subsides with exercise	Prolonged and not usually as quickly relieved by rest or taking NTG
Associated signs and symptoms	During anginal attack: dyspnea, anxiety, diaphoresis, cool clammy skin	Similar to stable angina pectoris	Similar to stable angina pectoris but symptoms may be more prominent and may persist; may be associated with nausea
PHYSICAL EXAMINATION			
	Normal during asymptomatic periods; during anginal attacks, increased HR, pulsus alternans, and transient abnormal findings including precordial bulge and atrial and ventricular gallops (S_3, S_4)	Similar to stable angina pectoris	Similar to stable angina pectoris; may also demonstrate irregular pulse, hypotension, or signs of LV dysfunction

From Canobbio MM: *Cardiovascular disorders: Mosby's clinical nursing series,* St Louis, 1990, Mosby–Year Book.

Assessment
Observations/findings

Chest pain or pressure: mild to severe aching; sharp, tingling, or burning sensation or pressure, described as heavy, squeezing; heartburn or tight chest lasting 5 to 30 min
Precipitating factors
  Physical or emotional stress
  Exposure to temperature extremes such as cold
  Eating a heavy meal
Alleviating factors
  Termination of precipitating factors
  Taking nitroglycerin (NTG) tablets
Associated signs and symptoms
  Diaphoresis
  Lightheadedness
  Palpitations
  Shortness of breath (SOB)
Anxiety
Indigestion
Skin: pallor, diaphoresis
Respiration: shortness of breath
Cardiac: tachycardia; pulsus alternans; atrial and/or ventricular gallops (S_3, S_4)

Laboratory/diagnostic studies (Table 2-2)

Cardiac enzymes: CPK-MB, LDH
Electrocardiographic (ECG) changes recorded during episodes of pain
Exercise stress test (EST): changes during chest pain
Echocardiography
Thallium 201 scintigraphy
Radionuclide blood pool imaging with technetium 99m
Coronary angiography

Potential complications

Myocardial infarction
Heart failure

Medical Management

Medications
  Nitrates: short and long acting
  Beta-adrenergic blocking agents
  Calcium antagonists
  Analgesics, sedatives
Oxygen therapy
Diet: low saturated fat, low cholesterol, low sodium
Percutaneous transluminal coronary angiogram (PTCA)
Surgical management
  Coronary artery bypass graft

Nursing diagnoses/interventions/evaluation

■ **NDX:** Pain (chest) related to imbalance of myocardial oxygen supply and demand

Maintain rest during episodes of pain

Assess pain: location, duration, radiation, and onset of new symptoms
Administer oxygen as indicated
Assess and record description of pain
Obtain 12-lead ECG during anginal pain episodes
Monitor for signs of associated symptoms
Monitor BP and apical pulse during episode of pain
Administer medications as indicated; assess and record response
Maintain diet as ordered; if chest pain occurs during eating, advise small feedings rather than two or three large meals

Expected outcome/evaluation

Patient verbalizes relief of pain
  Appears relaxed and verbalizes a sense of calm

■ **NDX:** Knowledge deficit related to lack of information about disease process

Assess level of understanding
Explain atherosclerotic process and its different clinical manifestations
Discuss contributing risk factors and importance of modification (see box on p. 79)
Discuss management and nature of chest pain; assist in identifying precipitating factors
Discuss allowances and limitations
  Avoid isometric-type activity: heavy lifting and pushing
  Exercise regularly; encourage regular home exercise program
  Avoid sexual activities when fatigued; if chest pain occurs during sexual activity, stop and take nitrates if ordered; if pain persists or extreme fatigue occurs, report symptoms to physician
Self-management during episodes of pain
  Stop activity and rest
  Take nitrates as ordered
  Report to physician if pain persists longer than 20 min or diaphoresis and SOB appears
Diet as ordered; avoid caffeine intake
Discuss importance of not smoking and avoiding use of all tobacco products
Explain importance of controlling any coexisting diseases that may aggravate atherosclerotic process: hypertension, diabetes, hyperlipidemia
Explain importance of weight control; avoid obesity
Explain role that stress plays in aggravating heart disease; need to identify stress-producing factors; methods of stress management using relaxation techniques
Discuss medications: name, dosage, time of administration, purpose, and side effects

Expected outcome/evaluation

Patient verbalizes understanding of precipitating factors contributing to chest discomfort

Text continued on p. 85.

TABLE 2-2. Laboratory and Diagnostic Studies

Diagnostic test	Findings			
	Stable angina pectoris	Variant (Prinzmetal's) angina	Unstable angina pectoris	Myocardial infarction
Electrocardiogram (ECG)	Changes usually seen during anginal episodes; 50%-70% of patients have normal ECG during pain-free episodes; ischemia determined by horizontal ST segment or downsloping with depression of >1 mm; T wave inversion represents impaired repolarization caused by ischemia	Ischemia appears as ST elevation during anginal attack but regresses as pain subsides; ECG changes may be seen before patient complains of chest pain or may be recorded in absence of pain; A-V conduction defects may occur, particularly when right coronary artery is involved, and include Mobitz type II and complete A-V block; ventricular irritability such as premature ventricular contractions, ventricular tachycardia, or fibrillation can occur, particularly during ischemic attack	Ischemia determined by horizontal ST segment or downsloping with depression of >1 mm; T wave inversion represents impaired repolarization caused by ischemia; ventricular irritability, such as premature ventricular contractions, ventricular tachycardia, or fibrillation	Changes are evolutionary and indicate progression of infarction; in acute stage, ST elevations with subsequent T wave inversion and Q wave formation; Q waves indicate necrosis and are considered pathologic if they are 0.04 second or greater in duration, 0.4 mm or greater in depth, or present in leads that do not normally have Q waves; ST elevations reflect myocardial injury that interferes with polarization of cells, are seen in leads facing injured area, and return to normal (isoelectric) within days; ST elevations beyond 4-6 wk should raise suspicion of ventricular aneurysm; infarction location determined by identifying leads that demonstrate characteristic ECG changes; such leads are those with positive terminals that face injured site of heart; reciprocal changes, seen in leads that face opposite surface of damaged heart, are absence of Q wave, increase in R wave amplitude, depressed ST segment, upright tall T wave *RV infarction:* ST elevation in right precordial leads (V_1, V_3R-V_6R). V_4R-V_6R may be more sensitive indicators
Laboratory tests Enzymes	No elevation; checked to rule out MI	No elevation; checked to rule out MI	No elevation; checked to rule out MI	**Onset / Peak / Return to normal** SGOT 6-12 hr / 36 hr / 3-4 days; CPK-MB 4-12 hr / 24 hr / 3-4 days; LDH (isoenzyme) 24-48 hr / 3-6 days / 8-14 days; LDH_1 to LDH_2, ratio > 1.0
Complete blood count (CBC)	No elevation; checked to rule out anemia-induced angina	No elevation; checked to rule out anemia-induced angina	No elevation; checked to rule out anemia-induced angina	Elevated WBC and ESR reflect tissue necrosis
Glucose	No elevation	No elevation	No elevation	Transiently elevated owing to adrenergic response
Lipid levels (triglycerides, cholesterol, high- and low-density lipids)	Checked to determine any lipoprotein abnormalities	Checked to rule out presence of atherosclerotic process	Checked to determine any lipoprotein abnormalities	Checked to determine any lipoprotein abnormalities; total cholesterol and HDL may drop 48 hours after admission

From Canobbio MM: *Cardiovascular disorders: Mosby's clinical nursing series,* St Louis, 1990, Mosby–Year Book.

Continued.

TABLE 2-2. Laboratory and Diagnostic Studies—cont'd

Diagnostic test	Findings			
	Stable angina pectoris	Variant (Prinzmetal's) angina	Unstable angina pectoris	Myocardial infarction
Chest x-ray examination	Normal	Normal	Normal; may show signs of cardiomegaly or signs of left ventricular failure	Same as unstable angina
Exercise stress test (EST)	Chest pain; horizontal ST segment or downsloping of 1 mm or more; failure of systolic blood pressure to rise or drop; ST elevations	Normal stress test done to differentiate between variant and classic angina; ST elevation with or without associated chest pain occasionally develops	As in stable angina pectoris; should not be done until patient has been stable and pain free for 24 hours	Not done in presence of documented MI, low-level test may be performed before discharge from hospital
Echocardiography	Limited use, but performed after EST may detect wall motion abnormalities		2-dimensional: may show transient abnormalities of ventricular wall motion	Identifies area of abnormal regional wall motion; aids in detecting complications associated with acute MI: papillary dysfunction, septal rupture; visualizes LV thrombus *RV infarction:* dilated RV, abnormal RV wall motion
Thallium 201 scintigraphy	Ischemic areas appear as "cold" areas, reflecting reduced thallium uptake; when ischemia relieved, "cold" areas show normal thallium uptake	Ischemic "cold" areas may be demonstrated once involved coronary artery has been identified	Similar to stable angina pectoris	Similar to stable angina pectoris
Radionuclide blood pool imaging with technetium 99m			Positive findings suggest recent (previous) minor degrees of subendocardial necrosis or infarction	Confirms myocardial damage by localizing and permitting estimation of size of transmural infarction; must be done within 2-6 days after acute infarction; determines wall motion abnormalities; permits estimation of ventricular function by determining ejection fractions
Magnetic resonance imaging (MRI)				Differentiates ischemic, infarcted, and normal myocardial tissue; used in early detection of MI to assess areas of perfusion and to detect jeopardized or vulnerable tissue
Cardiac catheterization and coronary angiography	Determines number and location of obstructive lesions, "graftability" of artery distal to obstructive lesion, and ventricular function	Distinguishes spasm in normal coronary arteries from those with severe obstructive lesions; intravenous injection of ergonovine maleate provokes coronary artery spasm in patients with variant angina	As in stable angina pectoris; used in conjunction with PTCA	Generally not performed as diagnostic procedure during acute period unless done in conjunction with intracoronary thrombolysis

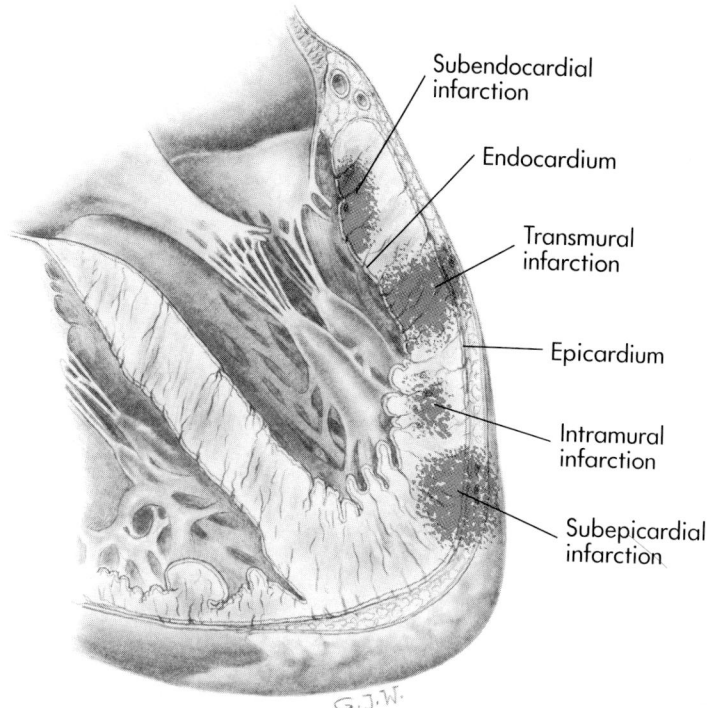

FIGURE 2-8. Location of infarctions in the ventricular wall. (From Thelan LA, Davis JK, and Urden LD: *Textbook of Critical Care Nursing: diagnosis and management*, St Louis, 1990, Mosby–Year Book.)

Identifies own risk factors

Patient verbalizes appropriate actions to take for pain control

Additional Nursing Diagnoses to Consider

Anxiety related to perceived biological threat and pain

ACUTE MYOCARDIAL INFARCTION (AMI)

Complete occlusion of the coronary artery and/or its branches, resulting in myocardial ischemia and necrosis (Figure 2-8)

Assessment

Observations/findings

Severe, crushing chest pain
  Precordial
  Substernal
  Unrelated to exertion or respiration
Diaphoresis
Skin
  Cold
  Clammy
  Pale
Shortness of breath
Faintness
Indigestion; nausea
Decreased BP
Tachycardia
Elevated temperature

Anxiety
Restlessness
Behavioral responses
  Denial
  Depression
Heart sounds
  S₃ gallop
  Pericardial friction rub
  Murmurs
Right ventricular infarction
  Increased jugular venous distension
  Peripheral edema
  Liver tenderness

Laboratory/diagnostic studies (see Table 2-2)

Elevated enzymes
  Creatine phosphokinase (CPK-MB, CPK)
  LDH
  SGOT
  Elevated ESR
  Elevated WBC
ECG changes (Figure 2-9)
  ST segment elevation
  T wave depression, inversions
  Q waves
  Dysrhythmias, heart block
Echocardiography: ventricular wall motion abnormalities
Radionuclide blood pool studies: thallium, technetium
  Localization of infarct area
  Ventricular function

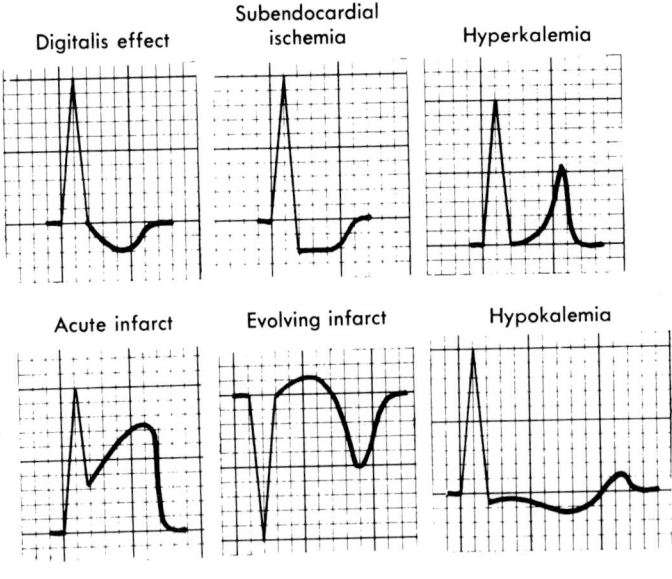

FIGURE 2-9. ST-T segment changes. (From Goldberger AL, Goldberger E: *Clinical electrocardiography: a simplified approach,* ed 4, St Louis, 1990, Mosby–Year Book.)

Magnetic resonance imaging
Angiography

Potential complications

Heart failure
Cardiogenic shock
Extension of MI
Pulmonary/systemic emboli
Pericarditis
Rupture
   Ventricular
   Papillary muscle
Ventricular septal defect
Valvular dysfunction
Ventricular aneurysm
Postmyocardial infarction syndrome (Dressler's)

Medical Management

Coronary care unit (CCU) admission
Oxygen therapy: 2 to 4 L/min
Parenteral fluids
Diet: low saturated fat, low sodium, low cholesterol
Cardiac monitor
Medications
   Pain management
   Sedatives
   Antiarrhythmics
   Beta-adrenergic blocking agents
   Vasodilators
   Antiplatelets
   Calcium antagonist
Intraaortic balloon pump (IABP)
Hemodynamic monitoring; SV_{O_2}

Myocardial reperfusion
   Percutaneous transluminal coronary angiography
   Thrombolytic therapy
Surgical reperfusion: coronary artery bypass graft

Nursing diagnoses/interventions/evaluation

■ **NDX:** Pain (chest) related to myocardial ischemia or necrosis

Maintain bedrest for first 24-30 hr and as indicated; position patient comfortably
Assess and record description of pain and factors that aggravate pain; determine if influenced by respiration or body position
Administer oxygen as ordered
Administer drug therapy as ordered; assess and record response
Obtain BP, pulse, and respiration during pain episode
Initiate nonpharmacologic measures to relieve pain: relaxation techniques, guided imagery, quiet, restful environment

Expected outcome/evaluation

Patient verbalizes absence of pain and appears relaxed

■ **NDX:** Potential alteration in cardiac output related to electrical factors (dysrhythmias), decreased myocardial contractility, and structural defects

Maintain bedrest
Assess and report signs of decreased cardiac output
   Decreased BP, increased heart rate
   Decreased urine output

Fatigue and weakness

Cool, pale, clammy skin

Assess and monitor BP, T, R, and apical pulse q2h to 4h or as indicated by clinical status

Monitor and record ECG continuously to assess rate and rhythm q2h to 4h as indicated

Obtain and compare 12-lead ECG as ordered

Administer oxygen therapy as ordered

Auscultate breath and heart q1h to 2h or as indicated

Monitor serial serum enzymes

Monitor PAP, PCWP, or CVP as indicated

Monitor intake and output q2h to 4h

Maintain parenteral fluids as ordered

Administer medications as ordered

Provide diet as tolerated; avoid use of caffeine

Avoid straining such as Valsalva maneuver; use stool softeners or laxatives

Expected outcome/evaluation

Cardiac output remains stable or improved

Patient demonstrates hemodynamic stability

Vital signs and urine output are within normal values

Patient is able to perform activities of daily living

■ **NDX:**   Anxiety related to perceived or actual threat to biologic integrity

Assess for signs and verbal expressions of anxiety

Initiate comfort measures such as a quiet, restful environment and relaxation techniques, e.g., visual imaging, soft rhythmic music

Minimize contact with stressful stimuli, such as other anxious patients

Use calm, reassuring voice

Discuss and orient patient to CCU environment and equipment

Administer sedation as indicated

Stay with patient during periods of highest anxiety, offering reassurance

Give simple explanations regarding care and procedures

Encourage expression of feelings; permit crying

Permit family member to assist patient whenever possible

Expected outcome/evaluation

Patient's anxiety level is reduced

Patient appears relaxed and verbalizes sense of calm

■ **NDX:**   Knowledge deficit related to lack of information about disease process

Assess level of understanding and degree of readiness to learn

Review physician's explanation of heart condition

Extent of infarction

Associated complications

Dysrhythmias

Angina

Postmyocardial infarction syndrome

Nature of disease process

Risk factors involved and methods of modification (p. 79)

Precipitating factors of angina

Explain importance of planned rest periods

Discuss importance of activity limitations as related to healing process; that healing takes approximately 6 to 8 weeks

Discuss importance of controlling any coexisting disease that may aggravate recovery

Hyperlipidemia

Hypertension

Diabetes

Explain importance of weight control

Explain stress management: need to control stress-producing events and activities

Review limitations and allowances of activity

Check with physician for walking and exercise limitations

Avoid or modify activity after heavy meals, alcohol consumption, periods of emotional stress, or in extremes of temperature

Discuss importance of encouraging independence in self-care activities

Discuss importance of communication with significant other

Explain need to deal with feelings about possible role change and sexual activity

Discuss signs and symptoms of an extending MI vs. angina

Extending MI: chest pain, shortness of breath, perspiration, weakness not relieved by medication or rest, pain not always associated with physical exertion

Angina: chest pain or pressure is usually relieved by rest and/or vasodilators; pain is usually associated with physical or emotional strain

Explain importance of calling physician if chest pain lasts longer than 20 min (if pain is associated with other symptoms, call physician immediately)

Explain importance of maintaining low-sodium, low-cholesterol, low-lipid, and low-calorie diet as ordered

Explain need to avoid use of caffeine products, such as coffee, certain teas, and cola drinks

Explain need to avoid use of tobacco products, such as cigarettes, cigars, and chewing tobacco

Explain importance of dietary limitations (if no specific diet is ordered, limit intake of eggs, cream, butter, and foods high in animal fat; modify or restrict salt intake)

Explain need to rest after meals (avoid exercising up to 2 hr after heaving meals)

Explain names of medications, dosages, times of administration, purposes, and side effects

Explain need to avoid taking over-the-counter medications without checking with physician

Explain need to avoid constipation and straining

Explain need to avoid sitting in same position for long periods

Explain need to exercise at regular intervals; encourage home exercise program (p. 120)

Explain importance of checking with physician with regard to resuming sexual activity, traveling, and driving automobile

Explain need to avoid isometric-type activity: heavy lifting and pushing

Explain need to monitor daily activities (space activities with periods of rest; stop when fatigued; avoid rushing)

Expected outcome/evaluation

Knowledge level is increased

Patient verbalizes increased understanding of disease process and health care management; identifies own risk factors

Patient verbalizes appropriate actions regarding pain management and medications

VASODILATOR DRUGS

Pharmacologic agents that improve cardiac performance through relaxation of blood vessels; effect occurs through direct action on vascular smooth muscles or indirectly through interference with the neurogenic process (Table 2-3)

Assessment
Observations/findings

Arterial pressure

Heart rates

Hemodynamic measurements

Cardiac output (CO)

Pulmonary capillary wedge pressure (PCWP)

Pulmonary artery diastolic pressure (PADP)

Peripheral vascular resistance (PVR)

Dysrhythmias

Liver function

Laboratory studies

Drug levels

Electrolytes

Clinical indications

Congestive heart failure (CHF)

Cardiogenic shock

Angina

Hypertension

Sodium Nitroprusside (Nipride)

A rapid-acting drug that causes relaxation of arterial and venous smooth muscle; decreases venous return and LVEDP; used in treatment of hypertensive crisis to lower BP and in CHF and cardiogenic shock to reduce afterload

Hemodynamic Effects

CO: increases

BP: decreases

PVR: decreases

HR: increases

Left ventricular end-diastolic pressure (LVEDP): decreases

Method of Administration

IV

Onset of action: immediate

Duration: effect stops within 10 min of stopping infusion

TABLE 2-3. Potential Complications of Vasodilator Drugs Commonly Used for the Treatment of Heart Failure

Nitroprusside	Phentolamine	Nitroglycerin, nitrates	Hydralazine	Prazosin	Nifedipine	Captopril
Hypotension	Hypotension	Hypotension	Hypotension	Hypotension	Hypotension	Hypotension
Nausea, vomiting	Nausea, vomiting	Headache	Nausea, vomiting	Nausea, vomiting	Nausea	Proteinuria
Mental confusion	Tachycardia	Methemo-globinemia	Drug fever	Fluid retention	Headache	Loss of taste
Cyanide poisoning		Tolerance	Skin rash	Weight gain	Fluid retention	Neutropenia
Thiocyanate toxicity			Lupus syndrome		Chest pain	
Lactic acidosis			Fluid retention			
Hypothyroidism			Weight gain			
Vitamin B_{12} deficiency			Peripheral neuropathy			
Methemoglobinemia						

Modified from Bassie BM, Chatterjee K: *Med Clin North Am* 63(1):34, 1979.

Usual Dosage

IV: 0.5 to 10 µg/kg/min

NOTE: Given in intensive care area where continuous hemodynamic monitoring can be done; may be given alone or with dopamine

Acute Care

Obtain baseline readings before administration
    CO
    PVR
    PADP
    PCWP
    BP
    HR
Determine parameters to be achieved
Wrap IV solution in foil because of light sensitivity
Change solution q4h; dilute medication with 5% dextrose in water—do not use saline or bacteriostatic water for reconstitution
Assess arterial pressure and/or cuff BP q5min when beginning infusion, then q15min as ordered
Infuse solution using volumetric infusion pump
Monitor BP closely; avoid if diastolic BP <60 mm Hg
Assess for side effects that may indicate overdosage
    Headache, dizziness, ataxia
    Restlessness
    Diaphoresis
    Weak pulse
    Palpitations
    Dyspnea
    Nausea, vomiting
Secure IV site; check for tissue sloughing and necrosis
Monitor thiocyanate levels

Nitrates

Drugs that cause arterial and venous dilation, reduce venous return, and cause a decrease in LVEDP and PAP; used in treatment of CHF and angina pectoris

Hemodynamic Effects

CO: no change; decreases
BP: decreases
PVR: decreases
LVEDP: decreases
HR: increases

Methods of Administration

Oral
Sublingual
Topical (ointment, transdermal patches)

Usual Dosage
Nitroglycerin tablets

Sublingual: gr 1/400, 1/200, 1/150, 1/100
    Onset of action: 1 to 2 min

Duration: 30 min

Nitroglycerin transdermal patch disk

Topical: 2.5 to 15.0 mg over 24 hr
    Onset of action: 1 hr
    Duration: 6 to 24 hr

Nitroglycerin ointment 2%

Topical: 1 to 2 inches
    Onset of action: 15 to 30 min
    Duration: 4 to 6 hr

Isosorbide dinitrate

Oral: 5 to 30 mg
    Onset of action: 15 min
    Duration: 90 min
Chewable: 5 to 10 mg
    Onset of action: 2 to 5 min
    Duration: 3 to 4 hr
Sublingual: 2.5 to 10 mg
    Onset of action: 30 min
    Duration: 4 hr

Side Effects

Headaches: varying intensity
Dizziness
Tachycardia
Orthostatic hypotension
Flushing
Palpitations
Nausea, vomiting
Hypersensitivity reaction
Burning under tongue with sublingual tabs

Patient Teaching/Discharge Planning

Ensure that patient and/or significant other knows and understands
    Name of medication, purpose, dosage, and side effects
    Need to avoid sudden changes in body position (e.g., standing up)
    Need to lie down if dizziness occurs
    That patient may take aspirin or acetaminophen if headache occur; need to report to physician if not relieved
    Need to take medication on time; importance of not interrupting dose (prn nitrates may be taken prophylactically before anticipated stress-producing activity, e.g., long walks, climbing stairs or hills)
    Need to avoid alcoholic beverages
    That cotton needs to be removed from medication container
    Need to store medications in cool dark place in airtight container (drugs lose potency when exposed to light, moisture, and heat)
    Need to check expiration date and replace supply q3 months

Procedure for sublingual administration

Read label carefully; do not confuse with oral or chewable tablets

Burning sensation indicates fresh tablets

Wet tablet with saliva and place under tongue; stop activity and rest until tablet is absorbed or pain relieved

If tablet is taken for angina, may repeat q5min for maximum of 3 doses; keep record of doses taken

If no relief occurs within 15 min, notify physician or go to nearest emergency room

Procedure for topical administration

Clean area of skin to be used; remove any traces of previous application

Select hairless or shaved area of skin for best absorption of medication: upper arms, chest, thigh, abdomen, forehead, back

Procedure for chewable tablets

Read label carefully; do not confuse chewable tablets with oral or sublingual ones

Chew tablets thoroughly before swallowing

Procedure for oral administration

Read label carefully; do not confuse with chewable or sublingual tablets

Take on empty stomach 30 min before meals or 1 to 2 hr after meals

Hydralazine

A drug that causes vascular smooth muscle relaxation; action is principally arterial; used in treatment of hypertension and in CHF by reducing afterload

Hemodynamic Effects

CO: increases
BP: decreases
SVR: decreases
LVEDP: no change
HR: increases

Methods of Administration

Oral
    Onset of action: 20 to 45 min
    Duration: 3 to 6 hr
IV
    Onset of action: 5 to 15 min
    Duration: 2 to 6 hr
IM
    Onset of action: 10 to 30 min
    Duration: 2 to 6 hr

Usual Dosage

CHF

Orally: 50 to 100 mg tid/qid
Hypertension
    Orally: 10 to 50 mg qid
    IM: 20 to 40 mg q4h to 6h
    IV: 20 to 40 mg q4h to 6h

Side Effects

Headache
Dizziness
Tachycardia
Dysrhythmias
Angina
Palpitations
Sodium retention
Nausea, vomiting, diarrhea
Lupus erythematosus
    Fever
    Rash
    Muscle and/or joint aches

Prazosin

A drug that causes arterial and venous relaxation by blocking alpha-adrenoreceptors; reduces systemic arterial pressure and venous return; used in treatment of hypertension and in CHF to decrease afterload

Hemodynamic Effects

CO: increases
BP: decreases
SVR: decreases
LVEDP: decreases
HR: no increase

Methods of Administration

Oral
    Onset of action: 2 hr
    Duration: up to 24 hr
Usual dosage
    Initial dose: 1 mg tid
    Maintenance dose: 3 to 20 mg/day
    Maximum dose: 20 mg/day

Side Effects

Dizziness
Headache
Drowsiness, weakness
Orthostatic hypotension
Depression
Palpitations
Blurred vision
Dry mouth
Nausea, vomiting
Abdominal cramps
Constipation
Priapism
Syncope

Nifedipine

A potent arterial vasodilator with mild negative inotropic effect used in treatment of coronary artery spasm (Prinzmetal's variant angina), stable and unstable angina, and hypertension; acts as an afterload reducing agent in CHF

Hemodynamic Effects

CO: increases
BP: decreases
SVR: decreases
LVEDP: decreases
HR: increases

Method of Administration

Oral
Usual dosage
　CHF: 10-20 mg tid
　Stable angina; Prinzmetal's: 10 mg bid to qid (maximum 80 mg/24 hr)
　Unstable angina: 10 mg q24h (maximum 60 mg/24 hr)
　Hypertension: 10 mg bid

Side Effects

Dizziness
Lightheadedness
Swelling of ankles and feet
Flushing
Headache
Nausea

Captopril

An inhibitor of angiotension-converting enzyme that results in arteriolar dilation and diminished sympathetic activity

Hemodynamic Effects

CO: increases
BP: decreases
SVR: decreases
LVEDP: decreases
Heart rate: no change

Method of Administration

Oral
　Onset of action: 60 to 90 min
　Duration of action: 6 to 12 hr
Usual dosage
　CHF: 12.5 bid/tid
　Hypertension: 25 mg tid; may increase up to 450 mg/day

Side Effects

Skin rash with or without itching
Fever
Dizziness
Lightheadedness
Swelling of face, mouth, and hands
Irregular pulse
Neutropenia
Metallic taste

Patient Teaching/Discharge Outcome

Ensure that patient and/or significant other knows and understands
　Name of medication, purpose, dosage, and side effects
　That patient may develop dizziness with first dose; if loss of consciousness occurs, need to notify physician to reduce dosage
　Need to lie down if dizziness occurs
　Need to avoid sudden changes in body position (e.g., standing up)
　Importance of not discontinuing medication because of side effects; need to notify physician

INFECTIVE ENDOCARDITIS

An inflammatory process involving the endothelium of the heart, including the cardiac valves (Figure 2-10)

Assessment
Observations/findings

Recurrent temperature elevation
　Acute: 102° to 104° F (39° to 40° C)
　Subacute: 102° F (39° C)
Alternating chills and diaphoresis; may occur at night
Malaise
Arthralgia
Signs of embolization
　Petechia
　　Conjunctiva
　　Palate, buccal mucosa

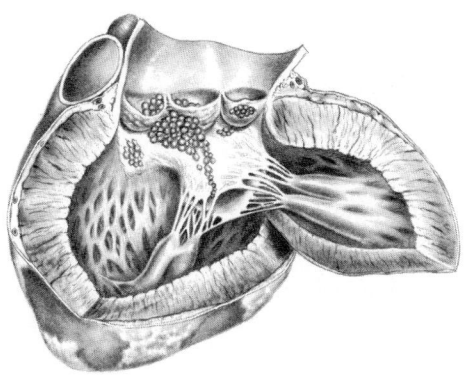

FIGURE 2-10. Endocarditis. (From Canobbio MM: *Cardiovascular disorders: Mosby's clinical nursing series,* St Louis, 1990, Mosby–Year Book.)

Extremities
Osler's nodes
"Café-au-lait" complexion
Anorexia
Weight loss
Headache
Splenomegaly
Heart sounds
Early: usually normal
Late: murmurs

Laboratory/diagnostic studies

Positive blood cultures
CBC
Normocytic, normochromic anemia
Elevated ESR
Leukocytosis
Rheumatoid factor: positive in patients with infection 6 weeks or longer
Echocardiogram: presence of vegetation or abscesses; valve involvement; LV dysfunction
Electrocardiogram: atrial fibrillation or flutter
Radionuclide studies
Galluim 67 citrate

Potential complications

Cardiac
Abscesses
Valvular heart disease
Heart failure
Myocarditis
Embolization
Cerebral
Renal
Splenic
Coronary
Mycotic aneurysms

Medical Management

Parenteral therapy
Medications
IV antibiotics
Antipyretics: salicylates
Analgesics
Anticoagulation

Nursing diagnoses/interventions/evaluation

 NDX: Alteration in nutrition: less than body requirements related to biologic factors (fever, infection)

Monitor daily caloric intake
Offer high-calorie and high-protein supplemental feedings
Consult with dietitian regarding nutritional requirements
Ensure patient comfort during meals

Expected outcome/evaluation

Nutritional status is maintained or improved
Age-appropriate, sex-appropriate body weight is achieved or maintained
Patient verbalizes appetite improved

■ **NDX:** Diversional activity deficit related to prolonged hospitalization (4 to 6 weeks)

Assess for diversional deficit; differentiate from progression of disease process
Encourage patient to explore diversional activities, such as reading, puzzles, and out-of-hospital passes
Initiate occupational therapy if indicated
Encourage daily structured exercise program

Expected outcome/evaluation

Patient engages in identifiable inpatient diversional activities

■ **NDX:** Altered body temperature related to infectious process

Assess for dehydration: diaphoresis, poor skin turgor, dry mucous membrane
Obtain temperature q4h to 8h as indicated
Monitor fluid intake and output q8h, noting water loss resulting from perspiration
Encourage fluid intake as tolerated
Administer antibiotics as ordered, ensuring they are given on time
Administer antipyretics as ordered
Monitor laboratory reports on CBC with differential and blood cultures
Monitor IV sites for redness and swelling; change site q48h

Expected outcome/evaluation

Inflammatory process has cleared
Patient demonstrates normal body temperature
Skin is warm and dry

■ **NDX:** Potential alteration in cerebral tissue perfusion related to embolization

Assess for signs of embolization each shift and prn; report positive signs to physician immediately
Perform neurological checks every shift or as indicated by patient's condition
Administer anticoagulant therapy as ordered
Instruct patient about need to continue with anticoagulants, if ordered, to prevent future embolic episode

Expected outcome/evaluation

Cerebral tissue perfusion is maintained
Patient is alert and oriented
No signs of embolization is present

TABLE 2-4. Recommended Antibiotic Coverage for Endocarditis Prophylaxis

Drug	Dosing regimen†‡§
RECOMMENDED STANDARD PROPHYLACTIC REGIMEN FOR DENTAL, ORAL, OR UPPER RESPIRATORY TRACT PROCEDURES IN PATIENTS WHO ARE AT RISK*	
Standard regimen	
Amoxicillin	3.0 g orally 1 h before procedure; then 1.5 g 6 h after initial dose
Amoxicillin/penicillin–allergic patients	
Erythromycin	Erythromycin ethylsuccinate, 600 mg, or erythromycin stearate, 1.0 g., orally 2 h before procedure; then half the dose 6 h after initial dose
Clindamycin	300 mg orally 1 h before procedure and 150 mg 6 h after initial dose
ALTERNATE PROPHYLACTIC REGIMENS FOR DENTAL, ORAL, OR UPPER RESPIRATORY TRACT PROCEDURES IN PATIENTS WHO ARE AT RISK‡	
Patients unable to take oral medications	
Ampicillin	Intravenous or intramuscular administration of ampicillin, 2.0 g, 30 min before procedure; then intravenous or intramuscular administration of ampicillin, 1.0 g, or oral administration of amoxicillin, 1.5 g, 6 h after initial dose
Ampicillin/amoxicillin/penicillin–allergic patients unable to take oral medications	
Clindamycin	Intravenous administration of 300 mg 30 min before procedure and an intravenous or oral administration of 150 mg 6 h after initial dose
Patients considered high risk and not candidates for standard regimen	
Ampicillin, gentamicin, and amoxicillin	Intravenous or intramuscular administration of ampicillin, 2.0 g, plus gentamicin, 1.5 mg/kg (not to exceed 80 mg), 30 min before procedure; followed by amoxicillin, 1.5 g, orally 6 h after initial dose; alternatively, the parenteral regimen may be repeated 8 h after initial dose
Ampicillin/amoxicillin/penicillin–allergic patients considered high risk	
Vancomycin	Intravenous administration of 1.0 g over 1 h, starting 1 h before procedure; no repeated dose necessary
REGIMENS FOR GENITOURINARY/GASTROINTESTINAL PROCEDURES§	
Standard regimen	
Ampicillin, gentamicin, and amoxicillin	Intravenous or intramuscular administration of ampicillin, 2.0 g, plus gentamicin, 1.5 mg/kg (not to exceed 80 mg), 30 min before procedure; followed by amoxicillin, 1.5 g, orally 6 h after initial dose; alternatively, the parenteral regimen may be repeated once 8 h after initial dose
Ampicillin/amoxicillin/penicillin–allergic patient regimen	
Vancomycin and gentamicin	Intravenous administration of vancomycin, 1.0 g, over 1 h plus intravenous or intramuscular administration of gentamicin, 1.5 mg/kg (not to exceed 80 mg), 1 h before procedure; may be repeated once 8 h after initial dose
Alternate low-risk patient regimen	
Amoxicillin	3.0 g orally 1 h before procedure; then 1.5 g 6 h after initial dose

From JAMA—The Journal of the American Medical Association, 264: Copyright 1990, American Medical Association.
* Includes those with prosthetic heart valves and other high risk patients.
† Initial pediatric doses are as follows: amoxicillin, 50 mg/kg; erythromycin ethylsuccinate or erythromycin stearate, 20 mg/kg; and clindamycin, 10 mg/kg. Follow-up doses should be one half the initial dose. *Total pediatric dose should not exceed total adult dose.* The following weight ranges may also be used for the initial pediatric dose of amoxicillin: <15 kg, 750 mg; 15 to 30 kg, 1500 mg; and >30 kg, 3000 mg (full adult dose).
‡ Initial pediatric doses are as follows: ampicillin, 50 mg/kg; clindamycin, 10 mg/kg; gentamicin, 2.0 mg/kg; and vancomycin, 20 mg/kg. Follow-up doses should be one half the initial dose. *Total pediatric dose should not exceed total adult dose.* No initial dose is recommended in this table for amoxicillin (25 mg/kg is the follow-up dose).
§ Initial pediatric doses are as follows: ampicillin, 50 mg/kg; amoxicillin, 50 mg/kg; gentamicin, 2.0 mg/kg; and vancomycin, 20 mg/kg. Follow-up doses should be half the initial dose. *Total pediatric dose should not exceed total adult dose.*

CARDIAC CONDITIONS/PROCEDURES FOR WHICH ENDOCARDITIS PROPHYLAXIS IS RECOMMENDED/NOT RECOMMENDED*

ENDOCARDITIS PROPHYLAXIS RECOMMENDED

Prosthetic cardiac valves, including bioprosthetic and homograft valves

Previous bacterial endocarditis, even in the absence of heart disease

Most congenital cardiac malformations

Rheumatic and other acquired valvular dysfunction, even after valvular surgery

Hypertrophic cardiomyopathy

Mitral valve prolapse with valvular regurgitation†

ENDOCARDITIS PROPHYLAXIS NOT RECOMMENDED

Isolated secundum atrial septal defect

Surgical repair without residua beyond 6 mo of secundum atrial septal defect, ventricular septal defect, or patent ductus arteriosus

Previous coronary artery bypass graft surgery

Mitral valve prolapse without valvular regurgitation†

Physiologic, functional, or innocent heart murmurs

Previous Kawasaki disease without valvular dysfunction

Previous rheumatic fever without valvular dysfunction

Cardiac pacemakers and implanted defibrillators

The American Heart Association. Reprinted from JAMA—The Journal of the American Medical Association, Dec. 12, 1990, 264, Copyright 1990, American Medical Association.

* Cardiac conditions listed for which endocarditis prophylaxis is recommended/not recommended are not meant to be all-inclusive.

† Individuals who have a mitral valve prolapse associated with thickening and/or redundancy of the valve leaflets may be at increased risk for bacterial endocarditis, particularly men who are 45 years of age or older.

DENTAL OR SURGICAL PROCEDURES FOR WHICH ENDOCARDITIS PROPHYLAXIS IS RECOMMENDED/NOT RECOMMENDED*

ENDOCARDITIS PROPHYLAXIS RECOMMENDED

Dental procedures known to induce gingival or mucosal bleeding, including professional cleaning

Tonsillectomy and/or adenoidectomy

Surgical operations that involve intestinal or respiratory mucosa

Bronchoscopy with a rigid bronchoscope

Sclerotherapy for esophageal varices

Esophageal dilatation

Gallbladder surgery

Cystoscopy

Urethral dilatation

Urethral catheterization if urinary tract infection is present†

Urinary tract surgery if urinary tract infection is present†

Prostatic surgery

Incision and drainage of infected tissue†

Vaginal hysterectomy

Vaginal delivery in the presence of infection†

ENDOCARDITIS PROPHYLAXIS NOT RECOMMENDED‡

Dental procedures not likely to induce gingival bleeding, such as simple adjustment of orthodontic appliances or fillings above the gum line

Injection of local intraoral anesthetic (except intraligamentary injections)

Shedding of primary teeth

Tympanostomy tube insertion

Endotracheal intubation

Bronchoscopy with a flexible bronchoscope, with or without biopsy

Cardiac catheterization

Endoscopy with or without gastrointestinal biopsy

Cesarean section

In the absence of infection for urethral catheterization, dilatation and curettage, uncomplicated vaginal delivery, therapeutic abortion, sterilization procedures, or insertion or removal of intrauterine devices

The American Heart Association. Reprinted from JAMA—The Journal of the American Medical Association, Dec. 12, 1990, 264, Copyright 1990, American Medical Association.

* This table lists selected procedures but is not meant to be all-inclusive.

† In addition to prophylactic regimen for genitourinary procedures, antibiotic therapy should be directed against the most likely bacterial pathogen.

‡ In patients who have prosthetic heart valves, a previous history of endocarditis, or surgically constructed systemic-pulmonary shunts or conduits, physicians may choose to administer prophylactic antibiotics even for low-risk procedures that involve the lower respiratory, genitourinary, or gastrointestinal tracts.

■ **NDX:** Knowledge deficit related to lack of information disease process

Discuss symptoms of recurrence to report to physician
Fatigue
Elevated temperature
Chills
Weight loss
Just not feeling well
Discuss need to avoid persons with infections, especially upper respiratory infection (URI), and to report symptoms (e.g., cold, flu, cough) to physician
Explain importance of avoiding fatigue; need to plan rest periods before and after activity
Discuss importance of reporting to physician any event that may predispose to bacteremia
Dental or gum therapy
Surgical procedures
Medical procedures
Childbirth
Trauma
Furuncles
Explain need to maintain good oral hygiene: daily care and regular visits to dentist
Explain importance of ongoing outpatient care
Discuss name of medication, dosage, times of administration, purpose, and side effects
Explain significance of prophylactic antibiotic therapy before procedures that predispose to bacteremia (Table 2-4)

Expected outcome/evaluation

Patient demonstrates understanding of factors contributing to endocarditis, need for antibiotic prophylaxis, symptoms to report to physician

VALVULAR HEART DISEASE

An acquired or congenital disease involving the heart valves being maintained in a closed or open position: Most common types are aortic or mitral stenosis and aortic or mitral regurgitation (Figure 2-11) (Table 2-5).

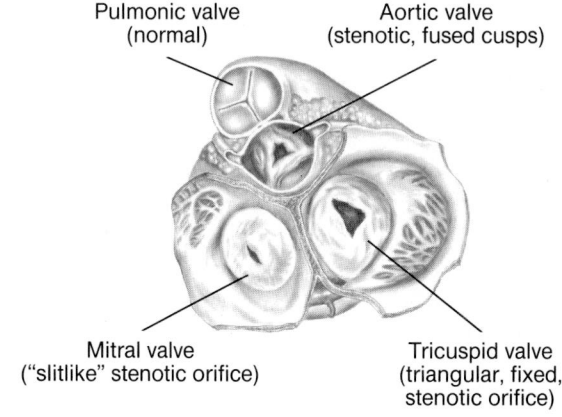

Pulmonic valve (normal)

Aortic valve (stenotic, fused cusps)

Mitral valve ("slitlike" stenotic orifice)

Tricuspid valve (triangular, fixed, stenotic orifice)

FIGURE 2-11. Valvular heart disease. (From Canobbio MM: *Cardiovascular disorders: Mosby's clinical nursing series,* St Louis, 1990, Mosby–Year Book.)

TABLE 2-5. Common Valvular Disorders: Adult Onset

Aortic stenosis	Mitral stenosis	Aortic regurgitation	Mitral regurgitation
OBSERVATIONS			
DOE	DOE	Dyspnea	Dyspnea
Syncope	Fatigue	Awareness of strong pulsations of heart	Fatigue
Fatigue	Decreased tolerance to exercise	Excessive sweating	Exercise intolerance
Angina pectoris	Orthopnea	Skin warm, flushed, and damp	Orthopnea
Decreased pulse pressure	PND	Dizziness	Palpitations
Carotid pulse	Cough	Neck pain	
Slow with long upstroke	Hemoptysis	Head bobbing (DeMusset's sign)	
Small quality to pulse		Pulses	
		Visible arterial pulsations in neck	
		Bisferiens pulse	
		Water-hammer (Corrigan's) pulse	
		Widened pulse pressure to greater than 80 mm Hg	
Apical impulse: strong, sustained during systole	Apical impulse: tapping quality	Apical impulse: forceful, sustained, displaced downward and outward	Apical impulse; large, laterally displaced
Systolic thrill			

Continued.

TABLE 2-5. Common Valvular Disorders: Adult Onset—cont'd

Aortic stenosis	Mitral stenosis	Aortic regurgitation	Mitral regurgitation
OBSERVATIONS—cont'd			

Heart sounds
  Moderate: crescendo-decrescendo, rough, harsh systolic murmur heard over aortic area
  Decreased aortic second sound
	Heart sounds
	  Loud first heart sound; low-pitched rumbling diastolic murmur with an opening snap heard at apex
		Heart sounds
		  Decrescendo: high-pitched blowing heard at left sternal border
		  Systolic ejection sound
		  Diastolic murmur
			Heart sounds
			  Holosystolic systolic murmur heard at apex
			  First heart sounds diminished
			  Splitting of second heart sound
			  Third heart sound

POTENTIAL COMPLICATIONS			
Endocarditis Systemic emboli	Endocarditis Systemic emboli: brain, extremities, abdomen	Endocarditis	Endocarditis Rupture of chordae tendineae; systemic emboli
DIAGNOSTIC FINDINGS			

ECG
  Left ventricular hypertrophy (LVH)
  Conduction defects
    Left anterior hemiblock
    Left bundle branch block (LBBB)
    Complete heart block
  Dysrrhythmias: atrial fibrillation
	ECG
	  P waves notched or peaked in I, II, III, and AVF
	  Atrial fibrillation
	  Right ventricular hypertrophy (RVH)
		ECG
		  Normal
		  Septal Q waves V_5, V_6
		  LVH
			ECG
			  Nonspecific ST segment and T wave abnormalities
			  LVH
			  P waves abnormalities
			  Atrial dysrrhythmias: premature atrial contractions (PACs), atrial fibrillation

Chest x-ray examination: enlargement of LV; calcification of aortic valve	Chest x-ray examination: enlargement of LA, RV, right atria (RA), and pulmonary trunk; calcification of mitral valve	Chest x-ray examination: enlargement of LV; dilation of aorta	Chest x-ray examination: enlargement of LA, LV
Hemodynamic changes: elevated left atrial (LA) and LV pressures	Hemodynamic changes: elevated pressures—LA, pulmonary artery (PA), and RV	Hemodynamic changes: elevated left ventricular end-diastolic pressure (LVEDP)	Hemodynamic changes: elevated LA and PA pressures and PCWP

Assessment

Observations/findings

NOTE: Observations and care listed are for moderate-to-severe forms of valvular heart disease

General complaints
  Fatigue
  Malaise
  Shortness of breath
DOE
  Anorexia
  Sleep disorders: PND, orthopnea, nocturnal sweats
  Palpitations
  Heart sounds
    Murmurs (Figure 2-12)
    S_3, S_4

Laboratory/diagnostic studies

ECG
  Atrial, ventricular hypertrophy

  Dysrhythmias: atrial fibrillation, flutter
  Conduction defects: bundle branch blocks
Echocardiogram: decreased excursion of leaflets; chamber enlargement; dilation
Chest x-ray examination
  Cardiomegaly
  Pulmonary vascular congestion
  Valve calcification
Cardiac catheterization

Potential complications

Infective endocarditis
Embolism
  Brain
  Lungs
Left ventricular (LV) failure
Right ventricular (RV) failure
Dysrhythmias
Rupture of papillary muscles or chordae tendineae
Pulmonary edema

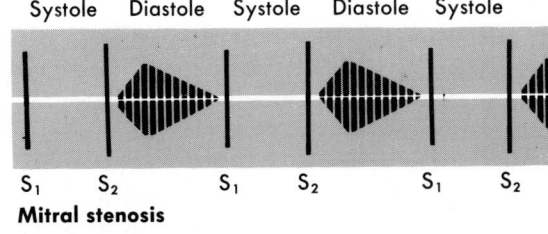

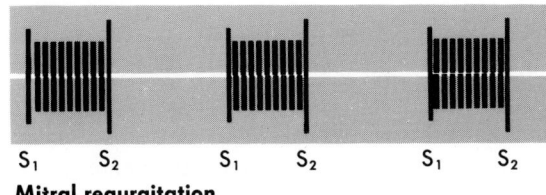

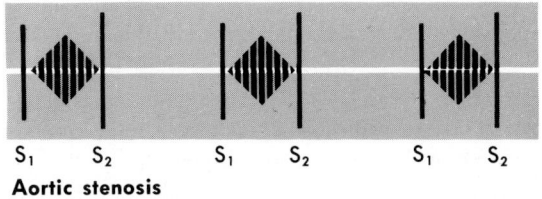

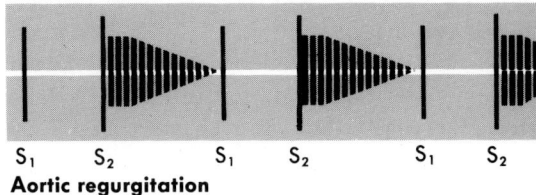

FIGURE 2-12. Valvular heart disease murmurs. (From Guzzetta C, Dossey B: *Cardiovascular nursing: bodymind tapestry.* St Louis, 1985, CV Mosby.)

Medical Management

Medications
   Antibiotics
   Antiarrhythmics
   Diuretics
   Analgesics
   Anticoagulants
Sodium restriction
Cardiac monitoring
Cardioversion
Hemodynamic monitoring
Percutaneous balloon catheter dilation (balloon angioplasty)
Surgical management
   Commissurotomy
   Valvotomy
   Valvuloplasty
   Valve replacement

Nursing diagnoses/interventions/evaluation

■ **NDX:** Decreased cardiac output related to mechanical factors (preload, afterload) secondary to valvular dysfunction

Establish baseline assessment of cardiovascular status
Maintain bed rest as ordered; elevate head of bed 30 to 40 degrees
Monitor BP, T, and R with apical pulse q4h or as indicated
Auscultate breath sounds q4h to 6h
Auscultate heart sounds q6h to 8h; record presence or absence of murmurs, or gallop sounds
Monitor cardiac rhythm for changes from baseline; record any dysrhythmia
Administer medications as ordered
Monitor intake and output
Restrict and monitor dietary intake of sodium

Limit and/or modify activity during acute phase
   Avoid fatigue; maintain planned rest periods
   Perform active or passive ROM exercises to extremities qid

Expected outcome/evaluation

Patient demonstrates stable or improved cardiac output
   Reports improvement of symptoms
   Lungs are clear
   Vital signs and urine output are within normal limits
   Patient is able to perform activities of daily living (ADLs)

■ **NDX:** Fluid volume excess related to cardiac decompensation

Assess and monitor intake and output; report output of <30 ml/hr or intake greater than output on daily basis
Auscultate heart sounds (S_3, S_4) and breath sounds q4h to 8h
Assess for increase or decrease in jugular venous pressure
Weigh daily using same amount of clothing and at same time of day
Administer diuretics and vasodilator therapy as ordered
Restrict sodium and fluids as indicated
Monitor electrolytes, chemistries, Hgb, and Hct

Expected outcome/evaluation

Patient's fluid balance is restored
   Lung sounds clear
   S_3, S_4 absent
   Ideal body weight is achieved

■ **NDX:** Activity intolerance related to diminished cardiac reserve

Assess and monitor for signs of activity intolerance

Check BP, HR, and respiration before and after activity, report HR >20 bpm above resting HR, marked increase in BP, or complaints of dyspnea, chest pain, diaphoresis, or excessive fatigue

Maintain on bed rest or on chair rest as indicated

Identify factors known to cause fatigue

Space treatments and procedures to allow for periods of uninterrupted rest; provide periods of rest throughout day and evening

Implement measures that will improve activity tolerance by minimizing fatigue (e.g., toileting via bedside commode rather than bedpan; up in chair with legs elevated rather than complete bed rest

Increase activity level as indicated by condition; assess activity tolerance and activity progression

Expected outcome/evaluation

Activity level improved
> Patient reports being able to participate in ADL; denies SOB
> HR, BP, R within normal limits

■ **NDX:** Knowledge deficit related to lack of information disease process

Assess level of understanding

Explain nature and cause of disease process

Discuss importance of reporting signs and symptoms of
> Heart failure
>> Increased fatigue
>> Tachypnea
>> Orthopnea
>> Cough
> Infective endocarditis
>> Elevated temperature
>> Malaise and anorexia
>> Chills alternating with diaphoresis

Discuss importance of reporting to physician any event that may predispose to bacteremia
> Dental or gum manipulation
> Genitourinary procedures
> Drainage of abscesses
> Presence of skin boils
> Gynecological procedures
>> Childbirth
>> Dilation and curettage (D & C)
>> Therapeutic abortion
>> Tubal ligation

Explain importance of notifying dentist, urologist, and gynecologist of valvular heart disease

Provide instruction to women regarding appropriate choice of contraceptives: to avoid oral contraceptives and intrauterine devices; explain importance of obtaining counseling regarding pregnancy before conception

Explain need to maintain good oral hygiene, daily care, and regular visits to dentist

Explain need to avoid fatigue; to plan rest periods before and after activity

Instruct patient in measures that will minimize fatigue
> Bathing: shower with chair rather than tub bath
> Avoid prolonged periods of standing, use stool to lean against when cooking, ironing

Instruct patient about importance of prophylactic antibiotic therapy to prevent endocarditis (see Table 2-4)

Discuss name of medication, dosage, times of administration, purpose, and side effects

Explain need to avoid taking over-the-counter drugs without checking with physician

Explain importance of ongoing outpatient care

Expected outcome/evaluation

Patient
> Verbalizes understanding of disease, precautions to take
> Identifies physical limitations
> Reports taking prescribed medication

Additional Nursing Diagnoses to Consider

Potential for injury (cerebral) related to interruption of arterial blood flow secondary to embolization

PERICARDITIS

An inflammatory process involving the parietal and visceral layers of the pericardium and outer myocardium

Assessment
Observations/findings

Substernal chest pain
> Precordial
> May radiate to shoulder or neck
> Severe, sharp
> Increases with inspiration
> Relieved by sitting up and leaning forward

Increased systemic venous pressure

Pericardial friction rub: scratchy sound in time with heartbeat

Dyspnea

Elevated temperature

Chills alternating with diaphoresis

Restlessness

Nausea

Muscle aches

Anxiety

Fatigue

Orthopnea

Pericardial effusion

Laboratory/diagnostic studies

ECG
> Elevated ST segment in LV leads: V_5, V_6, I, II, aV_L and aV_F
> T wave inversion (late stage)

Low-voltage QRS complex in presence of pericardial effusion

Dysrhythmias

Blood studies

Leukocytosis (increased WBC)

Increased ESR; elevated viral titers

Chest x-ray examination: normal or symmetrically enlarged cardiac silhouette

Echocardiogram: presence of pericardial effusion

Radionuclide blood pool scanning

Technetium label macroaggregated albumin and Thallium: confirms presence of pericardial effusion

Magnetic resonance imaging (MRI): visualizes pericardium, can differentiate acute from chronic pericarditis

Potential complications

Cardiac tamponade

Heart failure

Medical Management

Medications

Nonsteroidal antiinflammatory agents: indomethacin

Analgesics, antipyretics: aspirin

Corticosteroids

Pericardiocentesis

Surgical procedures

Pericardial window

Pericardiectomy

Nursing diagnoses/interventions/evaluation

■ **NDX:** Pain (chest) related to pericardial inflammation

Assess and record quality of chest pain

Maintain bed rest

Position for comfort

Elevate head 45 degrees

Provide padded overbed table

Administer pain medications as ordered

Expected outcome/evaluation

Patient's chest pain is relieved

■ **NDX:** Anxiety related to perceived or actual threat to biological integrity

Assess level of anxiety and degree of understanding, noting verbal and nonverbal expressions

Provide supportive care

Remain with patient if anxious

Encourage communication with significant other

Explain procedures and treatments thoroughly

Ensure quiet environment; reduce external stimuli

Use calm, reassuring voice

Expected outcome/evaluation

Patient's anxiety level is reduced; appears calm

■ **NDX:** Potential decreased cardiac output related to reduced ventricular filling

Assess and monitor for signs of cardiac tamponade

Check for pulsus paradoxus, narrowing pulse pressure, respiratory filling of neck veins

Monitor BP, T, R, and apical pulse q4h as indicated

Place on cardiac monitor during acute phase, checking rhythm q1h to 2h

Obtain 12-lead ECG as ordered

Auscultate heart sounds for presence of pericardial friction rub q6h to 8h

Administer medications as ordered

Prepare for pericardiocentesis when ordered

Expected outcome/evaluation

Patient's

Cardiac output and hemodynamic stability maintained

Vital signs within normal limits

Negative for pulsus paradoxus

■ **NDX:** Knowledge deficit related to lack of information about disease process

Explain underlying cause and disease process

Discuss symptoms of recurrence to report to physician

Increasing fatigue

Elevated temperature

Difficult respirations

Chest pain

Explain that symptoms may continue up to 2 weeks but notify physician if symptoms do not diminish or if they increase

Explain need to avoid persons with infections, especially upper respiratory infections, and to report symptoms (e.g., cold, flu, cough) to physician

Explain need to avoid overexertion and heavy lifting; alternate periods of activity with rest

Explain importance of ongoing outpatient care

Discuss medications: name, dosage, time of administration, purpose, and side effects

Explain need to avoid taking over-the-counter medications without checking with physician

Expected outcome/evaluation

Patient's level of understanding is increased

Patient identifies signs and symptoms to report to physician

Patient verbalizes knowledge of disease

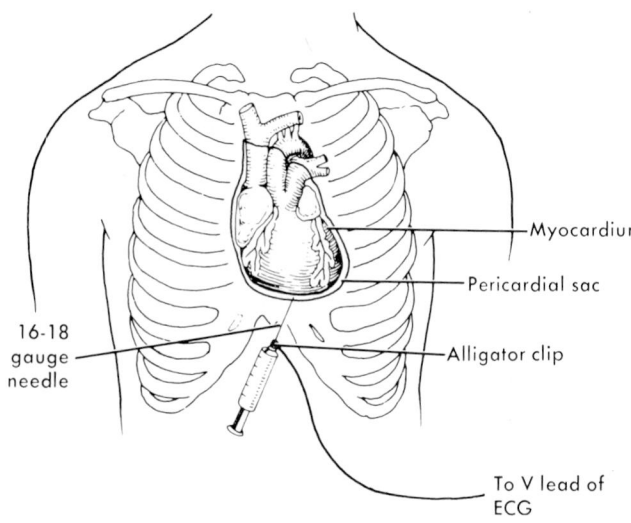

FIGURE 2-13. Pericardiocentesis. (From Budassi SA, Barber J: *Emergency nursing: principles and practice,* St Louis, 1980, CV Mosby.)

PERICARDIOCENTESIS

Withdrawal of blood or fluid from the pericardial sac via percutaneous needle puncture (Figure 2-13)

Preparation

Reinforce physician's explanation of procedure
Obtain signed consent
Maintain NPO 4 to 6 hr before procedure when possible
Elevate head of bed 20 to 30 degrees as ordered
Obtain 12-lead ECG and rhythm strip; connect ECG unipolar lead to needle using alligator clip
Obtain laboratory studies as ordered: CBC, PT, PTT, platelets
Administer oxygen by mask or cannula as ordered
Obtain and record baseline arterial pressures, as well as paradoxic pulse and pulse pressure
Maintain parenteral fluids as ordered
Obtain necessary equipment as ordered
  ECG machine
  Needles: No. 16 spinal
  Syringes: 30 cc and 50 cc
  Three-way stopcock
  Sterile drapes
Administer medications as ordered
  Atropine
  Lidocaine
  Sedatives
Maintain defibrillator and emergency drugs at bedside
Provide emotional support

Assessment During and After Procedure
Observations/findings

Level of consciousness
ECG

ST elevations
Increased PR interval
Arterial pressure
Right atrial pressure (RAP)
Pericardial aspirate
  Amount
  Color
  Turbidity
  Blood
Respirations

Potential complications

Puncture of coronary artery, ventricle, or lung
Dysrhythmias
Ventricular fibrillation
Laceration of lung
Pneumothorax
Cardiac tamponade

Postprocedure Care

Maintain bed rest
Assess BP, R, and apical pressure q15min for 1 hr, then q4h as ordered
Monitor arterial pressures; check for decreased pulse pressure or pulsus paradoxus q15min for 1 hr, then q4h as ordered
Maintain NPO as ordered
Auscultate heart sounds q2h to 4h
Observe for recurrence of tamponade; be prepared to repeat pericardiocentesis or surgical intervention
Continue ongoing care for specific disease process

CARDIAC TAMPONADE

Rapid accumulation of fluid or blood within the pericardial cavity that results in restriction of diastolic filling

Assessment
Observations/findings

Distended neck veins with inspiratory rise in venous pressure (Kussmaul's sign)
Decreased systolic BP; narrowing pulse pressure; pulsus paradoxus >10 mm Hg
  Decreased heart sounds
  Pericardial friction rub
  Anxiety and restlessness
  Tachypnea
  Tachycardia: weak, absent peripheral pulses
  Skin
    Cyanotic
    Dusky
    Pale
Posture: Patient sits upright or leans forward
Abdominal pain
Hemodynamic findings
  Decreased CO

Elevated RAP
Elevated CVP
Lowered left atrial pressure (LAP)

Laboratory/diagnostic studies

Echocardiogram: pericardial effusion; paradoxic septal motion
ECG
Tachycardia
Nonspecific ST and T wave changes
Diminished voltage, altering voltage of both P wave and QRS
Dysrhythmias
Chest x-ray examination: enlarged cardiac silhouette (globular shape); lung fields clear
Blood pooling scanning
Magnetic resonance imaging (MRI): to show loculated effusions
Right heart catheterization: decreased ventricular filling pressures, elevated RAP

Potential complications

Heart failure
Cardiogenic shock
Cardiac arrest

Medical Management

NPO
Parenteral fluids
Pericardiocentesis
Medications
Inotropic, chronotropic
Corticosteroids
Antiarrhythmics
Twelve-lead electrocardiogram
Maintain defibrillator and emergency drugs at bedside
Surgery
Pericardiectomy

Nursing diagnoses/interventions/evaluation

■ **NDX:** Decreased cardiac output related to restricted ventricular filling

Assess for and estimate degree of pulsus paradoxus and increased JVP
Maintain bed rest; elevate head of bed 45 degrees
Place patient on cardiac monitor; check rhythm strip qh
Monitor arterial pressure, pulse pressure, pulse volume, ECG, and level of consciousness q5min to 15 min
Administer parenteral fluids as ordered
Administer medications as ordered
Assist with pericardiocentesis

Expected outcome/evaluation

Patient demonstrates hemodynamic stability
Negative for pulses paradoxus

Vital signs within normal limits
Jugular venous detension decreases

■ **NDX:** Anxiety (moderate to severe) related to perceived and/or actual threat to biology integrity

Assess level of anxiety, noting both verbal and nonverbal expressions
During this period, remain with patient, offering realistic assurances; use simple explanations
Ensure quiet environment, reduce external stimuli as much as possible

Expected outcome/evaluation

Patient's anxiety level is reduced; appears relaxed

HEART FAILURE

Inability of the heart to increase cardiac output sufficiently to meet the body's metabolic demand

Assessment
Observations/findings
GENERAL

Fatigue
Effort intolerance
Anorexia
Cachexia
Nausea and/or vomiting
Tachypnea
Dyspnea
Nocturia
Tachycardia
Pulsus alternans
Gallop rhythms (S_3, S_4)
Peripheral cyanosis
Anxiety
Restlessness
Crackles, rhonchi
Cheyne-Stokes respiration
Respiratory assessment
Drug toxicity
Digitalis toxicity
Hypokalemia
Dysrhythmias

LEFT VENTRICULAR FAILURE

Shortness of breath
Restlessness
Dyspnea, exertional and/or at rest
PND
Orthopnea
Tachypnea
Cough: dry, unproductive
Hemoptysis
Elevated BP

Tachycardia
Pulsus alternans
Left ventricular gallop: S_3
Hypoxemia
Crackles, rhonchi
Cyanosis

RIGHT VENTRICULAR FAILURE

Increased venous pressure (rise in "a" and "v" waves)
Distended neck veins
Edema: firm, pitting
    Peripheral extremities
    Sacrum
    Genitalia
Ascites
Right upper quadrant abdominal tenderness
Hepatosplenomegaly; hepatojugular reflex
Diaphoresis
Weight gain
Right ventricular gallop: S_3
Decreased urine output
Anorexia

Laboratory/diagnostic studies

GENERAL

Serum
    Hct, Hgb
    BUN, creatinine
    Electrolytes
        Hyponatremia
        Hyperkalemia
        Hypokalemia
    Bilirubin: hyperbilirubinemia
    Enzymes: SGOT, SGPT, LDH
    PT
    Albumin
    Glucose
    Arterial blood gases
Urine
    Specific gravity
    Protein
    Creatinine
    Sodium
ECG
Chest x-ray examination
Echocardiogram
MUGA
Hemodynamic monitoring
Pulmonary function tests

LEFT VENTRICULAR FAILURE

ECG: left ventricular hypertrophy (LVH), left atrial hypertrophy (LAH), dysrhythmias
Increased PCWP
Decreased CO
Chest x-ray examination

Chest x-ray examination
    Redistribution of pulmonary flow to upper lobes
    Kerley B lines
    Pleural effusion
    Increased cardiac shadow
Pulmonary function tests
    Decreased vital capacity (VC), residual volume, and total lung capacity

RIGHT VENTRICULAR FAILURE

ECG: right ventricular hypertrophy (RVH), right atrial hypertrophy (RAH)
Elevated RA, RV pressure
Elevated CVP
Chest x-ray examination
    Generalized enlargement of cardiac shadow

Potential complications

Pulmonary edema
Embolic phenomenon
Pulmonary infarction
Cardiogenic shock

Medical Management

Bed rest
Low-sodium diet
Medications
    Diuretics
    Vasodilators
    Beta-blocking agents
    Inotropic drugs
    Morphine sulfate
Oxygen therapy
Cardiac monitor
Hemodynamic monitoring
SVO_2
Intra-aortic balloon pump (IABP)
Ventricular assist devices (VAD)

Nursing diagnoses/interventions/evaluation

■ **NDX:** Decreased cardiac output related to mechanical factors (preload, afterload, or contractility)

Assess and monitor BP, apical pulse, HR, and respirations, q4h or as indicated
Maintain bed rest as indicated; elevate head of bed 30 to 60 degrees; lean patient forward on padded overbed table
Monitor cardiac output q4h to 6h as ordered
Monitor and record hemodynamic parameters as indicated
Administer medications as ordered
    Digitalis
    Dobutamine
    Amrinone
    Milrinone

Monitor for signs of drug toxicity; monitor drug levels

Maintain quiet environment

Restrict activities as indicated by condition

Provide bedside commode

Implement measures that avoid fatigue

Plan rest periods between procedures

Have patient rest before and after meals

Maintain planned rest periods

Provide emotional support; offer simple explanations

Expected outcome/evaluation

Patient will have improved cardiac output as evidenced by

Vital signs within acceptable limits for age

HR CO, PCWP within acceptable limits

Urine output increased

Activities tolerance is increased

■ **NDX:** Alteration in fluid volume: excess related to compromised regulatory mechanism

Assess and monitor for increase or decrease in jugular venous pressure

Auscultate chest for breath and heart sounds (S_3, S_4) q4h to 8h

Maintain parenteral fluids by microdrip when ordered; avoid rapid and excessive hydration; use concentrated IV infusion to decrease volume administration when possible

Administer diuretics and vasodilator therapy as ordered; observe for effect and toxicity

Measure intake and output

Record output qh; report output of less than 30 ml/hr

Estimate diaphoretic fluid loss

Weigh patient daily at same time with same clothing and scale; report increase of 500 g/day or greater

Monitor BUN and electrolytes

Maintain sodium-restricted diet as ordered

Maintain fluid restrictions; assist patient with planning distribution of fluids over waking hours

Expected outcome/evaluation

Patient exhibits no signs of fluid overload as evidenced by

Absence of edema

Weight loss, return to baseline

Lung sounds clear; heart sounds: no S_3, S_4

No signs of increased jugular venous pressure

■ **NDX:** Impaired gas exchange related to alveolar-capillary membrane changes caused by increased pulmonary capillary pressure

Assess and monitor for changes in respiratory function

Monitor serial arterial blood gases

Auscultate lung sounds q4h

Monitor chest x-ray examinations for changes

Monitor hemodynamic parameters: PAP, PCWP as indicated

Elevate head of bed; have patient lean forward on padded overbed table; reposition q2h to 4h as indicated

Administer oxygen therapy as ordered; prepare for intubation and assisted mechanical ventilation if required

Provide humidified inspired air as ordered

Instruct patient to cough and deep breathe

Administer medications as ordered

Morphine

Rapid-acting diuretics

Instruct patient to avoid smoking or using tobacco products

Provide brief explanations of all treatments and procedures

Expected outcome/evaluation

Patient demonstrates improved gas exchange as evidenced by

Effortless breathing

Improved respirations

Lungs clear on auscultation

PO_2 and PCO_2 levels within normal limits

■ **NDX:** Potential impaired skin integrity related to impaired circulation and metabolic state

Assess skin integrity and bony prominences daily for signs of redness, scaling, breaks, or ulcerations

Initiate measures to maintain skin integrity

If on bed rest turn and reposition q2h

Provide alternative preventive devices

Alternating pressure mattress

Air pressure beds (Clinitron)

Prevent and eliminate pressure and friction; position pillows or other supports between pressure areas to avoid two skin areas touching

Assist patient out of bed frequently or as ordered

Administer skin care q2h

Keep skin clean and dry

Massage bony prominences q2h to 4h, using lanolin-based lotion

NOTE: To prevent skin excoriations do not massage reddened area

Initiate decubitus care at first signs of tissue breakdown or ulceration (p. 1)

Expected outcome/evaluation

Demonstrates maintenance of skin integrity as evidenced by

Skin intact

Warm and dry, normal color

Signs of healing over areas of breakdown

■ **NDX:** Alteration in nutritional status: less than body requirements related to impaired absorption of nutrients secondary to decreased cardiac output

Observe daily for signs of malnutrition and cardiac cachexia
- Dry body weight 20% or more under the ideal for age, height, and frame
- Decreased triceps skinfold measurements
- Stomatitis
- Anorexia
- Increasing fatigue and weakness
- Decreased serum albumin, transferrin, iron-binding capacity, BUN
- Lack of interest in food

Determine patient's baseline weight
- Weigh patient daily at same time with same clothing and scale

Administer oral hygiene 2qh to 4h

Administer medications to relieve nausea and/or vomiting; arrange medication schedule so it does not interfere with mealtime

Maintain diet as ordered; consult with dietitian to evaluate nutritional status and to assist in selection of foods
- Do not force patient to eat
- Tempt appetite with food preferences compatible with diet restrictions and cultural values
- Remove unsightly and odorous items from room during mealtime
- Serve small, frequent meals
- Supplement with high-calorie foods

Initiate caloric count if nutritional status fails to improve

Initiate tube feedings or parenteral nutrition as indicated

Expected outcome/evaluation

Patient demonstrates adequate nutritional status as evidenced by
- Dry body weight that is improved or normal for age and body build
- Improved appetite
- Good skin turgor, increased muscle mass

■ **NDX:** Activity intolerance related to weakness secondary to decreased cardiac output

Assess and monitor for signs of activity intolerance

Check BP, HR, and respiration before and after activity

Maintain patient on bed rest or on chair rest with feet elevated as indicated

Identify factors known to cause fatigue, restrict and/or limit activities as indicated, e.g., number of visitors and their length of stay

Space treatments and procedures to allow for periods of uninterrupted rest; provide periods of rest throughout day and evening

Implement measures that will improve activity tolerance by minimizing fatigue, e.g., bathing in shower with chair rather than self-bathing; using bedside commode rather than bedpan

Increase activity level as indicated; assess activity tolerance and activity progression

Expected outcome/evaluation

Patient
- Demonstrates improved activity tolerance
- Verbalizes improved energy to perform activities of daily living (ADLs)
- ECG, BP, HR, and respiratory rate within acceptable limits during and after activity

■ **NDX:** Knowledge deficit related to lack of information about disease process and self-care management

Assess level of understanding

Discuss nature and cause of disease process and underlying cause

Discuss importance of pacing activities to avoid overexertion and fatigue
- Alternate exercise and other activities with rest periods
- Use energy-saving techniques (e.g., sitting to brush hair and prepare foods)

Discuss importance of maintaining prescribed diet and fluid amounts; need to avoid food high in sodium
- Instruct patient to read labels for sodium content before buying
- Provide information on alternative ways to season foods
- Refer to dietitian as necessary

Discuss need to avoid persons with infections, especially upper respiratory infections

Discuss importance of daily weighing at same time with same amount of clothing

Review symptoms of early heart failure to report to physician
- Decreased exercise tolerance
- Shortness of breath
- Dyspnea on exertion (DOE)
- Paroxysmal nocturnal dyspnea (PND)

SHOCK SYNDROME: CAUSES/ETIOLOGIES

HYPOVOLEMIC SHOCK

Loss of blood volume (hemorrhage, GI bleeding, wounds)

Loss of plasma volume (dehydration, burns, peritonitis)

CARDIOGENIC SHOCK

Acute myocardial infarction

Septal rupture

Other causes (pulmonary emboli, cardiac surgery, tamponade)

VASOGENIC SHOCK

Sepsis

Immune-mediated reactions (anaphylaxis)

Deep anesthesia effects

Persistent cough
Swelling of extremities
Sudden weight gain of more than 3 lb (6.6 kg) in a 24-hr period
Nocturia
Explain importance of not smoking
Discuss medications: name, dosage, time of administration, purpose, and side effects (see Vasodilator Drugs, p. 88)
Explain importance of avoiding extreme temperature changes
Explain importance of ongoing care

Expected outcome/evaluation

Patient verbalizes an increased knowledge level regarding disease process, diet, medications, and activity allowances and limitations

SHOCK

A clinical syndrome in which blood flow to the tissues is insufficient to sustain normal cell metabolism, resulting in a generalized decrease in perfusion to vital body function (see box on p. 104 and Table 2-6)

hypovolemic shock ("cold" shock) Deficient return of venous blood to the heart caused by external losses of blood plasma or extracellular fluid or caused by internal sequestration of plasma

vasogenic (warm shock) Shock syndrome that results in massive vasodilation from an increase in total vascular capacity; most common form is sepsis, but may occur as a result of other factors, including anaphylactic reactions

cardiogenic shock Shock caused by inadequate tissue perfusion that results from impaired LV function

Assessment
Observations/findings
HYPOVOLEMIC SHOCK

Syncope
Vertigo

TABLE 2-6. Early and Late Signs of Shock Syndrome

Signs	Early	Late
Blood pressure	↓ Pulse pressure ↑ Diastolic pressure	↓ Systolic pressure
Urine output	↓ Urine sodium concentration ↑ Urine osmolality	↓ Urine volume
Acid-base changes	↑ Respiratory alkalosis Metabolic alkalosis	Metabolic acidosis
Tissue perfusion	Occasionally warm, dry skin Slight restlessness	Cold, clammy skin Cloudy sensorium

From *Shock* 1976, The Upjohn Company. Reproduced with permission of The Upjohn Company.

Restlessness
Anxiety
Decreased or falling BP: determined by patient's baseline pressure
Narrowed pulse pressure
Hemodynamics
    Interarterial pressure
        Early: normal
        Late: decreased
    Decreased PAP, PCWP
    Decreased CO
    Decreased CVP (<3 cm H_2O pressure)
    Normal or slightly increased
Low SVO_2
Flat neck veins
Collapsed peripheral veins
Tachycardia: weak, thready pulse
Tachypnea: shallow respirations
Extreme weakness
Altered levels in mental status
    Lethargy
    Semiconsciousness
    Coma
Circumoral pallor
Conjunctival pallor
Lip cyanosis
Skin
    Pale
    Cool
    Clammy
    Cyanotic
    Mottling of extremities
Subnormal temperature
Excessive thirst
Nausea, vomiting
Renal status
    Urinary output below 30 ml/hr
    Elevated serum creatinine
    Elevated serum urea nitrogen
    Low urine sodium (<20 mEq/L)
Internal or external circulating blood volume loss
    Hemorrhage
        Postsurgical
        Gastrointestinal (GI)
        After trauma
    Plasma volume losses
        Burns
        Excessive diarrhea, vomiting

VASOGENIC SHOCK

Fainting
Vertigo
Restlessness
Anxiety
Early stage
    Normal or slightly decreased BP

Decreased or normal SVR
  Hemodynamics
    Decreased or normal PCWP
    Greatly increased CO
  Warm skin
  Tachycardia: bounding pulse
Late stage
  Decreased BP
  Increased peripheral vascular resistance
  Decreased CO
  Decreased PCWP
  Increased SVR
  Metabolic acidosis
  Tachycardia
  Low SVO_2
Excessive thirst
Nausea, vomiting
Tachypnea: see Respiratory Assessment (p. 186)
Temperature
  Subnormal
  Elevated
Altered level of consciousness
  Lethargy
  Semiconsciousness
  Coma
Skin
  Pale
  Cool
  Clammy
  Cyanotic
Renal status
  Urinary output below 30 ml/hr
  Elevated serum creatinine
  Elevated serum urea nitrogen
Wounds
  Swelling, redness
  Abnormal secretions
  Generalized urticaria, pruritus

CARDIOGENIC SHOCK

Restlessness
Anxiety
Decreased or falling BP; determined by patient's baseline
  pressure
Hypotension: systolic pressures <90 mm Hg
Left ventricular pressures
  Increased LVEDP
  Increased LAP
  Increased PCWP
Cardiac output
  2.2 L/min
  Decreased ejection fraction
  Decreased cardiac index
Increased SVR: >1600 dyne/sec/cm^{-5}

Elevated RV filling pressures
  Presence of jugular vein distension
  Increased CVP: above 15 cm H_2O pressure
  Positive hepatojugular reflex
Tachycardia
  Thready radial pulse
  Diminished or absent peripheral pulses
Presence of S_3, S_4 gallops or murmurs
Increased SVO_2
Respiratory distress
  Tachypnea
  Orthopnea
  Hypoxia
Alteration in level of consciousness
  Apathy
  Lethargy
  Semiconsciousness
  Coma
Skin
  Pale
  Cool
  Clammy
  Cyanosis
Temperature
  Subnormal
  Elevated
Excessive thirst
Nausea, vomiting
Renal status
  Urinary output below 20 ml/hr
  Elevated serum creatinine
  Elevated serum urea nitrogen
ECG changes
  Ischemic changes
  Dysrhythmias
  Ventricular fibrillation
Pain
  Chest
  Abdominal

Laboratory/diagnostic studies
HYPOVOLEMIC SHOCK

Electrolytes
Chemistries
Arterial blood gases
Specific gravity

VASOGENIC SHOCK

Cultures
  Blood
  Sputum
  Urine
WBC
ESR

Chest x-ray examination
Clotting profile

CARDIOGENIC SHOCK

Serum
  Arterial blood gases
  Chemistries
  Electrolytes
  Drug levels
  Cardiac enzymes
ECG
Chest x-ray examination
MUGA
Echocardiogram
Radionuclide ventriculography

Potential complications
HYPOVOLEMIC SHOCK

Heart failure

VASOGENIC SHOCK

Adult respiratory distress syndrome (p. 225)
Disseminated intravascular coagulation
Multisystem failure

CARDIOGENIC SHOCK

Metabolic acidosis
  Increased serum lactate levels
  Decreased pH
Electrolyte imbalances
Myocardial ischemia: elevated enzymes
Heart failure
Pulmonary edema
Adult respiratory distress syndrome (p. 223)
  Diminished breath sounds
  Pulmonary congestion

Medical Management

Admission to cardiac intensive care unit
Cardiac monitor
Hemodynamic monitoring
Assisted mechanical ventilation
Oxygen therapy
Medications
  Vasodilators, sodium nitroprusside
  Sympathomimetics: dopamine, dobutamine
  Osmotic diuretics
  For vasogenic shock: epinephrine, antihistamine, hydrocortisone
Parenteral therapy
  Blood replacement
  Plasma volume expanders
  Fluid challenges
Ventricular assist devices (VAD)
  IABP

Nursing diagnoses/interventions/evaluation

■ **NDX:** Alteration in tissue perfusion (cerebral, cardiopulmonary, peripheral) related to decreased cardiac output

Assess for signs and symptoms reflecting impaired tissue perfusion
Maintain complete bed rest; flat supine position; position extremities to facilitate circulation
Maintain parenteral therapy as ordered: whole blood, plasmanate, volume expanders
Measure intake and output qh
Connect indwelling urethral catheter to closed gravity drainage system; notify physician if urinary output is less than 30 ml/hr
Measure all body fluid loss; estimate loss in dressings or perineal pads
Administer medications as ordered
Assess for effects of drug therapy and signs of toxicity
Maintain NPO or clear liquid as ordered
Check R, apical pulse, and femoral pulse q15min and prn
Monitor PAP and PCWP q1h to 2h as ordered
Monitor intraarterial pressure q1h to 2h; check peripheral arm BP q15min if arterial line is not in place
Monitor cardiac output as ordered
Check CVP reading qh and prn
Apply pressure to control bleeding if necessary
  Pressure dressing
  Direct pressure
  Gastric tube with balloon
  Traction to urethral catheter
Apply shock trousers as ordered; patient may arrive in trousers
Prepare medications to control bleeding if ordered
  Vitamin K
  Protamine sulfate
Prepare for surgery
  Resuturing of the bleeding site
  Removal of ruptured organ or resection of bleeding site
  See General Preoperative Care/Teaching (p. 27)
Avoid routine nursing functions during acute phase
Keep patient warm and dry

Expected outcome/evaluation

Tissue perfusion is maintained
  Blood pressure is within normal limits
  Urine output is normal
  Skin warm and dry
  Peripheral pulses >2T

■ **NDX:** Decreased cardiac output related to mechanical factors (preload, afterload, and myocardial contractility)

Maintain position best suited to promote optimal ventilation; elevate head of bed 30 to 60 degrees

Avoid routine nursing functions
Maintain complete bed rest
Maintain NPO
Initiate IV: maintain an open vein
Monitor ECG continuously
Measure intake and output qh
  Maintain parenteral fluids as ordered
  Connect indwelling urethral catheter to closed gravity drainage system; notify physician if urinary output is less than 30 ml/hr
Check BP, R, apical pulse, and femoral pulse q15min and prn
Monitor LAP, PAP, and PCWP q1h to 2h as ordered:
Measure and calculate CO, CI
Monitor intraarterial pressure to 2h as ordered
Monitor cardiac output as ordered
Calculate systemic vascular resistance as ordered:

$$\frac{\text{Mean aortic pressure} - \text{Mean right atrial pressure (mm Hg)}}{\text{Cardiac output (L/min)}}$$

Check CVP reading qh and prn
Check axillary temperature qh
Administer oxygen as ordered prn
Administer medications as ordered
  To decrease afterload and O_2 consumption
    Vasodilators
    Corticosteroids
    Adjust flow rate according to BP response
  To increase myocardial contractility and reduce peripheral vascular resistance (PVR)
    Sympathomimetics
    Vasodilators
    Adjust flow rate according to BP response
Administer plasma volume expanders as ordered; adjust flow rate according to PAP and PCWP readings
Keep patient warm and dry
Auscultate heart sounds q2h to 4h
Prepare for and monitor intraaortic balloon counterpulsation as ordered; assess cardiac response
Restrict and plan activities; provide rest periods between procedures
Avoid constipation, straining, or rectal stimulation; give stool softeners or laxatives as ordered

Expected outcome/evaluation

Patient demonstrates improved cardiac output as evidenced by
  Vital signs within normal limits
  CO and PCWP within normal limits
  Improved mentation

■ **NDX:** Impaired gas exchange related to increased pulmonary capillary permeability

Assess respiratory pattern noting rate and depth of respirations

Auscultate lungs q1h to 2h
Monitor serial arterial blood gases
Monitor SVo_2; report if SVo_2 <60%
Administer oxygen as ordered
Suction as ordered to ensure patent airway
Assist and teach patient to cough and deep breathe q1h to 2h

Expected outcome/evaluation

Patient demonstrates improved ventilation as evidenced by
  Effortless breathing
  Clear lungs
  Po_2 and Pco_2 levels within normal limits

■ **NDX:** Anxiety/fear related to actual or potential biological threat

Determine patient's source of fear and anxiety
Explain all procedures and treatments; offer brief explanations
Remain with patient to offer reassurance
Anticipate needs
Maintain quiet, nonstressful environment
Allow family or significant other to remain with patient as condition permits
Encourage verbalization of needs and fears of dying
Maintain calm and reassuring manner

Expected outcome/evaluation

Patient verbalizes decrease in anxiety level

CARDIAC SURGERY (OPEN-HEART PROCEDURE)*

cardiac surgery Care depends on whether the operation is an open-heart procedure, requiring use of the cardiopulmonary bypass machine, or a closed-heart procedure that does not require use of the bypass machine

Classification of Cardiac Surgery

CLOSED-HEART SURGERY

Patent ductus arteriosus (PDA)
Coarctation of aorta
Palliative pulmonary shunts
  Blalock/Taussig
  Potts
  Glenn
Closed mitral commissurotomy

---

*The standard for postoperative care of the patient with open-heart surgery can be used in either cases of open-heart or closed-heart procedures. The patient with closed-heart surgery will usually require less specialized equipment with decreased frequency of nursing functions; however, such a patient may have complications that would also be seen with open-heart surgery (e.g., atelectasis and hypertension).

OPEN-HEART SURGERY

Atrial septal defect (ASD)
Ventricular septal defect (VSD)
Transposition of great vessels
Tetralogy of Fallot
Truncus arteriosus
Tricuspid atresia
Aortic stenosis
Coronary artery bypass graft (CABG)
Ventricular aneurysm
Mitral commissurotomy
Mitral valve replacement
Aortic valve replacement
Aortic aneurysm
Fontan procedures for complex congenital heart defects
Cardiac transplantation

Preoperative Care

Assessment

Observations/findings

Level of consciousness
See Respiratory Assessment (p. 186)
Emotions
    Anxiety: adaptive vs. maladaptive
    Euphoria
    Depression
    Denial
    Fear
BP, T, P, and R
Skin
    Color
    Turgor
    Temperature
Peripheral circulation
Heart sounds
    Murmurs
    Rubs
    Gallops
Breath sounds: abnormal
    Decreased breath sounds
    Rales
    Crackles
    Wheezes
Smoking history
Weight and height
Activity tolerance
Medications being taken
    Cardiac medications
    Anticoagulants/antiplatelets
    Antiarrhythmics
    Birth control pills

Laboratory/diagnostic studies

ECG: acute changes, increase in dysrhythmias
    12-lead
    Rhythm strip

Chest x-ray examination
    Cardiomegaly
    Pulmonary vascular congestion
CBC: Hgb, Hct
Blood type and cross match
Coagulation studies: PT, PTT, and platelets
Electrolytes
BUN
Creatine
Urinalysis
Pulmonary function
    VC
    Tidal volume
    Minute ventilation

Preoperative Teaching

Assess level of understanding
Involve family or significant other in care and instructions
Reinforce physician's explanation regarding
    Operative procedure
    Location, type and length of incision(s)
    Length of time anticipated for recovery
Explain preoperative procedures
    Skin preparation: shaving, antiseptic bath or shower
    Visits from anesthesiologist and respiratory therapist
Check if dental clearance was given (dental checks should
    be done 10 to 14 days before operation)
Explain and review postoperative procedures and routines
    of CCU or ICU
    How special unit will differ from regular unit
    Types of noises to be experienced
    Visiting privileges
    Usual length of stay in unit
    Pain to be experienced and availability of medications
        as needed
    Method of communication while intubated
    Disorientation that may occur resulting from medica-
        tions and/or lack of sleep
Assess patient's awareness, emotional status, and fears re-
    garding
    Surgical procedure
    Heart-lung machine
    Short-term and long-term outcomes
    Possible disabilities
    Previous surgical experiences
Report any *acute* changes in emotional status
    Anxiety
    Depression
    Fear of dying
Instruct patient on simple relaxation techniques such as
    guided imagery
Introduce patient to unit staff who will be providing care
    postoperatively
When possible, introduce patient and family to CCU or
    ICU, explaining equipment to be used
    Cardiac monitor

Hemodynamic monitor
Drainage tubes
Pacing wires, pacemaker
Respirator
Nebulizer
Oxygen administration
IV therapy
  Blood transfusions
  Replacement fluids
Review postoperative medications, particularly those that will be long term, such as anticoagulants
Review procedures for and stress importance and purpose of
Turning
Coughing
Deep breathing
Incentive spirometry
Foot and leg exercises
Practice these procedures 1 to 2 days before operation
Withhold medications as ordered (e.g., anticoagulants)
Refer to spiritual advisor or social service worker as indicated

Postoperative Care
Assessment
Observations/findings
GENERAL

Neurological: level of consciousness
Pulmonary
  Respirations
    Quality
    Rate
    Character
  Breath sounds: equal or decreased
    Dullness
    Crackles
    Rhonchi
  Chest drainage
    Amount
    Quality
    Color
Cardiovascular
  Hemodynamic parameters
    Arterial BP
    HR, rhythm
    LAP, LVEDP, PCWP
    CVP
  Heart sounds
    Rubs
    Murmurs
  Arterial pulses
    Quality
    Rate
    Rhythm
    Equality
Skin
  Color
  Turgor
  Temperature
ECG: check for presence of acute changes or dysrhythmias
Pacemaker: settings
Renal
  Intake and output
  Urine output
    Amount
    Color
    Specific gravity
    Osmolality
  Electrolytes
  BUN, creatinine
Gastrointestinal
  Nasogastric tube drainage
    Amount
    Color
  Absence or presence of bowel sounds
  Abdominal tone
    Flat
    Distended
    Tenderness
  Incision(s), location
    Midsternotomy
    Submammary
    Leg

VALVE REPLACEMENT

Type of valve replaced
  Heterograft
  Mechanical
  Homograft
Valve sounds: normal
  Mechanical: opening, closing clicks
  Heterograft, homograft: produces no clicks
Valve dysfunction: occurrence of new regurgitant-type murmur
  Obstruction
  Perivalvular leak
  Rupture
Anticoagulation therapy (p. 148)
Endocarditis

CORONARY ARTERY GRAFT

Graft site
  Saphenous vein
  Mammary artery

CONGENITAL HEART DISEASE REPAIR

Type of repair: palliative, corrective
Use of conduits, grafts, baffles

Laboratory/diagnostic studies

CBC, chemistries, electrolytes, platelet function, PT, PTT

Arterial blood gases

Chest x-ray examination

Potential complications

GENERAL

Cardiovascular
  Dysrhythmias
    Premature ventricular contractions (PVCs)
    Ventricular tachycardia
    Atrial fibrillation
    Atrial flutter
    Asystole
    Complete heart block
  Fluid volume excess
    Dyspnea, orthopnea
    Increased JVD
    Lung sounds: crackles
    Heart sounds: S_3, S_4
    Elevated PAP, LAP, and PCWP
  Low CO syndrome
    Restlessness
    Lethargy
    Skin: cool, pale, peripheral cyanosis
  Tachycardia
  Decreased arterial pressure
  Decreased urine output
  Increased PCWP and LAP
  Increased SVR
  Hypertension
  Hemorrhage
    Increased drainage through chest tubes
    Presence of bright red drainage
    Adults: blood loss >150 ml/hr
    Children: blood loss >5 ml/kg/hr
    Decreased Hct
    Hypotension
  Pericarditis
  Cardiac tamponade
  Shock
    Cardiogenic
    Hypovolemic
  Heart failure
  Endocarditis
  Postpericardiotomy syndrome
  Venous thrombosis
Pulmonary
  Atelectasis
  Pneumonitis
  Respiratory acidosis
  Pleural effusion
  Tension pneumothorax
  Respiratory failure

Neurological
  Altered level of consciousness
  Postpump psychosis
    Restlessness
    Agitation
    Confusion
    Combativeness
    Visual and auditory disturbances
    Transient perceptual disorientation
  Cerebral embolism; CVA (p. 404)
Renal
  Electrolyte imbalance
    Hyponatremia
    Hypokalemia
  Metabolic
    Acidosis
    Alkalosis
  Hypovolemia
    Decreased BP
    Tachycardia
    Low PAP
    Oliguria
Gastrointestinal
  Stress ulcers
  Paralytic ileus
Systemic infection: elevated temperature

VALVE REPLACEMENT

Disintegration of prosthesis
Vegetations from resected valve

MITRAL VALVE REPLACEMENT

Brain embolism
Supraventricular tachyarrhythmias
  Atrial tachycardia
  Rapid atrial fibrillation
Low CO syndrome

TRICUSPID VALVE REPLACEMENT/AORTIC VALVE REPLACEMENT

Conduction defects
Subendocardial necrosis

CORONARY ARTERY BYPASS GRAFT

Acute myocardial infarction
Ventricular dysrhythmias
  PVC
  Ventricular tachycardia
Low CO syndrome
Graft failure
  Angina

CONGENITAL HEART DISEASE REPAIR

Conduction defects
Atrial dysrhythmias
Conduit obstruction
Patch leaks

Medical Management

Admission to cardiac intensive care unit
Oxygen therapy with mechanically assisted ventilation
Cardiac monitor
Hemodynamic monitoring
SVO_2 monitoring
Medications
  Narcotics, analgesics
  Antihypertensives
  Antiarrhythmics
  Inotropic agents
    Dopamine
    Dobutamine
    Digoxin
  Vasodilators
  Anticoagulants
  Electrolytes
Parenteral therapy
  Blood replacement
  Plasma expanders
  Colloids
Pacemaker insertion
Intraaortic balloon pump (IABP)
Ventricular assist devices (VAD)

Nursing diagnoses/interventions/evaluation (adults)

■ NDX: Impaired gas exchange related to hypoventilation and/or ventilation/perfusion abnormalities

Assess and monitor respiratory function while patient is on ventilator
Maintain patent airway
Administer oxygen and assisted ventilation as ordered
Elevate head of bed to 45 degrees
Assess quality and rate of R
Monitor FIO_2 tidal volume to yield arterial PO_2 of about 100 mm Hg
Obtain and monitor arterial blood gases as ordered; observe for and report signs of respiratory alkalosis or acidosis
Monitor SVO_2 as indicated
Auscultate lung sounds q1h to 2h
Suction q1h to 2h; hyperoxygenate 1 to 2 min before procedures; monitor and record any dysrhythmias
Assist and teach patient to turn; percuss chest and reposition q2h
Encourage patient to turn, cough, and deep breathe q1h to 2h in absence of endotracheal tube
Have patient use high-humidity face mask after extubation
Obtain serial chest x-rays q4h to 6h as ordered

Expected outcome/evaluation

Patient demonstrates adequate ventilation as evidenced by

Effortless breathing
Absence of respiratory complications
Clear, equal, and bilateral breath sounds
PO_2 and PCO_2 within normal limits

■ NDX: Decreased cardiac output related to mechanical factors (altered preload, afterload, contractility, heart rate) or electrical instability

Assess and monitor for signs of decreased CO
Maintain bed rest with head of bed elevated 45 degrees
Assess BP, apical pulse, and peripheral pulses q15 min to 30min for 2h, then qh as ordered, reporting
  Systolic BP: drop of 20 mm Hg
  Systolic BP <80 or >180 mm Hg
  Diastolic BP >100 mm Hg
  Decreased amplitude in pulses
  Pulse rate <60 or >100 beats/min
Monitor PAP, PCWP, arterial pressure, and SVO_2 q15min during immediate postoperative period, decreasing frequency as clinical status stabilizes
Calculate CO and SVR as ordered
Check temperature on admission, q1h × 6, then q4h
Initiate rewarming procedures
  Blankets
  Heat lamp
Auscultate heart sounds q2h to 4h
Monitor urine output q1h; report outputs <30 ml/h
Administer fluids, blood products, and medications as ordered
Perform laboratory studies q4h to 6h as ordered
  Cardiac enzymes, CPK-MB, SGOT, LDH
  Electrolytes and potassium levels (checked more frequently)
  Hgb, Hct
Initiate IABP or VAD as ordered
Avoid valsalva maneuvers, such as caused by constipation
  Bedside commode
  Stool softeners
  Mild laxative
Record dysrhythmias
  Monitor and record ECG rhythm strips qh; measure rate plus PR, QRS, and QT intervals
  Assess and record any dysrhythmias during procedure and report to physician
  Monitor for fluid and electrolyte disturbances
  Obtain blood studies q4h to 6h or as indicated: electrolytes, potassium
  Connect pacemaker when ordered; check rate and milliamperes (MA)
  Administer antiarrhythmic agents as ordered
  Administer medications: to increase myocardial contractility, to decrease SVR, to control dysrhythmias

Expected outcome/evaluation

Patient demonstrates improved cardiac output as evidenced by
Vital signs within normal limits
CO, LVEDP, and PCWP within acceptable limits
Increased activity tolerance

■ **NDX:** Injury potential: hemorrhage related to surgically induced fibrinolysis and/or inadequate reversal of heparin

Assess and monitor for clinical signs of excessive bleeding
Perform blood studies q4h to 6h as ordered
Hgb, Hct
Coagulation: PT, PTT, platelet count
Measure chest drainage qh; report drainage in excess of 150 to 200 ml/hr
Administer transfusions, platelets, and plasma expanders as ordered
Administer drugs to correct coagulopathy
Protamine sulfate
6-aminocaproic acid (Amicar)
Epsilon aminocaproic acid (EACA)
Vitamin K
Check dressings q1h to 2h
Note drainage: amount, color, and consistency
Change as indicated

Expected outcome/evaluation

Patient demonstrates stable hemostasis as evidenced by
Progressive decrease in chest tube drainage
Stable or improved Hct, Hgb

■ **NDX:** Ineffective breathing pattern related to decreased lung expansion

Assess rate and quality of respiration
Observe and maintain patency of chest tubes; record drainage amount and color q1h to 2h and prn
Auscultate chest for diminished breath sounds q1h to 2h and later q4h to 6h
Encourage patient to cough and deep breathe q1h to 2h
Assist and encourage patient to use incentive spirometry
Administer oxygen therapy as ordered

Expected outcome/evaluation

Patient demonstrates fully expanded lung
Bilateral equal excursion
Full and clear breath sounds

■ **NDX:** Potential for infection related to compromised host defense and environmental exposure

Monitor suture sites for local redness, drainage, and swelling

Assess rectal, oral, or axillary temperature q2h as indicated
Change incisional dressings daily
Administer antibiotics as ordered
Change IV and pressure lines and dressings according to protocol
Remove urethral catheter when patient awakens or as soon as possible
Obtain laboratory studies as indicated
CBC with differential
Blood and urine cultures

Expected outcome/evaluation

Patient shows no signs of infection
Afebrile
Wounds: no signs of irritation or redness

■ **NDX:** Fluid volume excess related to expanded extracellular fluid volume and to postoperative sodium and water retention

Assess for signs of fluid volume excess
During rewarming, monitor filling pressures RAP, LAP, and PAP q5min, then q30min to 60min
Inspect for increased JVD and dependent edema
Maintain parenteral fluids as ordered
Limit fluid intake as indicated
Titrate according to LAP, PCWP, and CVP
Know appropriate fluid allowances
CABG: 2000 ml/24 hr
Valve replacement: 1000 to 1500 ml/24 hr
Congenital heart defect surgery after bypass
60 ml/kg for first 10 kg body weight
30 ml/kg for next 10 kg body weight
15 ml/kg for remainder of weight
Maintain NPO
Measure intake and output; record color and specific gravity of urinary drainage
Weigh patient daily; same time of day with same amount of clothing (weight change of 1 kg indicates loss or gain of 2.2 lb)
Restrict sodium: 2 g sodium/day

Expected outcome/evaluation

Patient demonstrates baseline level of consciousness
Exhibits no signs of fluid overload
Absence of edema, no jugular venous distension (JVD)
Weight loss, return to baseline

■ **NDX:** Alteration in thought process related to biophysiological changes (cerebral hypoxia, age, metabolic alterations, CNS depressants, sleep deprivation)

Assess LOC and neurological signs q15min to 30min for

2 hr, then qh or as indicated

Deal with any personality or psychological changes

    Use reality orientation

    Offer explanations of all procedures

    Administer sedatives as ordered

    Reorient patient to time of day and surroundings

    Use simple, clear sentence structure

    Anticipate needs

    Maintain quiet environment; minimize external stimuli as much as possible

    Remain with patient

Allow family to visit and participate in care when possible

Provide assurance of daily progress

Maintain patient safety; use soft restraints

Expected outcome/evaluation

Patient regains baseline level of consciousness

    Arouses easily

    Clear mentation

    Oriented to time, place, situation

■ **NDX:** Knowledge deficit related to lack of information about health care and follow-up management care

General

Assess level of understanding

Review nature and type of operative procedure, emphasizing precautions and complications associated with surgery

Discuss changes in body image and sexuality

Discuss activity limitations and allowances

Explain need to ambulate to tolerance, to avoid excessive physical exertion, to avoid lifting heavy objects or performing isometric exercises; to restrict driving first 4 to 6 weeks

Instruct patient to increase activity gradually to avoid fatigue

Discuss importance of avoiding fatigue and avoiding sitting for long periods of time

Explain that sexual activity may be contraindicated for 2 to 4 weeks; need to check with physician when it is feasible to resume

Discuss medications: name, dosage, time of administration, purpose, and side effects

Explain need to avoid taking over-the-counter medications before checking with physician

Discuss diet as ordered

    Refer to dietitian for specific diets

    Restrict salt intake

Discuss symptoms to report to physician

    Shortness of breath

    Swelling of hands and legs

Explain importance of wearing medical alert band if patient has (is taking)

    Prosthetic valve

    Pacemaker (p. 134)

    Anticoagulants (p. 148)

Explain need to avoid persons with infections, especially upper respiratory infections

Discuss symptoms of wound infection to report to physician

    Chest discomfort

    Elevated temperature

    Rapid, irregular pulse

    Chills

    Anorexia

    Redness

    Pain

    Swelling

    Drainage

Explain care of incision

Discuss importance of ongoing care

Discuss importance of contacting spiritual advisor or social worker as necessary

Valve replacement

Provide instruction regarding anticoagulation therapy

    Mechanical valves: life-long therapy

    Heterografts: 3 to 6 months as ordered

Explain importance of reporting to physicians signs and symptoms of endocarditis

    Elevated temperature

    Chills, diaphoresis

    Anorexia

Discuss importance of reporting to physician any event that may predispose to bacteremia

    Dental and gum manipulation

    Genitourinary procedures

    Gynecologic procedures (D & C)

    Childbirth

    Skin boils, infective acne

Discuss importance of notifying all physicians, dentists, urologists, and obstetricians of valve replacement before any treatments

Discuss need to maintain good oral hygiene

    Daily care

    Regular visits to dentist

    NOTE: Patient should wait 6 weeks after surgery before seeing a dentist

Explain significance of prophylactic antibiotic therapy before procedures that predispose to bacteremia

Expected outcome/evaluation

Patient verbalizes understanding of clinical status and demonstrates skills and understanding of home health management

CARDIAC TRANSPLANTATION

Assessment

Observations/findings

Rejection

Mild to moderate: usually no clinical symptoms

Severe: weakness, fatigue, malaise, anorexia, nausea and vomiting, decreased urine output, weight gain, peripheral edema, distended neck veins, increased jugular pulsations, decreased perfusion, cool pale skin, diminished pulses, diaphoresis, confusion, restlessness, pulmonary venous congestion, DOE, cough, tachycardia

S_3, S_4

Shock state

Cardiac arrest

Potential complications

Infection: cytomegalovirus (CMV)

Obstructive coronary atheroscleroses

Laboratory/diagnostic studies

ECG: atrial dysrhythmia (e.g., PAC, atrial fibrillation)

NOTE: With cyclosporine, these ECG changes may not be seen

Chest x-ray examination: increased C-T ratio (cardiomegaly)

Echocardiogram: thickening of LV, decreased LV function, contractility

Endomyocardial biopsy (EMB)

Lymphocytes (findings vary with degree of rejection)

Mild, occasional WBCs

Moderate: myocyte necrosis

Severe: perivascular infiltration of lymphocytes, interstitial edema, myocyte, necrosis

Increased CPK-MB, SGOT, LDH

Medical Management

NOTE: Postoperative care is similar to that for any patient who has had cardiac surgery (p. 108)

Strict reverse isolation

EMB: 1 week for 1 month, progressing to twice a week for 2 months

Diet: low saturated fat, cholesterol, sodium restriction (2g)

Medications

Cyclosporine (Sandimmune)

Azathioprine (Imuran)

Antithymocyte globulin (ATG)

Orthoclone (OKT$_3$, Ortho)

Corticosteroids

Prednisone

Methylprednisone (Medrol, Depo-Medrol, Solu-Medrol)

Antihistamines

Acetaminophen

Nursing diagnoses/interventions/evaluation

■ **NDX:** Potential for injury (rejection) related to noncompliance with prescribed medical regimen

Assess and evaluate patient for understanding of prescribed lifelong therapy

Encourage discussion regarding anticipated changes in lifestyle that may have a positive or negative effect

Ensure that patient is aware that skipping cyclosporine will result in rejection

Review prescribed medical treatment and drug therapy

Anticipate and allow questions regarding prescribed therapy

Expected outcome/evaluation

Patient demonstrates no signs of rejection;

No new change(s) in EMB results

No clinical signs of rejection

■ **NDX:** Potential for infection related to immunosuppressive drug therapies

Assess and monitor for signs of infection

Take temperature every 4 hours

Obtain cultures as indicated: sputum, throat, urine, any suspicious drainage in wounds

Obtain and evaluate CBC; chest x-ray examination as indicated (NOTE: laboratory values may be altered if steroids are taken)

Minimize or avoid use of invasive lines and/or procedures: IVs, indwelling catheters

Change IV tubing, bags, and dressings each day using strict aseptic techniques

Avoid placing patient in room with another patient who is at risk for infection

Institute reverse isolation for staff and visitors according to institutional protocol

Minimize number of visitors; restrict visitors with signs of infections, e.g., colds, herpes simplex

Expected outcome/evaluation

Patient demonstrates no signs of infection

Baseline temperature maintained

CBC, urinalysis, cultures within normal limits

■ **NDX:** Knowledge deficit related to lack of information about self-care management

Discuss and review signs and symptoms of rejection

Emphasize importance of keeping scheduled EMB appointments

Discuss lifelong need to take medications and need to take them exactly as prescribed; caution patient *never to stop* taking cyclosporine and to notify physician if dose is skipped

Review signs and symptoms of infection: elevation of baseline temperature, early signs of sore throat, cold, flu

Discuss need to reduce risks of infection by avoiding individuals with infections or contagious diseases, avoiding large crowds

Discuss importance of lifelong follow-up: clinic visits, EMB appointments, and periodic stress test

Discuss activity allowances and limitations; instruct patient to check with physician before engaging in strenuous or competitive activities or sports

Discuss importance of daily weighing and reporting of more than 2 pounds weight gain in 24 hours

Expected outcome/evaluation

Patient's knowledge level is increased

Patient verbalizes understanding of postoperative care; need for continuous follow-up, allowances and limitations, medications, and signs to report to physician

Additional nursing diagnoses to consider

Potential decreased cardiac output related to severe rejection

POSTCARDIAC INJURY SYNDROME

A group of signs and symptoms that occur after injury to the myocardium or pericardial cavity, which are thought to be due to an immune response or hypersensitivity reaction to pericardial injury

postcardiotomy syndrome After cardiac surgery (usually 7 to 10 days after surgery)

postmyocardial infarction syndrome (Dressler's syndrome) A late-appearing autoimmune response to myocardial necrosis; symptoms usually appear 3 to 6 weeks after MI

Assessment
Observations/findings

Elevated temperature
Diaphoresis
Chest discomfort or pain
Pericardial friction rub
Dyspnea
Malaise
Arthralgias
Anxiety
   Worry
   Fear of consequences

Laboratory/diagnostic studies

Leukocytosis
Increased ESR

Chest x-ray examination: pleural effusions
Echocardiogram: pericardial effusion

Potential complications

Pericarditis
Cardiac tamponade

Medical Management

Medications
   Analgesics
   Antipyretics
   Antiinflammatory agents

Nursing diagnoses/interventions/evaluation

■ **NDX:**   Chest-pain–related pericardial irritation

Assess quality of chest pain
Encourage bed rest; position patient for comfort
   Elevate head of bed 45 degrees
   Provide padded overbed table
Auscultate heart sounds q6h to 8h
Administer medications as ordered
   Analgesics
   Antiinflammatory agents
   Antipyretics

Expected outcome/evaluation

Patient verbalizes absence of chest pain
Activity level returns to normal

■ **NDX:**   Anxiety related to perceived threat to health status

Explain that syndrome commonly occurs after trauma or injury to heart and pericardial cavity and may clear up without specific treatment
Discuss symptoms to report to physician
   Elevated temperature
   Chest pain
   Chills, diaphoresis
   Difficult respirations
Explain need to avoid fatigue; to alternate periods of activity with rest
Discuss name of medication, dosage, times of administration, purpose, and side effects

Expected outcome/evaluation

Patient demonstrates reduced level of anxiety
   Verbalizes insight into causes of symptoms and appropriate actions to take for signs and symptoms
   Appears calm

CARDIAC REHABILITATION

Physical and psychologic restoration of the patient with heart disease to an enjoyable and productive life as ef-

ficiently as possible; suggested for patients with angina, cardiomyopathy, pacemakers, and congenital heart disease and for patients recovering from myocardial infarction, valve surgery, and coronary artery bypass surgery*

Inpatient Program

Assessment

Observations/findings

CRITERIA FOR TERMINATING EXERCISE

Symptoms during activity and/or 30 min after activity or exercise session
Severe dyspnea
Chest pain
Vertigo
Diaphoresis
Fatigue

---

*Definition from *Guidelines for cardiac rehabilitation centers,* June 1985, copyright the American Heart Association Greater Los Angeles Affiliate.

Leg claudication
Disorientation or confusion
Palpitations
Heart rate
   Increase greater than 20 to 25 beats/min during activity or exercise
   Appearance of irregular rhythm
On telemetry: during exercise and rest periods
   ST elevation of 3 mm or more
   ST segment depression of 2 mm
   Multiple premature ventricular contractions (PVCs)

Activity progression program

Follow physician's orders for progressive activity program
Initiate program using a predeveloped in-hospital exercise program (Table 2-7)
Assess patient's progress on a daily basis and plan activity levels for the day (done by rehabilitation team and/or charge nurse and physician)
Increase activity levels gradually until discharge date

TABLE 2-7. Cardiac Rehabilitation Program: Inpatient Activity (Myocardial Infarction)*

Level	Self-care activities	Position	Exercises	Repetitions	Education
Level I (1 to 1.5 MET†)	1. Absolute bed rest, complete bed bath 2. Begin feeding self while sitting with head of bed elevated to 45 degrees and arms supported 3. Turn self	1. Supine *Advance to:* Supine 2. Supine	a. Passive ROM: all extremities (excluding shoulders in acute MI) b. Active exercises: all extremities except shoulders as tolerated Deep breathing exercises: all levels	5 times 3 times	
Level II (1.5 to 2.5 MET [except bedside commode])	4. Bed rest 5. Feed self, wash face and hands, brush teeth, and shave in bed 6. Bedside commode (3 MET) 7. Up in chair 20-30 minutes bid 8. Light recreational activity such as reading, writing	3. Supine	Active plantar and dorsiflexion ankle exercises qid		
Level III (1.5 to 3 MET)	9. In bed, patient assists with self-bath (not legs or back) 10. Patient stands and vital signs are taken 11. May walk to bathroom with help 12. Walk to chair and sit 15 to 30 minutes tid	4. Supine Sitting	a. Advance active exercises to include neck rotation and shoulder flexion to 90 degrees as tolerated b. Active exercises: all limbs including shoulder flexion to 180 degrees c. Knee extension and hip flexion	5 times 5 times 3 times	Begin education a. Energy conservation b. Body mechanics c. Concepts of heart anatomy and physiology

Adapted from *Guidelines for cardiac rehabilitation centers,* June 1985, copyright the American Heart Association Greater Los Angeles Affiliate.
*Recommended levels and times are for average patients and must be individualized.
†MET: metabolic equivalent: the amount of oxygen consumed per kilogram of body weight per minute at rest. Approximately 3.5 cc kg/min.

Continued.

TABLE 2-7. Cardiac Rehabilitation Program: Inpatient Activity (Myocardial Infarction)—cont'd

Level	Self-care activities	Position	Exercises	Repetitions	Education
Level III—cont'd		*Advance to:*			
		5. Supine	a. Active exercises: all extremities	7 times	
		Sitting	b. Knee extension and hip flexion	7 times	
		Sitting	c. Shoulder flexion to 90 degrees	7 times	

Level IV (3 MET)	13. Same as 9
	14. Begin dressing self (gown and pajamas)
	15. If vital signs stable, see 10, walk to bathroom for toilet use only
	16. Sit in chair 2 to 3 times a day 30 to 60 min with assistance
		6. Supine
		Sitting
		7. Supine
			a. Exercise 5a
			b. Exercise 5b
			Instruct patient to perform independent exercise 3 times a day (patient to take own pulse)
				7 times
				7 times
				5 times
					d. Begin instruction in self heart rate measurement
					e. Discuss inpatient activity: importance of pacing, rest, relaxation
					f. Dietary assessment and referral if appropriate
					g. Begin discussion of:
					  Signs and symptoms
					  Risk factors
					  Medication
					  Warning signs
					  Sexual counseling
					  Activity progress

Level V	17. Sponge bathe self, sitting in bathroom (nurse bathes back) 18. Up in room and chair ad lib 19. Ambulate in hall 5 to 10 min with telemetry bid		Active exercises 5a, b, c; walk slow pace one half length of corridor (50 feet) with telemetry		
Level VI (3 to 4 MET)	10. Sit-down shower 21. Wash hair while seated 22. Shave, apply makeup in sitting position 23. Sit for meals 24. Full bathroom privileges 25. Up and about in room 26. Ambulate in hall 5 to 10 min bid with telemetry	8. Supine 9. Sitting 10. Walk 11. Ascend 12.	Active exercise 5a Active exercise 5b Increase distance walked, as tolerated, using moderate pace Three to six stair steps as tolerated May transport to cardiac rehabilitation center for low-level activity or test	5 to 7 times 7 times	Complete home instruction a. Diet b. Medications c. Activity allowances and limitations
Level VII (4 to 5 MET)	27. Same as level VI with addition of walking in hall 150 feet, advancing as tolerated 28. Evaluate any special requirements for home activities	13.	Continue stairs and ambulation as tolerated		
Level VIII	29. Same as level VI and VII, advancing in frequency, distance, and time	14.	Establish progressive home activity program		

Avoid exercises
  After meals; allow 1 hr
  In the presence of dysrrhythmias
  In the presence of CHF
Begin exercise program while patient is on telemetry
Record and report any signs or symptoms of shortness of
  breath, fatigue, or nausea if they occur during or up to
  24 hr after exercise
Obtain the following baseline information before activity
  On telemetry
    ECG rhythm strip, noting rate and rhythm
    Resting BP, P, and R, noting rate, rhythm, and qual-
      ity
    Atrioventricular (AV) block
    Paroxysmal atrial tachycardia
  BP
    Drop of 15 to 20 mm Hg when patient stands
    Decrease in pulse pressure
    Increase in systolic-diastolic pressures: greater than
      20 mm Hg

Medical Management

Prescription for inclusion to program
Prescription for activity order

Interventions

MI
  Maintain bed rest for first 3 to 4 days except for use of
    bedside commode
  Progress to chair rest
  Avoid prolonged bed rest
CABG
  Maintain bed rest for first 1 to 2 days postoperatively
    or as ordered by physician
  Start activity levels within 24 hr or as ordered by phy-
    sician
  Off telemetry obtain resting BP, P, and R, noting rate,
    rhythm, and quality
Assist patient with performing activity
Obtain peak exercise heart rate
Obtain the following information during and 2 min after
  exercise
  On telemetry
    ECG rhythm strip toward end of activity, noting rate,
      rhythm, and ST segment changes or arrhythmias
    Postexercise heart rate
  Off telemetry
    BP and heart rate at 1 and 2 min intervals at end of
      exercise and at any signs of fatigue, pain, or short-
      ness of breath
Observe and report patient's tolerance

Patient Teaching/Discharge Outcome

Ensure that patient and/or significant other knows and
  understands

Normal function of the heart
Nature and causes of coronary heart disease
Importance of identifying risk factors and need to mod-
  ify or eliminate personal risk factors
  Family history of heart disease
  Patient history of heart disease
  Diabetes
  High blood pressure
  Overweight
  High cholesterol and/or triglyceride level
  Smoking
  Sedentary job and/or lifestyle
  Stressful lifestyle
Dietary restrictions and limitations
Importance of maintaining weight control
Importance of verbalizing any questions and feelings
  regarding presence of heart disease
Importance of verbalizing any feelings of anxiety and
  fear regarding sexual impotency, return to work, and
  death
Warning signs and symptoms of overexercising to report
  to physician
  Excessive fatigue
  Chest discomfort
  Muscle pain
  Dizziness
  Shortness of breath
  Palpitations
Physician's explanation of prescribed exercise program,
  allowances, and limitations
Need to avoid isometric (static) activities and/or ex-
  ercises (e.g., pushing heavy objects, doing pushups,
  or carrying heavy objects)
Importance of taking and recording heart rate before and
  after exercise, noting rate and rhythm
Importance of reporting heart rate increase of greater than
  20 to 25 beats/min
Recommended limitations and allowances for first 2 weeks
  after discharge
  Avoid heavy lifting and pushing
  Refrain from extensive housework and gardening
  Avoid sitting in same position for longer than 2 hr
  Plan regular rest periods for at least twice a day
  Avoid vigorous arm and shoulder exercises, especially
    those that require arms to be held above shoulders
    (e.g., washing windows or painting house)
  Space activities, alternating activity with rest period
  Avoid exercising at the following times
    After meals; wait 1 hr
    When feeling very tired
    When suffering from a cold or other illness
  Stop activity at onset of warning signs and rest
Importance of avoiding sexual activity for at least 2 weeks
  (check with physician when feasible to resume; once
  resumed, avoid after eating heavy meals, drinking al-

coholic beverages in excess, or becoming emotionally stressed)

Need to avoid travel by car, bus, airplane, or train without first checking with physician

That all walking and exercise activities must be preceded by warm-up exercises (i.e., stretching and knee bends)

Prescribed Exercise Program

INITIAL POSTDISCHARGE ACTIVITIES FOR CARDIOVASCULAR RECONDITIONING

Continue predischarge activities; actively exercise all extremities, including shoulder flexion and knee extension

Distance walking

Week after discharge	Total distance (mile)	Time (min)
1	0.25	8 to 10
2	0.25	5
3	0.5	15
4	1.0	30

Adjust speed and time to maintain heart rate at less than 100 beats/min

Record all exercise sessions, noting distance, time, and resting and peak heart rates (see chart below)

Exercise record: Target heart rate: __ beats/min

Date	Resting heart rate	Distance	Time	Peak heart rate	Comment
1-3-91	80	¼ mile	5 min	100	No complaints

Follow all exercise sessions with a cooling down period

CARDIOVASCULAR RECONDITIONING PROGRAM

Ordered approximately 6 to 8 weeks after discharge (done by physician)

Follow prescription for exercise determined by treadmill stress test before start of program

ECG RHYTHMS

Rhythms of Sinus Origin

Rhythms originating in the sinus (sinoatrial; SA) node (Located in the right atrium near the opening of the superior vena cava, the sinus node functions as the normal pacemaker of the heart)

Assessment

General complaints
  Palpitations

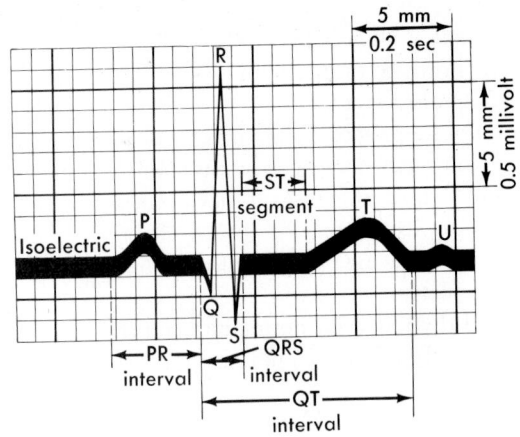

FIGURE 2-14. Normal ECG complex.

Dizziness
Lightheadedness
Chest pain
Syncope
Skin
  Pallor
  Diaphoresis
Heart rate
  Normal with ectopy
  Tachycardia
  Bradycardia
Heart rhythm
  Normal or irregular
Hypotension

Laboratory/diagnostic studies

12-lead ECG
24-hour ambulatory ECG
Electrophysiologic (EP) studies
Signal average (SA) electrocardiogram

NORMAL SINUS RHYTHM (Figure 2-16)
Assessment
Observations/findings

Rhythm: regular
Rate: 60 to 100 beats/min
P wave: normal configuration, one before each QRS
PR interval: 0.12 to 0.20 sec
QRS complex: 0.06 to 0.10 sec

Medical Management

None indicated

SINUS BRADYCARDIA (Figure 2-17)

A sinus rhythm of less than 60 beats/min; etiology—may be normal or occur in response to drugs or increased vagal tone

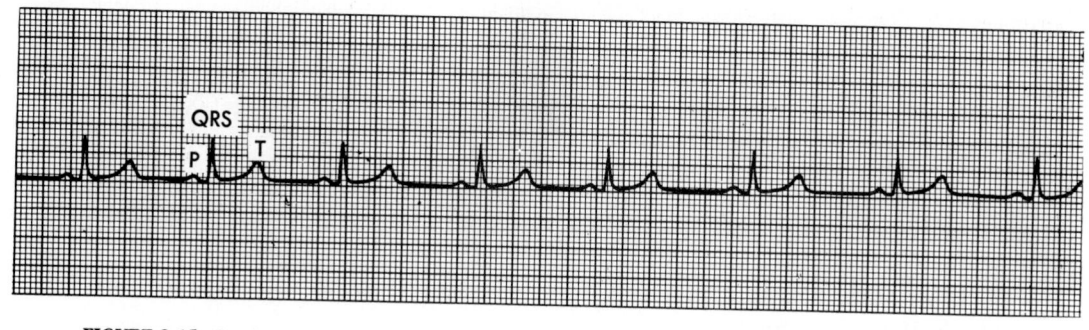

FIGURE 2-15. Cardiac cycle. Basic cardiac cycle (P = QRS = T). (From Goldberger AL, Goldberger E: *Clinical electrocardiology: a simplified approach*, ed 4, St Louis, 1990, Mosby–Year Book.)

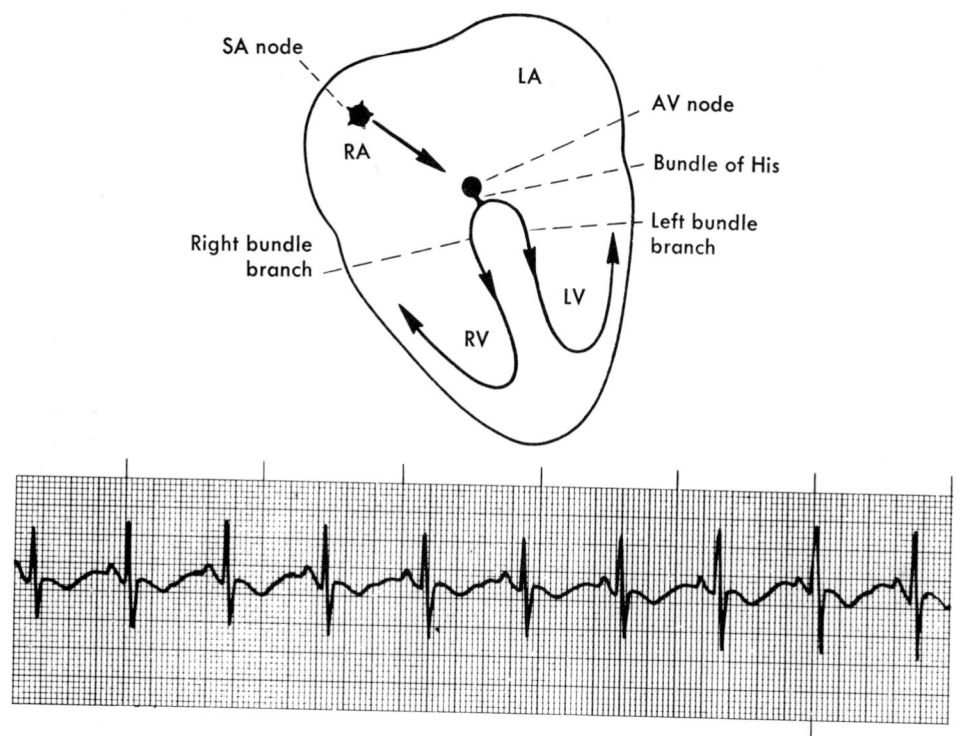

FIGURE 2-16. Normal sinus rhythm. (From Andreoli KG et al: *Comprehensive cardiac care*, ed 6, St Louis, 1987, CV Mosby.)

TABLE 2-8. Meaning and Significance of ECG Intervals*

Description	Duration	Significance of disturbance
PR interval: from beginning of P wave to beginning of QRS complex; represents time taken for impulse to spread through the atria, AV node, His bundle, bundle branches, and Purkinje fibers, to a point immediately preceding ventricular activation	0.12 to 0.20 sec	Disturbance in conduction, usually in AV node, His bundle, or bundle branches, but can be in atria as well
QRS interval: from beginning to end of QRS complex; represents time taken for a depolarization of both ventricles	0.06 to 0.10 sec	Disturbance in conduction in bundle branches and/or in ventricles
QT interval: from beginning of QRS to end of T wave; represents time taken for entire electrical depolarization and repolarization of the ventricles	0.36 to 0.44 sec	Disturbances usually affecting repolarization more than depolarization, such as drug effects, electrolyte disturbances, and rate changes

From Andreoli K et al: *Comprehensive cardiac care*, ed 6, St Louis, 1987, CV Mosby.
*Heart rate influences the duration of these intervals, especially that of PR and QT.

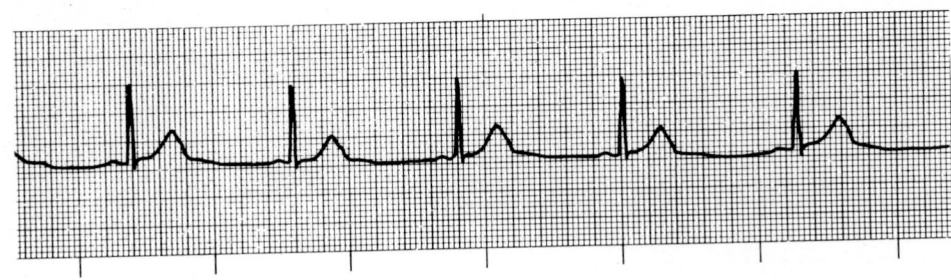

FIGURE 2-17. Sinus bradycardia. (From Andreoli K et al: *Comprehensive cardiac care,* ed 6, St Louis, 1987, CV Mosby.)

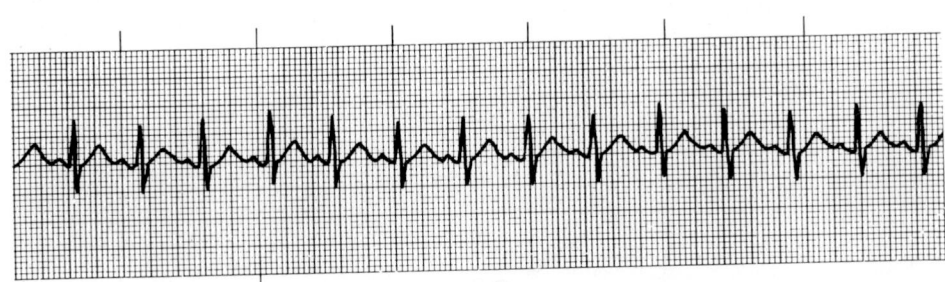

FIGURE 2-18. Sinus tachycardia. (From Andreoli K et al: *Comprehensive cardiac care,* ed 6, St Louis, 1987, CV Mosby.)

Assessment
Observations/findings

Faintness
Dizziness
Syncope
Rhythm: regular
Rate: below 60 beats/min
P wave: normal configuration, one before each QRS
   PR interval: 0.12 to 0.20 sec
   QRS complex: 0.06 to 0.10 sec

Medical Management

None indicated unless patient is symptomatic
Medications
   Atropine
   Isoproterenol
   Pacing: atrial, ventricular

Interventions

Check BP and apical pulse q4h and prn
Monitor cardiac activity; check rhythm strips q6h to 8h
  and prn
Administer oxygen therapy as ordered

Patient Teaching

Ensure that patient and/or significant other knows and
  understands
   How to take radial pulse
   Pacemaker insertion (p. 134), if indicated

SINUS TACHYCARDIA (Figure 2-18)

*A sinus rhythm of greater than 100 beats/min; causes—
drugs, exercise, emotions, fever, increased sympathetic
stimulation*

Assessment
Observations/findings

Fatigue
Shortness of breath
Rhythm: regular
Rate: 100 to 160 beats/min
P wave: normal configuration, one before each QRS
PR interval: 0.12 to 0.20 sec
QRS complex: 0.06 to 0.10 sec

Medical Management

Treatment of underlying factors
Carotid sinus massage

Interventions

Administer medications as ordered
Check BP, R, and apical pulse q4h to 6h and prn
Administer oxygen therapy as ordered
Initiate measures to decrease work of heart: rest, avoidance
  of caffeine intake

SINUS DYSRHYTHMIA (Figure 2-19)

*An irregular sinus rhythm; is normally found in children
and young adults; causes—respiratory variation*

II

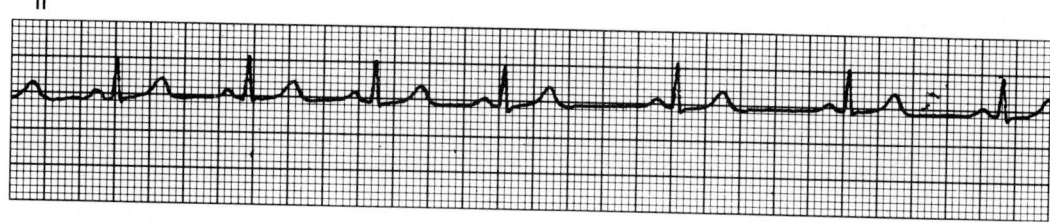

FIGURE 2-19. Sinus dysrhythmia. (From Conover MB: *Exercises in diagnosing ECG tracings,* ed 3, St Louis, 1984, CV Mosby.)

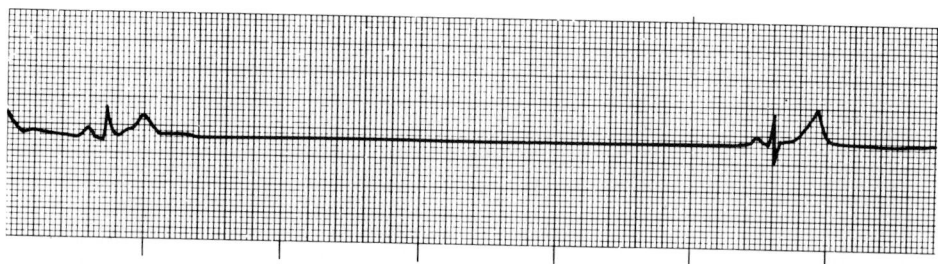

FIGURE 2-20. Sinus arrest. (From Andreoli K et al: *Comprehensive cardiac care,* ed 6, St Louis, 1987, CV Mosby.)

Assessment
Observations/findings

Rhythm: irregular
Rate: 60 to 90 beats/min; may increase with inspiration and decrease with expiration
P wave: normal configuration, one before each QRS complex
PR interval: 0.12 to 0.20 sec
QRS complex: 0.06 to 0.10 sec

Medical Management

None indicated

SINUS ARREST (Figure 2-20)

A rhythm in which a sinus impulse is not generated; causes—drugs, coronary artery disease, increased vagal tone, SA node disease

Assessment
Observations/findings

Dizziness
Syncope
Rhythm: irregular during periods of arrest
Rate: variable
P wave: absent during periods of arrest
PR interval: absent during periods of arrest
QRS complex: absent during periods of arrest

Potential complications

Ventricular standstill

Medical Management

Medications: atropine
Cardiac pacing
Parenteral fluids
Cardiopulmonary resuscitation (CPR)

Interventions

Monitor cardiac activity; check rhythm strips q4h to 6h and prn
Maintain bed rest as indicated
Check BP, R, and apical pulse q4h to 6h and prn
Administer oxygen therapy as indicated

Rhythms of Atrial Origin

Supraventricular or atrial rhythms that originate outside the SA node and above the bundle of His

PREMATURE ATRIAL CONTRACTIONS (PACs, APCs)
(Figures 2-21 and 2-22)

premature atrial contractions *Ectopic beats generated outside the SA node; causes—anxiety, ingestion of tobacco or caffeine, electrolyte imbalance, hypoxia, drug toxicity*

Assessment
Observations/findings

Palpitations: skipped beats
Anxiety
Dizziness
Rhythm: irregular in presence of PACs

II

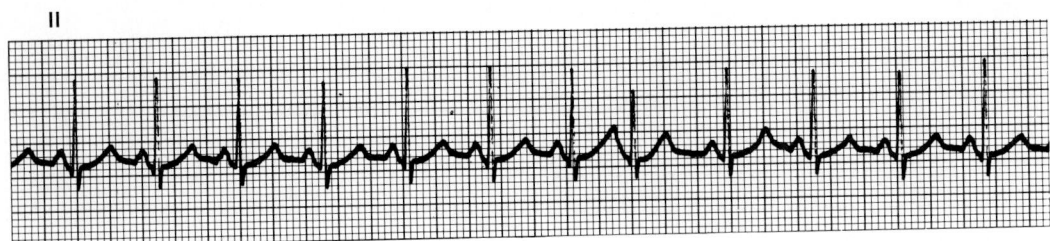

FIGURE 2-21. Premature atrial contraction. (From Conover MB: *Exercises in diagnosing ECG tracings,* ed 3, St Louis, 1984, CV Mosby.)

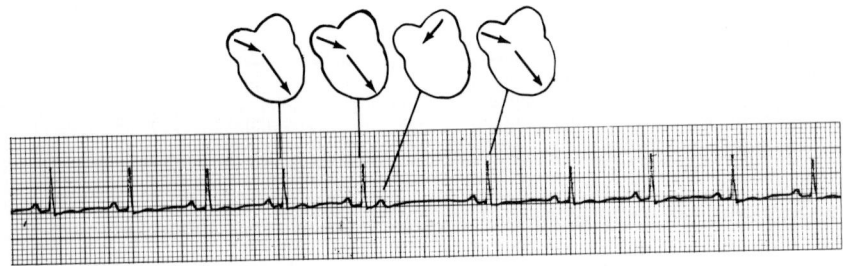

FIGURE 2-22. Nonconducted premature atrial contraction (PAC). (From Conover MB: *Understanding electrocardiography: arrhythmias and the 12-lead ECG,* ed 4, St Louis, 1984, CV Mosby.)

II

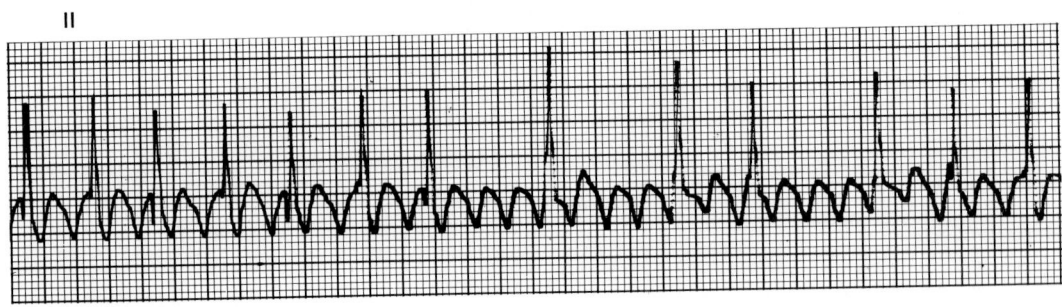

FIGURE 2-23. Atrial flutter. (From Conover MB: *Exercises in diagnosing ECG tracings.* ed 3, St Louis, 1984, CV Mosby.)

Rate: variable, may be normal or irregular in presence of ectopic beats

P wave: premature P wave is distorted; may be inverted or fused on preceding T wave

PR interval: may be prolonged

QRS complex: may be normal or may show abnormal conduction in ectopic beat; no QRS will follow if P wave is blocked

Potential complications

Atrial fibrillation

Laboratory/diagnostic studies

Holter monitor examination

Medical Management

Treatment of underlying disease; none indicated for occasional PACs

Medications: antiarrhythmics

Interventions

Monitor cardiac activity; check rhythm strips 4qh to 6h and prn

Check BP, R, and apical pulse q6h to 8h

Restrict caffeine and nicotine as ordered

ATRIAL FLUTTER (Figure 2-23)

A rapid, regular ectopic atrial rhythm with characteristic "flutter" waves; causes—most forms of cardiac disease

V₁

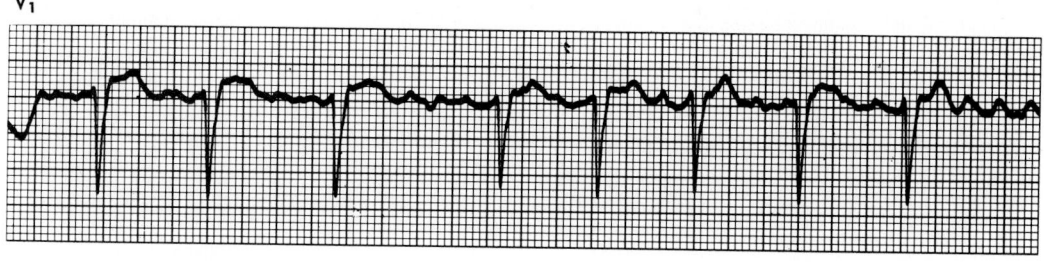

FIGURE 2-24. Atrial fibrillation. (From Conover MB: *Exercises in diagnosing ECG tracings,* ed 3, St Louis, 1984, CV Mosby.)

Assessment

Observations/findings

Tachycardia
Tachypnea
Palpitations
Shortness of breath
Rhythm
  Atrial: regular
  Ventricular: may be regular or irregular
  Emboli
Rate
  Atrial: 250 to 350 beats/min
  Ventricular: 100 to 150 beats/min
  PR interval: unmeasurable
  P wave: absent; rhythm shows F waves in sawtooth
    shape
  QRS complex: usually normal

Potential complications

Emboli
CHF
Shock

Medical Management

Treatment of underlying disease
Cardioversion
Carotid massage
Medications
  Antiarrhythmics
  Digitalis preparations
Atrial pacing
12-lead ECG

Interventions

Monitor cardiac activity; check rhythm strips q4h to 6h
  and prn
Check BP, R, and apical pulse q2h to 4h
Maintain bed rest as indicated
Administer oxygen therapy as ordered

ATRIAL FIBRILLATION (Figure 2-24)

*A rapid, irregular, ectopic atrial rhythm with characteristic "fibrillatory" activity; causes—coronary artery dis-*ease (CAD), valvular heart disease, hypertension, increased left atrial size in the elderly*

Assessment

Observations/findings

Palpitations
Faintness
Tachycardia
Irregular pulse
Pulse deficit (apical and radial pulses)
Chest discomfort
Nausea
Rhythm: irregular
Rate
  Atrial: 350 beats/min
  Ventricular: 90 to 100 beats/min
PR interval: unmeasurable
P wave: absent; rhythm shows "f" waves that are seen as
  undulations
QRS complex: usually normal

Potential complications

Mural thrombi
CHF
Shock

Medical Management

Medications: antiarrhythmics
Cardioversion
12-lead ECG

Interventions

Monitor cardiac activity; check rhythm strips 4qh to 8 h
  and prn
Check BP, R, and apical pulse q4h to 6h and prn
Administer oxygen therapy as ordered

SUPRAVENTRICULAR TACHYCARDIA (SVT) (Figure 2-25)

*An ectopic atrial rhythm that is regular and may start
  and stop abruptly, originating above AV node;
  causes—precipitated by sympathetic stimulation (e.g.,
  emotion, caffeine, tobacco, fatigue, excessive alcohol
  intake)*

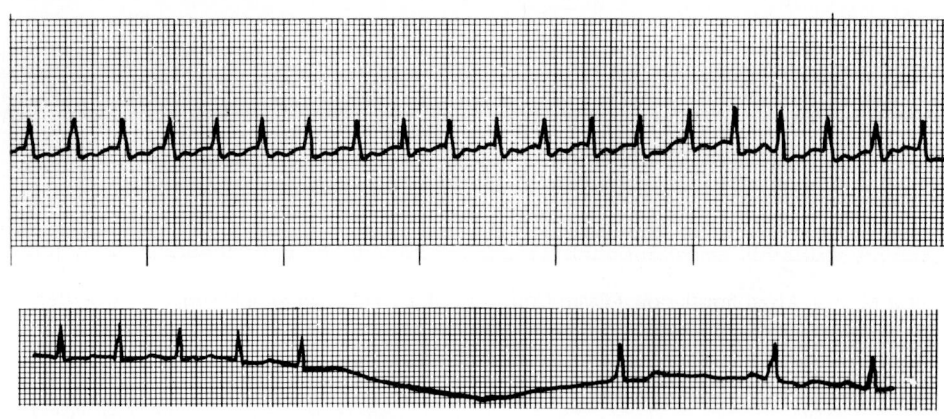

FIGURE 2-25. Supraventricular tachycardia (SVT) (From Andreoli KG et al: *Comprehensive cardiac care,* ed 6, St Louis, 1987, CV Mosby.)

Assessment
Observations/findings

Palpitations
Shortness of breath
Lightheadedness
Hypokalemia
Chest pain or discomfort
Abdominal discomfort
Tachycardia of short or prolonged duration
Rhythm: usually regular
Rate: 150 to 250 beats/min
P wave: normal or buried in QRS or T wave; may not be visible
PR interval: usually normal
QRS complex: usually normal

Laboratory/diagnostic studies

Holter monitor examination

Potential complications

CHF
Shock

Medical Management

Carotid massage
Medications
    Antiarrhythmics
    Vagotonic preparations
Potassium replacement as indicated
Cardioversion
Atrial or ventricular pacing
12-lead ECG
Treat underlying etiology

Interventions

Monitor cardiac activity; check rhythm strips q4h to 6h and prn
Administer oxygen therapy as ordered

Check BP, R, and apical pulse q2h to 4h
Maintain bed rest as indicated
Check serum potassium level if patient is taking digitalis preparations
Maintain quiet environment

Rhythms of Ventricular Origin

Rhythms that occur as either escape or reentry (overdrive) rhythms arising within the ventricles

PREMATURE VENTRICULAR CONTRACTIONS (PVCs)
(Figures 2-26 and 2-27)

Premature beats arising in the ventricles below the bundle of His; may be a forerunner of ventricular tachycardia and ventricular fibrillation; causes—increased sympathetic stimulation (e.g., caffeine, tobacco, emotion), most forms of heart disease, electrolyte imbalance

Assessment
Observations/findings

Palpitations
Precordial pain
Dizziness
Faintness
Momentary loss of consciousness
Rhythm: irregular
Rate
    Atrial: normal
    Ventricular: may be normal or rapid
P wave: does not precede premature beat; premature beat is usually followed by complete compensatory pause
PR interval: unmeasurable
QRS complex: premature beat is wide and bizarre in appearance, lasting longer than 0.12 sec

Laboratory/diagnostic studies

12-lead ECG
Holter monitor examination

II

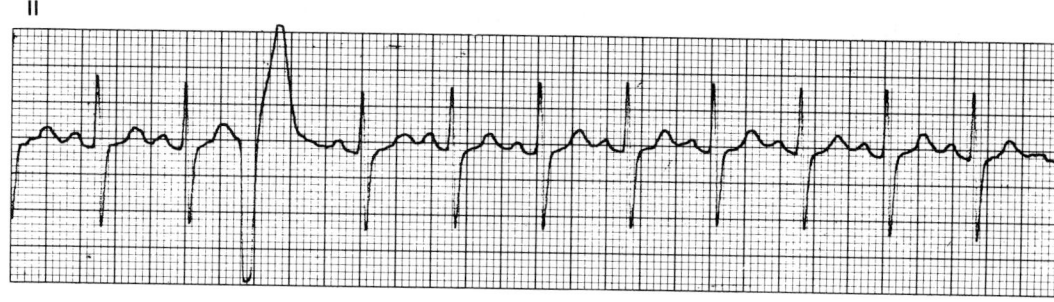

FIGURE 2-26. Premature ventricular contraction (PVC). (From Conover MB: *Exercises in diagnosing ECG tracings,* ed 3, St Louis, 1984, CV Mosby.)

V₁

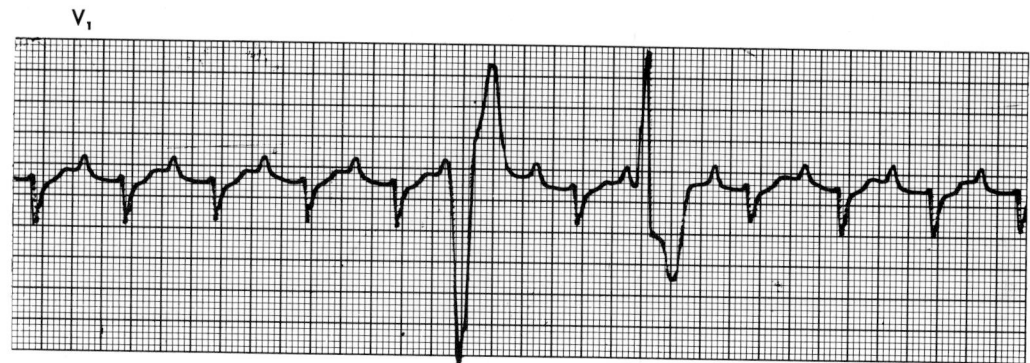

FIGURE 2-27. Multifocal premature ventricular contractions (PVCs). (From Conover MB: *Exercises in diagnosing ECG tracings,* ed 3, St Louis, 1984, CV Mosby.)

V₁

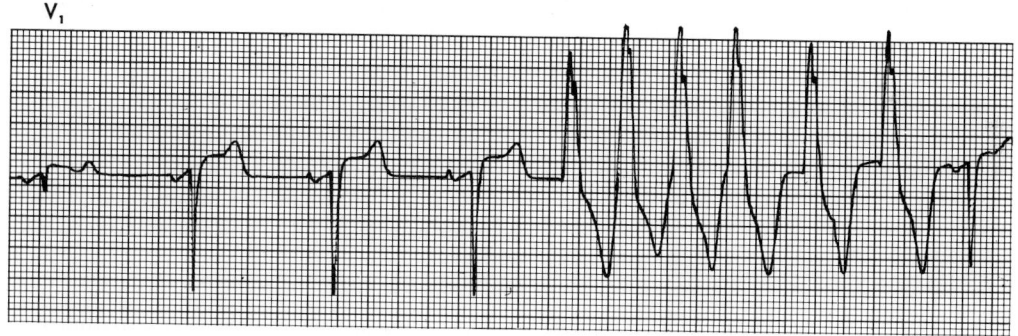

FIGURE 2-28. Ventricular tachycardia. (From Conover MB: *Exercises in diagnosing ECG tracings,* ed 3, St Louis, 1984, CV Mosby.)

Potential complications

Ventricular tachycardia
Ventricular fibrillation

Medical Management

Treatment of underlying disease
Medications: antiarrhythmics
12-lead ECGs for
   Multifocal PVCs
   R on T phenomenon
   Coupling or paired PVCs
   Six or more PVCs/min

Interventions

Monitor cardiac activity; check rhythm strips 4qh to 6h
   and prn; report if more than 6 PVCs/min or if they
   occur close to preceding T waves
Monitor BP, R, and apical pulse q4h to 6h and prn
Administer oxygen therapy
Restrict caffeine, nicotine, and hot and cold fluids

VENTRICULAR TACHYCARDIA (Figure 2-28)

Three or more consecutive PVCs; causes—ischemic heart disease, significant chronic heart disease, drug toxicity

Assessment
Observations/findings

Anxiety
Palpitations
Dizziness
Precordial discomfort
Cyanosis
Confusion
Syncope
Altered level of consciousness
Rhythm: usually regular
Rate: ventricular; 150 to 200 beats/min
P wave: absent; may be retrograde to atria
PR interval: unmeasurable
QRS complex: wide and bizarre in configuration, lasting more than 0.12 sec

Potential complications

Heart failure
Ventricular fibrillation

Medical Management

Antiarrhythmic agents

Interventions
Immediate care

Apply direct current (DC) countershock
Administer medications as ordered: lidocaine bolus and drip
Initiate CPR as indicated
Initiate parenteral fluids as ordered
Take 12-lead ECG as ordered
Monitor BP, R, and apical pulse q15min to 30min as indicated
Administer oxygen as indicated

Ongoing care

Monitor cardiac activity; check rhythm strips q4h to 6h and prn
Monitor BP, R, and apical pulse q2h to 4h and prn, decreasing frequency as condition stabilizes

Administer medications as ordered
    Antiarrhythmics
    Sedatives
Maintain bed rest as indicated

VENTRICULAR FIBRILLATION (Figure 2-29)

Disorganized electrical activity of ventricles, which leads to abrupt cessation of effective blood flow; causes—severe heart disease, drug toxicity

Assessment
Observations/findings

Anxiety
Palpitations
Dizziness
Cyanosis
Precordial pain
Nausea, vomiting
Shortness of breath
Syncope
Absence of pulse
Rhythm: irregular
Rate: >210 beats/min; no beat-to-beat count
P wave: not seen; absent atrial activity
QRS complex: wide undulations; wandering, irregular baseline

Interventions
Immediate care

Cough CPR if patient is awake and able to cough
Apply DC countershock
Administer CPR; usually indicated
Administer medications as ordered
Initiate parenteral fluids as ordered
Take 12-lead ECG as ordered
Administer oxygen with assisted ventilation as ordered
Monitor BP, R, and apical pulse q15min to 30min

Ongoing care

Monitor cardiac activity; check rhythm strips q1h to 2h, decreasing frequency as condition stabilizes

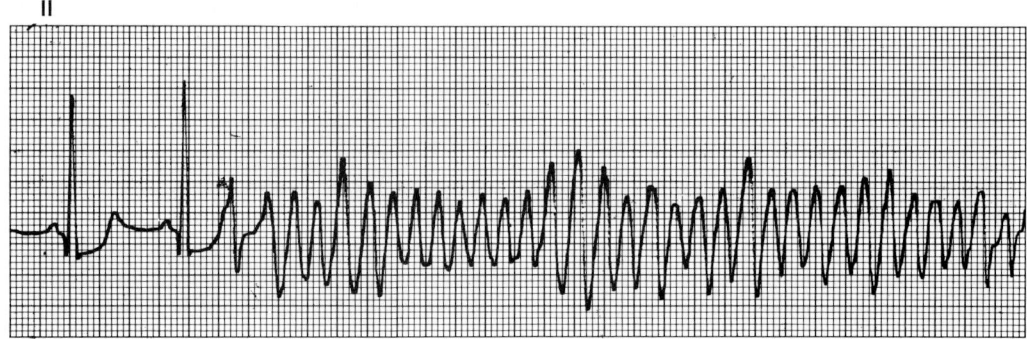

FIGURE 2-29. Ventricular fibrillation. (From Conover MB: *Exercises in diagnosing ECG tracings,* ed 3, St Louis, 1984, CV Mosby.)

Monitor BP, R, and apical pulse q1h to 2h and prn

Maintain bed rest as indicated

Keep defibrillator and emergency cart at bedside until condition stabilizes

TORSADES DE POINTES (POLYMORPHOUS VENTRICULAR TACHYCARDIA) (Figure 2-30)

Atypical ventricular tachycardia occurring in the setting of delayed repolarization (prolonged QT interval); causes—drug toxicity such as quinidine; electrolyte imbalance

Assessment

Observations/findings

Palpitations

Faintness

Syncope

Rhythm: regular or irregular

Rate: ventricular, 150 to 300 beats/min

PR interval: not measurable

QRS complex: wide and bizarre in configuration, lasting >0.12 sec; amplitude and direction of QRS complex will vary

QT interval during baseline rhythm: >0.46 sec or >33% of baseline

T wave during baseline: very broad and flat

Potential complications

Ventricular fibrillation

Sudden death

Medical Management

Correction of underlying cause if identifiable (e.g., drug toxicity; quinidine, procainamide, amiodarone)

Correction of electrolyte imbalance: hypokalemia, hypomagnesemia

Medications (avoid drugs that prolong QT intervals, e.g., quinidine, Norpace)

Overdrive pacing: rate set at 80 to 120 beats/min

Cardioversion

Left stellate ganglionectomy

Interventions

Monitor cardiac activity; check rhythm strips q2h to 4h and prn, decreasing frequency as condition stabilizes

Monitor BP, P, and apical pulse q4h to 6h and prn

Atrioventricular (AV) Block

A conduction disturbance involving the AV junction, which normally functions as a bridge between the atria and ventricles

FIRST-DEGREE AV BLOCK (Figure 2-31)

A consistent delay in impulse conduction throughout the AV node; causes—digoxin toxicity, ischemic heart disease, hyperkalemia

Assessment

Observations/findings

Rhythm: regular

Rate: 60 to 90 beats/min

P wave: normal configuration; one before each QRS

PR interval: prolonged, greater than 0.20 sec

QRS complex: 0.06 to 0.10 sec

Medical Management

Medications

    Atropine

    Isoproterenol

Interventions

Monitor cardiac activity; check rhythm strips q4h to 6h and prn

Check BP, R, and apical pulse q4h to 6h and prn

Discontinue use of digitalis preparation or quinidine as ordered

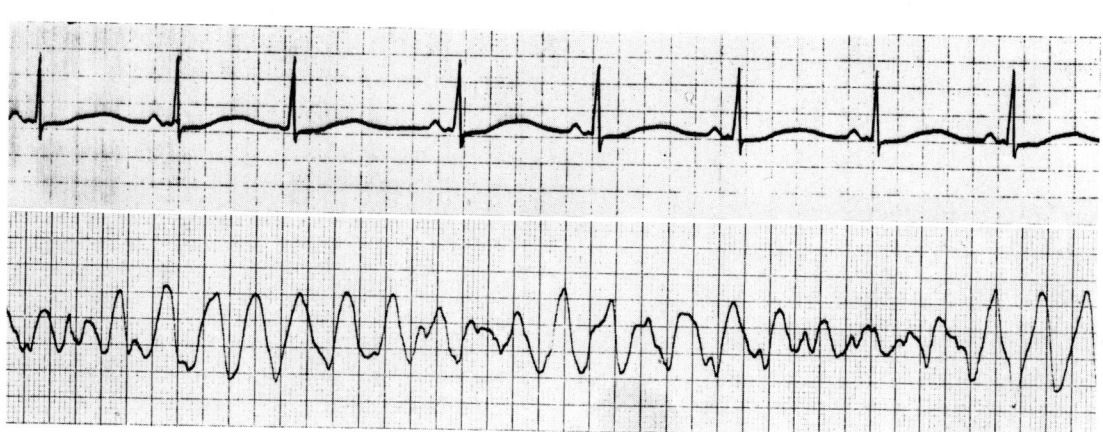

FIGURE 2-30. Torsades de pointes. Sinus rhythm. T waves are flat, and QT interval is prolonged. (Courtesy Dr Daniel H Schwartz. From Goldberger E: *Textbook of clinical cardiology,* St Louis, 1982, CV Mosby.)

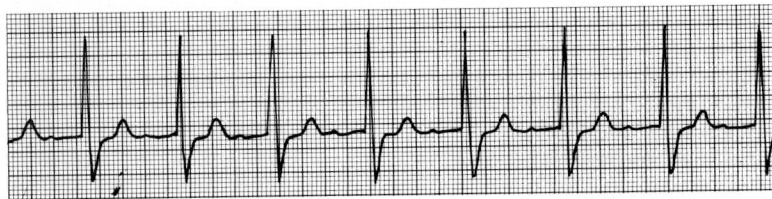

FIGURE 2-31. First-degree AV block. (From Conover MB: *Understanding electrocardiography: arrhythmias and the 12-lead ECG,* ed 4, St Louis, 1984, CV Mosby.)

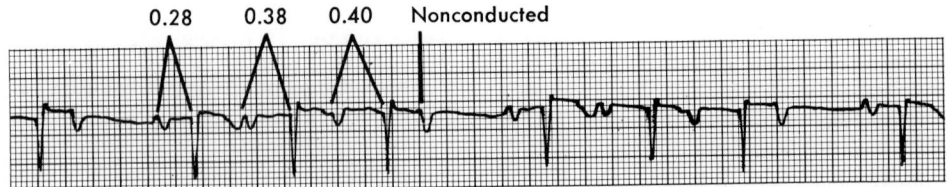

FIGURE 2-32. Second-degree AV block: Mobitz type I (Wenckebach phenomenon) with narrow QRS complex. (From Conover MB: *Understanding electrocardiography: arrhythmias and the 12-lead ECG,* ed 4, St Louis, 1984, CV Mosby.)

Check serum levels of digitalis preparation and potassium as indicated

Observe for changes in PR interval and measure

SECOND-DEGREE AV BLOCK

An AV conduction disturbance characterized by nonconducted P waves and classified as type I or type II; causes—digoxin toxicity, ischemic heart disease

Assessment
Observations/findings

Rhythm: regular
Rate
   Atrial: regular
   Ventricular: irregular
P wave: may show one or more nonconducted P waves
PR interval: progressive prolongation of PR interval until one impulse is completely blocked
QRS complex: 0.06 to 0.10 sec

Laboratory/diagnostic studies

Serum drug levels
His bundle recording

Potential complications

Angina
Heart failure
Complete AV block
Asystole

Medical Management

Medications
   Atropine
   Isoproterenol
Temporary cardiac pacing

Interventions

Monitor cardiac activity; check rhythm strips q2h to 4h
Monitor BP, R, and apical pulse q4h to 6h and prn

Mobitz Type I (Wenckebach Phenomenon)
(Figure 2-32)

Causes—digoxin toxicity, inferior wall myocardial infarction (MI), rheumatic fever

Assessment
Observations/findings

Rhythm
   Atrial: regular
   Ventricular: irregular
Rate
   Atrial: > ventricular
P wave: may have multiple P waves before each QRS
PR interval: becomes progressively prolonged (greater than 0.28 sec) until one P wave is blocked; cycle will then be repeated
QRS complex: 0.06 to 0.10 sec; RR interval will shorten until QRS complex is dropped

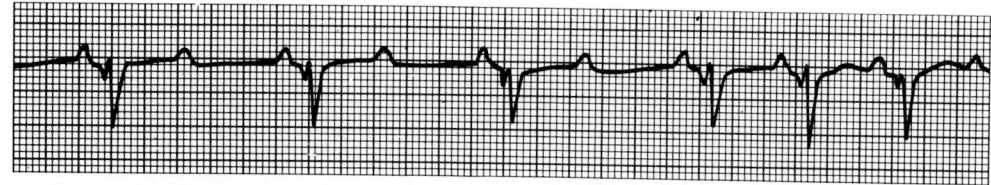

FIGURE 2-33. Second-degree AV block: Mobitz type II. (From Conover MB: *Exercises in diagnosing ECG tracings,* ed 3, St Louis, 1984, CV Mosby.)

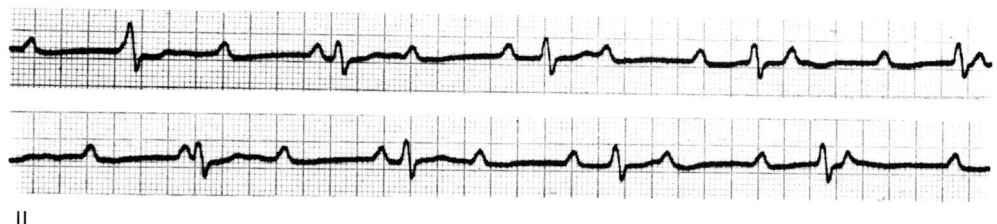

II

FIGURE 2-34. Third-degree (complete) AV block. (From Andreoli KG et al: *Comprehensive cardiac care,* ed 6, St Louis, 1987, CV Mosby.)

Medical Management

Medications
    Atropine
    Isoproterenol

Interventions

Withdraw use of digitalis preparation as ordered
Check serum levels of digitalis preparation and potassium as indicated

Mobitz Type II (Figure 2-33)

Causes—digitalis toxicity, anterior MI

Assessment
Observations/findings

Dizziness
Weakness
Rhythm
    Atrial: regular
    Ventricular: irregular
Rate
    Atrial: 60 to 90 beats/min
    Ventricular: will vary according to degree of block
P wave: may have multiple P waves before each QRS
PR interval: remains constant and may be greater than 0.20 sec
QRS interval: usually normal or slightly prolonged

Potential complications

Complete AV block
Asystole

Medical Management

Cardiac monitor
Medications
    Atropine
    Isoproterenol
Temporary or permanent cardiac pacing

THIRD-DEGREE HEART BLOCK (COMPLETE) (Figure 2-34)

Atria and ventricles are controlled by independent pacemakers
Causes—chronic conduction defect disease, digoxin toxicity, ischemic heart disease, congenital heart disease

Assessment
Observations/findings

Bradycardia
Syncope
Altered level of consciousness
Angina
Seizure activity
Rhythm: regular; atrial and ventricular rhythms act independently of each other
Rate
    Atrial: 60 to 90 beats/min
    Ventricular: 25 to 45 beats/min
P wave: multiple P waves that occur independently of QRS
PR interval: unmeasurable
QRS complex
    Normal if impulse originates above bifurcation of bundle of His (rate = 40-60/min)

II

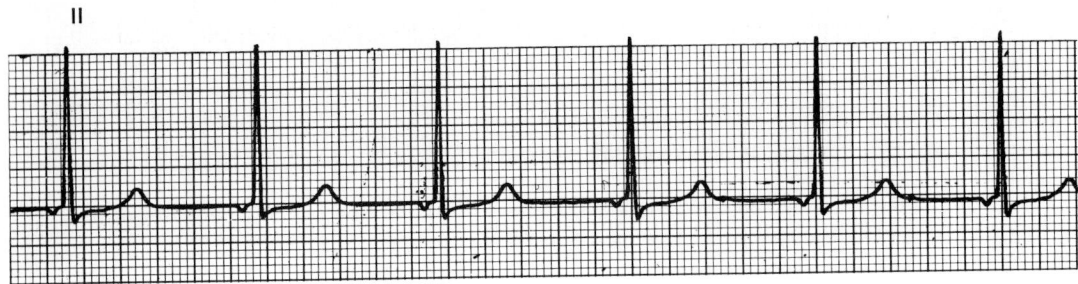

II

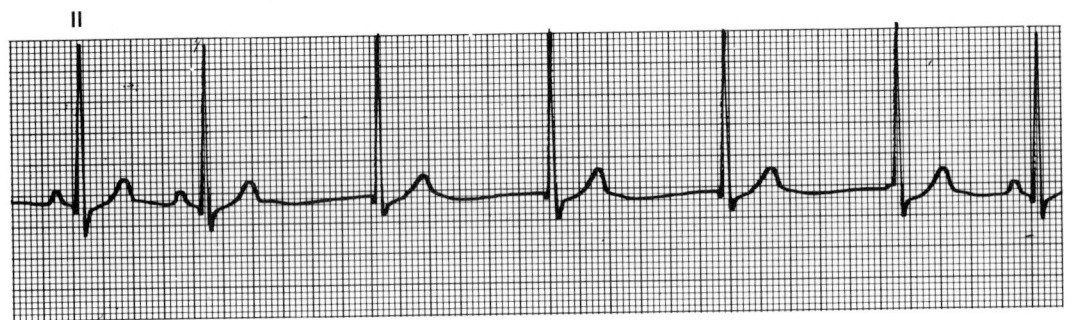

FIGURE 2-35. Junctional escape rhythms. (From Conover MB: *Exercises in diagnosing ECG tracings,* ed 3, St Louis, 1984, CV Mosby.)

Greater than 0.12 sec of impulse originates below bifurcation (rate = 15-40/min)

Potential complications

Heart failure
Shock
Ventricular fibrillation
Asystole

Medical Management

Transvenous cardiac pacing
Medications
  Atropine
  Isoproterenol
12-lead ECG

Interventions

Monitor cardiac activity; check rhythm strips q2h to 4h
  or as needed
Monitor BP, R, and apical pulse q2h to 4h and prn
Administer oxygen therapy as ordered
Maintain bed rest as indicated

Atrioventricular Junctional Rhythms

Dysrhythmias that originate at the AV junction; may include premature, escape, and accelerated junctional rhythm; causes—digitalis toxicity, MI, hypoxia, hyperkalemia, tricuspid valve surgery, rheumatic fever, SA node pathology

AV JUNCTIONAL ESCAPE (Figure 2-35)
Assessment
Observations/findings

Dizziness
Faintness
Heart block
Rhythm: regular
Rate: 40 to 60 beats/min
P wave: may precede or follow QRS; inverted in lead II
PR interval: not measurable
QRS complex: 0.06 to 0.10 sec; may be slightly abnormal

Medical Management

Treatment of underlying disease
Medications
  Atropine
  Isoproterenol
Ventricular pacing
12-lead ECG as ordered

Interventions

Monitor cardiac activity; check rhythm strips q4h to 6h
Check serum levels of digitalis preparation and potassium
  as indicated

Wolff-Parkinson-White Syndrome (Ventricular Preexcitation) (Figure 2-36)

Preexcitation of the ventricles over an accessory AV pathway: cause—congenital heart disease

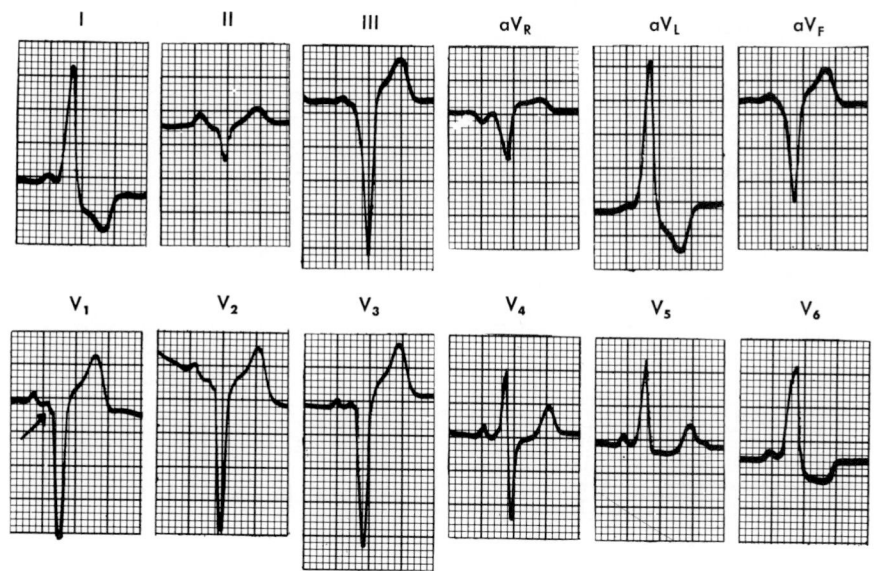

I   II   III   aV_R   aV_L   aV_F

V_1   V_2   V_3   V_4   V_5   V_6

FIGURE 2-36. Characteristic triad of Wolff-Parkinson-White (WPW) pattern: wide QRS complex, short PR interval, and delta wave (arrow in lead V₁). (From Goldberger AL, Goldberger E: *Clinical electrocardiography: a simplified approach,* ed 4, St Louis, 1990, Mosby−Year Book.)

Assessment

Observations/findings

Rhythm: regular
Rate: regular
P wave: normal configuration; one before each QRS
PR interval: less than 0.12 sec
QRS complex: when following shortened PR interval, complex is widened and distorted, exhibiting delta waves

Laboratory/diagnostic studies

Holter monitor examination
Electrophysiological studies

Potential complications

Atrial tachycardia
Atrial fibrillation

Medical Management

Valsalva maneuver; eyeball pressure
Medications as ordered
    Calcium channel−blocking agents
    Beta-adrenergic−blocking agents
Cardioversion

Interventions

Monitor cardiac activity as indicated; check rhythm strips q4h to 6h; report any changes in rhythm to physician

ECG Rhythms

Nursing Diagnoses/Interventions/Evaluation (General)

■ **NDX:**   Anxiety related to altered heart action

Assess level of anxiety and degree of understanding
Provide continuous explanation for various monitoring devices in use and procedures
Remain with patient during periods of heightened anxiety
Offer realistic assurances
Promote physical rest to decrease cardiac workload
Administer sedation as ordered

Expected outcome/evaluation

Patient's anxiety level is reduced
    Patient appears calm
    Verbalizes fears and concerns, asks questions

■ **NDX:**   Knowledge deficit related to lack of information regarding disease process

Assess level of understanding
Explain purpose of treatment and equipment
Reinforce physician's explanation of rhythm disturbance and associated symptoms to report
Discuss need to exercise to tolerance and/or as ordered
Explain purpose and demonstrate method of taking pulse
Describe dietary restrictions as ordered; need to avoid caffeine and nicotine

Normal T wave

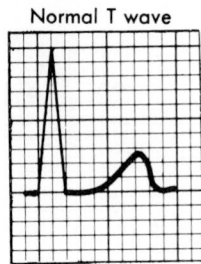

Nonspecific ST-T changes

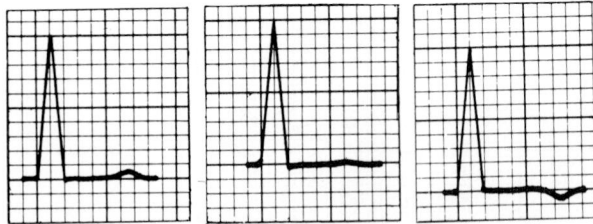

FIGURE 2-37. Miscellaneous ECG changes. (Flattening of T wave or slight T wave inversion are abnormal but relatively nonspecific changes.) (From Goldberger AL, Goldberger E: *Clinical electrocardiography: a simplified approach,* ed 4, St Louis, 1990, Mosby—Year Book.)

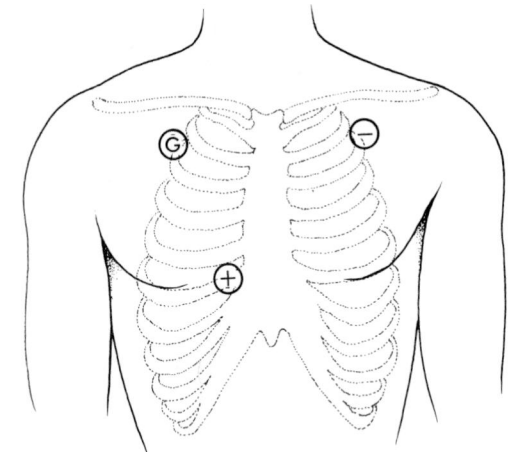

FIGURE 2-38. MCL. Modified V₁ monitoring lead.

Discuss medication: name, dosage, time of administration, purpose, and side effects
Need to avoid taking over-the-counter medications without checking with physician
Importance of ongoing patient care
Pacemaker care when indicated

Expected outcome/evaluation

Patient demonstrates understanding regarding dysrhythmia
    Verbalizes any food or drug restrictions
    Demonstrates pulse-taking procedure

PACEMAKER INSERTION

pacemaker An electronic device used to electronically stimulate the myocardium to control or maintain the heart rate

Preprocedure Teaching

Reinforce physician's explanation of procedure
    How pacemaker functions
        To optimize cardiac function
        To restore and/or maintain AV synchronization
    Indications
        To control bradyarrhythmias
        To control tachyarrhythmias
        To control ventricular fibrillation
    Type or mode to be used
        Temporary

        Permanent
    Method insertion
        Transvenous
        Transthoracic
        Epicardial
Ensure that patient and/or significant other knows and understands
    Procedure, duration of procedure, where it will be performed (operating room vs. procedure room), equipment that will be used (e.g., fluoroscopy), and type of anesthesia
Importance of restricting activities for 4 to 6 hr in order to avoid lead dislodgment
Importance of performing passive ROM exercises to extremities postoperatively
Importance of being closely monitored postoperatively
Signs and symptoms of pacemaker malfunction
    Faintness
    Dizziness
    Dyspnea
    Twitching
        Pectoral muscles
        Abdominal muscle
    Hiccups
    Chest pain

Postprocedure Assessment
Observations/findings
TEMPORARY PACEMAKER (Figure 2-39)

Heart rate based on preset pacemaker setting
Pacemaker unit (Figure 2-40)
    Firing at preset rate
    Output threshold (milliamperes)
    Sensing needle
    Terminal connections
Electrical grounding

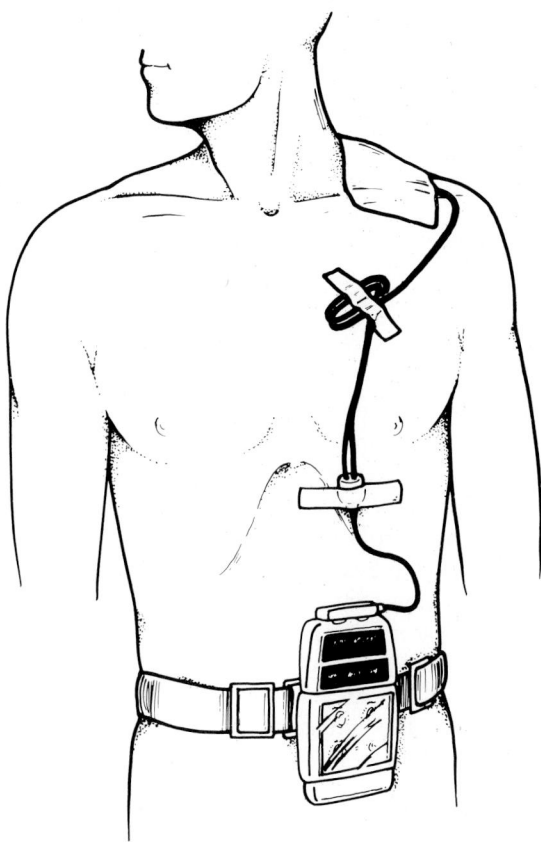

FIGURE 2-39. Temporary external pacemaker.

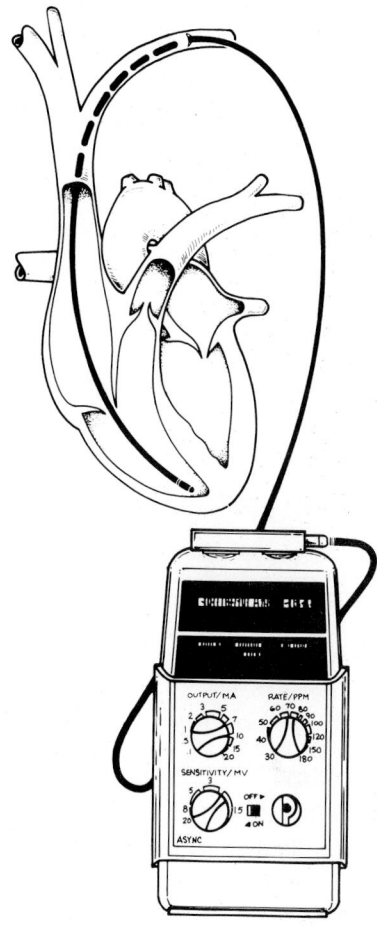

FIGURE 2-40. Temporary pacemaker unit: transvenous approach.

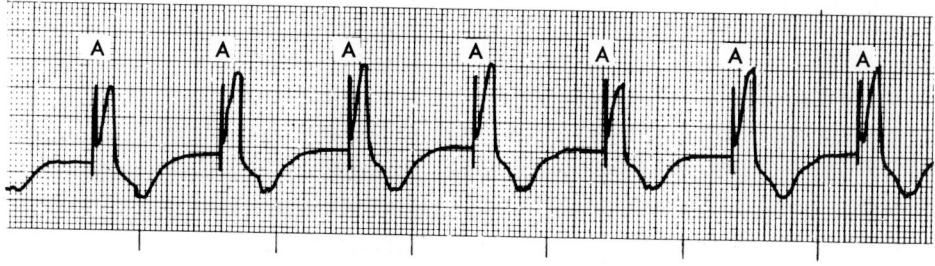

FIGURE 2-41. Ventricular pacemaker, **A,** Pacemaker spikes. (From Andreoli K et al: *Comprehensive cardiac care,* ed 6, St Louis, 1987, CV Mosby.)

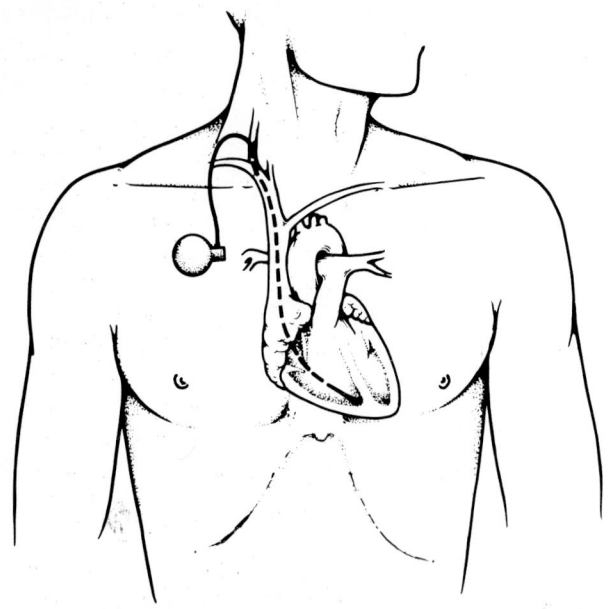

FIGURE 2-42. Permanent pacemaker.

ECG pattern (Figure 2-41)
  Pacemaker artifact
  Capturing
  Patient's underlying rhythm
Battery failure
  Loss of capture
  Failure to sense
  Sensing needle: not moving

PERMANENT PACEMAKER

Pacemaker unit (Figure 2-42)
  Heart rate: based on preset pacer rate
  Location of pulse generator
  Mode (see box above)
    Ventricular inhibited (demand): VVI
    AV sequential: DVI
    Atrial triggered: VDD
    Universal: DDD
  Programmable
    Pacer rate
    Output (milliamperes)
    Sensitivity (to PQRS complex)
    Mode
      Atrial
      Ventricular

Potential complications

Pacemaker dysfunction
  Syncope
  Decreased BP
  Pallor or cyanosis
  Bradycardia

PERMANENT PACEMAKER MODE	
CHAMBER SENSED	**MODE OF RESPONSE**
A—atrium	I—Inhibited
V—ventricle	T—Triggered
D—dual	D—Dual
0—none	R—Reserve
	0—None

Fatigue
Shortness of breath
ECG pattern changes
Absent pacemaker artifact
No ventricular response, absence of QRS complex after
  pacemaker artifact
Competition; presence of pacemaker response complex
  and patient's own complex
Runaway pacemaker; pacemaker artifact appears at several hundred per minute
Catheter dislodgment
  Change in QRS configuration
  Loss of artifact on ECG
  Failure to sense
  Hiccups
  Muscle twitching: chest, abdomen
Stokes-Adams syndrome
  Hypotension
  Vertigo
  Fainting
  Convulsions
  Coma
Cardiac dysrhythmias
  PVCs
  Ventricular tachycardia
Site of insertion
  Discoloration
  Pain
  Swelling
  Bleeding
Perforation
  Hiccough
Infection of incisional site
  Elevated temperature
  Redness
  Discoloration
  Pain, swelling
  Fluid collection, drainage
Cardiac tamponade

Medical Management

Cardiac monitor
Pacemaker
  Heart rate setting

Threshold (milliamperes)
Medications
    Analgesics

Nursing diagnoses/interventions/evaluation

■ **NDX:** Potential for decreased cardiac output related to pacemaker dysfunction secondary to displacement or breakage of pacing catheter, infection, or bleeding

Assess patient and pacemaker unit for proper functioning
Maintain bed rest as ordered
Place patient on cardiac monitor
Monitor BP, T, and R q4h; check apical pulse q1h to 2h for 7 hr, then q4h
For temporary pacemaker
    Check settings: output, sensing, and rates
    Immobilize and secure extremity
Check rhythm strips on return to unit, q4h, and prn, noting pacemaker function and rate
Examine site of insertion q2h to 4h; report any excessive bleeding to physician
Continue with immediate postoperative care and decrease frequency of nursing functions as patient's condition improves
Increase activity as tolerated and ordered
Change dressing daily as ordered, using aseptic technique

Expected outcome/evaluation

Patient demonstrates stable cardial output; pacemaker unit functioning as programmed

■ **NDX:** Potential for injury related to noncompliance

Permanent pacemaker

Assess level of understanding and degree of readiness to learn
Ensure that patient and/or significant other knows pacemaker model, date of insertion, location of pacer generator, and pacer rate
Demonstrate method of caring for pacemaker
Demonstrate changing of dressing
Demonstrate taking of pulse for 1 min; give patient range of normal rates and instruct to report to physician if pulse is less than set range (i.e., < 5 beats/min below set rate)
Deal with behavioral changes such as denial
Discuss living with pacemaker, assist patient to adjust to any limitations and explain that pacemaker will eliminate feelings of faintness and fatigue
Discuss signs of pacemaker failure
    Pulse < 60 beats/min or < 5 beats/min below set rate
    Dizziness
    Faintness
    Palpitations
    Hiccups

MANAGEMENT OF PACEMAKER EQUIPMENT

TEMPORARY PACEMAKER

Ground all equipment
Secure all terminal connections
Avoid use of electrical equipment such as shavers
Insulate exposed pacemaker wires by enclosing pacemaker and connections with rubber glove
Avoid wetting pacemaker
Apply soft restraints prn

PERMANENT PACEMAKER

Avoid exposure to electrical equipment that causes electromagnetic interference (EMI) such as diathermy and ungrounded equipment
Ground all equipment
Apply soft restraints prn

Chest pain
Discuss method of reporting pacemaker failure
    Telephone monitoring
    Notifying physician
Discuss signs of infection around pacemaker generator
    Fever
    Heat
    Pain
    Swelling
Discuss medications: name, dosage, times of administration, purpose, and side effects
Explain need to avoid taking over-the-counter medications without checking with physician
Review prescribed diet
Explain importance of ongoing outpatient care: pacemaker clinic, use of transtelephonic system
Discuss need to maintain activities as ordered
    Avoid traveling for at least 3 months after insertion
    Discuss type of employment and make adjustments in work accordingly
    Resume sexual activity as tolerated
    Avoid engaging in body contact sports such as baseball, football, and basketball
Discuss need to wear nonrestrictive clothing over site of pacemaker
Discuss electrical safety
    Avoid working with radar or electrical equipment such as diathermy motors that may cause electromagnetic interference
    Ground home appliances so that they have little or no effect on permanent pacemakers
    Wear medical alert band
    Carry pacemaker card with information regarding type

of pacemaker, set rate, date of implantation, and name of physician

Inform dentist of pacemaker before any extensive dental work

Expected outcome/evaluation

Patient demonstrates an understanding of home health care

Demonstrates pulse taking

Verbalizes electrical sources that may interfere with pacemaker function

Verbalizes signs of pacemaker failure and actions to take

Demonstrates no complications

AUTOMATIC IMPLANTABLE CARDIOVERTER-DEFIBRILLATOR (AICD)

A self-contained automatic device that is capable of identifying and treating recurrent ventricular tachy-cardia (RVT) and fibrillation

Preoperative instruction

Review purpose and basic function of AICD device, implantation procedure, and postoperative care

Review surgical approaches that may be used (thoracotomy, median sternotomy, subxiphoid)

Describe the AICD device, discussing signs and symptoms associated with defibrillation discharge

Assessment

Malfunction of AICD

Dizziness, lightheadedness, palpitations, loss of consciousness

Infection of pulse generator pocket site

Redness, swelling head; fluid drainage, skin irritation

Elevated temperature

Potential complication

Atelectasis

Pericarditis

Laboratory/diagnostic studies

ECG: transient episodes of supraventricular tachycardia, nonsustained ventricular tachycardia

EP studies

Medical Management

NOTE: Postoperative care is similar to that given any patient after cardiac surgery (p. 108)

Cardiac monitor

Hemodynamic monitor

Medications

Antiarrhythmic agents

Nursing diagnoses/interventions/evaluation

■ **NDX:** Potential decreased cardiac output related to recurrent ventricular dysrhythmias

Assess and monitor HR and rhythm, BP, and level of consciousness

Determine if AICD is in inactive or active mode

Administer medications as ordered

Defibrillate and initiate CPR as indicated

Instruct patient in cough CPR; to be used when feeling dizzy or lightheaded or when experiencing palpitations

Expected outcome/evaluation

Patient demonstrates electromechanical stability

Baseline rhythm is maintained

No further episodes of syncope are reported

AICD shows appropriate discharge response during magnet testing

■ **NDX:** Fear of sudden death related to anticipated shock and/or to frequency of RVT episodes

Assess level of understanding, encouraging patient to verbalize feelings regarding AICD

Provide information to correct any misperceptions

Assist patient to identify source(s) of fear

Offer brief explanations of the "shock", that it has been described as a thump or kick; that it is brief, lasting less than 1 second; that the shock usually will not be felt by another person touching the patient, and if it is, the energy felt would be like a tingle

Refer to AICD support groups

Expected outcome/evaluation

Patient's fear level is reduced

Patient is able to verbalize fears and concerns regarding AICD unit, asks appropriate questions regarding self-care, participates in patient teaching activities

■ **NDX:** Knowledge deficit related to lack of information about self-management regarding self-care management

Assess level of understanding, include family or significant other in discussion

Review basic function of AICD device, signs and symptoms associated with shock

Discuss importance of recording and/or notifying physician each time patient receives a shock

Describe signs and symptoms of AICD malfunction, (e.g., inappropriate shocks) and need to notify physician

Explain need for regular follow-up magnet testing to evaluate battery life

Explain need to protect implantation site; avoid tight clothing such as belts, girdles

Discuss need to avoid strong magnetic fields that may activate AICD device (e.g., radio and television stations, electrical power plants)

Assure patient that normal household appliances (e.g., microwave ovens) will not interfere with AICD unit

Discuss need to maintain activities as ordered

Advise patient to avoid heavy lifting and dangerous sports

Advise patient to resume sexual activity as tolerated

Inform patient to avoid metal detectors in airport

Teach patient how to take peripheral pulses

Explain need to carry AICD identification and to wear medical-alert bracelet at all times

Encourage family members to be certified in CPR

Instruct patient in cough CPR

Provide personal AICD manual offered through manufacturer

Expected outcome/evaluation

Patient's knowledge level is increased and self-care skills are demonstrated

Patient verbalizes understanding of AICD unit, follow-up care, activity allowances and limitations, frequency of medical follow-up, signs and symptoms to report, pulse taking, skin care, and how to inactivate AICD

Additional nursing diagnosis to consider

Potential for injury related to sudden loss of consciousness

CARDIAC CATHETERIZATION

An invasive cardiac procedure; assists in detection and localization of intracardiac problems, determines intracardiac measurements, and shows visualization of the cardiac chambers; performed with patient under local anesthesia

Preprocedure Teaching

Involve family or significant other in care and instruction

Assess level of understanding

Reinforce physician's explanation of purpose of procedure

Review routine preparation for procedure
 Arm or leg shave and preparation
 Medication for sedation may be ordered
 No food or water 6 to 12 hr before procedure

Review sensations to be experienced during procedure
 Palpitations
 Warm, flushed feeling during injection of dye
 Desire to cough
 Feeling of falling if rotated from side to side

Review sensations to be expected after procedure
 Soreness at insertion site
 Possible backache from lying on table for 1 to 3 hr
 Fatigue

Stress importance of bed rest and immobility of extremity after procedure

Postprocedure Assessment
Observations/findings

Hematoma at site of insertion
 Neck
 Antecubital fossa
 Inguinal
Vasospasm of affected extremity
 Numbness
 Tingling
 Cyanosis
 Loss of pulse

Potential complications

Ventricular dysrhythmias
Syncope
Allergic reaction to dye
Nausea, vomiting
Decrease or fall in BP
Thrombus
 Pain at incision site
Thrombophlebitis
Cardiac perforation
Myocardial ischemia
Local infection
Cardiac tamponade

Postprocedure Care

Assess BP, T, R, apical pulse, and peripheral pulses, noting quality q15min for four times, then qh for 4 hr, then as ordered

Maintain bed rest for 6 to 8 hr after procedure or as ordered
 Elevate head of bed 20 to 30 degrees
 Keep extremity immobile for 2 to 4 hr after procedure as ordered
 Maintain sandbag over puncture site as ordered

Obtain 12-lead ECG as ordered

Monitor cardiac activity as ordered; check rhythm strips q4h and prn

Examine dressing at site of insertion q2h to 4h, noting amount and color of drainage; change qd and prn

Reinforce dressing as necessary

Inspect surrounding skin
 Redness or discoloration
 Swelling
 Irritation

Control pain as ordered

Ambulate as tolerated

Instruct patient to report any signs of pain, swelling, or discoloration of puncture site

Continue ongoing care for underlying disease process

PERCUTANEOUS TRANSLUMINAL CORONARY ANGIOPLASTY (PTCA)

An invasive nonsurgical procedure using a balloon-tipped catheter to restore patency of coronary artery by compressing atheromatous plaques within the artery

Preprocedure Teaching

Assess level of understanding and emotional status: fears of procedure and possible necessity of cardiac surgery

Involve family or significant other in care and instruction

Reinforce physician's explanation of purpose of procedure, desired outcome, and associated risks

Explain need to follow directions regarding administration and withholding of medications

Encourage verbalization and questions

Explain that procedure is similar to cardiac catheterization, identifying any previous negative experiences; procedure may last 45 min to 1½ hr

Review routine preparation for procedure

   Skin prepared for coronary bypass surgery

   Medication for sedation may be ordered

   No food or water for at least 8 hr before procedure

Explain sensations to be expected

   During procedure

      Palpitations

      Warm, flushed feeling during injection of dye

      Possible chest discomfort during balloon inflation

   After procedure

      Soreness at insertion site

      Possible backache from lying on table for 3 to 5 hr

      Fatigue

Stress importance of bed rest and immobility of extremity after procedure

Stress importance of drinking fluids for first 6 to 8 hr to wash out contrast material

Explain and review postprocedure procedures

   Need to be admitted to CCU for 24 hr for observation

   Routines of CCU

   Visiting privileges

   Equipment to be used

      Temporary pacing electrode

      Cardiac monitor

      Oxygen administration

      IV therapy

NOTE: Cardiac surgical team must be on standby during procedure; see Cardiac Surgery on p. 108 for brief explanation of differences in patient care after cardiac surgery

During procedure intraaortic balloon pump must be available on standby

Preparation

Obtain informed consent

Maintain NPO 8 hr before procedure

Withhold anticoagulation therapy 1 to 2 days before procedure

Administer medications as ordered

   Salicylates and dipyridamole may be ordered 2 days before procedure

   Nitrates

   Beta-blocking agents may be decreased

   Calcium antagonists

   Sedation

Obtain baseline data

   CBC

   Electrolytes

   BUN, creatinine

   Blood type and crossmatch

   Coagulation studies

   ECG

   Chest x-ray

Postprocedure Assessment
Observations/findings

Chest pain or pressure

ECG changes

   ST elevations, depressions

   Ventricular dysrhythmias

Shortness of breath

Skin

   Pale

   Diaphoretic

Hypotension

Hematoma at site of insertion

Vasospasm of affected extremity

   Numbness

   Tingling

   Cyanosis

   Loss of pulse

Dysrhythmias

Behavioral response

   Anxiety

   Fear

Laboratory/diagnostic studies

CBC

Coagulation studies: PTT

Serum potassium and sodium

Cardiac enzymes: CPK

BUN, creatinine

12-lead ECG

Potential complications

Failure to dilate coronary artery

Abrupt coronary occlusion

MI

Bleeding

Rupture or dissection of coronary artery

   Cardiac tamponade

MI
Shock
Cardiac arrest
Cannulated extremity
Ischemia
Thrombosis formation
Renal hypersensitivity to contrast material

Medical Management

Admission to CCU for 24 to 48 hr
Bed rest
Cardiac monitor
Parenteral fluids
Medications
Heparin infusion
Nitrates
Calcium channel blockers
Aspirin
Dipyridamole

Nursing diagnoses/interventions/evaluation

■ **NDX:** Potential alternation in tissue perfusion: peripheral related to hematoma, thrombus formation, secondary to arterial cannulation

Assess pulses distal to site, noting quality, q15min for four times, decreasing frequency as ordered; note skin color, temperature
Observe for diminished pulses in extremity distal to cannulation site; report decreased or absent pulses immediately to physician
Maintain bed rest for 6 to 8 hr in flat position until arterial and venous sheaths are removed; when sheaths are removed maintain 5 to 10 lb sandbag over cannulation site
Inspect cannulation site for swelling, tenderness, discoloration, warmth, and drainage
Keep extremity immobile for 2 to 4 hr after procedure
Inspect dressing at site of insertion q2h to 4h, noting amount and color of drainage
Reinforce dressing as necessary
Inspect surrounding skin
Redness or discoloration
Swelling
Irritation
Administer antiplatelets as ordered
Monitor coagulation studies, reporting prolonged PTT to physician

Expected outcome/evaluation

Patient maintains adequate peripheral tissue perfusion
Pulse is full and bounding
Cannulation site: color is good, there are no signs of tenderness or swelling

■ **NDX:** Potential decrease in cardiac output related to myocardial ischemia or dysrhythmias

Assess for signs of diminished CO
Monitor BP, R, and apical pulse q15min for 1 hr, then q30min for 1 hr, then qh for 6 hr, then as ordered
Monitor cardiac activity, check rhythm strips q4h and prn, observing for signs of ischemia or dysrhythmias
Obtain 12-lead ECG during episodes of chest pain; observe for and report any signs of ischemic change or dysrhythmias
Auscultate chest for heart and lung sounds q4h for 24 hr
Monitor intake and output; report output of less than 30 ml/hr or inability to void within first 4 hr
Administer medications as ordered

Expected outcome/evaluation

Patient maintains good cardiac output
Vital signs are stable
Urine output is good
Mentation is clear

■ **NDX:** Knowledge deficit related to lack of information regarding postprocedure care
NOTE: Refer to p. 82 for education for patients with angina pectoris
Assess level of understanding
Reinforce physician's explanation of postprocedure results
Review allowances and limitations of activity
Avoid heavy lifting and pushing
Ambulate at regular intervals
Explain importance of calling physician if chest pain occurs, lasting longer than 20 min
Discuss medications: name, dosage, time of administration, purpose, and side effects
Explain importance of taking antiplatelet medications as ordered
Explain importance of ongoing outpatient care
Refer to standard for angina pectoris for patient teaching regarding
Chest pain
Risk factors
Exercise, activities

Expected outcome/evaluation

Patient's knowledge level is increased
Knows signs and symptoms to report, activity allowances and limitations
Verbalizes understanding of medications

Additional nursing diagnosis to consider

Anxiety related to perceived biological threat

THROMBOLYTIC THERAPY

Infusion of thrombolytic agents to promote clot lysis, restore coronary blood flow, and limit myocardial ischemia

Preprocedure teaching

Assess level of understanding and anxiety level

Involve family or significant other in care and instruction

Reinforce physician's explanation of purpose of procedure, desired outcome, and associated risks

Describe procedure to be performed

Intracoronary: similar to cardiac catheterization, may last 1 to 2 hours; sensations that may occur: pressure during insertion of catheter but no discomfort with infusion

Intravenous: usually in emergency department or in CCU; infusion administered over 3-hour period

Explain and review intraprocedure and postprocedure routines

Monitoring in CCU

Visiting privileges

Equipment to be used

Cardiac monitor

Oxygen administration

IV therapy

Explain need for bed rest during and after administration and need for frequent blood sampling to monitor clotting times

Instruct patient to inform nurse if chest pain develops

Preparation

Obtain informed consents as required: thrombolytic therapy, cardiac catheterization, PTCA, and CABG surgery

Obtain baseline laboratory data

To determine hemostatic status: CBC with platelets, PT, fibrinogen, fibrin split-product labels

To determine degree of myocardial injury: CPK-MB

Blood type and cross match, electrolytes, BUN creatinine

Obtain diagnostic data

12-lead ECG

Chest x-ray examination

Establish two to three patent IV lines

Administer medications as ordered

Lidocaine may be given prophylactically

Postprocedure Assessment
Observations/findings

Successful myocardial reperfusion

Abrupt cessation of chest pain

ECG changes: return of ST elevations to baseline

Dysrhythmias: sinus bradycardia, AV block with hypotension, ventricular tachycardia

Isoenzyme: early peaking of CPK-MB (within 12 hours of onset of symptoms)

Bleeding/hemorrhage:

Surface bleeding: oozing from puncture or catheter insertion site, gingival bleeding, ecchymoses

GI: hematemesis, tarry stools, positive occult blood

Coronary artery reocclusion

Chest pain

ECG: ST-T wave changes

Dysrhythmias

Skin

Pale

Diaphoretic

Clammy

Hypotension

Tachycardia

Anxiety

Laboratory/diagnostic studies

CBC

Serum fibrinogen levels

PTT

CPK-MB

Potential Complications

Bleeding

Hemorrhage: GI, intracranial

Myocardial ischemia or infarction

Medical Management

Admission to CCU

Bed rest

Cardiac monitoring

Hemodynamic monitoring

Arterial pressure, PA, PWCP

PTCA

Medications

During procedure

Thrombolytic agents

Streptokinase (SK)

Urokinase (UK)

Tissue plasminogen activator (t-PA)

Anisoylated plasminogen-SK activator complex (APSAC)

Diphenhydramine

Heparin

After procedure

Heparin

Nursing diagnoses/interventions/evaluation

■ **NDX:** Potential fluid volume deficit related to bleeding/hemorrhage secondary to thrombolysis-induced coagulopathy

Assess for signs and symptoms of surface or internal bleeding

Monitor BP, HR according to unit protocol during first hour, decreasing frequency as condition stabilizes

Inspect puncture sites every 15 min; apply manual pressure when removing IV catheters

Initiate measures that prevent disruption of vascular integrity and/or keep venous or arterial puncture and injections to a minimum

Instruct patient to avoid vigorous toothbrushing

Avoid removing IV or arterial lines during first 24 to 48 hours or as indicated by specific agents

Use heparin lock for IV access or blood sampling

Monitor PTT valves

Expected outcome/evaluation

Patient demonstrates no signs of bleeding
  Hemostasis is reestablished
    Coagulation studies are within acceptable limits
    No signs of surface or internal bleeding
    Vital signs are WNL

■ **NDX:** Potential decrease in cardiac output related to reperfusion dysrhythmias

Assess and record ECG changes during and after thrombolytic therapy

Assess and monitor BP, HR, respiration, and hemodynamic response to reperfusion dysrhythmias as they appear

Administer antiarrhythmic medictions as ordered; keep medications and defibrillator at bedside

Expected outcome/evaluation

Patient maintains good cardiac output
  ECG remains in stable or normal rhythm
  Reperfusion dysrhythmias are controlled or absent
  Vital signs remain stable

■ **NDX:** Potential for pain (chest): related to decreased myocardial tissue perfusion secondary to reocclusion of coronary artery

Assess and monitor complaints of chest pain, noting patient's nonverbal expressions, compare with preprocedural chest pain complaints

Obtain 12-lead ECG during episode of chest pain, comparing with baseline ECG taken after thrombolysis; report any changes

Maintain on bed rest

Monitor BP, HR, respiration

Administer analgesia: morphine sulfate

Prepare for possible catheterization, repeat thrombolysis, PTCA

Expected outcome/evaluation

Patient verbalizes absence of chest pain

■ **NDX:** Knowledge deficit related to lack of information about postprocedure care

NOTE: See p. 82 for patient education after an AMI

HEMODYNAMIC MONITORING

Method of evaluating filling pressure of left ventricle, cardiac output, and intraarterial pressure (Figure 2-43)

pulmonary artery pressure (PAP) and pulmonary capillary wedge pressure (PCWP) An indirect method of measuring left ventricular filling pressure using a flow-directed pulmonary artery catheter; cardiac output right atrial (RA) and mixed venous sampling may also be obtained via catheter (Figures 2-44 to 2-46)

Preprocedure Teaching

Reinforce physician's explanation of procedure, duration, and equipment that will be used

Explain importance of immobilizing extremity

Attach cardiac monitor to patient; record baseline rhythm strip

Equipment Preparation

Check integrity of balloon catheters before insertion; record amount of air needed for inflation

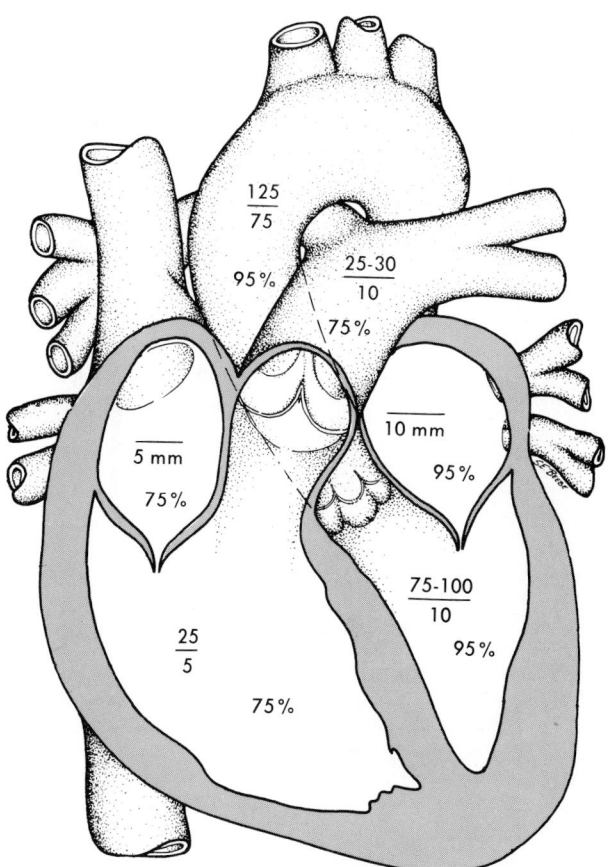

FIGURE 2-43. Normal pressures and percentages of oxygen saturation in heart chambers and great vessels.

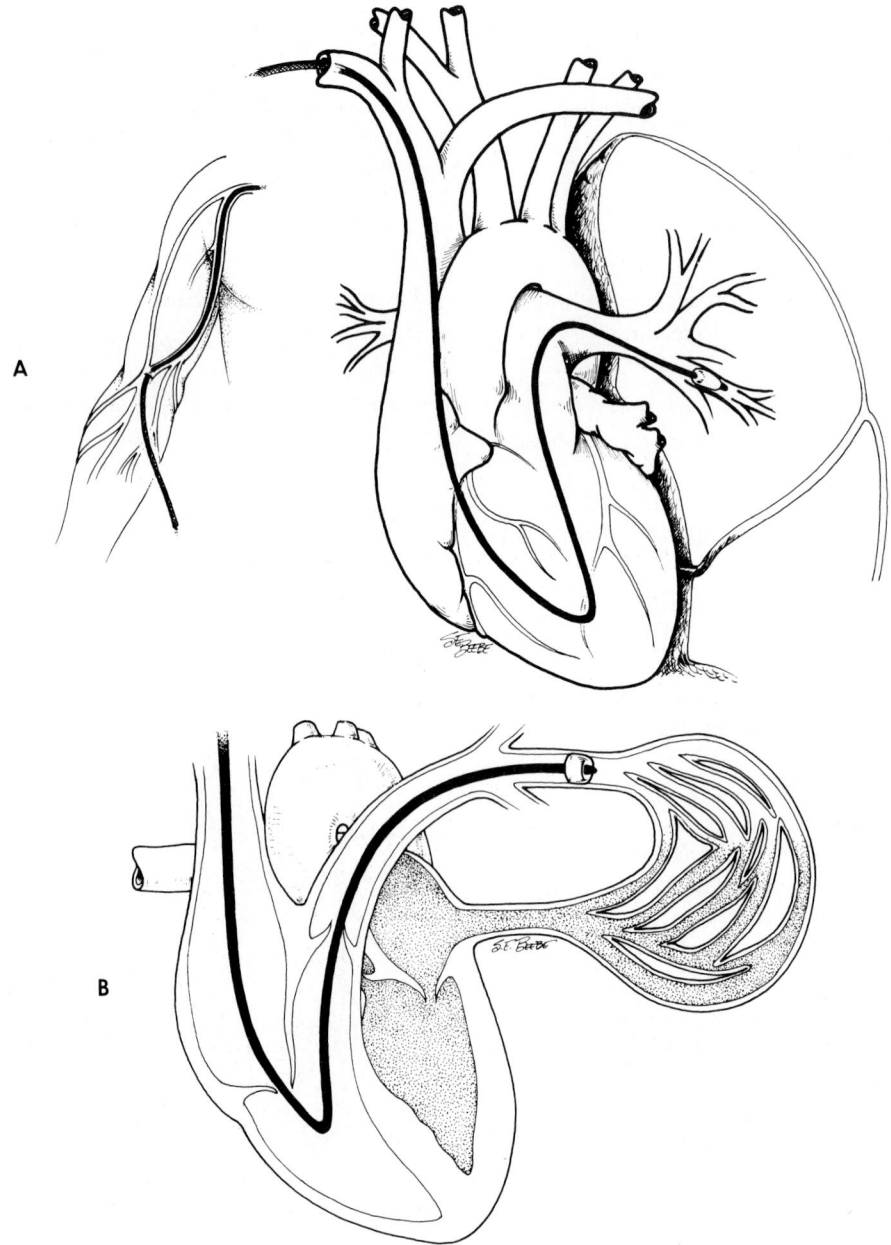

FIGURE 2-44. Swan-Ganz catheter. **A,** Placement of flow-directed catheter via superior vena cava. **B,** Balloon inflated and wedged in pulmonary artery.

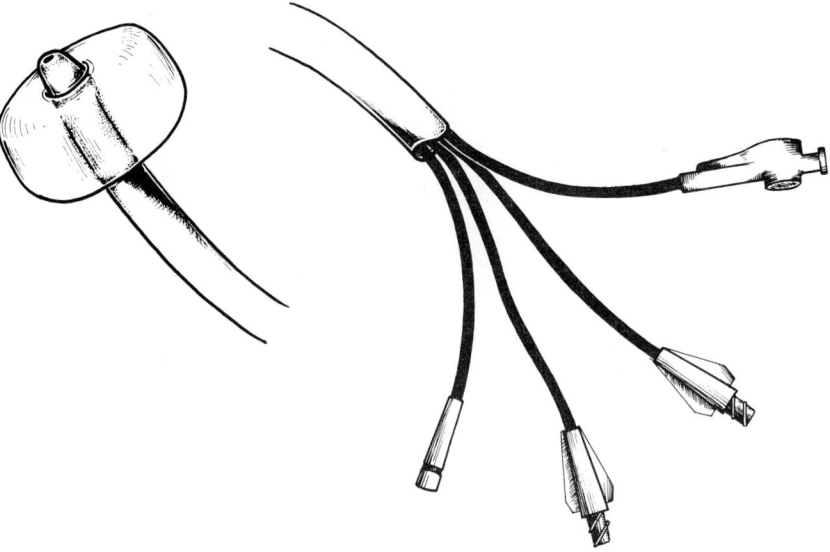

FIGURE 2-45. Triple-lumen, balloon-tipped pulmonary catheter (Swan-Ganz).

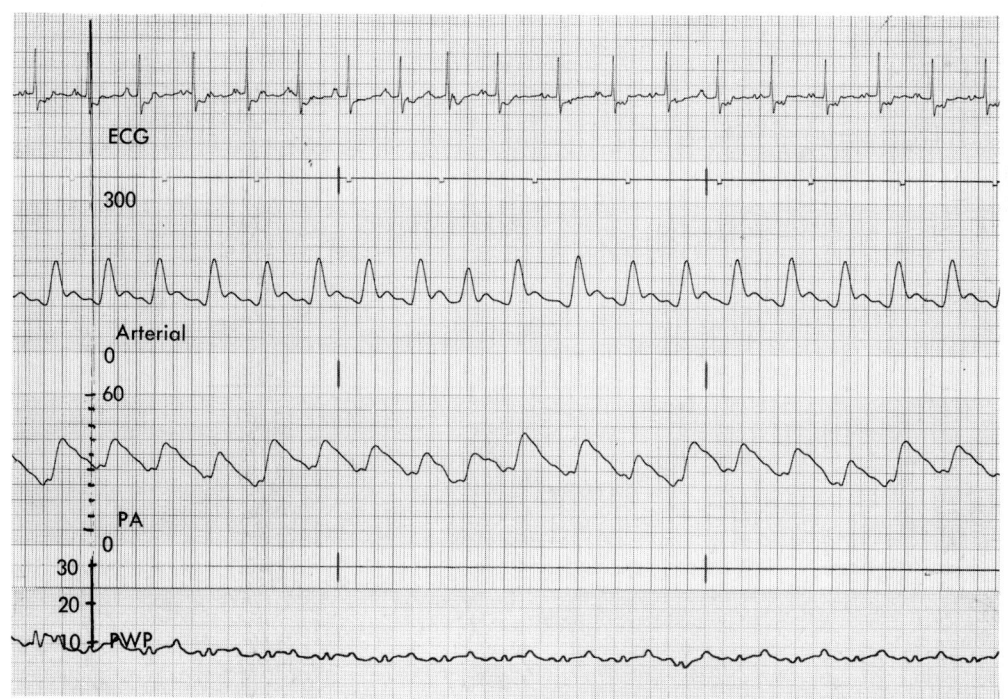

FIGURE 2-46. Pressure wave forms. Electrocardiogram *(ECG)*, arterial pressure, pulmonary artery pressure *(PAP)* and pulmonary capillary wedge pressure *(PCWP)*.

Postion transducer to level of right atrium

Calibrate all equipment before insertion
  Transducer
  Recording display unit
  Monitor

Have 100 mg IV bolus of lidocaine and defibrillator at bedside during insertion

Be aware that insertion must be done under sterile conditions

Assessment

Observations/findings

Normal pressures
RA: 5 mm Hg
PA: 25 to 30/10 to 15 mm Hg
PCWP: 10 to 12 mm Hg

DURING INSERTION

Ventricular irritability
Pneumothorax (with subclavian insertion)

POSTINSERTION

Catheter insertion site
  Infection
    Inflammation
    Redness

Thrombosis
Tenderness
Swelling
Edema
Endocarditis
Septicemia

Potential complications

Decreased circulation
    Numbness, absence of pulses to distal extremity
    Coolness, pallor, cyanosis of extremity
Blood loss
  Decreased BP
  Blood in tube and at insertion site
Pulmonary infarction (for pulmonary catheters)
  Chest pain
  Dyspnea
  Hemoptysis
  Tachypnea
  Dysrhythmias
    PVCs
    Ventricular tachycardia
Embolus (air or thromboembolus)
  Tachypnea
  Dyspnea
  Chest pain

TABLE 2-9. Problems Associated with Pressure Wave Forms

Observations	Etiologic factors	Interventions
Loss of wave form on oscilloscope	Displacement of catheter	Reposition patient; notify physician
Loss of PAP; PCWP is displayed on monitor	Self-wedging	Instruct patient to cough Obtain x-ray examination
Loss of PCWP	Displaced into PAP; balloon rupture	Use diastolic of PAP: *Do not attempt to rewedge*
Decreased amplitude of wave form	Damping caused by	
	Clot in catheter	Flush lines: *Do not force if resistance is met*
	Air bubbles	Check all connections for air leaks; flush air bubbles
	Kinking of catheter	Notify physician
	Occluded catheter	Reposition patient; have patient cough
	Tip against artery wall	
Loss of PCWP; no resistance with inflation	Rupture of balloon	Seal off balloon lumen: *Do not allow any injection of air*
Air bubbles in pressure lines Damping of wave form Inaccurate reading	Air leak in system	Check all connections and secure Remove all air or change flush system
Artifacts and inadequate pressure readings	Respiratory interference	Record pressure at end exhalation
	Handling of pressure equipment during readings	Check for possible equipment interference with tubing during readings
	Inaccurate calibration of equipment	Check for possible equipment interference with tubing during readings
	Faulty equipment	Check electrical system for grounding Check calibration of and level to RA of transducer Check all equipment for proper functioning

Catheter displacement
  Change in wave form morpholopy (Table 2-9)
  Dampening of wave form
Rupture of balloon
  Absence of resistance to inflation
  Failure of PA line to wedge
  Blood backup in balloon line

FLUSH SYSTEM

For continuous flush via pressure transfer pack
Pressure maintained at 300 mm Hg or as ordered by manufacturer
Heparinized solution (500 U/500 ml 0.9 normal saline solution or 1 unit of heparin/ml of solution)

PRESSURE LINES

Patency
Complications
  Air bubbles
  Blood in tubing
Slow blood return from catheter

PRESSURE TRANSDUCER

Air bubbles
Cracks
Foreign material
  Blood
  Dust particles

DISCONTINUATION

Extravasation of blood
Thrombi formation
Sepsis

Interventions

Check patency of lines, tubings, and connections q4h to 8h
Check pressure in transfer pack sq4h to 6h
Flush all lines q1h to 2h
Check calibration of transducer q8h or as indicated by manufacturer, never apply direct pressure to diaphragm of transducer
Relevel transducer as patient position is changed
  Keep level with right atrium
  Record position in which readings are taken
Change pressure line tubing, pressure bag, and manifold q48h
Change dressing qd
Record ECG rhythm strip q6h

Pulmonary artery pressures (PAP, PCWP)

Check that balloon is deflated except when testing PCWP
Record pressure reading q4h to 6h as dictated by patient's condition

Take readings at end-exhalation in presence of respiratory variation
Blood should not be withdrawn rountinely from PA line
Parenteral fluids should not be administered routinely through PA line

Cardiac output–thermodilution method

A method of measuring cardiac output using a triple-lumen flow-directed pulmonary catheter, the proximal lumen is used for injection of an iced or room temperature solution (5 to 10 ml); cardiac output is 5 L/min

Prepare equipment; if using iced injectate, allow 45 to 60 min
Follow manufacturer's manual regarding preparation of computer readout
Calibrate all equipment before procedure
Check integrity of catheter before injecting solution
Use aseptic technique in injection of solution
Inject 10 ml rapidly over 4 sec; record amount of injectate on intake and output

Arterial lines

Measure arterial blood pressure directly as ordered
Check connections q2h for tightness
Do not leave patient unattended, especially when restless; use soft restraints as indicated
Record pressure reading q4h as indicated by patient's condition
Check indirect arterial pressure q6h to 8h and record
Check circulation of extremity q2h; observe for changes in color, warmth, pulses, and nail beds
Flush lines before and after withdrawing blood specimens
Measure output of blood samples for replacement in pediatric patients
Change stopcocks qd
Remove dead-space fluid in tubing before removing blood specimens for analysis
Never use force to flush or irrigate a line that is resistant
Notify physician of
  Early signs of inflammation; swelling at insertion site
  Coolness or cyanosis of extremity
  Clotted pressure line
  Absence of pulses

Discontinuation of pressure lines

Maintain direct manual pressure over site for 5 to 10 min after removal of all catheters
Have lidocaine bolus with defibrillator at bedside during removal of pulmonary catheters
Check insertion site and pulses of extremity q2h to 4h for 24 hr
Check and observe for dysrhythmias, emboli, and infection for 24 hr after withdrawal of lines

ANTICOAGULANT THERAPY

anticoagulant Medication administered to prevent or treat arterial or venous thrombosis; used in treatment of pulmonary embolism, cerebral embolism, and valvular heart disease, and with a heart valve prosthesis

Assessment

Observations findings

Therapeutic serum levels
    Warfarin: protime—1.5 to 2 × control
    Heparin: partial thromboplastin time (PTT)—2 to 3 × control
Hematuria
Pain
    Abdominal
    Flank
Tarry stools
Hematemesis
Epistaxis
Bleeding gums
Hemoptysis
Subcutaneous bleeding
Ecchymosis
Hematoma
Joints
    Pain
    Immobility
Site of incision
    Bleeding
    Immobility
Neurological changes
Increased menstrual flow
Medications
    Potentiate anticoagulation
    Retard anticoagulation

Interventions

Administer parenteral heparin as ordered
    Use heparin lock if ordered
    Give heparin at exact time ordered
    Give dosage over a period of 1 min
    Never skip doses
    Do not remove heparin lock for 2 hr after last dose
    Maintain continuous heparin infusion if ordered
    Never hang more than 4 hr dose at one time; observe rate q30min
    Administer subcutaneous heparin as ordered, rotating sites
    Corrdinate all laboratory work; avoid multiple punctures
    Maintain manual pressure for at least 3 min after venous punctures
    Check puncture sites qh
    Monitor BP and P q4h to 8h

Avoid taking rectal temperature
Administer IM medications cautiously; apply manual pressure to injection sites until bleeding stops
Have protamine sulfate or phytonadione (Aqua-Mephyton) available
Administer routine medications cautiously; may potentiate or retard anticoagulation

Warfarin

Patient Teaching/Discharge Outcome

Ensure that patient and/or significant other knows and understands
    Name of medication, dosage, time of administration, purpose, and side effects
    Need to avoid taking over-the-counter medications without checking with physician; to read labels of all medications
        Cold prescriptions with aspirin
        Laxatives
        Vitamins
    Need to avoid aspirin (acetylsalicylic acid) without physician's order
    Need for diet with moderate-to-low fat content without abundance of dark, leafy green vegetables; to avoid excessive use of alcohol
    Importance of having laboratory work done as ordered and of contacting physician for possible dosage change
    General side effects: anorexia, nausea, vomiting, abdominal cramps, dermatitis, and urticaria
    Signs of bleeding to report to physician
        Hematuria
        Vomiting
        Elevated temperature
        Pain in joints, swelling
        Epistaxis
        Bleeding gums
        Easy bruisability
        Increased menstrual flow
        Abdominal pain
    Safety precautions to prevent injury
        Avoid vigorous nose-blowing and toothbrushing
        Avoid use of sharp-edge instruments such as razors
        Refrain from water-jet tooth cleaners; use soft-bristled toothbrush
        Refrain from engaging in dangerous hobbies or contact sports
        Wear shoes and slippers at all times
    Importance of avoiding pregnancy while on medication; need to report to physician if pregnancy is suspected
    Need to avoid use of intrauterine device (IUD) for birth control
    Importance of ongoing outpatient care
    Need to carry medical alert or identification care with name of medication

Need to inform physician when planning to travel in order to
    Obtain extra medications
    Arrange laboratory test

Subcutaneous Heparin Injection
Assessment
Observations/findings

Subcutaneous bleeding
    Hematoma
    Bruises
    Intraabdominal bleeding
        Pain
        Rigid, tender abdomen
    Tarry stools
    Bleeding gums
    Epistaxis
    Hematemesis
    Hemoptysis
    Hematuria
    Injection sites
        Inflammation
        Bruises
        Tenderness
    Increased menstrual flow
    Allergic reactions
        Itching
        Urticaria
        Redness
    Joints
        Pain
        Immobility
    Pain
        Flank
        Abdominal

Patient Teaching/Discharge Outcome
General guidelines

Ensure that patient and/or significant other knows and understands
    Name of medication, dosage, time of administration, purpose, and side effects
    Importance of giving heparin injections at exact time designated
    Importance of not skipping any doses; keep record of all missed doses
    Need to avoid taking over-the-counter medications without checking with physician
        Aspirin
        Salicylates
    Need to avoid drinking alcoholic beverages while on heparin therapy
    Importance of having laboratory work done as ordered
    Signs of bleeding to report to physician
        Bleeding gums

        Joint pain
        Epistaxis
        Hematuria
        Tarry stools
        Increased menstrual flow
        Easy bruisability
    Safety precautions to prevent injury
        Avoid vigorous nose-blowing
        Avoid vigorous toothbrushing
        Avoid use of sharp-edged instruments such as razors
        Refrain from engaging in dangerous hobbies or contact sports
    Importance of preventing pregnancy while on medication; need to report to physician if pregnancy is suspected
    Need to avoid use of IUD for birth control
    Importance of taking correct dosage at correct time
Demonstrate and explain purpose of each step of heparin therapy
    Preparation for injection
    Rotation of injection sites
    Action of heparin
    Care of equipment
Have patient repeat steps verbally and then perform procedure
Positively reinforce proper performance of procedure and correct errors
Leave equipment at bedside for practice: syringe (1 to 2 ml with needle (25-gauge, ½ to ⅝ inch), vial of sterile water, alcohol swabs, and flat sponge or orange
Arrange to have equipment that will be used at home available
Have patient continue procedure with supervision while in hospital

Preparation of injection

Ensure that patient and/or significant other demonstrates
    Handwashing technique
    Preparation of syringe and needle using sterile technique
    Withdrawal of exact heparin dosage
    Ability to maintain sterile technique throughout procedure

Site of injection

Ensure that patient and/or significant other knows and understands
    Importance of using subcutaneous fatty tissue and avoiding bruised areas, hematomas, incisions, or scarred tissue and the area within 5 cm (2 inches) of umbilicus
    Importance of rotating site of injection with every dose of heparin to prevent bleeding or tissue damage
    Importance of recording site of each injection

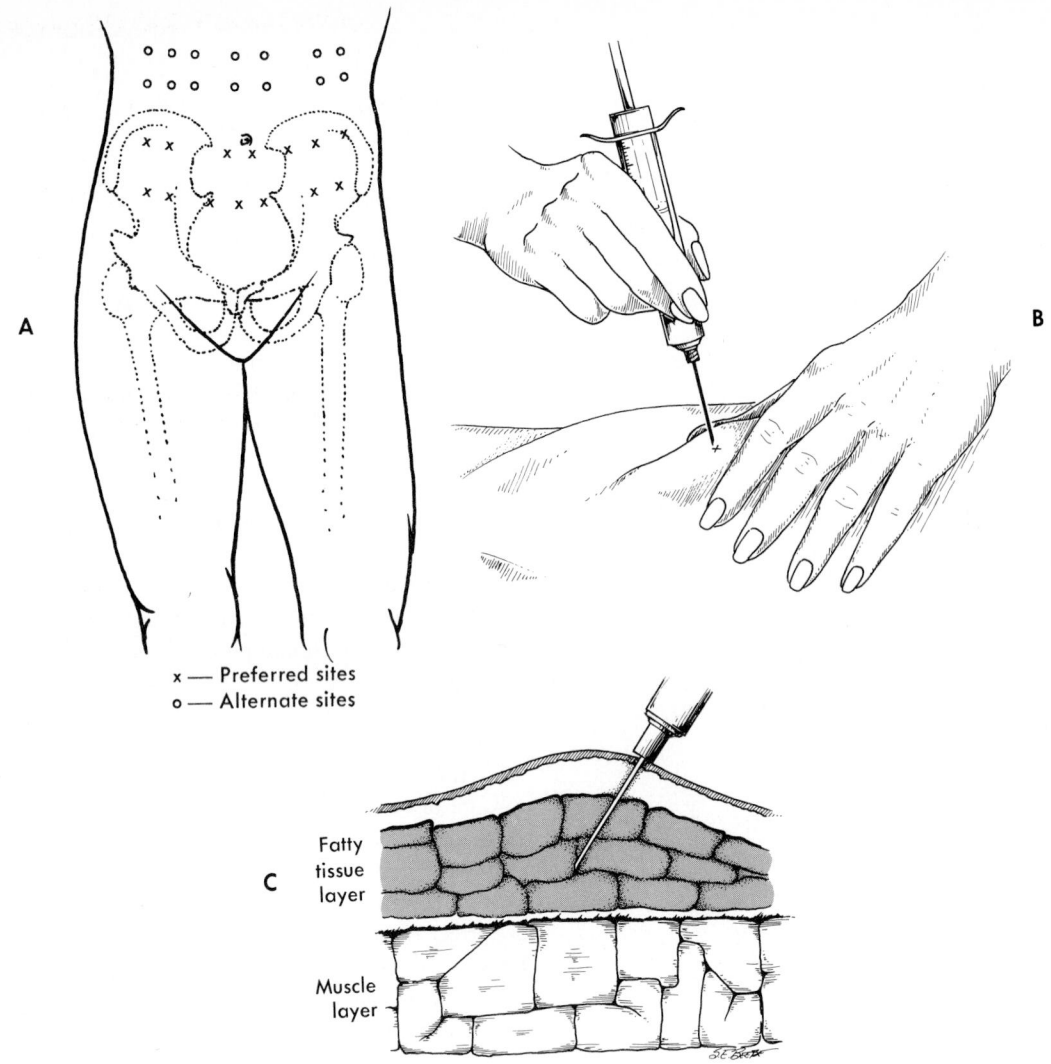

FIGURE 2-47. Subcutaneous heparin injection. **A,** Sites to be used. **B,** Pinching skin to form a flat roll between fingers. **C,** Injection into fatty tissue layer.

Injection

Ensure that patient and/or significant other demonstrates injection technique

    Select injection site (Figure 2-47, A)

    Prepare skin by cleaning with alcohol

    Hold syringe filled with correct heparin dosage like a pencil or a dart

    Pinch up skin, forming a fat roll between fingers (Figure 2-47, B)

    Insert needle at 45-degree angle and quickly push it into subcutaneous tissue up to hub of syringe; may need to guide patient's hand at this point (Figure 2-47, C)

NOTE: Do not pull back on plunger

Inject medication slowly

Withdraw needle; gently release skin as needle is removed

Press area gently; avoid rubbing or massaging area

Record date, time, site, and dosage of each injection on home record (see following)

Heparin Home Record*			
Date	**Time**	**Site**	**Dosage**
1/22/91	6:30 AM	Right upper side	5000 U
	2:30 PM	Left upper side	5000 U
	10:30 PM	Right lower side	5000 U
1/23/91			
1/24/91			

*Physician's order—5000 U heparin injected every 8 hr.

BIBLIOGRAPHY

Abels LF: *Mosby's manual of critical care,* St Louis, 1979, CV Mosby.

Allen JA, Throm L: Percutaneous transluminal coronary angioplasty: a new alternative for ischemic heart disease, *Crit Care Nurse* 2(1):24, 1982.

American Heart Association: *Guidelines for cardiac rehabilitation,* ed 2, Los Angeles, 1982, American Heart Association, Greater Los Angeles Affiliation.

American Heart Association: *Standards and guidelines for cardiopulmonary resuscitation and emergency cardiac care,* JAMA 225:2841, 1986.

American Nurses' Association, Division of Medical-Surgical Nursing Practice, and American Heart Association, Council on Cardiovascular Nursing: *Standards of cardiovascular nursing,* Kansas City, MO, 1981, American Nurses' Association

Andreoli K et al: *Comprehensive cardiac care,* ed 6, St Louis, 1987, CV Mosby.

Braunwald E, ed: *Heart disease: a textbook of cardiovascular medicine,* Philadelphia, 1988, WB Saunders.

Budassi SA, Barber JM: *Emergency nursing: principles and practice,* ed 2, St Louis, 1985, CV Mosby.

Canobbio MM: *Cardiovascular disorders,* St Louis, 1990, Mosby–Year Book.

Canobbio MM: Cardiovascular system. In Thompson JM et al: *Mosby's manual of clinical nursing,* ed 2, St Louis, 1989, Mosby–Year Book.

Cobey JC, Covey JH: Chronic leg ulcers, *Am J Nurs,* 74:258, 1974.

Conover MH: *Exercises in diagnosing ECG tracings,* ed 3, St Louis, 1984, CV Mosby.

Conover MH: *Pocket guide to electrocardiography,* ed 2, St Louis, 1990; Mosby–Year Book.

Costrini NV, Thomson WM: *Manual of medical therapeutics,* ed 22, Boston, 1977, Little, Brown.

Dasling MC et al: Surgery of the aorta, CCQ 8:25, 1985.

Doyle B: Nursing challenge: the patient with end stage heart failure. In Kern LS: *Cardiac critical care,* Rockville, Md, 1988, Aspen Publishers.

Doyle JE: Treatment modalities in peripheral vascular disease, *Nurs Clin North Am* 21(2):241, 1986.

Fardy PA et al: *Cardiac rehabilitation: implication for the nurse and other health professionals,* St Louis, 1980, CV Mosby.

Foreman MD: Arterial prosthetic graft infections: the pathophysiologic basis of nursing care, *Focus Crit Care* 12:23, 1985.

Fowkes WC, Hunn VK: *Clinical assessment for the nurse practitioner,* St Louis, 1973, CV Mosby.

Gershan JA, Jiricka MK: Percutaneous transluminal coronary angioplasty: implications for nursing, *Focus Crit Care* 11:28, 1984.

Giles ID: Principles of vasodilator therapy for left ventricular congestive heart failure, *Heart Lung* 9(2):271, 1980.

Goldberger AL, Goldberger E: *Clinical electrocardiography: a simplified approach,* ed 4, St Louis, 1990, Mosby–Year Book.

Goldberger E: *Textbook of clinical cardiology,* St Louis, 1982, CV Mosby.

Guzzetta EE, Dossey DM: *Cardiovascular nursing: bodymind tapestry,* St Louis, 1984, CV Mosby.

Harris L, et al: The cardiovascular effects of caffeine post-myocardial infarction, *Circulation* 72(Suppl III):116, 1985.

Herman JA: Nursing assessment and nursing diagnosis in patients with peripheral vascular disease, *Nurs Clin North Am* 21:219, 1986.

Isaacson J et al: Post pump psychosis, *Crit Care Nurse* 14:83, 1982.

Jamieson SW et al: Heart transplantation for end-stage ischemic heart disease: the standard experience, *Heart Transplant,* 3:224, 1984.

Johanson BC et al: Standards for critical care, St Louis, ed 3, 1988, CV Mosby.

Joint National Committee: The 1984 Report of the National Committee on Detection, Evaluation, and Treatment of High Blood Pressure, *Arch Intern Med* 144:1045, 1989.

Katsaros C, Bobb J: Shock—the critical hour, *JEN* 4:45, 1978.

Khan MIG: *Manual of cardiac drug therapy,* London, 1984, Baillière Tindall.

Kim HS, Chung EK: Torsades de pointes: polymorphous ventricular tachycardia, *Heart Lung* 12(3):296, 1983.

King O: *Care of the cardiac surgical patient,* St Louis, 1975, CV Mosby.

Kossowsky WA, Lyon AF, and Spain DM: Repraisal of the postmyocardial infarction Dressler's syndrome, *Am Heart J* 102:(5):954, 1981.

Lasater MG: Torsades de pointes: etiology and treatment, *Focus Crit Care* 13(5):17, 1986.

Loan T: Nursing interaction with patients undergoing coronary angioplasty, *Heart Lung* 15(4):369, 1986.

Long GD: Managing the patient with abdominal aortic aneurysm, *Nursing '78* 8:20, 1978.

Lundin DV: You can inject heparin subcutaneously, *RN* 41:51, 1978.

Massey JA: Diagnostic testing for peripheral vascular disease, *Nurs Clin North Am* 21:207, 1986.

Massie BM, Chatterjee K: Vasodilator therapy of pump failure complicating acute myocardial infarction, *Med Clin North Am* 63:25, 1979.

McCarthy JJ, Williams LR: Femoral artery reconstruction, *CCQ* 8:39, 1985.

McCauley K, Weaver TE: Cardiac and pulmonary disease: nutritional implications, *Nurs Clin North Am* 18(1):81, 1983.

Michaelson C: Bedside assessment and diagnosis of acute left ventricular failure. In Canobbio M, ed: Issues in cardiology, *CCQ* 4(3):1, 1981.

Miller DC, Roon AJ: *Diagnosis and management of peripheral vascular disease,* Menlo Park, Calif, 1982, Addison-Wesley Publishing.

Moore K, Maschak BJ: How patient education can reduce the hazards of anticoagulation, *Nursing '77* 7:24, 1977.

Moore SJ: Pericarditis after acute myocardial infarction: manifestations and nursing implications, *Heart Lung* 3(3):551, 1979.

Nurse's Reference Library: *Drugs,* Horsham, Pa, 1982, Intermed Communications.

Ott BB: Percutaneous transluminal coronary angioplasty and nursing implications, *Heart Lung* 11(4):294, 1982.

Painain GA et al: Cardiac transplantation: indications, procurement, operation and management, *Heart Lung* 14:484, 1985.

Parsonnet V et al: A revised code for pacemaker identification: pacemaker study group, *Circulation* 64:60A, 1981.

Reid CL et al: Infective endocarditis: improved diagnosis and treatment, *Current Probl Cardiol* 10:6, 1985.

Riedinger MS, Shellock FG: Technical aspects of the thermodilution method for measuring cardiac output, *Heart Lung* 13(3):215, 1984.

Sadler D: *Nursing for cardiovascular health,* East Norwalk, Conn, 1984, Appleton-Century-Crofts.

Sexton DL: The patient with peripheral arterial occlusive disease, *Nurs Clin North Am* 12:89, 1977.

Spann JF: Pericarditis: diagnosis and complications. In *Chest pain: problems in differential diagnosis,* vol 6, Kansas City, Mo, 1981, Biomedical Marion Laboratories.

Spillall JA: Office diagnosis of occlusive arterial disease, *J Cardiovasc Med,* p 107, 1984.

Swearingen PL et al: *Manual of critical care: applying nursing diagnosis to adult critical illness,* ed 2, St Louis, 1991, Mosby–Year Book.

Thelan L et al: *Textbook of critical care nursing: diagnosis and management,* St Louis, 1990, Mosby–Year Book.

Tikian AG, Daily EK: *Cardiovascular procedures: diagnostic techniques and therapeutic procedures,* St Louis, 1986, CV Mosby.

Underhill S et al: *Cardiac nursing,* ed 2, Philadelphia, 1989, JB Lippincott.

Webb PH: Neurological deficit after carotid endarterectomy, *Am J Nurs* 79(4):654, 1979.

Weiland AP, Walker WE: Physiologic principles and clinical sequelae of cardiopulmonary bypass, *Heart Lung* 15(1):34, 1986.

Whitman G, Hicks LE: Major nursing diagnosis, following cardiac transplantation, *J Cardiovas Nurs* 2:1, 1988.

Young JR: Thrombophlebitis and chronic venous insufficiency, *Geriatrics* 28:63, 1973.

3
CHAPTER

Hematologic System

HEMATOLOGIC ASSESSMENT*

General

Age
Sex
Ethnic background
Cultural background
Appearance
  Stated age equals appearance
  Pallor
  Facial flushing
  Profuse perspiration
  Signs of pain
  Dehydration
  Abnormal body posture, movements, or gait
  Activity level
Vital signs
  T, P, R, or BP changes
  Height and weight changes

Integumentary System

Skin and mucous membranes
  Complaints of
    Pruritus
    Easy bruisability
    Lesions, cuts, infections that do not heal
  Pallor
  Cyanosis
  Plethora
  Erythema
  Jaundice
  Petechiae
  Ecchymosis
  Purpuric lesions
  White patches
  Telangiectasis
  Rashes
  Subcutaneous nodules
  Infiltrates
  Vesicles
  Nonhealing lesions
  Increased skin temperature
  Drainage
  Ulcers
  Diaphoresis
  Turgor
  Note distribution of abnormalities

Nails
  Brittle
  Ridges
  Flattened
  Spoon shaped
  Clubbed
  Loosened
Hair
  Texture
  Growth patterns
Eyes
  Edema
  Redness
  Inflammation
  Infection
  Enlarged/engorged vessels
  Vessel tortuosity
  Infiltration
  Hemorrhage
  Cataracts
  Position
  Alignment

Gastrointestinal System

Complaints of
  Nausea
  Vomiting
  Dysphagia
  Anorexia
  Weight loss
Mouth
  Red mucous membranes
  Bleeding of gums and mucosa
  Stomatitis
  Purpura
  Telangiectasis
  Tonsillar hypertrophy
  Gingival hypertrophy
  Ulcers
Tongue
  Complaints of pain
  Appearance
    Beefy
    Swollen
  Texture
    Absence of papillae
    Furrows
  Color: red

*See Table 3-1 on p. 156 for possible assessment conclusions.

Abdomen
  Splenomegaly
  Hepatomegaly
Frank, occult bleeding in stool

Cardiovascular System

Complaints of
  Palpitations
  Shortness of breath
  Fatigue
    After exertion
    All the time
  Angina
Murmurs
Dysrhythmias
Tachycardia
Extremities
  Color
  Response to temperature changes

Respiratory System

Orthopnea
Tachypnea
Dyspnea
Rhythm
Excursion
Breath sounds change

Musculoskeletal System

Range of motion (ROM)
Joints/bones
  Swelling
  Pain
  Stiffness
Romberg's sign
Soft tissue
  Edema
  Hematoma
  Abscess

Genitourinary System

Hematuria
Incontinence
Impotence
Heavy menses

Neurological System

Complaints of
  Headache
  Numb, tingling extremities
  Paresthesia
  Weakness
  Frequent napping
  Sleeplessness
Behavior/mood changes
Changes in attention span and responses

Pertinent Background Information

CONCURRENT DISEASES OR CONDITIONS

Frequent illness
Infectious processes
Blood transfusion/component therapy
Multiple allergies
Asthma
Bleeding tendency
Hemorrhage
Renal, cardiovascular, or liver disorders
Cancer

PREVIOUS SURGERY OR ILLNESS

Gastric ulcers
Gastric surgery
Hepatic surgery
Cardiac surgery
Renal surgery
Radioactive exposure and irradiation
Exposure to chemical agents
Recurrent infectious processes: frequent sore throats, etc.

FAMILY HISTORY

Cancer
Blood dyscrasias, anemias
Immune disorders
Allergies
Rh incompatibility

SOCIAL HISTORY

Smoking
Alcohol use
Increased stress
Occupation; exposure to toxic substances
Environmental factors
Diet
  Recent changes
  Cultural or religious restrictions
  Decreased protein intake
  Fad diets

MEDICATION HISTORY

Immunizations
Prescription medications
  Present medications
  Previously taken medications (e.g., chloramphenicol)
Over-the-counter medications
Home remedies
Use of other drugs

Diagnostic Aids

LABORATORY STUDIES (see Figures 3-1 and 3-2)

Complete blood cell count (CBC)
White blood cell count (WBC)/differential
Hematocrit (Hct)
Hemoglobin (Hgb)

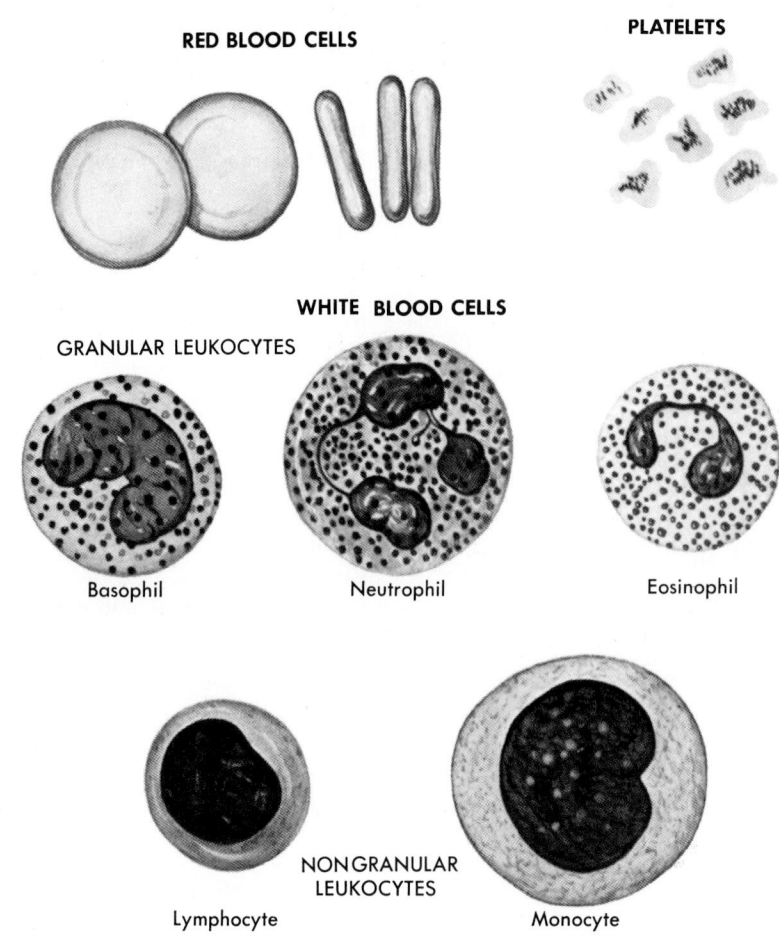

RED BLOOD CELLS

PLATELETS

WHITE BLOOD CELLS

GRANULAR LEUKOCYTES

Basophil

Neutrophil

Eosinophil

NONGRANULAR
LEUKOCYTES

Lymphocyte

Monocyte

FIGURE 3-1. Human blood cells. (From Anthony CP, Kolthoff NJ: *Textbook of anatomy and physiology,* ed 12, St Louis, 1987, CV Mosby.)

Reticulocyte count
Platelet count
Mean corpuscular volume (MCV)
Mean corpuscular hemoglobin concentration (MCHC)
Mean corpuscular hemoglobin (MCH)
Bleeding time
Prothrombin time (PT)
Partial thromboplastin time (PTT)
Thrombin time
Activated partial thromboplastin time
Sedimentation rate
Electrophoresis of serum proteins
Immunoelectrophoresis of serum proteins
Total protein
Fibrinogen
Electrolyte values
Bilirubin level
Direct/indirect Coombs' test
Factor assay
Total iron-binding capacity

Serum iron level
Ferritin titers
Sideroblasts
Gastric analysis
Schilling test
Human lymphoctye antigens (HLA)
Sickle-cell test

OTHER PROCEDURES

Biopsies
   Bone marrow
   Lymph nodes
   Spleen
   Liver
Chest and abdominal x-ray examinations
Computed tomography (CT) scans
   Bone
   Liver
Intravenous pyelogram (IVP)

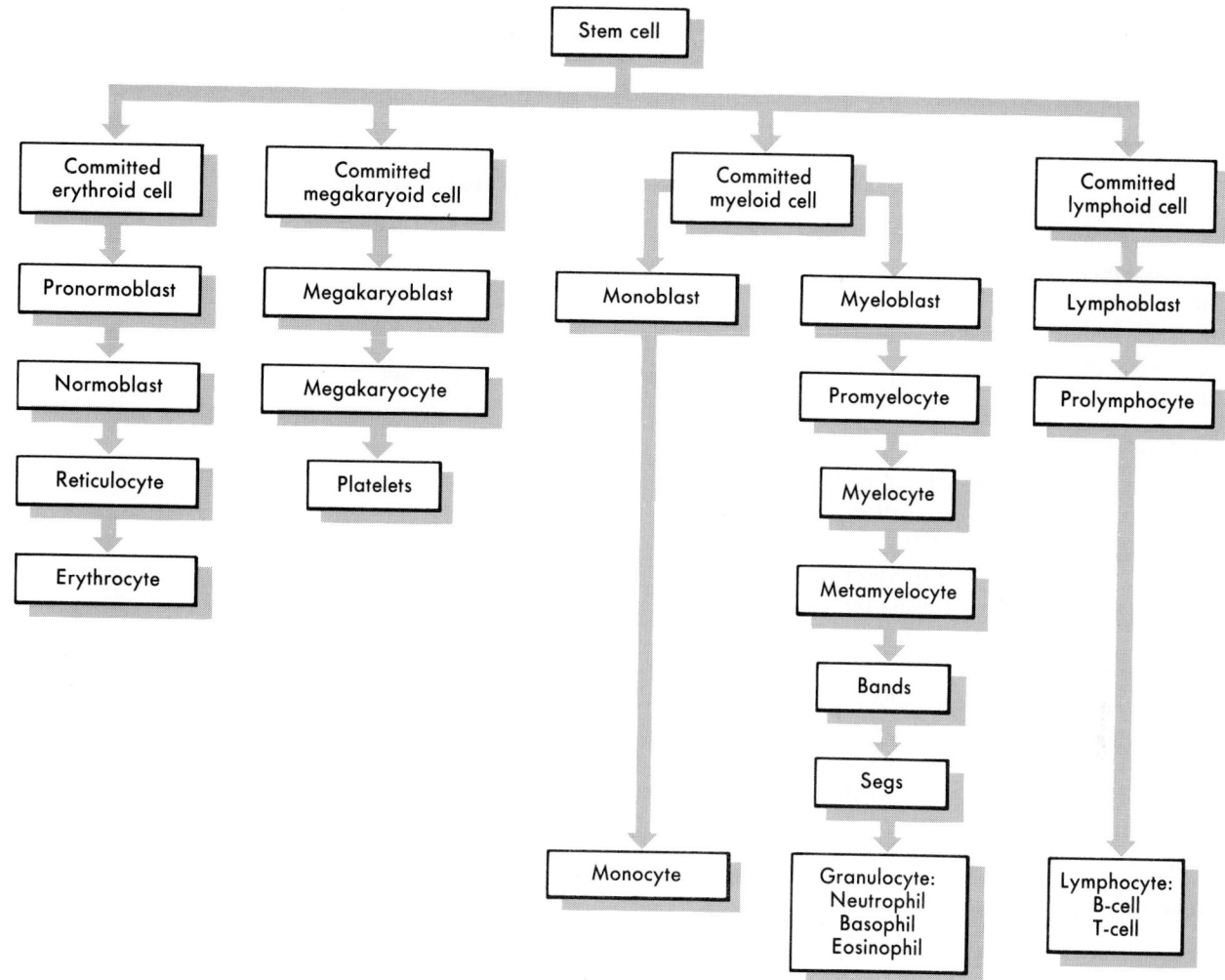

FIGURE 3-2. Formation and maturation of blood cells. All circulating blood cells originate from a common stem cell. (From Beare PG, Myers IL: *Principles and practice of adult health nursing,* St Louis, 1990, Mosby–Year Book.)

PERNICIOUS ANEMIA (HYPERCHROMIC MACROCYTIC ANEMIA)

Defective red blood cell production caused by lack of the intrinsic factor essential for absorption of vitamin B$_{12}$ (deficiency of vitamin B$_{12}$ causes gastric, intestinal, and neurologic abnormalities)

Assessment

Observations/findings

Central nervous system
 Fatigue
 Weakness
 Paresthesia of hands and feet
 Impaired fine finger movement
 Disturbed coordination and position sense; loss of vibratory sense; ataxia
 Positive Romberg's and Babinski's signs
 Disturbances in vision, taste, and hearing
 Irritability
 Poor memory
 Impaired judgment
 Depression
Gastrointestinal
 Tongue: beefy red, smooth, painful
 Nausea, vomiting
 Anorexia
 Flatulence
 Diarrhea
 Constipation
 Weight loss
Cardiovascular
 Palpitations

Tachycardia
Wide pulse pressure
Dyspnea
Orthopnea
Integumentary
  Skin: waxy, pale to bright lemon-yellow
  Sclera: slight jaundice
  Lips and gums: verypale
Increased susceptibility to infection
Family history of disease
Ethnic background: primarily Northern European
Age: usually between 50 and 60
Previous surgery: gastrectomy

Laboratory/diagnostic studies

Hemoglobin may be reduced to 4 to 5 g/100 ml
Decreased red blood cell count (RBC)
Elevated MCV, MCHC, MCH
RBCs of variable, abnormal size (anisocytosis)
RBCs of variable abnormal shape (poikilocytosis)
Serum $B_{12} < 0.1$ µg/ml
Decreased Schilling test
Bone marrow aspiration: erythroid hyperplasia, increased
  megaloblasts, and few normally developing RBCs
Decreased WBC
Gastric analysis: absence of free hydrochloric acid after
  pengastrin or histamine injection
Upper GI series: atrophy of gastric mucosa

Potential complications

Cardiomegaly
Congestive heart failure (CHF)

Gastritis
Paralysis
Paranoia
Hallucinations, delusions
Infection, usually genitourinary

Medical Management

Vitamin B_{12} replacement therapy
Iron replacement, initially
Antifungal, analgesic mouth rinse
Vital signs, pulse pressure monitoring

Nursing diagnoses/interventions/evaluation

■ **NDX:** Activity intolerance related to imbalance between oxygen supply and demand

If patient is on bed rest
  Maintain position of comfort
  Perform active or passive ROM exercises qid
  Assist with ADLs and ambulation to conserve energy
Plan undisturbed rest periods to conserve energy and permit performance of activities patient desires
Monitor pulse and respiratory rate qid and during activities
Assess adverse responses to activities: tachycardia, dysrhythmias, dyspnea, etc.
Set goals with patient to increase activities as symptoms of intolerance decrease
Explain that activity tolerance will increase with therapy

Expected outcome/evaluation

Patient performs ADLs without evidence of exertional

TABLE 3-1. Approach to Hematologic Disorders; Various Clues That may be Found*

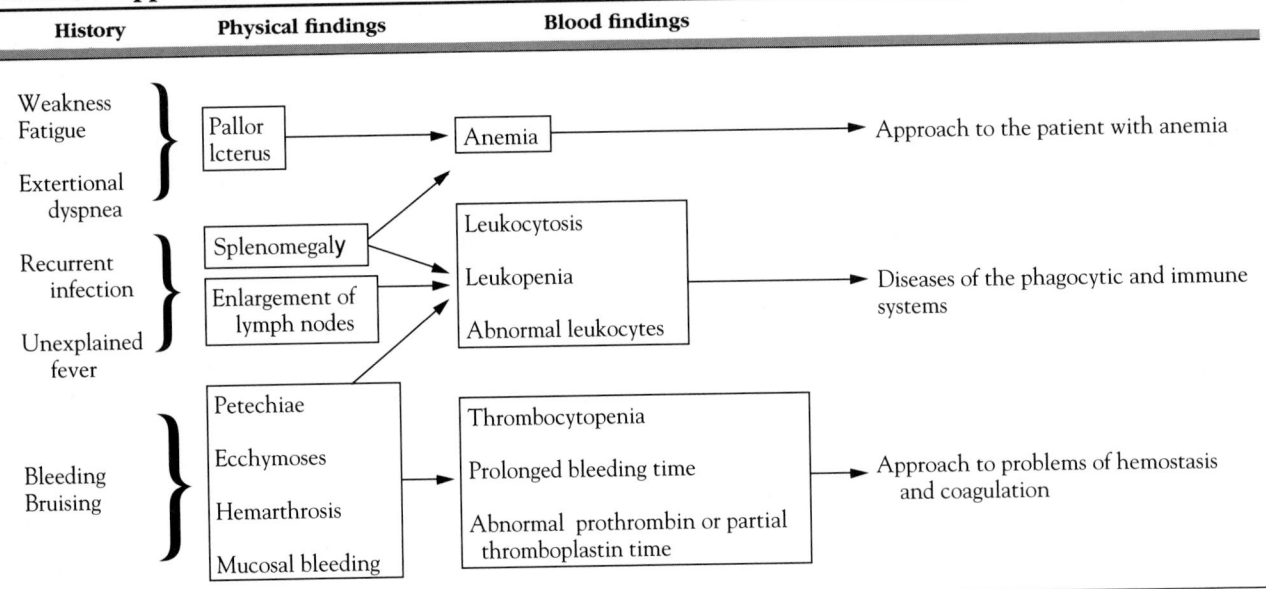

History	Physical findings	Blood findings	
Weakness / Fatigue / Extertional dyspnea	Pallor / Icterus	Anemia	Approach to the patient with anemia
Recurrent infection / Unexplained fever	Splenomegaly / Enlargement of lymph nodes	Leukocytosis / Leukopenia / Abnormal leukocytes	Diseases of the phagocytic and immune systems
Bleeding / Bruising	Petechiae / Ecchymoses / Hemarthrosis / Mucosal bleeding	Thrombocytopenia / Prolonged bleeding time / Abnormal prothrombin or partial thromboplastin time	Approach to problems of hemostasis and coagulation

From Wintrobe MM et al: *Clinical hematology,* Philadelphia, 1981, Lea & Febiger.
*Features in the history, physical examination, or preliminary blood examination that can guide the examiner toward the solution of a clinical problem.

dyspnea or tachycardia; activity level is progressing to preillness state

■ **NDX:** Altered nutrition: less than body requirements, related to achlorhydria, anorexia, and diarrhea

Monitor intake and output q8h
Weigh daily; same time, scale, and clothing
  Report 2% decrease in weight
Provide foods and fluids to 2500 ml of patient's choice
  Avoid foods that are GI irritants; spicy, flatus-forming foods and those with caffeine
Provide six small feedings or between-meal nourishment to enhance appetite
Assist with meals when necessary to conserve energy
Present food attractively arranged
Encourage visitors of patient's choice to remain during meals
Monitor and record character, amount, color, and frequency of stools; administer antidiarrheal medication as indicated

Expected outcome/evaluation

Patient's weight is increasing toward normal for patient. Patient is taking balanced diet with fluids to 2000 ml; intake and output are balanced

■ **NDX:** Altered oral mucous membrane related to nutritional imbalance

Assess oral cavity q8h
Administer oral hygiene q2h and before and after meals
Use dilute mouthwash or normal saline mouth rinse
Choose brush or sponge cleaners depending on severity of oral alteration and patient's tolerance
Use water-soluble jelly on lips
For severe oral discomfort, medicate with topical analgesics 30 min before meals
Have patient avoid irritating, hard-to-chew foods
Encourage fluids; iced liquids or popsicles may be soothing

Expected outcome/evaluation

Patient's oral mucosa, especially tongue, is moist and pink; no report of discomfort

■ **NDX:** Potential for injury related to risk of sensory-motor deficits

Maintain safe environment
Provide safety measures when needed: side rails up, bed in low position if patient is on bed rest
Assess for absence of neurological deficit before ambulation
Remind patient to call for assistance when needed

Remove obstacles and keep furniture in place when patient is ambulatory
Have patient use support-type slippers or shoes, walkers, canes, or other assistive devices when needed
Assess skin integrity bid
Ensure that bath/shower water will not burn and that oral fluids are of moderate temperature
Provide warmth through use of extra blankets or layers of clothing; avoid use of heating devices
Keep articles out of bed and prevent wrinkles
Avoid use of restrictive clothing and shoes

Expected outcome/evaluation

Patient does not sustain an injury because of sensory-motor deficits

■ **NDX:** Potential for infection related to risk of increased susceptibility secondary to decrease in WBC

Assess for signs of infection q8h
Have patient avoid contact with infectious persons
Instruct patient in handwashing technique and when to perform
Teach patient to turn, cough, and deep breathe q4h
Encourage ambulation as soon as patient is able
Give fluids to 2500 ml/day unless contraindicated
Provide undisturbed rest and sleep periods

Expected outcome/evaluation

Patient exhibits no evidence of infection in any body system

■ **NDX:** Knowledge deficit related to lack of exposure to accurate information regarding medication, disease process, nutrition, and activities

Medication

Explain need to take vitamin B_{12} on ongoing basis; teach method for administration, name of medication, dosage, time of administration, purpose, and side effects
Instruct patient to avoid over-the-counter medications without checking with physician

Disease process

Instruct patient to observe and report symptoms of recurrence to physician; explain that symptoms will recede with continuing therapy (check with physician for symptoms that may be irreversible)
Arrange for visits by public health nurse if needed
Instruct patient to continue follow-up care with physician and laboratory

Nutrition

Explain need to maintain balanced diet and fluid intake

Activity requirements

Explain need to increase activities gradually to desired level as tolerated

Instruct patient to assess pulse rate and rhythm during activity/exercise and to stop if dysrhythmia is apparent

Explain need to avoid fatigue, to maintain planned rest periods

Instruct patient to use safety precautions when needed

Expected outcome/evaluation

Patient and/or significant other verbalizes understanding of home and follow-up care and demonstrates method for medication administration and assessment of pulse

IRON DEFICIENCY ANEMIA (HYPOCHROMIC, MICROCYTIC ANEMIA)

Defective red blood cell production resulting from depletion of iron stores in the body needed to synthesize hemoglobin

Assessment
Observations/findings

Neuromuscular
    Weakness
    Fatigue
    Vertigo
    Headache
    Inability to concentrate
    Irritability
    Numb, tingling extremities
Gastrointestinal
    Heartburn
    Anorexia
    Pica
    Glossitis
    Stomatitis
    Dysphagia
    Flatulence
    Vague abdominal pains
    Poor skin turgor
    Poor nutrition; inadequate iron intake
    Weight loss
    Chronic diarrhea
    Gastrectomy
    Chronic malabsorption syndrome
Cardiovascular
    Palpitations
    Tachycardia
    Functional systolic murmur
    Dizziness
    Tachypnea
    Dyspnea on exertion
    Sensitivity to cold
    Ankle edema

Integumentary
    Pale skin, mucous membranes
    Blue or pearl-white sclera
    Brittle, spoon-shaped fingernails
Chronic blood loss
    Gastrointestinal (GI) bleeding
    Heavy menses

Laboratory/diagnostic studies

Serum iron <55 mm/100 ml
Iron-binding capacity >350 µg/100 ml
Hgb: 6 to 10 g/100 ml; rings 6.2 to 6.8 µm in diameter
Decreased MCV
Decreased MCHC
Decreased MCH
Poikilocytosis marked
Reduced reticulocytes
Bone marrow studies: depleted or absent iron stores; normoblastic hyperplasia

Potential complications

Chest pain
Cardiomegaly
Hemoglobinuria

Medical Management

Iron therapy, orally or parenterally
Diet high in iron-rich foods
Antifungal, anesthetic-type mouth rinse
Ascorbic acid
Stool softeners, laxatives

PRECAUTIONS IN IRON THERAPY ADMINISTRATION

ORAL

Use straw to prevent staining teeth

IM

Use second needle after withdrawing solution from ampule to avoid staining tissue
Use Z-tract method of injection
Inject 0.5 ml of air before removing needle from tissue

IV

Administer test dose
Remain with patient to assess for symptoms of shock
Use small gauge needle
Cover solution with dark plastic

Nursing diagnoses/interventions/evaluation

■ **NDX:** Altered nutrition: less than body requirements, related to gastrointestinal involvement

Provide six small feedings if easily fatigued

Provide foods of patient's preference and according to condition of oral mucosa; be certain that patient receives all required nutrients

Serve trays attractively arranged; remove uneaten, undesired food immediately

Assist with cutting foods, opening containers, and pouring liquids to conserve energy for eating

Have family visit during meals to provide company and assistance when necessary

Administer iron therapy as ordered (see box above)

Administer ascorbic acid if ordered

Avoid constipation: increase fluids and bulky foods

Weigh patient daily at same time with same clothing and scale

Expected outcome/evaluation

Weight is increasing toward patient's normal range; balanced diet and fluids are maintained

■ **NDX:** Altered oral mucous membrane related to nutritional imbalance

Assess oral cavity q8h

Administer oral hygiene q4h and before and after meals

Choose soft-bristled brush or sponge cleaners, depending on severity of oral alteration and patient's tolerance

Use dilute mouth wash or normal saline mouth rinse

Use water-soluble jelly on lips

Medicate with topical analgesics 30 min before meals for oral discomfort

Avoid irritating hard-to-chew foods

Expected outcome/evaluation

Patient's oral mucosa is pink and moist; reports no discomfort

■ **NDX:** Potential for injury related to risk of hypoxia as evidenced by vertigo, numbness, or tingling of extremities

Provide a safe environment free of obstacles

Add warmth with extra bedclothes, warm robes, etc., when needed; avoid use of uncontrolled-temperature heating devices

Instruct patient to sit at side of bed and then stand before walking to determine whether dizziness is present

Direct patient to call for assistance with ambulation when needed

Assist with hygiene and other care to prevent injury

Avoid very hot liquids at meal or bath time

Teach patient risk factors and precautions to prevent injury

Expected outcome/evaluation

Patient verbalizes precautions to prevent injury and exhibits no injuries

■ **NDX:** Altered thought processes related to hypoxia as evidenced by decreased concentration and irritability

Evaluate cognitive functioning q8h

Plan care with patient to promote consistency and sense of calmness

Encourage verbalization of concerns about ability to concentrate; assure patient that this will improve with therapy

Inform patient of each step of activity or instruction; do not overload with many, varied instructions at one time

Avoid completing sentences for patient; listen with patience

Provide diversional activities related to patient's ability to concentrate e.g., music of preference, etc.

Expected outcome/evaluation

Patient exhibits increased concentration when performing ADLs and other scheduled activities; signs of irritability are absent

■ **NDX:** Activity intolerance related to imbalance between oxygen supply and demand

Monitor vital signs (BP, P, and R) qid, during and after activity

Assess response to activity

Plan with patient so the desired activities can be performed without exertion

Assist with ADLs, when necessary, to conserve energy

Provide uninterrupted rest periods to maintain energy level

Increase patient activities in small increments until tolerance level is reached

Expected outcome/evaluation

Patient's activity level is progressing to pre-illness state. Performs ADLs without evidence of tachycardia or dyspnea

■ **NDX:** Knowledge deficit related to lack of exposure to accurate information regarding disease process, medication, nutrition, and activities permitted

Medication

Discuss medications: name, dosage, time of administration, purpose, and side effects to report (nausea, vomiting, diarrhea, or constipation)

Explain need to continue iron therapy even though feeling well

Discuss color of stools expected and explain need and methods to avoid constipation

Explain reason for not taking oral iron medication with milk or antacids

Demonstrate method for parenteral administration of iron

Nutrition

Explain importance of maintaining a balanced diet high in iron-rich foods and liquids

Explain importance of monitoring weight weekly

Disease process

Discuss signs and symptoms of recurrence to report to health provider

Activity

Explain importance of increasing exercise and activities to tolerance, alternating with periods of rest

Discuss how to prevent injury through assessment of self-help and ambulation abilities; discuss symptoms that indicate assistance is needed or activities should be decreased

Expected outcome/evaluation

Patient and/or significant other verbalizes home care instructions and demonstrates parenteral administration of medication if applicable

HEMOLYTIC ANEMIA

A disorder characterized by a rapid rate of erythrocyte destruction; ability of the bone marrow to increase the production of erythrocytes determines the extent of anemia present; may occur with inherited or acquired red blood cell disorders, or in response to toxic agents or drugs, infectious disease, or trauma

Assessment
Observations/findings

Inherited RBC disorder
  Fatigue
  Shortness of breath
  Jaundice
  Urine changes
Trauma/infectious disease
  Chills
  Fever
  Weakness
  Jaundice

Irritability
Headache
Nausea
Vomiting
Abdominal pain
Diarrhea
Decreased urinary output
Acquired RBC disorder
  Headache
  Fatigue
  Shortness of breath
  Jaundice
  Nocturnal hemoglobinuria
  Abdominal pain
  Splenomegaly
  Venous thrombosis

Laboratory/diagnostic studies

Increased reticulocyte count
Normocytic anemia
Decreased hematocrit
Increased RBC fragility
Shortened erythrocyte life span
Increased bilirubin

Potential complications

Renal failure
Hemoglobinuria

Medical Management

Elimination of causative factors
Management of primary condition (trauma, e.g., burns; infectious disease)
Parenteral fluids
Washed PRC transfusions
Whole blood transfusions (for rapid, severe hemolysis)
Osmotic diuretics
Corticosteroids
Antidiarrheals
Antiemetics

Nursing diagnoses/interventions/evaluation

■ **NDX:** Fluid volume deficit (2) related to vomiting, diarrhea, and/or hemorrhage

Monitor intake and output q8h; report imbalances

Weigh patient daily at same time with same clothing and scale; report changes of 2% to 3% of original weight

Monitor vital signs and mental status q4h

Assess skin turgor and peripheral pulses q8h

Monitor character, amount, color, and frequency of vomitus or stools

Monitor parenteral fluids, electrolytes, and blood transfusions when administered

Administer antidiarrheals and antiemetics as ordered

Be prepared to collaborate with physician in managing underlying cause

Assess type and amount of foods and liquids tolerated

Provide clear liquid diet to reduce nausea: juices, carbonated beverages, flavored ice popsicles, progressing to balanced diet as symptoms abate

Force fluids to 2500 ml/day unless contraindicated

Enlist patient's assistance

    Provide fluids of choice and temperature

    Offer small amounts frequently (makes taking fluids less of a chore)

    Serve attractively

Arrange for quiet rest periods before meals

Expected outcome/evaluation

Patient's vital signs are stable with balanced intake and output; peripheral pulses are present; extremities are warm with good color and turgor

 NDX: Activity intolerance related to imbalance between oxygen supply and demand, as evidenced by fatigue, weakness, and shortness of breath

Plan with patient so that desired activities can be performed without exertion

Assist with ADLs when necessary to conserve energy

Provide uninterrupted rest periods to maintain energy level

Increase activities patient performs in small increments until tolerance level is reached

Monitor vital signs qid, during and after activities; instruct patient to stop activity if adverse response appears

Assess response to activity; note positive advances

Advise significant others to encourage and assist patient with continuing efforts

Expected outcome/evaluation

Patient's activity level is progressing to pre-illness state; performs ADLs without evidence of tachycardia or dyspnea

 NDX: Pain related to headache and abdominal pain

Maintain environment free of stress

Assess pain: predisposing factors, intensity, frequency, duration, and effective methods of control used by patient; use pain rating scale

Place patient in position of comfort

Change position qh; assist with ROM exercise if helpful

Consider diversional, relaxation, or imagery measures

Administer pain relief medications as ordered at patient's request; assess effectiveness

Expected outcome/evaluation

Patient verbalizes feelings of increased comfort and reports no headache or abdominal pain

■ **NDX:** Potential for impaired skin integrity related to risk of mechanical factors: scratching related to jaundice or pruritus

Assess condition of skin q8h

Monitor laboratory values daily

Administer skin care daily and as needed

    Soothing baths: sodium bicarbonate or oatmeal

    Avoid skin dryness; apply lotions to slightly moist skin

    Cool sponge baths or tub soaks may be beneficial

Keep clothing light with no constrictions

Elevate bedclothes with bed cradle

Keep bed wrinkle-free

Provide linen laundered in nondetergents

Advise patient to avoid scratching; instead, apply pressure or use cool applications

Expected outcome/evaluation

Patient's skin remains intact and moist without evidence of scratching

■ **NDX:** Knowledge deficit related to lack of exposure to accurate information regarding disease process, activity/hygiene, and diet and fluids

Disease process

Instruct patient about type of hemolytic condition

    Hereditary RBC deficiency: patient is susceptible to hemolysis after ingestion of chemical oxidants; family members should be screened

    Response to trauma or infectious disease

        Explain that primary condition will be treated

        Discuss symptoms of recurrence to report

    Acquired RBC deficiency

        Explain that this may be induced by infection, immunization, iron products, or plasma in whole blood transfusions

        Discuss symptoms of recurrence to report

Explain need for ongoing follow-up care

Activity/hygiene

Explain importance of increasing activities daily

Explain need to plan and maintain regular rest and sleep periods

Teach pulse taking and assess any respiratory effort during activities

Instruct patient to decrease activity level if adverse signs appear

Instruct patient to use assistance from others to conserve energy when needed

Explain need to perform daily skin care; discuss products to use to increase comfort, prevent injury, and decrease itching

Diet and fluids

Explain importance of taking at least 2500 ml of fluids each day unless contraindicated

Explain importance of eating a balanced diet and using supplements when necessary

Instruct patient to notify physician or nurse if intake or output decreases significantly as indicated by change in weekly weight

Expected outcome/evaluation

Patient and/or significant other verbalizes understanding of home care and follow-up instructions and demonstrates methods of taking pulse and measuring weight

SICKLE CELL ANEMIA AND CRISIS

A genetic disease that occurs in individuals with a defective hemoglobin molecule (HbS); this defect results in a major rearrangement, and rigid, elongated, crescent-shaped or sickle-shaped cells when oxygen tension is decreased; the microcirculation becomes slowed, and cells adhere to epithelium and clump, causing occlusion and infarction; crisis occurs when a critical point is reached and hemolysis occurs; sickle cell anemia is the most prevalent of the congenital hemolytic anemias and causes a shortened life span

Assessment
Observation/findings

Neurological
    Elevated temperature
    Irritability
    Headaches
Cardiac
    Fatigue
    Tachycardia
    Murmurs
    Dysrhythmias
    Chest pain
    Cardiomegaly
Respiratory
    Dyspnea at rest or with exertion
    Chest pain
GI system
    Vomiting
    Anorexia
    Jaundice
    Hepatomegaly
    Splenomegaly (infant) to impalpable caused by autosplenectomy
Musculoskeletal
    Joint swelling
    Aching bones
Integumentary
    Pallor
    Leg ulcers above ankle
Renal
    Polyuria
    Hematuria
    Enuresis
Increased susceptibility to infection
Infant/child
    Dactylitis
    Failure to thrive
    Impaired growth and development with delayed puberty
Painful crisis
    Severe pain
        Abdomen
        Chest
        Back
        Joints
        Bones
        Muscles
    Increased jaundice
    Dark-colored urine
    Low-grade temperature
Aplastic crisis
    (Associated with infection, usually viral)
        Temperature elevated to 104° F (40° C) or 100° F (37.8° C) for 2 days
        Pallor
        Lethargy
        Sleepiness
        Possible coma
        RBC hemolysis with bone marrow depression
Sequestration crisis (6 mo-2 yr)
    Massive entrapment of RBCs in spleen and liver
    Pallor
    Progressive lethargy
    Hypovolemic shock

Laboratory/diagnostic studies

Sickle-turbidity test—presence of HbS
Hemoglobin electrophoresis
    HbS only indicates sickle cell anemia
Decreased RBC
Elliptocytosis
Nucleated RBC (normoblasts)
Hemoglobin 5-10 g/100 ml
Decreased hematocrit
Decreased ESR
Increased WBC
Increased platelet count
Increased reticulocytes
Increased bilirubin

Potential complications

Cerebral vascular accidents
Subarachnoid hemorrhage
Pulmonary infarction
Massive liver necrosis

Renal failure
Myocardial infarction
Congestive heart failure
Osteomyelitis
Retinopathy
Priapism
Gallstones
Severe infections

Medical Management

Rigorous hydration using parenteral fluids
Oxygenation
Bed rest
Analgesics
Antipyretics
Antibiotics to treat existing infections, if any
Transfusion of packed RBCs
Exchange transfusions for aplastic, hyperhemolytic, and sequestration crises

Nursing diagnoses/interventions/evaluation

■ **NDX:** Potential altered tissue perfusion; cardiopulmonary, cerebral, renal, GI, and/or peripheral related to risk of exchange problems caused by sickling of RBCs or interruption of flow resulting from thrombus formation

Monitor and document vital signs and auscultate chest for heart and breath sounds q2h
  Report changes immediately
Monitor and document level of consciousness and mental status q2h
Maintain bed rest
Position for maximum respiratory excursion
Assess effectiveness of oxygen therapy when administered
Maintain a stress-free environment conducive to rest
  Group required activities; omit routine care when possible
  Control visitors as desired by patient
  Provide uninterrupted periods of time
Assist with care needs; turning, coughing, deep-breathing, elimination, etc., to reduce oxygen need
Monitor administration of packed RBCs carefully to avoid reaction and circulatory overload
Check peripheral pulses q4h
Monitor skin color, turgor, presence of breaks, etc.
Position extremities to maintain circulation and support
Teach and assist with ROM; support joints with movement
Keep warm and dry
Avoid constrictive clothing and bed clothes
Measure and record intake and output q4h to 8h
Monitor and document nausea and vomiting; hematuria, etc.
Weigh daily at same time with same scale and clothing

Provide and encourage intake of fluids of choice to 2500 ml daily
Collaborate with physician to determine parenteral fluid needs; administer carefully, monitoring for overload
Provide small feedings to enhance appetite
  Assist as needed to reduce energy expenditure

Expected outcome/evaluation

Patient's vital signs are stable; oriented and alert; skin is warm, dry, intact with good turgor; is taking diet and fluids; weight is stable, and output is equal to intake

■ **NDX:** Pain related to tissue hypoxia as evidenced by swelling of joints; back, abdominal, or chest pain

Assess pain location, duration, intensity using pain rating scale
Protect painful joints with pillows
Apply warm soaks to joints prn for comfort
Maintain anatomical alignment
Administer back and pressure point care q2h
Move patient using slow gentle movements
Administer analgesics orally or by constant intravenous patient-controlled infusion (PCA) as ordered; assess effectiveness
  Slowly titrate until maximum pain control is achieved
Give analgesics to *prevent* pain
Teach alternate pain relief measures; relaxation, imagery, music therapy, etc.

Expected outcome/evaluation

Patient's posture and face are relaxed; verbalizes comfort

■ **NDX:** Potential for impaired skin integrity related to risk of impaired circulation

Inspect skin for redness, lesions, swelling, or drainage q8h
Keep skin clean and dry
Cleanse with mild soap, rinse well, dry thoroughly
Apply protective cream after bathing and position change
Keep bed linens wrinkle-free and nonconstrictive
Use pull sheet to move patient when on bed rest
Reposition q2h; avoid high Fowler's position for more than 1 hour
Collaborate with physician to determine care for skin breaks and lesions
Assess effectiveness of ordered treatment in 48 hr; discuss with physician if no improvement noted

Expected outcome/evaluation

Patient's skin is warm and dry with good color; breaks, lesions, etc. are healing

NDX: Potential for infection related to risk of inadequate cellular response

Monitor vital signs and breath sounds q4h

Assess for signs of infection in all systems q8h

Administer antipyretics and antibiotics when ordered; assess effectiveness

Use cooling measures carefully to prevent chilling

Prevent exposure to personnel and/or visitors who exhibit signs of infection

Place patient in reverse isolation when ordered

Collaborate with physician to ensure fluid and dietary needs are met

Obtain culture of areas suspected of infection after discussion with physician

Expected outcome/evaluation

Patient's vital signs are stable and within normal limits for patient; there is no evidence of infection

Additional nursing diagnoses to consider

Self-esteem disturbance related to physical, lifestyle, or role losses

Social isolation related to disease process

Sexual dysfunction related to disease process

Other self-perceptual, role, or coping diagnoses

■ **NDX:** Knowledge deficit related to lack of exposure to accurate information regarding preventive measures, home care, and follow-up needs

Discuss need to avoid conditions that precipitate crisis

Infections

Dehydration

Activities that may cause an increase in oxygen requirement: flying in unpressurized planes, high altitudes, cold weather, vasoconstrictive drugs

Explain nutrition requirements and importance of eating a well-balanced diet with fluids to 2000 ml each day; avoid iced drinks and foods

Discuss importance of maintaining relationships with others and participating in meaningful activity and work

Teach that balancing exercise/activity with adequate rest is important

Use stress reduction methods daily

Instruct patient to maintain good hygiene

Teach signs and symptoms of infection to report to physician or nurse; need to avoid exposure to infectious persons, to treat early symptoms, and to have early childhood and yearly immunizations

Instruct about signs and symptoms of recurrence to report to physician

Complaints of pain

Persistent low-grade temperature

Decreased fluid intake

Decreased appetite

Increased lethargy or sleeping

Teach name of medication, purpose, side or toxic effects, time and frequency of administration

Explain that it is necessary to tell all health care givers about disease

Wear medical alert bracelet and keep follow-up appointments

Explain that childbearing may cause some risks to females and refer for gynecologic consultation

Refer family for genetic counseling and psychological counseling when appropriate

Expected outcome/evaluation

Patient verbalizes understanding of conditions that may precipitate a crisis, home care, and follow-up instructions

APLASTIC ANEMIA

Anemia, aplastic or hypoplastic, resulting from destruction of or injury to the bone marrow stem cells or bone marrow matrix; exposure to toxins, specifically large doses of radiation, benzene, metabolites, alkylating agents, chloramphenicol, or sulfonamides, may cause pancytopenia (bone marrow failure with granulocytopenia, thrombocytopenia, and anemia)

Assessment
Observations/findings

Anemia

Waxlike pallor

Fatigue

Weakness

Failure to gain energy after rest

Dyspnea on exertion

Headache

Dizziness

GI disturbances

Irritability

Slowed thought processes

Confusion

Unsteady gait

Bleeding tendency

Petechiae

Ecchymosis; especially dependent areas, sites of pressure

Bleeding (see Table 3-2)

Gums

Nose

GI tract

Urinary tract

Vagina

Infection

Elevated temperature

Cold, flulike symptoms

Cough
Nonhealing cuts, lesions
Burning pain on urination
Frequent recent infections
History of exposure to chemical toxin radiation or, specific
medications

Laboratory/diagnostic studies

Erythrocytes
<1 million/mm^3
Normocytic
Normochromic
Reticulocytes: low
Leukocytes: <2000/mm^3
Granulocytes: reduced
Platelets: $<30,000$/mm^3
Serum iron: elevated
Iron binding capacity: normal if not bleeding
Coagulation tests: abnormal
Bone marrow: hypocellular, fatty marrow with few stem
cells (see box)

Potential complications

Hemorrhage
Cirrhosis
Diabetes
Heart failure
Blood reactions
Overwhelming infections

Medical Management

Elimination of identifiable cause
Blood transfusions
Packed cells
Platelets
Leukocytes, HLA matched
Splenectomy (rare)
Bone marrow transplant
Laboratory studies
Supportive care
Oxygen therapy
Corticosteroids
Antibiotics
Pain management
Monitoring of cardiac status

Nursing diagnoses/interventions/evaluation

■ **NDX:** Activity intolerance related to imbalance between oxygen supply and demand (anemia)

Position patient comfortably
Position with head elevated 30 degrees or position for
maximum chest expansion if respiratory difficulty occurs
Support with pillows

BONE MARROW STUDY

Bone marrow is obtained by aspiration or biopsy
to examine types and numbers of cells, maturation
level, and composition of supporting tissue; used for
diagnosis and treatment response

INDICATIONS

Evaluation of the hematolymphatic systems for
differential diagnosis of various anemias, neutropenia, leukemia, thrombocytopenia, immunoglobulin
disorders, lymphoma, or granulomatous disease

CARE

Inform patient that pressure will be felt with insertion of needle and some pain with aspiration; position for good visualization; apply pressure and
dressing at site; check BP, T, and R q30min × two;
maintain bedrest for 1 hr; assess site for bleeding,
hematoma, infection

Administer oxygen therapy as ordered
Take and record vital signs q4h to 8h
Assess respiratory and cardiac status q4h to 8h; report
tachycardia, irregular cardiac sounds, dyspnea, wheezes,
or rales
Assess neurological status q8h
Provide adequate periods of sleep and rest
Plan nursing activities to avoid interrupting sleep
Provide activity-free periods throughout the day for rest;
schedule examinations and tests carefully
Conserve patient's energy for desired activities
Assist with meal preparation
Assist with hygiene measures
Plan activities after rest periods
Maintain activity as tolerated
Perform passive or assist with active ROM exercises q4h
for patient on bed rest
Assist with ambulation
Handle patient gently
Determine activity tolerance
Check pulse rate
Note posture, respirations, and facial expression
Allow patient to set own pace
Observe safety precautions
Instruct patient to sit at side of bed before getting up;
change position slowly
Keep needed items close to patient

Expected outcome/evaluation

Patient's activity level is progressing to pre-illness level;
performs desired activities without evidence of weakness, tachycardia, or dyspnea

■ **NDX:** Potential alteration in tissue perfusion: cerebral, cardiovascular, gastrointestinal, renal, and/or peripheral related to risk of interruption of flow as evidenced by bleeding

Auscultate chest for heart and breath sounds q4h
Monitor cardiac status continuously
Monitor central venous pressure (CVP) q2h to 4h
Check BP, T, R, and apical pulse q4h
Assess sensorium and neurological status q4h to 8h
Check stools for bleeding
Measure intake and output; check urine for bleeding q4h to 8h
Assess skin and mucous membranes for extension or new sites of ecchymosis, hemorrhage, or hematoma q4h
If bleeding tendency or hemorrhage
  Use smallest gauge needles possible
  Consolidate laboratory work; use fingersticks when able
  Apply pressure to site of puncture 5 min and observe q15min for 1 hr
  Do not disturb clots
Do not take rectal temperature or administer rectal medications
Avoid scratching
Use soft-bristled toothbrush, towels, and nonabrasive soaps
Assist with walking when necessary to avoid bumps and falls
Keep patient warm
  Encourage use of warm robes, socks
  Provide extra blankets; avoid use of heating pads because of reduced sensation
Avoid constipation
  Increase fluids to 2500 ml/24 hr if permitted
  Add bulk to diet
  Use stool softeners or laxatives as ordered
Administer blood component transfusions as ordered
  If patient is not hemorrhaging, rate of transfusion is not to exceed 1 ml/kg body weight/hr; do not extend transfusion more than 4 hr
  The lower the Hgb, the slower the rate of transfusion
Administer platelets as ordered
  Assess for blood reactions
  Maintain balance sheet
  Monitor laboratory studies
Prepare for bone marrow transplantation when ordered

Expected outcome/evaluation

Patient's vital signs remain stable; there is no evidence of bleeding; skin and mucous membranes are warm and moist with good turgor

■ **NDX:** Altered nutrition: less than body requirements related to gastrointestinal disturbances

Assess amount and types of foods and liquids tolerated and desired
Provide diet high in vitamins and proteins; observe patient's preferences
Provide fluids of patient's choice to 2500 ml/day unless contraindicated
Measure intake and output q8h
Notify physician when intake and output are not equivalent and/or weight decreases by 2% to 3%
Weigh patient daily at same time with same clothing and scale
Arrange for quiet rest periods before meals
Eliminate distractions during mealtimes
Provide stress-free, no-hurry environment
Serve food attractively arranged
Assist with cutting of food and preparation for eating
Position patient and tray to reduce energy expenditure
Assist with meal or ask family or friends to remain during mealtime to assist as necessary
Small, frequent, high-calorie meals may be preferable

Expected outcome/evaluation

Weight is stable and/or increasing toward normal range for patient; takes a balanced diet and adequate fluids

■ **NDX:** Altered oral mucous membrane related to oxygen therapy and/or injury from microorganisms

Teach and assist patient with routine oral care
  Inspect and palpate lips, gums, and buccal mucosa gently q8h
  Clean teeth and rinse mouth each morning, after meals, and at bedtime
  Increase frequency of oral care to q2h with presence of lesions
  Choice of dental equipment will depend on state of oral cavity
    Soft-bristled toothbrush if there are no breaks or lesions
    Gauze or sponge-covered cleaners if there are breaks in skin or gums are bleeding
Assess patient's denture fit
  Avoid gumlike grips
  Keep dentures scrupulously clean
  Remove and clean before using mouth rinse
Keep patient's mouth moist
  Provide appealing, tepid liquids for sipping
  Flavored ice pops may be soothing
Keep lips moist; use water-soluble gel

Expected outcome/evaluation

Patient exhibits no oral lesions or healing of lesions is progressing

■ NDX: Anxiety related to changes in health, uncertainty about tests, treatment, and prognosis

Assess level of anxiety and understanding of disease process when appropriate

Assess past coping behavior

Visit frequently or have significant other remain with patient

Use touch, reassurance, and positive body language

Be sensitive to needs; listen to nonverbal clues

Plan care with patient to ensure meeting needs and expectations

Be consistent and provide care on time as planned; give explanations if delays are unavoidable

Speak clearly and concisely; allow patient time to complete requests and thoughts; do not anticipate and complete sentences

Provide atmosphere for discussion of fears and consequences of limited ability to carry out ADLs

Provide information about condition, procedures, and diagnostic studies

Encourage questions; answer clearly and consistently and clarify when necessary

Encourage communication with significant other

Provide diversional activities within limits of patient's energy level

Assess responses to activities and ventilation of feelings

Encourage use of adaptive coping measures

Provide access to others as requested: clergy, social worker, business associates, etc.

Expected outcome/evaluation

Patient expresses and discusses fears and anxiety regarding prognosis; discusses realistic future plans; seeks out resources and assistance as needed; shows infrequent or no symptoms of anxiety

■ NDX: Potential for infection related to inadequate cellular response caused by decreased leukocytes

Place in noninfectious environment

Reduce exposure to bacteria

    Explain and ensure that personnel and visitors follow handwashing procedure with povidone-iodine before entering room

    No one with infectious condition (cold, flu, cold sores, skin rash, etc.) may enter room

    Staff assigned to care for patient must not be assigned to care for patients who have infections

    Keep room clean

        Avoid any trash in room and bathroom

        Remove food and examination trays immediately after use

        Maintain furniture, fixtures, floor, and equipment free of dust and spills

    Ensure that no plants, flowers, fresh fruits, or vegetables are taken into room

    Ensure that allied health personnel (e.g., laboratory technicians) do not bring equipment into patient's room that has been in other areas of hospital

    If patient requires transportation, avoid using elevator with potentially infectious passengers present; gown and mask for patient may be required

Assess and record skin condition each shift

Provide mild, antibacterial, superfatted soap and soft cloths and towels for skin hygiene, daily and prn

Encourage mobility q2h

Turn and position immobile patient q2h to relieve pressure areas

Assess and record condition of perineum daily

Initiate and teach perineal care to be performed after each bowel movement; use ABDs, or very soft cloths; rinse and dry well

Prevent constipation and diarrhea

    Administer medications as ordered

    Avoid use of enemas and suppositories

Maintain skin integrity

    Avoid IM injections

    Observe IV, central line site q4h

        Change dressing daily if nonporous type is used, using aseptic technique

        Change IV tubing and bottles daily

        Avoid infiltrations that necessitate restarting IV

        Position IV site to prevent stress and movement at site of insertion

Consolidate laboratory work; clean skin with povidone-iodine scrub before puncture

Assess previous puncture sites each shift for signs of infection

    Assess and record condition of oral cavity each shift

    Monitor and record vital signs q4h; take temperature more frequently if trend is beginning

    Report temperature elevations immediately

    Institute comfort and cooling measures as indicated by condition

        Change linen and clothing to keep patient dry

        Administer antipyretics as ordered

        Prevent chilling; turn q2h

    Assess and record respiratory status q4h; report changes in breath sounds, cough, and sputum, increases in respiratory rate, or presence of sore throat immediately

    Assist and teach patient to turn, cough, and deep breathe q2h to 4h

    Monitor effects of oxygen therapy if administered

    Monitor intake and output; report urinary frequency, burning, or changes in character of urine

    Use voiding measures when indicated to avoid catheterization

    If catheterization is necessary

        Use strict aseptic technique for insertion

Perform catheter care each shift

Obtain cultures as ordered and monitor results: blood, urine, sputum, skin, drainage, etc.

Assess mental status shift; report changes

Monitor laboratory data daily; report changes

Expected outcome/evaluation

Patient exhibits no signs and symptoms of infection; lungs are clear; no skin or oral lesions noted; urine is clear; patient is oriented

■ **NDX:** Knowledge deficit related to lack of exposure to accurate information regarding nutrition, activity, and complications

Nutrition

Explain need to maintain balanced diet of preference and as tolerated; to use frequent, small feedings if preferred; to avoid foods that irritate oral mucous membranes

Explain need to take fluids of preference—at least 2500 ml/day unless contraindicated

Explain need to perform mouth care routinely before and after meals and prn; to report early signs of mouth lesions or those that do not heal; to use special mouth rinses as ordered

Demonstrate method of checking for and explain need to report signs and symptoms of mucositis

Explain need to weigh weekly with same amount of clothing and at same time of day

Activity

Instruct patient to alternate activities with rest periods to conserve energy

Explain need to increase activity gradually; to not become nonfunctional

Instruct patient on placing personal items at hand and furniture to prevent accidents

Demonstrate use of equipment to assist with ambulation when needed

Explain need to monitor activity tolerance (check pulse rate; if elevated or patient is feeling exhausted, rest, then continue)

Instruct patient to report symptoms to physician if no relief occurs with rest

Demonstrate oxygen therapy administration

Liters/minute ordered

Use of equipment: changing tank, cleansing or replacement of cannula

Bleeding

Discuss signs and symptoms of bleeding to be reported to physician in any of the following areas

Skin

Oral

Nasal

Rectal

Stomach

Cerebral

Urinary tract

Discuss emergency plan to follow if spontaneous hemorrhage occurs

Have emergency numbers on hand

Call paramedics

Go to nearest emergency facility

Explain importance of telling dentist and other medical personnal about disease process and low platelet count

Explain importance of maintaining safe, clutter-free environment

Explain importance of avoiding over-the-counter medications, especially those containing acetylsalicylic acid (i.e., aspirin) without checking with physician

Instruct patient to avoid use of sharp objects whenever possible

Instruct patient to avoid harsh coughing and blowing of nose

If cough persists, notify physician

Take cough medication as ordered

Explain need to avoid activities and sports that may cause injury

Explain need to avoid constipation through diet, fluids, and stool softeners

Explain importance of ongoing outpatient care

Routine laboratory appointments

Return physician and nurse appointments

Ensure that patient and/or significant other demonstrates

Method for applying pressure to bleeding site

Apply dressing or clean material directly over site

Apply pressure for 5 min

Apply ice in covered plastic bag over site once bleeding stops

Check site for further bleeding q15min for 1 hr

Method for testing stool and urine for occult blood

Infection

Discuss signs and symptoms of infection to report to physician or nurse

Explain importance of avoiding persons who may be infectious or who may have potentially contagious conditions, as well as persons who have been recently vaccinated and crowds

Explain need to avoid multiple sexual partners

Explain need to wash hands after using bathroom before eating, or before performing any care procedures or food preparation

Discuss importance of preventing injury to skin

Use electric razor

Handle knives and sharp objects carefully

Wear protective gloves when gardening and when using strong household cleaning solutions

Wear broad-brimmed hat and sun screen when in sun

Avoid going barefoot
Wear warm clothing and boots in cold weather
Avoid cutting cuticles, corns, or calluses
Wear padded gloves when using oven
Explain need to perform oral hygiene periodically throughout day and importance of daily hygiene, including perineal and rectal care
Explain importance of drinking up to 2500 ml of fluid each day unless contraindicated; need to avoid using common drinking fountain
Explain need to maintain clean home environment and to handle food properly
Explain need to avoid contact with pets or other animals
Demonstrate method for taking and recording temperature
Demonstrate procedure for caring for very small cuts or breaks in skin

Expected outcome/evaluation

Patient verbalizes understanding of home and follow-up care and demonstrates handwashing, skin, and mouth care, use of oxygen equipment, taking temperature, and testing urine and stool for occult blood

POLYCYTHEMIA

An increase in the number of circulating erythrocytes
polycythemia vera A chronic disorder in which overproduction of myelocytes and thrombocytes, as well as erythrocytes, occurs with a resulting increase in blood viscosity, blood volume, and hemoglobin concentration
secondary polycythemia A compensatory response to hypoxemia, which may result from chronic obstructive pulmonary disease (COPD), congenital heart disease, or prolonged exposure to low oxygen content (high altitude)
relative polycythemia A result of decreased plasma volume; erythrocyte level is normal or decreased

Assessment
Observations/findings

Skin
  Dusky, red-purple (rubor) appearance: face, mucous membranes, and hands
  Pruritus
  Urticaria
Cardiovascular
  Hypertension
  Intermittent claudication
  Chest pain
  Thrombus
  Emboli
  Bleeding
Central nervous system
  Headache
  Dizziness
  Tinnitus

Lassitude
Paresthesia
Bleeding
Respiratory: dyspnea with exertion
Gastrointestinal
  Epigastric distress
  Feeling of fullness
  Thirst
  Flatulence
  Constipation
  Weight loss
  Bleeding
  Hepatosplenomegaly (polycythemia vera)
Eyes
  Blurred vision
  Diplopia
  Engorged veins: fundus, retina
Musculoskeletal: symptoms of gout

Laboratory/diagnostic studies

RBC: 7 to 12 million/mm^3
Hgb: 8 to 25 g/100 ml
Hct: >60%
Coagulation studies: abnormal
Myelocytosis
Thrombocytosis } polycythemia vera
Hyperuricemia

Potential complications

Thromboses in any system
  Myocardial infarction (MI)
  Cerebrovascular accident (CVA)
  Gangrene: digits
Hemorrhage in any system
Congestive heart failure (CHF)
Hypertension
Peptic ulcer
Leukemia

Medical Management

Phlebotomy, apheresis therapy
Fluid replacement
Myelosuppressive therapy
  Radioisotopes
  Alkylating agents
Secondary, relative polycythemia: treatment of underlying disease or condition; environmental change

Nursing diagnoses/interventions/evaluation

■ **NDX:** Altered tissue perfusion: cardiopulmonary, cerebral, gastrointestinal, and/or peripheral related to interruption of blood flow as evidenced by bleeding

Report early signs or symptoms of bleeding to physician

Monitor BP, T, R, apical pulse, and neurological status q4h to 6h

Auscultate chest for breath and heart sounds q4h to 6h

Assist and teach patient to turn, cough, and deep breathe q4h

Ambulate as soon as possible

Check peripheral pulses and color and temperature of extremities q4h to 6h

Auscultate abdomen for bowel sounds q4h to 6h

Assess skin and mucous membranes q4h to 6h

Avoid invasive procedures when possible

Consolidate laboratory procedures; use smallest gauge needles possible; observe for bleeding at venipuncture sites; apply pressure over site for 5 to 10 min or until bleeding stops

Encourage communication with significant other

Provide information about condition and progress; answer questions consistently; promote other stress-reduction activities

Prepare for phlebotomy or apheresis therapy as ordered

    Explain procedure

    Check vital signs before and after procedure

    Assess for untoward responses during procedure: vertigo; cold, clammy skin; tachycardia; hypotension

    Instruct patient to sit for 10 to 15 min and then stand for 3 to 5 min before attempting ambulation

Expected outcome/evaluation

Patient's vital signs are stable; there is no evidence of bleeding

■ **NDX:** Altered protection related to abnormal coagulation

Assess and report signs/symptoms of thrombus formation: mental, cardiac, respiratory, GI, GU status, extremities

Maintain position for comfort and for maximum respiratory excursion when on bed rest

    No knee gatch

    Active or passive ROM exercises q2h to 4h

    Padded footboard for exercises

    Change position qh

    Avoid restrictive clothing; use bed cradle when necessary

Keep patient warm and dry to prevent vasoconstriction

Avoid sitting for long periods; instruct patient not to cross legs when sitting or lock knees when standing and to use well-fitting, not tight, slippers or shoes

Arrange furniture and provide good lighting so patient can avoid bumps and falls when ambulating

Instruct patient to call for assistance if needed

Instruct patient to call if sudden pain occurs, such as in chest, head, extremities; dysuria

Collaborate with physician in managing acute onset of thrombus formation

Expected outcome/evaluation

Patient verbalizes understanding of instructions to notify about pain onset; oriented; no evidence of cardiac, pulmonary, GI, or GU involvement; color and temperature of extremities remain unchanged

■ **NDX:** Altered nutrition: less than body requirements related to inability to digest or absorb nutrients as evidenced by epigastric distress, feelings of fullness

Assess amount of food or fluids patient can take before feeling full

Provide small feedings of nutritious foods and liquids to patient's tolerance; low-sodium, low-purine diet may be ordered; avoid gas-forming, acidic foods

Remind patient to eat slowly and chew well

Provide fluids of choice to 2500 ml/day

Monitor intake and output q8h

Have snacks available but out of sight if this contributes to distress

Vary texture of foods and liquids to enhance appetite

Provide time for oral hygiene before and after meals; assist when necessary

Arrange rest periods before meals and assist with preparations to conserve energy

Serve meals attractively arranged

Arrange for vistors of patient's preference to enhance social aspect of mealtime

Encourage ROM exercises or ambulation between meals

Weigh patient daily at same time with same clothing and scale

Expected outcome/evaluation

Weight is progressing toward normal for patient; patient is taking a balanced diet with fluids to 2000 to 2500 ml/day

■ **NDX:** Pain related to chronic disease as evidenced by joint pain or headache

Assess location, duration, and severity of pain using pain scale

Monitor effectiveness of analgesics when administered

Joint pain

Place patient in position of comfort; support joints anatomically with pillows or pads

Change position qh; assist with ROM exercise

Avoid restrictive clothing; use bed cradle

Use alternate comfort measures: distraction, imagery, etc.

Headache

Maintain quiet environment

Provide uninterrupted rest periods

Encourage fluid intake

Provide hot or cold compresses of patient's choice

Expected outcome/evaluation

Patient verbalizes absence of headache; manages activities without discomfort; posture and face are relaxed

 NDX: Potential for impaired skin integrity related to risk of mechanical factors: scratching caused by pruritus, urticaria

Assess condition of skin and mucous membranes q4h to 8h

Administer skin care q4h to 6h; provide soothing, cool baths with oil or bicarbonate of soda

Provide unrestrictive clothing that is not rough; clothing laundered with nondetergents may be needed

Keep bedclothes wrinkle-free to prevent irritation

Keep nails short and manicured to prevent scratches

Use distraction and socialization to increase comfort

Administer medications as ordered; assess effectiveness

Expected outcome/evaluation

Patient's skin is clear with good color; there is no evidence of urticaria

Additional nursing diagnoses to consider

Activity intolerance related to immobility caused by joint pain or generalized weakness caused by anemia

Potential for injury related to risk of sensory dysfunction

 NDX: Knowledge deficit related to lack of exposure to accurate information regarding disease process, complications, activity, nutrition, and medication

Disease process

Discuss symptoms of recurrence or progression of disease and complications to report to physician

Demonstrate how to check skin and peripheral pulses

Explain importance of regular follow-up care

Complications

Discuss trauma prevention

Avoid restrictive clothing

Wear well-fitting shoes

Keep home and work area free of clutter

Use assistive devices when needed

Use caution when performing oral hygiene

Avoid sports and hobbies that may cause injury

Handle equipment and sharp objects carefully

Avoid extremes in environmental temperature

Activity

Instruct patient to balance rest and activity periods

Instruct patient not to cross legs when sitting or lock knees when standing; explain need to change position and exercise extremities q30 min

Explain need to plan regular exercise program

Nutrition

Explain importance of well-balanced diet; low-sodium or low-purine diet may be ordered

Instruct patient to take at least 2500 ml of fluid daily unless contraindicated

Discuss foods to avoid: gas-forming, acidic foods

Medication

Teach name of medication, dosage, time of administration, purpose, and side effects

Instruct patient to avoid taking over-the-counter medications without checking with physician

Expected outcome/evaluation

Patient and/or significant other verbalizes understanding of home care and follow-up instructions and demonstrates method for checking pulses

THROMBOCYTOPENIA

A bleeding disorder in which the number of platelets is reduced; defective or diminished production of platelets may be caused by bone marrow infiltration, aplastic anemia, myelosuppressive drugs, radiation, or viral infections; increased peripheral destruction may be caused by immune drug sensitivities or autoantibodies that sensitize platelets.

Assessment
Observations/findings

Mild to excessive bleeding

Skin: easy bruising, petechiae, ecchymosis

Epistaxis

Gum bleeding, blood-filled bullae

"Coffee ground" vomitus or hematemesis

Blood-streaked sputum

Hematuria

Guaiac-positive stool

Heavy menses

Cerebral: headache, slurred speech, malaise

Numb, painful extremities

Family history of bleeding

Laboratory/diagnostic studies

Platelets <100,000/mm^3

Prolonged bleeding time

Normal coagulation time

Decreased Hgb

Increased capillary fragility

Bone marrow: increased number of megakaryocytes in ITP

Potential complications

Hemorrhage
Loss of consciousness

Medical Management

Treatment of underlying cause or removal of precipitating
agent
Corticosteroids
Immunosuppressive therapy
Plasmapheresis
Platelet or fresh blood transfusions
Splenectomy
Analgesics

Nursing diagnoses/interventions/evaluation

■ **NDX:** Altered protection related to abnormal blood
profile (thrombocytopenia)

Maintain bed rest when bleeding
Position patient comfortably
Support with pillows
Avoid pressure to any area of body; use foam or gel
pads, sheepskin, air mattress, and heel and elbow
guards
Protect from sheet burns; use turn-and-lift sheet to
move patient in bed
Check BP, T, P, and R qid
Auscultate chest for breath sounds each shift
Assess neurological status q2h to 4h when applicable
Check stool and urine for bleeding daily
Assess skin and mucous membranes for bleeding q4h to
8h
Monitor laboratory studies
Administer care to sites of puncture
Consolidate laboratory work
Use fingersticks when possible
Apply pressure at least 5 to 10 min after puncture or
until bleeding stops
Observe site for bleeding or hematoma q15min for four
times
Clean area with povidone-iodine swab before veni-
puncture
Place bacteriostatic ointment at site
Use sterile technique when changing dressings daily
Observe site q1h to 2h for redness, pain, swelling, or
infiltration
Avoid trauma to prevent bleeding
Protect patient from falls and bumping into or dropping
objects; arrange furniture and equipment conve-
niently; pad bed rails if necessary; assist with ambulation when necessary
Avoid use of constrictive clothing; use bed cradle to
prevent tight bedclothes
Use soft towels and cloths for bathing; avoid vigorous
skin care

Advise patient to avoid straining at stool to prevent
increasing intracranial pressure; use stool softeners or
laxatives as ordered to prevent constipation
Provide soft-bristled toothbrush; avoid use of nonelec-
tric razors
Advise patient not to cough to avoid increased intracranial pressure
Administer platelet blood transfusions when ordered; administer platelets quickly through recommended tubing
to prevent destruction
Administer corticosteroid therapy and immunosuppressive
therapy as ordered (ITP)
Avoid use of antihistamines, phenothiazines, aspirin, and
nonsteroidal, antiinflammatory agents in ITP
Prepare for plasmapheresis when ordered
Administer medications (penicillin, sulfinpyrazone, ace-
tylaslicylic acid, dipyridamole, or antihistamines) to inhibit platelet function as ordered in TTP
Prepare for splenectomy if ordered

Expected outcome/evaluation

Patient's vital signs are stable; there is no evidence of
bleeding or bruising in new sites; urine and stool test
negative for bleeding; neurological and respiratory systems exhibit no symptoms of bleeding

■ **NDX:** Altered oral mucous membrane related to physical injury as evidenced by blood-filled bullae

Assess integrity of oral mucous membrane q4h
Administer careful oral hygiene before and after meals and
q2h to 4h
Use soft-bristled toothbrush; avoid brushing area with
bullae
Rinse mouth with dilute mouthwash or irrigate if pa-
tient is unable to do so
Maintain diet of preference or as ordered; avoid use of
hard, spicy, or difficult-to-chew foods to prevent trauma
Provide fluids of choice to 2500 ml daily unless contrain-
dicated; iced liquids may be more comforting
Measure intake and output q8h
Weigh patient daily at same time with same clothing and
scale

Expected outcome/evaluation

No bullae are noted in oral cavity; patient is taking a
balanced diet with fluids; weight is stable

■ **NDX:** Pain related to physical agent resulting from
nerve pressure secondary to bleeding

Assess pain (location, duration, intensity [use pain scale],
and predisposing factors) q4h to 6h
Position patient for comfort; use pillows or other support
as needed

Provide bed cradle to prevent constriction by bedclothes
Provide warm or cold applications as patient desires
Place articles within patient's reach
Use alternate pain relief measures: relaxation, music therapy, guided imagery, touch, etc.
Manage visitors according to patient's wishes
Monitor effectiveness of analgesics when administered

Expected outcome/evaluation

Patient manages activities without pain or discomfort; face and posture remain relaxed

■ **NDX:** Knowledge deficit related to lack of exposure to accurate information regarding disease process, nutrition, activity, and medication

Disease process

Demonstrate method to assess for bleeding
Discuss signs and symptoms of recurrence to report to physician: continuous headache, coughing red-streaked sputum, persistent abdominal pain, vomiting frank blood or "coffee ground" material, increased areas of petechiae or ecchymosis, blood-filled bullae in oral cavity, blood in urine or stools
Demonstrate methods of checking for blood in stool and urine
Instruct patient to notify physician when contemplating pregnancy or when pregnancy is first suspected
Caution patient never to donate blood
Explain need to prevent trauma by
  Avoiding constipation through diet, fluids, and use of stool softeners or laxatives if needed; avoiding vigorous nose-blowing or coughing; avoiding contact sports or other hazardous hobbies
  Careful movements and careful handling of objects that may cause bleeding
  Use of nonabrasive skin and mouth care products
Explain importance of notifying all health care providers of diagnosis and keeping follow-up appointments

Nutrition

Explain importance of regular oral hygiene; discuss products to use or avoid; demonstrate method for daily inspection
Explain need to maintain balanced diet with adequate hydration; discuss foods to avoid to prevent trauma

Activity

Explain need to balance rest and activity periods; to increase activity as comfort increases; to use assistance when needed to prevent injury

Medication

Teach name of medication, dosage, time of administration, purpose, and side effects

Teach how to read contents of over-the-counter medications, avoiding those that contain acetylsalicylic acid (antihistamines, phenothiazines, or nonsteroidal antiinflammatory agents in ITP)

Expected outcome/evaluation

Patient and/or significant other verbalizes understanding of home care and follow-up instructions; demonstrates method to detect any bleeding, including checking stool and urine; demonstrates oral hygiene and skin care measures

DISSEMINATED INTRAVASCULAR COAGULATION (DIC)

Overstimulation of the normal coagulation process associated with underlying conditions such as snakebite, septicemia, severe hypotension, neoplasms, hemolysis, obstetric emergencies, acidosis, cancer chemotherapy, transplant rejection, and extensive burns, trauma, or surgery; the initial accelerated clotting process consumes large amounts of coagulation factors in the formation of fibrin clots; the fibrinolytic system is then activated to lyse fibrin clots into fibrin degradation products; the activity of these products and the depletion of plasma coagulation factors result in hemorrhage

Assessment
Observations/findings

Abnormal bleeding in all systems and at sites of invasive procedures (see Table 3-2)
  Skin and mucous membranes
    Diffuse oozing of blood or plasma
    Petechiae
    Palpable purpura: initially chest and abdomen
    Hemorrhagic bullae
    Subcutaneous hemorrhage
    Hematoma
    Tape burns
    Acral cyanosis*
  GI system
    Nausea, vomiting
    Guaiac-positive emesis/nasogastric aspiration and stools
    Severe abdominal pain
    Increasing abdominal girth
  Renal system
    Hematuria
    Oliguria
  Respiratory system
    Dyspnea
    Tachypnea
    Blood-tinged sputum
  Cardiovascular system
    Increasing hypotension

TABLE 3-2. Signs and Symptoms of Blood Loss

Volume lost		
ml	%TBV*	Clinical signs
500	10	None; occasionally vasovagal syncope in blood donors
1000	20	At rest there may be no clinical evidence of volume loss; a slight postural drop in BP may be seen; tachycardia with exercise
1500	30	Resting supine BP and P may be normal; neck veins flat when supine; postural hypotension; exercise tachycardia
2000	40	Central venous pressure, cardiac output, and arterial blood pressure below normal even when supine and at rest; air hunger, rapid thready pulse, cold clammy skin
2500	50	Lactic acidosis, severe shock, death

From Wintrobe MM et al: *Clinical hematology*, Philadelphia, 1981, Lea & Febiger.
*Total blood volume.

Postural hypotension
Increasing heart rate
Absence of peripheral pulses
Central nervous system
    Changing level of consciousness
    Restlessness
    Vasomotor instability
Musculoskeletal system
    Pain: muscles, joints, back
Bleeding to hemorrhage
    Surgical incisions
    Postpartum uterus
    Eye fundus: visual changes
    Invasive procedure sites: injection, IV, arterial catheters and chest or nasogastric tubes, etc.

Laboratory/diagnostic studies

Serial studies
    PT >15 sec
    Fibrinogen <160 mg/ml
    Fibrin degradation products (FDP) >1/8
    Platelets <100,000/mm³
With significant liver disease
    PT >25 sec
    Fibrinogen <125 mg/ml
    FDP >1/64
    Platelets <50,000
Decreased factor assays: V, VII, VIII, X, XIII
PTT >60 to 80 sec
Decreased Hct without clinical bleeding
Schistocytes noted on CBC
Respiratory acidosis

*Slightly blue, gray, or dark purple discoloration of the extremities

Potential complications

Shock
Acute tubular necrosis
Focal gangrene
Pulmonary edema
CHF
Convulsions
Coma
Failure of major organ systems

Medical Management

Treatment of underlying disorder
Anticoagulant therapy: heparin IV
Fresh frozen plasma, platelets, clotting factors, other blood products, and parenteral fluids
Thrombolytic therapy
Oxygen therapy

Nursing diagnoses/interventions/evaluation

■ **NDX:** Altered tissue perfusion: renal, cerebral, cardiopulmonary, gastrointestinal, or peripheral related to interruption of flow as evidenced by bleeding

Maintain venous access using strict aseptic technique
Administer IV heparin and fresh frozen plasma, platelets, and other blood products as ordered; assess response and/or reactions
Perform exchange transfusion as ordered for neonates
Observe for bleeding at venipuncture site or clotting at end of catheter; apply pressure dressing if needed
Monitor FDP titers and report to physician for heparin dosage changes
    NOTE: PTT and Lee-White test are prolonged in DIC and are not reliable indicators of heparin therapy
Monitor arterial pressure, ECG, BP, T, P, and R q30min to 60min; report progressive decrease in BP, increase in heart rate, and elevated temperature
Assess neurological status q30min to 60min; report changes
Auscultate chest for heart and breath sounds qh; report abnormal changes immediately
Monitor arterial blood gases; report acidotic states immediately
Monitor effects of oxygen therapy when administered
Assess for increased bleeding and/or new sites of hemorrhage in all body systems; report changes immediately
Measure intake and output qh; report decreasing output or <30 ml/hr; weigh dressings and linen when hemorrhage occurs
Assist patient with turning and deep breathing qh; avoid vigorous coughing
Measure abdominal girth when GI bleeding is suspected
Administer careful skin care as needed; do not disturb

clots; use lift sheet to prevent bruising and abrasions; use heel and elbow padding; support joints anatomically

Apply Gelfoam or thrombin dressings to areas with frank bleeding or those that continue to ooze

Provide oral hygiene q2h to 4h; avoid vigorous toothbrushing; use soft-bristled toothbrush, cotton swabs, and dilute mouth rinse or saline

Weigh patient daily at same time with same clothing and scale

Protect from trauma

Pad side rails if necessary

Avoid constrictive bedclothes; use bed cradle if needed

Clip nails to prevent scratching

Avoid invasive procedures when possible

Use caution when suctioning or inserting tubes and lines

Apply pressure to site for 5 to 10 min or until bleeding stops if IM injections are necessary, or when removing IV catheters; observe q10min to 15min; apply pressure dressing if appropriate

Expected outcome/evaluation

Patient's vital signs are stable; there is no further evidence of bleeding; past sites of bleeding are resolving

■ NDX: Pain related to tissue trauma

Assess location, quality, and intensity of pain; use pain rating scale

Place patient in position of comfort; provide support with pillows to prevent stress on body parts

Assist with care when patient is actively bleeding or experiencing discomfort

Maintain quiet environment

Provide adequate periods of rest; cluster activities and diagnostic studies, when possible, according to patient's tolerance

Assist patient with alternate comfort measures such as music therapy, imagery, or other distractions

Administer analgesics as ordered; assess effectiveness

Expected outcome/evaluation

Patient verbalizes no discomfort; body posture and face are relaxed

■ NDX: Anxiety related to threat of death

Assess level of patient's fears and understanding of current condition when appropriate

Maintain calm, nonstressful environment

Prepare family/significant other for patient's appearance

Remain with patient or have significant other stay with patient; use touch, reassurance, and positive body language

Provide information about condition, procedures, and diagnostic studies in language understood by patient

Encourage questions; answer clearly and consistently and clarify when necessary

Note positive progress in physical condition when appropriate

Provide atmosphere conducive to discussion and expression of feelings, worries, fears, and loss

Be sensitive to needs; listen to nonverbal clues

Maintain and assist with coping strategies

Provide access to others to assist patient: clergy, psychologist, social worker, etc.

Expected outcome/evaluation

Patient verbalizes understanding of condition; participates in care; uses positive coping measures; symptoms of anxiety are absent

NOTE: See primary condition for patient teaching and discharge planning

SPLENECTOMY

Surgical removal of the spleen to treat traumatic injuries or blood dyscrasias in which hypersplenism occurs (the spleen produces leukocytes, lymphocytes, monocytes, and plasma cells; it also destroys nonfunctional red blood cells and platelets, stores blood, and assists in maintaining hemopoiesis; the spleen indiscriminantly sequesters normal red blood cells and platelets, thereby removing them from the circulation when hypersplenism occurs)

Assessment
Postoperative observations/findings

Cardiovascular
  Bleeding
  Tachycardia
  Thrombosis
Respiratory
  Splinting with respiration
  Decreased breath sounds
  Tachypnea
  Atelectasis
  Subdiaphragmatic abscess
Gastrointestinal
  Character and amount of gastric drainage
  Nausea, vomiting
  Dehydration
  Abdominal distension
Infection
  Elevated temperature
  Site of incision
    Redness
    Swelling
    Draining
    Dehiscence

Laboratory/diagnostic studies

Elevated thrombocyte level
Bleeding and clotting times: normal
Electrolytes

Potential complications

Hemorrhage
Infection
Paralytic ileus
Shock

Medical Management

Incentive spirometer
Nasogastric tube
Parenteral therapy
Pain management
Management of complications

Nursing diagnoses/interventions/evaluation*

■ **NDX:** Potential for ineffective breathing pattern related to risk of decreased lung expansion caused by anesthetic and/or site of incision

Assess respiratory effort, breath sounds, and rate q4h for 48 hr, then q8h
Position patient to decrease respiratory effort
Assist and teach patient to turn, cough, and deep breathe q2h to 4h; support incision
Teach patient to use incentive spirometer q4h
Assist with ambulation as soon as possible

Expected outcome/evaluation

Patient's lungs are clear; respiratory excursion is adequate

■ **NDX:** Pain related to surgical procedure

Assess pain location, frequency, intensity, and duration; use pain rating scale
Assist patient with assuming position of comfort; support as necessary
Collaborate with physician to establish analgesic schedule and dosage to obtain maximum effectiveness; increased frequency usually required during immediate postoperative period
Teach alternate methods of pain relief; relaxation, imagery, music, etc.
Administer pain medication before performing activities, thereby increasing compliance with:
Coughing and deep breathing
ROM exercises
Early periods of ambulation and self-care activities
If pain increases, assess for other factors (e.g., complications, exacerbation of primary condition)

Expected outcome/evaluation

Patient verbalizes feelings of increased comfort; performs activities without limitation; body posture and face are relaxed

■ **NDX:** Potential fluid volume deficit (2) related to risk of loss of fluid through nasogastric drainage

Maintain NPO as ordered
Connect nasogastric sump tube to low, intermittent suction apparatus as ordered
Do not change position of tube
Maintain tube patency
Check drainage q2h to 4h; report excessive bleeding
Assess skin turgor q8h
Measure intake and output q8h; report imbalance
Weigh patient daily at same time with same clothing and scale

Expected outcome/evaluation

Patient's intake equals output; mucous membranes are moist; skin turgor is good

■ **NDX:** Potential for altered pattern of urinary elimination related to risk of anesthesia and/or indwelling urinary catheter

Observe voiding: frequency, amount, color, odor, discomfort, distension, q4h to 8h
Insert catheter when ordered for retention or overflow voiding; perform daily catheter care
Institute voiding measures as needed; when catheter is removed; obtain midstream culture

Expected outcome/evaluation

Patient voids without difficulty and has no signs of infection

■ **NDX:** Constipation related to lack of dietary fiber and fluids caused by NPO status

Auscultate abdomen for bowel sounds q8h; report return of bowel sounds
Begin oral liquids, progressing to regular diet when ordered after return of bowel sounds; note tolerance
Encourage fluids to 2500 ml/day unless contraindicated
Administer Harris flush q6h prn for distension if ordered
Monitor for first bowel movement after surgery; give stool softeners or enemas as ordered

Expected outcome/evaluation

Patient takes regular diet and fluids to 2500 ml/day; has had soft-formed bowel movement

---

*See also standard for primary condition, General Preoperative Care/Teaching (p. 27), and Care of Patient in Recovery Room (p. 28).

■ **NDX:** Potential altered tissue perfusion: gastrointestinal and/or peripheral related to risk of interruption of flow caused by bleeding or thrombosis

Monitor BP, P, R, CVP, and T q4h for 48 hr, then q8h
Assess for signs of bleeding or thrombosis q4h to 8h
Check dressing for bleeding q2h to 4h for 48 hr
    Reinforce as necessary
    Report excessive bleeding to physician
Change dressing daily and prn; observe healing process; report early signs of infection when present
Position patient comfortably; assist with turning q2h; avoid knee gatch or pillows under knees
Assist with and teach active or perform passive ROM exercises q4h
Provide correct-size antiembolic stockings when ordered
Plan uninterrupted rest and sleep periods to avoid fatigue
Assist with ambulation as necessary
    Avoid sitting for long periods
    Walk in place when standing

Expected outcome/evaluation

Vital signs are within patient's normal limits; peripheral pulses are palpable; color and patient's temperature of extremities are normal; incision is healing

■ **NDX:** Knowledge deficit related to lack of exposure to accurate information regarding self-care, activities, and nutrition

Self-care

Instruct patient to shower daily, to dry incision well
Teach patient to observe for and report increased pain, swelling, redness, or drainage
Emphasize importance of not applying creams, lotions, or powders to incision
Instruct patient to support incision, if needed, when deep breathing and coughing
Emphasize need for follow-up care

Activities

Explain need to increase ambulation and activities each day and to plan regular, uninterrupted rest periods
Explain need to exercise extremities routinely; demonstrate ROM and breathing exercises
Instruct patient to avoid sitting for long periods; explain importance of not crossing legs
Instruct patient to avoid heavy lifting and contact sports for 6 to 8 weeks or as directed by physician

Nutrition

Instruct patient to maintain well-balanced diet, taking 2500 ml of liquids daily
Instruct patient to report inability to tolerate food or liquids, nausea, any vomiting, diarrhea, or constipation

Expected outcome/evaluation

Patient and/or significant other verbalizes understanding of home care and follow-up instructions and demonstrates incision care, breathing, and ROM exercises

APHERESIS THERAPY

Selective removal of blood or blood components for therapeutic goals; types of apheresis—procedures are named depending on the blood component to be removed (Table 3-3)

GENERAL CARE OF PATIENT RECEIVING THERAPEUTIC APHERESIS
Assessment

Assess for appearance of complications during procedure (see Table 3-3)
Continue required assessment for primary condition

Preapheresis care

Reinforce physician's explanation of procedure; include significant other
Obtain written consent after physician has explained procedure
Assess patient's existing condition and note routine and special nursing care requirements for primary condition
Check preapheresis laboratory values
Take and record vital signs and standing and lying BP
Assess patient's heart and lung sounds
Administer medications and fluids as ordered
NOTE: Wear protective gloves and gowns when handling blood components, needles, and centrifuge equipment

Interventions

NOTE: Procedure is performed by a specifically qualified operator

During procedure

Assess vital signs, heart and breath sounds qh
Measure intake and output
Monitor infusions and rates qh
Administer routine medications
Continue care for primary condition

Postapheresis care

If antecubital veins are used for access
    Never use for other venipunctures
    Apply warm soaks qid
    Teach arm-strengthening exercises
If arteriovenous fistula is used for access
    Check patency daily
    Never use for venipunctures
    Never take BP in that extremity; no IM injections in same extremity
    See standard of care for primary condition

TABLE 3-3. Therapeutic Apheresis Procedures

Considerations	Plasmapheresis	Plateletpheresis	Leukapheresis	Erythrocytapheresis
Indications	Hemolytic anemia (AIHA) acute ITP, nonrelapsing TTP, Guillain-Barré syndrome, myasthenia gravis, renal transplant rejection syndrome, Goodpasture's syndrome, systemic lupus erythematosus, rheumatoid arthritis, multiple myeloma, biliary cirrhosis, hyperlipidemia, hypercholesterolemia, cancer conditions in which plasma substances interfere with immune system	Thrombocytosis	Chronic lymphatic leukemia, rheumatoid arthritis, multiple sclerosis	Acute, severe sickle cell disease, polycythemia vera
Preapheresis laboratory/ diagnostic studies	Total albumin and protein, K, Mg, Ca, CBC, Hgb, Hct, platelet count, PT, activated PTT, hepatitis-associated antigen/ VDRL, cold agglutinins, liver/renal function tests, HBSAg if history of hepatitis	Platelet count, CBC, Hgb, PT, activated PTT, cold agglutinins, liver and renal function tests, HBSAg if history of hepatitis	CBC, differential, Hgb, Hct, platelet count, PT, activated PTT, cold agglutinins, liver/renal function tests, HBSAg if history of hepatitis	CBC, Hbg, platelet count, PT, in activated PTT, cold agglutinins, liver/renal function tests, HBSAg if history of hepatitis
Complications	Electrolyte imbalance (hypocalcemia, hypokalemia), hypothermia, hypovolemia, fluid overload, vasovagal reaction, thrombus or air embolus, oliguria or anuria, shock	Air embolus, reaction from anticoagulation: (citrate) tingling chills, seizures, hypotension, hemolysis, bleeding, fluid overload	Air embolus, reaction from anticoagulation: (citrate) tingling chills, seizures, hypotension, hemolysis, bleeding, fluid overload	Hypovolemia, hemolytic transfusion reaction
Usual volume removed	2-4 L	1000 ml, depending on platelet count		
Replacement therapy	Volume removed replaced with normal saline and albumin or fresh frozen plasma (replaces Ig and coagulation factors but increases risk of hypersensitivity and hepatitis)	Albumin 5% add 0.9% NS or plasmanate	Albumin 5% add 0.9% NS or plasmanate	Amount removed replaced with washed, frozen or WBC-poor RBCs
Usual length of each treatment	2-3 hr usually, dependent on volume to be removed	2-4 hr	3-4 hr	Varies with condition being treated
Usual length of therapy	Six treatments	Varies with primary condition	18-20 treatments, depending on rate of cell proliferation	Varies with primary condition
Usual schedule of treatments	Every other day or every day to total required dependent on antigen/ complement levels	Varies with condition, continued until platelet count is at desired level	Three times week 1, two times week 2, then 1 time a week thereafter to total required	Varies with primary condition

Patient Teaching

Ensure that patient and/or significant other demonstrates
  Care of venous or arteriovenous fistula
  Extremity exercises to perform daily
Ensure that patient and/or significant other knows and understands
  Signs and symptoms of bleeding and infection to report to physician
  To avoid exposure to persons with infections, especially URIs
See standard of care for primary condition

BLOOD TRANSFUSIONS

Assessment
Observations/findings

Venipuncture site
  Pain
  Warmth
  Redness
  Swelling
  Leakage at insertion site
Position of extremity
Blood
  Type and Rh factor (Table 3-4)
  Flow rate
  Amount

Potential reactions (Table 3-5)

Hemolysis
  Elevated temperature
  Decreased BP
  Hemoglobinuria
  Hematuria
  Chills
  Pain
Circulatory overload
  Shortness of breath
  Lung congestion: rales, rhonchi
  Frothy sputum
Pyrogenic reaction
  Sudden chilling
  Elevated temperature
  Headache
Allergic reaction
  Urticaria
  Laryngeal edema
  Asthmatic wheezing
Blood-borne infections: hepatitis, CMV, AIDS, etc.

Pretransfusion care

Select equipment needed for venipuncture according to hospital policy, procedure, and physician's order
Prepare equipment and normal saline solution

Obtain blood no more than 30 min before administration; check blood according to hospital policy, ensuring that correct patient receives type-specific blood
Obtain baseline T, P, R, and BP
Prepare venipuncture site

Care during transfusion

Flush blood tubing with normal saline solution before starting transfusion
Remain with patient for at least 15 min (or 50 ml) after starting blood; check vital signs and compare to baseline
Discontinue blood immediately if transfusion reaction occurs, call physician, change blood tubing, maintain patent IV, and follow hospital procedure

Posttransfusion care

Apply pressure to venipuncture site
Apply adhesive bandage and/or dressing as indicated
Change blood tubing after transfusion
Observe for reaction 1 hr after infusion of blood
Record whether a reaction occurred

Patient teaching

Ensure that patient and/or significant other knows and understands
  Importance of maintaining position of extremity
  Importance of reporting symptoms of reaction
  Rash
  Flushed feeling
  Chills
  Shortness of breath
  Chest pain
Importance of not regulating flow rate

TABLE 3-4. Blood and Blood Components

Product	Description	Indication(s)	Action	Administration
Red blood cells, packed (PRC)	Concentrated red blood cells that remain after plasma is separated	To improve oxygen-carrying capacity of the blood (hemolytic anemia in aplastic crisis, chronic hypoplastic anemia, leukemia, lymphoma, and other malignant diseases with bone marrow failure; exchange transfusions; surgery; shock; conditions in which sudden changes in blood volume are not tolerated	Increases oxygen-carrying capacity; elevates Hct (3% if unit of PRC has Hct of 70%-80%)	See blood administration standard; administer through a filter; regulate flow to 25 ml/hr for 15 min; remain with patient; observe for reaction; if no reaction, regulate flow to 100-200 ml/hr in adult with no cardiac failure or elevated CVP and in infants and children regulate flow to 2-6 ml/kg/hr; add sodium chloride to PRC before administration when ordered; *no other solution or medication may be added to red cells*
Red blood cells, leukocyte poor	Concentrated red cells with leukocytes removed, usually by continuous flow centrifuge or washing	See PRC; severe febrile transfusion reactions caused by antileukocyte or antiplatelet antibodies; candidates for transplantation	See PRC	See PRC
Red blood cells, frozen	Glycerol added to red cells to protect cell from hemolysis while suspended in hypertonic solution when frozen; glycerol is removed before administration	See PRC; hypersensitivity reactions to plasma components such as IgA	See PRC	See PRC
Whole blood	Plasma and red blood cells; may or may not contain other cells and factors; dependent on length of time transpired after collection; unit usually contains 520 ± 45 ml of anticoagulated blood with Hct of about 40%	Restoration of decreased blood volume caused by hemorrhage or trauma in which more than 25% of volume is lost	Restores blood volume and increases oxygen-carrying capacity	Administer through a filter; remain with patient until 25-50 ml transfused, usually 15-30 min; observe for transfusion reactions; if no reaction, adjust flow rate to administer complete unit within 4 hr; warm unit no higher than 37°C using special coils when refrigerated blood needs to be administered quickly

Continued.

TABLE 3-4. Blood and Blood Components—cont'd

Product	Description	Indication(s)	Action	Administration
Whole blood, modified		Hypovolemic shock	Increases oxygen-carrying capacity and provides volume without adding platelets, which release serotonin (a vasoconstrictor)	See whole blood
Whole blood with antihemophilic factor (factor VIII) removed	Prepared by removing factor VIII, using heparin in initial collection, or converting a previously collected unit of blood containing a citrate anticoagulant	Exchange transfusion in the adult	Provides volume without contributing to coagulation ability	See whole blood
Plasma	Plasma prepared from single donor unit of fresh blood	Burns; traumatic shock; replacement of certain coagulation factors	Provides plasma coagulation factors	Administer unit in less than 1 hr in hypovolemic patient; in normovolemic patient, administer at rate of 5-20 ml/kg
Plasma, fresh-frozen	Plasma prepared from single donor unit of fresh blood; it is frozen within 6 hr of collection	Source of fibrinogen and factors V and VIII	See plasma; 1 U usually contains approximately 400 mg fibrinogen, 200 U factors VIII and IX, and other stable and labile coagulation factors	Thaw frozen plasma in 37°C water bath with gentle agitation; *do not warm*; administer through a filter; *never add* medications or fluids
Plasma, liquid	Plasma prepared from single donor unit within 5 days after collection; stored frozen	Factor VII, IX, X, XI, and XIII deficiencies or abnormalities	Replacement of factors VII, IX, X, XI, or XIII	See plasma, fresh-frozen
Cryoprecipitated antihemophilic factor (factor VIII)	Preparation containing factor VIII is obtained from a single unit of blood; contains approximately 80 U factor VIII, and 200 mg fibrinogen in 15 ml of plasma	Hemophilia A; von Willebrand's disease (factor VIII deficiency)	Provides high concentrations of factor VIII and fibrinogen	Thaw in warm water bath at 37°C with gentle agitation; administer through filter rapidly within 6 hr after thawing if container not entered; 2 hr after thawing if container entered
Leukocyte concentrate	Leukocytes, platelets, and erythrocytes in varying amounts in 200-500 ml of plasma collected by apheresis; a compatible HLA donor is usually preferred (not identical donor whose use as a tissue donor is anticipated)	Bacterial sepsis not responsive to antibiotic therapy in presence of neutropenia; chronic granulomatous disease when bone marrow recovery is foreseen and temperature elevated for 24-48 hours	Provides granulocytes to more effectively control infection	Administer irradiated leukocytes to prevent engraphment and possible GVHD; regulate rate of flow to give 250-850 granulocytes/μl/M², usually 1 U/day is ordered; slow rate of transfusion at appearance of elevated T wave, chills, and urticaria; stop transfusion when symptoms of transient pulmonary infiltrate appear

Continued.

TABLE 3-4. Blood and Blood Components—cont'd

Product	Description	Indication(s)	Action	Administration
Platelet concentrate (random or single donor)	Platelets separated from whole blood suspended in plasma; collection from single donor preferred	Hemorrhage caused by thrombocytopenia; prevention of potential hemorrhage in bone marrow suppression caused by chemotherapy; abnormalities in platelet function	Corrects hemostatic deficit in thrombocytopenia and abnormally functioning platelets; I U usually increases platelet count 5000/ml in 70 kg adult	Administer through a filter (*never* a microaggregate filter); regulate flow rate to assure administration of total unit in less than 20 min
Normal serum albumin, USP 25% solution hyperoncotic (Note: 5% solution is osmotically equal to plasma)	Derived from pooled venous plasma; contains 25 g normal serum albumin/100 ml	Hypoproteinemia; burns; shock caused by trauma, hemorrhage	Increases oncotic pressure; increases circulating volume by drawing 5 times the infused volume of albumin into circulation unless patient is dehydrated; reduces hemoconcentration and blood viscosity	Administer at flow rate <2-3 ml/min to prevent rapid rise in BP, circulatory embarrassment, or pulmonary edema
Hespan, Hetastarch	A synthetic colloid derived from a waxy starch composed of amylopectin; it has a molecular weight suitable for use as a plasma expander; Hespan is 6% Hetastarch in 0.9% sodium chloride injection	An adjunct in treatment of hemorrhagic shock, burns, and septic shock	Volume expansion resulting from albumin-like properties; Increases ESR when added to whole blood, thereby improving efficacy of granulocyte collection	For hemorrhagic shock, administer at 20 ml/kg/hr, slower rate usually ordered for other indications; contraindications; severe bleeding disorders, severe CHF, renal failure, increased PT or PTT times

TABLE 3-5. Reactions to Transfusion of Blood and Blood Components

Product	Type of reaction	Onset	Observations	Nursing actions
Red blood cells (RBCs), all preparations	Febrile nonhemolytic	Initiation of transfusion to 24 hr post-transfusion	Chills, elevated temperature, headache, nausea, vomiting	Check and record baseline T, P, R, and BP; slow infusion; notify physician; administer antipyretic or antihistamines as ordered; check and record T, P, and R q15min; saline-washed RBCs: frozen, thawed, washed RBCs or leukocyte filter may be ordered to decrease reaction
	Febrile hemolytic	Immediately to 30 min after initiation of transfusion or when 25-50 ml infused	Restlessness, anxiety, precordial oppression, elevated T to 105°F (40.6°C), tachycardia, tachypnea, flushed face, back and thigh pain, generalized tingling, chills, nausea, vomiting, shock, disseminated intravascular coagulation (DIC), renal failure, oliguria, hematuria, anuria	Stop transfusion immediately; change IV tubing; initiate normal saline at 4-6 ml/hr; cap blood tubing with sterile needle or cap; report symptoms to physician and blood bank; recheck identifying blood numbers with patient's numbers; monitor and record T, R, and cardiac rate and rhythm q10-15min; measure and record urine output with each voiding or q½h; send first specimen to lab for testing; report output less than 15 ml/30 min or presence of bleeding; ensure that blood samples are drawn for testing; the following are usually ordered: Hgb, haptoglobin level, methemalbumin, bilirubin, differential agglutination, serologic studies, renal function tests, and aerobic and anaerobic cultures; complete transfusion record, send discontinued blood, tubing, and record to lab for testing; administer medications and fluids IV as ordered; diuretics, oxygen, electrolytes, and heparin may be ordered; prepare for dialysis
Whole blood	Allergic reaction to plasma proteins	Within 30 min after initiating transfusion	Mild reaction; chills, elevated temperature, backache, pain in legs	Check and record baseline T, P, R, and BP; stop infusion; initiate slow (4-6 ml/hr) infusion of saline using new sterile IV tubing; notify physician and blood bank; monitor T, P, R, and BP q 10-15min; ensure that blood specimen is drawn for testing; return remainder of blood product, tubing, and transfusion record to blood bank; indicate observations on transfusion record; usually red cells without IgA will be ordered for administration; oxygen, steroids, vasopressors, or epinephrine may be ordered for anaphylactic shock; prepare for resuscitation
		Immediately to 30 min after initiation of transfusion	Moderate-to-severe reaction: erythematous rash, urticaria, dyspnea, wheezing, hypotension, intestinal hyperperistalsis, anaphylactic shock	
		During transfusion to several days after	Urticaria, swelling of lymph nodes, sore throat	Slow transfusion rate; report observations to physician; administer antihistamines as ordered; blood obtained from a fasting donor may be ordered if reaction is severe

Continued.

TABLE 3-5. Reactions to Transfusion of Blood and Blood Components—cont'd

Product	Type of reaction	Onset	Observations	Nursing actions
	Circulatory overload	During transfusion to 24 hr after	Sharp cough, precordial pain, back pain, dyspnea, cyanosis, increased venous pressure, distended neck veins, productive cough, frothy sputum, pleural rales	Slow transfusion rate; report observations to physician; continue rate of flow as ordered; usually 2 ml/kg/hr; monitor T, P, R, BP, and CVP q15-30min; see CHF (p. 835)
	Febrile (hemolytic)	See RBC	See RBC	See RBC
	Febrile (WBC and/or platelet antibodies)	See leukocyte concentrate	See leukocyte concentrate	See leukocyte concentrate
Massive transfusions of red blood cells or whole blood	Metabolic hyperkalemia and citrate toxicity with acid citrate dextrose (ACD) anticoagulant	Citric acid elevations of 100 mg/100 ml	Tremors, prolonged QT segment on ECG, hypocalcemia, acidosis then alkalosis, cardiac arrest if citric acid levels higher	When massive transfusions required, transfusion products with citrate-phosphate dextrose (CPD) anticoagulant usually ordered; monitor and record T, R, and cardiac function q10-15min; ensure that blood samples are drawn for electrolytes, calcium, pH, CO_2, bicarbonate levels; administer calcium gluconate IV as ordered; administer oral or rectal cation exchange resins as ordered for hyperkalemia
	Pulmonary infiltrates	During transfusion	Chills, elevated temperature, tachycardia, nonproductive cough, dyspnea, respiratory distress syndrome (p. 225)	Stop blood immediately; change tubing; institute normal saline IV at 4-6 ml/hr; monitor and record T, P, R, and BP; auscultate chest for breath and heart sounds; report observations to physician; see respiratory distress syndrome (p. 225)
	Bleeding tendency caused by dilutional effect	Transfusion volume equal to blood volume of patient	Bleeding in any body system, thrombocytopenia, coagulation abnormalities	Report observations to physician immediately; check and record T, P, R, and BP q10-15min; monitor cardiac function continuously; auscultate chest for heart and breath sounds q15-30min; administer platelet concentrate, fluids, and medications as ordered; manage hemorrhage as indicated and ordered
	Pulmonary air embolus	During transfusion	SOB, chest pain, cyanosis, syncope, hypotension, shock	Stop transfusion immediately; place patient on left side; administer oxygen as ordered; monitor vital signs, CVP q15min; see pulmonary embolus (p. 211)
Leukocyte concentrate	Acute reaction	Immediately	Elevated temperature, chills	Slow transfusion; monitor and record T, P, R, and BP q15-30min; auscultate chest for breath and heart sounds q15-30min; report observations to physician; see respiratory distress syndrome (p. 225); medicate with Demerol when ordered
	Transient pulmonary infiltrate		Retrosternal constriction, pallor, cyanosis, tachycardia, cough	
	GVHD			Usually only irradiated leukocytes are administered for prevention of GVHD

Continued.

TABLE 3-5. Reactions to Transfusion of Blood and Blood Components—cont'd

Product	Type of reaction	Onset	Observations	Nursing actions
Platelets	Febrile; usually caused by infusion of incompatible leukocytes contaminating platelet preparations	Immediately to 12-24 hr posttransfusion	Chills, hives, flushing	Check and record T, P, R, and BP q15-30min; administer medications when ordered; reaction usually self-limiting; patient may develop antibodies and destroy platelets in subsequent transfusions; check platelet count 1 hr after transfusion
Plasma	Similar to whole blood	Similar to whole blood	Similar to whole blood	Similar to whole blood
Whole blood with factor VIII removed	Bleeding caused by heparin used as anticoagulant; reactions as in whole blood	During and after transfusion when large volumes administered; see whole blood	Bleeding in any body system See whole blood	Report observations to physician immediately, check and record T, P, R, and BP; monitor cardiac status continuously; administer protamine sulfate as ordered; measure and record urinary output See whole blood
Normal serum albumin	Reactions are rare	During administration	Chills, elevated temperature, nausea	Slow transfusion rate; report observations to physician; check and record T, P, R, and BP q15-30 min
	Circulatory overload/bleeeding during rapid infusion	During transfusion	Rising or elevated BP, circulatory overload, pulmonary edema; new areas of bleeding appear in hemorrhagic shock	Monitor rate of infusion carefully; slow rate of transfusion; report observations to physician; check and record T, P, R, and BP q10-15min; monitor cardiac status continuously; auscultate chest for heart and breath sounds q15-30min; observe closely for new sites of bleeding

BIBLIOGRAPHY

American Association of Blood Banks: Blood transfusions outside the hospital, *Am J Nurs* 486, 1989.

Birdsall C, Carpenter K, and Considine R: How is autotransfusion done? *Am J Nurs* 108, 1988.

Daeffler RJ: Potential for bleeding. In Daeffler RJ, Petrosino BM: *Manual of oncology nursing practice: nursing diagnosis and care*, Rockville, Md, 1990, Aspen Publishers.

Doenges ME, Jeffries MF, and Moorhouse MF: *Nursing care plans: nursing diagnosis in planning patient care*, Philadelphia, 1990, FA Davis.

Griffin JP: The bleeding patient, *Nurs '86* 34, 1986.

Gulanick M et al: *Nursing care plans: nursing diagnosis and treatment*, ed 2, St Louis, 1990, Mosby–Year Book.

Guyton AC: *Textbook of medical physiology*, ed 6, Philadelphia, 1986, WB Saunders.

Huntoon MB: The hematologic system. In Armstrong ME et al, eds: *McGraw-Hill handbook of clinical nursing*, New York, 1979, McGraw-Hill.

Ihde JK, Jacobsen WK, and Briggs BA: *Principles of critical care*, Philadelphia, 1987, WB Saunders.

Kaiser Permanente Hospital, Southern California Permanente Medical Group: *Policy and procedure manual, 1989: blood transfusion therapy.*

Kim MJ, McFarland GK, and McFarlane AM: *Pocket guide to nursing diagnosis.* ed 3, St Louis, 1989, CV Mosby.

Kinney MR et al, eds: *AACN clinical reference for critical care nursing*, ed 2, New York, 1988, McGraw-Hill.

Pagana KD, Pagana TJ: *Diagnostic testing and nursing implications*, ed 3, St Louis, 1990, Mosby–Year Book.

Schechter N, Berrien FB, and Katz S: PCA for adolescents in sickle cell crisis, *Am J Nurs* 719, 1988.

Simmonson GM: Caring for patients with acute myelocytic leukemia, *Am J Nurs* 304, 1988.

Thompson JM et al: Mosby's *manual of clinical nursing*, ed 2, St Louis, 1989, CV Mosby.

Ulrich C, Canale S, and Wendell S: *Nursing care planning guides: a nursing diagnosis approach*, ed 2, Philadelphia, 1990, WB Saunders.

Weintrobe MM et al: *Clinical hematology*, ed 8, Philadelphia, 1981, Lea & Feibiger.

Westphal RG, Kasprisim DO: *Current status of hemapheresis: indications, technology and complications*, Arlington, 1987, American Association of Blood Banks.

4
CHAPTER

Respiratory System

RESPIRATORY ASSESSMENT

Subjective Data

Cough
Pain
  Chest
  Abdomen
Wheeze
Shortness of breath
How many pillows used
Amount of exercise tolerated
Fever
Chills
Rapid breathing
Tiring easily
Change in voice
Dizziness
Sweating
Swelling of feet and hands

Objective Data

Anxious facies
DOE (dyspnea on exertion)
Flaring nostrils
Red, swollen nose
Nasal discharge
Color
  Cyanosis
    Lips
    Circumoral area
    Nail beds
    Gums
    Earlobes
    Soles of feet
    Palms of hands
  Pallor
  Ashen
  Gray
  Cherry red
  Red
  Reddish blue
Confusion, restlessness
Hallucinations
Cough
  Onset and duration
  Characteristics

Dry hacking, barking, congested
  Severity
  Nonproductive
  Productive
  Sputum
  Characteristics: color, odor, consistency
Hemoptysis
Stridor
Wheeze
Assuming upright position: orthopnea
Clubbing of extremities: nail beds
Use of accessory muscles of respiration
Telegraphic speech pattern—short, choppy sentences
Eyes
  Engorged veins
  Papilledema
Elevated temperature
Diaphoresis
Anorexia
Weight
  Obese
  Gain
  Loss
Ascites
Rash
Respirations (Tables 4-1 and 4-2)
  Bradypnea
  Tachypnea
  Long expiratory phase
  Irregular
  Asymmetric
  Periods of apnea
  Cheyne-Stokes
  Shallow
  Pursed-lip breathing
  Biot's
  Kussmaul's
  Apneustic
  Hyperventilation
Retractions
  Suprasternal
  Supraclavicular
  Substernal
  Intercostal
Cardiac status
  Elevated BP

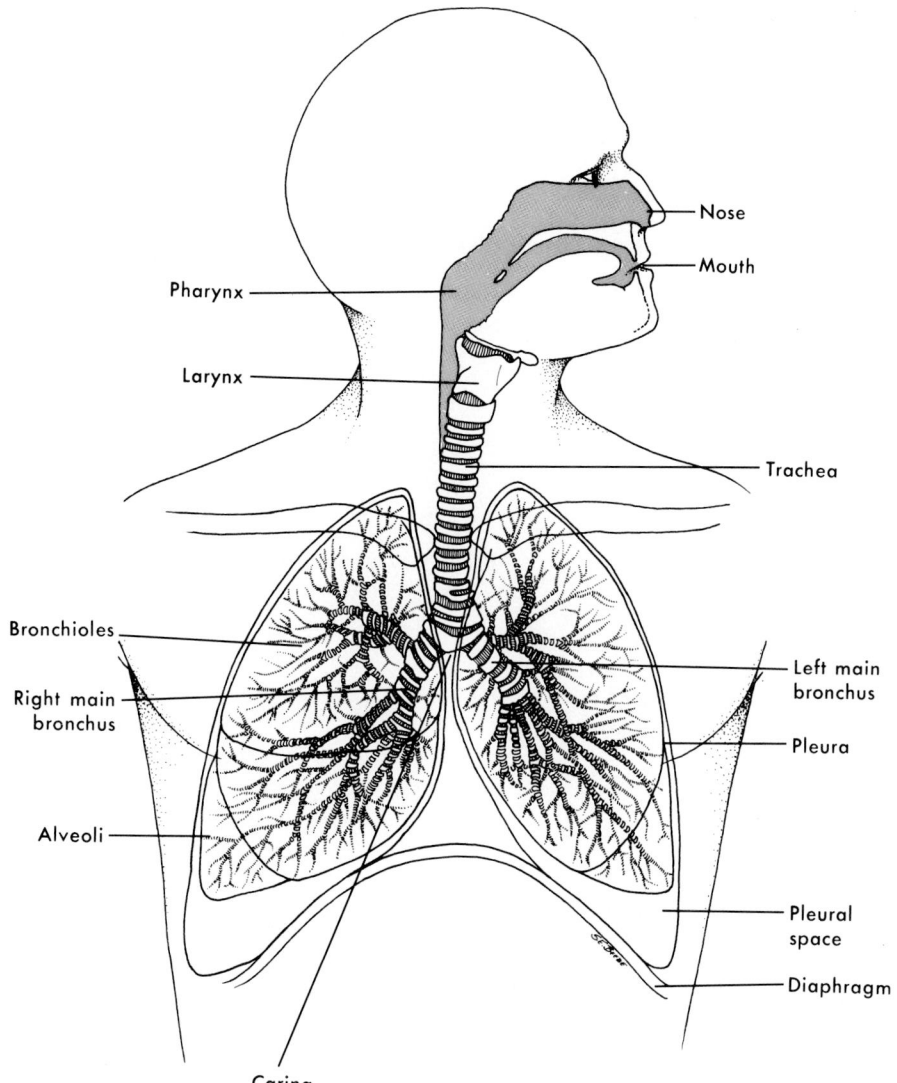

FIGURE 4-1. Respiratory system.

TABLE 4-1. Patterns of Respiration

Type		Characteristics
Normal respirations		Rate Rhythm, regular
Cheyne-Stokes respiration		Periods of apnea alternating with series of respiratory cycles Rate and amplitude of successive respiratory cycles increase to a maximum and then decrease until terminated by period of apnea
Biot's respiration		Variation of Cheyne-Stokes respiration in which periods of apnea alternate irregularly with periods of breaths of equal depth
Sighing respiration		Deep audible sighs that interrupt normal respiratory rhythm
Painful respiration		Interruption of normal respiratory rhythm caused by pain; breathing frequently becomes shallow during interruption
Ataxic respiration		Gross irregularity in rate, rhythm, and depth of respiration; also referred to as meningitic respirations

Modified from Abels LF: *Mosby's manual of critical care*, St Louis, 1979, CV Mosby.

TABLE 4-2. Normal Respiratory Findings

Area of concern	Normal adult findings	Variations in child	Variations in older adult
General appearance	Appears relaxed Breathing is quiet and easy without apparent effort Facial expressions and limb movements are relaxed		
Breathing pattern	Diaphragmatic-thoracic pattern is smooth and regular May have occasional sighing respirations Breathing is quiet and passive	Abdominal and nasal breathing during childhood until 6 to 7 years of age, then change to adult pattern Newborns may demonstrate Cheyne-Stokes breathing until 3 to 4 weeks of age	Pattern is same as for adults, but calcification at rib articulation points may decrease chest expansion

Respiratory rate	12-20 resp/min
	Ratio of pulse to respirations is 4:1
		Newborn: 30-50 resp/min
		  1 yr: 20-40 resp/min
		  3 yr: 20-30 resp/min
		  6 yr: 16-22 resp/min
		  10 yr: 16-20 resp/min
		  17 yr: 14-20 resp/min	

Skin	Appears well oxygenated; no cyanosis or pallor present Palpation of skin and chest wall reveals smooth skin and a stable chest wall; there are no crepitations, bulging, or painful spots	Babies may become mottled if left uncovered	
Nail bed, nail configuration	Minimal angulation between base of nail and finger No thickening of distal finger width		
Chest wall configuration	Symmetrical, bilateral muscle development A:P to transverse ratio is 1:2 to 5:7; larger than these ratios is considered to be barrel chest Straight spinal processes Downward and equal slope of ribs; costal angle 90 degrees or less	Newborns have rounded chest wall configuration; by 6 years of age, A:P ratio should be 1:2	Kyphosis is a common finding in elderly persons; there is dorsal scoliosis with slight tracheal deviation; this may also cause a slight increase in A:P to transverse ratio
Tracheal position	Midline and straight directly above the suprasternal notch		May be slightly deviated if kyphosis is present

From Thompson JM et al: *Mosby's manual of clinical nursing*, ed 2, St Louis, 1989, CV Mosby.

Tachycardia
Bradycardia
Sinus dysrhythmia
Congestive heart failure (CHF)
  Crackles
  Rhonchi
  Jugular venous distention
  Edema
  Abdominal distention and pain
  Hepatosplenomegaly
Thoracic examination
  Scoliosis
  Kyphosis
  Kyphoscoliosis
  Pectus excavatum (funnel chest)
  Pectus carinatum (pigeon chest)
  Barrel chest
  Unequal shoulder height

Palpation
  Thoracic expansion
  Fremitus (vocal/tactile)
  Tracheal deviation
  Crepitus
Percussion
  Resonance
  Hyperresonance
  Tympany
  Dullness
  Flatness
Auscultation (Table 4-3)
  Decreased or absent breath sounds
  Crackles
  Rhonchi
  Wheezing
  Friction rubs
  Pectoriloquy

TABLE 4-3. Breath and Voice Sounds: Normal and Abnormal

Breath and voice sounds	Characteristics	Findings
NORMAL		
Vesicular	Heard over most of lung fields; low pitch; soft and short expirations	Low pitch, soft expirations
Bronchovesicular	Heard over main bronchus area and over upper right posterior lung field; medium pitch; expiration equals inspiration	Medium pitch, medium expirations
Bronchial	Heard only over trachea; high pitch; loud and long expirations	High pitch, loud expirations
ABNORMAL		
Bronchial when heard over peripheral lung fields	High pitch; loud and long expirations	
Bronchovesicular sounds when heard over peripheral lung fields	Medium pitch with inspirations equal to expirations	
Adventitious	Crackles: discrete, noncontinuous sounds *Fine crackles* (rales): high-pitched, discrete, noncontinuous crackling sounds heard during the end of inspiration (indicates inflammation or congestion)	
	Medium crackles (rales): lower, more moist sound heard during the midstage of inspiration; not cleared by a cough	
	Coarse crackles (rales): loud, bubbly noise heard during inspiration; not cleared by a cough	
	Wheezes: continuous musical sounds; if low pitched, may be called rhonchi *Sibilant wheeze:* musical noise sounding like a squeak; may be heard during inspiration or expiration; usually louder during expiration	
	Sonorous wheeze (rhonchi): loud, low, coarse sound like a snore heard at any point of inspiration or expiration; coughing may clear sound (usually means mucus accumulation in trachea or large bronchi)	
	Pleural friction rub: dry, rubbing, or grating sound, usually caused by the inflammation of pleural surfaces; heard during inspiration or expiration; loudest over lower lateral anterior surface	

From Thompson JM et al: *Mosby's manual of clinical nursing*, ed 2, St Louis, 1989, CV Mosby.   *Continued.*

TABLE 4-3. Breath and Voice Sounds: Normal and Abnormal—cont'd

Breath and voice sounds	Characteristics	Findings
RESONANCE OF SPOKEN VOICE		
	Bronchophony: using diaphragm of stethoscope, listen to posterior chest as patient says "ninety-nine"	Negative response: muffled "nin-nin" sound heard Positive response: clear, loud "ninety-nine" response heard because the lung tissue is consolidated
	Whispered pectoriloquy: listen to posterior chest as patient whispers "one, two, three"	Negative response: muffled sounds heard Positive response: clear "one, two, three" is heard because of lung consolidation
	Egophony: listen to posterior chest as the patient says "e-e-e"	Negative response: muffled "e-e-e" sound heard Positive response: sound of *e* changes to an a-a-a sound because of consolidation

Bronchophony
Egophony

Pertinent Background Information

CONCURRENT DISEASES OR CONDITIONS

Cancer
Heart disease
Renal disease
Liver disease
Ascites
Polycythemia
Obesity
Hypertension
Guillain-Barré syndrome
Myasthenia gravis or other neurologic disease affecting respiratory function

PSYCHOLOGIC RESPONSES

Response to stress
Methods of coping
Response to pain
Relationships with others

PREVIOUS RESPIRATORY CONDITION/MEDICAL HISTORY

Asthma
Bronchitis
Emphysema
Tuberculosis
Fibrocystic disease
Premature birth
Previous operations

FAMILY HISTORY

Heart disease
Hypertension
Diabetes
Obesity
Pulmonary disorders

SOCIAL HISTORY

Smoking (past and present): packs per day times how many years
Alcohol use
Exercise and activity levels
Occupation
    Current and previous
Sleep patterns
Environmental factors: exposure to dust, fumes, asbestos, or chemicals
Recent exposure to infections
Travel out of country
Available family support

MEDICATION HISTORY

Prescription medications
Over-the-counter medications

Diagnostic Aids

Chest x-ray examination
Complete blood cell count (CBC)
Arterial blood gases (ABGs)
Serum electrolytes
Electrocardiogram (ECG)
Sputum evaluation
    Amount
    Color, odor, viscosity
    Culture and sensitivity
Throat or nasopharyngeal culture
Pulmonary function tests
    Tidal volume (V_T)
    Minute volume (V_E)
    Vital capacity (VC)
    Forced vital capacity (FVC)
    Forced expiratory volume (FEV)
    Functional residual capacity (FRC)
    Inspiratory reserve volume (IRV)
    Residual volume (RV)
    Inspiratory capacity (IC)
    Expiratory reserve volume (ERV)

Total lung capacity (TLC)
Gastric washings
Skin tests
Sweat test
Bronchoscopy
Bronchograms
Lung biopsy
Lung scans
Scalene node biopsy
Aortography
Pulmonary angiography
Tomography
Fluoroscopy
Barium swallow
Computed tomography (CT) scan
Pulmonary echograms
Body plethysmography
Thoracentesis

THERAPEUTIC BRONCHOSCOPY

*Direct visual examination of the trachea and tracheo-
bronchial tree by means of a bronchoscope; the flexible
fiberoptic bronchoscope is commonly used because it is
better tolerated by the patient and allows better visualization of distal airways*

Purpose/Indications

Collect secretions for laboratory examinations
Obtain tissue for biopsies
Locate and biopsy tumors
Diagnose hemoptysis, lesions, or masses
Remove foreign bodies or mucous plug secretions
Treat lung abscesses, pneumonia, or aspiration

Preparation

Explain procedure to patient
Maintain NPO for 6 hr before procedure
Manage pain with sedation as indicated; assess effective-
ness of pain relief measures
Provide emotional support (patient may be fearful of dis-
comfort and/or possible findings)
Remove dentures
Place patient in sitting or supine position as directed
Instruct patient to breathe in and out of nose with mouth
open during procedure
Fiberoptic bronchoscope is inserted through nose or
mouth
Rigid bronchoscope is inserted through mouth

Postbronchoscopic Assessment
Observations/findings

Difficulty in breathing
Stridor
Nasal flaring
Suprasternal and/or supraclavicular retractions
Hemoptysis

Hypotension
Tachycardia
Tachypnea
Cyanosis
Nausea, vomiting
Absence of gag and cough reflex
Hoarseness
Throat pain
Chest pain

Potential complications

Crepitus and/or subcutaneous emphysema
Absence of breath sounds
Pneumothorax

Immediate Postbronchoscopic Care

Check BP, P, and R q15min for four times, then q2h to
4h and prn
Assist and teach patient to
Not eat or drink until gag reflex returns
Maintain bed rest; elevate head of bed 45 degrees
Dispose of tissue after coughing
Understand importance of not smoking
Manage pain as indicated; assess effectiveness of pain
relief measure(s)
Establish means of communication
Call bell within reach
Pad and pencil or Magic Slate*
Auscultate chest for breath sounds q2h to 4h and prn
Report absent or diminished breath sounds to physician
Perform postural drainage as ordered
Perform oropharyngeal suctioning prn
Administer oxygen as ordered

Convalescent Care

Check BP, T, P, and R q8h and prn
Assist and teach patient to
Gargle with warm saline solution q2h to 4h as indicated
Maintain position of comfort
Progress from liquids to diet as tolerated; avoid ex-
tremely hot foods

Patient Teaching/Discharge Outcome

Ensure that patient and/or significant other knows and
understands
Importance of not driving self home if procedure is done
on an outpatient basis
Importance of maintaining liquid or soft diet as ordered
until throat pain disappears
Importance of forcing fluids to 3000 ml daily unless
contraindicated by patient's condition
Need to avoid extremely hot foods and liquids
Need to avoid smoking
Symptoms to report to physician
Chest pain

*Registered trademark of Western Publishing Co., Inc., Racine, Wis.

Difficulty in breathing
Inability to swallow
Importance of ongoing outpatient care
Name of medication, dosage, time of administration, purpose, and side effects
Need to avoid taking over-the-counter medications without checking with physician
Importance of avoiding persons with upper respiratory infections (URIs)

THORACENTESIS

Puncture of the chest wall with a large-gauge needle to remove air or fluid from the pleural space

Preparation

Auscultate chest for breath sounds
Obtain chest x-ray examination as ordered by physician
Obtain baseline BP, T, P, and R
Administer sedation as ordered
Prepare local anesthetic as ordered
Position patient on edge of bed with feet supported; head and arms should be resting on overbed table; if patient is unable to sit on edge of bed, have patient lie on unaffected side with head of bed elevated and arm raised over head
Provide emotional support
Obtain signed informed consent

Preprocedure Teaching

Ensure that patient and/or significant other knows and understands
Procedure to be performed
Importance of remaining immobile during procedure
Importance of not coughing during procedure
That sensations of pain and/or pressure are to be expected

Assessment During and After Thoracentesis
Observations/findings
DURING PROCEDURE

Chest tightness
Difficulty in breathing
Tachypnea
Tachycardia
Vertigo
Hypotension
Cyanosis
Diaphoresis
Pallor
Anxiety

POSTPROCEDURE

Difficulty in breathing
Chest pain
Uncontrollable cough

Hemoptysis
Decreased BP
Tachycardia
Tachypnea
Absent or diminished breath sounds
Crepitus
Hyperresonance
Diminished chest wall movement on affected side
Distended neck veins
Cyanosis
Elevated temperature
Deviation of larynx and trachea

Potential complications

Mediastinal shift
Pneumothorax
Pulmonary edema

Immediate Postprocedure Care

Check BP, P, and R q15min for four times, then q2h to 4h and prn
Check temperature q4h for 24 hr
Apply adhesive bandage or dressing to site of puncture
Check dressing q15min to 30min
Turn patient on unaffected side for 1 hr, then to position of comfort
Manage pain as indicated; assess effectiveness of pain relief measure(s)
Administer oxygen as ordered
Measure and record total amount of fluid removed; note color and character
Auscultate breath sounds q2h for two times; then q4h for 24 hr
Report diminished or absent breath sounds and/or audible rales to physician
Obtain chest x-ray examination as ordered by physician

Ongoing Care

Continue with immediate postprocedure care and decrease frequency of nursing functions as patient's condition improves
Change dressing prn
Assist and teach patient to
Turn and deep breathe q2h to 4h
Ambulate as tolerated
Maintain diet as ordered

Patient Teaching/Discharge Outcome

Ensure that patient and/or significant other knows and understands
Importance of deep breathing q2h to 4h
Importance of maintaining a well-balanced diet
Importance of forcing fluids to limit allotted for patient's condition
Importance of not smoking
Importance of avoiding persons with URIs

Name of medication, dosage, time of administration, purpose, and side effects

Need to avoid taking over-the-counter medications without checking with physician

Symptoms to report to physician
  Difficulty in breathing
  Chest pain
  Vertigo
  Elevated temperature
  Diaphoresis
  Uncontrollable cough
  Hemoptysis
Importance of ongoing outpatient care

ASPIRATION OF SECRETIONS

Preprocedure Assessment
Observations/findings

Restlessness
Wheezing
Inability to expectorate
Difficulty in breathing
Tachycardia
Crackles
Rhonchi over large airways
Decreased breath sounds
Cyanosis

Preprocedure Teaching

Explain procedure to patient
Discuss what is expected of patient during procedure
Demonstrate suction equipment
Assist and teach patient to cough and deep breathe before procedure

Assessment During Procedure
Observations/findings

Tachycardia
Hypoxemia
Trauma to airway; bloody aspirate
Bronchospasm
Aspirate
  Color
  Consistency
  Amount
Cyanosis
Tachypnea
Dyspnea
Nausea

Potential complications

Hypotension
Sudden hypertension
Hypoxemia
Bradycardia
Cardiac dysrhythmias

Atrioventricular (AV) heart block
Premature ventricular contractions (PVCs)
Cardiac arrest

Care During Procedure

Auscultate breath sounds
Maintain sterile technique
Use vented or Y catheter
Choose correct catheter to prevent airway occlusion and/or trauma; should be half diameter of airway
  General guide
    Adult: 12 to 18 French
    Child: 6 to 12 French
    Infant: 5 to 6 French
Hyperoxygenate and hyperinflate patient's lungs for four to five breaths × 1 min
Avoid use of force when inserting catheter
Apply suction only while removing catheter; do not exceed 10 sec
Rotate catheter while removing; avoid moving catheter up and down while suctioning
Suction pressure must not exceed
  Adult: 120 to 150 mm Hg
  Child: 100 to 120 mm Hg
  Infant: 60 to 100 mm Hg
Release suction every 10 sec; ventilate patient for four or five breaths or longer if necessary as soon as suction has been released
Use separate sterile catheter for tracheal suctioning if catheter has already been used for oral suctioning
Assess patient for
  Adequate chest expansion
  Changes in skin color: lips, earlobes, fingertips
  Increased restlessness
  Increased pulse rate
  Cardiac dysrhythmias
  Bronchospasm
If bronchospasm, bradycardia, PVCs, or AV block occurs, stop suctioning immediately and ventilate and hyperoxygenate patient
Observe aspirate: if purulent or colored, obtain specimen for culture

Postprocedure Assessment
Observations/findings

Breath sounds
  Crackles
    Decreased
    Increased
  Rhonchi over large airways
    Decreased
    Increased
Arterial blood gases: decreased PaO_2
Elevated temperature
Bronchospasm
Tachycardia
Cyanosis

Immediate Postprocedure Care
General

Auscultate breath sounds; prepare to repeat suctioning procedure as indicated

Return oxygen concentration to setting ordered by physician

Check apical pulse and/or record ECG rhythm strip

Assist and teach patient to deep breathe after suctioning procedure

Specific

Oropharyngeal and nasopharyngeal suction

Avoid nasopharyngeal suctioning if patient has a spinal fluid leak or epistaxis

Elevate head of bed 45 degrees

Suction mouth and throat and discard catheter

Lubricate sterile catheter with water-soluble lubricant or water and insert into nares for suctioning

NASOTRACHEAL SUCTION

Avoid nasotracheal suction if patient has a spinal fluid leak or epistaxis

Elevate head of bed 60 to 90 degrees

Hyperoxygenate and hyperinflate patient's lungs for four to five breaths before suctioning

Lubricate sterile catheter with water-soluble lubricant or water and insert through nostril to pharynx

Have patient cough or deep breathe and pass catheter into trachea

Suction no more than 10 sec at a time

Hyperoxygenate and hyperinflate patient's lungs for four or five breaths after suctioning

Return oxygen to setting ordered by physician

ENDOTRACHEAL OR TRACHEOSTOMY SUCTION

Be aware that a coudé (curved-tip) catheter may be used in an attempt to suction left mainstem bronchus in certain disease states

Hyperoxygenate and hyperinflate patient's lungs for four or five breaths before suctioning

Suction oropharynx and discard catheter

Suction endotracheal tube or tracheostomy tube with a sterile catheter

Suction no more than 10 sec at a time

Hyperoxygenate and hyperinflate patient's lungs for four or five breaths after suctioning

Return oxygen to setting ordered by physician

OXYGEN THERAPY

Use of oxygen to relieve hypoxemia and avoid hypoxia; oxygen flow rate and concentration should be regulated to maintain PaO_2 between 60 mm Hg and 100 mm Hg

Preprocedure Assessment
Observations/findings

Hypoxemia
$PaO_2 < 60$ mm Hg
$PaCO_2 > 42$ mm Hg
Respiratory
Cyanosis
Tachypnea
Dyspnea
Shallow respiration
Neurological
Drowsiness
Disorientation
Restlessness
Decreased attention span
Impaired judgment
Delirium
Decreased long-term and short-term memory
Nausea
Nasal flaring
Muscle weakness
Retractions
Cardiovascular
Hypotension
Sudden hypertension
Bradycardia
Tachycardia
Cardiac dysrhythmias

Preprocedure Teaching

Explain procedure to patient
Demonstrate equipment to be used

Assessment During Procedure
Observations/findings

Respiratory depression
Somnolence
Substernal pain with deep inspiration
Arterial blood gases
PaO_2
$PaCO_2$
pH
Tidal volume
Vital capacity (VC)
Elevated temperature
Tachycardia
Psychosocial problems
Anxiety
Depression
Dependence

Potential complications

Oxygen toxicity: time and dose related
Decreased lung compliance
Reduced VC
Sore throat

Cough
Diminished breath sounds
Crackles
CNS toxicity
   Nausea
   Anxiety
   Numbness
   Muscular twitching
Substernal pain with deep inspiration
Circulatory depression: falling central venous pressure (CVP)
Visual impairment
   Tearing eyes
   Papilledema

Care During Procedure
General

Assess patient for signs of hypoxemia

Maintain patent airway

Assist and teach patient to maintain position best suited for optimal lung expansion; head of bed usually elevated 45 to 90 degrees

Initiate and maintain oxygen flow rate and concentration with humidification as ordered; have portable oxygen tank and/or extension tubing available if oxygen is to be used continuously and patient is ambulatory or needs to be transported

Monitor BP, T, R, and apical pulse q15min for 4 hr, then q2h to 4h if stable

Assess level of consciousness q15min for 4 hr, then q2h to 4h if no change

Auscultate breath sounds q2h to 4h; report diminished or absent breath sounds or audible crackles and rhonchi to physician

Administer oral and nasal hygiene q2h to 4h

Assist and teach patient to turn, cough, and deep breathe q2h to 4h

Provide emotional support; remain with patient if acutely anxious

Continue other nursing functions required for primary disease process

Avoid high-flow rate and concentration of oxygen for patients who require some degree of hypoxemia to maintain respirations

Monitor arterial blood gases as ordered

NOTE: Oxygen toxicity can occur with oxygen concentrations of 50% or higher administered for 24 to 48 hr; symptoms include tachypnea, substernal pain, and dizziness; physiologic effects include atelectasis, ciliary dysfunction, and nitrogen washout; in carbon dioxide retainers, hypoventilation, somnolence, and apnea may occur with minimal elevations in PaO_2

General precautions

Provide humidification with oxygen administration

Always use sterile equipment when administering oxygen; change connecting tubing, humidification equipment, masks, and nasal cannulas q24h

Do not allow smoking while oxygen is in use

Do not permit oil, grease, or other combustible material to come in contact with cylinders, regulators, gauges, valves, or fittings

Administer oxygen only with a safely functioning and properly fitting regulating device

Cylinders
   Secure safely to prevent from falling
   Transport only in proper carrier
   Maintain valve in closed position when not in use
   Open valve slowly to full open position when using

Care with use of various devices
NASAL CATHETER

Check catheter patency before insertion

Lubricate catheter with water-soluble lubricant

Avoid kinking or twisting tubing

Position catheter so it cannot be seen when patient's tongue is depressed

Tape securely to nose

Remove catheter q6h to 8h

Reinsert new catheter in opposite nostril if possible

Assess patient for abdominal distention

NASAL CANNULA (PRONGS)

Useful for providing approximately 24% to 44% oxygen at flow rates of 1 to 6 L/min (Flow >6 L/min does not deliver more oxygen)

Ensure proper positioning; avoid kinking or twisting, which impedes oxygen flow

Apply water-soluble lubricant to nares

Evaluate patient for pressure sores or nasopharyngeal irritation

Reposition q2h

Clean equipment daily

SIMPLE OXYGEN MASK

Can deliver 40% to 60% oxygen at flow rates of 6 to 10 L/min (rate lower than 5 L/min with face mask can lead to carbon dioxide retention in dead space of mask)

Choose correct size for patient

Remove mask periodically for a few seconds
   Dry patient's face
   Observe for pressure areas

Use face mask only with artificial airway in unconscious patient

Have nasal cannula available for patient to use while eating

PARTIAL REBREATHING MASK WITH RESERVOIR BAG

Used for higher oxygen concentrations (40% to 60%) at flow rates of 8 to 12 L/min

Select correct size for patient

Ensure proper positioning of mask

Apply mask as patient exhales

Avoid twisting or kinking bag

Avoid letting bag totally deflate when patient is inhaling; increase oxygen flow rate if necessary

Remove mask periodically for a few seconds
  Dry patient's face
  Observe for pressure areas
  Apply water-soluble lubricant to lips

Have nasal cannula available for patient to use while eating

Monitor arterial blood gases

Observe for signs of oxygen toxicity

NONREBREATHING MASK WITH RESERVOIR BAG

Provides 60% to 90% oxygen at flow rates of 6 to 15 L/min

Select correct size for patient

Ensure proper positioning of mask

Avoid letting bag totally deflate

Avoid twisting bag

Ensure that all rubber flaps stay in place

Remove mask periodically for a few seconds
  Dry patient's face
  Observe for pressure areas
  Apply water-soluble lubricant to lips

Observe patient for signs of oxygen toxicity; monitor arterial blood gases as ordered

Have a nasal cannula available for patient to use while eating

VENTURI MASK

Provides 24% to 50% oxygen at 3 to 8 L/min flow rate

Select correct size for patient

Ensure proper positioning; avoid kinking of tubing and blockage of oxygen intake parts, which alter FIO_2

Maintain oxygen flow rate as ordered by physician

Monitor arterial blood gases

Remove mask periodically for a few seconds
  Dry patient's face
  Observe for pressure areas
  Apply water-soluble lubricant to lips

Rid tubing of excessive moisture prn

Have nasal cannula available for patient to use while eating

HUMIDITY AND AEROSOL THERAPY

Valuable in loosening thick secretions and in the delivery of medications; aerosol and humidity devices used to provide humidity when artificial airways are being used are as follows

jet nebulizers *Hand-held nebulizers commonly used to provide medicated aerosol treatment; these are large-reservoir nebulizers for continuous aerosol treatment with or without supplemental oxygen*

ultrasonic nebulizers *Can be given to patients breathing on their own or installed into ventilator circuits; treatments generally last 20 to 30 min*

humidifiers *Used to prevent humidity deficit when artificial airways are in use; the most commonly used are the bubble humidifiers in conjunction with low-flow oxygen devices*

Assessment
Observations/findings

PATIENT

Respirations
  Quality
  Rate
  Depth
Breath sounds
  Crackles
  Diminished or absent
Secretions
  Amount
  Color
  Character
Fluid overload

EQUIPMENT

Oxygen concentration ordered

Oxygen concentration delivered

Heat control

Connecting tubing patent; free from excess moisture

Ongoing Care
Patient

Maintain patent airway

Monitor patient as frequently as indicated by disease or patient's condition during treatment

Suction as indicated

Auscultate breath sounds q2h to 4h; report absent or diminished breath sounds to physician

Position patient comfortably

Dry face of moisture as indicated

Assist and teach patient to turn, cough, and deep breathe q2h to 4h

Equipment

Use sterile distilled water in nebulizer; check water level in reservoir q4h—when adding water, empty reservoir, then refill to correct level

Free tubing of excess moisture q2h to 3h and prn

Check heat control q2h to 4h

Maintain temperature between 95° and 97.8° F (35° and 36.6° C)

Change mask, adaptors, and tubing q24h

Secure and allow sufficient tubing for turning

CHRONIC OBSTRUCTIVE PULMONARY DISEASE (COPD), CHRONIC OBSTRUCTIVE LUNG DISEASE (COLD)

Chronic condition associated with a history of emphysema (Figure 4-2), asthma, chronic bronchitis (see box), bronchiectasis, cigarette smoking, or exposure to

DISEASES CONTRIBUTING TO DEVELOPMENT OF COPD

Chronic bronchitis

Mucosal swelling and inflammation of the bronchial mucous membrane with excessive mucus secretion in bronchial tree

Assessment
Observations/findings

Shortness of breath
Cough
  Persistent
  Productive
Sputum (morning)
  Thick, tenacious, copious
  Mucopurulent
Breath sounds
  Scattered
  Moist crackles
  Rhonchi
Wheezing respirations
Bronchospasm
Cyanosis, "blue bloater"

Laboratory/diagnostic findings

Arterial blood gases
  Decreased PaO_2
  Increased $PaCO_2$
  Respiratory acidosis
Sputum secretions
  Increased polymorphonuclear
    neutrophil leukocytes
Chest x-ray examination
  Increased peribronchial markings
    at both bases
  Increased cardiac size
Pulmonary function tests
  Decreased FEV_1/FVC ratio
  Increased residual volume
  FRC: may be normal in pure
    bronchitis

Emphysema

Destruction of elastic tissues of the alveolar walls, causing a reduced expiratory flow rate and overinflated alveoli; a progressive disease that is irreversible

Assessment
Observations/findings

Shortness of breath
Difficulty in breathing
Respirations
  Tachypnea
  Shallow
  Prolonged expiratory phase
Use of accessory muscles
  Intercostals
  Neck
  Shoulder
Cough: may be productive
Pursed-lip breathing
Orthopnea
Thoracic changes
  Barrel chest
  Unequal chest expansion
  Increased AP chest diameter
  Skin color: usually normal, "pink
    puffer"
Cachexia
Anorexia
Weight loss
Breath sounds
  Distant
  Expiratory wheezes
Hyperresonance
Weakness
Fatigue

Laboratory/diagnostic findings

Arterial blood gases
  Decreased PaO_2; normal or increased $PaCO_2$
  pH within normal limits if compensation has occurred
Chest x-ray examination
  Hyperlucent lung fields; small, narrow heart; increased AP diameter; low, flat diaphragm, widened intercostals
  Apical bullae are common
  Decreased vascular markings
Pulmonary function tests
  Increased total lung capacity
  Increased residual volume, FRC
Blood chemistry: α_1-antitrypsin

Bronchiectasis

Chronic dilation of a bronchus or bronchi, secreting large amounts of purulent sputum

Assessment
Observations/findings

Cough: paroxysms in early morning
Sputum
  Profuse (up to 200-300 ml/day)
  Purulent
  Foul odor
Wheezes
Shortness of breath
Prolonged expiration
Hemoptysis
Nasal stuffiness
Breath sounds
  Crackles
  Rhonchi
Recurrent infection, pneumonia
Elevated temperature
Chronic sinusitis

Laboratory/diagnostic findings

Chest x-ray examination
  Usually normal
  Air fluid levels and infiltrates may
    be seen in advanced diffuse disease
Bronchography
Sputum examination: staphylococci, streptococci, and pseudomonas commonly seen on sputum smears and cultures
Pulmonary function tests
  Normal or slightly decreased lung volumes
  Decreased flow rates
Arterial blood gases: mild decrease in PaO_2 and $PaCO_2$ are common

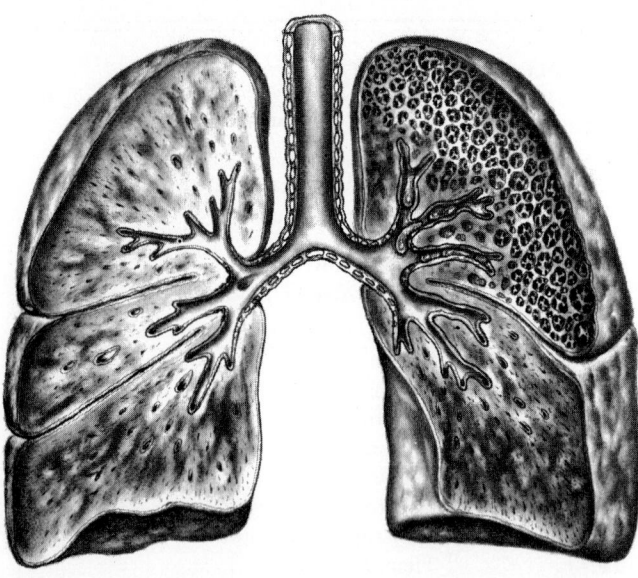

FIGURE 4-2. Lobar emphysema. (From Wilson SF and Thompson JM: Respiratory disorders, *Mosby's clinical nursing series,* St Louis, 1990, Mosby—Year Book.)

air pollution; there is persistent airway obstruction that progressively increases

Assessment
Observations/findings

Audible expiratory wheeze
Prolonged expirations with considerable effort
Pursed-lip breathing
Use of accessory muscles of respiration
Increased AP diameter of chest (barrel chest)
Breath sounds
   Diminished breath sounds
   Crackles
   Rhonchi
Bronchospasm
Restlessness
Fatigue
Anorexia
Weight loss
Cough
   Productive/unproductive
   Hacking, ineffective
Amount and character of sputum
Malaise
Cardiac
   Hypotension
   Tachycardia
   Dysrhythmia
Pulsus paradoxus
Carbon dioxide retention
   Restlessness
   Confusion
   Somnolence

Loss of memory
Psychosocial problems
   Anxiety
   Fear of death
   Fear of suffocation

Laboratory/diagnostic studies

ABG studies
   Alveolar-arterial (A-a) oxygen gradient: widened
   Decreased PaO_2, pH
   Increased PCO_2
Chest x-ray examination
   Flattened diaphragm
   Increased AP diameter
   Hyperinflation of lungs
Pulmonary function studies
   Decreased FEV, FVC, FEV_1/FVC ratio
Sputum specimen analysis
CBC: polycythemia if chronically hypoxic
Serum electrolytes
ECG: atrial dysrhythmia low voltage, right axis deviation in advanced disease

Potential complications

Dysrhythmias
Acute respiratory failure
Cardiac failure
Cor pulmonale
   Peripheral edema
   Hepatomegaly
   Cyanosis
   Distended neck veins
   Loud P_2
   Murmur of tricuspid regurgitation
Polycythemia
Peptic and esophageal reflux

Medical Management

Oxygen therapy
Artificial airway/mechanical ventilation as required
Chest physiotherapy
Serial ABG assessment
Medications
   Bronchodilators
   Antibiotics
   Corticosteroids
   Diuretics
   Influenza vaccinations
   Cardiotonics
Parenteral fluids
Restriction of smoking

Nursing diagnoses/interventions/evaluation

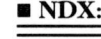 **NDX:** Ineffective airway clearance related to tracheobronchial obstruction and/or secretions

---

CONTROLLED COUGH TECHNIQUE

1. *Maximal inhalation*—an effective cough is contingent on filling the lungs and airways distal to the mucus so that the succeeding forced exhalation will propel the mucus up to the airways. Maximal inhalation also increases airway caliber; as a result, it is more likely that the air will pass distal to partially obstructing mucus or foreign matter.
2. *Hold breath 2 seconds*—this step permits the patient to prepare for exhalation and allows distribution of the inhaled air to the lung's periphery.
3. *Cough twice*—the first cough will loosen mucus; the second will propel the mucus. Further coughing may use excessive oxygen and energy at a time when the lung volume has already been expelled with the first two coughs, and the effort is thus wasted.
4. *Pause*—just long enough to regain control.
5. *Inhale by sniffing*—sniffing is recommended, because a deep inhalation through the mouth may drive loose mucus back down into the airways.
6. *Rest.*

Adapted from Thelan LA, Davie JK, Urden LD: *Textbook of critical care nursing: diagnosis and management,* St Louis, 1990, CV Mosby.

Auscultate lungs q1h to 2h and prn for rhonchi, crackles, or wheezing
Assess secretions, noting quantity, color, consistency, and odor
Assess hydration status: skin turgor, mucous membrane, q2h I&O
Increase fluid intake to 2000 ml/day unless contraindicated
Encourage incentive breathing with large tidal volumes
Assist and teach patient to turn and cough q2h; position for optimal coughing: upright and flexed forward
Assist with and monitor chest physiotherapy: postural drainage, percussion
Provide periods of rest between treatments
Teach controlled cough techniques (see box at left)
Instruct patient in breathing retraining techniques: pursed-lip, diaphragmatic breathing (see box below)
Provide humidification via mask, vaporizer
Suction nasopharyngeal airway or artificial airway as indicated
Administer medications as ordered
  Bronchodilators
  Antibiotics

Expected outcome/evaluation

Patient maintains a patent airway as evidenced by
  Improved breath sounds

BREATHING RETRAINING TECHNIQUES

PURSED-LIP BREATHING

- With mouth closed, inhale through nose.
- Exhale through mouth with lips "pursed" (lips in a whistling or kissing position).
- Make exhalation at least twice as long as inhalation (2 seconds in, 4 seconds out).

RATIONALE

Explain to the patient that this maneuver keeps airways open longer during exhalation and evacuates trapped air. The procedure for pursed-lip breathing can be used, along with diaphragmatic breathing, during episodes of shortness of breath.

DIAPHRAGMATIC BREATHING

Have the patient place two fingers just below the xiphoid process and push in with his or her fingers while sniffing gently. Explain that the movement felt at the fingertips is the diaphragm moving as he or she sniffs and that this muscle requires exercise so that it can increase the efficiency of breathing.

TECHNIQUE

- Place one hand on chest, one hand on abdomen.
- Inhale, pushing abdominal hand outward.
- Exhale slowly (through pursed lips), allowing abdominal hand to fall inward.
- Chest hand should remain still.

RATIONALE

Explain that this maneuver saves energy because the diaphragm uses oxygen more efficiently than the accessory muscles and that this technique retrains the diaphragm to assume the work of breathing. Diaphragmatic breathing is useful in terminating episodes of acute shortness of breath but should also be incorporated into a regular routine of muscle retraining.

From Thelan LA, Davie JK, Urden LD: *Textbook of critical care nursing: diagnosis and management,* St Louis, 1990, CV Mosby.

Cough produces thinned secretions
Normal rate and depth of respirations
Absence of dyspnea and cyanosis
Blood gases within acceptable levels

■ **NDX:** Altered nutrition: less than body requirements, related to decreased oral intake and increased metabolic demand associated with dyspnea, anorexia, and fatigue

Assess nutritional status: weigh daily, monitor dietary intake
Record oral intake using calorie counts
Monitor albumin and lymphocyte levels
Place in high Fowler's position at meals to reduce dyspnea
Encourage rest periods before meals to reduce fatigue
Provide liquid-to-soft, high-protein diet
    Administer supplementary feedings
    Provide attractive meals
Provide small, frequent meals to decrease abdominal pressure on diaphragm
Encourage significant others to bring patient's favorite foods
Administer oral hygiene before meals
Weigh patient daily at same time with same clothing and scale

Expected outcome/evaluation

Patient's nutritional status is maintained or improved as evidenced by weight remaining stable and within or moving toward normal range for patient's height, age, and build
Patient's food intake is increased
Albumin and lymphocytes within normal limits (WNL)

■ **NDX:** Impaired gas exchange related to alveolar capillary membrane changes

Assess respirations qh; note quality, rate, and use of accessory muscles
Auscultate breath sound q1h to 2h; note area of abnormal sounds
Assess level of consciousness, somnolence, confusion, reporting any changes
Observe color, odor, and amount of secretions
Maintain bed rest in quiet environment during exacerbation of symptoms
Elevate head of bed 45 to 90 degrees
    Allow patient to assume position of comfort to ease work of breathing
    Padded overbed table may be helpful for patient's comfort
Administer humidified oxygen per nasal catheter or cannula at low flow as ordered
Observe for signs of cyanosis

Monitor BP, T, and apical pulse q2h to 4h and prn
Monitor ABGs
Assist and teach patient to turn, cough, and deep breathe q2h; note type of cough and color and character of sputum
Collect sputum for culture as ordered
Allow absolutely no smoking
Administer medications as ordered
    Bronchodilators
    Antibiotics

Expected outcome/evaluation

Patient maintains adequate gas exchange as evidenced by
    Improved mental status, skin color
    Blood gases within acceptable levels for patient
    Clear breath sounds

■ **NDX:** Anxiety/fear related to change in health status

Assess level of anxiety (mild, moderate, severe); identify any misperceptions of illness or treatment
Assess usual coping skills
Provide quiet, nonstressful environment
Provide emotional support
    Remain with patient during anxious periods
    Be aware of subjective statements of patient
    Encourage patient to ask questions and to verbalize fears and concerns
    Limit visitors during periods of heightened anxiety as necessary
    Plan care to provide frequent rest periods
    Avoid "you brought it on yourself" attitude
    Encourage verbalization of fear and anxiety
    Explain all procedures and treatment
    Introduce support groups available to patient and family (e.g., Better Breathing Clubs of American Lung Association)

Expected outcome/evaluation

Patient experiences a decrease in fear and anxiety as evidenced by
    Relaxed facial expression
    Verbalization of feeling less anxious
    Verbalization of understanding hospital routines, procedures, and disease process

■ **NDX:** Activity intolerance related to imbalance between oxygen supply and demand

Assess level of response to activities (Table 4-5)
    Monitor HR and respiration during and after activity
Plan care to provide optimal rest
Instruct patient on energy conservation measures (e.g., perform activities such as bathing, shaving in sitting position; rest between activities)

Encourage use of pursed-lip breathing during activities

Provide O₂ therapy as indicated

Monitor for signs of extreme fatigue, chest pain, or diaphoresis during and after activity

Assist and teach patient progressive exercise conditioning (e.g., ROM exercises)

Encourage participation in pulmonary rehabilitation program (see p. 204)

Expected outcome/evaluation

Patient demonstrates an increased tolerance for activity as evidenced by ability to resume ADLs without extremes of fatigue or dyspnea

■ **NDX:** Knowledge deficit related to lack of information about disease process and home care management

Assess patient level of understanding regarding disease process and prescribed home care management

Encourage questions and discussion

Explain importance of maintaining optimal respiratory function by taking medications, by not smoking, and by avoiding those who smoke

Provide detailed instruction in use of any oxygen or respiratory equipment to be sent home with patient

Initiate contact with Visiting Nurses Association (VNA)

Determine need for home care nursing

Instruct patient and family on cleaning of all home respiratory equipment; refer to respiratory therapy department as indicated

Explain need to avoid respiratory irritants

Dust

Fumes

Smoke

Perfume

Aerosol sprays

Cold temperatures

Explain need to avoid persons with infections, especially URIs

Explain importance of ongoing outpatient care

Discuss symptoms to report to physician immediately

Elevated temperature

Sore throat

Increase in sputum production

Change in color of sputum

URI

Increased difficulty in breathing

Decreased activity tolerance

Decreased appetite

Increased use of IPPB and oxygen

Explain need to keep warm and avoid chilling

Explain importance of influenza immunization if ordered

Explain importance of environmental control

Avoid dry air by using humidifier

Be aware that some patients tolerate high humidity poorly

Keep free of irritating factors

Avoid emotional stress; teach stress reduction techniques

Provide warm house (75° to 80° F [23.8° to 26.6° C])

Explain importance of activity and rest

Exercise to tolerance

Need to limit activity on days of high air pollution

Plan rest periods during day

Rest before and after meals if shortness of breath increases at mealtimes

Breathe deeply and slowly during periods of activity

Understand own lifestyle and avoid waste of energy

Discuss medications: name, dosage, time of administration, purpose, and side effects

Explain need to avoid taking over-the-counter medications without checking with physician

Demonstrate use of bronchodilator nebulizers if ordered

Use tid or qid

Take one or two deep inhalations

Release medication only one or two times with each use

Watch for side effects such as tachycardia

Avoid overuse

Explain need to wear medical alert band identifying chronic obstructive lung disease

Explain need to maintain high-calorie diet as indicated; to force fluids to 2000 to 3000 ml/day unless contraindicated

Explain need to avoid constipation and straining

Ensure that patient and/or significant other demonstrates

Deep-breathing exercises: pursed-lip breathing

Positions for postural drainage if needed

Use of ventilator if applicable

Use of oxygen equipment if applicable

Expected outcome/evaluation

Patient demonstrates understanding of disease process and home care management as evidenced by

Verbalizing signs and symptoms to report

Regular attendance at doctor's appointment

Discussing lifestyle changes necessary to accommodate disease process

Increased activity tolerance

Verbalizing principles of home management including use of respiratory equipment

Decreased admissions to hospital

Additional nursing diagnoses to consider

Sleep pattern disturbance related to frequent coughing and difficulty breathing

Potential for infection related to ineffective airway clearance and increased risk factors (chronic disease, steroid therapy)

Sexual dysfunction related to activity intolerance secondary to chronic disease

ASTHMA

A reversible obstructive disease characterized by increased reactivity of the trachea and bronchi to stimuli, manifested by wheezing and dyspnea; narrowing is due to a combination of bronchospasm, mucosal swelling, and increased secretions

Assessment
Observations/findings

Sudden onset of respiratory distress
  Prolonged expiratory wheeze
  Short inspiratory period
  Intercostal and sternal retraction
  Use of accessory muscles of respiration
  Air hunger
  Crackles
Breath sounds
  Wheezes
  Decreased
  Absent
Assumes upright sitting position; leans forward
Diaphoresis
Tachycardia
Distended neck veins
Cyanosis
  Circumoral area
  Nail beds
Hard, dry cough; productive cough is difficult
Altered level of consciousness
Hypoxemia
Hypotension
Pulsus paradoxus >10 mm
Dehydration
Increased anxiety
  Fear of suffocation
  Fear of death

Laboratory/diagnostic studies

Arterial blood gases
  Mild decrease in PaO_2 and $PaCO_2$: common between attacks
  Decreased PaO_2, increased PaO_2 with severe attacks
Chest x-ray examination
  Normal between attacks
  Hyperinflation with attacks
Skin testing (extrinsic asthma)
Pulmonary function tests
  Normal or increased lung volumes
  Decreased flow rates; improvement with bronchodilators
WBC and sputum examination
  Sputum and blood eosinophilia are common
  Serum IgE levels are elevated in extrinsic asthma

Potential complications

Pulmonary edema
Respiratory failure
Status asthmaticus
Pneumonia

Medical Management

Oxygen therapy with humidification
Fluid management
Artificial airway and ventilatory support if necessary
Medications
  Bronchodilators (Table 4-4): parenteral, aerosols, oral
    Sympathomimetics
    Theophylline
    Steroids
    Antibiotics

Nursing diagnoses/interventions/evaluation

■ **NDX:** Anxiety related to difficulty in breathing, fear of suffocation, and/or fear of recurrent attacks

Assess level of anxiety (mild, moderate, severe)
Assess usual coping skills
Provide emotional support
  Remain with patient during acute attack
  Anticipate patient's needs
  Provide quiet reassurance
  Maintain quiet environment
Implement relaxation techniques: guided imagery, muscle relaxation
Explain procedures; encourage questions
Maintain planned rest periods
  Pace and plan ADLs
  Discourage talking if extremely dyspneic
  Limit visitors as necessary
  Encourage frequent rest periods

Expected outcome/evaluation

Patient demonstrates a reduction in fear and anxiety as evidenced by
  Relaxed facial expression
  Verbalization of feeling less anxious
  Vital signs within normal parameters

■ **NDX:** Ineffective airway clearance related to excessive tenacious secretions and bronchospasm

Assess sputum for color, tenacity, and amount
Auscultate breath sounds q1h to 2h for wheezes, crackles, or rhonchi
Assess respirations noting quality and rate
Observe skin color and temperature q2h
Monitor arterial blood gases
Monitor level of consciousness; report changes to physician
Position to level of comfort and to optimize breathing

Elevate head of bed 60 to 90 degrees
Support back with pillows
Provide well-padded overbed table to lean over
Place side rails up for safety and support
Place humidifier or steam vaporizer at bedside as ordered
Administer low flow of oxygen by nasal catheter as ordered (Avoid oxygen mask, which increases sensation of suffocation)
Administer IPPB as ordered
Initiate and/or assist with chest physiotherapy
Administer medications as ordered

Epinephrine preparations
Aminophylline
Antihistamines
Expectorants
Adrenal corticosteroids
Isoproterenol or cromolyn nebulization; avoid using isoproterenol and aminophylline together (can cause arrest)
Force fluids as ordered to keep secretions thin
Collect sputum for culture as ordered
Suction prn

TABLE 4-4. Bronchodilators

Generic name	Brand names	Availability	Adult dosage range
SYMPATHOMIMETICS			
Albuterol	Proventil, Ventolin	Tablets: 2, 4 mg Aerosol: 90 µg	PO: 2-4 mg 3-4 times daily Inhale: 2 inhalations every 4-6 hours
Ephedrine	Ephedrine	Tablets: 25 mg Capsules: 25, 50 mg Syrup: 11, 20 mg/5 ml Injection: 25, 50 mg/ml	PO: 25-50 mg every 3-4 hours SC, IM, IV: 25-50 mg
Epinephrine	Primatene, Vaponefrin, Bronkaid Mist	Nebulization: 1:100 Aerosol: 0.2, 0.25, 0.3 mg Injection: 1:200, 1:100	See manufacturer's recommendations
Ethylnorepinephrine	Bronkephrine	2 mg/ml	SC or IM: 0.5 ml
Isoetharine	Bronkosol, Beta-2, Bronkometer	Nebulization: 0.125, 0.2, 0.5, 1% Aerosol: 0.61%	See manufacturer's recommendations
Isoproterenol	Isuprel, Aerolone, Norisodrine	Nebulization: 0.25, 0.5, 1% Aerosol: 0.2, 0.25% Injection: 0.2 mg/ml SL: 10, 15 mg tabs	See manufacturer's recommendations
Metaproterenol	Alupent, Metaprel	Tablets: 10, 20 mg Syrup: 10 mg/5 ml Aerosol: 225 mg Nebulization: 5%	See manufacturer's recommendations
Terbutaline	Brethine, Bricanyl	Tablets: 2.5, 5 mg Injection: 1 mg/ml	PO: 5 mg every 6 hours SC: 0.25 mg; repeat, if needed, in 30 minutes
XANTHINE DERIVATIVES			
Aminophylline		Tablets: 100, 200 mg Elixir: 250 mg/15 ml Liquid: 105 mg/5 ml Suppositories: 250, 500 mg Injection: 250, 500 ml Others	See manufacturer's recommendations
Dyphylline	Dilor, Dyflex, Lufyllin	Tablets: 200, 400 mg Liquid: 100 mg/5 ml Elixir: 100, 160 mg/15 ml Injection: 250 mg/ml	PO: 15 mg/kg, 5 times daily IM: 250-500 mg slowly
Oxtriphylline	Choledyl	Tablets: 100, 200 mg Elixir: 100 mg/5 ml Syrup: 50 mg/5 ml	200 mg 4 times daily
Theophylline	Bronkodyl, Elixophyllin, Theolair, others	Tablets: 125, 200, 225, 300 mg Capsules: 50, 100, 200, 250 mg Elixir: 80 mg/15 ml Liquid: 80 mg/15 ml Syrup: 80 mg/15 ml Suspension: 300 mg/15 ml Others	9-20 mg/kg/24 hours in 4 divided doses

Modified from Clayton BD, Stock YN: *Basic pharmacology for nurses*, ed 9, St Louis, 1989, CV Mosby.

Expected outcome/evaluation

Patient maintains a patent airway as evidenced by
Improved breath sounds
Normal rate and depth of respirations
Absence of dyspnea
Absence of cyanosis
Blood gases within normal range

■ **NDX:** Ineffective breathing pattern related to decreased lung expansion during acute attack

Assess for signs and symptoms of ineffective breathing: shallow respirations, diaphroesis, dyspnea, use of accessory muscles
Monitor vital signs and arterial blood gases
Place patient in high Fowler's position for maximal chest expansion
Administer oxygen therapy as ordered
Maintain patent airway
Suction prn
Administer medications as ordered

Expected outcome/evaluation

Patient maintains an effective breathing pattern as evidenced by
Normal rate, rhythm, and depth of respirations
Absence or reduction of dyspnea
Blood gases within acceptable range for patient

■ **NDX:** Knowledge deficit related to lack of information about self-care management

Assess level of understanding regarding disease process and self-care management during severe attacks
Explain importance of preventing future attacks
Avoid known irritants
Avoid stressful situations
Express anxieties and fears
Encourage communication with significant other and/or family
Provide adequate humidity
Nonflowering plants can increase humidity 5% to 10%
Humidifiers are helpful (provide instructions on use of humidifiers and need to keep clean)
Avoid persons with infections especially URIs
Do not smoke; avoid persons who smoke
Explain importance of breathing exercises such as pursed-lip breathing
Discuss importance of exercising to tolerance
Avoid fatigue
Plan rest periods
Explain importance of diet and fluids
Eat balanced, nutritious meals
Force fluids to 2000 to 3000 ml/day unless contraindicated

Avoid gaining weight
Explain importance of ongoing outpatient care
Discuss symptoms to report to physician
URI
Flu
Elevated temperature
Discuss medications: name, dosage, time of administration, purpose, and side effects
Demonstrate proper use of inhalers and maintenance of containers
Explain need to wear medical alert band identifying asthma
Discuss importance of taking medications as ordered

Expected outcome/evaluation

Patient demonstrates knowledge of health care management as evidenced by verbalization of principles of self-care related to disease process

PULMONARY REHABILITATION

An inpatient or outpatient program designed to increase exercise tolerance in COPD patients while educating them to understand and assist in the management of their disease; components generally include physical therapy, respiratory therapy, exercise conditioning, medications, and education

Admission Criteria

Symptomatic pulmonary disease (Table 4-5)
Dyspnea
Cough
Wheezing
Sputum production

PULMONARY REHABILITATION PROGRAM: SUGGESTED CLASS CONTENT

Orientation to rehabilitation program
Anatomy and physiology of pulmonary system
Nutrition
Effects of stress and emotions on lung disease
Coping with chronic lung disease
COPD, specific diseases
Medications
Effect of COPD on family and friends
Oxygen, IPPB treatments
Principles of exercise
Relaxation techniques
Breathing exercises: pursed-lip breathing and diaphragmatic breathing
Energy conservation techniques
Postural drainage
Prevention of infection
Stop smoking sessions
Discussions on sexuality

TABLE 4-5. COPD Disability Scale

Class	Observations/findings
Class I	No significant restriction of normal activities, but dyspnea on strenuous exertion
Class II	No dyspnea with essential activities of daily living; dyspnea on climbing stairs and in other climbs but not on level walking; employability limited to sedentary occupations
Class III	Dyspnea with some activities of daily living (e.g., showering, dressing), but can perform all such activities without assistance; able to walk at own pace for a city block, but cannot keep up while walking with normal others of the same age
Class IV	Dependent on others in some activities of daily living; not dyspneic at rest, but dyspneic with minimal exertion
Class V	Dyspneic at rest; dependent on assistance from others for most activities of daily living

From Hodgkin J, Zorn E, and Connors G, eds: *Pulmonary rehabilitation: guidelines to success*, Stoneham, Mass, 1984, Butterworth Publishers. Adapted from Moser KM et al: Results of a comprehensive rehabilitation program, *Arch Intern Med* 140:1596, 1980.

Chest pain
Patient motivation
Restricted ADLs
No underlying condition that would interfere with the program (psychosis, alcoholism, drug abuse)
Medically stable: no signs of CHF, uncontrolled dysrhythmias, or myocardial infarction (MI) in previous 6 months
Adequate financial/insurance status
Family support system

Exclusion Criteria

Terminal cancer
Heart failure
Stroke
Alcoholism, active
Drug abuse
Organic brain disease
End-stage COPD

Inpatient Program (see box on p. 204)

Assessment

Observations/findings

Heart rate
  Increase of 30 beats/min above resting rate with activity
  Heart rate less than 50 during activity
  Consistent drop in heart rate of more than 10 beats/min during activity
ECG rhythm: presence of irregular rhythm
Blood pressure
  Increase of 20 mm Hg above normal
  Diastolic increase of more than 10 to 15 mm Hg
  Systolic drop to below 90 at rest; diastolic below 40

Symptoms during activity

Dyspnea
Dizziness
Fatigue
Pain
Palpitations
Diaphoresis

Indicators of energy expenditure during activity

Arterial oxygen saturation values
PaO_2
Oxygen consumption rate

Indicators of ventilatory response during activity

Minute ventilation
Respiratory rate
Carbon dioxide production

Ongoing Care

Activity progression program
  Follow physician activity prescription
  Initiate exercise program
Evaluate daily progress and plan activity levels
Maintain progressive increase in activities until discharge
Monitor ECG and respiratory parameters
Record and report any signs or symptoms of shortness of breath (SOB), fatigue, or nausea during or after exercise
Assist patient in performing ADLs and monitor HR, R, and BP 1 min and 4 min after activity (response to activity should return to preactivity level within 5 min; if it does not, monitor every 2 min until pretest levels are reached)
Observe, record, and report patient's tolerance

Discharge Evaluation

Self-care/ADL skills
Equipment needs for the home
Weekly schedule of exercise and rest
Assessment of level of knowledge
Knowledge of agency referral sources

Benefits of Pulmonary Rehabilitation Program

Reduced symptoms
Decreased anxiety and depression
Improved ability to perform ADLs
Increased exercise tolerance
Reduced hospital admissions/days/cost of care
Improved quality of life

PNEUMONIA/PNEUMONITIS

Inflammation of the lung parenchyma caused by bacteria, viruses (Table 4-6), chemicals, smoke inhalation, dust, allergens, and aspiration of gastric contents; lung tissue is consolidated as alveoli fill with exudate (Figure 4-3)

TABLE 4-6. Bacterial and Nonbacterial Causes of Pneumonia/Pneumonitis

Pathogen	Persons at risk	Complications
BACTERIAL		
Streptococcus pneumoniae (pneumonococcus) Gram positive Accounts for 80% to 90% of cases	Infants Elderly Alcoholics People with debilitating diseases (diabetes mellitus, sickle cell)	Meningitis Emphysema Pericarditis Impaired liver function
Klebsiella pneumoniae Gram-negative bacilli	Alcoholics Patients with diabetes mellitus or COPD	Lung abscess Emphysema Necrotizing pneumonitis Respiratory failure 25% to 50% mortality
Staphylococcus aureus Gram-positive diplococcus Accounts for 10% of cases in hospitalized patients and 1% of cases in unhospitalized patients	Infants Elderly As complication of influenza As secondary infection after surgery	Necrotizing infections Lung abscess 15% to 50% mortality
Haemophilus influenzae (Type B) Gram-negative bacillus Accounts for 1% of cases	Children under 10 years Persons with COPD or immune disease	Bronchiolitis
Legionella pneumophila (Legionnaires' disease) Gram negative	Older adults Smokers Persons with lung diseases	Hypotension Respiratory failure Shock 15% mortality
Pseudomonas aeruginosa Gram-negative bacilli	Hospitalized patients: endotracheal intubation, respiratory inhalation therapy Burns	70% mortality
NONBACTERIAL		
Mycoplasma (Mycoplasma pneumoniae)	School age children Young adults Spreads within family	Interstitial infections
Pneumocystis (Pneumocystis carinii pneumonia) Protozoan organism	Patients with AIDS, bone and renal transplant	Respiratory failure
Viral infleunza A	Elderly Symptoms may begin 1 week after viral infection	Secondary bacterial infection Respiratory failure
Aspiration pneumonia Nonbacterial Bacterial aspiration	Patients with LOC, impaired gag or cough reflex	With aspirated material: Atelectasis Pulmonary edema Hemorrhage Necrosis

Assessment (see box)
Observations/findings

Difficult and painful respirations
   Pleuritic pain
   Shortness of breath and grunting
   Tachypnea
Breath sounds over area of consolidation
   Diminished, progressing to absent
   Crackles
   Rhonchi
   Egophony
Asymmetrical chest movements

Chills and fever (102° to 106° F [38.8° to 41.1° C]); delirium
Diaphoresis
Anorexia
Malaise
Productive, tenacious cough
   Incessant, painful
   Copious amounts of green-yellow sputum progressing to pink or rusty
Restlessness
Cyanosis
   Circumoral area

OBSERVATIONS/FINDINGS OF VIRAL AND BACTERIAL PNEUMONIA

Viral

Symptoms

Usually mild at onset
Headache

Sudden onset of chills followed by fever
Cough early nonproductive
Sputum (late)
    Purulent
    Blood tinged
Myalgia

Photophobia
Anorexia
Nausea

Laboratory/diagnostic studies

Sputum examination: Gram stain and culture; influenza
    A, BC, varicella cytomegalovirus, adenovirus

Blood cultures
WBC normal or low, elevated lymphocytes
Elevated antibody titers
Arterial blood gases: hypoxemia
Chest x-ray examination
    Bronchopneumonic infiltrates

Bacterial

Symptoms

Sudden onset of high fever and shaking chills
Streptococcal pneumonia: afternoon, evening temperature; diaphoresis
Pleuritic chest pain
Cough
Sputum
    Rust colored or greenish

Breath sounds
    Crackles
    Friction rub

Cyanosis

Laboratory/diagnostic studies

Sputum examination: Gram stain and culture streptococcal, pneumococcal, staphylococcal, *Haemophilus influenzae*
Blood cultures
WBC leukocytes with shift to left

Arterial blood gases: hypoxemia
Chest x-ray examination
    Patchy areas of consolidation and infiltrates

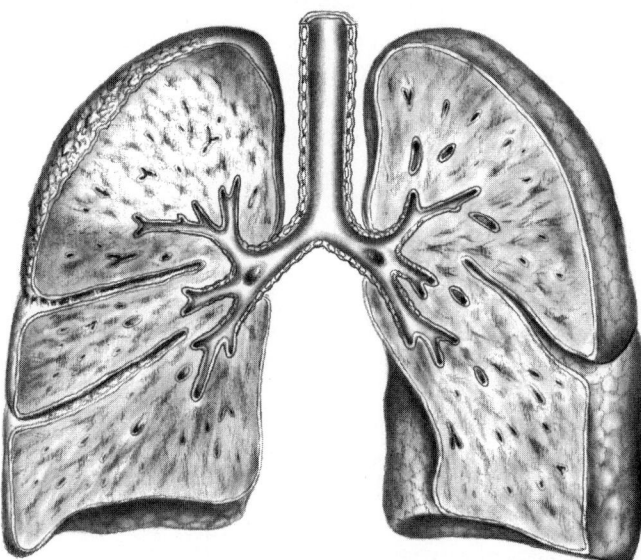

FIGURE 4-3. Pneumococcal pneumonia. Lobar pneumonia (right upper lobe). (From Wilson SF and Thompson JM: Respiratory disorders, *Mosby's clinical nursing series,* St Louis, 1990, Mosby—Year Book.)

Nail beds
Tachycardia
Psychosocial problems
    Disorientation
    Anxiety
    Fear of death

Laboratory/diagnostic studies

Chest x-ray examination: patchy or diffuse infiltrates
    Pleural effusion
Sputum examination: Gram stain and culture
WBC count
Leukocytosis
Blood culture
Serologic studies: titers, cold agglutinins
Arterial blood gases
    PaO_2 <80 mm Hg
Transtracheal aspiration
Bronchoscopy

Potential complications

Atelectasis
Empyema
ARDS

Superinfection pericarditis
Lung abscess

Medical Management

Fluid management
Parenteral therapy
Oxygen therapy
Chest physiotherapy
Artificial airway or mechanical ventilation support
Medications
    Antipyretics
    Antibiotics
    Antimicrobials

Nursing diagnoses/interventions/evaluation

■ **NDX:** Impaired gas exchange related to lung consolidation with decrease in effective lung surface

Auscultate breath sounds q2h to 4h
Assess respiratory pattern, noting quality and rate
Monitor mental status and LOC
Observe color, odor, and amount of secretions
Provide humidified oxygen per mask or nasal catheter as ordered; maintain continuous vaporizer at bedside
Position patient to optimize breathing
Administer oxygen therapy as ordered
Assist and teach patient to turn, cough, and deep breathe q2h to 4h
Initiate or assist with chest physiotherapy
Assist with use of incentive spirometry
Administer medications as ordered
    Antibiotics
    Expectorants
Pace activities to patient's tolerance
Monitor ABGs, CBC, and serum osmolality
Encourage fluid intake as tolerated
Assist with administration of mechanical ventilation as indicated

Expected outcome/evaluation

Patient maintains adequate gas exchange as evidenced by
    Usual mental status
    Usual skin color
    Blood gases are within acceptable range

■ **NDX:** Ineffective airway clearance related to increased tracheobronchial secretions secondary to inflammatory process

Assess secretions, noting quantity, color, consistency
Assess hydration status: skin turgors, mucous membranes, 24-hr intake
Auscultate breath sounds for crackles, rhonchi, friction rubs q2h to 4h
Assist patient with use of incentive spirometry

Perform nasopharyngeal or nasotracheal suctioning prn
Force fluids as ordered to help liquefy secretions
Assist and teach patient to turn, cough, and deep breathe q2h to 4h
Monitor laboratory reports and serial chest x-ray examinations
Position patient to optimize breathing and coughing
Provide humidification as indicated

Expected outcome/evaluation

Patient maintains an effective breathing pattern as evidenced by
    Normal rate, rhythm, and depth of respirations
    Clear lungs
    Decreased dyspnea
    Blood gases within normal range
    Cough that has subsided

■ **NDX:** Alteration in body temperature related to infectious process

Assess body temperature: measure temperature and pulse q4h; increase frequency during periods of chilling
Monitor skin color and temperature
Collect blood cultures and sputum cultures as ordered; monitor reports daily
Administer prescribed antipyretics as indicated
Encourage oral fluids as ordered
Administer cooling procedures as indicated: tepid sponge bath

Expected outcome/evaluation

Patient demonstrates no signs of elevated temperature as evidenced by
    Temperature WNL (35.8° to 37.3° C)
    No signs of shivering, flushing
    Pulse WNL

■ **NDX:** Pain: in chest related to inflammation of lung parenchyma

Assess and monitor quality of pain, noting any changes
Assist patient in chest splinting techniques during coughing episode
Administer medications to treat cough
Administer analgesics as ordered
    Be aware of potential for depression of respiratory function
    Evaluate effectiveness
Provide additional comfort measures to ease pain
Plan rest periods
    Bed rest
    Quiet environment; soft or low light
    Avoid unnecessary talking if necessary
    Limit visitors as necessary

Expected outcome/evaluation

Patient experiences decreased pain as evidenced by
Verbalization of pain relief
Relaxed facial expression and body movements
Improved breathing pattern
Effective cough

■ **NDX:** Potential alteration in nutrition: less than body requirements related to decreased oral intake secondary to increased metabolic needs associated with fever and infectious process

Assess and monitor daily food intake
Identify factors contributing to anorexia
Nausea/vomiting
Fever
Pain
Initiate measures to correct aggravating factors
Administer antiemetics, antipyretics, analgesics
Weigh daily and compare to admission weight
Remove sputum containers during mealtimes
Provide small frequent meals
Have family members bring patient's favorite foods
Schedule respiratory treatments 1 hour before mealtimes
Administer oral hygiene every 2 to 4 hours and after any enemas

Expected outcome/evaluation

Patient maintains balanced nutritional status as evidenced by
Baseline weight maintained or reestablished
Daily caloric intake equaling nutritional requirement

■ **NDX:** Knowledge deficit related to lack of information about self-care management

Assess level of understanding regarding disease process
Explain importance of avoiding transmission of disease
Turn head away when coughing and cover mouth with tissue
Use tissue once only
Dispose of tissue in waste container
Explain importance of gradual convalescence
Limit exercise and activity to tolerance
Plan two or three rest periods during day
Avoid fatigue
Explain importance of postural drainage and deep breathing exercises; continue deep-breathing exercises qid for 6 to 8 weeks
Explain importance of maintaining diet as tolerated
Avoid high-calorie diet if overweight
Force liquids to 3000 ml daily unless contraindicated
Explain need to avoid recurrence of disease
Keep warm
Avoid chilling
Avoid persons with infections, especially URIs

Receive influenza vaccine as ordered
Explain need to use vaporizer or humidifier at home
Explain importance of ongoing outpatient care
Discuss symptoms to report to physician
Elevated temperature
Diaphoresis
Difficulty in breathing
Persistent cough
Cold or flu
Discuss medications: name, dosage, time of administration, purpose, and side effects
Explain need to avoid taking over-the-counter medications without checking with physician
Ensure that patient and/or significant other demonstrates methods of postural drainage

Expected outcome/evaluation

Patient demonstrates knowledge of self-care management principles as evidenced by verbalization of those principles indicating understanding of disease process, compliance with treatment regimen, and isolation procedures as necessary

PULMONARY EDEMA

Abnormal accumulation of fluid in the alveoli caused by an increase in pulmonary microvascular pressure, usually a result of abnormal cardiac function

Assessment
Observations/findings

Respiratory distress
Labored, noisy breathing
Orthopnea
Nasal flaring
Tachypnea: shallow, moist respirations
Breath sounds
Crackles: in dependent parts of lung initially, extending progressively upward
Cough: pink, frothy sputum
Bounding pulse
Hoarseness
Anxiety
Confusion
Restlessness, thrashing about
Tachycardia: thready pulse
Diaphoresis
Pallor
Cyanosis
Heart failure (see p. 101)

Laboratory/diagnostic studies

Arterial blood gases: variable
Early: respiratory alkalosis
Late: respiratory acidosis and hypoxemia
Chest x-ray examination

Bilateral interstitial (Kerley B lines are common) and alveolar infiltrates
ECG
  Tachycardia
  Dysrhythmias
Pulmonary capillary wedge pressure (PCWP)
  14 to 20 mm Hg: mild
  25 to 30 mm Hg: moderate to severe
Protein concentration of edema fluid

Potential complications

Respiratory failure
Respiratory/cardiac arrest

Medical Management

O_2 therapy: high flow by Venturi mask
Parenteral therapy
Intake and output
Hemodynamic monitoring
Cardiac monitor
Rotating tourniquets and/or phlebotomy may be used
Medications
  Morphine
  Diuretics
  Cardiotonics
  Bronchodilators
Mechanical ventilatory support

Nursing diagnoses/interventions/evaluation

■ **NDX:** Impaired gas exchange related to alveolar-capillary membrane changes

Assess respirations, noting rate, depth, and use of accessory muscles
Assess level of consciousness and mental status
Auscultate breath sounds qh
  Decreased breath sounds
  Crackles
Elevate head of bed 60 to 90 degrees with lower extremities dependent
Monitor ABGs; intraarterial line may be required because of frequent need of samples
Monitor serial chest x-rays, noting signs of improvement or exacerbation
Administer medications to relieve bronchospasm and respiratory effort as ordered
Administer oxygen therapy as ordered
Administer IPPB as ordered (p. 237)
Check BP, R, and apical pulse qh and prn
Assist and teach patient to cough and deep breathe qh and prn
Maintain bed rest during acute phase

Expected outcome/evaluation

Patient has adequate gas exchange as evidenced by
  Demonstrated effortless breathing

Lungs clear to auscultation
Hemodynamic stability
Blood gases within normal range

■ **NDX:** Anxiety related to perceived biological threat (fear of suffocation)

Assess degree of anxiety (mild, moderate, severe)
Provide emotional support
  Remain with patient
  Reassure that treatments will relieve symptoms
  Reduce environmental stimuli
  Explain procedures and treatments thoroughly
  Use short, simple sentences
  Use calm, reassuring voice
Position to level of comfort: high Fowler's position with padded overbed table
Plan rest periods
Encourage patient to verbalize fears and concerns
Administer morphine sulfate to calm patient

Expected outcome/evaluation

Patient demonstrates decreased anxiety as evidenced by
  Verbalization of reduced anxiety
  Demonstration that treatment is understood
  Decreased use of tranquilizers and/or pain medication

■ **NDX:** Knowledge deficit related to lack of information about disease process and home care management

Assess level of understanding regarding disease process and contributing factors
Provide instruction regarding disease process and home care management
Explain need to exercise to tolerance
  Avoid strenuous exercise
  Plan frequent rest periods
Explain need to maintain a low-sodium diet as ordered
Explain importance of not smoking
Explain importance of ongoing outpatient care
Discuss symptoms to report to physician
  Sudden weight increase
  Decreased urinary output
  Swollen feet and ankles
  Chest pain
  Difficulty in breathing
  Persistent cough
Discuss medications: name, dosage, time of administration, purpose, and side effects
Provide instruction in use of any oxygen or respiratory equipment sent home with patient

Expected outcome/evaluation

Patient demonstrates knowledge of self-care management as evidenced by

Verbalization of principles of home management including respiratory therapy
Demonstration of understanding of disease process
Stating of symptoms to report to physician
Ability to name medications with purpose, dose, and times

Additional nursing diagnoses to consider

Fluid volume excess related to left ventricular dysfunction (see Heart Failure, p. 101)
Ineffective breathing related to tracheobronchial secretions
Activity intolerance related to imbalance between oxygen supply and demand

PULMONARY EMBOLISM

Occurs when the pulmonary artery or one of its branches is partially or completely occluded; damage to the lung depends on the number of clots and the extent of obstruction to pulmonary circulation

Assessment
Observations/findings

Dyspnea
Sudden, severe substernal pain
Shortness of breath
Restlessness
Apprehension
Diaphoresis
Cyanosis, pallor
Tachypnea
Tachycardia
Hypotension
Hemoptysis (rare)
Cough
Breath sounds
  Decreased
  Crackles
  Pleural friction rub

Laboratory/diagnostic studies

Chest x-ray examination
  Unilateral elevated diaphragms
  Atelectasis
  Hyperlucent lung fields
  Unilateral pleural effusion
  Interstitial infiltrates
Arterial blood gases
  Decreased PaO_2 (<80 mm Hg)
  Decreased $PaCO_2$ (<40 mm Hg)
  Elevated pH (>7.45 mm Hg)
ECG
  Right ventricular strain
  Right axis deviation
  Incomplete right bundle branch block (RBBB)

Atrial fibrillation
Lung (ventilation/perfusion) scan
Pulmonary angiogram
Serum assays
  Elevated LDH, elevated bilirubin
  Fibrin split products (FSP)/fibrin degradation tests
Prothrombin time (PT), partial thromboplastin time (PTT)
Pattern of abnormal perfusion in area of ventilation
  Intraarterial filling defects
  Pulmonary artery obstruction(s)

Potential complications

Extended/recurrent pulmonary embolism
Pulmonary infarction
Atelectasis
Pulmonary hypertension
RV failure
Cor pulmonale
Decreased cardiac output
Shock
Cardiopulmonary arrest

Medical Management

Bed rest
Oxygen therapy
Cardiac monitor
Medication
  Anticoagulants
    Heparin
    Coumadin
  Fibrinolytic enzymes
    Streptokinase
    Urokinase
  Vasopressors
  Analgesics/sedatives
Parenteral fluids
Surgical therapy
  Insertion of umbrella filter for multiple emboli

Nursing diagnoses/interventions/evaluation

■ **NDX:** Impaired gas exchange related to ventilation/perfusion abnormalities

Assess, monitor for, and report signs of hypoxemia and respiratory distress
Assess quality and rate of R q2h to 4h and prn
Administer oxygen as ordered; intubation and assisted ventilation may be indicated
Monitor BP, R, and apical pulse q1h to 2 h and prn
Auscultate breath sounds q2h to 4h
Maintain bed rest during acute phase; turn and deep breathe q2h to 4h
Elevate head of bed to promote optimal breathing
Monitor arterial blood gases as ordered
Monitor and document any changes in mental status

Expected outcome/evaluation

Patient experiences adequate O_2/CO_2 exchange as evidenced by
ABGs within normal range
Reporting exhibiting no signs of respiratory distress
Normal breath sounds

 NDX: Potential for injury: bleeding related to increased risk of bleeding from anticoagulant therapy

Observe for signs and symptoms of bleeding
Stools: occult and frank bleeding
Hematuria
Sputum
Bleeding of gums
Bruising of skin
Monitor PT and clotting functions or coagulation factors daily as ordered
Administer anticoagulants as ordered
Do not administer aspirin-containing products
Provide antiembolic stockings as ordered
Avoid constipation and straining; use stool softeners or mild laxatives

Expected outcome/evaluation

Patient experiences no bleeding or extension of embolism as evidenced by
Normal clotting parameters
Absence of blood in stool, urine, sputum, or other sites

NDX: Anxiety related to fear of perceived threat (suffocation) and/or actual threat to biological integrity

Assess verbal and nonverbal signs and symptoms of anxiety/fear; encourage questions
Provide emotional support; maintain quiet environment
Remain with patient during periods of heightened anxiety
Explain procedures and treatments; use simple explanations

Expected outcome/evaluation

Patient experiences a reduction in anxiety as evidenced by
Relaxed facial expression
Verbalization of feeling less anxious
Decreased use of sedatives and/or tranquilizers
Verbalization of an understanding of routines and treatments

NDX: Knowledge deficit regarding health care management

Assess level of understanding regarding disease process and home management

Provide information on prevention for patients at risk for pulmonary embolism
Review strategies to prevent venous pooling
Avoid sitting or standing for long periods of time
Elevate legs while sitting
Do not cross legs
Use antiembolic stockings if ordered
Perform regular exercise such as walking
Discuss symptoms to report to physician
Sudden, sharp chest pain
Bloody sputum
Difficulty breathing
Discuss medications: name, dosage, time of administration, purpose, and side effects
Explain need to avoid taking over-the-counter medications without checking with physician
Explain need to check for bleeding in urine, stools, and sputum if sent home on anticoagulants (see Anticoagulant Therapy, p. 148)
Explain need to exercise to tolerance with planned rest periods
Explain need to avoid constipation and straining
Explain importance of ongoing outpatient care
Explain importance of not smoking
Explain need to wear medical alert band identifying use of anticoagulants

Expected outcome/evaluation

Patient demonstrates an understanding of home care management principles; verbalizes management principles of the disease process

Additional nursing diagnosis to consider

Alteration in tissue perfusion related to interruption of arterial blood flow secondary to pulmonary embolism

PULMONARY HYPERTENSION

An elevation of mean pulmonary artery pressure (MPAP) greater than 20 mm Hg

Assessment
Observations/findings

Dyspnea on exertion (DOE) and at rest
Tachypnea
Breath sounds
Distant
Decreased at periphery
Crackles
Cyanosis
Right ventricular (RV) failure (Figure 4-4)
Distended jugular veins
Right ventricular heave
Loud accentuated P_2
RV diastolic gallop

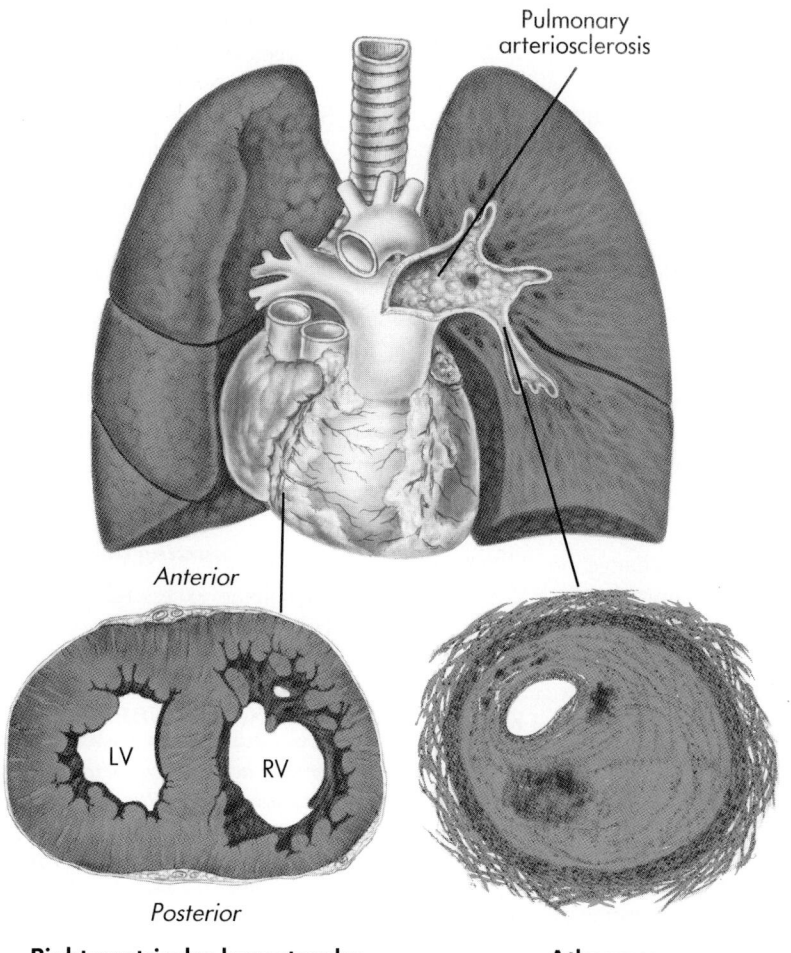

Pulmonary
arteriosclerosis

Anterior

LV   RV

Posterior

Right ventricular hypertrophy   **Atheroma**

FIGURE 4-4. Right ventricular phytrophy. (From Wilson SF and Thompson JM: *Respiratory disorders, Mosby's clinical nursing series,* St Louis, 1990, Mosby—Year Book.)

Murmur of tricuspid insufficiency
Peripheral edema
Chest pain

Laboratory/diagnostic studies

Chest x-ray examination
  Enlarged pulmonary artery
  Diminished diaphragmatic excursions
  RV dilation or hypertrophy
ECG
  Right axis deviation
  RBBB
Echocardiogram
  Enlarged RA, RV
  Diminished wall motion
  PV malfunction
Cardiac catheterization
  Elevated PA systolic and diastolic pressure with normal PCWP
  Decreased CO

ABGs
  PaO_2 60 mm Hg
  $PaCO_2$ will vary depending on cause

Medical Management

Oxygen therapy
Hemodynamic monitoring
Cardiac monitoring
Medications
  Vasodilator
    Prostacyclin
    Hydralazine
  Calcium channel blockers
  Diuretics
  Digitalis (used for biventricular failure)
Lung transplantation

Nursing diagnoses/interventions/evaluation

■ **NDX:** Impaired gas exchange related to alveolar-capillary membrane changes

Assess and monitor rate and quality of respirations

Assess skin color, use of accessory muscles

Auscultate breath sounds noting increase or decrease of rhonchi, crackles; report significant changes

Position patient in semi-Fowler's position to optimize lung expansion

Monitor serial ABGs; report signs of progressive hypoxemia

Administer oxygen therapy as ordered

Monitor chest x-ray examinations

Assist and instruct patient to cough and deep breathe, assess need to suction at regular intervals

Monitor progressive activity intolerance

Plan regular rest periods

Administer vasodilator as ordered

Expected outcome/evaluation

Patient maintains adequate gas exchange
ABGs are within acceptable limits
Lung sounds are improved

■ **NDX:** Activity intolerance related to fatigue and dyspnea secondary to increased work of breathing

Assess degree of reported activity intolerance; observe respiratory rate in response to activities

Assist and instruct patient to plan frequent rest periods; to plan rest periods between activities

Monitor signs of progressive deterioration in performing ADLs; report to physician

Provide oxygen therapy as indicated

Assist patient to identify energy-saving methods while performing ADLs, e.g., shower chair, sitting while shaving

Instruct and encourage patient to use adaptive breathing techniques

Expected outcome/evaluation

Patient reports ability to perform ADLs and verbalizes a decrease in fatigue

■ **NDX:** Knowledge deficit related to lack of understanding regarding disease process and self-care management

Assess level of understanding regarding pulmonary hypertension, identifying any misconceptions

Provide patient and significant others with information regarding disease process, signs and symptoms to report
Decreased activity tolerance
Changes in color, consistency of sputum
Increased cough
Swelling of legs, ankles, or abdomen

Discuss action to take during episodes of fatigue and/or dyspnea

Discuss importance of spacing heavy workloads and resting between activities

Teach energy-saving procedures
Shower chair; sitting while shaving, combing hair, dressing, cooking

Discuss importance of taking prescribed medications, name, dosage, purpose, time of administration, and side effects

Discuss importance of not smoking or using nicotine products

Provide instruction on adaptive breathing techniques

Expected outcome/evaluation

Patient demonstrates understanding regarding disease process, verbalizes signs and symptoms to report, demonstrates adaptive breathing techniques

Additional nursing diagnosis to consider

Fluid volume excess related to biventricular failure (see Heart Failure, p. 101)

PULMONARY TUBERCULOSIS

A chronic acute or subacute infectious disease caused by the tubercle bacillus, Mycobacterium tuberculosis, *most commonly affecting the alveolar structure of the lung; clinical presentation varies from asymptomatic with only a positive skin test to extensive pulmonary and systemic involvement*

Assessment
Observations/findings

Low-grade fever, night sweats

Headache

Tachycardia

Anorexia

Weight loss

Malaise

Fatigue

Cough: (nonproductive at first)
Blood-streaked sputum
Mucoid or mucopurulent sputum

Lymph nodes
Inflamed
Painful

Crackles over apex of lung

Pleuritic chest pain

Irregular menses

Laboratory/diagnostic studies

Skin testing
PPD (5 units of purified protein derivative)
Mantoux test: PPD or OT (old tuberculin, injected intradermally with pressure gun)
Tine test: OT pressed into skin with tine unit

Gastric washings

Sputum cultures: positive for M. *tuberculosis* within 2 to 3 weeks if active

Chest x-ray examination

Calcification at original site, enlarged hilar lymph nodes, and infiltrates if extension of original site has occurred

Pleural effusion or cavitation

CAUTION: Other lung abnormalities (pneumonia, tumors) can look like tuberculosis

Fiberoptic bronchoscopy

Needle biopsy of pleura

WBC: leukocytosis

Potential complications

Atelectasis

Hemoptysis

Pneumothorax

Recurrence

Miliary tuberculosis

Tuberculosis pericarditis, peritonitis, meningitis, lymphadenitis

Medical Management

Antiinfective agents

Primary drugs

Isoniazid (INH)

Ethambutol

Rifampin

Streptomycin

Secondary drugs

Paraaminosalicylic acid (PAS)

Pyrazinamide

Ethambutol

Analgesics

High-protein, high-carbohydrate diet

Respiratory isolation as necessary

Report to Board of Health for follow-up on family and contacts

Surgical therapy

Drainage of lung abscess

Lung resection

Nursing diagnoses/interventions/evaluation

■ **NDX:** Ineffective breathing pattern related to mucopurulent secretions and poor cough effort

Assess quality and depth of respirations, use of accessory muscles; record any changes

Assess quality of sputum: color, odor, consistency

Auscultate breath sounds q4h

Position patient to optimize breathing: semi-Fowler's or high Fowler's position

Assist and teach patient to turn, cough, and deep breathe q2h to 4h

Instruct patient to splint chest for more effective and productive cough

Provide frequent rest periods, avoid fatigue, and exercise to tolerance

Monitor T, P, and R q4h

Administer medications as ordered

Encourage fluid intake

Expected outcome/evaluation

Patient maintains an effective breathing pattern

Normal rate, rhythm, and depth of respirations

Decreased dyspnea

■ **NDX:** Potential for infection transmission related to insufficient knowledge of risk of pathogen

Discuss importance of maintaining respiratory isolation; avoid direct contact with sputum

Teach patient to cough into tissues

To turn head with coughing

To dispose of tissues properly

To use mask if unable to follow directions

Instruct patient to collect and care for sputum cultures as ordered

Teach patient importance of not stopping antituberculosis medications until directed to do so by physician

Expected outcome/evaluation

Patient has decreased potential for transmission of disease as evidenced by failure of patient contacts to convert to positive skin test

■ **NDX:** Alteration in nutrition: less than body requirements related to fatigue, anorexia, and/or dyspnea

Obtain admission weight and monitor daily

Assess nutritional status on a regular basis; consult with dietitian

Monitor percentage of meals eaten

Maintain high-protein, high-carbohydrate diet with small, frequent feedings

Assess for additional causes of malnutrition (e.g., depression)

Monitor albumin and lymphocytes

Place in high Fowler's position at meals to reduce dyspnea

Encourage rest periods before meals to reduce fatigue

Provide frequent small feedings

Encourage significant others to bring patient's favorite food

Expected outcome/evaluation

Patient maintains an adequate nutritional status

Weight remains stable and within normal range for patient's height, age, and build

■ **NDX:** Knowledge deficit related to lack of information about disease process and home care management

Assess level of understanding regarding disease process; identify any fears or misconceptions

Explain nature of disease and purpose of treatment and procedures

Explain importance of good hygiene and handwashing (coughing into tissues, use of mask if unable to follow directions, how to dispose of tissues, to turn head if coughing, and to avoid direct contact with sputum)

Explain importance of maintaining high-protein, high-carbohydrate diet; need to force fluids to 2000 to 3000 ml unless contraindicated

Explain importance of maintaining respiratory isolation until necessary medication levels are obtained

Explain importance of exercise, frequent rest periods, and avoiding fatigue

Explain importance of avoiding close contact with others until advised by physician

Explain need to avoid crowds and persons with URIs

Explain importance of ongoing outpatient care

Discuss symptoms to report to physician

   Hemoptysis

   Chest pain

   Difficulty in breathing

   Hearing loss

   Vertigo

Discuss medications: name, dosage, time of administration, purpose, and side effects

Explain need to avoid taking over-the-counter medications without checking with physician

Discuss importance of not stopping medication without physician's approval

Expected outcome/evaluation

Patient demonstrates increased level of knowledge regarding self-care

   Verbalizes those principles indicating understanding of self-care management

PNEUMOTHORAX

Collection of air or gas in the pleural space, causing the lung to collapse; may be partial or total collapse; open or communicating pneumothorax (sucking wound) occurs as result of an open chest wound that permits entry of air; spontaneous (closed) can be due to rupture of a bleb or bullae on the surface of the lung; or may be iatrogenically induced (e.g., thoracentesis)

Tension pneumothorax An opening through the pleura that allows air to pass into the pleura on inspiration; however, the air cannot exit on expiration; this produces a shift in the affected lung and mediastinum

---

ASSESSMENT/FINDING OF TENSION PNEUMOTHORAX AND HEMOTHORAX

Tension pneumothorax	Hemothorax
Assessment	**Assessment**
Observations/findings	***Observations/findings***
Respiratory distress: sudden, severe	Difficulty in breathing
Use of accessory muscles of respiration	Hyperresonance on percussion
Tachycardia	Distant to absent breath sounds on affected side
Cyanosis	Asymmetric chest movements
Tachypnea	Hypovolemic shock if blood loss is severe
Hypotension	Tachypnea
Chest pain	Tachycardia
Restlessness and agitation	Hypotension
Paradoxic chest movement	Anxiety
Tracheal and mediastinal shift: toward unaffected side	Restlessness
Breath sounds	Pallor
Absent (affected side)	Pain
Diminished (unaffected side)	
Distant heart sounds	***Laboratory/diagnostic studies***
Subcutaneous emphysema	Chest x-ray examination
	Blunting of costophrenic angles
Laboratory/diagnostic studies	Hazy appearance over lower chest
Chest x-ray examination: complete lung collapse, mediastinal or tracheal shift to unaffected side	Hematocrit/hemoglobin

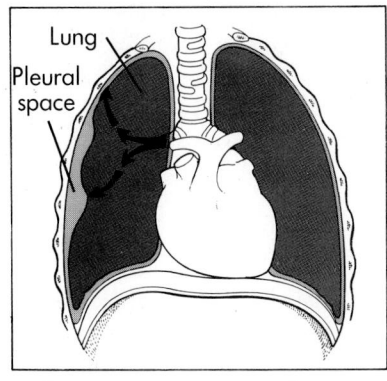

Spontaneous pneumothorax

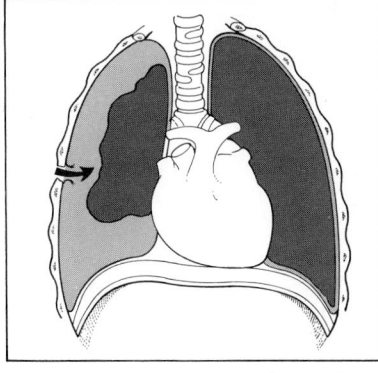

Traumatic pneumothorax

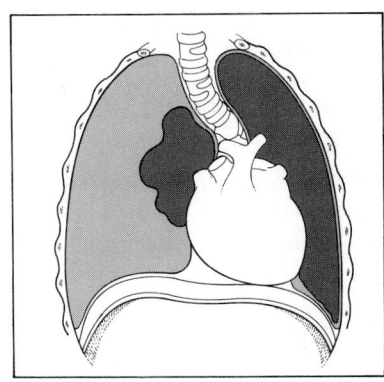

Tension pneumothorax

FIGURE 4-5. Spontaneous, traumatic, and tension pneumothorax. (From Wilson SF and Thompson JM: Respiratory disorders, *Mosby's clinical nursing series,* St Louis, 1990, Mosby—Year Book.)

FIGURE 4-6. Hemothorax. (From Wilson SF and Thompson JM: Respiratory disorders, *Mosby's clinical nursing series,* St Louis, 1990, Mosby—Year Book.

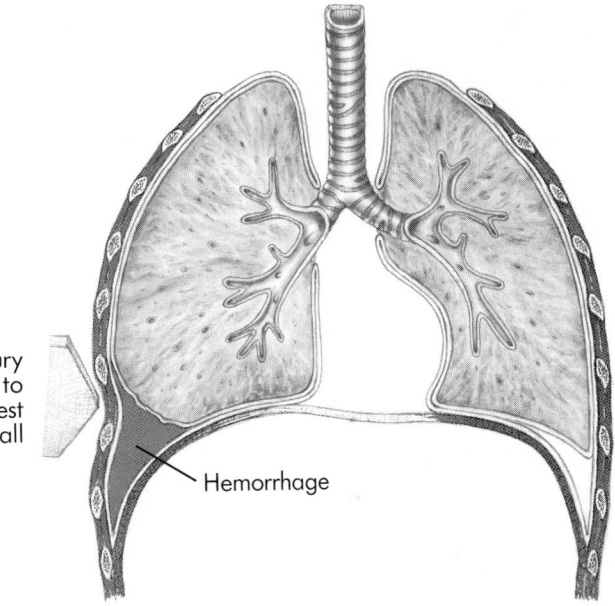

toward the unaffected side (tension pneumothorax is a medical emergency) (see box and Figure 4-5)

Hemothorax *Blood in the pleural space, causing the lung to partially or totally collapse; often appears as a complication of chest trauma and after chest surgery (see box and Figure 4-6)*

NOTE: symptoms and treatment depend on size of pneumothorax:

$<15\%$, small

15% to 60%, moderate

$>60\%$, large

Assessment

Observations/findings

Sudden, sharp chest pain radiating to shoulder or arm of affected side

Anxiety

Diaphoresis

Tachycardia

Cyanosis

Dyspnea

Tachypnea

Absent or decreased breath sounds on affected side

Hyperresonance to percussion over affected thoracic space

Decreased or absent chest wall motion

Pleural pain

Hypotension

Laboratory/diagnostic studies

Chest x-ray examination

Unequal lung expansion

Mediastinal shift to affected side

Arterial blood gases

Decreased PaO_2

Decreased pH

Increased $PaCO_2$

Potential complications

Decreased cardiac output

Respiratory failure

ARDS

Infection
Cardiac arrest

Medical Management

Chest tube insertion
Oxygen therapy
Parenteral therapy
Blood transfusion (hemothorax)
Mechanical ventilation with PEEP

Nursing diagnoses/interventions/evaluation

■ **NDX:** Ineffective breathing pattern related to inadequate chest expansion (air/fluid accumulation)

Assess quality, rate, and depth of respirations, reporting any changes
Note chest wall movement and position of trachea
Auscultate breath sounds q2h to 4h
Reassure and try to calm patient
Place patient in a position to ensure optimal respiration; in a sitting position, with head of bed elevated 60 to 90 degrees
Administer oxygen per nasal cannula at 2 to 6 L/min as ordered unless contraindicated
Assist with insertion of chest tube (see Chest tubes, p. 229)
Administer oxygen and IPPB as ordered
Monitor BP, T, R, and apical pulse q2h to 4h
Assist and encourage patient to
    Turn and deep breathe q2h to 4h: diaphragmatic, segmental breathing; instruct patient to suppress cough
    Avoid stretching, reaching, or sudden movements
Provide emotional support; remain with patient during periods of heightened anxiety
Continue with acute care and decrease frequency of nursing functions as patient's condition improves

Expected outcome/evaluation

Patient maintains an effective breathing pattern as evidenced by
    Normal rate, rhythm, and depth of respirations
    Chest x-ray examinations show full expansion
    Breath sounds are clear with full aeration

■ **NDX:** Impaired gas exchange related to decreased oxygen supply

Assess for signs and symptoms of hypoxemia
Monitor ABG results
Observe for signs of increased work of breathing
Observe for unequal lung expansion
Administer supplemental oxygen as ordered; assist with endotracheal intubation and mechanical ventilation as indicated

Monitor function and patency of chest tube
Provide periods of rest to decrease oxygen demand

Expected outcome/evaluation

Patient maintains adequate gas exchange as evidenced by
    Usual mental status
    Usual skin color
    Blood gases within normal range

■ **NDX:** Pain: chest related to biological factors (tissue trauma) and physical factors (chest tube insertion)

Assess for presence of pain (verbal and nonverbal)
Administer analgesic as prescribed
Assess effectiveness of pain relief measures
Medicate patient before breathing/coughing exercises
Instruct patient on splinting techniques
Secure chest tubes to limit movement and resulting irritation

Expected outcome/evaluation

Patient experiences decreased pain as evidenced by
    Verbalizes pain relief
    Relaxed facial expression and body positioning
    Improved breathing pattern
    Increased activity

■ **NDX:** Knowledge deficit related to lack of information about self-care management

Assess level of understanding regarding disease process and contributing factors
Explain importance of maintaining diet as ordered; need to force fluids to 2000 to 3000 ml daily unless contraindicated
Explain need to exercise to tolerance; to avoid fatigue and to plan rest periods
Explain importance of avoiding strenuous activity or exercise, especially contact sports
Explain importance of not smoking
Explain need to avoid persons with infections, especially URIs
Explain importance of ongoing outpatient care
Discuss symptoms to report to physician
    Cold
    Sore throat
    Flu
    Elevated temperature
    Cough
    Sudden, sharp chest pain
    Difficulty in breathing
    Any redness, pain, swelling, or tenderness of puncture wound

Discuss medications: name, dosage, time of administration, purpose, and side effects

Ensure that patient and/or significant other demonstrates care of chest puncture wound (see Chest tubes, p. 229)

Expected outcome/evaluation

Patient demonstrates increased level of knowledge regarding self-care as evidenced by verbalization of principles of self-care management

---

THORACIC EMPYEMA

Pus in the pleural cavity caused by underlying infections of the lung, such as pneumonia or lung abscess, occurring after thoracic surgery or resulting from penetrating chest wounds

Assessment

Observations/findings

Difficulty in breathing
Orthopnea: mild to severe
Localized chest pain
    Constant
    Only during inspiration
Nasal flaring
Asymmetrical chest expansion
Decreased or absent breath sounds over affected area
Productive cough
Malaise
Fatigue
Elevated temperature
Tachycardia
Tachypnea

Laboratory/diagnostic studies

Chest x-ray examination
    Unilateral/bilateral pleural effusions
Thoracentesis
Examination of pleural fluid
    Fluid cell count/differential
        Specific gravity
        pH < 7.2 mm Hg
    Cytologic examination
ABGs: PaO_2 < 70 mm Hg; $PaCO_2$ and pH within normal limits

Potential complications

Pneumothorax
Pneumonia
Bronchopleural fistula

Medical Management

Chest tube insertion
    Irrigation of pleural cavity
Thoracentesis
Thoracic drainage

Intrapleural aspiration and instillation of medications
Thoracotomy if necessary
High-protein, high-carbohydrate diet
O_2 therapy as necessary
Medications
    Antibiotics
    Antipyretics
    Analgesics
Fluid management

Nursing diagnoses/interventions/evaluation

■ **NDX:**   Ineffective breathing pattern related to decreased lung expansion secondary to pus in the pleural space

Assess respirations, noting changes in rate, depth, and quality

Assess chest movement, noting signs of asymmetry

Auscultate breath sounds q2h to 4h

Place patient in a sitting position, with head of bed elevated 60 to 90 degrees

Administer oxygen per nasal cannula at 2 to 6 L/min as ordered unless contraindicated

Assist with insertion of chest tube (see p. 229)

Administer oxygen and IPPB as ordered

Monitor BP, T, R, and apical pulse q2h to 4h

Administer medications as ordered

Review serial chest x-ray and ABGs as ordered

Assist and teach patient to
    Deep breathe q2h to 4h; position onto affected side; use diaphragmatic, segmental breathing
    Encourage use of incentive spirometer (see p. 234)
    Perform passive and active ROM exercises to extremities q4h

Encourage coughing: assist patient to splint affected side when coughing

Avoid stretching, reaching, or sudden movements

Expected outcome/evaluation

Patient maintains an effective breathing pattern as evidenced by
    Normal rate, rhythm, and depth of respirations
    Decreased dyspnea
    Blood gases within normal range

■ **NDX:**   Pain: chest related to biological factors (tissue trauma) and physical factors (chest tube insertion)

Assess for presence of pain (verbal and nonverbal)
Administer analgesic as prescribed
Assess effectiveness of pain relief measures
Medicate patient before breathing/coughing exercises
Instruct patient on splinting techniques
Secure chest tubes to limit movement and resulting irritation

Expected outcome/evaluation

Patient experiences decreased pain
  Verbalizes pain relief
  Relaxed facial expression and body positioning
  Improved breathing pattern
  Increased activity

■ **NDX:** Knowledge deficit related to lack of information about disease process and self-care management

Assess level of understanding of disease process
Discuss symptoms to report to physician
  Difficulty in breathing
  Chest pain on inspiration
  Elevated temperature
  Persistent cough
  Coughing up foul-smelling sputum
Explain importance of avoiding persons with URIs
Discuss symptoms of a cold or flu to report to physician
Discuss importance of coughing and deep breathing
Explain need to exercise to tolerance
  Plan rest periods
  Avoid fatigue
Explain importance of ongoing outpatient care
Explain importance of influenza vaccination as ordered
Discuss medications: name, dosage, time of administration, purpose, and side effects
Explain need to avoid taking over-the-counter medications without checking with physician

Expected outcome/evaluation

Patient demonstrates increased levels of knowledge regarding self-care as evidenced by verbalization of principles of self-care management

Additional nursing diagnosis to consider

Impaired gas exchange related to alveolar-capillary membrane changes

ATELECTASIS

Collapse of alveoli or airless condition of the lung caused by mucous plugs, excessive secretions, compression of lung tissue by tumors, effusions, or pneumothorax, or shallow breathing

Assessment
Observations/findings

Elevated temperature
Breath sounds
  Absent or decreased over affected area
  Crackles
  Egophony and bronchophony
Tachypnea
Tachycardia
Labored breathing

Shortness of breath
Nasal flaring
Anxiety
Restlessness
Asymmetrical chest movement on inspiration

Laboratory/diagnostic studies

Arterial blood gases
  Decreased PaO_2
  Normal or decreased $PaCO_2$
  Significant atelectasis: increased $PaCO_2$
Chest x-ray examination
  Elevated diaphragm on affected side
  Shift of trachea mediastinum toward affected side if large area is atelectatic
  Narrow rib spaces

Potential complications

Pneumonia
Pneumothorax

Medical Management

Oxygen therapy as needed
Chest physiotherapy
IPPB/incentive spirometry
High tidal volume and/or PEEP for intubated patient
Bronchoscopy
Nutritional support
Fluid management
Medications
  Antipyretics
  Bronchodilators
  Antibiotics

Nursing diagnoses/interventions/evaluation

■ **NDX:** Impaired gas exchange related to compressed lung tissue

Assess for signs of hypoxemia: labored breathing, tachypnea, restlessness, pallor
Assess LOC
Auscultate breath sounds q2h to 4h
  Check quality and rate of respirations
  Note area of lung without breath sounds
Assist and instruct patient to turn, cough, and deep breathe q1h to 2h and prn
Assist and teach patient to perform postural drainage qid and prn; clapping may be ordered
Assist or initiate chest physiotherapy
Perform nasotracheal suction as indicated
Administer nebulization as ordered
Administer oxygen and/or IPPB as ordered
Instruct and encourage patient to use incentive spirometer as ordered
Encourage early ambulation as soon as possible

Monitor BP, T, and apical pulse q4h

Monitor arterial blood gases as ordered

Administer medication as ordered

   Antipyretics

Expected outcome/evaluation

Patient's gas exchange is improved

   ABGs within acceptable limits

   Lungs clear to auscultation

   Normal rate and rhythm of respiration

■ **NDX:**   Knowledge deficit regarding disease process and health care management

Assess level of understanding regarding disease process

Instruct patient in coughing and deep breathing techniques; teach patient to splint chest when coughing

Instruct patient in use of incentive spirometer and how frequently to use if continued at home

Explain need to avoid persons with infections, especially URIs

Explain importance of not smoking

Explain importance of ongoing outpatient care

Discuss symptoms to report to physician

   URI

   Flu

   Difficulty in breathing

   Persistent cough

   Elevated temperature

Explain importance of exercising to tolerance; need to avoid fatigue and to plan rest periods

Discuss medications: name, dosage, time of administration, purpose, and side effects

Explain need to avoid taking over-the-counter medications without checking with physician

Expected outcome/evaluation

Patient demonstrates understanding of health care management of disease process as evidenced by

   Use of incentive spirometer as ordered

   Ambulation as directed by health team

   Verbalization of principles of health care management

PLEURAL EFFUSION

Excessive amount of nonpurulent fluid in the pleural space; between visceral and parietal layer

Assessment
Observations/findings

Related to underlying disease and may be asymptomatic if effusion is small

Shortness of breath

Respiratory difficulty

Breath sounds

   Diminished or absent over affected area

   Egophony over effusion area

   Pleural friction rub

Localized chest pain

Asymmetrical chest expansion

Elevated temperature

Fatigue

Cough

Laboratory/diagnostic studies

Chest x-ray examination

   Blunting of costophrenic angle

   Partially obscured diaphragm

   Complete "white out" (opaque densities) of involved area in large effusions

Thoracentesis

Pleural biopsy

Cytologic examination of fluid

Gram stain, culture and sensitivity of pleural fluid

Potential complications

Pneumothorax

Pneumonia

Empyema

Medical Management

Bed rest

Chest tube insertion (see p. 229)

Thoracentesis

Medications

   Antibiotics

Fluid management

Nitrogen mustard installation or tetracycline via chest tube

Nursing diagnoses/interventions/evaluation

■ **NDX:**   Ineffective breathing pattern related to decreased lung expansion secondary to fluid accumulation in the pleural space

Assess rate, depth and quality of respirations

Auscultate chest q2h to 4h

Maintain bed rest; assist patient to assume position of comfort

See Thoracentesis (p. 192) and/or Chest tubes (p. 229) if ordered

Monitor BP, T, P, and R q4h and prn

Administer medications as ordered

Assist and teach patient to

   Turn, cough, and deep breathe q2h to 4h

   Encourage incentive breathing

   Splint chest when coughing

   Perform active ROM exercises to all extremities q2h to 4h

Use blow bottles or incentive spirometry

Increase activity as tolerated

Expected outcome/evaluation

Patient maintains an effective breathing pattern
   Normal rate, rhythm, and depth of respirations
   Decreased dyspnea
   Chest x-ray examination clear

■ **NDX:**   Knowledge deficit related to lack of information
            about disease process

Assess level of understanding regarding disease process
Discuss symptoms to report to physician
   Difficulty in breathing
   Chest pain
   Elevated temperature
   Persistent cough
Explain need to exercise to tolerance
   Plan rest periods
   Avoid fatigue
Instruct and encourage patient to cough, deep breathe to
   maintain lungs well aerated
Explain importance of ongoing outpatient care
Explain importance of avoiding persons with URIs
Discuss symptoms of a cold or flu to report to physician
Explain importance of influenza vaccination as ordered
Discuss medications: name, dosage, time of administra-
   tion, purpose, and side effects
Explain need to avoid taking over-the-counter medica-
   tions without checking with physician

Expected outcome/evaluation

Patient demonstrates understanding of disease process and
   principles of self-care management as evidenced by verbalization of principles of self-care management

FLAIL CHEST

*Chest cage abnormality usually resulting from crushing
chest injury where multiple fractures of ribs have occurred*

Assessment
Observations/findings

Sharp chest pain
Difficulty in breathing
Respirations
   Shallow
   Paradoxical chest wall movement
   Splinting
Tachypnea
Tachycardia
Cyanosis
Decreased breath sounds
Mediastinal and tracheal shift
Sputum

Copious
Blood tinged

Laboratory/diagnostic studies

Chest x-ray examination
   Atelectasis
   Pneumothorax
   Evidence of fractured ribs
Arterial blood gases
   Decreased PaO_2
   Increased $PaCO_2$
Pulmonary function tests: decreased lung volumes

Potential complications

Tension pneumothorax
Hemothorax
Pulmonary edema
Cardiac tamponade
Respiratory arrest
Shock

Medical Management

O_2 therapy
Chest tube insertion
Intubation and mechanical ventilation
Medications
   Pavulon
   Curare
   Antibiotics
   Pain management

Nursing diagnoses/interventions/evaluation

■ **NDX:**   Potential for ineffective breathing pattern re-
            lated to unstable chest wall movement

Maintain bed rest; assist patient in assuming position for
   comfort; do not turn patient onto flailed side
Understand that endotracheal tube (p. 231) or trache-
   ostomy (p. 232) may be ordered
Place on continuous mechanical ventilation (p. 235) as
   ordered
   Positive-pressure ventilator
   Volume-cycled ventilator
   Respirations may be controlled by ventilator
Understand that chest tubes may be ordered (p. 229)
Monitor BP, P, and R q1h to 2h and prn
Auscultate breath sounds q1h to 2h and prn
Report decreased or absent breath sounds to physician
Perform oropharyngeal suctioning prn
Monitor arterial blood gases as ordered
Turn and reposition patient q2h to 4h and prn
Maintain body alignment
Assist and teach patient to deep breathe q2h to 4h and
   prn in absence of tracheostomy or endotracheal tube;
   do not splint chest manually when deep breathing

Continue acute care management but decrease frequency of nursing functions as patient's condition improves

Administer IPPB with humidification as ordered

Assist and teach patient to use incentive spirometer as ordered

Expected outcome/evaluation

Patient maintains an effective breathing pattern
  Normal rate, rhythm, and depth of respirations
  Decreased dyspnea
  Blood gases within normal range
  Breath sounds clear

■ **NDX:** Pain: chest related to trauma

Assess for verbal and nonverbal signs of pain

Manage pain as indicated; assess effectiveness of pain relief measure(s)

Prepare for possible intercostal nerve block

Establish means of communication of pain
  Call bell within reach
  Pad and pencil or Magic Slate

Explain all procedures thoroughly, using calm, reassuring voice

Expected outcome/evaluation

Patient experiences decreased pain as evidenced by
  Verbalization of pain relief
  Relaxed facial expression and body positioning
  Improved breathing pattern
  Increased activity

■ **NDX:** Knowledge deficit related to lack of information about health care management

Assess level of understanding regarding disorder, causes, treatment, and procedures

Discuss symptoms to report to physician
  URI
  Shortness of breath
  Persistent cough
  Persistent chest pain

Explain importance of exercising to tolerance; avoid overexertion, excessive sports and activities

Explain importance of ongoing outpatient care

Discuss medications: name, dosage, times of administration, purpose, and side effects

Explain need to avoid taking over-the-counter medications without checking with physician

Expected outcome/evaluation

Patient demonstrates knowledge and skill in self-care as evidenced by verbalization of principles required for self-care management

RESPIRATORY FAILURE

Inability of the respiratory system to maintain normal oxygenation of blood (hypoxia: $PaO_2 < 50$ mm Hg) and/or elimination of carbon dioxide ($PaCO_2 > 50$ mm Hg) resulting from problems with ventilation, diffusion, and/or perfusion
  Type I *Hypoxia without hypercapnia*
  Type II *Hypoxia and hypercapnia*
  Type III *Hypoventilation with hypercapnia*

Assessment
Observations/findings

Respiratory distress
  Nasal flaring
  Tachypnea or bradypnea
  Retractions
  Use of accessory muscles of respiration
Labored breathing
  Air hunger
  Diaphoresis
  Cyanosis
Breath sounds
  Crackles
  Rhonchi
  Wheeze
Increased respiratory secretions
Headache
Altered level of consciousness
  Anxiety
  Restlessness
  Confusion
  Drowsiness
Impaired motor function; asterixis
Papilledema
Cardiovascular
  Tachycardia
  Hypertension
  Dysrhythmias
    Atrial
    Ventricular
  Decreased cardiac output
    Restlessness
    Lethargy
    Tachycardia
Decreased urinary output

Laboratory/diagnostic studies

Arterial blood gases
  Hypoxemia
    Mild: PaO_2 <80 mm Hg
    Moderate: PaO_2 <60 mm Hg
    Severe: PaO_2 <40 mm Hg
  Increased or decreased $PaCO_2$, depending on stage of failure

Chest x-ray examination: documents underlying pathology and/or progressive disease process

Hemodynamic findings: Type I: increased PCWP

Chest x-ray examination: depends on underlying cause of failure

ECG

May show evidence of right-sided heart strain

Dysrhythmias

Potential complications

ARDS

Deterioration from type I to type II

Cardiac failure

Barotrauma

Medical Management

Oxygen therapy

Low-flow oxygen delivery: Venturi masks or nasal prong

Mechanical ventilatory support with constant positive airway pressure (CPAP) or PEEP

Nebulized inhalation

Chest physiotherapy

Hemodynamic/cardiac monitoring

Parenteral therapy

Medications

Bronchodilators

Steroids

Nutritional support as needed

Nursing diagnoses/interventions/evaluation

■ **NDX:** Ineffective breathing pattern related to decreased lung expansion

Assess rate, depth, and quality of respirations, and breathing pattern

Assess vital signs and level of consciousness qh and prn

Be aware that endotracheal tube may be inserted (see p. 231) or tracheostomy done (see p. 232) if $PaCO_2$ is over 50 mm Hg or PaO_2 is less than 60 mm Hg

Adminsiter oxygen with assisted ventilation and humidification as ordered

Monitor and record arterial blood gases as indicated: assess for downward trend in PaO_2 or upward trend in $PaCO_2$

Be aware that continuous mechanical ventilation (see p. 235) is indicated if $PaCO_2$ is over 60 mm Hg, $PaCO_2$ increases at a rate of 5 mm Hg or more per hour, PaO_2 cannot be maintained at 60 mm Hg or higher, or patient manifests increased fatigue or mental depression, or secretions become difficult to control

Auscultate breath sounds qh

Maintain bed rest with head of bed elevated 30 to 45 degrees to optimize breathing

Encourage coughing and deep breathing; assist patient to splint chest during coughing

Instruct patient to use pursed-lip and diaphragmatic breathing

Expected outcome/evaluation

Patient maintains an effective breathing pattern

Normal rate, rhythm, and depth of respirations

Decreased dyspnea

Blood gases within normal range

■ **NDX:** Ineffective airway clearance related to obstructed airway and poor ventilation secondary to retention of secretions

Assess rate and quality of respirations

Auscultate breath sounds q2h

Assess, monitor, and record amount, consistency, and color of secretions

Assist and teach patient to turn, cough, and deep breathe

Encourage use of incentive spirometry (see p. 238)

Instruct patient in controlled coughing techniques

Position patient

Assist and teach patient to perform postural drainage as ordered

Administer oxygen therapy as indicated

Provide airway humidification

Maintain adequate fluid intake

Suction secretions if necessary

Use sterile technique

Hyperoxygenate and/or hyperinflate patient's lungs for four or five breaths before and after procedure

Observe cardiac monitors for dysrhythmias during procedure

Administer medications as ordered

Bronchodilators

Mucolytic agents

Expected outcome/evaluation

Patient maintains a patent airway as evidenced by

Improved breath sounds

Normal rate and depth of respirations

Ability to expectorate secretions

Blood gases within normal range

■ **NDX:** Impaired gas exchange related to ventilation-perfusion abnormalities secondary to hypoventilation

Assess for signs and symptoms of hypoxia and hypercapnia

Assess BP, P, apical pulse, and level of consciousness qh and prn; report changes in level of consciousness to physician

Monitor and record serial arterial blood gases, assessing for upward trend in $PaCO_2$ or downward trend in PaO_2

Assist with administration of mechanical ventilation as indicated; assess need for CPAP or PEEP

Auscultate for diminished breath sounds qh

Review daily chest x-ray examination, noting improvement or deterioration

Monitor cardiac rhythm

Administer parenteral fluids as ordered
Administer drugs as ordered
　Bronchodilators
　Antibiotics
　Steroids
Evaluate ADLs in relation to decreased oxygen demands

Expected outcome/evaluation

Patient maintains adequate gas exchange
　Lungs clear
　Usual skin color
　Blood gases within normal range for predicated age

■ **NDX:** Anxiety/fear related to perceived and actual biological threat (inability to breathe)

Assess level of anxiety (mild, moderate, severe)
Encourage patient and family to verbalize fears and concerns, and to ask questions regarding procedures and condition
Explain procedures and treatments using simple sentences
Instruct patient on energy conservation techniques
　Pursed-lip breathing
　Diaphragmatic breathing
Use calm, reassuring manner
Monitor vital signs

Expected outcome/evaluation

Anxiety level is reduced
　Appears calm and relaxed
　Able to verbalize fear

Additional nursing diagnoses to consider

Potential for infection: risk factors: invasive procedures, inadequate primary defenses, chronic disease
Sleep pattern disturbance related to sensory alteration: illness, disrupted circadian rhythms

ADULT RESPIRATORY DISTRESS SYNDROME (ARDS)

Nonspecific result of acute injury to the lung, characterized by a group of symptoms that include decreased compliance of the lung, noncardiac pulmonary edema, and refractory hypoxemia (Figure 4-7); etiology is diverse and includes shock, chest trauma, aspiration, fat embolism, and massive viral pneumonia; end result is a uniform hyaline membrane development that leads to gas exchange abnormalities; mortality is 50% to 60%

Assessment
Observations/findings

Early phase
　Anxiety
　Dyspnea

　Tachypnea
　Restlessness
　Cough
　Clear breath sound
Late phase
　Grunting respirations
　Use of accessory muscles of respiration
　Color
　　Pallor
　　Cyanosis
　Diaphoresis
Breath sounds
　Crackles
　Rhonchi
Tachycardia
Confusion

Laboratory/diagnostic studies

Arterial blood gases
　Decreased PaO_2 that is unresponsive to increasing FIO_2
　Decreased $PaCO_2$ initially; then elevated $PaCO_2$ in later stages
　pH initially > 7.45 mm Hg; as ARDS worsens, pH < 7.35 mm Hg
CBC
Chest x-ray examination
　Early: normal
　Late
　　Diffuse bilateral pulmonary infiltrates
　　"White out" on x-ray film, giving ground-glass appearance
Pulmonary artery pressures (PAP, PCWP)
　Early: normal
　Late: elevated
Pulmonary function tests
　Decreased VC, MV, FRC
　Decreased pulmonary compliance of >50 m/cm H_2O
Increased shunt fraction $(\dot{Q}s\text{-}Qt) >15\%$ to 20% (normal 3% to 4%)
Increased lactic acid levels

Potential complications

Dysrhythmias
Low cardiac output
Renal failure
Infection/sepsis
Barotrauma
Disseminated intravascular coagulation (DIC)

Medical Management

Oxygen therapy
Intubation with ventilator support; use of CPAP, PEEP
Parenteral therapy
Nutritional support

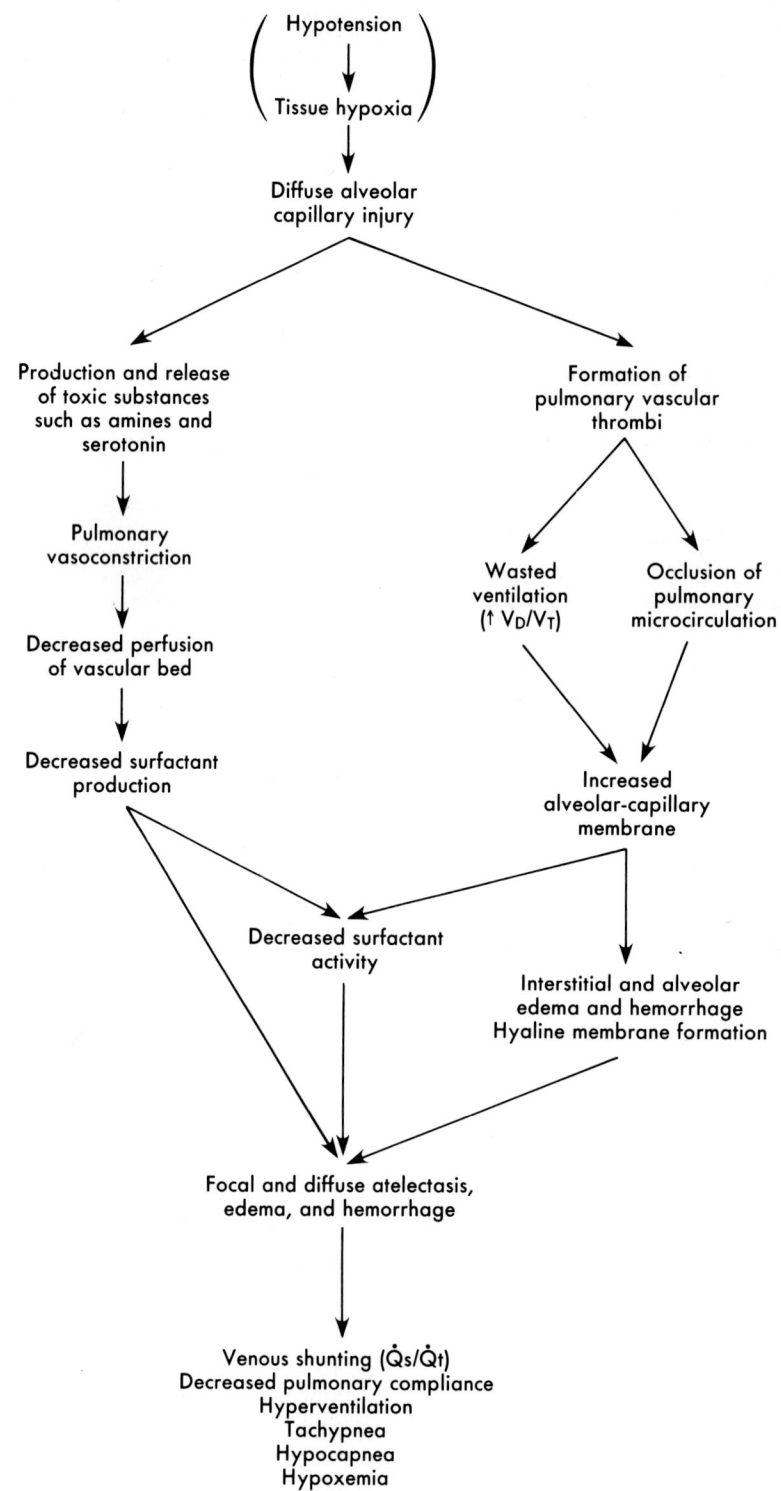

FIGURE 4-7. Proposed pathogenesis for ARDS. (From Thompson, JM et al: *Clinical nursing*, St Louis, 1986, CV Mosby.)

Medications
  Sedation
  Steroids
  Heparin
  Diuretics
Cardiac monitor
Hemodynamic monitoring

Nursing diagnoses/interventions/evaluation

■ **NDX:** Impaired gas exchange related to ventilation/perfusion abnormalities

See Respiratory Failure (see p. 223)
See standard of care for primary condition
Assess and monitor rate, quality, and depth of respirations
Assess for signs of respiratory distress
Auscultate breath sounds for crackles and wheezes
Place patient on volume-cycled ventilator with positive end-expiratory pressure (PEEP) or continuous positive airway pressure (CPAP) as ordered; PEEP is contraindicated in patients with chronic obstructive pulmonary disease (COPD)
Administer oxygen therapy, monitoring FIO_2
Assess arterial blood gases; monitor for increases or decreases of PaO_2 and $PaCO_2$
Monitor lactic acid levels
Administer parenteral fluids and electrolytes as ordered by physician
Monitor BP, P, and R qh; assess level of consciousness qh and prn
Suction secretions if crackles or rhonchi are present
Administer corticosteroids and diuretics as ordered by physician
Assess PAP and PCWP qh
Measure and record urinary output qh
Maintain bed rest with head of bed elevated 30 to 45 degrees
Reposition from side to side q1h to 2h

Expected outcome/evaluation

Patient maintains adequate gas exchange as evidenced by
  Return to baseline: level of consciousness, skin color, respirations
  Blood gases within acceptable range

■ **NDX:** Ineffective airway clearance related to excessive secretions secondary to interstitial edema

Assess and monitor rate and quality of respirations
Assess characteristics of secretions
Auscultate for breath sounds qh
Review serial chest x-ray examinations
Assist and teach patient to turn, cough, and deep breathe if crackles or rhonchi are auscultated
Suction secretions as indicated

If patient is intubated, hyperoxygenate and hyperinflate patient's lung for four or five breaths before and after procedure
Observe cardiac monitor for dysrhythmias during suctioning procedure
Assist and teach patient to perform postural drainage as ordered
Administer bronchodilators and expectorants as ordered

Expected outcome/evaluation

Patient's airway is patent
  Normal rate, rhythm, and depth of respirations
  Breath sounds clear
  Secretions are diminished/absent

Additional nursing diagnosis to consider

Altered nutrition: less than body requirements related to insufficient intake vs. increased metabolic demand

See standard of care for primary condition
See Volume-cycled positive pressure ventilators (p. 236)

THORACOTOMY, LOBECTOMY, PNEUMONECTOMY

thoracotomy *Surgical incision of the chest wall*
lobectomy *Removal of one or more lobes of the lung*
pneumonectomy *Removal of an entire lung*

Preoperative Care

See General preoperative care/teaching (p. 27)

Postoperative assessment
Observations/findings

Patent airway
Respiratory distress
Labored breathing
Use of accessory muscles of respiration
Tachypnea
Shallow respirations
Dyspnea
Tachycardia
Breath sounds
  Present/Absent
  Crackles, rhonchi
Elevated temperature
Hemoptysis
Crepitus
Chest pain
Cyanosis
Mediastinal shift
Incision
  Redness
  Pain

Swelling
Drainage
Arm contracture: operative side

Laboratory/diagnostic studies

Chest x-ray examination
Arterial blood gases
ECG

Potential complications

Pulmonary embolism
Pulmonary edema
Hemorrhage
Atelectasis
Tension pneumothorax
Infection
Bronchopleural fistula

Medical Management

O_2 therapy
Intubation and ventilator support
NPO until stable
Fluid and electrolyte therapy
Medications
  Analgesics
Chest tube insertion

Nursing diagnoses/interventions/evaluation

■ **NDX:** Potential for ineffective breathing pattern related to pain secondary to surgical incision

Assess and monitor respiratory rate; note use of accessory muscles
Assess chest symmetry
Assess severity and quality of pain
Administer oxygen as ordered
Elevate head of bed 60 to 90 degrees
Assist and teach patient to turn, cough, and deep breathe qh
  Do not turn to unaffected side when pneumonectomy is done
  Pad area around chest tube when turned to operative side
  Splint chest to assist with coughing
  Administer IPPB as ordered
  Assist and teach patient to use incentive spirometer
Provide emotional support
Auscultate breath sounds q2h; report diminished or absent breath sounds on unaffected side to physician
Monitor ABGs
Check function of chest tube
Administer pain medications as indicated

Expected outcome/evaluation

Patient maintains an effective breathing pattern
  Normal rate, rhythm, and depth of respirations

Decreased dyspnea
Blood gases within acceptable range
Clear breath sounds

■ **NDX:** Impaired physical mobility (arm on affected side) related to incisional pain and edema

Consult with physical therapy department to obtain ROM exercises
Assist and teach patient to exercise to tolerance
  Ambulate as ordered
  Plan rest periods q1h to 2h
Begin ROM exercises, starting with passive ROM and progressing to active ROM
Encourage patient to rotate arm 360 degrees as ordered
Document progress
Medicate for pain as needed

Expected outcome/evaluation

Patient has full range of motion of affected side by discharge date
  Is able to rotate arm in full 360-degree circles

■ **NDX:** Knowledge deficit related to lack of information about self-care management

Assess level of understanding regarding surgical procedure
Explain need to continue coughing and deep breathing qid at home
Explain need to avoid smoking
Explain importance of exercising to tolerance
  Increase amount of exercise gradually
  Adjust activities according to degree of fatigue experienced
  Plan rest periods
Explain that some numbness, pain, or heaviness in operative area is expected; it is caused by interruption of intercostal nerves and is usually temporary
Explain need to avoid persons with URIs
Explain importance of ongoing outpatient care
Discuss symptoms to report to physician
  Persistent dyspnea
  Cough
  Elevated temperature
  URI
  Redness
  Pain
  Swelling
  Drainage from incision
Discuss medications: name, dosage, time of administration, purpose, and side effects
Explain need to avoid taking over-the-counter medications without checking with physician
Ensure that patient and/or significant other demonstrates care of incision

Expected outcome/evaluation

Patient demonstrates understanding of self-care management as evidenced by verbalization of principles of self-care management

CHEST TUBES

Drainage tubes placed in the pleural space and attached to a water seal drainage system and/or suction to remove air and/or fluid and allow expansion of the affected lung

Indications: pneumothorax/hemothorax, pleural effusion, empyema, postoperative thoracotomy

Assessment
Observations/findings
PATIENT

Chest drainage
  Amount
  Color
  Character
Dyspnea
Labored breathing
Tachypnea
Tachycardia
Nonsymmetrical chest expansion
Breath sounds on affected side
  Diminished
  Absent
  Crackles
  Rhonchi
Crepitus

EQUIPMENT

Patency of tube(s) and water seal drainage system
Continuous fluctuation of water in water seal drainage system
Water level in water seal drainage system
Stability and security of water seal drainage system
Amount of added suction applied to water seal drainage system

Ongoing care
PATIENT

Position patient on affected side with head of bed elevated 45 to 60 degrees after insertion of chest tube
Explain purpose of chest tube(s)
Monitor and record BP, T, P, and R q4h and prn
Monitor and record amount, color, and character of drainage q2h to 4h; report drainage in excess of 100 ml/hr to physician
Manage pain as indicated; assess effectiveness of pain control measure(s)
Check chest tube site(s) and surrounding area q2h to 4h for crepitus and air leaks
Assist and teach patient to turn, cough, and deep breathe q2h

Splint chest when coughing
Pad area around chest tube(s) when patient is turned to operative side
Assist and teach patient to perform active or passive ROM exercises to extremities q2h to 4h
Ambulate patient as indicated
Auscultate breath sounds q2h to 4h; report diminished breath sounds in unaffected lung to physician
Change dressing as ordered

EQUIPMENT

Tape connecting tubing and secure chest tube to thorax securely
Maintain pressure if patient is on added suction as ordered
Inspect tubing for kinking and obstruction
Keep water seal drainage system lower than patient's chest at all times
Secure connecting tubing and chest tube(s) to avoid tension and allow freedom of movement
Observe fluctuation of water in water seal drainage system; if patient is breathing spontaneously, fluid level rises during inhalation and falls during exhalation
Change water seal drainage system as indicated; never allow drainage to fill collection unit
Have petroleum jelly gauze at bedside for emergency use
Keep two rubber-tipped hemostats at bedside at all times to clamp chest tube if disconnection occurs
Clamp chest tube(s) only under the following circumstances
  When disconnecting closed water seal drainage system to change collection unit
  If closed water seal drainage system breaks or integrity is disrupted for any reason

Patient Teaching

See standard of care for primary condition
Ensure that patient and/or significant other knows and understands
  Purpose of chest tube(s), function, and care
  Importance of turning, coughing, and deep breathing
  Importance of keeping closed water seal drainage system below level of patient's chest when sitting or ambulating
  Importance of not placing tension on chest tube(s)
  Need to report difficulty in breathing and chest pain to nurse and/or physician
Ensure that patient understands importance of and demonstrates coughing and deep breathing

Removal of Chest Tube
Interventions

Place patient in a sitting position
Instruct patient to take a deep breath and hold it until chest tube(s) is (are) removed by physician
Assist physician in applying pressure dressing to chest tube site

Instruct patient to breathe normally

Auscultate chest for breath sounds q4h for 24 hr; report diminished or absent breath sounds to physician

Monitor respirations and drainage from pressure dressing

Patient Teaching/Discharge Outcome

See standard of care for primary condition

Ensure that patient and/or significant other knows and understands

Importance of reporting any sudden chest pain, difficulty breathing, redness, pain, swelling of puncture site

Importance of coughing and deep breathing

Importance of exercising to tolerance; avoiding strenuous activity or exercise; checking with physician when to resume

Need to avoid contact with any person with URI

Need to avoid crowds

Importance of not smoking

ARTIFICIAL AIRWAYS

Oral (Oropharyngeal) Airway

An artificial airway that extends from the lips to the pharynx, displacing the tongue anteriorly; oral airway is usually temporary, removed once patient regains consciousness or when more permanent airway is required for ventilation

Nasal (Nasopharyngeal Airway)

An artificial airway that extends from the nares to the pharynx (Figure 4-8)

Assessment
Observations/findings

Level of consciousness
Difficulty in breathing
Airway obstruction
  Restlessness

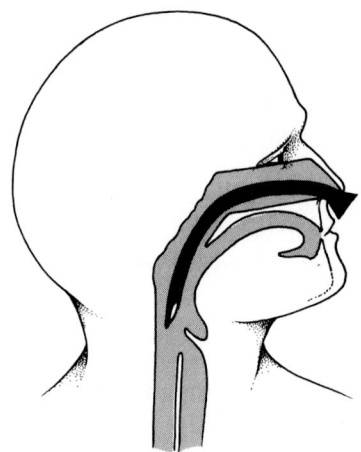

FIGURE 4-8. Nasopharyngeal airway.

Stridor
Labored breathing
Retractions
  Intercostal
  Suprasternal
  Supraclavicular
  Nasal flaring
Cyanosis or pallor
Tachycardia
Breath sounds
  Crackles
  Rhonchi
  Decreased
Secretion incrustations
Airway ports
  Patent or occluded
Oral airway
  Gagging
  Mouth infections
  Oral lacerations or pressure sores
  Position of tongue
  Position of head and neck
Nasal airway
  Mouth breathing
  Pressure sores on nares
  Position of head and neck
Complications
  Oral airways: airway obstruction, aspiration

Ongoing Care
General

Assess airway for patency and proper size of airway
Auscultate chest for breath sounds q2h and prn
Suction oropharynx or nasopharynx as indicated
Administer oxygen as ordered
Tape airway to prevent slippage or dislodgment
Monitor P and R q4h and prn; note quality of respirations
Administer oral hygiene q4h to 8h and prn

Oral airway

Assess level of consciousness
Ensure that tongue is not between teeth and airway
Maintain patient on side to decrease possibility of aspiration; if in supine position and gagging or vomiting occurs, turn head to side
Change airway daily
Reposition airway q1h to 2h if flange of airway contacts lip
Apply cream, petroleum, or water-soluble jelly to lips to prevent mucosal drying and cracking

Nasal airway

Change airway q72h, alternating nares if possible
Clean nares q8h and prn
  Use cotton-tipped applicator with saline solution

Apply water-soluble lubricant to nares
Assess need for humidification via face mask in long-term use
Use soft restraints if indicated
Establish means of communication when necessary
Call light within reach
Pad and pencil or Magic Slate at bedside

Removal of airway

Assess level of consciousness
Suction before removal
Remain with patient for 15 min after removal
Assess for any signs of respiratory distress
Monitor vital signs, noting any changes in rate and quality of respirations
Auscultate chest for breath sounds q15min to 30min for three times then q2h to 4h as ordered

Patient Teaching

Explain purpose of airway as indicated
Explain need to avoid mouth breathing

Endotracheal Tube

An artificial airway that extends from the nose or mouth into the trachea (Figure 4-9)
Indications
Upper airway obstruction
To protect airway from aspiration
To remove secretions from central airways
To provide mechanical ventilation

Assessment
Observations/findings
PATIENT

After insertion
Correct position of tube
Bilateral breath sounds

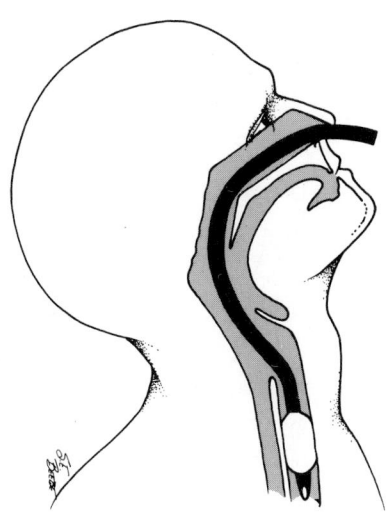

FIGURE 4-9. Endotracheal tube.

Incorrect placement
Right mainstem bronchus: unilateral (right) breath sounds; decreased breath sounds on left
Carina: persistent coughing
Esophagus: absent breath sounds
Respiratory distress: cyanosis, tachypnea, restlessness, tachycardia, decreased PaO_2, increased $PaCO_2$
Crackles
Rhonchi over large airways
Level of consciousness
Pressure sores/infection on nares, ears
Anxiety

COMPLICATIONS

Tracheal injury
Tracheal ulceration
Tracheal bronchial fistula
Aspiration
Dysrhythmias
Gag reflex
Pressure sores on nares, ears
Equipment
Tube and cuff size
Hard vs. soft cuff
Inflation pressure
Inflated cuff
Minimal leak technique (MLT) pressure 20 to 25 mm Hg
Minimal occlusion volume (MOV) technique pressure not >20 mm Hg or 25 cm H_2O
Deflated cuff
Tube placement should be assessed by chest x-ray examination: tube tip should be 5 ± 2 cm above carina
Humidification with room air or oxygen

Ongoing Care

Maintain patent airway
Auscultate chest for breath sounds qh; report decreased or absent breath sounds to physician
Suction secretions when crackles and/or rhonchi over large airways are heard
Observe color of aspirate: if purulent or colored, obtain specimen for culture
Irrigate with normal saline solution if ordered
Check position of tube q½h to 1h to prevent slippage into right or left mainstem bronchus
Obtain chest x-ray examination after insertion in order to ascertain position of tube
Keep hand-held resuscitator with adaptor at bedside
Assess respirations for quality and rate qh
Be aware that respirations are usually maintained on a continuous mechanical ventilator
Use air or oxygen blow-by if indicated
Be certain cuff is inflated while patient is on ventilator
Maintain inflated cuff with either a minimal leak or minimal occlusion volume technique

Test pressure in inflated cuff q2h to 4h: cuff pressure should remain below 20 mm Hg

Deflate cuff when patient is off ventilator for long periods of time; suction mouth and trachea before deflating cuff

Monitor ABGs as indicated

Assess level of consciousness qh; establish means of communication if patient is conscious

Call bell within reach

Pad and pencil or Magic Slate at bedside

Provide emotional support; explain all procedures

Administer oral hygiene q1h to 2h

Clean nares gently around endotracheal tube q8h and prn; use cotton-tipped applicator with saline solution; apply water-soluble lubricant to nares

Provide oropharyngeal airway or bite-block if patient bites on endotracheal tube

Apply soft restraints as necessary if patient is restless

Provide humidification to endotracheal tube when patient is off ventilator

CARE DURING/AFTER EXTUBATION
Assessment
Observations/findings

Level of consciousness

Gag reflex

Respiratory distress

Laryngeal spasm

Dyspnea

Noisy breathing

Use of abdominal or accessory muscles

Ongoing Care

Assess whether patient is able to maintain spontaneous respirations at a rate sufficient to maintain normal arterial blood gases

Auscultate chest for breath sounds

Assess level of consciousness

Elevate head of bed 45 to 90 degrees

Preoxygenate and hyperinflate patient's lungs for four or five breaths

Suction oropharynx and/or nasopharynx

Suction endotracheal tube

Instruct patient to take a deep breath

Deflate cuff at peak of deep breath

Remove tube quickly as patient exhales, using a smooth, slightly downward motion

Administer humidified oxygen

Instruct patient to cough and deep breathe

Auscultate chest for breath sounds q15min for four times, then q1h to 2h; report absent or diminished breath sounds to physician

Monitor BP, R, and apical pulse q15min for four times, then q1h to 2h

Monitor arterial blood gases as ordered

Assess for signs of stridor and/or laryngospasm

Prepare for reinsertion of endotracheal tube if laryngospasm occurs or if patient is unable to maintain adequate respiratory rate

Administer oral hygiene

Provide emotional support

Remain with patient as much as possible

Explain that sore throat, hoarseness, and dysphagia are common after extubation and will resolve in a few days

Encourage patient to minimize talking for a few hours

Provide a pad and pencil or Magic Slate

Have call light within reach

Patient Teaching

Explain all procedures whether patient appears conscious or not; orient patient to date, time, and place

Explain why patient is unable to talk and that it is only a temporary condition

Establish means of communication

Call bell within reach

Pad and pencil or Magic Slate at bedside

Emphasize importance of turning and coughing up secretions

TRACHEOSTOMY

Insertion of a tube into the trachea through a surgical incision (tracheotomy) (Figure 4-10)

Preoperative Care

See General preoperative care/teaching (p. 27)

Teach as much of the following as possible

Provide emotional support

Explain purpose of tracheostomy

Remain with patient as much as possible

Speak calmly and act unhurried

Involve family or significant other in care and instructions

Demonstrate

Tracheostomy tube

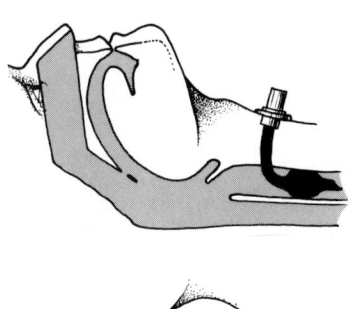
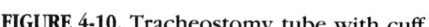

FIGURE 4-10. Tracheostomy tube with cuff.

Cleaning equipment

Suctioning equipment; explain suctioning procedure

Determine if patient can read and write English or another language

Determine if patient can hear

Explain that patient will not be able to talk postoperatively

Have pad and pencil or Magic Slate at bedside

Have picture cards available if patient is unable to write

Explain that patient may be in critical care area after operation; tour critical care area with patient and family

Review means of contacting nurse

Call light

Tap bell

Postoperative Assessment
Observations/findings
PATIENT

Position of tracheostomy

Cuff

Present

Inflated

Deflated

Bilateral expansion of chest

Sputum

Amount

Character

Stoma

Pain

Swelling

Drainage

Anxiety

Fear of suffocation

Helplessness

Hemorrhage

Airway obstruction

Restlessness

Tachycardia

Tachypnea

Noisy respirations

Wheezing

Stridor

Pallor

Cyanosis

Subcutaneous or mediastinal emphysema

Pneumothorax

Injury to thyroid, laryngeal nerve

Complications of tracheostomy

Stomal infection

Stomal hemorrhage

Excessive cuff pressure

Infection

Elevated temperature

Purulent aspirate

EQUIPMENT

Tracheostomy tube

Size

Type: cuffed vs. uncuffed

Tubes used for weaning from mechanical ventilation

Fenestrate tube

Tracheostomy buttons

Immediate Postoperative Care

See Care of patient in recovery room (p. 28)

Maintain patent airway

Administer humidification to tracheostomy

Suction prn; need for suctioning is determined by auscultation of chest for breath sounds qh

Suction when crackles and rhonchi over large airways are heard

Use sterile technique when suctioning secretions

Hyperoxygenate and hyperinflate patient's lungs for four or five breaths before suctioning

Clean inner cannula (if present) q2h to 4h and prn

Avoid occluding airway with bed linen or when turning patient

Tape tracheostomy obturator to head of bed

Have standby tracheostomy tube available: same size and type

Have hand-held resuscitator with adaptor at bedside

Elevate head of bed 45 to 60 degrees; prevent forward flexion of neck

Remove pillow if necessary

Place small towel under shoulder area

Administer oxygen or mechanical ventilation as ordered; see appropriate standard

If a cuffed tracheostomy tube is used

Maintain inflated cuff with either minimal leak or minimal occlusive volume technique; test pressure in inflated cuff q2h to 4h; cuff pressure should remain below 20 mm Hg

Use a low-pressure—cuffed tube

Auscultate chest for breath sounds q2h to 4h; report diminished or absent breath sounds to physician

Monitor BP, P, R, and rectal temperature q4h for 48 hr, then qid

Maintain NPO

Assess stoma and neck q2h to 4h as indicated; report a constant ooze, subcutaneous emphysema

Assist and teach patient to turn, cough, and deep breathe q2h

Ongoing Care

Continue with immediate postoperative care and decrease frequency of nursing functions as patient's condition improves

Maintain diet as ordered

Assess swallowing ability

NOTE: Feedings may begin with nasogastric tube until swallowing ability returns

Begin feedings with semisolid foods (e.g., gelatin)

Inflate cuff before feedings and leave inflated for 30 min after each feeding

Test swallowing reflex with gelatin; have suctioning equipment available

Observe for signs of aspiration and tracheoesophageal fistula

Cleanse skin around stoma q4h and prn

    Wash with hydrogen peroxide

    Rinse with saline solution

    Pat dry

    Change and secure tracheostomy ties prn

Place 4 × 4 inch gauze under tracheostomy tube

Perform tracheostomy care

    Postintubation: q4h for 2 days

    Routine care: q8h and prn

Be aware that physician may change tracheostomy tube daily using progressively smaller sizes

If tracheostomy is permanent, begin to demonstrate tracheostomy care while patient watches in mirror

Establish means of communication

    Have pad and pencil or Magic Slate available

    Avoid asking questions that require "yes" or "no" answers

    Wait for patient to write answer; do not anticipate end of sentence

    Read statements aloud

    Encourage patient to communicate feelings

Provide emotional support

    Encourage communication with significant other; help visitors and staff not to exclude patient from conversation or talk exclusively to one another

    Remain with patient as much as possible

    Answer call light promptly

    Deal with fear of suffocation and helplessness

Decannulate tracheostomy as ordered

    Be aware that a fenestrated tube may be used for decannulation process

    Partially cork tracheostomy tube

        Make sure cuff is deflated throughout procedure

        Observe patient for respiratory obstruction

    Progressively increase size of cork until tracheostomy is completely occluded; notify physician when patient is able to tolerate complete occlusion of tracheostomy for 24 hr

If tracheostomy is long term or permanent provide means of communication

    Pad and pencil

    Magic Slate

    Call light within reach

    Tap bell

Initiate instruction on

    Care of tracheostomy and stoma; discuss and demonstrate; provide mirror

    Handwashing procedure

Suctioning procedure before tracheostomy care: use clean procedure, not sterile

Care of inner cannula: clean procedure, not sterile

Changing of tracheostomy ties

Cleansing skin around stoma bid

    Use hydrogen peroxide

    Rinse with water

    Pat dry

Understand that patient may not be motivated to participate initially

Have patient shower daily

    Direct spray below neck

    Cover tracheostomy with waterproof material

Refer to Visiting Nurses Association, other home health agency, or self-help groups in area

Patient Teaching/Discharge Outcome

Ensure that patient and/or significant other knows and understands

    Care of tracheostomy tube and stoma

    Importance of clean not sterile technique

        Gloves not necessary unless another person is cleaning tracheostomy

    Tracheostomy dressings are not recommended unless excessive secretions

    Importance of reporting signs and symptoms of skin irritation, infection, or changes in secretions

    Importance of maintaining diet as ordered

    Force fluids to 3000 ml/day unless contraindicated

    Need to shower daily

    Wear shield over stoma

    Use shower hose

    Direct spray below neck

    Avoid getting soap into stoma

    Need for male patients to shave with electric razor or safety razor; avoid getting lather into stoma

    Need to exercise to tolerance but no swimming; to plan rest periods

    Need to keep stoma covered at all times; to wear clothing with high neckline, scarves, and jewelry

    Importance of covering stoma when coughing; need to report persistent cough to physician

    Importance of not smoking

    Need to wear medical alert band identifying neck breather

    Importance of not using aerosol sprays around patient

    Need to use commercial humidifier or pan of water on stove to add to comfort

    Importance of ongoing outpatient care

    Need to avoid persons with URIs

    Need to report any respiratory distress to physician

    Name of medication, dosage, time of administration, purpose, and side effects

    Need to avoid taking over-the-counter medications without checking with physician

CONTINUOUS MECHANICAL VENTILATION

A method of providing ventilatory support for those patients who are unable to spontaneously maintain adequate oxygenation of the blood, with or without carbon dioxide retention; two categories of ventilators are positive pressure (volume-cycled or pressure-cycled) and negative pressure (iron lung, cuirass), not commonly used; examples of a volume-cycled positive-pressure ventilator are the Bird Mark 7 and Bennett PR2; on the other hand, the Bennett MA-1, Emerson, Bourns Bear 1, Ohio 560, and Engstrom are pressure-cycled positive-pressure ventilators

Care of Patient on Continuous Mechanical Ventilation

Assessment
Observations/findings

Position of airway
  Endotracheal tube
  Tracheostomy
Patency of airway
Respiratory distress
  Tachypnea
  Tachycardia
  Restlessness
  Apprehension
  Diaphoresis
  Pallor
  Cyanosis
Breath sounds
  Diminished
  Absent
  Crackles
  Rhonchi
Respiratory acidosis (acidemia)
  Decreased pH: below 7.4 mm Hg
  Elevated PaCO₂: above 45 mm Hg
Respiratory alkalosis (alkalemia)
  Increased pH: above 7.4 mm Hg
  Decreased PaCO₂: below 35 mm Hg
Hypoxemia
Sputum
  Amount
  Color
  Consistency
Atelectasis
Psychosocial problems
  Anxiety
  Dependence on ventilator

Potential Complications

Disconnection from ventilator
Acid-base imbalance
Respiratory infection
Oxygen toxicity (time and dose related)
  Diminished breath sounds
  Crackles
  Decreased lung compliance
  Decreased VC
  Decreased PaCO₂ while using same oxygen concentration
  Changes on chest x-ray examination
  Visual impairment
  Papilledema
Fluid and electrolyte imbalance
  Dehydration
  Positive water balance
Decreased cardiac output
Pneumothorax
Barotrauma
GI bleeding

Acute Care

Assess quality and rate of respirations
Assess for bilateral chest movement
Ensure that respirations are in phase with the ventilator
Maintain patent airway
  Suction prn; determine need for suctioning by auscultating chest for breath sounds qh—suction when crackles or rhonchi are present
    Hyperoxygenate and hyperinflate lungs for four or five breaths before suctioning secretions
    Use sterile technique when suctioning patient
    Place respirator attachment on sterile towel while suctioning patient
  Keep hand-held resuscitator with adaptor at bedside
See Tracheostomy (p. 232)
See Endotracheal tube (p. 231)
Administer medications as ordered
  Sedatives
  Morphine sulfate
  Neuromuscular blocking agents
Monitor arterial blood gases as indicated
Assess BP, R, and apical pulse q1h to 2h
Check rectal temperature q4h
Auscultate breath sounds q1h to 2h, reporting any changes indicating progressive disease
Maintain position of optimal ventilation; elevate head of bed 60 to 90 degrees; turn q1h to 2h and prn, alternating postural drainage positions
Have patient sigh q15min or as ordered
Measure ventilator settings q4h to 8h or as indicated; readjust as indicated
  FIO₂; measure after suctioning
  Tidal volume (V_T)
  Airway pressure
  Sigh rate: usually 1 ½ to 2 times the V_T
Maintain temperature in inspiratory tubing between 89.6° and 95° F (32° and 35° C)

Check ventilatory alarms
Administer parenteral fluids as ordered
Provide nutritional support
　Assess nutritional status daily
　Administer tube feedings, total parenteral nutrition as ordered
Provide emotional support
　Remain with patient as much as possible
　Answer call light promptly
　Establish means of communication: pad and pencil or Magic Slate
　Allow patient sufficient time to communicate thoughts and feelings
　Maintain nonstressful environment
　Be calm, confident, and unhurried when caring for patient
　Encourage communication with significant other

Ongoing Care: Subacute

Continue with acute care and decrease frequency of nursing functions as patient's condition improves
Wean patient off respirator as ordered
　Obtain baseline respiratory rate, VC, and tidal volume
　Explain weaning process thoroughly
　Remain with patient during weaning process
　Monitor R and apical pulse q5min to 15min after removal from ventilator
　Place on ventilator immediately if respiratory distress occurs
　Be prepared to repeat weaning process several times if necessary

Convalescent Care

See standard of care for primary condition

Patient Teaching

Ensure that patient and/or significant other knows and understands
　Purpose of ventilator
　Importance of breathing with ventilator
　Importance of coughing up secretions
　Importance of artificial airway
　Need to avoid placing any tension on airway; to never touch airway with hands
　Need to communicate in writing

Pressure-Limited Positive-Pressure Ventilator

Delivers a volume of air until a preset pressure is reached; used primarily for IPPB treatments in the adult population

Assessment/Care of Equipment

Attached to gas source
Connecting tubing
　Patent

Free of excessive moisture
Air leaks
　Cuff of endotracheal tube
　Cuff of tracheostomy
Patent airway
Adequate humidification
　Nebulizer
　Heated humidification
Temperature of inspired gas
Settings as ordered
　Respiratory rate: should not be less than 12/min
　Oxygen concentration: air mix control
　Inspiratory pressure control
　Apnea control
　Sensitivity control

Ongoing Care

Maintain inspiratory rate and respiratory pressure as ordered
　Patent airway
　System free of leaks
　Connective tubing patent and free of excessive moisture
Be aware that inspiratory positive pressure ventilators may not have alarm systems
Remain with patient as much as possible
Determine respiratory rate, oxygen concentration, and inspiratory pressure setting by arterial blood gases
Establish flow sheet
　Record ventilator settings
　Record laboratory values
Maintain oxygen concentration as ordered; measure FIO_2 q8h and prn
Maintain respiratory rate as ordered
　Measure tidal volume q8h and prn
　Auscultate chest for breath sounds qh
Provide humidification
Make sure that equipment continues to cycle when cuff is deflated
Have patient sigh q15min or as ordered; use hand-held resuscitator
Change connecting tubing, nebulizer, and humidification system q24h; replace with sterile equipment

Volume-Cycled Positive-Pressure Ventilator

Delivers breathing gas at a predetermined volume; once the desired volume has been delivered; the ventilator will cycle and patient will passively exhale

Assessment/Care of Equipment

Electrical system
　Plugged in
　Alarms on
Connecting tubing
　Patent
　Free of excessive moisture
Air leaks

Cuff of endotracheal tube
Cuff of tracheostomy
Patent airway
Adequate humidification
Heated humidification
Nebulizer
Temperature of inspired gas
Settings as ordered
Flow rate
Inspiratory pressure
Tidal volume
Positive end-expiratory pressure (PEEP)
Continuous positive airway pressure (CPAP)
Ventilator rate: should not be less than 12/min
Oxygen concentration
Sigh pressure
Sigh volume
Number of sighs per hour
Ventilatory mode
Control
Assist
Assist-controlled
Synchronized intermittent mandatory ventilation (SIMV or IMV)

Ongoing Care

Maintain tidal volume as ordered
Patent airway
System free of leaks
Connective tubing patent and free of excessive moisture
Determine ventilator settings by arterial blood gases
Establish flow sheet
Record ventilator settings
Record laboratory values
Maintain oxygen concentration as ordered (determined by PaO_2); measure FIO_2 q8h and prn
Maintain respiratory rate as ordered
Provide heated humidification
Remove excessive water in tubing
Have patient sigh q15min or as ordered; sigh pressure and volume as ordered
Avoid turning alarm system off
Measure tidal volume q8h and prn
Test alarm system q8h
Change connecting tubing, nebulizer, and humidification q24h; replace with sterile equipment

INTERMITTENT POSITIVE PRESSURE BREATHING (IPPB)

intermittent positive pressure ventilator *A ventilator that delivers breathing gas until equilibrium is established between the patient's lungs and the ventilator; depends on pressure buildup in the patient's lungs rather than on time or volume; a valve mechanism shuts off the gas flow when the pressure has been* reached and patient exhales passively; should be used only after less expensive modalities have been tried

Pretreatment Assessment
Observations/findings

BP
Pulse
Color
Respiratory effort
Breath sounds

Preparation

Observe BP and apical pulse before treatment
Auscultate chest for breath sounds
Place patient in sitting position
Prepare machine
Secure all tubing connections
Place medication or saline solution in nebulizer
Set pressure and oxygen concentration as ordered
Control nebulizer to produce fine mist

Preprocedure Teaching

Explain procedure and what is expected of patient
Concentrate on using diaphragm
Breathe at normal rate through mouth
Allow machine to fill lungs to desired volume
Prolong expiration
Purse lips around mouthpiece

Assessment During Treatment
Observations/findings

Respiratory rate
Chest expansion
Sudden respiratory distress
Hyperventilation
Circumoral numbness
Tingling of fingers
Dizziness
Fatigue
Nervousness
Tachycardia
Chest pain
Function of equipment

Ongoing Care

Take pulse one or two times during treatment
Remain with patient during initial treatment
Stop treatment if sudden respiratory distress or chest pain occurs
Have patient deep breathe slowly one or two times during treatment
Have patient cough one or two times during and after treatment
Check pressure gauge and adjust flow to avoid negative inspiratory pressure
Administer oral hygiene after treatment

Patient Teaching/Discharge Outcome

Ensure that patient and/or significant other knows and understands

Need to follow physician's instructions regarding use of IPPB

Need to cough during and immediately after treatment

Importance of using saline solution or medication in nebulizer

Symptoms of respiratory distress to report to physician

Need to stop treatment if dizziness, nervousness, chest pain, rapid pulse, or sudden respiratory distress occurs during treatment

Importance of avoiding persons with URIs

Symptoms of URI to report to physician

Importance of ongoing outpatient care

Name of medication, dosage, time of administration, purpose, and side effects

Need to avoid taking over-the-counter medications without checking with physician

Ensure that patient and/or significant other demonstrates

Preparation of machine for treatment

Use of machine during treatment

IPPB procedure

Coughing techniques

Care of equipment

INCENTIVE SPIROMETER

A mechanical device that assists patient in maintaining maximal inspiratory effort; effective when used by postoperative patients to prevent development of atelectasis and pneumonia; more physiologic and less hazardous than IPPB as it depends only on the patient's inspiratory effort (not on electricity, batteries, or gas)

Assessment
Observations/findings
PATIENT

Presence or absence of pain

Motivation

Weakness

Hyperventilation
Dizziness
Lightheadedness
Numbness around mouth and nose
Tingling in fingers and toes

Cough
Productive
Nonproductive

Breath sounds
Diminished
Absent
Crackles
Rhonchi over large airways

EQUIPMENT

Type of device
Tidal volume

Ongoing Care

Patient must be alert and cooperative

Assess degree of pain present
Administer analgesics as ordered
Assess effectiveness of pain relief measure(s)

Elevate head of bed 60 to 90 degrees or have patient sit in chair

Assist and teach patient to use incentive spirometer
Exhale slowly
Place mouthpiece in mouth between teeth
Close lips tightly around mouthpiece
Inhale through mouth only, taking a slow, deep breath
Hold breath for 3 to 5 sec
Remove mouthpiece from mouth
Exhale slowly

Repeat procedure 10 to 20 times qh

Caution patient not to breathe too rapidly

Observe for signs of hyperventilation; stop use of incentive spirometer if dizziness or lightheadedness occurs

Assist and teach patient to cough after using incentive spirometer

Auscultate chest for breath sounds q4h
Assist and teach patient to cough if crackles or rhonchi are heard
Report diminished or absent breath sounds to physician

Monitor patient's progress q4h

Increase tidal volume as patient tolerates it

Patient Teaching

Ensure that patient and/or significant other knows and understands

Purpose of incentive spirometer

Importance of using it 10 to 20 times qh

Importance of holding breath for 3 to 5 sec

Need to inhale through mouth

Importance of not exhaling into apparatus

Importance of reaching desired tidal volume

Importance of coughing after using apparatus

Ensure that patient demonstrates
Use of incentive spirometer
Coughing productively

BIBLIOGRAPHY

Abels L: *Critical care nursing: a physiologic approach*, St Louis, 1986, CV Mosby.

Berte J: *Critical care: the lung*, ed 2, East Norwalk, Conn, 1986, Appleton-Century-Crofts.

Bransetter RD: The adult respiratory distress syndrome, *Heart Lung* 15:155, 1986.

Brenner B: *Comprehensive management of respiratory emergencies*, Rockville, Md, 1985, Aspen Publishers.

Clayton DB, Stock YN: *Basic pharmacology for nurses*, ed 9, St Louis, 1989, Mosby–Year Book.

Davido J: Pulmonary rehabilitation, *Nurs Clin North Am* 16(2):275, 1981.

Farzan S: *A concise handbook of respiratory diseases*, Reston, Va, 1985, Reston Publishing.

Halloway NM: *Nursing the critically ill adult*, Menlo Park, Calif, 1988, Addison-Wesley Publishing.

Hodgkin J, Zorn E, and Connors G: *Pulmonary rehabilitation: guidelines to success*, Boston, 1984, Butterworth Publishers.

Hopp L: Ineffective breathing related to decreased lung expansion, *Nurs Clin North Am* 22:193, 1987.

Kenner CV, Guzzetta CE, and Dossey BM: *Critical care nursing: body-mind-spirit*, Boston, 1985, Little, Brown.

Kim MJ, McFarland GK, and McLane AM: *Pocket guide to nursing diagnoses*, ed 4, St Louis, 1990, Mosby–Year Book.

Kinney MR, Packa DR, and Dunbar SB: *AACN's clinical reference for critical-care nursing*, ed 2, New York, 1988, McGraw-Hill.

Lehrer S: *Understanding lung sounds*, Philadelphia, 1984, WB Saunders.

Luckmann J, Sorensen K: *Medical-surgical nursing*, ed 3, Philadelphia, 1987, WB Saunders.

McDonald BR: Validation of three respiratory nursing diagnosis: ineffective airway clearance, ineffective breathing pattern, and impaired gas exchange, *Nurs Clin North Am* 20:697, 1985.

McDonald G: Symposium on respiratory care: a home care program for patients with chronic lung disease, *Nurs Clin North Am* 16:259, 1981.

Murray J: *The normal lung: the basis for diagnosis and treatment of pulmonary diseases*, ed 2, Philadelphia, 1986, WB Saunders.

Op'T Holt T: *Assessment-based respiratory care*, New York, 1986, John Wiley & Sons.

Perry AG et al: *Shock: comprehensive nursing management*, St Louis, 1983, CV Mosby.

Peterson G: Symposium on respiratory care: application and assessment of oxygen therapy, *Nurs Clin North Am* 16:241, 1981.

Robinson S, Russo R, eds: Providing respiratory care, *Nursing '83* 13:1983.

Sweetwood H: *Nursing in the intensive respiratory care unit*, New York, 1979, Springer Publishing.

Tisi G: *Pulmonary physiology in clinical medicine*, ed 2, Baltimore, 1985, Williams & Wilkins.

Ulrich S, Canale S, and Wendell S: *Nursing care planning guides*, Philadelphia, 1986, WB Saunders Co.

Wade J: *Comprehensive respiratory care*, ed 3, St Louis, 1983, CV Mosby.

Weinberger S: *Principles of pulmonary medicine*, Philadelphia, 1986, WB Saunders.

Wilkins R, Shelden R, and Krider S: *Clinical assessment in respiratory care*, ed 2, St Louis, 1990, Mosby–Year Book.

Wilson S, Thompson JM: *Respiratory disorders*, St Louis, 1990, Mosby–Year Book.

Zschoche D, ed: *Mosby's comprehensive review of critical care*, ed 3, St Louis, 1986, Mosby–Year Book.

5
CHAPTER

Digestive System

GASTROINTESTINAL ASSESSMENT

Subjective Data

Mouth, gums, tongue, lips
  Painful
  Tender
Dysphagia
Eructation
Anorexia, weight loss
Indigestion
Pyrosis (heartburn)
Fullness after eating
Pain, discomfort after certain foods
Nausea, vomiting; regurgitation without vomiting
Abdomen
  Painful
  Tender
  Cramping
Fatigue
Change in eating or bowel habits
Change in color, character, or frequency of stools or urine
Constipation
Diarrhea
Hemorrhoids
Painful defecation
Use of laxatives or enemas
Change in skin color or texture; rash or itching
Edema of extremities

Objective Data

General appearance
Vital signs
  BP, P, and R
    Lying
    Sitting
    Standing
Temperature
Weight
Urinary output, color, amount, specific gravity
Allergies
Mouth
  Stomatitis
  Condition and color of tongue, gums, mucous membrane, and teeth
  Halitosis
  Saliva production: increased or decreased

Abdomen
  Distention, rigidity, ascites
  Increased abdominal girth
  Symmetry
  Hepatomegaly
  Keloid tissue, scars
  Visible peristalsis
  Bowel sounds
    Present
    Absent
  Visible palpable masses; hernia(s)
  Presence of ostomies
Perianal area
  Hemorrhoids
  Color and condition of area
  Odor
  Color, consistency, and frequency of stools
Sclera: jaundice
Skin
  Jaundice
  Turgor
  Pruritus
  Spider angioma
  Purpura
  Palmar erythema
  Peripheral edema
  Distended, tortuous blood vessels
  Abdominal striae

Pertinent Background Information
CONCURRENT DISEASES OR CONDITIONS

Carcinoma
Cardiovascular disease (hypertension)
Alcoholism
Endocrine disorders
Severe burns
Psychological problems
Drug abuse
Neurological conditions
Epistaxis

PREVIOUS SURGERY OR ILLNESS

Inflammatory bowel disease
Carcinoma
Gastrointestinal (GI) surgery
  Cholecystectomy

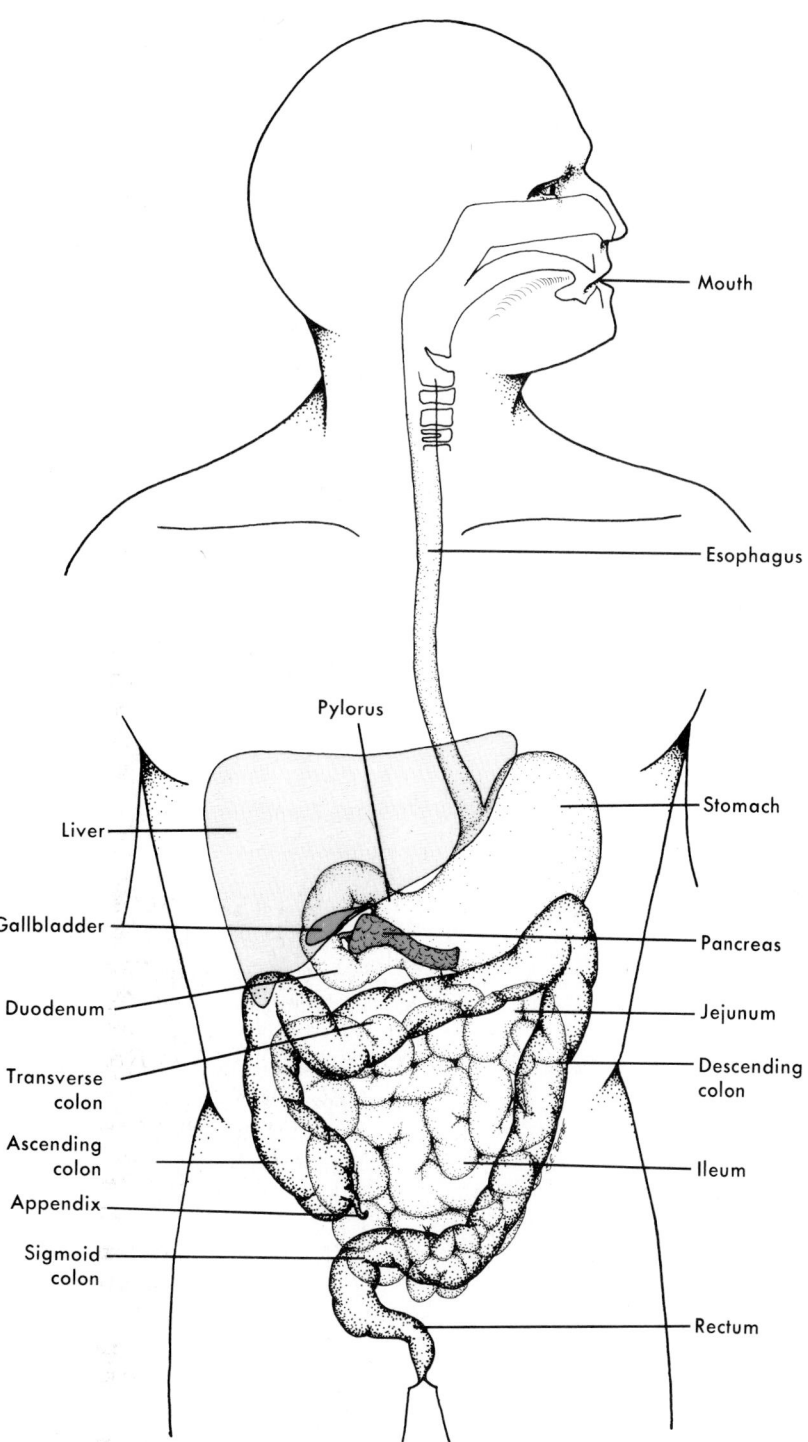

Mouth

Esophagus

Pylorus

Liver

Gallbladder

Duodenum

Transverse colon

Ascending colon

Appendix

Sigmoid colon

Stomach

Pancreas

Jejunum

Descending colon

Ileum

Rectum

FIGURE 5-1. Digestive system.

Gastric surgery
Ostomies
Other abdominal, pelvic, or rectal surgeries
Hepatitis
Cirrhosis
Pancreatitis
Diabetes mellitus

FAMILY HISTORY

Carcinoma
GI-related disease
Diabetes mellitus

SOCIAL HISTORY

Alcohol, tobacco use
Cultural food use; eating habits
Personality type: tense, stressful
View of life's work

MEDICATION HISTORY

Antacids
Laxatives, cathartics
Anticholinergics
Steroids
Antidiarrheals
Antiemetics
Tranquilizers
Sedatives
Antihypertensives
Barbiturates
Antibiotics
Acetylsalicylic acid
Hydrogen receptor antagonists (Tagamet, Zantac)

Diagnostic Aids

LABORATORY STUDIES

Complete blood cell count (CBC)
Alkaline phosphatase level
Bilirubin level
  Serum
  Urine
  Feces
Serum glutamic oxaloacetic transaminase (SGOT)
Serum glutamic pyruvic transaminase (SGPT)
5-Nucleotidase
Lactic acid dehydrogenase (LDH)
Prothrombin time (PT)
Amylase level
  Serum
  Urine
Blood urea nitrogen (BUN)
Stool examination
  Occult blood
  Fat
  Protein
  Parasite, ova

Secretin stimulation test
Serum lipase, cholinesterase levels
Serum calcium level
Serum ammonia level
Serum gastrin level, parietal cell antibodies
Serum α-fetoprotein
Sulkowitch's urine test
Serum albumin level
Total protein level
Serum glucose level
Serum electrolyte profile
Serum carotene test
D-Xylose tolerance test
Lactose intolerance test
Schilling's test
Albumin-globulin (A/G) ratio
Urobilinogen level
Galactose tolerance test
Insulin tolerance test
Hollander test
Carcinoembryonic antigen (CEA)

PROCEDURES

Endoscopy and biopsy
  Esophageal
  Gastric
  Duodenal
Cine-esophagogram
Motility studies
Radioisotope scintiscan
Basal secretion
Gastric acid stimulation test
Esophageal manometry
Contrast radiography
Hypotonic duodenography
Radionuclide imaging
Computed tomography (CT) scan
Ultrasonography
Upper GI series
Small bowel series
Barium enema or swallow gastrography
Barium air-contrast studies
Cholecystography
Intravenous cholangiography
T tube cholangiography
Biopsy
  Liver
  Rectum
  Colon
  Small bowel
Digital rectal examination
Sigmoidoscopy
Colonoscopy
Proctoscopy
Fluoroscopy
Complete abdominal x-ray examination

Bernstein test
Gastric cytology
Percutaneous transhepatic cholangiography
Celiac and mesenteric arteriography
Superior and inferior mesenteric angiogram
Scans
    Liver, spleen
    Pancreas, gallbladder
Splenoportography
Endoscopic retrograde cholangiopancreatography (ERCP)
Magnetic resonance imaging (MRI)

Esophagus

ESOPHAGEAL STRICTURE, ESOPHAGITIS, ACHALASIA, DIVERTICULOSIS

stricture *Narrowing of the wall of the esophagus (usually lower two thirds); most commonly resulting from reflux esophagitis, chemical ingestion, sliding hiatal hernia, or neoplastic infiltration*

esophagitis *Acute or chronic inflammation caused by gastroesophageal reflux, trauma, bacteria, chemical ingestion, hiatal hernia, or overindulgence in alcohol and/or spices*

achalasia *Disruption or absence of peristaltic action in the lower two thirds of the esophagus and failure of the cardiac sphincter to relax on swallowing*

diverticulosis *Saclike protrusion in the esophageal wall, usually of a congenital nature*

Assessment
Observations/findings

Midsternal or substernal pain; may radiate to back, neck, and arms
Discomfort after eating, when bending, or when in supine position
Sore throat
Nocturnal choking
Pyrosis (heartburn)
Regurgitation without vomiting
Weight loss
Eructation
Dysphagia
Hematemesis

Laboratory/diagnostic studies

Endoscopy with biopsy, cytology, and/or dilation
Barium swallow esophagogram
Splash down time
Chest radiological study
Manometry
CBC and electrolytes
Bernstein test

Potential complications

Aspiration pneumonia
Esophageal obstruction
Malnutrition
Esophageal perforation

Medical Management

High-calorie diet according to tolerance
Antacids
Calcium-blocking agents, Isordil, Procardia
Topical liquid anesthetics
Stool softeners
Antibiotics

Nursing diagnoses/interventions/evaluation

■ **NDX:** Altered nutrition: less than body requirements related to dysphagia

Assess ability to swallow
Provide small, frequent meals
Teach patient to chew food well and to eat slowly
Encourage patient to sit up during and after meals
Encourage fluids with meals
Avoid extremes in food temperatures
Measure intake and output
Administer liquid topical anesthetic before meals to decrease dysphagia
Encourage fluid intake to 2500 ml/24 hr if not contraindicated
Provide high-fiber foods if tolerated to assist in elimination
Monitor CBC, electrolytes
Weigh patient daily at same time with same clothing and scale
Discourage smoking

Expected outcome/evaluation

Patient's
    Calorie and fluid intake is optimal
    Electrolytes are within normal limits
    Weight is maintained

■ **NDX:** Potential for aspiration related to impaired swallowing

Assist and teach patient to cough and deep breathe q4h
Monitor breath sounds q4h
Elevate head of bed 30 to 45 degrees after meals and at bedtime
Avoid supine position
Provide planned rest periods
Assist with feeding as needed
Administer oral hygiene qid

Expected outcome/evaluation

Patient
    Demonstrates correct coughing and breathing techniques
    Presents normal breath sounds

■ **NDX:** Pain related to esophageal inflammation and/or heartburn

Provide calm, nonstressful environment
Reinforce physician's explanation of disease process
Administer and monitor antacids for effectiveness/side effects
Provide soothing back rubs
Change patient's position in small ways to promote comfort
Encourage activities and self-care to decrease discomfort

Expected outcome/evaluation

Patient
Reports a decrease in heartburn
Maintains activities at optimal level
Reports no pain or discomfort after eating

■ **NDX:** Knowledge deficit related to lack of information about home and follow-up care

Discuss with patient and/or significant other the importance of diet and diet restrictions
Explain need to avoid foods that cause dysphagia
Provide and review high-calorie, high-protein diet instruction sheet if applicable
Encourage increased fluid intake
Advise patient to avoid tobacco, aspirin, and phenylbutazone
Advise elevating head while sleeping
Discuss methods for avoiding stress
Advise bending and stooping should be avoided
Discuss methods of avoiding constipation
Recommend high-fiber foods if tolerated
Encourage natural laxatives
Increase patient's activities to tolerance
Discuss medications: name, dosage, time of administration, purpose, and side effects
Explain importance of follow-up care with physician
Discuss symptoms of recurrence or progression of disease to report to physician

Expected outcome/evaluation

Patient
Demonstrates understanding of prescribed diet regimen
Verbalizes medication schedule accurately
Seeks information concerning care
Identifies signs of recurrence to report to physician

BLEEDING ESOPHAGEAL VARICES

A condition usually associated with cirrhosis and portal hypertension in which the small esophageal veins become distended and rupture as a result of the increased pressure in the portal system; may be controlled medically, but surgery (portacaval shunt) is often required

Assessment
Observations/findings

Character, frequency, and amount of hematemesis
Respiratory distress
Altered vital signs
Restlessness
Aspiration of emesis
Disorientation
Confusion
Dehydration
Electrolyte imbalance
Abdominal distention
Anxiety
Melena
Jaundice

Laboratory/diagnostic studies

Esophagoscopy
Esophageal arteriogram
CBC, platelets, PT, arterial blood gases, electrolytes
Blood alcohol
SGOT, SGPT, LDH, alkaline phosphatase
Liver function tests
Guaiac stools for blood

Potential complications

Aspiration pneumonia
Hemorrhage
Shock
Hepatic coma
Death

Medical Management

NPO
Esophagogastric tube with suction and pressures to be maintained
Gastric lavages
Parenteral fluids with electrolytes
Fresh whole blood
Indwelling urinary catheter with hourly measurements
Orotracheal suctioning
Oxygen therapy
Central venous pressure (CVP) line or Swan-Ganz catheter
Arterial blood gases
Saline enemas
Vasopressin (Pitressin), neomucin, vitamin K, lactulose
Analgesics, usually phenobarbital
Histamine receptor antagonists (Tagamet, Zantac)
Esophageal sclerotherapy
Surgical intervention (see Portacaval Shunt, p. 299)
Diet, activity

Nursing diagnoses/interventions/evaluation

■ **NDX:** Potential for aspiration related to esophagogastric tube, impaired swallowing

Maintain bed rest in quiet environment
  Position patient on side during vomiting episodes
  Elevate head of bed 30 degrees
Perform orotracheal suctioning prn
Auscultate chest for breath sounds qlh to 2h
Administer oxygen therapy by mask or catheter
Assist and teach patient to turn and deep breathe qh; instruct not to cough
Administer oral hygiene qlh to 2h; keep mouth and nares well lubricated

Expected outcome/evaluation

Patient
  Presents normal breath sounds
  Manages secretions adequately
  Demonstrates turning and deep breathing exercises accurately

 NDX: Alteration in tissue perfusion: cardiopulmonary, cerebral, gastrointestinal, renal, peripheral related to hypovolemia

Gastrointestinal

Monitor bowel sounds and measure abdominal girth q2h; report changes to physician
Monitor stools for melena
Maintain esophagogastric tube
  Sengstaken-Blakemore tube (p. 249)
  Linton tube (p. 249)
Monitor character and amount of gastric drainage q1h to 2h
Administer lavages via tube
Maintain NPO

Cardiopulmonary

Assess for signs of hypovolemia, tachycardia, tachypnea, cold clammy skin
Replace blood as needed
Monitor breath sounds
Provide oxygen prn
Maintain parenteral fluids with electrolytes, using large-bore catheter
Monitor hemoglobin (Hgb), hematocrit (Hct), serum electrolytes, and PT
Monitor CVP line or Swan-Ganz catheter
Monitor arterial blood gases
Monitor BP, R, and apical pulse q15min to 30min
Take rectal temperature q2h while esophagogastric tube is in place

Renal

Maintain urinary catheter to gravity drainage
Measure intake and output qh; if urine output is less than 30 to 50 ml/hr, report to physician
Monitor specific gravity of urine
Monitor serum pH, BUN, and creatinine

Cerebral

Assess level of consciousness and mental acuity
Establish baseline neurological assessment

Peripheral

Monitor pedal pulses
Encourage active/passive ROM exercises
Maintain warmth of extremities
Apply antiembolic hose
Elevate legs to increase venous flow
Monitor medication administration; observe for effectiveness/side effects
  Antibiotics
  Vitamin K
  Vasopressin
  Antacids

Expected outcome/evaluation

Patient's
  Gastric drainage is clear or clearing
  Vital signs are normal
  Electrolytes are within normal limits
  Intake and output are balanced
  Pedal pulses are palpable
  Skin is warm and dry
  Mental acuity is normal

■ **NDX:** Pain related to invasive procedures and therapeutic treatments

Maintain position of comfort within limits of ongoing treatments
Administer skin care and back rubs q2h to 4h to promote comfort
Keep patient warm and dry
Perform passive (ROM) exercises q4h
Assess pain intensity level
  Medicate according to pain scale
  Provide diversional activities where possible
  Provide alternate pain management techniques
  Assess effectiveness of pain relief measures
Increase activity as tolerated

Expected outcome/evaluation

Patient
  Reports reduction in pain/discomfort
  Demonstrates relaxed affect

■ **NDX:** Anxiety related to uncertainty and threat to bodily health

Remain with patient at onset of bleeding as much as possible
  Use restraints if applicable
  Keep side rails up

Monitor mental acuity
Plan care to provide rest periods
Orient patient to place, date, and time frequently
Explain each procedure as much as time allows
Reinforce physician's explanation of disease process
Maintain nonstressful environment
    Dim lights when possible
    Discourage loud talking and noises
Encourage verbalization of fears and anxieties
Promote relaxation techniques
Discuss past successful coping behaviors
Involve in care as much as possible
Promote family/significant other support

Expected outcome/evaluation

Patient
    Expresses understanding of cause of anxiety
    Demonstrates ability to cope independently with stress

■ **NDX:**   Knowledge deficit related to lack of information
            about home and follow-up care

Explain diet restrictions on carbohydrates, fats, and proteins
Consult dietitian for low-roughage diet plan
Discuss importance of avoiding alcohol
Explain about available counseling
    Alcoholics Anonymous
    Al-Anon, Al-Ateen
    Chemical dependency agencies
Instruct patient in a mild exercise-to-tolerance program
    with planned rest periods
Reinforce physician's explanation of effects of alcohol on
    disease process
Discuss medications: name, purpose, dosage, time of administration, and side effects; caution patient not to
    take over-the-counter medications without checking
    with physician; especially aspirin compounds
Explain symptoms of recurrence or progression to report
    to physician
Discuss importance of follow-up care with physician

Expected outcome/evaluation

Patient
    Demonstrates understanding of relationship of alcohol
        to disease
    Seeks information about counseling
    Expresses knowledge of diet and activity regimen
    Verbalizes medication schedule accurately

ESOPHAGEAL SURGERY

Surgery performed when medical management of esophageal disorders such as diverticulitis, perforation, and hiatal hernia has been unsuccessful; for carcinoma of the esophagus, an esophagogastrectomy is usually performed—approach may be thoracic or abdominal

Assessment
Observations/findings

Decreased breath sounds
Splinting with respirations
Tachypnea
Bradypnea
Function of chest tubes (thoracic approach)
Character and amount of gastric drainage and urine output
Location and character of pain

Laboratory/diagnostic studies

CBC and electrolytes
Chest radiological study

Potential complications

Respiratory distress
Electrolyte imbalance
Gastroesophageal anastomosis leak
Hemorrhage
Shock
Tracheoesophageal fistula
Suture line infection
Pheumothorax (thoracic approach)
Pneumonia

Medical Management

Analgesics
NPO
Parenteral fluids with electrolytes
Whole blood
Nasogastric tube and urinary catheter
Orotracheal suction
Oxygen per mask or catheter
Chest tubes (thoracic approach)
Incentive spirometer
Gastrostomy tube and type of feeding if appropriate
Diet, activity

Nursing diagnoses/interventions/evaluation

■ **NDX:**   Potential for aspiration related to anesthesia
            and nasogastric tube

Assess ability to swallow
Auscultate chest for breath sounds q2h to 4h
Elevate head of bed 35 to 45 degrees
Teach and assist patient to turn, cough, and deep breathe
    q2h to 4h; splint chest as needed
Maintain oxygen and/or use incentive spirometer qh
Perform orotracheal suctioning prn

Expected outcome/evaluation

Patient
    Presents normal breath sounds
    Performs turning, deep breathing adequately

■ **NDX:** Fluid volume deficit (2) related to abnormal fluid loss, NPO state, and nasogastric tube

Maintain NPO; assess for signs of dehydration
Maintain parenteral fluids with electrolytes
Monitor serum electrolytes
Measure intake and output
Monitor vital signs q4h
Maintain nasogastric tube or gastrostomy tube to intermittent suction or gravity drainage
Monitor placement of nasogastric tube; tape in place; if tube is dysfunctional, notify physician; *do not reposition*
Monitor character and amount of gastric drainage q8h
Monitor wound for excessive drainage/bleeding prn; report excess to physician
Encourage movement of legs, feet to promote venous return; do not gatch knees
After nasogastric tube removal
  Initiate oral fluids in small amounts
  Progress to soft, bland diet as tolerated
  Report pain, retching, or vomiting to physician
For gastrostomy tube: administer tube feedings (p. 32)

Expected outcome/evaluation

Patient's
  Intake and output are balanced
  Electrolytes are within normal limits
  Vital signs are normal

■ **NDX:** Pain related to surgical intervention

Assess type, location, and intensity of pain
Administer analgesics to maintain comfort; assess effectiveness of pain relief measures
Turn and change position q2h to 4h
Provide back rubs and skin care to promote comfort
Maintain planned rest periods
Splint incision when coughing
Discuss alternate pain management techniques

Expected outcome/evaluation

Patient
  Reports reduction in or absence of pain
  Demonstrates more relaxed affect

■ **NDX:** Potential for ineffective individual coping related to surgical procedure and possible changes in lifestyle

Reinforce physician's explanation of surgical procedure and expected outcome
Encourage and allow time for verbalization of concerns; involve significant others
Discuss stress management techniques; breathing, relaxation, imagery, etc.

Explain nursing care plan and all procedures
Assess present coping patterns; assist patient with identifying alternative and positive ways of coping
Explain needed changes in lifestyle in nonthreatening and positive manner

Expected outcome/evaluation

Patient
  Demonstrates progress in developing positive attitudes toward needed changes in lifestyle
  Uses family/significant others for support group

■ **NDX:** Knowledge deficit related to lack of information about home care needs

Provide and discuss diet and dietary restrictions
  Eat small, frequent meals
  Chew foods well and eat slowly
  Drink water with meals
  Elevate head of bed at night
  Explain procedure for gastrostomy feedings (p. 32)
Discuss need to avoid smoking
Explain importance of balancing activity and rest
Discuss need to aavoid constipation with natural laxatives
Demonstrate wound and dressing care
Explain signs of wound infection and fistula formation
Reinforce stress management techniques
Discuss importance of follow-up care with physician

Expected outcome/evaluation

Patient
  Verbalizes understanding of diet and activity regimen
  Demonstrates adequate wound care
  Understands signs of infection to report to physician

ENDOSCOPY: ESOPHAGEAL, GASTRIC, DUODENAL

Insertion of a fiberoptic scope into the esophagus, stomach, or duodenum to determine pathological conditions and/or obtain tissue specimens for diagnostic studies; also used to remove foreign bodies (Figure 5-2)

Preendoscopy Care

Encourage and allow time for verbalization of fears and concerns
Reinforce physician's explanation of procedure
Maintain NPO
Remove dentures and partial plates
Administer oral hygiene
Administer premedications

Postendoscopy Assessment
Observations/findings

Level of consciousness and vital signs
Swallow and gag reflexes present

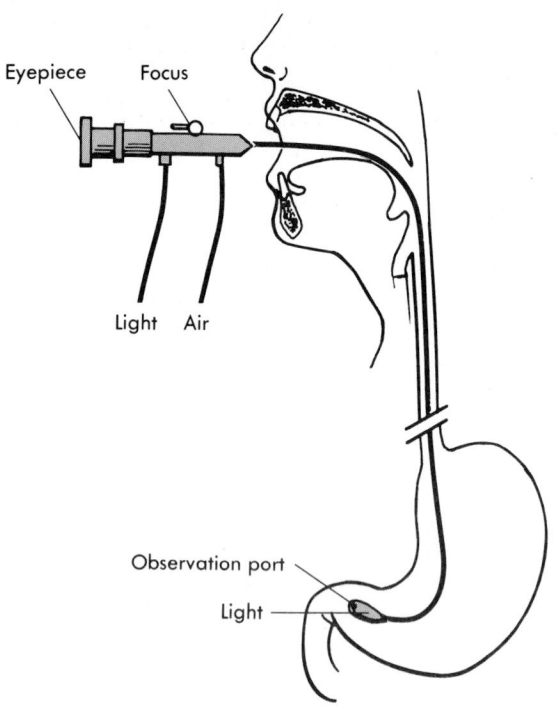

Eyepiece   Focus

Light   Air

Observation port

Light

FIGURE 5-2. Stomach may be visualized by means of a fiber-scope. (From Phipps WJ, Long BC, Woods NF et al: *Medical-surgical nursing and clinical practice,* ed 4, St Louis, 1991, Mosby–Year Book.)

Respiratory rate and depth
Hoarseness
Sore throat

Potential complications

Respiratory distress
Esophageal, gastric, or duodenal perforation
　Dysphagia
　Subcutaneous crepitus in neck
　Extreme pain: increases with respirations or neck or
　　shoulder movement
　Hematemesis

Interventions

Assist and teach patient to turn and deep breathe q2h
Administer warm saline gargles prn
Provide warm liquids until patient is able to swallow with-out discomfort, then diet as tolerated
Administer oral hygiene prn
Explain signs/symptoms to report to physician; increased pain, bleeding, difficulty breathing
Discuss deep-breathing exercises and oral hygiene
Encourage ongoing outpatient care

SENGSTAKEN-BLAKEMORE TUBE OR LINTON TUBE

Sengstaken-Blakemore tube *Nasoesophagogastric tube with three lumens and two pressure balloons: two lu-*

mens are used to inflate the balloons, and the third is for gastric drainage; used to control esophageal hemorrhage (Figure 5-3, A*)*
Linton tube *Three-lumen nasogastric tube for control of gastric hemorrhage: two lumens suction esophageal and gastric contents and the third lumen inflates the gastric balloon (Figure 5-3,* B*)*

Preinsertion Assessment and Care

Assess patient's ability to swallow and mouth breathe; maintain patent airway
Explain purpose of tube and procedure
Observe amount and color of emesis after stomach con-tents have been aspirated
Check tube for patency of each lumen and strength of balloon(s)
　Tube should not be over 1 year old
　Use sphygmomanometer for balloon inflation of Sengs-taken-Blakemore tube
　Use 50 cc syringe for balloon inflation of Linton tube
　Lubricate and chill tube according to instructions

Postinsertion Care
Observations/findings
SENGSTAKEN-BLAKEMORE TUBE

Tube is inserted through nose into stomach
Balloons are inflated to 20 to 40 mm Hg each or as ordered (Figure 5-3, A)
Lumens are securely clamped and labeled from each bal-loon
Gastric suction tube is labeled and attached to intermit-tent suction apparatus
Traction (¼ to 1 lb) is applied to gastric balloon as ordered
Tube is securely taped to nose or traction sponge

LINTON TUBE

Tube is inserted through nose into stomach
Gastric tube and esophageal tube are labeled and con-nected to separate intermittent suction apparatuses
Balloon is inflated with 100 to 200 cc of air or as ordered, and lumen is securely clamped and labeled
Tube is taped to traction sponge and traction applied

Interventions

Maintain prescribed balloon pressure
Release traction, deflate balloon(s) q8h-12h to avoid ne-crosis of tissues
Irrigate only gastric lumen of tubes
Tape tube comfortably, securely to cheek to prevent pres-sure on oral/nasal tissues

Potential complications

Respiratory distress
Aspiration pneumonia
Chest pain
Abdominal distention

Stomach

ANOREXIA NERVOSA/BULIMIA NERVOSA

anorexia nervosa *A disorder characterized by emacia-*
tion occurring as a result of self-inflicted starvation;
etiology appears to be primarily psychological, but it
may include underlying organic factors
bulimia nervosa *An eating disorder characterized by ex-*
cessive overeating and use of laxatives, diuretics, and
self-induced vomiting to purge intestinal tract of food
(binge-purge syndrome)
Usual age: adolescence; predominantly females
Peak ages: 12 to 13 years; 19 to 20 years and into young
adulthood

Assessment
Observations/findings
USUAL FAMILY PROFILE

Middle- to upper-class socioeconomic level
Conservative philosophy, high personal standards
Often dependent, seductive relationship with a warm,
    passive father
Often dependent relationship with dominant, solicitous,
    chronically depressed mother
Family members closely fused
Personal boundaries not respected
Mind reading prevalent
Sense of independence sabotaged
Expressions of anger, anxiety, or aggressiveness blocked
Arguments not allowed
Togetherness prized
Loyalty exaggerated
Excellence as the standard
Anorectic seeks love and approval, becomes perfectionist,
    cannot achieve it, develops physical complaints
Family attention focuses on and reinforces weight loss and
    poor eating

PRODROMAL PERIOD

Increasing irritability
Eczema may develop
Abdominal discomfort
Headaches
Hyperactivity
Depression
Anxiety
Social withdrawal from friends
High level of investment in schoolwork and high-energy
    sports or high-stress employment
Often was previously overweight

ORGANIC SYMPTOMS

Severe weight loss
Secondary amenorrhea
Bradycardia
Lowered body temperature

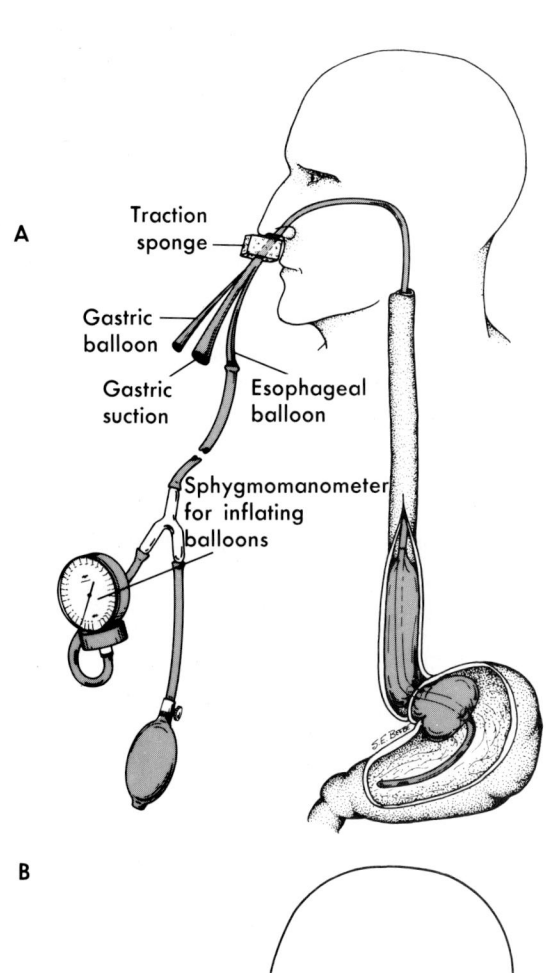
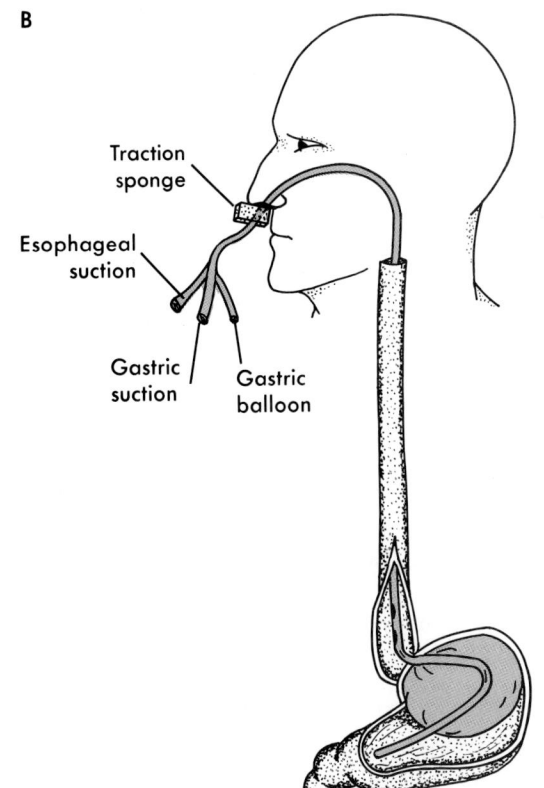

FIGURE 5-3. A, Sengstaken-Blakemore tube. **B,** Linton tube.

Decreased BP
Cold intolerance
Dry skin, poor turgor
Brittle nails
Lanugo hair
Decreased appetite
Feelings of satiety
Breasts atrophied
Axillary and pubic hair reduced
Sleep disturbances
Constipation
Increased susceptibility to infection

AFFECT/BEHAVIOR

Academically, professionally high achiever
Conforming behavior
Conscientious
Increased energy levels
Relentless pursuit of thinness and fear of fatness
Anorexia frequently precipitated by adolescent crisis
History of being overweight
Fear of developing feelings of sexuality
Disturbed body image of delusional proportions
    Defends emaciation as normal
    Feels rewarded by achieving and maintaining emaciated state
    Is fearful of weight gain
    Interprets others' concerns as attempts to make her fat
    Admires emaciated self in mirror
Inaccurate and confused perception and interpretation of inner stimuli
    Does not recognize signs of nutritional need
    Is unable to assess amount of food taken
    Derives pleasure from refusal of food
    Hides food; may secretly flush it down toilet
    May induce vomiting after eating
    May use laxatives to speed passage of food
    Is preoccupied with food and related activities; may plan and prepare meals for others, collect recipes, count calories, etc.
    Increases activity to counteract weight gain
    May conceal weights on body before weighing
    May hoard food, especially candy and nonnutritive foods
Paralyzing sense of ineffectiveness
    Behaves with defiance and rebellion but is overwhelmed by sense of ineffectiveness
    Feels she responds only to demands and wishes of others
    Doubts ability of, or right to, self-assertion

Laboratory/diagnostic studies

CBC with differential: leukopenia, lymphocytosis, anemia
Blood serum studies
    Hypoglycemia, hypocholesteremia, hypoproteinemia, hypokalemia, hyponatremia
        Decreased estrogen levels, elevated BUN

Urine studies: decreased urinary 17-ketosteroids, presence of ketones

Potential complications

Cardiac dysrhythmias

Medical Management

Determination of extent of nutritional deprivation
If severe, nasogastric feedings are ordered if food is refused by patient
Parenteral fluids with electrolytes/hyperalimentation for dehydration or life-threatening malnutrition
Behavior modification therapy
Daily weighing
Reference to psychotherapist with family therapy approach to care

Nursing diagnoses/interventions/evaluation

■ NDX: Altered nutrition: less than body requirements related to anorexia, self-induced vomiting, laxative abuse, and/or distorted perception of body

Allow choice of foods (low-calorie foods not allowed)
Structure mealtimes to a time limit (e.g., 40 min)
Diminish distractions (e.g., conversation, television) during mealtimes
State time to eat, present food, and state time limit; inform patient that if food is not consumed during a set time, alternate feeding methods will be necessary
If food not taken, initiate tube feedings, TPN as ordered in a matter-of-fact, nonpunitive manner; do not allow bargaining
Initiate alternate methods of feeding each time oral food is rejected; be consistent
Withdraw attention during mealtime if patient refuses to eat
Do not allow hoarding of food
Minimize attention paid to eating, or behavior will be reinforced

Behavior modification therapy

Patient obtains or loses privileges based on established desired weight gain per day
    Separation from family for a period is helpful
    Depriving of pleasurable activities
    Restricting nursing intervention to technical nature
    Social isolation
    Utilitarian communication, not supportive
    Rewarding patient only for weight gain
        Time with nurse
        Increased visitor time
        Social activities with other children
        Access to television, radio, stereo, and/or telephone
    Consistency of treatment should be maintained
One staff member per shift should have final word on decisions

Prevent manipulation of staff
   Set and maintain strict limits
   Communicate limits and consequences of exceeding those limits clearly and in nonpunitive manner
   Refer to Manipulative behavior (p. 22)
Obtain accurate weights
   Weigh patient daily before morning meal
   Weigh patient in gown only; prevent concealment of weights on body
   Establish allowable privileges if weight is gained
   Encourage feeling of responsibilty for weight gain

Expected outcome/evaluation

Patient
   Expresses understanding of nutritional needs
   Ingests caloric intake adequate to maintain normal weight
   Resumes normal eating pattern

■ **NDX:** Potential fluid volume deficit (2) related to dieting/purging

Monitor intake and output
   Keep records at nurses' station
   Observe as unobtrusively as possible
Monitor parenteral fluids with electrolytes/TPN as needed; accompany patient to bathroom to prevent emptying of IV fluids
Monitor vital signs as needed

Expected outcome/evaluation

Patient's
   Hydration is maintained adequately
   Intake and output are balanced

■ **NDX:** Disturbance in body image related to inaccurate perception of self as fat: poor self-esteem

Give positive support and praise for things well done
Foster successful experiences
Begin with tasks easily accomplished
Focus on positive traits
Encourage patient to verbalize thoughts
Have patient draw picture of self and discuss perception of self
Encourage good hygiene and grooming for feeling of well-being
Respond factually and consistently to patient's questions concerning diet and nutrition
Encourage and reinforce constructive physical activity, bedmaking, helping other patients

Expected outcome/evaluation

Patient
   Verbalizes positive thoughts of self
   Begins to perceive self as thin

■ **NDX:** Ineffective individual coping related to feelings of loss of control, fear of growing up and/or personalized response to family dysfunction

Encourage ventilation of feelings
Observe and record responses to stress
Encourage coming to staff when stressed
Discourage (withdraw your attention from) rituals or emotional associations with meals, food, etc.
Support patient's attempts at self-determination, especially when with family
Promote stress-reduction techniques
Encourage support of significant others

Expected outcome/evaluation

Patient
   Begins to exhibit positive coping skills
   Maintains weight during stressful periods
   Seeks appropriate support and resources

■ **NDX:** Ineffective family coping related to inability to communicate and inability to meet the needs of all family members

Encourage patient and family to verbalize thoughts, perceptions, and feelings
Point out areas where patient and family members disagree
Determine each family member's perception of what another has said to reinforce listening skills
Emphasize with patient and family members importance of using "I" and taking responsibility for self
With family members present, be patient's advocate and support attempts at self-determination
Redirect control conflicts between patient and parents/significant other away from food and onto issues related to curfews, school activities, job satisfaction, etc.
Refer family for ongoing psychiatric care

Expected outcome/evaluation

Patient
   Begins to recognize needs of others
   Identifies areas where needs and expectations are unmet
   Responds positively to provided support
   Seeks assistance as needed

■ **NDX:** Knowledge deficit related to lack of information about condition and poor coping skills

Reinforce nutritional guidelines and how to manage diet away from home
Discuss with patient the need to reassess caloric requirements q2wk to 4wk
Reinforce use of stress-management techniques
Promote regular exercise program
Encourage follow-up visits with physician, counselor

Expected outcome/evaluation

Patient
   Verbalizes need for changes in lifestyle to maintain normal weight
   Seeks sources of counseling to aid in changes
   Strives to maintain weight

PEPTIC ULCER DISEASE (GASTRIC AND DUODENAL)

gastric ulcer *Ulceration of gastric mucosa caused by a break in the mucosal barrier, allowing backwash of hydrochloric acid; causative factors include medications (aspirin, indomethacin), chemicals (tobacco, alcohol), stress, and heredity*

duodenal ulcer *Ulceration of duodenal mucosa caused by increased amounts of hydrochloric acid in the duodenum; causative factors include heredity, psychosocial stressors, and medications*

Assessment
Observations/findings
GASTRIC ULCER

Left to midepigastric pain; may radiate to back
Pain experienced 60 to 90 min after eating

DUODENAL ULCER

Right epigastric pain; may radiate to back or thorax; pain occurs 2 to 4 hr after eating
Pain may be unrelated to food intake
Pyrosis (heartburn)
Fullness after eating
Eructation
Nausea
Abdominal tenderness

Laboratory/diagnostic studies

Endoscopy with biopsy and cytology
Barium studies
Abdominal radiological studies
Gastric analysis
Hgb, Hct, blood pepsinogen, gastrin levels
Stool for melena

Potential complications

Electrolyte imbalance
Gastric, duodenal hemorrhage
Perforation
Pyloric stenosis
Shock

Medical Management

Analgesics
Aluminum-magnesium antacids: Delcid, Mylanta-II
Cimetidine (Tagamet)
Ranitidine (Zantac)
Sucralfate (Carafate)
Diet

Nursing diagnoses/interventions/evaluation

■ **NDX:**   Altered nutrition: less than body requirements related to discomfort after eating, anorexia

Assess patient's nutritional status: present diet, eating patterns, foods precipitating pain
Assess patient's medication history: aspirin, steroids, vasopressors
Monitor vital signs q4h
Monitor intake and output q8h
Maintain nonstressful environment
Provide diet in small, frequent meals
Monitor effectiveness/side effects of medications

Expected outcome/evaluation

Patient
   Tolerates diet without discomfort
   Maintains balanced intake and output

■ **NDX:**   Pain related to irritation, disruption of gastric mucosa

Assess pain; location, type, frequency, and duration; sudden severe pain may indicate gastric, duodenal perforation
Monitor effectiveness/side effects of analgesics/antacids
Provide diversional activities
Administer back rubs, changes in position
Discuss and teach relaxation techniques

Expected outcome/evaluation

Patient reports reduction in or absence of pain

■ **NDX:**   Knowledge deficit related to lack of information about home care and nutritional status

Discuss relationship of causative agents to peptic ulcer disease
Provide and review written instructions concerning medications, including name, purpose, dosage, time of administration, and side effects; instruct patient to take only antacids prescribed by physician and to avoid aspirin, steroids
Discuss dietary plan: importance of eating meals at regular times, necessity of not missing a meal, and benefits of small frequent meals; avoid coffee, tobacco, and alcohol
Explain signs and symptoms of perforation: extreme epigastric pain and hematemesis
Describe importance of nonstressful environment, especially at mealtime

Discuss methods of stress management: relaxation, exercise, meditation

Encourage follow-up care with physician

Expected outcome/evaluation

Patient
- Expresses understanding of causative relationship between certain foods and discomfort
- Demonstrates knowledge of dietary regimen
- Verbalizes symptoms to report to physician

GASTRIC BLEEDING

Condition in which ulceration of the mucosa has progressed to the vasculature of the stomach or duodenum; may be insidious or acute

Assessment
Observations/findings

Decreased blood pressure
Elevated pulse
Abdominal distention
Nausea, vomiting
Hematemesis
Melena
Hyperperistalsis
Abdominal tenderness, pain
Increased bowel sounds
Dehydration
Chills, fever
Anxiety/fear

Laboratory/diagnostic studies

Endoscopy
GI series
Stools for occult blood
CBC, electrolytes, BUN

Potential complications

Electrolyte imbalance
Gastric perforation
Hemorrhage
Shock

Medical Management

Analgesics
NPO
Nasogastric tube or Linton tube, depending on bleeding site
Parenteral fluids with electrolytes and vitamins
Whole blood or packed red blood cells (PBCs)
CVP line, Swan-Ganz catheter
Urethral catheter
Cimetidine intravenously
Antacids via nasogastric tube

Gastric lavage (norepinephrine bitartrate [Levophed] may be added to produce vasoconstriction)
Endoscopy: endoscope electrocoagulation
Vasopressin arterially
Surgical intervention: repair of resection

Nursing diagnoses/interventions/evaluation

■ **NDX:** Alteration in tissue perfusion: cardiopulmonary, gastrointestinal, and renal, related to hypovolemia

Cardiopulmonary

Auscultate chest for breath sounds q2h to 4h
Maintain bed rest with head elevated 30 degrees
Assess acuteness of bleeding and for signs of hypovolemia and shock
Monitor vital signs q15min to 30min until stable; take apical pulse
Maintain parenteral therapy: electrolytes, volume expanders, whole blood, packed cells
Monitor CVP line or Swan-Ganz line if appropriate

Gastrointestinal

Auscultate abdomen for bowel sounds q4h
Monitor for distention
Measure abdominal girth q4h
Monitor stools for melena
Maintain NPO
Monitor nasogastric tube and intermittent suction apparatus; measure gastric output q4h to 8h
- Irrigate with measured amounts of saline solution
Measure intake and output
Monitor electrolytes, Hgb, and Hct

Renal

Weigh patient daily, same time, scale, and clothes
Maintain indwelling urethral catheter; monitor hourly output; if output less than 50 ml/hr notify physician
Monitor urine pH and specific gravity
Monitor serum BUN, creatinine

Expected outcome/evaluation

Patient's
- Vital signs are normal
- Intake and output are balanced
- Gastric drainage is clear or is clearing

■ **NDX:** Altered nutrition: less than body requirements related to altered diet patterns, anorexia

When bleeding subsides and nasogastric tube is removed, initiate fluids in small amounts as tolerated
- Progress to blended or soft foods in small, frequent meals
- Continue monitoring intake, output, and stools for melena

Administer saline enemas to clear bowel of old blood
Avoid constipation with natural laxatives
Assess effectiveness/side effects of antacids, vitamin K, cimetidine

Expected outcome/evaluation

Patient
Tolerates diet well, and weight is stable
Tolerates medications

■ **NDX:** Pain related to disruption of gastric mucosa

Administer analgesics (e.g., morphine); meperidine is usually avoided because it can cause nausea and vomiting
Assess effectiveness of pain relief measures
Assist and teach patient to turn and deep breathe q2h to 4h
Administer back care and oral hygiene to promote comfort
Discuss and teach alternate pain relief measures
Change patient's position frequently to provide comfort
Keep patient warm and dry
Provide planned rest periods
Ambulate patient with assistance when tolerated to decrease discomfort

Expected outcome/evaluation

Patient
Expresses reduction in or absence of pain
Appears relaxed and comfortable

■ **NDX:** Anxiety related to altered health status

Maintain quiet environment
Explain all procedures and treatments
Encourage and allow time for verbalization of concerns
Assess level of anxiety/fear and current coping styles
Discuss alternative coping behaviors and stress management techniques
Encourage communication with significant other(s)

Expected outcome/evaluation

Patient
Demonstrates positive coping behaviors
Expresses a reduction in anxiety
Uses stress management techniques appropriately

■ **NDX:** Knowledge deficit related to lack of information on home care

Discuss nutritional plan, stressing importance of
Small, frequent meals at regular intervals
Chewing food well and eating slowly
Avoiding caffeine, alcohol, tobacco, and aspirin
Reinforce physician's explanation of relationship of causative factors to disease process

Reinforce stress management techniques
Provide medication instructions: name, dose, purpose, time of administration, and side effects; instruct patient to take only antacids prescribed by physician
Explain signs and symptoms of further bleeding: hematemesis, abdominal distention, tarry stools, fainting, dyspnea
Discuss importance of balancing exercise and rest periods
Encourage follow-up visits with physician

Expected outcome/evaluation

Patient
Verbalizes understanding of needed diet, medication regimen
Seeks information regarding stress management; uses it appropriately
Expresses knowledge of symptoms to report to physician

GASTRIC SURGERY

Surgery performed for medical emergencies such as gastric hemorrhage, perforation, obstruction, and carcinomas, or for ulcers that have not responded to medical management

Preoperative Assessment and Care

Assess respiratory status
Discuss and explain pain management
Reinforce physician's explanation of procedure
Teach patient to turn, deep breathe; methods of incisional splinting
Discuss placement of tubes, drains that may be present postoperatively
Insert nasogastric tube as ordered
Allow time for verbalization of concerns

Postoperative Assessment
Observations/findings

Splinting with respirations
Decreased breath sounds
Tachypnea
Bradypnea
Character and amount of gastric drainage
Nausea, vomiting
Urinary output
Abdominal distention

Laboratory/diagnostic studies

Hgb, Hct, electrolytes

Potential complications

Dehydration, anemia
Electrolyte imbalance
Atelectasis
Hemorrhage

Shock
Thrombophlebitis (p. 70)
Dumping syndrome (p. 256)
Paralytic ileus (p. 271)
Wound evisceration, infection
Postprandial hypoglycemia
Gastrojejunocolic fistula

Medical Management

NPO until bowel sounds return
Parenteral fluids with electrolytes until diet is allowed
Nasogastric suction
Analgesics
Antiembolic stockings
Diet and activity

Nursing diagnoses / interventions / evaluation

 NDX: Potential fluid volume deficit related to the risk
of hemorrhage; altered intake and nasogastric
tube suction

Maintain NPO; assess hydration status
   Maintain nasogastric tube to intermittent suction
      apparatus
   Monitor color and amount of gastric output q4h
   Do not reposition tube
   Maintain patency of tube by irrigation with measured
      amounts of saline *only* if ordered
   Note that after gastrectomy, drainage will be minimal
   Report excessive bleeding to physician
Monitor electrolytes, Hgb, and Hct
Maintain parenteral fluids with electrolytes
Measure intake and output
Weigh daily; same time, clothes, scale

Expected outcome / evaluation

Patient's
   Intake and output are balanced
   Hydration is adequately maintained

■ **NDX:**   Altered nutrition: less than body requirements
related to inability to ingest food after surgery

Auscultate bowel sounds and passage of flatus q8h
When bowel sounds return, administer small amounts of
   water via nasogastric tube as ordered
   Aspirate stomach 2 hr after last feeding of the day;
      contents should be < 100 ml, and no pain, disten-
      tion, or nausea should be present
   Report to physician if amount is > 100 ml and/or the
      above symptoms occur
Initiate oral fluids when nasogastric tube is removed
   Offer 5 to 10 ml of warm water qh as ordered
   Increase amounts until 90 to 120 ml is tolerated qh

Progress to small, frequent meals of soft foods; avoid milk
   since it may cause dumping syndrome
Discontinue feedings if pain, nausea, distention, or vomiting occur and notify physician
Continue measuring intake

Expected outcome / evaluation

Patient
   Tolerates increasing diet without discomfort
   Ingests adequate calories to maintain normal weight

■ **NDX:**   Ineffective breathing pattern related to location
of surgical incision

Assess respirations, observing for signs of distress
Maintain bed rest with head elevated 30 degrees to facil-
   itate breathing
Auscultate chest for breath sounds q4h
Assist and teach patient to turn, cough, and deep breathe
   q2h to 4h; provide support to incision
Administer incentive spirometer q4h
Provide pain medication before deep breathing exercises
   to reduce discomfort

Expected outcome / evaluation

Patient
   Demonstrates breathing techniques accurately
   Exhibits normal respirations

■ **NDX:**   Alteration in tissue perfusion: peripheral, cardiopulmonary, renal, related to hypovolemia

Peripheral

Check extremities for temperature, color, and sensation
Monitor pedal pulses q4h
Do not gatch knees
Apply antiembolic stockings
Encourage ROM leg exercises qh to promote venous return

Cardiopulmonary

Monitor vital signs q4h
Auscultate chest for breath sounds q4h
Monitor CVP/Swan-Ganz readings qh and prn
Monitor arterial blood gases

Renal

Measure intake and output qh; if output less than 30 ml/
   hr report to physician
Monitor urine specific gravity and serum BUN, creatinine

Expected outcome / evaluation

Patient's
   Vital signs are normal
   Urine output is adequate and balances with intake
   Laboratory values are within normal limits

■ NDX: Potential for infection related to surgical incision, inadequate primary defenses

Monitor dressings and incision for drainage and bleeding q4h
Change dressings prn and observe healing process
Observe for signs of wound infection; redness, drainage, pain, odor

Expected outcome/evaluation

Patient's
Incision is clean, dry, and intact
Wound is healing adequately

■ NDX: Pain related to surgical intervention

Assess location, type, and intensity of pain
Assess effectiveness of analgesics
Change position often and support with pillows to decrease discomfort
Administer skin care and back rubs q4h to promote comfort
Maintain quiet environment
Schedule rest periods between treatments
Discuss alternate pain relief measures

Expected outcome/evaluation

Patient
Reports a tolerable level of pain/discomfort
Appears more relaxed

■ NDX: Anxiety related to change in health status

Explain all procedures and treatments
Reinforce physician's explanation of surgical procedure and treatment
Encourage and allow time for verbalization of feelings
Assess present coping behaviors and support positive responses
Teach stress management techniques
Encourage communication with significant others

Expected outcome/evaluation

Patient
Expresses and identifies anxieties
Uses stress management techniques appropriately

■ NDX: Knowledge deficit related to lack of information about home care needs and follow-up instructions

Discuss and explain dietary plan and restrictions according to type of surgery performed
Eat small, frequent meals at regular intervals; avoid high-fiber foods, sugar, salt, caffeine, alcohol, milk, and tobacco

Take fluids between meals, not with meals
Eat slowly and chew foods well
Measure weight q2d to 4d
Provide instructions and demonstrate wound care; identify signs of wound infection
Reinforce importance of avoiding stressful situations, especially at mealtimes
Reinforce stress management techniques
Explain symptoms of dumping syndrome: epigastric pain, weakness, nausea, vomiting after eating
Discuss medications: name, dosage, time of administration, purpose, and side effects; instruct patient to avoid over-the-counter medications, especially those containing aspirin
Discuss importance of adequate rest and exercise with planned rest periods
Explain use of natural laxatives to avoid constipation
Encourage follow-up care with physician

Expected outcome/evaluation

Patient
Expresses understanding of needed dietary and medication regimen
Demonstrates ability to care for incision
Seeks out and uses stress management methods
Verbalizes understanding of symptoms to report to physician

DUMPING SYNDROME

Postgastrectomy syndrome caused by loss of the pyloric valve, allowing food and fluid to pass too rapidly into the small bowel; appears 1 to 3 weeks after surgery

Assessment
Observations/findings

Time of onset of symptoms: usually around mealtime
Epigastric fullness
Nausea, vomiting
Abdominal distention
Malaise
Profuse diaphoresis
Palpitations
Vertigo
Tachypnea
Decreased BP
Increased bowel sounds
Urge to defecate

Potential complications

Syndrome becomes chronic
ECG changes

Medical Management

Diet
Anticholinergics, pectin powder
Surgery to alter dumping rate

Nursing diagnoses/interventions/evaluation

■ **NDX:**   Potential altered nutrition: less than body requirements related to inability to absorb nutrients

Collaborate with physician and dietitian about diet
    Provide six small meals a day
    Do not give liquids with meals
    Provide dry foods such as toast, crackers, and cereals
    Provide diet low in carbohydrates and salt, moderate in fat, and high in protein
    Include foods containing pectin: citrus fruits, yellow vegetables, bananas, apples, apricots, cherries, beans
    Avoid extreme temperatures in foods
Administer pectin powder; thoroughly mix with water, since patient may experience a sense of oral dryness if mixture is not liquid enough
Provide liquids only between meals
Administer anticholinergics 30 min before meals; assess for effectiveness
Measure intake and output q8h
Position patient in recumbent position after meals to allow foods to pass more slowly into intestine

Expected outcome/evaluation

Patient
    Tolerates diet without experiencing discomfort, distention, or nausea
    Maintains weight and adequate nutritional status

■ **NDX:**   Knowledge deficit related to lack of information about disease process and management

Discuss importance of dietary plan, stressing small, frequent meals, foods to avoid, and foods to eat

Explain that syndrome is usually only temporary but its continuance needs to be reported to physician after 2 to 3 weeks
Instruct patient to lie down after meals and to avoid stressful situations, especially at mealtimes
Reinforce stress management techniques
Encourage follow-up visits with physician

Expected outcome/evaluation

Patient
    Verbalizes understanding of needed dietary regimen
    Expresses understanding of prescribed activities
    Demonstrates ability to manage stress with learned coping skills

SURGICAL INTERVENTION FOR OBESITY

Insertion of two rows of staples across upper one tenth of the stomach to reduce capacity and ensure early satiety; performed for patients highly motivated to lose weight and where medical management of obesity has been unsuccessful; three types of surgery are performed:
gastric bypass Anastomosis of jejunum to upper one tenth of the stomach, bypassing the remaining stomach (Figure 5-4, A)
gastroplasty/partitioning Small opening left in rows of staples, allowing small amounts of food to pass into stomach (Figure 5-4, B)
jejunoileal bypass End-to-end or end-to-side anastomasis of 10 to 14 inches of jejunum to terminal ileum; distal end of ileum is closed, and proximal end is either anastamosed to transverse colon (Figure 5-4, C), or to shortened jejunum (Figure 5-4, D)

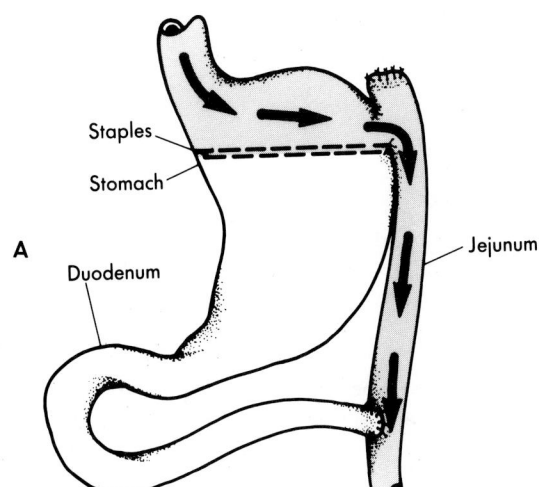

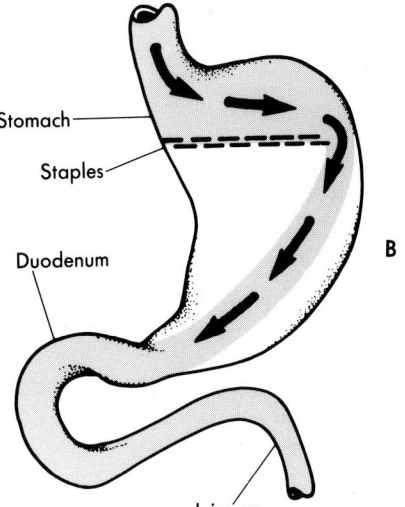

FIGURE 5-4. A, Gastric bypass. **B,** Gastroplasty/partitioning.

Continued.

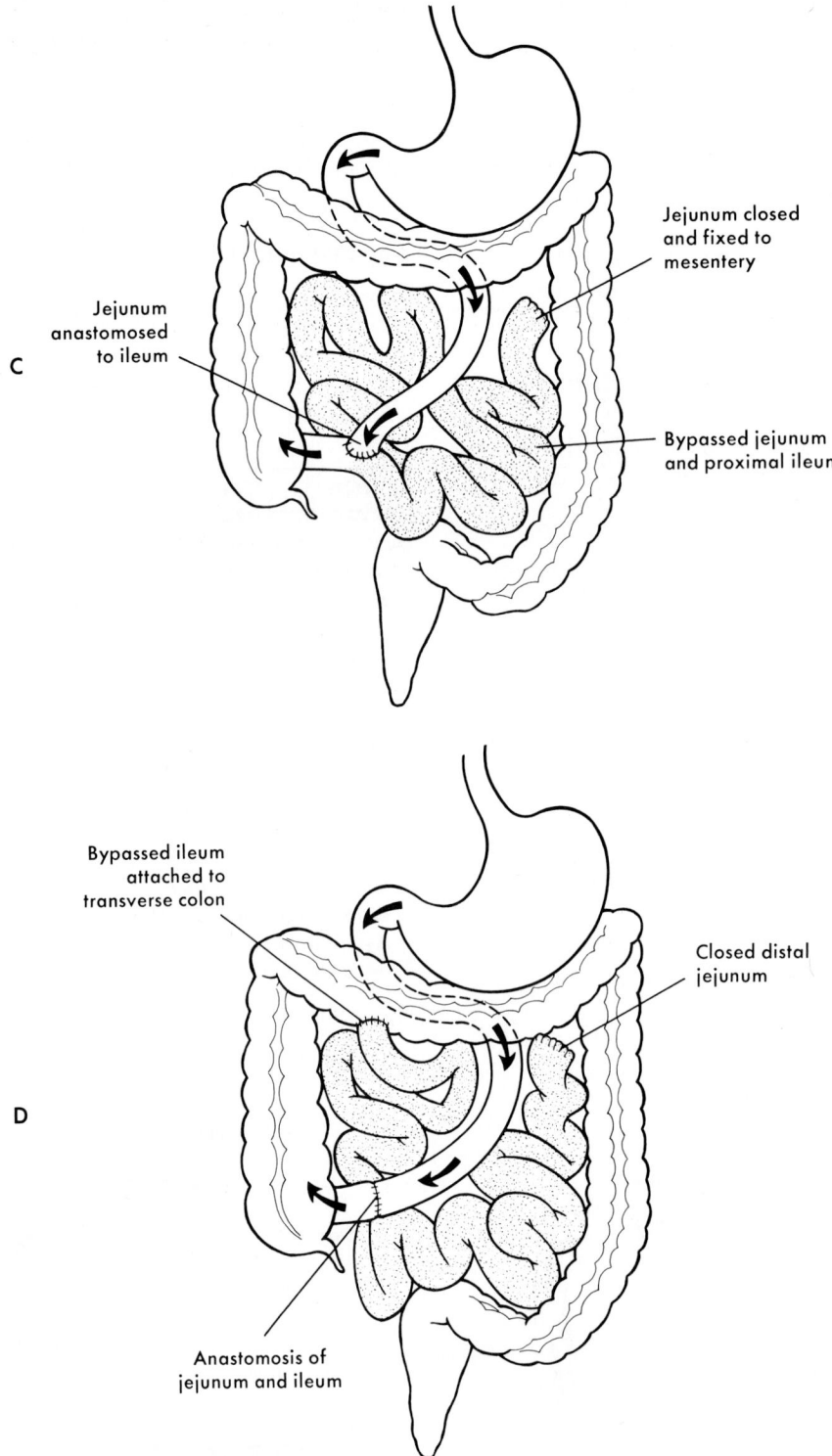

Jejunum closed
and fixed to
mesentery

Jejunum
anastomosed
to ileum

C

Bypassed jejunum
and proximal ileum

Bypassed ileum
attached to
transverse colon

Closed distal
jejunum

D

Anastomosis of
jejunum and ileum

FIGURE 5-4, cont'd. C, End-to-end jejunoileal anastomosis (type 1). **D,** End-to-end jejunoileal anastomosis (type 2). (**C** and **D** from Given BA, Simmons SJ: *Gastroenterology in clinical nursing,* ed 4, St Louis, 1984, CV Mosby.)

Preoperative Care
Assessment
Observations/findings

Nutritional history
  Previous eating patterns and types of foods eaten
  Present weight greater than 100 lb over ideal body
    weight
Medical history
  Absence of renal, cardiac, bowel, or liver disease
  No history of hypertension, diabetes, or arthritis
  No signs of upper respiratory infection (URI) or anemia
Psychological adjustment to procedure
  Motivation to lose weight
  Weight loss minimal or absent after many attempts
  Presence of positive coping behaviors

Laboratory/diagnostic studies

Renal and liver function studies
Abdominal and chest radiologic studies
Upper GI series
Cholecystogram
Intravenous pyelogram
Barium enema
Pulmonary function test
Serum glucose, insulin, cholesterol, triglycerides, creatinine, protein, iron, CBC, urinalysis
Baseline arterial blood gases

Medical Management

Preoperative medication
Parenteral fluids with heparin
Nasogastric tube and indwelling urethral catheter

Nursing diagnoses/interventions/evaluation

■ **NDX:** Anxiety related to hospitalization, procedures, surgery, and altered health status

Attempt to maintain nonstressful environment
Discuss stress management techniques
Orient patient to surroundings and provide comfortable armless chair
Encourage and allow time for verbalization of concerns
Assess coping skills and promote positive successful past behaviors
Reinforce physician's explanation of preoperative and postoperative care and surgical procedure
Perform activities in an unhurried manner, explaining each as it occurs
Encourage verbalization with significant other

Expected outcome/evaluation

Patient
  Expresses anxieties/concerns
  Exhibits positive coping skills

■ **NDX:** Knowledge deficit related to lack of information about preoperative and postoperative care

Discuss with patient and teach
  Use of trapeze bar and how to get in and out of bed
  Method for turning, coughing, and deep breathing with incisional support
  Use of inspiratory spirometer and diaphragmatic breathing procedure
  Procedure for sipping from a cup, 30 ml in 5 min
  Active ROM exercises, especially legs and feet
Explain that early ambulation (2 to 4 hr after surgery) will be required and trapeze bars will be in place
Explain that preoperatively a nasogastric tube and indwelling urethral catheter will be inserted
Discuss postoperative dietary management; small sips of water increasing to 30 to 60 ml as tolerated
Explain that IV line will be in place preoperatively and an anticoagulant will be administered
Discuss bowel preparation for jejunoileal bypass surgery

Postoperative Care
Assessment
Observations/findings

Location and character of pain
Splinting with respirations
Decreased breath sounds
Hypoventilation
Tachypnea
Character, color, and amount of
  Gastric drainage
  Urine output
  Wound drainage
Placement and patency of nasogastric tube
Pressure delivered by suction machine
Nausea, vomiting
Abdominal distention

Laboratory/diagnostic studies

Hgb, Hct, electrolytes
Chest radiological study

Potential complications

Dehydration
Electrolyte imbalance
Thrombophlebitis (p. 70)
Atelectasis
Anastomotic leak
  Tachycardia
  Referred abdominal pain to left shoulder
Peritonitis (p. 267)
Hemorrhage
Shock
Wound infection
Liver dysfunction, malabsorption syndrome (jejunoileal bypass)

Medical Management

Analgesics, heparin, antidiarrheals
Ambulation q2h to 3h
Parenteral fluids with electrolytes
Nasogastric tube to intermittent suction; irrigation schedule
Indwelling urethral catheter to gravity drainage
Incentive spirometer
Arterial blood gases, pulse oximetry
Diet, activity, rest
Antiembolic stockings

Nursing diagnoses/interventions/evaluation

■ **NDX:** Ineffective breathing pattern related to surgical incision, decreased lung expansion, anxiety, fatigue

Maintain bed rest with head elevated 30 degrees
Monitor respirations q1h to 2h; observe for shallow breathing, splinting, hypoventilation, and respiratory distress
Auscultate chest for breath sounds q2h
Provide incentive spirometer q2h
Place pads on side rails and encourage patient to use as arm rests (aids in lung expansion)
Encourage diaphragmatic breathing
Assist patient to turn, cough, and deep breathe q2h; support incision
Avoid abdominal binders

Expected outcome/evaluation

Patient
   Exhibits normal respirations
   Performs deep breathing exercises accurately

■ **NDX:** Potential alteration in tissue perfusion: cardiopulmonary, renal, and peripheral related to interruption of blood flow

Cardiopulmonary

Monitor vital signs q4h; take rectal temperatures while nasogastric tube in place
Monitor arterial blood gases, CVP or Swan-Ganz catheter, and pulse oximetry
Monitor Hgb and Hct
Assess heart/breath sounds

Peripheral

Monitor pedal pulses q2h, assess color, temperature of feet
Avoid elevating knee gatch
Check calves of legs for pain on dorsiflexion
Avoid sitting with legs in dependent or crossed position
Remove antiembolic stockings daily and inspect skin for pressure areas
Encourage leg and foot movement
Ambulate with assistance

Renal

Maintain indwelling urethral catheter to closed gravity drainage system
Monitor hourly urine output; if less than 30 to 50 ml/hr, notify physician
Measure intake and output

Expected outcome/evaluation

Patient's
   Vital signs are stable
   Urine output is normal
   Lower extremities are warm and of normal color

■ **NDX:** Potential fluid volume deficit related to gastric suction and/or electrolyte loss

Maintain NPO; assess for signs of dehydration
Monitor parenteral fluids with electrolytes
Monitor serum electrolytes, magnesium, and calcium
Measure intake and output
Maintain nasogastric tube to intermittent suction apparatus
   Note color, consistency, and amount of drainage
   Label tube: *"Do not reposition"*
   Mark tube where it enters nose and avoid placing tension on tube
Irrigate gently with 20 to 30 ml of normal saline q2h to 4h
Auscultate abdomen for bowel sounds q4h
Weigh patient daily at same time with same clothing and scale

Expected outcome/evaluation

Patient's
   Gastric output is minimal
   Electroytes are within normal limits
   Fluid volume is adequate for height and weight as evidenced by balanced intake and output

■ **NDX:** Potential for infection related to invasive surgical procedure and inadequate primary defenses

Observe incision and dressings q2h to 4h; reinforce or change dressings prn
Monitor incision for signs of wound infection
Maintain dressings securely; avoid taping too tightly
Keep skin clean and dry
Monitor temperature q4h

Expected outcome/evaluation

Patient
   Exhibits clean, dry, and intact incision
   Presents normal temperature
   Exhibits no evidence of inflammation at or near the incision site

■ **NDX:** Pain related to surgical intervention

Assess location, intensity, and character of pain
Administer analgesics and assess effectiveness of relief measure(s)
Assess patency of nasogastric tube since obstruction of tube may cause pain
Medicate 20 to 30 min before procedures when possible
Monitor type of pain closely and observe for abdominal distention, tenderness, and fever
Change position slightly at frequent intervals to alleviate discomfort
Encourage alternate pain management measures

Expected outcome/evaluation

Patient
   Express tolerable level of pain
   Appears more relaxed

■ **NDX:** Altered nutrition: less than body requirements related to decreased size of stomach

Remove nasogastric tube, usually third to fourth day postoperatively
Provide 1 oz medication cup and assist patient with sipping 30 ml of water per hour (adequate hydration demands almost constant fluid intake)
Collaborate with dietitian regarding caloric intake and calorie counting
Progress to clear liquids, using 1 oz cup, until soft, high-protein, low-fat diet is tolerated
Assess tolerance of foods, fluids as they are introduced
Instruct patient to heed feeling of satiety to avoid nausea or vomiting

Expected outcome/evaluation

Patient
   Tolerates frequent feedings adequately
   Maintains desired weight loss

■ **NDX:** Diarrhea related to induced malabsorption

Provide diet high in bulk with moderate fluid intake
Observe for signs of dumping syndrome (p. 256)
Provide perianal care after bowel movement; apply protective ointments as needed
Observe frequency, color, amount, and consistency of stools
Administer antidiarrheals

Expected outcome/evaluation

Patient
   Expresses understanding of rationale for diet regimen
   Verbalizes factors causing diarrhea

Has bowel elimination that is returning to normal

■ **NDX:** Potential impaired tissue integrity related to obesity, fluid deficit

Monitor incision for healing, drainage
Administer frequent skin care, especially in folds or on pressure points
Provide special air/foam mattress as indicated
Promote frequent position changes to increase comfort; support incision
Administer frequent skin care, especially in folds and on pressure points
Provide special air/foam mattress as indicated
Promote frequent changes of position; support incision

Expected outcome/evaluation

Patient's
   Incision is healing and surrounding skin is clean, dry, and intact
   Skin integrity is maintained without evidence of any stage of dermal ulcer

■ **NDX:** Knowledge deficit related to lack of information about home care needs

Discuss importance of following eating regimen
   Eat and drink slowly and chew foods well
   Always sit up while eating or drinking
   Do not overeat: stomach will expand and void surgical procedure
   Eat small amounts of all food and heed satiety feeling
   Avoid drinking 30 min before and after meals
   Eat with family, significant other
   Use small plate and glass to make portions appear larger
   Do not snack between meals
   Avoid carbonated beverages
   Eat only two meals a day or as prescribed by physician
Explain importance of diet management
   Refer to nutritionist as indicated
   Have patient avoid high-calorie, high-carbohydrate foods and drinks
Maintain well-balanced, high-protein diet, 300 to 500 calories/day or as prescribed
Be accurate in measuring all food allowances
Use 30 ml medication cup or 1½ tablespoon measuring scoop
Maintain 1500 ml/day fluid intake
Add new foods to diet one at a time; intolerances can occur, especially with meat and chicken
   Discuss methods of processing foods with blender for gastroplasty patients
   Discuss availability of high-protein liquid supplements
Measure urine output daily
Keep accurate record of daily intake
Take chewable multivitamin daily

Weigh weekly because weight loss will be more noticeable
Instruct patient regarding rest and exercise
    Avoid heavy lifting and strenuous exercise
    Walk daily with goal of 1 to 2 miles/day within 4 weeks
    Maintain planned rest periods
Demonstrate incisional and perianal care
Explain symptoms to report to physician
    Elevated temperature
    Wound drainage
    Persistent nausea and/or vomiting
    Hematemesis
    Abdominal tenderness and/or pain
    Abdominal distention
    Urine output of less than 750 ml/day for 3 consecutive days
    Constipation or continuing diarrhea
Reinforce stress management techniques
Explain importance of not taking over-the counter medications without first consulting physician
Encourage follow-up visits with physician, nutritionist, including laboratory testing as ordered

Expected outcome/evaluation

Patient
    Verbalizes understanding of dietary regimen
    Expresses understanding of potential complications
    Seeks and uses stress management methods
    Demonstrates desire to initiate needed lifestyle changes

NASOGASTRIC TUBES

nasogastric tube *A tube that is used for gastric decompression, such as Levine or Salem sump (Figure 5-5), or for administration of food, fluid, or medication; a Levine tube must always be connected to intermittent suction; a Salem sump tube is usually connected to low, continuous suction (since it is air vented) but can also be connected to intermittent suction*

Preinsertion Assessment and Care

Assess patient's ability to swallow and mouth breathe
Assess nasal patency; observe for deviated septum, fracture
Check tube for patency

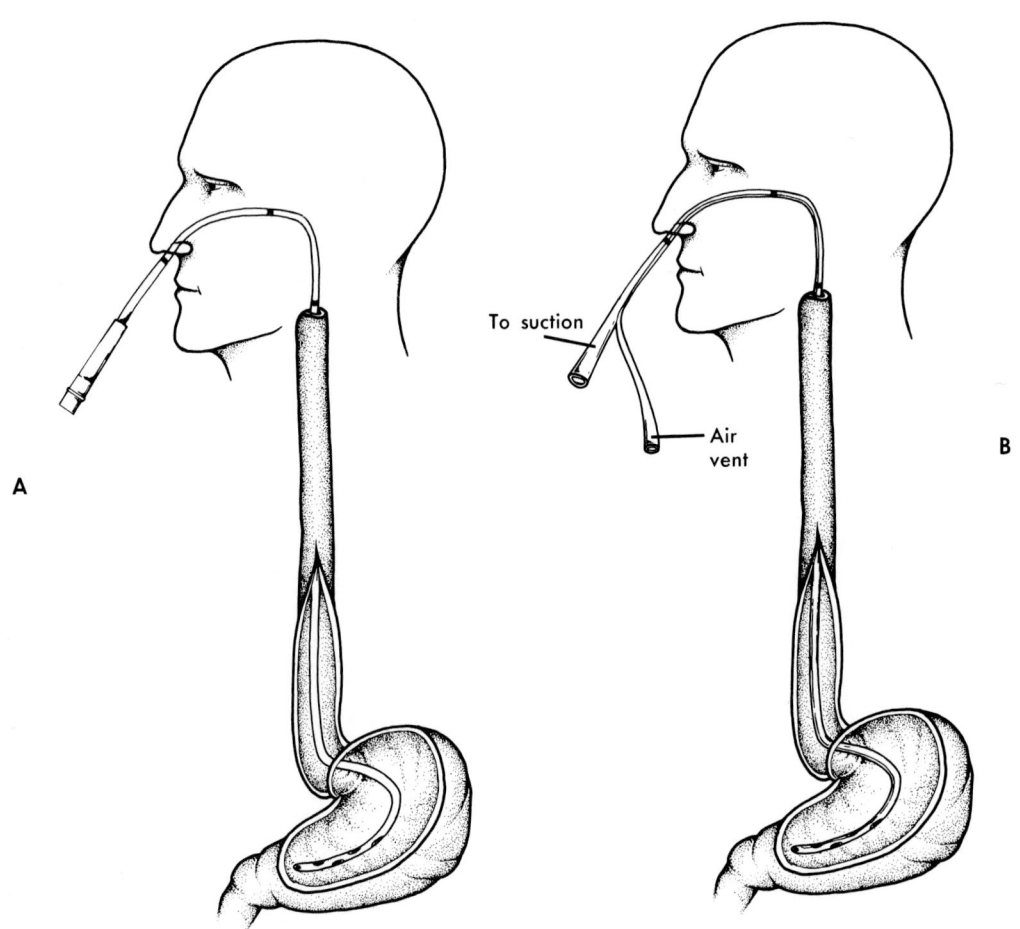

To suction

Air vent

A

B

FIGURE 5-5. A, Levine tube. **B,** Salem sump tube.

Lubricate and chill tube according to instructions
Explain purpose of tube and procedure

Postinsertion Assessment
Observations/findings

Character and consistency of gastric output
Patency of tube
Patency of sump if Salem tube is used
Placement for optimal drainage
Tube taped securely and comfortably to nose
Amount of pressure of suction apparatus
Nasal irritation

Potential complications

Dehydration
Electrolyte imbalance
Aspiration pneumonia

Interventions

Elevate head of bed 40 to 60 degrees
Maintain NPO
Monitor character, amount, and consistency of gastric contents q4h; monitor gastric pH; if pH is less than 3.5, notify physician
Auscultate stomach for placement of tube prn
Connect tube to low, intermittent suction apparatus as ordered; irrigate with measured amounts of normal saline solution as ordered
Salem sump tube
  Maintain patency of sump (air vent): keep opening higher than gastric tube and do not plug
  Sump tube may be irrigated, but instill 20 to 30 cc of air after irrigation to maintain patency
Avoid dislodgment: tape securely to nose and allow enough tube for freedom of movement
Apply lip balm or lubricant to nares and mouth prn
Check tape holding tube prn; observe for reddened area

ESOPHAGOSTOMY, GASTROSTOMY, DUODENOSTOMY-JEJUNOSTOMY MANAGEMENT

esophagostomy *A surgically constructed stoma used to drain saliva and other secretions in patients with esophageal carcinoma, stricture, dysphagia, or atresia; may be used to administer tube feedings for these conditions; this procedure is similar to gastrostomy except a longer catheter is used; the stoma may be permanent or temporary (Figure 5-6)*
gastrostomy *A surgically constructed stoma or opening for a catheter in patients with esophageal carcinoma, stricture, trauma, atresia, and dysphagia; used for tube feedings or decompression and drainage; the ostomy is usually permanent, whereas the catheter is either temporary or permanent (see Figure 5-6)*
duodenostomy-jejunostomy *Surgical incision for placement of a catheter for the feedings or decompression*

and drainage in patients when oral intake is prohibited or after gastrointestinal-esophageal surgery; may be permanent or temporary (see Figure 5-6)

Assessment
Observations/findings

Type and patency of stoma or catheter
Placement of dressing or stoma appliances
Length of catheter from incision to distal end
Taping of catheter
Pressure delivered by low, intermittent suction apparatus
Placement of closed gravity drainage system, clamp, or other collecting device
Character, color, and amount of drainage
Skin integrity around catheter or stoma
Condition of lips and mouth
Weight
Urinary output and specific gravity
Abdominal distention
Diminished bowel sounds
Character and color of stool

Potential complications

Dehydration
Nausea, vomiting
Electrolyte imbalance
Aspiration pneumonia
Wound infection
Hemorrhage/shock

Interventions

Measure intake and output q8h
For catheters
  Check color and consistency of drainage q4h; measure amount q8h
  Maintain catheter to suction apparatus or gravity drainage
  Measure length of catheter q8h
  Tape securely to abdomen or neck; allow sufficient tubing for freedom of movement
For ostomy
  Monitor dressings and observe for drainage, color, and consistency
  Place stoma appliance over ostomy
When bowel sounds return or drainage is less than 300 to 500 ml/24 hr
  Clamp catheter or cover ostomy
  Instruct patient in signs of retention and bowel obstruction
    Nausea
    Abdominal distention
    Abdominal pain
  If these symptoms occur, notify physician immediately, unclamp catheter, and connect to gravity drainage system
Initiate tube feedings as indicated (p. 32)

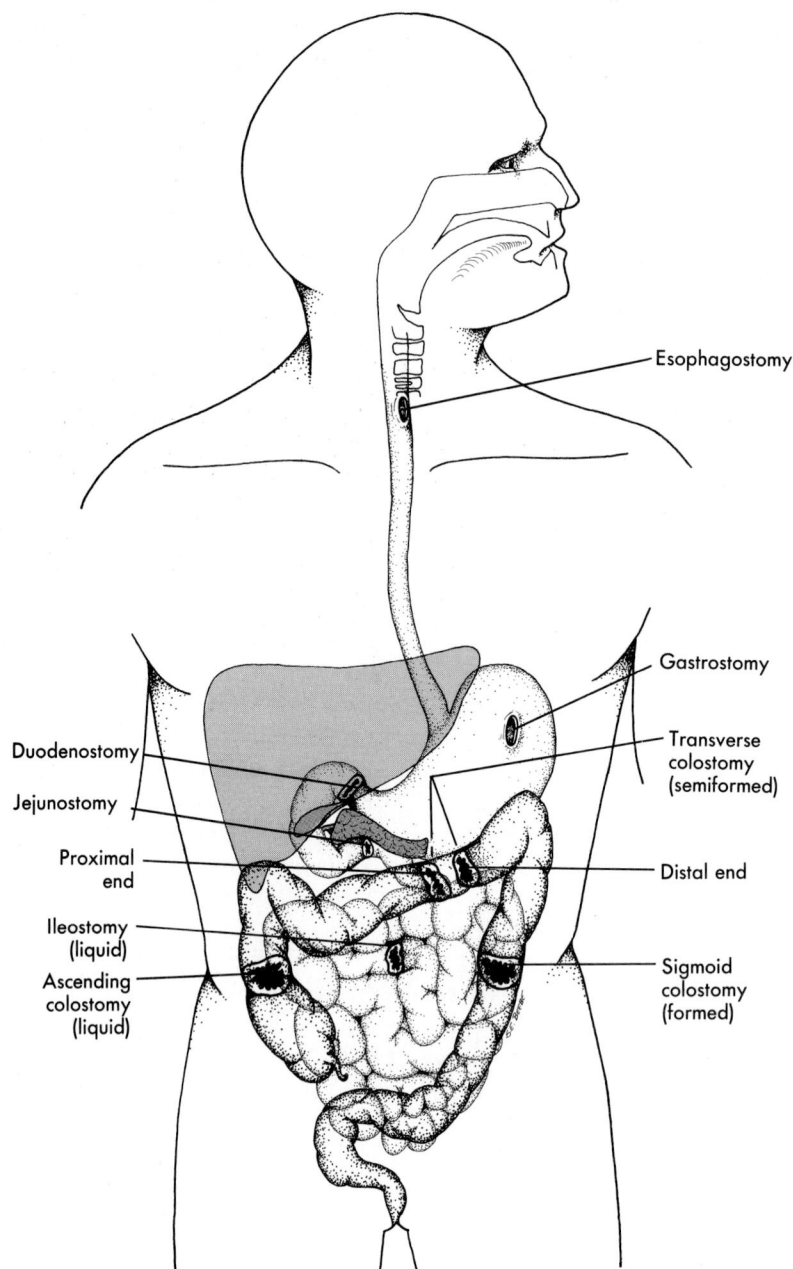

FIGURE 5-6. Types of ostomies and viscosity of fecal material from ileostomy and large intestine ostomies.

Provide skin care around surgical site q4h to 8h
 Wash area gently with soap and water
 Rinse and pat dry
 Apply skin barrier as needed (p. 283)
 Reapply dressings and appliance prn
Discuss with and demonstrate to patient and significant other procedure of tube feeding and tube feeding preparation, as well as amount and times of feeding (p. 32)
Discuss and demonstrate ostomy care (p. 283) and skin care around the tube sites

Demonstrate dressing change procedure
Explain importance of weighing q2d to 3d
Provide information on symptoms of bowel obstruction and wound infection
Demonstrate medication preparation via tube feeding; discuss name, dose, purpose, time of administration, and side effects
Encourage follow-up appointments with physician

Intestine

INFLAMMATORY BOWEL DISEASE: REGIONAL ENTERITIS (CROHN'S DISEASE) AND ULCERATIVE COLITIS

regional enteritis Chronic, recurrent nonspecific inflammation of the entire intestine, usually the terminal ileum, involving the mucosa and surrounding musculature and leading to deep fissure formation

ulcerative colitis Inflammatory intestinal disease of unknown cause, usually affecting the mucosal lining of the colon; may be mild, chronic, or acute

Assessment
Observations/findings

Regional enteritis: cramplike abdominal pain; often in right lower quadrant with frequent diarrhea containing melena and/or steatorrhea

Ulcerative colitis: colicky abdominal cramps; pain is usually minimal; diarrheal stools are frequent and contain mucus, melena, and pus

Anorexia

Weight loss

Fever

Nausea, vomiting

Generalized malaise

Increased peristalsis

Emotional instability

Laboratory/diagnostic studies

Barium studies of intestine

Sigmoidoscopy, colonoscopy

Biopsy

Radiological study of abdomen

Serum iron, decreased

Serum electrolytes, decreased potassium

Albumin, decreased

Liver function tests

Hematologic studies, anemia, leukocytosis

Stools for melena

Potential complications

Electrolyte imbalance

Dehydration, malnutrition, anemia

Intestinal obstruction, perforation

Hemorrhage, shock

Fistula, peritonitis

Perianal abscess, fistula, fissure

Depression

Medical Management

Anticholinergics

Immunosuppressants

Psyllium

Corticosteroids

Antibiotics

Antidiarrheals

Sedatives, analgesics

Parenteral fluids, elemental diet, TPN (depending on severity of disease)

Nasogastric suction; NPO

Sitz bath

Activity, rest, diet

Surgical interventions: ileostomy, colostomy, resection

Nursing diagnoses/interventions/evaluation

■ **NDX:** Potential fluid volume deficit related to abnormal fluid loss (diarrhea)

Maintain NPO; assess hydration status

Maintain parenteral fluids with electrolytes and vitamins

Monitor for signs of circulatory overload

Measure intake and output q8h

Monitor electrolytes

Weigh patient daily at same time with same clothing and scale

Monitor vital signs q4h; avoid rectal temperature

Expected outcome/evaluation

Patient's

Vital signs are stable

Hydration is adequate as evidenced by normal skin turgor and moist mucous membranes

Intake and output are balanced

■ **NDX:** Diarrhea, related to inflammation of bowel

Maintain bed rest

Assess and monitor stools for amount, frequency, consistency, and color

Monitor stools for occult blood

Auscultate abdomen for bowel sounds q8h

Measure abdominal girth q8h

Monitor effectiveness and side effects of antidiarrheal, antibiotic, and steroid therapy

Balance rest with activity

Provide odor-free environment; keep covered bedpan within easy reach; empty, clean, and return promptly

Monitor for signs of bowel perforation; fever, tachycardia, lethargy, pain

Expected outcome/evaluation

Patient

Expresses reduction in frequency of stools

States stool returning to normal consistency

■ **NDX:** Altered nutrition: less than body requirements related to diarrhea and altered absorption

Assess nutritional status and assist patient with identifying irritating foods

Provide diet high in calories, protein, and minerals; low in residue, fat, and fiber
   Prepared elemental diets are available
   TPN as indicated
   Six small meals are beneficial
Encourage patient to participate in meal planning
Maintain intake record and avoid foods that cause cramping, diarrhea
Encourage patient to eat slowly, chew well, and take small bites
Serve food attractively in a well-ventilated room
Monitor Hgb and Hct

Expected outcome/evaluation

Patient
   Maintains normal weight
   Presents laboratory values that are within normal limits

■ **NDX:** Potential impairment of tissue integrity related to risk of fluid/nutritional deficit

Assess perirectal area for inflammation, abscess, or fistula
Administer perirectal skin care after each bowel movement
   Wash gently with soap and water
   Pat dry and apply soothing protective ointments
Administer sitz baths
Provide skin care to bony prominences as needed
Provide frequent position changes

Expected outcome/evaluation

Patient's
   Perirectal tissue remains clean and intact
   Skin turgor and color are normal

■ **NDX:** Pain related to bowel inflammation and irritation

Assess character, intensity, and location of pain
Assess effectiveness/side effects of sedatives, analgesics, and rectal suppositories and ointments
Change patient's position frequently and administer back rubs to relieve discomfort
Provide diversional activities and frequent rest periods
Ambulate patient with assistance as tolerated
Encourage and teach alternate pain management methods

Expected outcome/evaluation

Patient
   Demonstrates a more relaxed affect
   Verbalizes a tolerable level of pain

■ **NDX:** Ineffective individual coping related to multiple stressors and needed lifestyle changes

Assess present and past coping patterns

Provide time for and encourage communication with significant other
Establish a supportive relationship with patient and/or significant other
   Explain all procedures and treatments
   Involve patient and/or significant other in plan of care and realistically reinforce physician's explanation of disease process
Maintain quiet and nonstressful environment
Encourage use of stress management techniques
Provide undisturbed rest periods
Accept patient's dependency and encourage independent activities as strength returns
Provide information about support groups*

Expected outcome/evaluation

Patient
   Expresses feelings/concerns more readily
   Demonstrates understanding of needed lifestyle changes
   Exhibits appropriate coping skills and behaviors

■ **NDX:** Sexual dysfunction related to altered body function and lack of knowledge

Explore patient's knowledge of sexuality and current sexual practices and behaviors
Explain to patient and/or significant other that sexual activity needs to be curtailed only while perineal area is inflamed or fistulas or abscesses are present
Explain that after ostomy surgery, sexual activity can be normal following healing of incision; explain need to avoid excessive pressure on ostomy site
Encourage patient and significant other to read about alternative sexual positions and techniques
Explain that odor may be controlled by changing ostomy appliance before sexual activity
Provide supportive and private environment

Expected outcome/evaluation

Patient
   Expresses understanding of needed changes in sexual practices
   Verbalizes feelings and concerns

■ **NDX:** Knowledge deficit related to lack of information about home care needs

Provide instructions in diet management, stressing foods to avoid: raw fruits and vegetables, alcohol, chocolate, and gas-producing foods
Discuss importance of introducing new foods one at a time
Discuss importance of avoiding stress during meals; need to chew food well and eat slowly
Demonstrate procedure for perineal care for inflammation, abscess, and/or fistula and for washing and drying area

---

*United Foundation for Ileitis and Colitis; United Ostomy Association.

after each bowel movement

Demonstrate ostomy and periostomy care if appropriate (see Ostomy Care, p. 283)

Explain causal relationship of stress to disease process and symptoms of recurrence or progression of disease to report to physician

Provide information about medications, including name, dosage, purpose, time of administration, side effects, and interactions; explain need to avoid over-the-counter medications unless discussed with physician first

Encourage follow-up appointments with physician

Expected outcome/evaluation

Patient

Verbalizes understanding of disease process, dietary regimen

Seeks out and uses positive learned coping abilities

Strives to initiate needed lifestyle changes

PERITONITIS

Inflammation of the peritoneal cavity caused by infiltration of intestinal contents from such conditions as a ruptured appendix, gastric or intestinal perforation or trauma, and anastomotic leaks

Assessment
Observations/findings

Abdominal pain and rigidity over area of inflammation

Rebound tenderness

May refer to shoulder

Abdominal distention

Anorexia

Nausea, vomiting

Decreased-to-absent bowel sounds

Failure to pass flatus or stool

Chills, fever

Tachycardia

Hypotension

Leukocytosis

Anxiety

Thoracic breathing: rapid, shallow

Fecal emesis

Laboratory/diagnostic studies

CBC, electrolytes

Radiological examination of abdomen

Peritoneal aspiration

Potential complications

Electrolyte imbalance

Dehydration

Metabolic acidosis

Respiratory alkalosis

Shock

Medical Management

Parenteral fluids with electrolytes, antibiotics, and vitamins

Analgesics

Nasogastric suction, NPO

Arterial blood gases

Central venous lines

Oxygen therapy, incentive spirometer

Peritoneal lavage with antibiotics

Surgical intervention

Nursing diagnoses/interventions/evaluation

■ **NDX:** Alteration in fluid volume (2) related to increased blood flow to peritoneum, vomiting, and/or gastrointestinal perforation

Maintain NPO; assess hydration status

Monitor vital signs and CPV qh or prn; observe for signs of shock

Maintain parenteral fluids with electrolytes, antibiotics, and vitamins

Weigh daily; same time, clothes, and scale

Measure intake and output q8h; measure urine output hourly; if less than 30 to 50 ml/hr notify physician

Assist with peritoneal aspiration/lavage

Monitor electrolytes, blood gases, Hgb, and Hct

Perform passive or assist with and teach active ROM exercises q4h

Expected outcome/evaluation

Patient's

Hydration is adequate as evidenced by normal skin turgor and moist mucous membranes

Vital signs are stable

Intake and output are balanced

■ **NDX:** Ineffective breathing pattern secondary to abdominal pain and distention

Assess respiratory status; monitor for shallow, rapid respirations

Maintain bed rest in quiet environment with head elevated 35 to 45 degrees

Monitor oxygen therapy or incentive spirometer

Assist and teach patient to turn and cough q4h and deep breathe q1h to 2h

Auscultate chest for breath sounds q4h

Expected outcome/evaluation

Patient

Exhibits normal respirations and breath sounds

Demonstrates ability to perform breathing exercises

■ **NDX:** Altered nutrition: less than body requirements related to vomiting and lack of intake

Monitor nasogastric tube or naso-oral intestinal tube; connect to low, intermittent suction apparatus
    Monitor character, amount, color, and odor of drainage
    Provide frequent oral and nasal hygiene
Measure abdominal girth q4h
Monitor for passing of flatus
Auscultate abdomen for bowel sounds q8h
Monitor TPN as indicated
When bowel sounds return and nasogastric-intestinal tube is removed, provide clear liquid diet as tolerated
If surgery is performed, see Intestinal surgery (p. 273)

Expected outcome/evaluation

Patient
    States absence of nausea/vomiting
    Tolerates diet adequately

■ **NDX:** Pain related to inflammation and distention

Assess type, location, and severity of pain
Administer analgesics only after diagnosis has been made
Assess effectiveness of pain relief measures
Maintain position of comfort to minimize stress on abdomen and change patient's position frequently
Provide planned rest periods
Discuss and teach alternate pain management techniques

Expected outcome/evaluation

Patient
    Verbalizes a tolerable level of pain
    Exhibits improving ability to use alternate pain relief measures

■ **NDX:** Anxiety related to situational crisis

Assess anxiety level (p. 13)
Assess present coping skills
Encourage and allow time for verbalization of feelings
Explain all treatments and procedures
Reinforce physician's explanation of illness and treatment
Assist with and teach relaxation techniques
    Provide periods of undisturbed rest
    Encourage support of family/significant others

Expected outcome/evaluation

Patient
    Expresses feelings and concerns and understands positive ways of coping
    Appears more relaxed and comfortable

SHORT BOWEL SYNDROME

Malabsorption that follows small bowel resection; severity depends on the amount and portion of small bowel removed

Assessment
Observations/findings

Frequent, watery diarrhea; may contain fat
Rapid dehydration resulting from malabsorption
Rapid weight loss
Weakness
Purpura, generalized bleeding
Anemia
Malabsorption of fat and fat-soluble vitamins (A, E, D, K)

Laboratory/diagnostic studies

Barium enema
Serum studies: iron, vitamins B_{12} and A, calcium, folate, magnesium, electrolytes, CBC, carotene, cholesterol
PT (increased)
Stool for fat and culture
Lactose tolerance, D-lactate level, xylose tolerance

Potential complications

Malnutrition
Electrolyte imbalance
Osteoporosis, osteomalacia
Night blindness
Tetany
Confusion, stupor

Medical Management

Antidiarrheals
Anticholinergics
Antibiotics
Antacids
Vitamins
Histamine receptor antagonists (cimetidine)
TPN, parenteral fluids (p. 36)
Elemental diet progressing to low-lactose, high-calorie diet

Nursing diagnoses/interventions/evaluation

■ **NDX:** Fluid volume deficit (2) related to profuse diarrhea and fluid loss

Monitor parenteral fluids with electrolytes and vitamins
Assess for signs of dehydration and shock; check level of consciousness q2h
Monitor vital signs q2h to 4h
Measure intake and output q8h
Weigh patient daily at same time with same clothing and scale
Monitor serum electrolytes, Hgb, and Hct

Expected outcome/evaluation

Patient's
    Vital signs are normal
    Intake and output are balanced

Skin turgor is adequate

Electrolytes are within normal limits

■ **NDX:** Diarrhea related to decreased intestinal absorption

Assess effectiveness/side effects of antidiarrheals, antacids, histamine receptor antagonists

Monitor stools for color, consistency, amount, and frequency

Provide perineal care after each bowel movement; keep environment free from odor

Auscultate abdomen for bowel sounds q4h

Expected outcome/evaluation

Patient's

Stools are less frequent

Stool consistency is more normal

■ **NDX:** Altered nutrition: less than body requirements related to loss of absorptive surface of intestine

Maintain TPN as indicated

Monitor urine for sugar and acetone qid

Monitor blood glucose

Observe central IV line for infection

Institute elemental diet (Vivonex, Precision LR), usually when weight gain is apparent and diarrhea is less frequent

Administer diet through nasogastric tube or orally, depending on patient's appetite: 300 to 350 ml/q2h

When given orally, provide a straw as the taste may be unpalatable to some patients

Discuss with and assist patient and significant other with accepting nutritional plan, as it may be necessary for a long period of time

Assess effectiveness and monitor side effects of antacids and anticholinergics

Expected outcome/evaluation

Patient

Maintains weight at level normal for patient

Demonstrates understanding of changes needed in dietary regimen

■ **NDX:** Knowledge deficit related to lack of information about home care needs

Provide and discuss written information about nutritional plan, usually low-lactose, high-calorie; introduce milk slowly and observe tolerance

Instruct patient and/or significant other concerning signs and symptoms to report to physician: nausea, vomiting, diarrhea, or other intestinal problems

Provide and discuss written instructions for home TPN if applicable; arrange for home health care visits (p. 36)

Discuss medication: name, dosage, purpose, time of administration, and side effects

Encourage follow-up visits with physician

Expected outcome/evaluation

Patient

Verbalizes understanding of disease process, nutritional plan, and potential complications

Expresses knowledge of medication schedule

INTESTINAL OBSTRUCTION

Blockage of the intestinal tract, which inhibits the passage of fluids, flatus, and food; may be mechanical or functional

Causes
Mechanical

Adhesions

Strangulated hernia

Abscess

Carcinoma

Volvulus

Intussusception

Obstipation

Functional

Paralytic ileus

Spinal cord lesions

Regional enteritis

Electrolyte imbalance

Uremia

Assessment
Observations/findings
SPECIFIC

Small bowel

Severe, cramplike abdominal pain, increasing with distention

Mild distention

Nausea

Vomiting; early contains undigested food and chyme; later vomitus is watery and contains bile; finally, dark and fecal

Rapid dehydration: acidosis

Large bowel

Mild abdominal discomfort

Severe distention

Latent fecal vomiting

Latent dehydration: rare acidosis

COMMON

Anorexia and malaise

Fever

Tachycardia
Diaphoresis
Pallor
Abdominal rigidity
Failure to pass stool or flatus rectally or per ostomy
Increased bowel sounds (early obstruction)
Decreased bowel sounds (later)
Urinary retention
Leukocytosis

Laboratory/diagnostic studies

Serum electrolytes, CBC, amylase
Barium enema
Radiological studies of abdomen

Potential complications

Dehydration
Electrolyte imbalance
Metabolic acidosis
Perforation
Shock

Medical Management

NPO
Nasointestinal suction
Surgical intervention: see Intestinal surgery (p. 273)
Parenteral fluids with electrolytes, antibiotics, and vitamins
Analgesics
Oxygen therapy

Nursing diagnoses/interventions/evaluation

■ **NDX:** Fluid volume deficit (2) secondary to nausea and vomiting, fever, and/or diaphoresis

Monitor vital signs and observe level of consciousness and for symptoms of shock
Maintain NPO; assess level of hydration
Monitor parenteral fluids with electrolytes, antibiotics, and vitamins
Monitor nasointestinal tube and low, intermittent suction apparatus
  Measure drainage output q8h
  Observe contents for color, consistency
Position patient on right side; then left side to facilitate passage into intestine; do not tape nasointestinal tube to nose until tube is in correct position
Monitor tube for advancement qh
Indwelling urethral catheter may be inserted; report output of less than 50 ml/hr to physician
Measure abdominal girth q4h
Monitor electrolytes, Hgb, and Hct
Prepare for surgery as indicated (p. 273)
If surgery is not performed, collaborate with physician and initiate oral fluids, either by clamping intestinal tube

for 1 hr and giving measured amounts of water or tea or giving these fluids after intestinal tube is removed
Open tube, if in place, at specified times as ordered, to estimate amount of absorption
Observe abdomen for discomfort, distention, pain, or rigidity and report to physician
Auscultate bowel sounds tid, 1 hr after meals; report absence of sounds to physician
Force fluids to 2500 ml/day unless contraindicated
Measure intake and output until adequate
Observe initial stool for color, consistency, and amount; avoid constipation

Expected outcome/evaluation

Patient's
  Vital signs are normal
  Intake and output are balanced

■ **NDX:** Pain related to distention, rigidity

Maintain bed rest in position of comfort; do not gatch knees
Assess location, severity, and type of pain
Assess effectiveness and monitor for side effects of analgesics; avoid morphine
Provide planned rest periods
Assist with and teach active or perform passive ROM exercises q4h
Change position frequently and administer back rubs and skin care
Auscultate bowel sounds; note increased rigidity or pain; give gentle enema if ordered
Provide and teach alternate pain relief measures

Expected outcome/evaluation

Patient
  Verbalizes decreased discomfort; states pain is at tolerable level
  Appears relaxed

■ **NDX:** Ineffective breathing pattern related to abdominal distention and/or rigidity

Assess respiratory status; observe for shallow, rapid breathing
Elevate head of bed 40 to 60 degrees
Monitor oxygen or incentive spirometer therapy
Assist and teach patient to turn and cough q4h and deep breathe qh
Auscultate chest for breath sounds q4h

Expected outcome/evaluation

Patient
  Demonstrates ability to perform breathing exercises
  Exhibits respirations that are deep and slow

■ **NDX:** Anxiety related to situational crisis and altered health status

Assess present coping behaviors and encourage use of past successful skills
Encourage and allow time for verbalization of anxieties and fears; provide quiet reassurance
Explain procedures and treatments and reinforce physician's explanation of illness, treatment, and prognosis
Maintain quiet, nonstressful environment
Encourage support of family and significant other

Expected outcome/evaluation

Patient
Expresses understanding of present illness
Demonstrates positive coping skills in dealing with anxiety

■ **NDX:** Knowledge deficit related to lack of information about home care needs

Discuss dietary management, stressing importance of eating slowly, chewing foods well, and eating at regular intervals
Explain need to avoid constipation
Use natural laxatives or stool softeners
Maintain fluid intake of 2500 ml/day
Increase activity as tolerated
Provide instructions on symptoms to report to physician: abdominal pain, cramps, distention, and/or nausea and vomiting
Encourage follow-up care with physician
If surgery was performed, see Intestinal surgery (p. 273)

Expected outcome/evaluation

Patient
Verbalizes understanding of disease process, dietary plan, and potential complications
Participates in treatment regimen

PARALYTIC ILEUS

Decrease in or absence of intestinal motility after intestinal or abdominal surgery or in connection with any severe metabolic disease; cause may be neuromuscular, resulting from lack of potassium, or gastrointestinal, resulting from gastric inactivity and air swallowing

Assessment
Observations/findings

Abdominal tenderness and distention
Absent or diminished bowel sounds
Nausea, vomiting
Lack of flatus
Decreased urinary output
Fever

Laboratory/diagnostic studies

Electrolytes (decreased potassium)
Abdominal radiography series

Potential complications

Dehydration
Electrolyte imbalance
Shock
Perforation of ileum
Peritonitis (p. 267)
Circulatory failure
Respiratory distress

Medical Management

NPO
Parenteral fluids with electrolytes
Nasointestinal, nasogastric aspiration
Oxygen therapy
Medications to promote peristalsis: dexpanthenol (Ilopan), bethanechol (Urecholine), neostigmine (Prostigmin), metoclopramide (Reglan)
Activity, diet
Enema, rectal tube

Nursing diagnoses/interventions/evaluation

■ **NDX:** Ineffective breathing pattern related to abdominal distention and rigidity

Maintain bed rest in position to facilitate respirations; do not gatch knees
Assess respiratory status
Auscultate chest for breath sounds q4h
Monitor oxygen therapy
Assist and teach patient to turn and cough q4h and deep breathe qh
Balance activity and rest
Monitor vital signs q4h
Ambulate when tolerated

Expected outcome/evaluation

Patient
Demonstrates ability to perform breathing exercises
Exhibits normal respirations and breath sounds

■ **NDX:** Fluid volume deficit (2) related to vomiting and distention

Maintain NPO; assess level of hydration
Maintain parenteral fluids with electrolytes
Maintain nasointestinal tube to low, intermittent suction apparatus (p. 282)
Do not tape tube to nose; position patient to facilitate passage of tube into intestine
Monitor advancement qh

Monitor character, amount, and color of intestinal drainage q4h; report any change in these to physician

Nasogastric tube may be inserted in lieu of intestinal tube; connect to low, intermittent suction apparatus

Tape securely to nose

Irrigate with measured amounts of normal saline

Monitor color and amount of drainage

Measure intake and output; report urine output of less than 30 ml/hr to physician

Monitor electrolytes

Collaborate with physician when intestinal or gastric output decreases and bowel sounds return to manage patient based on changing needs/status

Clamp tube

Administer liquids (warm tea, carbonated beverages) in measured amounts

Monitor for pain, distention, nausea, and cramps; unclamp tube if these signs occur

Remove tube and progress to previous diet

Continue measuring intake and output until adequate for patient

Expected outcome/evaluation

Patient's
  Vital signs are normal
  Hydration is normal as evidenced by skin turgor
  Intake and output are balanced
  Bowel sounds are normal
  Electrolytes are within normal limits

■ **NDX:** Constipation related to decreased intake

Assess effectiveness of and monitor for side effects of medication used to increase peristalsis

Auscultate abdomen for bowel sounds q4h; monitor for return of flatus and normal bowel elimination

Measure abdominal girth q4h

Promote high-fiber diet and increased fluid intake as tolerated

Encourage ambulation

Expected outcome/evaluation

Patient
  Understands causative factors of constipation
  Defecates soft, formed stool

■ **NDX:** Knowledge deficit related to lack of information about illness and its outcome

Reinforce physician's explanation of cause of paralytic ileus and that it is a temporary condition

Explain all procedures and treatments

Demonstrate technique for swallowing without ingesting air

Expected outcome/evaluation

Patient
  Verbalizes understanding of disease process
  Participates in treatment regimen

DIVERTICULAR DISEASE OF COLON

Herniation (pocket formation) along the mucosa of the large intestine caused by low-fiber diets and weakened intestinal wall (diverticulosis); an inflammatory process may occur when a diverticulum ruptures or feces become impacted in the diverticulum (diverticulitis)

Acute Diverticulitis

Assessment
Observations/findings

Cramplike pain and tenderness in left lower quadrant

Anorexia

Nausea

Low-grade fever

Irregular bowel function
  Constipation
  Diarrhea
  Mucus, blood in stool
  Increased flatulence
  Abdominal distention
  Decreased bowel sounds

Laboratory/diagnostic studies

Barium enema

Sigmoidoscopy, colonoscopy with biopsy

Ultrasonography

WBC, ESR (increased)

Urinalysis

Examination of surrounding organs (kidney, bladder) for possible involvement

Potential complications

Leukocytosis

Dehydration

Intestinal obstruction, perforation

Peritonitis

Fistula, abscess

Hemorrhage

Medical Management

Parenteral fluids with electrolytes and antibiotics

Nasogastric aspiration (severe vomiting, distention)

Analgesics, anticholinergics

NPO increasing to high-fiber diet

Surgical intervention (resection, colostomy)

Nursing diagnoses/interventions/evaluation

■ **NDX:** Potential fluid volume deficit related to vomiting, diarrhea, anorexia, risk of hypovolemia

Maintain NPO; assess level of hydration

Maintain parenteral fluids with antibiotics and electrolytes

Monitor electrolytes

Collaborate with physician, dietitian; when pain and fever subside, provide clear liquid diet and progress to soft diet until high-fiber diet can be tolerated

Encourage fluids to 2500 ml daily unless contraindicated

Assess and monitor amount of bleeding; check stools for occult or frank blood

Monitor vital signs q4h and Hgb, Hct as needed

Monitor blood transfusions or packed red blood cells

Assist with exercises of legs and feet q4h to increase venous return

Measure intake and output; report output of less than 30 ml/hr to physician

Expected outcome/evaluation

Patient's

Hydration is adequate as evidenced by normal skin turgor

Intake and output are balanced

Vital signs are within normal limits

■ **NDX:**   Constipation related to anorexia, low-fiber diet, and immobility

Monitor nasogastric tube and low, intermittent suction apparatus

Maintain tube patency

Irrigate with measured amounts of normal saline

Measure gastric output q8h

Auscultate abdomen for bowel sounds q4h

Measure abdominal girth q4h

Monitor stools for consistency, color, amount, and frequency

When nasogastric tube is removed, administer hydrophilic colloid laxative or psyllium (Metamucil) as tolerated

Expected outcome/evaluation

Patient

Tolerates increasingly high-fiber diet

Defecates soft and formed stool

■ **NDX:**   Pain related to inflammation, irritation of bowel

Maintain bed rest in position of comfort

Assess location, character, and severity of pain

Administer analgesics; avoid morphine; assess effectiveness of pain relief measures

Assist and teach patient to turn and deep breathe q2h; administer back rubs to promote comfort

Maintain planned rest periods

Change position frequently to prevent pressure and fatigue

Encourage and teach alternate pain management methods

Expected outcome/evaluation

Patient

Reports a tolerable level of pain

Appears relaxed

■ **NDX:**   Knowledge deficit related to lack of information about dietary management and home care needs

Provide written dietary instructions and discuss relationship of diet to disease process

Include listing of high-fiber foods: bran, fruits, vegetables, nuts

Explain importance of regular meals, eating slowly, and chewing well

Avoid large meals, extremely cold foods, and alcohol

Increase fluid intake to eight glasses/day unless contraindicated

Discuss importance of elimination

Establish regular bowel habits

Avoid constipation, straining, enemas, and harsh laxatives

Use psyllium (Metamucil) or high-fiber wafers or powder

Explain signs and symptoms of recurrence to report to physician

Encourage regular visits to physician

Expected outcome/evaluation

Patient

Verbalizes understanding of disease process, dietary plan, and potential complications

Participates in treatment to stabilize bowel elimination

INTESTINAL SURGERY

Any surgery performed on the intestine from the jejunum to the colon for such conditions as carcinoma, obstruction, acute enteritis or colitis, benign tumors, trauma, appendicitis, incarcerated hernia, and diverticulitis

Preoperative Assessment and Care

Assess respiratory status

Monitor potassium level

Prepare bowel

Low-residue, clear liquid diet

Magnesia preparations, antibiotics po

GoLytly bowel preparation

Enemas until clear; avoid depleting debilitated or elderly patients with multiple enemas at one time

Nasogastric/nasointestinal tube insertion

Provide patient with information regarding drains, tubes, etc., that may be present postoperatively

Teach patient to turn, cough, and deep breathe

Demonstrate methods for incisional support

Discuss importance of moving after surgery, especially feet and legs

Postoperative Assessment
Observations/findings

Character and amount
  Gastric or intestinal drainage
  Urinary output
  Ostomy drainage, if applicable
  Wound drainage
Nausea, vomiting
Abdominal distention
Placement of nasogastric tube
Location and type of pain
Decreased, shallow respirations
Decreased breath sounds

Laboratory/diagnostic studies

Electrolytes, Hgb, Hct
Urine culture after indwelling catheter is removed
Wound culture; suspected infection

Potential complications

Dehydration
Electrolyte imbalance
Atelectasis
Hemorrhage
Shock
Peritonitis
Paralytic ileus
Pulmonary embolus
Thrombophlebitis
Wound evisceration
Wound infection

Medical Management

Parenteral fluids with electrolytes
Nasogastric aspiration
Indwelling urethral catheter
NPO progressing to prescribed diet
Analgesics, antibiotics, vitamins
Patient-controlled anesthesia (p. 59)
Oxygen therapy
Activity, antiembolic stockings

Nursing diagnoses/interventions/evaluation

■ **NDX:** Ineffective breathing pattern related to place-ment of incision and/or pain

Assess respiratory status: type, frequency, and character of respirations
Elevate head of bed 35 to 45 degrees; do not gatch knees
Auscultate lungs for breath sounds q2h
Assist and teach patient to turn, cough q2h, and deep breathe qh; support incision
Provide incentive spirometer q2h
Administer pain medication before treatments as appli-cable

Expected outcome/evaluation

Patient
  Exhibits normal respiratory rate and rhythm
  Presents breath sounds that are clear

■ **NDX:** Potential for fluid volume deficit related to risk of increased fluid loss from gastric suction, diar-rhea

Maintain NPO, assess hydration status; skin turgor, moist mucous membranes, capillary refill
Maintain parenteral fluids with electrolytes, vitamins, and antibiotics
Monitor vital signs q2h to 4h
Monitor dressings for excessive drainage, hemorrhage
Monitor nasogastric/intestinal tube and low, intermittent suction
  Check color and consistency of drainage
  Irrigate with measured amounts of normal saline
Measure intake and output q8h and monitor for fluid shift; edema, weight gain, rales
Monitor serum electrolytes and urine specific gravity
Monitor indwelling urethral catheter and closed gravity drainage system
  Measure output hourly; if less than 30 to 50 ml/hr, report to physician
Perform guaiac test on stool for signs of intestinal bleeding
Observe for abdominal distention and monitor bowel sounds for 2 to 3 days postoperatively

Expected outcome/evaluation

Patient's
  Vital signs are normal
  Intake and output are balanced
  Hydration is adequate as evidenced by normal skin turgor

■ **NDX:** Pain related to surgical intervention

Maintain bed rest in quiet environment
Monitor location, character, intensity of pain
Assess effectiveness of pain relief measures and observe for side effects
Encourage patient to take pain medication as prescribed for 48 hr
Coordinate care to allow for planned rest periods
Change position frequently; administer back rubs
Discuss and teach alternate pain relief techniques as needed

Expected outcome/evaluation

Patient
  Reports a tolerable level of discomfort
  Appears more relaxed, comfortable

■ **NDX:** Potential impairment of tissue integrity related to increased risk of wound drainage, altered circulation, nutrition

Administer nasal and oral hygiene frequently and keep nares and mouth moist
Change dressings as needed; use nonallergenic tape or Montgomery straps
    Assess healing process
    Monitor drainage for signs of infection; culture as needed
    Keep skin around incision clean and dry
Provide splinting of incision when coughing to prevent dehiscence
Maintain permanency of tubes and catheters by taping comfortably and securely
Initiate a wound pouching system if drainage is profuse
Assess color and condition of stoma and peristomal skin integrity if applicable

Expected outcome/evaluation

Patient's
    Wound heals without incident
    Surrounding tissue is clean, dry, and intact

■ **NDX:** Alteration in bowel elimination related to surgical manipulation, immobility, altered nutritional intake

Assess preoperative bowel habits and nutritional intake; explain cause of alteration
Auscultate abdomen for return of bowel sounds q8h
Observe first postoperative bowel movement; assess color, consistency, amount, and frequency
Keep perineal area clean and dry
Assess rectal dressing and incision if abdominal-perineal resection was performed
Demonstrate and teach ostomy irrigation and appliance application if applicable (p. 283)

Expected outcome/evaluation

Patient
    Understands causative factors of altered elimination
    Defecates soft, formed stool

■ **NDX:** Altered nutrition: less than body requirements related to NPO status, nasogastric suction

Collaborate with physician, dietitian; after bowel sounds return and nasogastric/intestinal tube is removed or clamped, initiate clear liquids in measured amounts; observe for tolerance and discomfort or distention
Progress to soft or regular diet as tolerated
Monitor for malabsorption syndrome after surgery of small intestine: steatorrhea, diarrhea, weight loss

Weigh patient daily at same time with same clothing and scale
Monitor intake and output until adequate for age and weight

Expected outcome/evaluation

Patient
    Maintains normal weight
    Tolerates diet without discomfort

■ **NDX:** Knowledge deficit related to lack of information about home and follow-up care

Provide and discuss written dietary instructions and restrictions
Demonstrate dressing changes, wound care, aseptic technique
Discuss signs of wound infection; pain, redness, swelling, odor
Reinforce ostomy care if applicable (p. 283)
Explain importance of avoiding constipation and using natural laxatives or those prescribed
Discuss activities allowed, need for rest and mild exercise, and necessity of not lifting heavy objects (over 5 to 10 lb) for 6 to 8 weeks
Reinforce physician's explanation of surgical procedure and outcome expected
Discuss medications: name, dosage, purpose, time of administration, and side effects
Encourage follow-up visits with physician

Expected outcome/evaluation

Patient
    Verbalizes understanding of dietary regimen, disease process, and potential complications
    Demonstrates adequate ostomy care
    Expresses understanding of allowed activities

CONTINENT ILEOSTOMY (KOCK'S POUCH)

Surgical removal of the rectum and colon (proctocolectomy) with construction of an internal ileal reservoir, nipple valve, and stoma, allowing intermittent drainage of ileal contents; performed for patients with ulcerative colitis, familial polyposis, or existing ileostomy diversion (Figure 5-7)

Preoperative Care

Administer prescribed bowel preparation
    Oral antibiotics
    Mild laxatives
    Colonic irrigations
    Ileostomy irrigation
Bowel preparation will depend on
    Age and nutritional status
    Extent of disease process in colon

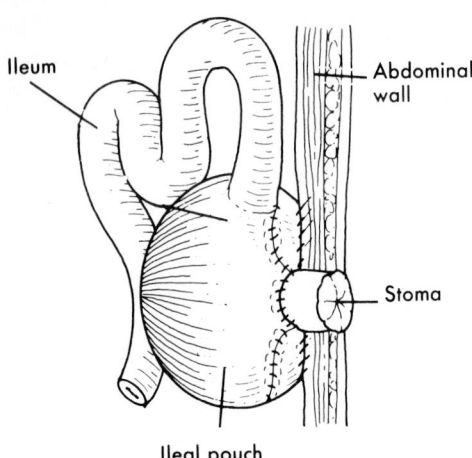

Ileum

Abdominal wall

Stoma

Ileal pouch

FIGURE 5-7. Continent ileostomy (Kock's pouch).

Presence of existing ileostomy
Stoma site selected
Insert nasogastric tube and indwelling urethral catheter as ordered
Involve enterostomal therapist in preoperative education
Reinforce physician's explanation of surgical procedure and postoperative care

Postoperative Assessment
Observations/findings

Patency and placement of plastic ileal reservoir catheter
Patency of nasogastric tube
Placement of suture holding catheter in place
Color and amount of
    Ileal reservoir drainage
    Gastric drainage
    Urine output
    Wound drainage
Color of stoma
Nausea, vomiting
Abdominal distention
Abdominal cramps
Diminished breath sounds

Laboratory/diagnostic studies

Electrolytes, Hgb, Hct

Potential complications

Electrolyte imbalance
Atelectasis
Intestinal obstruction, perforation
Peritonitis
Wound infection: stoma and rectum
Pouchitis
    Bloody diarrhea, fever
    Valve prolapse, leakage
    Pouch perforation

Medical Management

Parenteral fluids with electrolytes
Nasogastric/ileal reservoir aspiration
Irrigating solution
Indwelling urethral catheter
Sitz baths
Analgesics
Diet management
Activity

Nursing diagnoses/interventions/evaluation

■ **NDX:** Potential for ineffective breathing pattern related to pain and risk of decreased lung expansion

Assess respiratory status and respiratory rate q2h to 4h
Assist and teach patient to turn and cough q2h to 4h and deep breathe qh; support incision
Auscultate chest for breath sounds q4h
Provide incentive spirometer q1h to 2h
Elevate head of bed 30 to 45 degrees

Expected outcome/evaluation

Patient
    Exhibits normal respiratory rate and rhythm
    Presents clear breath sounds

■ **NDX:** Potential fluid volume deficit related to increased ileal output

Assess for dehydration
Maintain NPO
Maintain parenteral fluids with electrolytes
Measure intake and output q8h
Monitor vital signs q4h
Monitor nasogastric tube and low, intermittent suction apparatus; irrigate gently with measured amounts of normal saline q2h to 4h
Monitor indwelling urethral catheter and closed gravity drainage system; report output of less than 30 to 50 ml/hr to physician
Monitor serum electrolytes, Hgb, Hct, and urine specific gravity
Monitor for circulatory overload; tachycardia, neck vein distention, rales

Expected outcome/evaluation

Patient's
    Vital signs are stable
    Intake and output are balanced
    Hydration is adequate as evidenced by normal skin turgor

■ **NDX:** Potential impairment of tissue integrity related to acidity of ileostomy drainage and surgical procedure

Monitor dressings q1h to 2h for 24 hr; then q4h for 48 hr

Change dressings as needed; include rectal dressing

Place dressing around reservoir catheter to avoid tension and absorb drainage from stoma

Report excessive bleeding to physician

Monitor color of stoma (pink-red is normal); report any change to physician

Administer wound and stomal care prn

    Wash around stoma and wound with clear water, pat dry, and allow to air dry for 30 min

    Apply skin sealant around stoma to prevent irritation

    Assess healing process

Administer sitz baths tid to promote healing and comfort

Expected outcome/evaluation

Patient's

    Wounds are healing adequately

    Surrounding skin is clean, dry, and intact

■ **NDX:**   Alteration in bowel elimination related to ileostomy and ileal pouch reservoir

Monitor ileal reservoir catheter and closed gravity drainage system

Avoid placing tension on suture and catheter

Irrigate gently with 20 to 30 ml of normal saline q2h and prn as determined through collaboration with physician

Observe return flow: should equal amount instilled plus ileal contents

    Monitor color and consistency of drainage

Auscultate abdomen for bowel sounds q4h

Observe and monitor for signs of reservoir catheter obstruction

    Feeling of fullness in lower abdomen or around catheter

    Nausea, vomiting

    Increased pain or cramps

If symptoms of reservoir catheter obstruction occur, perform the following procedure, if ordered, after discussion with physician

    Gently irrigate catheter with 20 to 30 ml of normal saline

    If there is no outflow, carefully remove skin suture

    Retain suture around catheter since it marks length of insertion

    Gently irrigate with 20 ml of normal saline and rotate catheter clockwise until outflow begins

    If no results occur, notify physician immediately

Ileal catheter should remain in place 14 to 21 days to allow reservoir healing

Continue irrigations q2h to 3h with 30 to 40 ml of normal saline; contents will thicken as diet increases

Increase fluid intake to 3000 ml/day unless contraindicated

Provide grape and prune juice to keep ileal content thin

If plugging occurs, gentle milking of catheter and rotation

clockwise while irrigating may help; having patient cough and applying light pressure to lower abdomen may also help

Catheter may be removed, rinsed, and reinserted as ordered

Expected outcome/evaluation

Patient's

    Understanding of function of ileal pouch is clear

    Pouch remains patent, and output becomes more normal

■ **NDX:**   Altered nutrition: less than body requirements related to nasogastric aspiration and increased ileal output

Clamp or remove nasogastric tube as determined by collaboration with physician when bowel sounds return or bubbles appear in ileal catheter

Provide water and clear liquids as tolerated

Avoid carbonated beverages

Progress to soft, low-residue, low-fiber diet to prevent catheter plugging

Avoid gas-producing foods

Teach patient to chew foods well with mouth closed, to eat slowly, and to avoid talking while eating to prevent swallowing air

Have patient avoid drinking with straw

Consider patient's food preferences

Expected outcome/evaluation

Patient

    Demonstrates understanding of diet regimen

    Tolerates diet and weight remains stable

■ **NDX:**   Pain related to surgical intervention

Maintain bed rest in quiet environment

Assess location, intensity, and character of pain; severe gas pains are usually present postoperatively

Administer analgesics and monitor effectiveness of pain relief measures

Assist with and teach active exercises q4h, especially feet and legs

Coordinate care to provide planned rest periods

Discuss and teach alternate pain relief measures

Change position frequently; administer back rubs to promote comfort

Provide diversional activities

Ambulate with assistance

Expected outcome/evaluation

Patient

    Reports a reduction of pain

    Presents a more relaxed affect

■ **NDX:** Body image disturbance related to altered bowel function (ileostomy)

Encourage and allow time for verbalization of feelings and concerns; provide privacy

Encourage patient communication with significant other

Assess present coping behaviors and strengths

Offer praise for accomplishments in discussing, viewing, or exploring stoma

Introduce to enterostomal therapist and/or support group

Encourage patient to view stoma and catheter and discuss their positive aspects

Reinforce physician's explanation of procedure and treatment; clarify misconceptions

Expected outcome/evaluation

Patient

Demonstrates understanding of fears/concerns

Begins to accept ileostomy as part of body

Uses positive coping skills to incorporate body changes into lifestyle

■ **NDX:** Knowledge deficit related to lack of information about care of continent ileostomy, home care needs, and follow-up instructions

Assist and teach patient to care for ileal reservoir catheter when patient is physically and psychologically able

Involve patient and significant other in plan of care

Set and explain daily goals, with ultimate goal being total patient management

Phase I

Familiarize patient with anatomy and physiology of ileal reservoir

Explain that drainage will depend on food ingested and emphasize importance of high-liquid intake

Teach patient to irrigate catheter; use 50 ml syringe, normal saline, and 500 ml graduate

Instill 30 to 50 ml of normal saline

Measure outflow

Make certain all irrigating fluid is returned

Reconnect catheter to closed gravity drainage system

Phase II

When ordered, clamp catheter for 1 hr, then release for 30 min and reclamp

Irrigate prn with normal saline if outflow is thick

Teach patient procedure in small segments until mastered

Explain that purpose of clamping procedure is to gradually increase reservoir capacity

Explain that clamping time will increase by 15 to 30 min daily until 3 to 4 hr time is reached, usually in 5 to 6 days

Continue to connect catheter to closed gravity drainage system at night

See box below

Phase III

When ordered, remove catheter and teach patient reinsertion procedure using the following equipment and guidelines

Equipment

No. 28 plastic catheter with insertion tube

50 ml graduate

50 ml syringe

Normal saline

Water-soluble lubricant

Tissues

4 × 4 dressing

Nonallergenic tape

Guidelines

Have patient sit on side of bed

Remove dressings and catheter; disconnect catheter from drainage system

Rinse catheter with water and lubricate tip; place other end into graduate

Place graduate below stoma

Gently intubate stoma until resistance of nipple valve is felt (2 inches [5 cm])

Slide catheter through valve with gentle pressure to insertion line

If catheter meets resistance, do not force

Have patient lie down, relax, and take deep breaths

METHOD FOR INCREASING ILEAL RESERVOIR CAPACITY

- Leave catheter in pouch with continuous drainage for first 3 weeks
- Week 4

  Intubate and irrigate catheter every 2 hours during day

  Connect to gravity drainage at night

  Irrigate once at night
- Week 5

  Intubate every 3 hours and irrigate twice daily

  Connect to gravity drainage at night

  Irrigate once at night
- Week 6

  Intubate every 4 hours and irrigate twice daily

  Intubate at night only for discomfort or feeling of fullness
- Week 7 and thereafter

  Intubate pouch four times a day

  Irrigate once daily until return is clear

Modified from Thompson JM et al: *Mosby's Manual of Clinical Nursing,* ed 2, St Louis, 1989, CV Mosby.

Insert catheter through valve during exhalation

Drainage time is about 5 to 10 min unless fecal material is thick; irrigating with 30 ml of normal saline will thin material

Air bubbles in catheter are normal

When drainage is complete, remove catheter and wash with soap and water; rinse well and dry; store in plastic bag

Cleanse stoma and skin with warm water; pat dry and apply 4 × 4 dressing; secure with tape

Discuss importance of maintaining drainage schedule

Time between drainage periods will increase as reservoir capacity increases

Provide and discuss written schedule (see box on p. 278)

Provide needed equipment and information concerning where it may be purchased

Explain importance of diet regimen

Eat well-balanced low-residue diet

Avoid gas-producing foods: cabbage, cauliflower, carbonated beverages

Avoid foods that clog catheter: corn, nuts, mushrooms, lettuce, fruit peels

Eat at regular times, chew food well, eat slowly, and avoid straws

Maintain fluid intake of 2500 ml/24 hr; drink prune and grape juice to help liquefy drainage

Discuss signs and symptoms to report to physician

Inability to intubate stoma

Abdominal distention

Nausea, vomiting

Increased abdominal pain

Elevated temperature

Incontinence of stool and/or flatus (nipple valve dysfunction)

Explain need to wear nonirritating clothes until wound heals

Demonstrate care of surgical incisions

Encourage follow-up visits with physician

Expected outcome/evaluation

Patient

Demonstrates ability to care for reservoir; irrigation and clamping procedures

Verbalizes understanding of disease process, dietary plan, and potential complications

Demonstrates ability to use learned coping skills in dealing with stress

ILEOANAL RESERVOIR

A two-stage surgical procedure anastamosing the ileum to an ileal reservoir constructed at the anus, allowing normal bowel elimination without an ileostomy (Figure 5-8)

Stage I: Colectomy, Temporary Ileostomy, and Construction of Ileal Reservoir at Anus

Preoperative Assessment and Care

Reinforce physician's explanation of surgical procedure and expected outcome; clarify misconceptions

Contact enterostomal therapist for preoperative assessment

Monitor baseline vital signs

Prepare bowel as ordered: tap water enemas, oral antibiotics

Encourage and allow time for expression of concerns and feelings; promote positive aspects of surgical procedure

Explain possibility of nasogastric tube, indwelling urethral catheter, and presacral drainage tube exiting from abdomen postoperatively

Postoperative Assessment
Observations/findings

Location of ileostomy and presacral drain

Color, character, and amount of drainage

Incisional (abdominal and rectal) drainage

Gastric drainage

Ileostomy drainage

Presacral drain

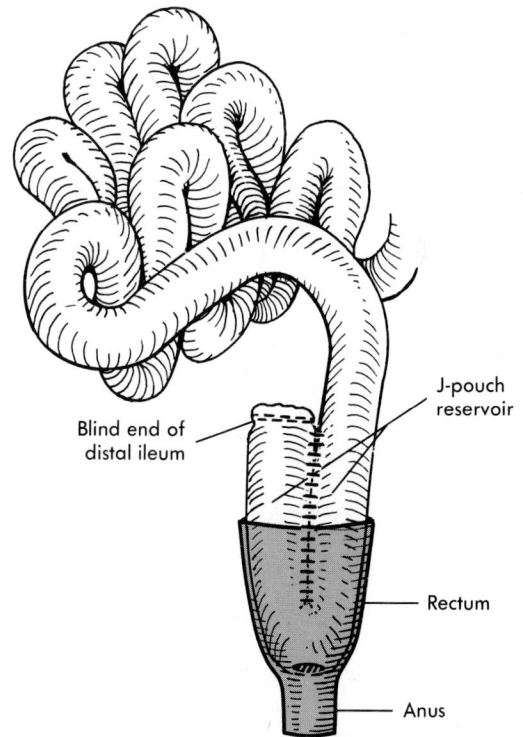

FIGURE 5-8. Ileoanal anastomosis with a valveless ileal reservoir. Side-to-side anastomosis of a J -loop of terminal ileum is incised at apex and anastomosed to anal sphincter; remaining rectal mucosa provides support. Defecation occurs through anus. (From Phipps WJ, Long BC, Woods NF et al: *Medical-Surgical Nursing: Concepts and clinical practice,* ed 4, St Louis, 1991, Mosby–Year Book.)

Skin integrity of ileostomy and rectal area
Urine output
Location, intensity, and character of pain

Laboratory/diagnostic studies

Electrolytes, CBC, urinalysis

Potential complications

Skin erosion from ileostomy
Reservoir abscess, ischemia, fistula
Intestinal obstruction, adhesions
Wound infection: pouchitis (inflammation of reservoir)
Cystitis, urinary retention
Phlebitis

Medical Management

Antidiarrheals, bulk-forming agents
Analgesics, antibiotics, dermatological creams
Parenteral fluids with electrolytes and vitamins
Nasogastric suction, NPO
Irrigation of reservoir
Presacral catheter drainage apparatus
Indwelling urethral catheter
Sitz baths
Diet, rest, ambulation, exercise

Nursing diagnoses/interventions/evaluation

■ **NDX:**   Potential fluid volume deficit related to risk of abnormal body fluid loss from ileostomy, gastric aspiration, and NPO status

Maintain NPO
Maintain parenteral fluids with electrolytes and vitamins
Monitor indwelling urethral catheter and closed drainage system; monitor hourly output for 12 hr; if less than 30 to 50 ml/hr, notify physician
Monitor nasogastric tube and low, intermittent suction apparatus; irrigate with measured amounts of normal saline to keep patent
Monitor ileostomy output; 800 to 1200 ml/24 hr is not uncommon
Monitor presacral catheter and closed gravity drainage system; monitor output q2h for 12 hr, then q4h
Calculate total intake and output q8h; assess for urinary retention and signs of dehydration
Monitor vital signs q2h until stable; then q4h
Weigh patient daily at same time with same clothing and scale
Monitor electrolytes, Hgb, and Hct
Collaborate with physician and, when nasogastric tube is removed, initiate liquids and progress to well-balanced diet as tolerated; monitor for tolerance of new foods as they are introduced

Expected outcome/evaluation

Patient's
Vital signs are stable

Intake and output are balanced
Ileostomy output is within normal limits
Electrolytes are within normal limits

■ **NDX:**   Potential impairment of tissue integrity related to ileostomy and rectal/anal drainage

Monitor perianal area for drainage and mucus; may be copious and odorous
Change dressings prn and clean area well; apply skin sealants and creams to promote healing, comfort, and skin integrity
Irrigate reservoir daily as ordered to remove mucus and other drainage and to prevent pouchitis
Provide absorbent pads to wear while ambulating or at night
Assist with and teach patient ileostomy and skin care (p. 283) as soon as tolerated physically and emotionally
Apply suitable appliance as soon as possible

Expected outcome/evaluation

Patient
Presents healing wounds, with surrounding skin clean, dry, and intact
Demonstrates increasing ability to manage ileostomy

■ **NDX:**   Knowledge deficit related to lack of information about home care management

Reiterate ileostomy care and appliance change; observe return demonstration
Stress importance of and demonstrate skin care of perianal area and ileostomy site
Demonstrate prescribed daily reservoir irrigation
Discuss and teach patient Kegel exercises (squeezing and relaxing perineal muscles) to increase anal sphincter tone
Reinforce physician explanation of stage II procedure and clarify misconceptions
Explain that Gastrografin film of reservoir will be taken in about 6 to 12 weeks to assess reservoir capacity and anatomic location
Explain that manometric studies of anal sphincter tone will also be performed
Stress importance of well-balanced diet, rest, and exercise
Instruct patient about signs and symptoms to report to physician: increasing diarrhea, drainage, foul odor from anus, abdominal distention, absence of feces
Promote follow-up visits with physician

Expected outcome/evaluation

Patient
Demonstrates ability to care for ileostomy and incisions
Verbalizes understanding of surgical procedure, treatment, dietary plan, and potential complications

Stage II: Ileostomy Closure and Anastomosis of Ileum to Anal Reservoir
Preoperative Assessment and Care

See Stage I (p. 279)
Presacral drainage tube is not usually in place, and enemas are not given
Irrigation of reservoir is usually ordered

Postoperative Assessment
Observations/findings

Location, intensity, and character of pain
Color, character, and amount of drainage
    Incisional drainage (abdominal)
    Gastric drainage
    Rectal drainage
Urine output
Skin integrity (perianal area)

Laboratory/diagnostic studies

Electrolytes, CBC, urinalysis

Potential complications

Reservoir abscess, ischemia, fistula
Skin erosion (perianal area)
Intestinal obstruction
Wound or reservoir infection
Cystitis, urinary retention
Phlebitis

Medical Management

Analgesics, antibiotics, antidiarrheals, dermatological creams, ointments
Parenteral fluids with electrolytes and vitamins
Nasogastric suction, NPO
Ileal reservoir irrigation
Indwelling urethral catheter
Diet, rest, ambulation, exercise
Sitz baths

Nursing diagnoses/interventions/evaluation

■ **NDX:**   Potential fluid volume deficit related to risk of abnormal body fluid loss from NPO status, nasogastric suction, and ileoanal reservoir

Maintain NPO; assess for signs of dehydration
Maintain parenteral fluids with electrolytes and vitamins
Monitor nasogastric tube and low, intermittent suction apparatus; irrigate with measured amounts of normal saline to keep patent
Monitor indwelling urethral catheter and closed gravity drainage system; monitor hourly output; if less than 30 to 50 ml/hr notify physician
Measure intake and output q8h
Monitor vital signs q4h
Weigh patient daily at same time with same clothing and scale

Monitor electrolytes, Hgb, Hct
Initiate voiding measures as needed after urethral catheter removal; observe for retention and signs of infection

Expected outcome/evaluation

Patient's
    Vital signs are stable
    Intake and output are balanced
    Weight remains stable
    Hydration is adequate as evidenced by normal skin turgor

■ **NDX:**   Potential for impaired skin integrity (perianal) related to diarrhea

Cleanse perianal area as needed with water or aluminum acetate (Domeboro solution) and soft cloth or cotton balls; dry thoroughly with hair dryer
Cover with skin barrier prn and use Tuck's pads
Administer sitz baths
Irrigate ileal reservoir daily and monitor return solution for blood, foul odor

Expected outcome/evaluation

Patient's
    Perianal wound is healing
    Surrounding skin is clean, dry, and intact

■ **NDX:**   Potential bowel incontinence related to ileal output and lack of sphincter control

Monitor bowel movements for frequency and consistency; will be frequent initially (10 to 20/day)
Collaborate with physician and provide well-balanced diet after nasogastric tube removal; introduce fresh fruits, spices, and dairy products one at a time to determine tolerance
Monitor for effectiveness/side effects of psyllium (Metamucil), diphenoxylate (Lomotil) to control diarrhea
Promote Kegel exercises qh to increase sphincter tone

Expected outcome/evaluation

Patient
    Defecates fewer and more formed stools
    Demonstrates ability to perform Kegel exercises

■ **NDX:**   Knowledge deficit related to lack of information about home care management

Stress importance of protecting perineal area
    After urinating or defecating cleanse area with water and dry thoroughly, using hair dryer when possible; take sitz baths prn
    Apply skin sealants, lotions, and dermatological creams prn

Avoid harsh, perfumed soaps and nylon underwear

Daily reservoir irrigation may be needed to prevent infection

Discuss bowel elimination; frequency will become less (6 to 10/day) and eventually drop to 3 to 4/day

Some incontinence may be noted at night; pads may be worn as protection

Psyllium (Metamucil) and loperamide (Imodium) will help avoid diarrhea

Use loperamide for only 48 hr; observe for abdominal distention

Provide information about diet and foods that cause diarrhea (spices, fresh fruit, and dairy products)

Instruct patient about signs and symptoms to report to physician: increasing diarrhea, drainage or foul odor from rectum, abdominal distention, absence of feces

Promote follow-up visits with physician

Expected outcome/evaluation

Patient

Verbalizes understanding of treatment and dietary plan, potential complications

Demonstrates ability to care for reservoir correctly

CARE OF NASO-ORAL INTESTINAL TUBE (CANTOR OR MILLER-ABBOTT TUBE)

Cantor or Miller-Abbott tube *An intestinal tube, 6 to 10 ft (2 to 3.3 m) in length, that is passed through the nose or mouth into the stomach and intestine; a balloon for mercury is attached to the distal end; used for decompression and drainage in patients with bowel*

obstruction or paralytic ileus; tube is advanced manually, by peristaltic action, by gravity and weight of mercury (Figure 5-9)

Preinsertion Assessment and Care

Reinforce physician's explanation of procedure and its purpose

Assess patient's ability to swallow and willingness to cooperate

Assess abdomen for

Size, shape, softness

Presence or absence of bowel sounds

Assess patient for presence of nausea, vomiting, and pain

Elevate head of bed 60 to 70 degrees; tilt head slightly forward to facilitate tube passage

Check tube for patency

Check that balloon is securely attached and test for leakage by inserting water into balloon via correct lumen with syringe

Prepare syringe with correct amount of mercury

Cantor tube: mercury is injected into balloon via lumen before insertion

Miller-Abbott tube: mercury is inserted into balloon via lumen after insertion

Ice tube according to procedure and lubricate with water-soluble jelly before insertion

Insertion Assessment

Heart rate and rhythm: dysrhythmias may occur as a result of vagal stimulation

Respiratory distress

Vomiting

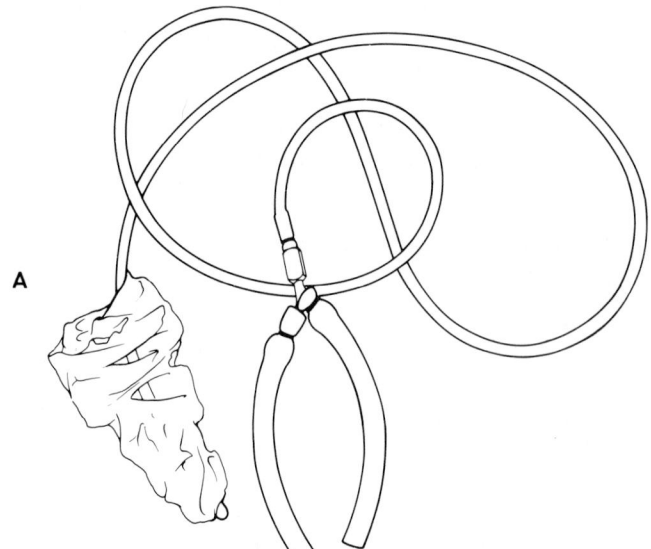
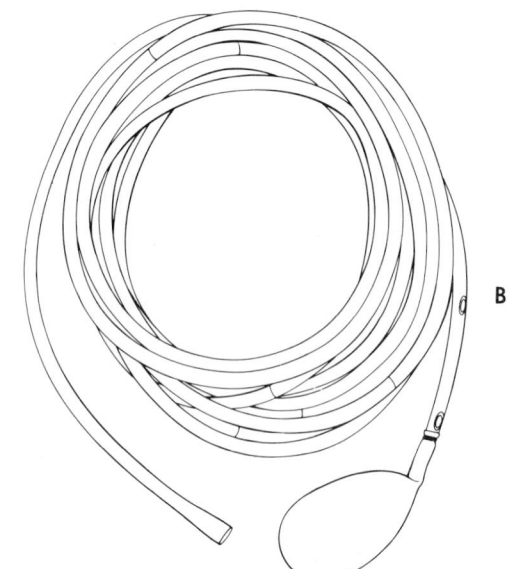

FIGURE 5-9. Intestinal tubes. **A,** Miller-Abbott tube. **B,** Cantor tube. (From Phipps WJ, Long BC, Woods NF et al: Medical-Surgical Nursing: Concepts and clinical practice, ed 4, St Louis, 1991, Mosby—Year Book.)

Postinsertion Assessment
Observations/findings

Nausea, vomiting
Character and amount of drainage
Accurate placement of tube in stomach
Pressure delivered by intermittent suction apparatus
Patency of tube
Position of patient and tube to facilitate passage of tube
Dysphagia
Sore throat
Abdominal distention, pain, or cramps
Increasing bowel sounds
Erosion of nares
Condition of mouth
Blockage of eustachian tube on insertion side

Potential complications

Dehydration
Electrolyte imbalance
Oliguria

Interventions

Maintain NPO; assess for signs of dehydration
Insert prescribed amount of mercury into correct lumen of Miller-Abbott tube and label "mercury"
Connect a nasointestinal tube to low, intermittent suction apparatus
Coil tube and pin to patient's gown; do not tape to nose; avoid placing tension on tube
Monitor color and consistency of intestinal drainage q4h
Irrigate tube gently with measured amounts of normal saline as ordered; if no return flow is obtained, include amount as intake
Measure abdominal girth and auscultate abdomen for bowel sounds q4h; report increasing girth measurements
Turn patient to right side, to back, to left side until tube passes into intestine
Advance tube, usually 3 to 4 inches at specified times; lubricate intestinal tube thoroughly before advancing it
When bowel sounds return and/or flatus or stool is passed and after discussion with physician
    Clamp tube for 2 to 4 hr
    Measure abdominal girth and observe for signs of distention, cramps, or nausea
    If these symptoms occur, unclamp tube and notify physician
    If patient tolerates clamping procedure, administer small, frequent, measured amounts of water and observe tolerance
    If patient tolerates fluids, tube is removed slowly, 2 to 3 inches at a time, or allowed to pass through rectum
    Provide clear liquid diet and progress to diet as tolerated
Maintain bed rest in position of comfort: usually head elevated 30 to 40 degrees

Administer oral hygiene q2h; provide lozenges or hard candy, if allowed, to stimulate salivation
Assess nares for irritation or dryness q2h; gently clean and apply lubricant as needed
Explain purpose of tube and appropriate anatomy and physiology
Discuss advancement of tube and how to avoid dislodgment
Discuss signs and symptoms to report to physician
    Ear pain or fullness on side of insertion
    Nausea or vomiting
    Increased abdominal pain or cramps
    Feeling of abdominal fullness or pressure

ILEOSTOMY, COLOSTOMY MANAGEMENT

ostomy Surgical opening into the intestine to provide temporary or permanent passage of feces; necessitated by carcinoma, inflammation, trauma, or obstruction below the site of the ostomy

Assessment
Observations/findings

Type of ostomy
    Ileostomy: usually permanent
    Colostomy: ascending, transverse, descending; may be temporary or permanent
Removal and closure of rectum
Level of patient's understanding of surgical procedure
Emotional status
    Acceptance of ostomy
    Understanding of ostomy function
    Ability to verbalize feelings
    Acceptance of body image change
Character, frequency, and amount of feces
Size, location, and color of stoma
Condition of skin around stoma
Appropriateness of appliance and size
Placement of stoma
Hydration

Laboratory/diagnostic studies

Electrolytes, Hgb, Hct

Potential complications

Leakage under appliance
Signs of wound infection
Electrolyte imbalance
Dehydration
Intestinal obstruction
Hemorrhage
Ostomy
Prolapse
Stricture
Retraction
Necrosis

Medical Management

Diet management
Corticosteroid aerosal spray, nystatin powder
Odor-control preparation

Nursing diagnoses/interventions/evaluation

■ **NDX:** Potential impairment of skin integrity (peristomal) secondary to ostomy drainage

Initiate peristomal care and apply ostomy appliance as soon postoperatively as possible
Measure stoma for correct appliance size at each appliance change; size should be ⅛ inch larger than stoma measurement
Change appliance prn and observe color, amount, and consistency of feces, and color of stoma and surrounding skin
Maintain peristomal skin integrity
  Wash with mild soap and water and rinse thoroughly with each appliance change; to avoid skin irritation, start with a drainable pouch
  Pat skin dry with towel and apply effective skin barrier (Skin Prep, Stomahesive, Releaseal)
NOTE: *Never place appliance directly on irritated skin*
Apply only clear appliance to facilitate monitoring stoma
Maintain a secure seal around stoma
Involve enterostomal therapist if available
Control odor with deodorant drops or bismuth/chlorophyll preparations

Expected outcome/evaluation

Patient
  Presents a healing wound, and surrounding skin is clean, dry, and intact
  Expresses understanding of ostomy function

■ **NDX:** Body image disturbance related to presence of ileostomy, colostomy

Assist patient and significant other in accepting ostomy
  Allow time for and encourage verbalization
  Answer all questions and explain treatments and procedures
  Provide care in a positive manner; avoid facial expressions connoting distaste
  Observe for signs of inappropriate denial, grief, or anger
  Provide privacy and a safe environment
Assess present coping patterns and explore strengths and resources
Encourage self-care and independence
Set goals with patient for
  Viewing stoma
  Discussing self-care

  Taking steps in performing self-care
Give positive reinforcement for each step taken

Expected outcome/evaluation

Patient
  Expresses feelings and concerns
  Demonstrates positive coping skills in dealing with presence of ostomy
  Views stoma; discusses and performs some steps of care

■ **NDX:** Sexual dysfunction related to ostomy and lack of knowledge

Assess stage of adaptation of patient to ostomy and explain its normalcy
Encourage communication with significant other and explain the need to share feelings
Explain that normal sexual activity can be resumed when allowed
Discuss methods of controlling odor, general hygiene
Provide information about alternative sexual techniques and positions
Encourage counseling if patient is unable to discuss sexuality

Expected outcome/evaluation

Patient
  Verbalizes understanding of the information provided about sexual activity
  Discusses feelings about sexuality with significant other

■ **NDX:** Potential for fluid volume deficit (2) related to risk of increased fluid loss (ileostomy)

Assess for dehydration
Monitor intake and output q8h
Monitor stools for frequent, high-volume output
  Notify physician if this occurs
Weigh daily, same time, clothes, and scale
Monitor vital signs q4h

Expected outcome/evaluation

Patient's
  Vital signs are stable
  Intake and output are balanced
  Weight remains stable
  Hydration is adequate as evidenced by normal skin turgor

■ **NDX:** Constipation (colostomy) or diarrhea (ileostomy) secondary to shortened bowel

Assess patient's previous bowel habits and lifestyle
Reinforce physician's explanation of surgical procedure and anatomy and physiology of ostomy

Colostomy feces will be more solid, whereas with ileostomy will be liquid to pasty

Colostomy may be irrigated to establish near-normal elimination; ileostomy should never be irrigated

Involve significant other when appropriate

Demonstrate irrigation procedure and have patient return demonstration until patient can perform it alone (see below)

Provide information on where to purchase equipment and symptoms of intestinal obstruction or stomal prolapse to report to physician

Collaborate with physician and dietitian for diet instructions, since each patient will differ in foods tolerated

Most ostomy patients are discharged on a general diet and given a list of foods that may cause gas or diarrhea

Follow these general rules

Ileostomates should have foods high in sodium and potassium: bananas, bouillon, citrus juices, tea, cola, rye flour, molasses

Ileostomates should avoid gas-producing foods, fried foods, highly seasoned foods, nuts, raisins, rich foods, and all raw fruits except bananas

Colostomates should avoid gas-producing foods such as cabbage, beans, corn, broccoli, and cauliflower if gas is uncomfortable or embarrassing

Each patient will have to use a trial-and-error method to establish which foods can be tolerated

Introduce new foods one at a time

Stress adequate nutritional and fluid intake

Stress eating slowly, chewing food well, and eating regular meals

Advise avoiding extremes in temperature of foods and carbonated beverages

Involve patient and/or significant other in meal planning

Auscultate abdomen for bowel sounds q8h; report absent sounds to physician

Discuss signs and symptoms of obstruction or stricture

Decreased drainage, constipation

Diarrhea

Cramps, abdominal distention

Nausea, vomiting

Expected outcome/evaluation

Patient

Expresses understanding of ostomy function

Begins to care for stoma and ostomy

■ **NDX:** Knowledge deficit related to unfamiliarity with ostomy, diet management, and home care needs

Explain and demonstrate stomal care step-by-step and have patient return demonstration

Discuss equipment used and where to purchase it; provide enough supplies to last a few days after discharge

Provide and explain written information on diet management

Provide information about outside support groups available and refer to home health care as needed

Discuss signs of wound infection, obstruction, prolapse, etc. to report

Encourage follow-up visits with physician

Expected outcome/evaluation

Patient

Demonstrates ability to perform ostomy care correctly

Verbalizes understanding of dietary regimen, potential complications, and available support groups

COLOSTOMY IRRIGATION

A procedure used by some colostomates to clear the bowel of fecal matter and to help establish an evacuation schedule; may not be applicable for all patients

Assessment
Observations/findings

Patient's emotional status

State of acceptance

Knowledge and understanding of procedure

Ability to comprehend

Tolerance of procedure

Size and color of stoma

Location of stoma(s)

Sigmoid colostomy

Descending colostomy

Hydration of patient

Temperature and amount of irrigating solution

Retention of irrigating solution; dehydrated patients may retain some fluid

Amount and character of return flow

Constipation

Diarrhea

Pain

Distention

Potential complications

Stoma constriction

Obstruction

Prolapse

Irrigating Procedure

Usually irrigations are ordered 7 to 10 days after surgery or whenever patient is ready psychologically and/or physically

Explain procedure and equipment

May be done every day or every other day

Use equipment that will be used at home

Demonstrate step-by-step

Assess patient's normal bowel habits

Involve patient in assisting with procedure as soon as physically and emotionally able

Use commode as soon as possible for irrigations to provide a more normal environment

Provide diversional activities after instillation of irrigating solution

During procedure observe these precautions

Have patient sit on commode when possible

Prepare 500 to 1000 ml of warm tap water

Remove all air in tubing

Hold bag at shoulder level or 12 to 18 inches above stoma

Apply irrigation sleeve over stoma; place end in commode

Insert lubricated cone tip gently into stoma; avoid using catheter, since it may cause intestinal perforation

Allow solution to run in slowly

Allow 45 min for return flow

Position change and/or abdominal massage will help if return is slow

Irrigation sleeve may be folded and clipped, and patient encouraged to ambulate

Stoma dilation may be ordered

Using glove, lubricate finger closest to size of stoma

Insert finger gently into stoma, *never* force

Rotate finger gently for 1 min to dilate

Involve significant other when appropriate

Demonstrate procedure and have patient return demonstration until patient can perform it unassisted

Provide information on where to purchase equipment and symptoms of obstruction or prolapse to report to physician

RECTAL SURGERY

Any surgery performed on the rectum, resulting from prolapse, polyps, thrombosed hemorrhoids, tumors, fistulas, or fissures

Assessment
Observations/findings

Character and amount of rectal drainage
Placement of drain
Character, intensity, and location of pain
Urinary output

Potential complications

Abdominal distention
Urinary retention
Hemorrhage
Infection

Medical Management

Analgesic, topical anesthetic ointment
Ice packs, sitz baths, warm compresses

Stool softeners
Diet progression

Nursing diagnoses/interventions/evaluation

■ **NDX:**   Pain related to surgical intervention

When on bed rest, turn side to side q2h

Administer analgesics as required; if ointments are ordered, test first for allergic reaction; assess effectiveness of pain relief measures

Have patient avoid supine position if possible; place pillows between knees while on side

Monitor effectiveness of warm, wet compresses or ice bag

Ambulate with assistance; provide Gelfoam or flotation pads for sitting; avoid rubber rings

Provide planned rest periods; have patient avoid sitting in chair for long periods of time

Administer analgesic before removing packing

Monitor sitz baths for effectiveness

Expected outcome/evaluation

Patient
Verbalizes increasing comfort level
Presents a more relaxed affect

■ **NDX:**   Constipation related to NPO status and painful defecation

Maintain NPO until nausea subsides

Provide low-residue, soft diet as tolerated

Encourage fluids to 2000 to 2500 ml/day unless contraindicated

Monitor for bowel sounds q shift

Administer stool softeners; encourage defecation as soon as urge occurs; provide privacy

Monitor effectiveness of stool softeners

Encourage activity and ambulation as soon as possible

Expected outcome/evaluation

Patient's
Bowel sounds are normal
Bowel movements are soft and formed

■ **NDX:**   Potential for altered urinary elimination pattern related to proximity of surgical procedure to bladder

Measure intake and output for 24 hr; observe for signs of urinary retention

Use voiding measures if necessary; run water nearby, pour warm water over lower abdomen, place hands in water, etc.

Assist patient with voiding: assist males to stand and void; females elevate head of bed or use commode

Promote and assist with ambulation to increase urge to void

Expected outcome/evaluation

Patient
    Reports urine is clear and pale yellow and of adequate amount
    Expresses ability to void without discomfort

■ **NDX:** Potential for risk of infection related to inadequate primary defenses

Monitor vital signs q4h
Observe dressings q2h to 4h; check for bleeding, drainage, odor, and packing
Change dressings prn; apply petroleum gauze
Cleanse perianal area after each bowel movement

Expected outcome/evaluation

Patient's
    Wound is healing adequately
    Surrounding tissue is clean, dry, and intact

■ **NDX:** Knowledge deficit related to lack of information about home care

Discuss importance of diet management
    Maintain low-residue diet for 1 week
    Increase roughage as tolerated
    Include fresh fruits
    Force fluids to 2500 ml daily unless contraindicated
Demonstrate care of incision and perirectal area
    Take sitz baths as ordered
    Use warm compresses
    Use petroleum gauze pads
    Cleanse perineal area well and dry thoroughly after each bowel movement
    Apply dressing
Discuss symptoms of wound infection and anal stricture to report to physician
Discuss maintaining soft bowel movements with use of stool softeners and natural laxative foods
Explain importance of avoiding heavy lifting and straining
Encourage follow-up visits with physician

Expected outcome/evaluation

Patient
    Verbalizes understanding of dietary plan, potential complications, and activity restrictions
    Demonstrates ability to perform incisional care accurately
    Participates in needed treatment program

Gallbladder

BILIARY OBSTRUCTION (STONES, INFECTION)

Obstruction of the common and/or cystic bile ducts caused by stones, which inhibits the drainage of bile and causes an acute inflammatory process to occur

Assessment
Observations/findings

Midepigastric colicky pain
Pain may radiate to shoulder
Nausea, vomiting
Chills
Fever
Dark, concentrated urine
Clay-colored feces
Weight loss
Tachycardia
Tachypnea
Abdominal distention

Laboratory/diagnostic studies

WBC (elevated over 12,000)
Serum bilirubin
Serum amylase
Ultrasound/radiological abdominal series
Biliary scintigraphy
Cholecystogram (for chronic cholecystitis only)
Chest radiological study (to rule out pneumonitis)
Prothrombin time (PT)

Potential complications

Jaundice
    Skin
    Sclera
Dehydration
Electrolyte imbalance
Bleeding tendencies (vitamin K deficiency)
Peritonitis if rupture occurs

Medical Management

Analgesics, antibiotics, antiemetics, anticholinergics, vitamin K
NPO
Nasogastric suction
Parenteral fluids with electrolytes
Diet and activity
Surgical intervention: cholecystectomy with exploration of common bile duct or cholecystotomy

Nursing diagnoses/interventions/evaluation

■ **NDX:** Potential for fluid volume deficit related to risk of abnormal loss of body fluids from NPO status, gastric suction

Maintain NPO, assess for signs of dehydration
Monitor vital signs q4h prn
Maintain parenteral fluids with electrolytes, vitamin K, antibiotics
Monitor nasogastric tube and low, intermittent suction apparatus; irrigate with measured amounts of normal saline prn
Auscultate abdomen for bowel sounds q8h

Measure intake and output q8h; note color and consistency of urine, stools, and gastric contents
Monitor serum electrolytes, PT
Observe for jaundice, pruritis, vitamin K deficiency
Monitor stools for clay color or return of bile
Monitor skin turgor q8h

Expected outcome/evaluation

Patient's
    Vital signs are stable
    Intake and output are balanced
    Electrolytes are within normal limits
    Hydration is adequate as evidenced by normal skin turgor

■ **NDX:**   Pain related to disease process, presence of stones, infection

Assess character, location, and intensity of pain
Administer analgesics (avoid morphine) and anticholinergics; assess effectiveness of pain relief measures
Maintain bed rest in position of comfort: usually head elevated 30 to 45 degrees; do not gatch knees
Teach alternate pain relief measures
Change position frequently in small ways to promote comfort

Expected outcome/evaluation

Patient
    Reports a reduction in pain intensity
    Appears more relaxed

■ **NDX:**   Altered nutrition: less than body requirements related to vomiting and decreased nutritional intake

After removal of nasogastric tube, collaborate with physician to initiate clear liquid diet and progress to low-fat, soft diet as tolerated
Monitor bowel sounds; observe for distention
Monitor serum BUN, albumin
Encourage fluids to 2500 ml/day unless contraindicated
Monitor for food intolerances
Provide quiet, nonstressful environment at mealtimes
Discuss food preferences
Encourage activity and ambulation
Weigh patient daily at same time with same clothing and scale

Expected outcome/evaluation

Patient
    Maintains desired weight
    Tolerates prescribed diet

■ **NDX:**   Knowledge deficit related to lack of information regarding home care needs

Provide information about increasing biliary distress and complications to report
On discharge, provide and discuss written dietary instructions on low-fat diet
    Avoid gas-producing foods
Advise patient and/or significant other to increase fat in diet slowly
Discuss need for weight loss if appropriate
Discuss importance of rest, especially after eating
Stress importance of activity to tolerance
Encourage follow-up visits with physician

Expected outcome/evaluation

Patient
    Verbalizes understanding of needed dietary plan, potential complications, and increasing biliary distress to report
    Participates in treatment plan

BILIARY SURGERY

Surgery of the gallbladder, such as cholecystectomy (removal of gallbladder), choledocholithotomy (removal of stones in common bile duct), or choledochojejunostomy (anastomosis of the common bile duct to the jejunum)

Assessment
Observations/findings

Respiratory distress
Diminished breath sounds
Splinting with respirations
Tachypnea
Bradypnea
Character and amount
    Gastric drainage
    Bile drainage (T tube)
    Drainage from incision
    Urinary output
Location, intensity, and character of pain

Laboratory/diagnostic studies

Electrolytes, Hgb, Hct

Potential complications

Dehydration
Electrolyte imbalance
Hemorrhage
Shock
Peritonitis (p. 267)
Jaundice (3 to 4 days postoperatively)
Signs of wound infection
Thrombophlebitis (p. 70)
Atelectasis
Pulmonary embolus (p. 211)

Medical Management

Analgesics, antibiotics, vitamin K
Nasogastric suction, NPO
Parenteral fluids with electrolytes
Oxygen therapy, incentive spirometer
Oral replacement of bile salts
T tube drainage and clamping
Diet, activity, rest

Nursing diagnoses/interventions/evaluation

■ **NDX:** Ineffective breathing pattern related to decreased lung expansion and pain

Assess respiratory status; observe for splinting and shallow, rapid breathing
Auscultate lungs for breath sounds q2h
Administer incentive spirometer q2h to 4h
Administer pain medication to assist patient to move and deep breathe
Assist and teach patient to turn and cough q2h and deep breathe qlh; support incision
Elevate head 20 to 30 degrees; do not gatch knees

Expected outcome/evaluation

Patient
    Demonstrates ability to turn, cough, and deep breathe
    Uses incentive spirometer correctly
    Exhibits normal respirations and breath sounds

■ **NDX:** Potential fluid volume deficit related to NPO status and risk of increased body fluid loss from nasogastric suction

Maintain NPO; assess for signs of dehydration
Maintain parenteral fluids with electrolytes and vitamin K
Monitor nasogastric tube and low, intermittent suction apparatus; irrigate prn to maintain patency with measured amounts of normal saline
Monitor intake and output q8h; observe for urinary retention
Monitor T tube and closed gravity drainage system if applicable; observe color and amount of drainage q8h; report drainage greater than 500 ml/24 hr to physician
Replace bile salts
Monitor serum electrolytes, Hct, and Hgb
Monitor stools for clay-colored feces and urine for presence of bile
Monitor for vitamin K deficiency
Weigh patient prn with same clothes and scale
Encourage movement of feet and legs to increase venous return

Expected outcome/evaluation

Patient's
    Intake and output are balanced
    Vital signs are stable

Hydration is adequate as evidenced by normal skin turgor

■ **NDX:** Potential for impaired tissue integrity related to T tube drainage, altered nutritional state, and invasive procedure

Monitor incision q2h for 8 hr, then q4h
Reinforce and change dressing prn
Report excess drainage or bleeding to physician
Cover "stab wound" drain with ostomy appliance or sterile dressing; change prn
Monitor vital signs q4h
Administer injections with small-gauge needle and apply more pressure longer
Provide swabs for oral hygiene if bleeding gums are noted
Assess patency of T tube q2h; observe for kinks in tubing
Anchor tubing to allow for freedom of movement
Assess skin around T tube q2h to 4h; clean prn with soap and water; rinse and pat dry
Apply petroleum jelly gauze or Skin Prep as needed to prevent irritation
Apply Montgomery straps as indicated to prevent adhesive burns
Observe skin and sclera for jaundice or pruritus
Provide distracting activities and remind patient not to scratch if pruritus is present
Collaborate with physician and clamp T tube after meals; observe for distention, cramps, and pain; unclamp T tube if symptoms occur and notify physician
Ambulate with assistance as tolerated

Expected outcome/evaluation

Patient's
    Wound is healing well
    Surrounding tissue is clean, dry, and intact

■ **NDX:** Pain related to surgical intervention

Assess location, type, and intensity of pain
Administer analgesics and assess effectiveness of pain relief measures
Maintain bed rest in quiet environment
Change position frequently; administer back rubs to promote comfort
Discuss alternate pain management techniques

Expected outcome/evaluation

Patient
    Reports a reduction of pain
    Appears relaxed and comfortable

■ **NDX:** Knowledge deficit related to lack of information about home care needs

Provide and review written diet instructions and restrictions; fats may be added as tolerated
Demonstrate care of incision and T tube (if applicable)

T tube requires draining of collection bag at prescribed times

Demonstrate record-keeping procedure

Explain signs/symptoms to report to physician; increased epigastric pain, dark urine, clay-colored stools, jaundice

Discuss importance of increasing activity to tolerance and planned rest periods

Explain that bowel movements may be loose for a while because of increased amount of bile

Encourage follow-up visits with physician

Expected outcome/evaluation

Patient

Expresses understanding of disease process, nutrition plan, and potential complications

Demonstrates ability to care for incision and T tube

BILIARY LITHOTRIPSY

Extracorporeal shock wave lithotripsy (ESWL) a noninvasive procedure performed under analgesia, using high-energy shock waves to disintegrate gallstones, allowing them to pass through the common bile duct into the intestine

Assessment
Observations/findings

Condition of skin at treatment site; redness, bruising, hematoma

Abdominal tenderness

Location and character of pain

Hematuria

Nausea, vomiting

Biliary colic; severe pain right upper quadrant

Laboratory/diagnostic studies

Preprocedure: lipase, amylase, bilirubin, creatinine, PT, PTT, Hgb, Hct, SGOT, SGPT

Oral cholangiogram

Potential complications

Retained fragments causing common duct obstruction

Jaundice, severe abdominal pain

Fever, nausea, vomiting

Acute cholangitis

Medical Management

Low-fat diet

Analgesics

Dicyclomine hydrochloride (Bentyl) for colic

Nursing diagnoses/interventions/evaluation

■ **NDX:** Ineffective breathing pattern related to decreased lung expansion

Assess respiratory status q4h to 8h

Monitor respirations for splinting and/or shallow, rapid breathing

Auscultate lungs for breath sounds q4h to 8h

Elevate head of bed 20 to 45 degrees

Assist and teach patient to deep breathe qh

Expected outcome/evaluation

Patient

Exhibits normal breath sounds

Demonstrates ability to perform breathing exercises correctly

■ **NDX:** Potential for fluid volume deficit related to risk of abnormal fluid loss from NPO status

Assess for signs of dehydration

Maintain parenteral fluids until fully reacted

Monitor vital signs q4h

Monitor intake and output q4h; observe for hematuria

Monitor for signs of jaundice

Encourage ambulation

Provide fluids to tolerance (2000 ml)

Provide low-fat diet as tolerated

Expected outcome/evaluation

Patient's

Vital signs are stable

Intake and output are balanced

Tolerance for low-fat diet is without discomfort

■ **NDX:** Pain related to corrective procedure and treatment

Assess location, intensity, and character of pain

Evaluate effectiveness of pain relief measures

Provide diversional activities

Change patient position frequently to promote comfort

Discuss alternate pain relief techniques

Notify physician if pain is severe and long lasting or does not respond to analgesics

Expected outcome/evaluation

Patient

Reports a decrease in pain or no pain

Presents a more relaxed affect

■ **NDX:** Knowledge deficit related to lack of information about home and follow-up care

Encourage returning to normal activities

Provide and review written dietary instructions

Low-fat diet to regular diet depending on tolerance

High-fat foods may cause discomfort; dicyclomine hydrochloride (Bentyl) usually relieves the pain

Discuss signs and symptoms to report to physician
  Severe nausea, vomiting
  Fever about 38°C (101°F)
  Severe abdominal pain, jaundice
Encourage follow-up visits with physician for ultrasonography and laboratory tests

Expected outcome/evaluation

Patient verbalizes understanding of diet plan, potential complications, and follow-up treatment plan

LAPAROSCOPIC, ENDOSCOPIC LASER CHOLECYSTECTOMY

Removal of the gallbladder without a surgical incision; four small punctures are made in the abdominal wall, and, with the use of a laparoscopic laser, the gallbladder is removed

Postoperative Assessment
Observations/findings

Respiratory function
Type, location, intensity of pain
Location of puncture wounds
Amount of drainage, bleeding
Nausea, vomiting

Laboratory/diagnostic studies

Electrolytes
Urinalysis

Potential complications

Hemorrhage
Bile leakage into abdominal cavity

Medical Management

Analgesics
Diet
Activity and exercise

Nursing diagnoses/interventions/evaluation

■ **NDX:** Ineffective breathing pattern related to decreased lung expansion

Maintain bed rest until fully reactive
Assess respiratory status including breath sounds q4h to 8h
Elevate head of bed 20 to 45 degrees
Assist and teach patient to deep breathe qh
Ambulate with assistance within 3 to 4 hr postoperatively

Expected outcome/evaluation

Patient
  Exhibits normal breath sounds
  Performs deep breathing qh

■ **NDX:** Potential for fluid volume deficit related to risk of abnormal fluid loss from NPO status, nausea, and vomiting

Monitor vital signs q4h
Assess for signs of dehydration
Provide clear liquids as tolerated
  Avoid carbonated beverages to prevent distention
Progress to regular or preprocedure diet as tolerated
Encourage fluids to tolerance unless contraindicated
Calculate intake and output q8h
  Collaborate with physician to correct discrepancies if present

Expected outcome/evaluation

Patient's
  Vital signs are stable
  Intake and output are balanced
  Skin turgor is good
  Tolerance of diet and fluids is good

■ **NDX:** Pain related to corrective procedure

Assess location, intensity, and character of pain
Assess effectiveness of analgesics; avoid IM medications as they can cause drowsiness and decreased mobility
Notify physician if pain is unrelieved, severe, or long lasting

Expected outcome/Evaluation

Patient
  Reports decreasing or absent pain/discomfort
  Presents a more relaxed affect

■ **NDX:** Potential for altered protection related to abnormal blood profile caused by hemorrhage

Monitor dressings for bleeding or bile drainage; change prn
Assess abdomen for distention or severe pain
Monitor vital signs q4h

Expected outcome/evaluation

Patient's
  Dressing remains dry without evidence of bleeding
  Vital signs are stable
  Abdomen remains soft and nondistended

■ **NDX:** Knowledge deficit related to lack of information about home and follow-up care

Discuss care of puncture sites and signs/symptoms to report to physician
  Wound drainage, redness, edema
  Abdominal distention

Nausea, vomiting

Increased pain

Instruct regarding prescribed activities, usually not limited after 2 to 3 days (usually discharged in 24 to 48 hr)

Discuss importance of maintaining diet and fluid intake

Expected outcome / evaluation

Patient

Verbalizes understanding of potential complications and follow-up treatment plan

Demonstrates care of puncture sites

T TUBE MANAGEMENT

*T **tube** A tube placed in the common bile duct to carry off excessive bile, decrease the amount of bile flowing into the intestine, and prevent backflow of bile into the liver when the common bile duct has been explored (Figure 5-10)*

Assessment
Observations / findings

Character, color, and amount of bile drainage; less than 500 ml/24 hr is within normal limits

Patency of tube

Leakage around tube

Tube taped securely to skin

Skin integrity around tube

Color, consistency, and frequency of stools

Potential complications

Jaundice: sclera, skin

Electrolyte imbalance

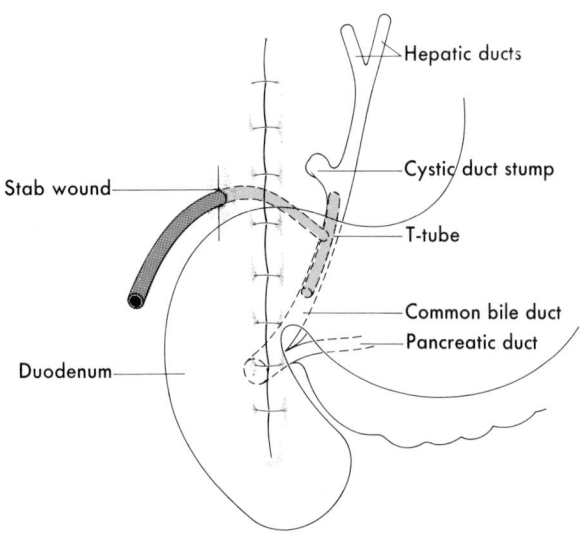

FIGURE 5-10. T tube. (From Beare PG, Myers JL: *Principles and practice of adult health nursing.* St Louis, 1990, Mosby–Year Book.)

Labels in figure:
Hepatic ducts
Cystic duct stump
T-tube
Stab wound
Common bile duct
Pancreatic duct
Duodenum

Abdominal distention

Fat-soluble vitamin (A, D, E, K) deficiency

Interventions

Connect T tube tubing to closed gravity drainage system placed well below incision

Secure connections with tape and allow enough tubing to allow for freedom of movement

Place rolled 4 × 4 pads under T tube at exit site and tape to skin to prevent tension

Monitor skin around T tube exit site; keep clean and dry; use Stomahesive wafer on Skin Prep to prevent irritation

Measure bile output q8h; report output of greater than 500 ml/24 hr to physician

Auscultate abdomen for bowel sounds q8h; report return to physician

Observe first stool for color, consistency, and amount; should be dark, clay color may indicate bile duct blockage

Collaborate with physician to clamp tube and observe for abdominal pain, distention, chills, fever, and nausea; if these occur, unclamp tube and notify physician

Increase time tube is clamped: usually before and after meals to facilitate digestion

Prepare for T tube cholangiogram (7 to 10 days postoperatively); T tube is removed after 24 hr if bile duct is patent

Demonstrate care of skin, drainage system, and incision

Discuss measuring and clamping procedure of T tube

Discuss symptoms to report to physician; pain, increased drainage, distention, fever

Encourage follow-up visits with physician

TRANSHEPATIC BILIARY DECOMPRESSION CATHETER MANAGEMENT

A multivented catheter inserted through the abdominal wall, liver, and common bile duct, and into the duodenum to allow bile to drain past the obstructed bile duct into the intestine; performed for hepatic dysfunction, biliary obstruction (jaundice), and inoperable malignancy of the biliary system

Assessment
Observations / findings

Location of catheter, type of drainage system

Character, color, and amount of drainage

Presence of stabilizing device or sutures

Decreasing jaundice and serum bilirubin

Color, frequency, and amount of stool and urine

Laboratory / diagnostic studies

Catheter usually inserted in radiology department

Postinsertion x-ray examination, cholangiography

Serum bilirubin, electrolytes

Stool for occult blood
Urine for bilirubin

Potential complications

Biliary sepsis
Bleeding or increased retrograde flow of bile
Catheter obstruction
Hyponatremia, electrolyte imbalance

Interventions

Maintain catheter with closed gravity drainage system; place stopcock between catheter and tubing; keep stopcock open

Monitor and measure amount of drainage q2h for 8 hr, then q4h; observe for increased amount of drainage; if more than 1500 ml/24 hr, notify physician immediately

Monitor catheter site for drainage, type of sutures, and dressing q2h to 4h; change dressing prn and apply antibacterial ointment

Collaborate with physician to irrigate catheter through external port of stopcock, closing off drainage bag

Aspirate a few milliliters to ascertain patency

Irrigate gently with prescribed amount of solution; this may be painful for patient, explain before procedure

Do not force irrigation if resistance is met; notify physician since catheter may be obstructed

After instillation open stopcock to allow irrigant to flow into drainage bag

Assess patient's tolerance and observe for increasing, continuous pain, cramping, or abdominal distention (peritonitis, catheter slippage)

Collaborate with physician to clamp catheter and observe patient for decreasing jaundice

Monitor stools, urine, skin, and sclera

Monitor serum bilirubin

Tape catheter comfortably to abdomen; cover with sterile dressing

Monitor electrolytes, especially for hyponatremia; observe for lethargy or altered mental status

Demonstrate and observe return demonstration for catheter irrigation and care

Provide and review written instructions for irrigating procedure

Discuss signs and symptoms of malfunction to report to physician

Fever, chills, weakness

Bleeding, increased bile output

Increasing jaundice, abdominal pain, distention

Dislodgment of catheter

Food particles in catheter drainage

Explain need for frequent visits to radiology department for evaluation of catheter position and function

Promote follow-up visits with physician

Liver

CIRRHOSIS: PORTAL, POSTNECROTIC, BILIARY

Liver disease characterized by the destruction of cells, progressive fibrosis, and eventual nodular formation that results from excessive alcohol intake (70% to 80% of patients), hepatitis, drug toxicity, biliary obstruction, metabolic disease, or congestive heart failure (CHF)

Assessment
Observations/findings

Anorexia
Nausea, vomiting
Weight loss or gain
Abdominal distention
Irregular bowel function
    Clay-colored stools
    Flatulence
    Melena
Ascites
Right upper quadrant pain
Elevated temperature
Pruritus
Decreased urinary output; dark urine
Generalized malaise/weakness
Foul breath
Spider angiomas
Jaundice; sclera, skin
Edema of extremities
Gynecomastia
Dysrhythmias, CHF, jugular venous distention
Clubbing of fingers
Dehydration
Altered mental status
History of substance abuse
History of hepatitis or biliary obstruction

Laboratory/diagnostic studies

Electrolytes
Serum bilirubin (elevated, jaundice)
SGOT, SGPT, LDH (elevated)
Serum albumin (decreased), ammonia (elevated)
CBC, prothrombin time (prolonged), urinalysis
Endoscopic retrograde cholangiopancreatography (ERCP) (common bile duct obstruction)
Esophagoscopy (varices) with barium esophagography
Liver biopsy, scans
Ultrasonography
Percutaneous transhepatic portography (visualizes portal venous system)
Paracentesis (ascites)

Potential complications

Electrolyte imbalance
Malnutrition

Pneumonia
Ascites
Oliguria
GI bleeding
Portal hypertension, esophageal varices, caput medusae (umbilical venous distention)
Hepatomegaly, splenomegaly
Coma

Medical Management

Diuretics, analgesics, antibiotics, lactulose (ammonia detoxicant)
Digestants (Cotazym, Kanulase), vitamins K and C, iron, thiamin, folic acid, antifibrinolytics
Stool softeners
Parenteral fluids with electrolytes
Fresh whole blood, fresh frozen plasma, or platelets
Nasogastric suction
Diet management according to disease process
Sodium and/or fluid restriction
Oxygen therapy, incentive spirometer

Nursing diagnoses/interventions/evaluation

■ **NDX:** Altered nutrition: less than body requirements related to inadequate diet, vomiting, and/or anorexia

Maintain bed rest in quiet environment
Provide small, frequent feedings of prescribed diet; amount of fat, carbohydrate, and protein will depend on patient's ability to metabolize these nutrients; salt may be restricted; monitor caloric intake using diary
Provide salt substitute
Assist and encourage patient to eat, and consider preferences in food choices
Provide oral hygiene prn, especially before meals

Expected outcome/evaluation

Patient
  Tolerates prescribed diet
  Demonstrates understanding of needed diet changes
  Gains optimum weight

■ **NDX:** Potential fluid volume deficit related to risk of increased loss of body fluids resulting from vomiting, fever, and nasogastric tube

Assess for dehydration
Monitor for jugular vein distention
Assess for dependent edema
Maintain NPO; maintain parenteral fluids with electrolytes and vitamins; restrict fluid intake as ordered
Measure intake, output, and abdominal girth q8h
Note consistency, color, and frequency of stools and urine
Monitor serum and urine electrolytes; observe for signs of sodium and/or potassium imbalance

Monitor vital signs q4h; observe for elevated temperature and dysrhythmias
Weigh patient daily at same time with same clothing and scale
Assess for effectiveness/side effects of diuretics

Expected outcome/evaluation

Patient's
  Vital signs are stable
  Intake and output are balanced
  Edema is decreasing; no jugular vein distention is present
  Electrolytes are within normal limits

■ **NDX:** Potential impairment of tissue integrity related to edema, dehydration, and/or jaundice

Assess skin for breaks, reddened areas, pruritus, and jaundice
Provide sheepskin with alternating pressure mattress as indicated
Administer skin care frequently; provide clean linen prn; use lotion and clip nails as needed; administer cholestyramine for pruritus
Provide perineal care after urination and bowel movement; apply lotions to prevent breakdown
Turn patient q2h and administer back care; change position slightly prn to promote comfort
Perform passive or assist with active ROM exercises q4h

Expected outcome/evaluation

Patient
  Demonstrates understanding of needed techniques to prevent skin impairment
  Participates in these activities
  Maintains tissue integrity

■ **NDX:** Potential for ineffective breathing pattern related to debilitated state and ascites

Elevate head of bed 45 to 60 degrees or as needed to maintain ventilation
Assist and teach patient to turn and cough q4h; deep breathe q½h
Auscultate lungs for breath sounds q4h
Assist and teach patient to use incentive spirometer q2h
Monitor blood gases
Assess for signs of hypoxia (altered mentation)

Expected outcome/evaluation

Patient's
  Blood gases are within normal limits
  Respirations and mental acuity are normal
  Breath sounds are clear

NDX: Potential for altered protection, hemorrhage related to risk of impaired blood coagulation or bleeding from portal hypertension

Monitor mucous membranes for signs of bleeding; avoid hard-bristled toothbrushes

Observe injection sites for prolonged bleeding; apply extra pressure and pressure bandage; use small-gauge needles

Monitor patient's use of razors and other objects

Avoid straining during bowel movement and forceful nose-blowing

Monitor PT and platelet count

Administer vitamin K and antifibrinolytic agents; assess for effectiveness/side effects

Observe for signs of bleeding; decreasing BP, increasing P, hematemesis, melena

Monitor vital signs, Hgb, Hct

Prepare for endoscopy if bleeding occurs

Monitor nasogastric tube and low, intermittent suction apparatus

    Measure gastric output qh and note color and consistency; irrigate, if ordered, with measured amounts of saline to maintain patency

Maintain parenteral fluids and/or transfusions

Administer vitamin K, vasopressin, and neomycin; avoid aspirin use

Expected outcome/evaluation

Patient

    Demonstrates understanding and ability to perform needed changes in activities

    Has absent or controlled bleeding

 NDX: Potential for altered thought processes as related to risk of increased serum ammonia and hepatic coma

Monitor frequently for changes in mental status, lethargy, drowsiness, and confusion

Monitor neurological status for decreased motor ability

Avoid use of sedatives, tranquilizers, and narcotics

Provide safe environment: side rails up and bed in low position

Monitor serum ammonia levels

Monitor for possible violent behavior

Reduce environmental stimulus

Acknowledge feelings of anger or fear

Assist patient to redirect aggressive behavior to an adaptive activity

Orient person to time and place as appropriate in each interaction

Teach and assist with stress-reduction techniques

Help to focus on accomplishing self-care activities; assist with ADLs as necessary only

Provide high-calorie, low-protein diet if mental deterioration occurs

Expected outcome/evaluation

Patient's

    Mental acuity is improving or normal

    Orientation to name, time, place is accurate

    Ability to focus on and accomplish ADLs increases

■ **NDX:** Knowledge deficit related to lack of information about home care management

Provide and discuss written dietary instructions from dietitian, listing amount of protein, carbohydrate, fat, and salt allowed

Discuss and teach stress management techniques

Discuss with patient importance of avoiding stress during meals and need to eat small, frequent meals

Provide information on community resources available for alcohol rehabilitation and assistance if applicable

Reinforce physician's explanation of relationship between alcohol and cirrhosis if applicable

Provide information about medications, including name, purpose, dosage, time of administration, and side effects; caution against using any medicine not prescribed by physician

Explain importance of rest and exercise, avoiding exposure to infection

Discuss skin care if pruritus persists

Discuss signs of progression of disease: hematuria, melena, abdominal distention, edema, fever, bleeding that does not subside, mental deterioration, personality changes

Encourage follow-up visits with physician

Ensure that significant other knows and understands symptoms of mental status change or behavior changes to report

Provide information about support groups in community

Expected outcome/evaluation

Patient

    Expresses understanding of disease process, needed dietary regimen, and potential complications

    Participates in own care; indicates willingness to alter lifestyle as needed.

VIRAL HEPATITIS

infectious Virus A (HAV); rapid onset of symptoms and destruction of liver cells caused by contaminated water or food; usually affects young adults

serum Virus B (HBV); slow onset of symptoms and destruction of liver cells caused by contaminated serum from needles and instruments; affects all age groups

non-A, non-B, Hepatitis C; little is known about this virus, but it manifests symptoms similar to HBV

Assessment
Observations/findings

Anorexia
Malaise

Headache
Tenderness and pain in right upper quadrant
Arthritic pain (HBV)
Elevated temperature (HAV)
Jaundice
  Pruritus
  Urticaria
  Sclera
  Clay-colored stools
  Dark urine
Nausea, vomiting
Diarrhea
History of IV drug use
History of accidental exposure to contaminated needles
  or instruments

Laboratory/diagnostic studies

Serum SGOT, SGPT, bilirubin (elevated)
Alkaline phosphatase, lactic dehydrogenase (elevated)
PT (elevated in severe hepatitis)
Stool and serology for HAV
Serum antigen/antibody tests for HBV
CBC, urinalysis, electrolytes
Liver biopsy

Potential complications

Decreased urinary output
Dehydration and electrolyte imbalance
Altered mental status
Hyperglycemia or hypoglycemia
Hepatic coma

Medical Management

Activity
Sedatives, antiemetics, antacids, vitamin K
Diet according to tolerance of protein, carbohydrates, and
  fat
Parenteral therapy with electrolytes and vitamins for vom-
  iting or GI bleeding
Nasogastric suction
Antihistamines and cholestyramine for pruritus

Nursing diagnoses/interventions/evaluation

■ **NDX:** Activity intolerance related to weakness or fatigue secondary to infection

Maintain bed rest in quiet environment; assist patient in
  assuming position of comfort; bathroom privileges may
  be allowed
Assist and teach patient to turn q2h and deep breathe
  q½h
Change position frequently to promote comfort
Administer sedatives; assess for effectiveness/side effects
Provide diversional activities
Assist with and teach active or perform passive ROM

exercises q4h while patient is in bed
Coordinate care to provide planned rest periods
Ambulate with assistance
Assess response to increased activity
Reinforce progress toward independence

Expected outcome/evaluation

Patient
  Expresses understanding of changes needed in activity
    levels
  Increases activities as strength returns

■ **NDX:** Altered nutrition: less than body requirements
secondary to anorexia, vomiting, altered intestinal absorption

Collaborate with physician, dietitian and provide soft
  diet, monitoring intake of protein, fat, and carbohydrates
Offer small, frequent meals, attractively prepared
Encourage fluids to 2500 ml/24 hr unless contraindicated;
  include fruit juices and carbonated beverages since they
  are easily digested
Assess for effectiveness/side effects of antacids and antiemetics; avoid Compazine and Thorazine
Weigh patient daily at same time with same clothing and
  scale
Provide oral hygiene prn, especially before meals
Monitor blood glucose

Expected outcome/evaluation

Patient
  Gains weight, progressing toward normal
  Tolerates prescribed diet

■ **NDX:** Potential fluid volume deficit related to risk of
excessive loss of body fluids resulting from vomiting, fever, diarrhea

Maintain NPO if vomiting and/or anorexia present
Maintain parenteral fluids with electrolytes and vitamin K
Assess for signs of dehydration; skin turgor, pedal pulses,
  etc.
Measure intake and output q8h
Monitor stool and urine for color, consistency, and fre-
  quency
Monitor for ascites, increasing jaundice, and mental de-
  terioration
Monitor vital signs, electrolytes, Hgb, Hct

Expected outcome/evaluation

Patient's
  Vital signs are stable
  Intake and output are balanced
  Skin turgor is normal

■ **NDX:** Potential for altered protection related to abnormal blood profile/coagulation

Assess for signs of bleeding: mucous membranes, injection sites, emesis, stool
Monitor coagulation studies
Use small-gauge needles for injections and apply increased pressure longer; rotate sites
Evaluate effectiveness of vitamin K administration

Expected outcome/evaluation

Patient is free of bleeding as evidenced by clear skin, absence of bleeding at gums and injection sites, no occult blood in urine and feces, normal coagulation studies

■ **NDX:** Potential for impaired skin integrity related to jaundice and ensuing pruritus

Administer frequent skin care; avoid soap or use super-fatted soap
Provide shower or bath with baking soda or starch; apply lotions
Assess effectiveness of cholestyramine
Offer frequent back rubs and changes in position
Encourage short fingernails or use of gloves

Expected outcome/evaluation

Patient
    Reports decreased pruritis/scratching
    Participates in activities to maintain skin integrity, skin is intact

■ **NDX:** Potential for infection related to inadequate secondary defenses and malnutrition

Establish and explain blood and body fluid precautions to prevent transmission to others
Ensure that all contacts are protected against hepatitis
Assess T and breath sounds q4h to 8h
Restrict visitors with infections, especially URIs
Provide nutritious diet with fluids to 2000 ml/24h

Expected outcome/evaluation

Patient
    Demonstrates understanding of precautions by following guidelines
    Maintains normal temperature, and respirations are clear with no other evidence of infection

■ **NDX:** Disturbance in self-concept related to disease process, hospitalization, and isolation

Encourage and allow time for communication of fears and concerns

Reinforce physician's explanation of disease process and treatment rationale
Explain purpose of isolation procedure to patient and/or significant other
Assess present coping patterns and be supportive and understanding
Encourage communication with significant other
Avoid making judgments about lifestyle
Promote bright colors (red, blue) in clothing to offset jaundice

Expected outcome/evaluation

Patient
    Uses adaptive coping measures as evidenced by discussion of feelings
    Uses diversional activities and maintains personal grooming

■ **NDX:** Knowledge deficit related to lack of information about disease process and transmission and home care management

Provide and discuss written diet instructions on amounts of protein, carbohydrate, and fat allowed; no alcohol for 1 year
Explain importance of rest and exercise
    Avoid heavy lifting, strenuous exercise, and contact sports
    Exercise to tolerance and get plenty of rest and sleep
Discuss techniques to prevent transmission
    HAV: perineal care, handwashing after toileting, and disinfection of soiled articles of clothing
    HAV and NANB: caution not to share razors or toothbrushes and to avoid serum or secretion contact with others
    Explain infectious nature of HAV, HBV, and non-B, and the need to avoid infecting others until laboratory values are normal; importance of not donating blood; need to avoid others with infections, especially URIs
    Provide information about drug rehabilitation program if appropriate
    Stress importance of follow-up medical care for 1 year
        Regular laboratory tests as ordered
        Routine follow-up care with physician
Encourage family members and friends to seek injection of gamma globulin, ISG, HBIG, hepatitis B vaccine
Discuss symptoms of recurrence to report to physician
Provide instructions about medication, including name, purpose, dosage, time of administration, and side effects; explain need to avoid medicines not prescribed by physician

Expected outcome/evaluation

Patient
    Verbalizes understanding of disease process, methods to

avoid transmission, needed lifestyle changes, dietary plan, and potential complications

Expresses willingness to participate in treatment at home

HEPATIC SURGERY

Surgical removal or repair of portions of the liver resulting from trauma or carcinoma

Preoperative Assessment and Care

Assess cardiovascular, respiratory, cerebral, and renal status; obtain baseline vital signs; observe for jaundice

Prepare bowel as ordered; enemas, oral antibiotics, magnesium preparations; keep enemas to a minimum to prevent dehydration

Insert nasogastric tube and/or indwelling urethral catheter as ordered; monitor aspirate and/or urine for color and consistency

Administer vitamin K and/or blood transfusions

Reinforce physician's explanation of surgical procedure and postoperative care; explain that chest tubes may be present

Provide emotional support to patient and/or significant others

Postoperative Assessment
Observations/findings

Placement of chest tubes and drainage apparatus if applicable
Character and amount of
    Chest drainage if applicable
    Gastric drainage
    Urinary output
    Wound drainage
Nausea, vomiting
Abdominal distention
Tachycardia
Tachypnea
Splinting of respirations
Decreased breath sounds
Elevated temperature

Laboratory/diagnostic studies

Serum electrolytes, albumin, liver function studies
Electrolytes, CBC, glucose, PT

Potential complications

Electrolyte imbalance
Decreased serum albumin levels
Hypoglycemia
Atelectasis (p. 220)
Pneumonia (p. 205)
Paralytic ileus (p. 271)
Hemorrhage

Shock
Subdiaphragmatic abscess
Jaundice
Ascites
Hepatic coma
Wound infection

Medical Management

Analgesics
Nasogastric suction, NPO
Parenteral fluids with electrolytes and vitamin K
Antibiotics, albumin, transfusions
Connection of chest tubes to underwater seal
Oxygen therapy, incentive spirometer
Urethral catheter drainage

Nursing diagnoses/interventions/evaluation

■ **NDX:** Ineffective breathing pattern related to invasive procedure, chest tube placement, and/or pain

Elevate head of bed 30 to 45 degrees; do not gatch knees

Assess placement of chest tubes and connect underwater seal to low, intermittent suction; monitor amount and color of aspirate q4h

Auscultate chest for breath sounds q2h; monitor respiratory rate and for signs of splinting

Assist and teach patient to turn and cough q2h and deep breathe q1½h; support incision; medicate for pain before procedure when possible

Provide incentive spirometer q1h to 2h

Expected outcome/evaluation

Patient
    Exhibits normal respirations
    Verbalizes understanding of need for breathing exercises
    Uses incentive spirometer routinely

■ **NDX:** Potential for fluid volume deficit related to risk of increased body fluid loss resulting from NPO status and/or nasogastric suction

Maintain NPO; assess hydration status

Maintain parenteral fluids with electrolytes and/or antibiotics

Monitor nasogastric tube and low, intermittent suction apparatus; irrigate gently with measured amounts of normal saline to maintain patency

Monitor urethral catheter and closed gravity drainage system; monitor output qh; report output of less than 30 to 50 ml/hr to physician

Measure intake and output q8h

Monitor vital signs q1½h until stable, then q4h

Encourage lower extremity movement to increase venous return

Monitor serum electrolytes, albumin, and glucose

Auscultate abdomen for bowel sounds q8h

Monitor for signs of hypoglycemia: nausea, shakiness, lethargy

Monitor mental acuity q4h

Expected outcome/evaluation

Patient's
Vital signs are stable
Intake and output are balanced
Electrolytes are within normal limits
Skin turgor is normal

■ **NDX:**   Potential for altered protection related to abnormal blood profile, altered clotting factors resulting from hemorrhage

Monitor dressings and incision q2h for drainage or bleeding; reinforce and change prn

Monitor for signs of bleeding; tachycardia, hypotension, cold, clammy skin

Assess for bleeding tendencies; mucous membranes, injection sites

Use small-gauge needles; apply increased pressure longer

Monitor Hgb, Hct, and clotting times

Assess for effectiveness/side effects of vitamin K administration

Expected outcome/evaluation

Patient's blood profiles (Hgb, Hct, clotting time) are within normal limits; there is no evidence of bleeding at sites of injection or wound

■ **NDX:**   Pain related to surgical intervention

Maintain bed rest in quiet environment

Assess type, intensity, and location of pain; use pain rating scale

Administer analgesics and assess effectiveness of pain relief measures; medicate as prescribed for first few postoperative days

Change position frequently; administer back rubs

Discuss alternate pain relief measures and techniques

Provide diversional activities

Encourage balanced activity/rest pattern

Expected outcome/evaluation

Patient
Reports a decrease in pain
Appears relaxed and comfortable

■ **NDX:**   Altered nutrition: less than body requirements related to NPO status, decreased energy

Collaborate with physician to remove or clamp nasogastric tube when bowel sounds return

Provide small amounts of water or clear liquids and monitor tolerance

Progress to soft diet as tolerated; amounts of fat, carbohydrate, and protein will depend on ability of liver to metabolize these nutrients

Measure intake and output

Administer oral hygiene prn; especially before meals

Encourage fluids to 2500 ml/day unless contraindicated

Weigh patient daily at same time with same clothing and scale

Expected outcome/evaluation

Patient's
Weight is maintained or is returning to normal
Prescribed diet is tolerated without discomfort

■ **NDX:**   Knowledge deficit related to lack of information about home care management

Provide and review written diet instructions with amounts of fat, carbohydrate, and protein allowed

Demonstrate care of incision and discuss signs of wound infection to report

Provide information about signs and symptoms to report to physician
Decreased mental acuity, lethargy
Abdominal distention, pain
Jaundice, dyspnea, fever

Discuss medications: name, dosage, purpose, times of administration, side effects, and importance of taking only medicines prescribed by physician

Discuss needed balance between activity and rest

Promote follow-up visits with physician

Expected outcome/evaluation

Patient
Expresses understanding of nutritional regimen, potential complications, and activity program
Demonstrates ability to care for incision

PORTACAVAL-SPLENORENAL SHUNTS FOR PORTAL HYPERTENSION

Procedures for correction of portal hypertension, which develops in patients with cirrhosis of the liver, subsequent bleeding esophageal varices and ascites are a result of obstruction of blood flow within the portal system

portacaval shunt *Blood flow is diverted from the liver by anastomosing the portal vein to the inferior vena cava; performed when obstruction is intrahepatic*

splenorenal shunt *Blood flow is diverted from the liver by anastomosing the splenic vein to the renal vein; performed when the portal vein is obstructed*

Preoperative Assessment and Care

Be aware that
Shunts are usually not performed on patients with active variceal bleeding because of increased surgical risk

Extensive preparation time may be required to physically and emotionally prepare patients for surgery

Assess respiratory, cardiovascular, and neurological status

Assess nutritional and integumentary status

Measure abdominal girth to assess presence or absence of ascites; assist with paracentesis when required

Monitor liver function studies, serum electrolytes, Hgb, Hct, and PT results

Administer prescribed medications

  Antibiotics

  Multivitamins

  Vitamin K

Provide diet with regulated amounts of protein, carbohydrates, salt, fat, and calories as ordered until NPO is required

Administer prescribed parenteral fluids with electrolytes

  TPN (p. 36)

  Transfusions (p. 179)

  Observe puncture site for bleeding

Insert nasogastric tube and indwelling urethral catheter as ordered; be aware that nasogastric tube may be inserted in operating room, since insertion may activate variceal bleeding

Discuss with and teach patient

  ROM exercises to extremities

  Method of turning, deep breathing, and coughing, and use of incentive spirometer

  That chest tubes may be in place postoperatively

Provide supportive environment

Reinforce physician's explanation of surgical procedure

Encourage and deal with verbalization of fears and anxieties

Encourage communication with significant other

Postoperative Assessment
Observations/findings

Placement of chest tubes and drainage apparatus

Character and amount of

  Chest drainage

  Gastric drainage

  Urinary output

  Wound drainage

Splinting of respirations

  Decreased breath sounds

  Tachypnea

  Difficulty in breathing

Mental alertness

Nausea, vomiting

Laboratory/diagnostic studies

Serum electrolytes, albumin, bilirubin, PT

Arterial blood gases

Chest radiography

Potential complications

Dehydration

Electrolyte imbalance

Atelectasis

Decreased serum albumin

Prolonged PT

Jaundice

Ascites

Peripheral edema

Hemorrhage

Shock

Hepatic coma

Wound infection

Medical Management

Analgesics, antibiotics, albumin, vitamin K, lactulose, antacids

Parenteral fluids with electrolytes or TPN

Nasogastric suction, NPO

Chest tube suction

Arterial blood gases

Oxygen therapy, incentive spirometer

Diet, activity

Nursing diagnoses/interventions/evaluation

■ **NDX:** Ineffective breathing pattern related to surgical incision, chest tube placement, and/or pain

Elevate head of bed 30 to 45 degrees; do not gatch knees

Monitor chest tubes and connect underwater seal to low, intermittent suction or as ordered (p. 229); monitor amount and color of aspirate q4h

Auscultate chest for breath sounds q2h; observe respiratory rate for signs of splinting

Monitor arterial blood gases

Provide incentive spirometer qh

Assist and teach patient to turn and cough q2h and deep breathe q½h; support incision

Expected outcome/evaluation

Patient

  Exhibits a normal respiratory rate and clear breath sounds

  Participates in breathing exercises

  Presents blood gases that are within normal limits

■ **NDX:** Potential for fluid volume deficit related to risk of abnormal fluid loss resulting from NPO status and/or nasogastric suction

Maintain NPO; assess for dehydration

Maintain parenteral fluids with electrolytes, vitamins, antibiotics, and/or salt-poor albumin

Monitor nasogastric tube and low, intermittent suction apparatus; irrigate with measured amounts of normal saline to maintain patency

Monitor urethral catheter and closed gravity drainage system; monitor hourly output; report output of less than 30 to 50 ml/hr to physician

Calculate intake and output q8h

Monitor vital signs q½h until stable, then q4h

Monitor serum electrolytes, albumin, and PT

Monitor urine specific gravity q2h to 4h

Auscultate abdomen for bowel sounds and measure abdominal girth q4h (some ascites may be normal)

Monitor ankles for edema (some edema is normal for 2 to 3 days); weigh prn

Monitor skin and sclera for jaundice

Encourage leg movement while in bed to promote venous return

Expected outcome/evaluation

Patient's

Vital signs are stable

Electrolytes are within normal limits

Intake is balanced with output

Skin turgor is good

■ **NDX:** Potential for altered protection related to abnormal blood profile (altered clotting factors) resulting from hemorrhage

Monitor incision and dressings for drainage or bleeding q2h; reinforce and change prn

Monitor nasogastric aspirate for bleeding; report any bleeding immediately to physician

Monitor Hgb, Hct, PT, and vital signs

Administer vitamin K; assess for effectiveness/side effects

Administer injections with small-gauge needle; apply more pressure for longer period

Observe mucous membranes for bleeding

Test stools and urine for occult blood qday

Expected outcome/evaluation

Patient

Presents clotting time within normal limits

Shows no evidence of bleeding at wound or injection sites, or in feces or urine

■ **NDX:** Potential for infection related to altered primary defenses resulting from invasive procedures

Maintain aseptic technique

Change dressings prn; observe for signs of infection and healing process; culture wound if indicated

Monitor temperature and WBC

Administer antibiotics and antipyretics; assess for effectiveness/side effects

Collect urine specimen for culture/sensitivity when indwelling catheter is removed

Expected outcome/evaluation

Patient's

Wound is healing adequately

Temperature and WBC are normal

Urine is clear and without evidence of infection

■ **NDX:** Potential for altered thought processes related to risk of physiological changes in liver function

Monitor mental acuity q4h; observe for confusion, lethargy, or inappropriate behavior

Monitor serum BUN, ammonia, and albumin levels

Orient patient to time and place at each interaction when appropriate; explain all procedures and treatments

Stimulate with diversional activities

Involve patient in care and decision making about care

Avoid analgesics that require liver metabolism: morphine, sedatives

Administer lactulose and monitor for effectiveness/side effects

Expected outcome/evaluation

Patient

Demonstrates appropriate reality orientation

Exhibits BUN and serum ammonia levels within normal limits

Participates in care as planned

■ **NDX:** Pain related to invasive procedure

Maintain bed rest in quiet environment

Assess type, intensity, and location of pain; use pain rating scale

Administer analgesics; avoid morphine and sedatives; phenobarbital or chloral hydrate is usually drug of choice

Assess effectiveness of pain relief measures

Discuss and teach alternate pain relief techniques

Change position frequently; administer back rubs; observe bony prominences for redness or breakdown

Ambulate with assistance when tolerated

Expected outcome/evaluation

Patient

Reports a decrease in level of pain

Appears rested and more relaxed

■ **NDX:** Altered nutrition: less than body requirements related to presurgical nutritional status, NPO status, and negative nitrogen balance

Monitor TPN if applicable; monitor urine for sugar and acetone q4h

Monitor serum glucose

Collaborate with physician to remove or clamp nasogastric tube when bowel sounds return

Provide small amounts of water and/or clear liquids and monitor tolerance

Progress to soft diet as tolerated; amount of fat, carbohydrate, and protein will be regulated according to liver metabolism

Provide frequent small meals; encourage to eat slowly and chew food well

Measure intake and output q8h

Encourage or restrict fluids as indicated

Weigh patient daily at same time with same clothing and scale; measure abdominal girth to ensure that weight gain is not ascites

Expected outcome/evaluation

Patient

Tolerates well-balanced diet

Demonstrates progressive weight gain to near normal

■ **NDX:** Knowledge deficit related to lack of information about disease process and home care management

Reinforce physician's explanation of disease process and treatments; discuss and clarify any misconceptions

Provide and review written diet instructions with amount of fat, carbohydrate, salt, and protein allowed; avoid alcohol and spicy foods

Maintain prescribed fluid intake

Eat slowly; chew foods well

Demonstrate: incisional care, measurement of abdominal girth, daily weight, method of record keeping, and stool testing with Hemastix

Discuss prescribed activities and rest; explain need to avoid heavy lifting and straining for a specified time

Discuss signs and symptoms to report to physician

Decreased mental acuity

Increased girth and weight

Peripheral edema, jaundice

Fever, nausea, vomiting

Tarry stools, hematuria

Provide instructions about medications, including name, purpose, dosage, time of administration, and side effects; explain importance of taking only medications prescribed by physician

Encourage follow-up care with physician

Expected outcome/evaluation

Patient

Verbalizes understanding of dietary regimen, potential complications, and medication schedule

Demonstrates ability to care for incision and follow treatment program at home

LIVER BIOPSY

Introduction of a special needle into the liver to obtain a specimen for pathological examination

Prebiopsy Care

Type and crossmatch for possible transfusion

Monitor baseline vital signs

Assess mental alertness and ability to cooperate

Explain procedure and follow-up care

Administer analgesics or sedatives as ordered

Monitor for allergy to local anesthetic

Teach patient how to inhale and hold breath during needle insertion

Monitor bleeding, clotting, and PT results; report abnormal results to physician

Postbiopsy Observations

Intraperitoneal, intrahepatic hemorrhage

Shock

Pneumothorax

Peritonitis

Interventions

Apply pressure to biopsy site for first 15 min after procedure

Maintain bed rest in supine position for 24 hr

Position patient on right side for first 6 hr to keep pressure at site

Monitor vital signs q15min for four times, then q30min for four times, then q4h or as ordered

Observe biopsy site q30min for bleeding, swelling, or increased pain

Monitor Hgb and Hct

Manage pain as indicated; epigastric pain or referred shoulder pain may occur

Report prolonged pain to physician

Administer vitamin K as ordered

Assist patient with eating and other activities as needed for 24 hr

Pancreas

ACUTE AND CHRONIC PANCREATITIS

acute pancreatitis Acute inflammatory disease in which autodigestion of the organ occurs as a result of obstruction of the pancreatic duct; exact cause is unknown, but various causative factors are thought to be excessive use of alcohol, stones, tumors, and trauma

chronic pancreatitis Chronic, progressive disease that may or may not follow acute pancreatitis; causative factors include gallbladder disease, carcinoma, and excessive use of alcohol; pancreas becomes fibrotic and necrotic, and enzyme action is markedly decreased or nonexistent

Assessment

Observations/findings

ACUTE PANCREATITIS

Severe pain in upper left quadrant: dull, unrelenting, boring

Increases in supine position

May radiate to shoulder and thoracic vertebrae

Mild abdominal distention, ascites

Nausea, vomiting

Fever, chills

Tachycardia, hypovolemia, hypotension

Respiratory impairment, dyspnea, splinting; adult respiratory distress syndrome (ARDS) may develop

Decreased urine output

Discoloration of abdomen and/or flanks

Jaundice

Hyperglycemia

CHRONIC PANCREATITIS

Intermittent epigastric pain: steady, boring, dull, or sharp
    Radiates to back
    Relieved when leaning forward

Nausea, vomiting

Weight loss

Diarrhea, steatorrhea

Malnutrition

Minimal jaundice

Fat-soluble vitamin deficiencies

Symptoms of diabetes mellitus

Laboratory/diagnostic studies
ACUTE PANCREATITIS

CBC, BUN, urinalysis, FBS

Arterial PO$_2$ less than 60 mm Hg

Serum calcium, albumin (decreased)

Serum LDH, SGOT, SGPT (increased)

Amylase: serum, urine, lipase (elevated)

CHRONIC PANCREATITIS

CBC, urinalysis

Alkaline phosphatase: elevated

Serum amylase, lipase: normal

ACUTE AND CHRONIC PANCREATITIS

Endoscopy

Serum glucose: elevated

Radiological abdominal films

Ultrasonography/CT scan

Upper GI series/cholangiography

Stool for fat

Potential complications

Electrolyte imbalance, hypocalcemia

Hyperglycemia

Respiratory, circulatory, renal failure

Paralytic ileus

Jaundice

Shock, hemorrhage

Medical Management

Analgesics, antacids, cimetidine, antibiotics, anticholinergics

Hemodynamic monitoring

Parenteral fluids with electrolytes, vitamins, serum albumin, and/or dextran

Nasogastric suction, NPO

Diet, activity, TPN

Digestants (pancreatic enzymes) for chronic pancreatitis

Insulin for hyperglycemia

Paravertebral block for pain management

Nursing diagnoses/interventions/evaluation

■ **NDX:** Potential for fluid volume deficit related to risk of abnormal body fluid loss resulting from vomiting, fever, and/or gastric aspiration

Maintain NPO, assess hydration status, skin turgor

Maintain parenteral fluids with electrolytes, vitamins, albumin, and antibiotics or TPN if indicated

Monitor nasogastric tube and low, intermittent suction apparatus; irrigate with measured amounts of normal saline; measure gastric output q4h

Auscultate abdomen for bowel sounds q4h
    Observe for distention, vomiting, and decreased sounds after nasogastric tube is removed

Monitor vital signs q2h to 4h; check apical pulse

Monitor CVP or Swan-Ganz catheter; monitor arterial blood gases and pulse oximetry

Monitor urine output qh; report output of less than 30 to 50 ml/hr to physician

Calculate intake and output q8h; report deficits

Monitor mental acuity for decreased sensorium

Monitor for calcium imbalance; tremors, twitching

Monitor electrolytes, glucose, liver function studies, PT, and calcium

Expected outcome/evaluation

Patient's
    Vital signs are stable
    Electrolytes are within normal limits
    Skin turgor is adequate
    Intake and output are balanced

■ **NDX:** Potential for infection related to inadequate primary defenses, nutrition imbalance

Monitor respiratory status: breath sounds, cough, sputum, shallow breathing, fluid collection

Assist and teach patient to turn and cough q2h and deep breathe q½h

Administer skin care and oral hygiene q2h to 4h; observe for reddened areas or breakdown

Observe for signs of jaundice: skin, sclera, urine

Monitor temperature for elevation; initiate cooling measures for temperature greater than 101° F (38.2° C)

Monitor urine for infection

Expected outcome/evaluation

Patient's
    Condition is afebrile
    Breath sounds are normal

Skin remains clean, dry, and intact

Urine is clear without signs of infection

■ **NDX:** Pain related to disease process

Maintain bed rest in quiet environment in position of comfort; no knee gatch

Assess type, intensity, and location of pain; assess effectiveness of pain relief measures

Avoid morphine; small, frequent doses of meperidine are beneficial

Medicate before pain becomes severe

Use pain rating scale

Teach alternate pain management techniques

Change position frequently; administer back rubs

Perform passive or assist with and teach active ROM exercises q4h to promote comfort

Coordinate care to provide for rest periods

Ambulate with assistance when allowed

Promote diversional activities

Expected outcome/evaluation

Patient

Verbalizes that pain is decreasing

Appears relaxed and comfortable

■ **NDX:** Altered nutrition: less than body requirements related to anorexia, vomiting, and/or decreased digestive enzymes

Monitor for presence of bowel sounds

Collaborate with physician, dietitian and provide liquid to soft diet when tolerated

Provide high-protein, high-carbohydrate, low-fat, or diabetic diet in small, frequent meals

Avoid coffee, tea, stimulants, and gas-producing foods

Monitor for food tolerances

Administer antacids, insulin, and anticholinergics; assess for effectiveness/side effects

Weigh patient daily at same time with same clothing and scale

Monitor stools for color, consistency, amount, frequency; test for presence of fat

Expected outcome/evaluation

Patient

Demonstrates progressive weight gain

Tolerates balanced diet

■ **NDX:** Knowledge deficit related to lack of information about home care management

Provide and review written dietary instructions

Reinforce causal relationship of alcohol use to pancreati-

tis; promote outside counseling with rehabilitation centers

Explain and teach about diabetes, blood testing, insulin therapy, and symptoms to report to physician

Discuss medications: name, schedule, dosage, purpose, and side effects; explain importance of taking only medicines prescribed by physician; promote discriminate use of narcotics

Encourage follow-up visits with physician

Expected outcome/evaluation

Patient

Verbalizes understanding of prescribed nutritional plan, signs of complications, and disease process

Participates in care and initiates needed lifestyle changes

PANCREATIC SURGERY

Surgery of the pancreas, including total pancreatectomy with or without islet cell autotransplant for chronic pancreatitis and carcinoma, subtotal pancreatectomy for islet cell tumor and carcinoma, and pancreatoduodenectomy (Whipple procedure) for carcinoma

Preoperative Assessment and Care

Assess respiratory, circulatory, and neurological status; take baseline vital signs; observe for abdominal distention and peripheral edema

Assess nutritional status and history of substance abuse

Provide nourishing diet as tolerated

Administer parenteral fluids, TPN, and/or blood transfusions as ordered

Insert nasogastric tube and/or indwelling urethral catheter as ordered

Provide emotional support and reinforce physician's explanation of surgical procedure; clarify misconceptions

Administer vitamin K, salt-poor albumin, and antibiotics as ordered

Explain and teach about possibility of insulin and pancreatic enzyme therapy postoperatively

Postoperative Assessment
Observations/findings

Hypotension

Patency of nasogastric tube

Character and amount of

Gastric drainage

Wound drainage

Urine output

Bile drainage if T tube is in place

Location and character of pain

Type of parenteral therapy equipment

CVP line

TPN line

Tachycardia
Splinting of respirations
Decreased breath sounds
Nausea, vomiting
Abdominal distention

Laboratory/diagnostic studies

Electrolytes, PT, FBS, Hgb, Hct
Arterial blood gases, pH, serum albumin
Serum and urine osmolalities

Potential complications

Oliguria
Dehydration
Electrolyte imbalance
Decreased serum albumin levels
Increased PT
Hyperglycemia
Hypoglycemia
Atelectasis
Pneumonia
Elevated temperature
Jaundice
Subdiaphragmatic abscess, intraperitoneal infection
Paralytic ileus
Gastric/wound hemorrhage
Shock
Wound infection

Medical Management

Analgesics, antibiotics, vasopressors, diuretics
Parenteral fluids with electrolytes, vitamins, and/or albumin
Blood transfusions
Nasogastric suction
Oxygen therapy, incentive spirometer
TPN
Stool softeners
Diet, activity

Nursing diagnoses/interventions/evaluation

■ **NDX:** Ineffective breathing pattern related to surgical incision, pain, and anesthesia

Elevate head of bed 30 to 45 degrees; no knee gatch
Monitor respiratory status q1h to 2h; observe for dyspnea and splinting
Auscultate chest for breath sounds q4h
Provide incentive spirometer qh
Monitor CVP and Swan-Ganz catheter, and check arterial blood gases and pH
Assist and teach patient to turn and cough q2h and deep breathe q½h; support incision and administer analgesics before procedure when possible

Expected outcome/evaluation

Patient
    Exhibits normal respiratory rate
    Performs deep breathing exercises correctly
    Presents normal breath sounds

■ **NDX:** Potential fluid volume deficit related to risk of abnormal body fluid loss resulting from nasogastric suction, NPO status, hypovolemia

Maintain NPO; assess hydration status
Maintain parenteral fluids with electrolytes, vitamins, and insulin
Monitor nasogastric tube and low, intermittent suction apparatus; irrigate with measured amounts of normal saline; measure output q4h
Monitor indwelling urethral catheter and/or T tube and closed gravity drainage system if applicable
Monitor urine output qh; report output of less than 30 to 50 ml/hr to physician; check for sugar and acetone q4h
Calculate intake and output q8h; report discrepancies and collaborate with physician to correct
Monitor vital signs qh until stable; report hypotension to physician
Encourage frequent movement of legs to promote venous return
Monitor electrolytes, glucose, and albumin levels
Auscultate abdomen for bowel sounds and measure girth q4h
Assess effectiveness/side effects of diuretics

Expected outcome/evaluation

Patient's
    Vital signs are stable
    Intake and output are balanced
    Laboratory studies are within normal limits
    Skin turgor is good

■ **NDX:** Potential for altered protection related to abnormal blood profile resulting from coagulation abnormalities and/or bleeding

Monitor incision and dressing q2h for bleeding or drainage; reinforce and change prn
Monitor character and color of gastric aspirate and bile drainage for blood
Observe skin, sclera, and urine for jaundice
    Provide measures to reduce itching and scratching if present
Monitor PT and liver function levels
Monitor transfusions and salt-poor albumin
Monitor Hgb and Hct

Expected outcome/evaluation

Patient
    Presents laboratory values within normal limits
    Shows no evidence of bleeding or jaundice

■ **NDX:** Potential for infection related to inadequate primary defenses

Maintain aseptic technique
Change dressings; observe for signs of infection and healing process
Monitor temperature q4h
Monitor and assess effectiveness of antibiotics and antipyretics
Collect urine specimen for culture/sensitivity when indwelling catheter is removed; initiate voiding measures when needed
Monitor breath sounds, signs of cough, sputum

Expected outcome/evaluation

Patient's
  Condition remains afebrile
  Wound is healing adequately
  Surrounding tissue is clear, dry, and intact
  Lungs are clear
  Urine shows no evidence of infection

■ **NDX:** Pain related to surgical intervention

Assess type, intensity, and location of pain
Administer analgesics before pain becomes severe and before treatments
Assess for effectiveness of pain relief measures
Change position frequently; administer back rubs
Discuss and teach alternate pain relief techniques
Provide skin care and oral hygiene q4h
Perform passive or assist with and teach active ROM exercises q4h
Ambulate with assistance when tolerated

Expected outcome/evaluation

Patient
  States that pain is decreasing
  Appears relaxed
  Demonstrates use of alternative pain relief measures

■ **NDX:** Altered nutrition: less than body requirements related to malnutrition preoperatively, NPO status, and/or anorexia

Continue with TPN as indicated
Auscultate abdomen for return of bowel sounds
Collaborate with physician, dietitian and provide water and other clear liquids in small amounts after removal of nasogastric tube; monitor tolerance
  Progress to soft diet or diabetic diet as tolerated; provide small, frequent meals; measure intake
Administer and assess for effectiveness/side effects of insulin and pancreatic enzymes

Monitor serum glucose
Continue monitoring blood for sugar
Clamp T tube when ordered and observe for signs of pain, distention, and nausea (see p. 292)
Weigh daily; same time, clothes, scale
Monitor color, consistency, frequency of stools
Use stool softeners to avoid constipation; discourage straining

Expected outcome/evaluation

Patient
  Tolerates prescribed diet/TPN
  Demonstrates progressive weight gain
  Presents serum glucose within normal limits

■ **NDX:** Knowledge deficit related to diabetes and lack of information about home care management

Provide and review written dietary instructions for regular or diabetic diet as needed
Demonstrate insulin administration and blood testing procedures (p. 332)
Discuss signs of hypoglycemia and hyperglycemia (p. 341)
Demonstrate care of T tube if applicable (p. 292)
Discuss medications: name, schedule, dosage, purpose, and side effects; explain importance of taking only medicines prescribed by physician and need to use narcotics discriminately
Explain incisional care and signs of wound infection
Provide information about outside sources available for substance abuse rehabilitation
Demonstrate management of TPN if applicable
Discuss use of stool softeners, natural laxatives to prevent constipation
Discuss symptoms to report to physician
  Increased abdominal pain, distention
  Fever, jaundice
  Nausea, vomiting
  Gastric bleeding, tarry stools
  Mucosal bleeding
  Hypoglycemia/hyperglycemia
  Complications of diabetes
Encourage follow-up visits with physician

Expected outcome/evaluation

Patient
  Expresses understanding of needed dietary regimen, potential complications, and medication schedule
  Demonstrates testing procedure and insulin administration correctly
  Demonstrates incisional care accurately
  Participates in treatment plan and expresses willingness to maintain plan after discharge

BIBLIOGRAPHY

Alltop SA: Teaching for discharge: gastrostomy tubes, *RN* 51(11):42, 1988.

Becker KL, Stevens SA: Performing in-depth abdominal assessment, *Nursing '88* 18(6):60, 1988.

Camp D, Otten N: How to insert and remove nasogastric tubes quickly and easily, *Nursing '90;* 20(9):59, 1990.

Carpentino LJ: *Handbook of nursing diagnosis,* Philadelphia, 1990, JB Lippincott.

Dalton-Loehner D, Connor PA: Beyond ileostomy: surgery for a normal life, *RN* 52(7):29, 1989.

Deters GE: Managing complications after abdominal surgery, *RN* 50(3):27, 1987.

DiIorio C, Price ME: Swallowing: an assessment guide, *Am J Nurs* 90(7):38, 1990.

Doenges ME et al: *Nursing care plans: guidelines for planning patient care,* ed 2, Philadelphia, 1989, FA Davis.

Edwards J, Krouse S: Helping the emergency colostomy patient through reality shock, *Nursing '87* 17(7):63, 1987.

Gauwitz DF: Endoscopic cholecystectomy: the patient-friendly alternative, *Nursing '90* 20(12):58, 1990.

Goodman L: Would your assessment spot a hidden alcoholic? *RN* 51(8):56, 1988.

Grochowski-Meize AR: When the dx is Crohn's disease, *RN* 54(2):52, 1991.

Gulanick M et al: *Nursing care plans,* ed 2, St Louis, 1990, CV Mosby.

Guzzetta CE et al: *Clinical assessment tools for use with nursing diagnoses,* St Louis, 1989, CV Mosby.

Hufler DR: Helping your dysphagic patient eat, *RN* 50(9):36, 1987.

Jurf JB, Clements L, and Llorente J: Cholecystectomy made easier, *Am J Nurs* 90(12):38, 1990.

Kim MJ et al: *Pocket guide to nursing diagnoses,* ed 3, St Louis, 1989, CV Mosby.

McConnell EA: Meeting the challenge of intestinal obstruction, *Nursing '87* 17(7):34, 1987.

McFarland GK, McFarlane EA: *Nursing diagnosis and intervention,* St Louis, 1989, CV Mosby.

Mertes JE: Action stat! G.I. bleeding, *Nursing '89* 19(8):37, 1989.

Munn NE: Acute abdomen, *Nursing '88* 18(9):34, 1988.

Munn NE: When the bile duct is blocked, *RN* 52(1):50, 1989.

Patras AZ, Paice JA, and Lanigan K: Managing G.I. bleeding—it takes a two track mind, *Nursing '88* 18(4):68, 1988.

Price MA, DiIorio C: Swallowing: a practice guide, *Am J Nurs* 90(7):42, 1990.

Rowland GA, Marks DA, and Torres WE: The new gallstone destroyers and dissolvers, *Am J Nurs* 90(11):1473, 1989.

Smith CE: Assessing bowel sounds, *Nursing '88* 18(2):42, 1988.

Starkey JF, Jefferson PA, and Kirby DF: Taking care of percutaneous endoscopic gastrostomy, *Am J Nurs* 88(1):42, 1988.

Thelan LA et al: *Textbook of critical care nursing,* St Louis, 1990, CV Mosby.

Thompson JM et al: *Mosby's manual of clinical practice,* ed 2, St Louis, 1989, CV Mosby.

Whiteman K et al: Liver transplantation, *Am J Nurs* 90(6):69, 1990.

Willis D, Harbit MD, and Julius LM: Gallstones: alternatives to surgery, *RN* 53(4):44, 1990.

Young ME, Flynn KT: Third-spacing: when the body conceals fluid loss, *RN* 51(8):46, 1988.

Endocrine System

ENDOCRINE ASSESSMENT

Subjective Data

Change in stamina and ability to perform activities of daily living (ADLs)
Fatigue
Numbness
Tingling
Paresthesia
Bone pain
Change in mental status
Irritable
Anxious
Nervous
Headache
Syncope
Anorexia
Nausea
Abdominal pain
Change in body proportions
Palpitations
Shortness of breath
Hoarseness
Change in secondary sex characteristics
Change in menstrual cycle
Impotence
Decreased libido
Dysuria

Objective Data

General appearance: body development, proportion
Vital signs: BP, P, R, T
Skin
  Temperature
  Turgor
  Hydration
    Dry, scaly
    Excessive perspiration
    Excessive oiliness
  Texture
    Fine, smooth
    Coarse, leathery
  Color
    Increased pigmentation

    Gums
    Breast
    Abdomen
    Creases
  Yellow pigmentation
  Flushed
  Pale
  Cyanotic
  Purple striae over areas of fat
Edema
  Face, eyelids
  Lower extremities
  Pitting, nonpitting
Lipodystrophy
Poor wound healing
Hair and nails
  Texture of nails
    Thick
    Brittle
    Thin
    Cracking
  Horizontal nail ridges
  Amount of hair
    Thin
    Increased
    Alopecia
  Distribution of hair
  Texture of hair
    Coarse, dry, brittle
    Fine, silky, soft
Musculoskeletal system
  Fat distribution
  Muscle mass distribution
  Buffalo hump
  Changes in height
  Extremities
    Weakness
    Twitching
    Tremors
    Spasms
    Tetany
    Ataxia
Central nervous system (CNS)
  Personality changes
    Complacent
    Dull

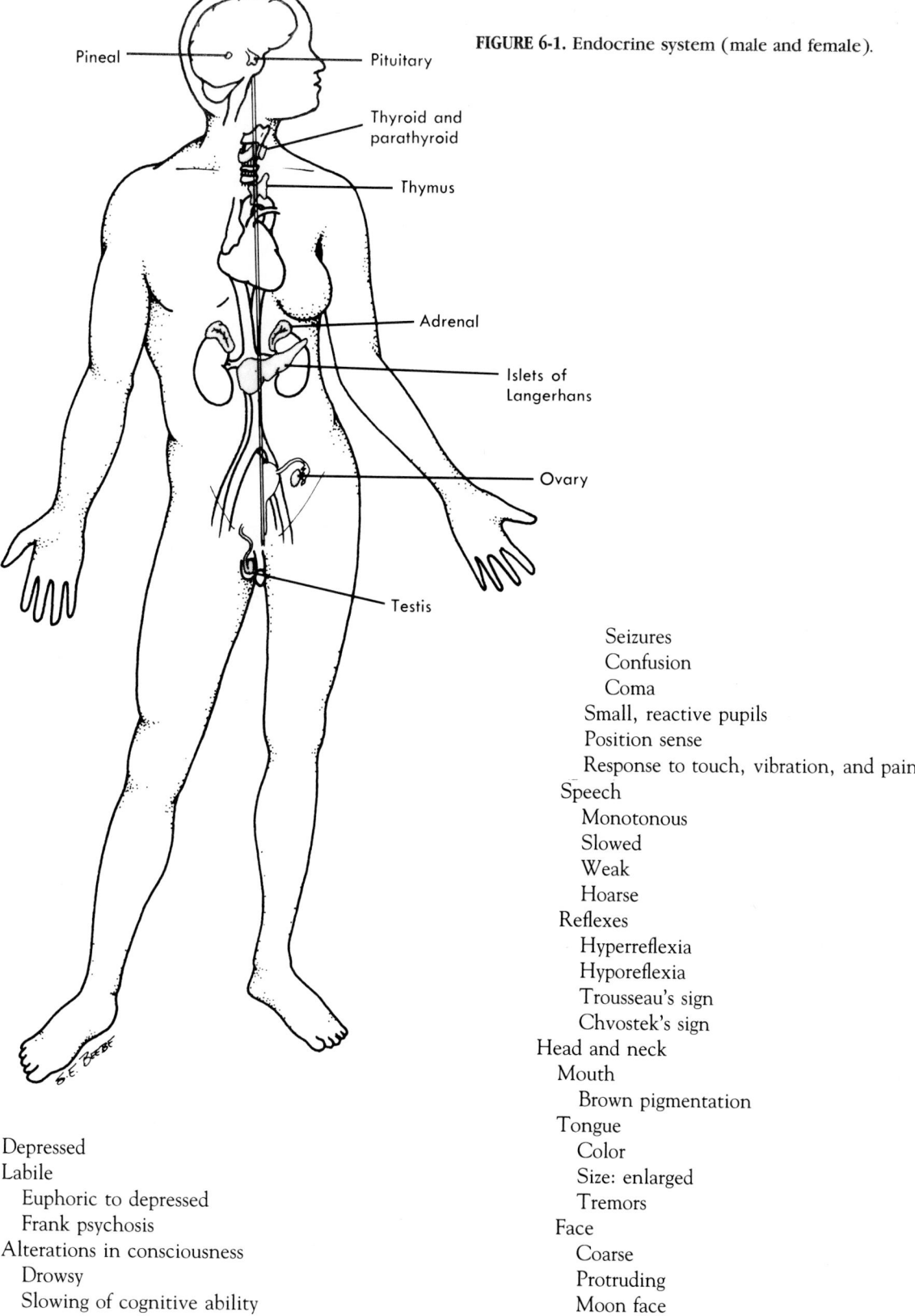

Pineal

Pituitary

Thyroid and parathyroid

Thymus

Adrenal

Islets of Langerhans

Ovary

Testis

FIGURE 6-1. Endocrine system (male and female).

Seizures
Confusion
Coma
Small, reactive pupils
Position sense
Response to touch, vibration, and pain
Speech
    Monotonous
    Slowed
    Weak
    Hoarse
Reflexes
    Hyperreflexia
    Hyporeflexia
    Trousseau's sign
    Chvostek's sign
Head and neck
    Mouth
        Brown pigmentation
    Tongue
        Color
        Size: enlarged
        Tremors
    Face
        Coarse
        Protruding
        Moon face
        Edema
            Wide, puffy eyes
            Wrinkled eyelids

Depressed
Labile
    Euphoric to depressed
    Frank psychosis
Alterations in consciousness
    Drowsy
    Slowing of cognitive ability
    Inappropriate response to questions
    Somnolence
    Stupor

TABLE 6-1. The Endocrine Glands

Name	Hormones	Function	Endocrine disorders
Pituitary			
Anterior	Somatotropin (growth hormone)	Promotes growth and retention of nitrogen for protein metabolism; maintains established lactation	Hypofunction Dwarfism Hyperfunction Acromegaly
	Thyroid-stimulating hormone (TSH)	Promotes bone growth and function of thyroid; controls release of thyroxine	Increased or decreased function of thyroid gland
	Adrenocorticotropic hormone (ACTH)	Promotes growth and function of adrenal cortex; controls release of glucocorticoid	Increased or decreased function of adrenal cortex
	Follicle-stimulating hormone (FSH)	Promotes development of ovaries, secretion of estrogen, and sperm maturation	Increased or decreased function of gonads
	Luteinizing hormone (LH)	Promotes maturation of ovaries, ovulation, and secretion of progesterone	
	Interstitial cell-stimulating hormone (ICSH)	Promotes secretion of testosterone	
	Prolactin (luteotrophic hormone)	Maintains corpus luteum; initiates secretion of milk and progesterone	Hyperprolactinemia
Posterior	Antidiuretic hormone (ADH)	Promotes reabsorption of water	Hypofunction Diabetes insipidus Hyperfunction SIADH
	Oxytocin	Contracts pregnant uterus	
Adrenal cortex	Glucocorticoids (Cortisol)	Regulates metabolism of carbohydrates, fats, protein; acts as an antiinflammatory agent	Hypofunction Addison's disease Hyperfunction Cushing's syndrome
	Androgens	Masculinization of females (axillary and pubic hair); supplements the testes as major source of androgens in males	Hypofunction Delay of secondary sex characteristics
	Mineralocorticoids (aldosterone)	Balances sodium, water, and potassium concentration; controls release of angiotensin	Primary aldosteronism
Medulla	Epinephrine Norepinephrine	Increases blood sugar, stimulates ACTH production, controls vasoconstriction	Pheochromocytoma
Islets of Langerhans	Insulin (beta cells)	Increases anabolism of carbohydrates; lowers blood glucose	Hypofunction Diabetes mellitus Hyperfunction Hyperinsulinism
	Glucagon (alpha cells)	Elevates blood glucose; increases fat metabolism (ketogenesis)	

TABLE 6-1. The Endocrine Glands—cont'd

Name	Hormones	Function	Endocrine disorders
Thyroid	Thyroxine (T_4) Triiodothyronine (T_3)	Regulates metabolic rate Influences growth and development	Hypofunction Cretinism Hypothyroidism (myxedema)
	Calcitonin	Decreases serum calcium levels, bone remodeling	Hyperfunction Hyperthyroidism (Graves' disease)
Parathyroid	Parathyroid hormone (PTH)	Activates bone calcification; increases serum calcium levels	Hypofunction Tetany
			Hyperfunction Hyperparathyroidism—reabsorption of bone and formation of renal calculi
Gonads	Estrogen and testosterone	Influences secondary sex characteristics; sexual functioning	Hypofunction Lack of or regression of sexual development
			Hyperfunction Abnormal sexual development
	Progesterone	Prepares and maintains pregnancy; develops mammary secretory tissue	

Broad, short, upturned nose
Enlarged lip and nose
Eyes
   Protruding eyeballs
   Drooping eyelids
   Cataracts
   Periorbital edema
   Ocular dysfunction
   Microaneurysms
   Hemorrhage
   Exudates
   Arteriolar narrowing
Thyroid
   Size
   Shape
   Symmetry
   Nodules
     Tenderness
     Systolic bruit
Gastrointestinal system
   Polyphagia
   Polydipsia
   Vomiting
   Diarrhea
   Constipation
   Dehydration
   Weight change
   Increased abdominal girth
   Obesity
Cardiovascular system

Tachycardia
Bradycardia
Hypotension
Hypertension
Arrhythmias
Cardiomegaly
Respiratory system
   Tachypnea
   Kussmaul's respirations
   Acetone breath
   Stridorous respirations
   Supraclavicular retractions
Renal system
   Polyuria
   Oliguria
   Anuria
   Enuresis
Reproductive system
   Female masculinization
   Changes in secondary sex characteristics
     Genital atrophy
     Breast atrophy

Pertinent Background Information
CONCURRENT DISEASES OR CONDITIONS

Cardiovascular disease
   Angina
   Hypertension
   Heart failure
   Pericardial effusion

Myocardial infarction
Intestinal obstruction
Pulmonary edema
Psychological problems/stress
Pathological fracture
Obesity

PREVIOUS SURGERY OR ILLNESS

Cancer
Pancreatic disease
Burns
Renal disease
Cardiovascular disease
Transplant
Sarcoidosis
Trauma
Oophorectomy
Neck surgery
Adrenalectomy
Hypophysectomy
Gestational diabetes
Irradiation
Meningitis
Encephalitis

FAMILY HISTORY

Diabetes mellitus
Thyroid disease
Hypertension
Pheochromocytoma
Rheumatoid arthritis

SOCIAL HISTORY

Physical environment
Psychological environment

MEDICATION HISTORY

Corticosteroids
Diuretics
Medication for sleep, nerves, and/or anxiety
Alcohol

Diagnostic Aids

LABORATORY STUDIES

T_3 serum triiodothyronine
T_3 resin uptake
T_4 serum thyroxine
Thyroid-stimulating hormone (TSH)
^{123}I or ^{125}I (radioactive iodine uptake)
Parathyroid hormone level (PTH)
Plasma adrenocorticotropic hormone (ACTH)
Plasma cortisol
Plasma ketones
Plasma testosterone or estrogen
Cholesterol
Triglyceride

Creatinine phosphokinase (CPK)
Catecholamine levels
Potassium
Sodium
Calcium
  Serum
  Urine
Phosphorus
Phosphate reabsorption test
pH
CO_2
Bicarbonate levels
Blood urea nitrogen (BUN)
Fasting blood sugar
Glucose tolerance test (GTT)
17-Hydroxycorticosteroids
17-Ketosteroids
Serum osmolality
Urine metanephrine
Urine specific gravity

PROCEDURES

X-ray examinations of bone
Water deprivation test
Thyroid scan/ultrasound
Thyroid stimulation test
Thyroid suppression test
Achilles tendon reflex recording
Twenty-four hour urine collections
Fractional urine testing
Chemstrip bG
Computed tomography (CT) scans
  Thyroid
  Adrenals
Adrenal angiography
Adrenal venography
Dexamethasone suppression test
ACTH stimulation test
Metyrapone test
Insulin tolerance test
Insulin stress test

HYPOTHYROIDISM: MYXEDEMA

hypothyroidism Lack of thyroid hormone in the adult resulting from removal or atrophy of the thyroid gland, hypofunction of the pituitary gland or the hypothalamus, or defective hormone biosynthesis
myxedema coma A severe form of hypothyroidism; develops after a prolonged period of untreated or uncontrolled hypothyroidism

Assessment
Observations/findings

Neurological
  Lethargy
  Slow, monotonous, slurred speech

Memory impairment
Slow cognition
Personality changes: complacent, dull, apathetic
Nystagmus
Night blindness
Perceptive hearing loss
Paresthesia
Intention tremor
Slowed deep tendon reflexes
Ataxia
Somnolence
Syncope
Musculoskeletal
  Muscle stiffness or aching
  Myalgia
  Arthralgia
  Fatigue
Cardiovascular
  Intolerance to cold
  Decreased sweating
  Low blood pressure, pulse, and temperature
  Narrow pulse pressure
  Diminished heart sounds
  Precordial pain
Respiratory
  Hoarseness
  Shortness of breath with mild exertion
Gastrointestinal/nutritional
  Unexplained weight gain
  Anorexia
  Constipation
  Abdominal distention
  Ascites
Sexual/reproductive
  Menorrhagia, metrorrhagia, amenorrhea
  Decreased libido
  Decreased fertility: spontaneous abortion
  Impotence
Integumentary
  Skin: pale, cold, dry, coarse, scaling
  Nonpitting edema: hands, feet, periorbital
  Upper eyelid droop
  Enlarged tongue and lips
  Coarse, thinning hair
  Nails: brittle, slow growing, thick

Laboratory/diagnostic studies

Electrocardiogram (ECG): low-voltage, nonspecific ST segment changes, prolonged PR interval, heart block, flat or inverted T wave
Decreased free T_4 and T_3
Decreased radioiodide uptake test (RAIU)
Decreased serum T_4 and T_3
Decreased serum sodium
TSH levels if used: low if secondary hypothyroidism; elevated if primary hypothyroidism

Increased serum: cholesterol, triglycerides, CPK, alkaline phosphatase
Increased protein in cerebrospinal fluid (CSF)
Arterial blood gases: hypoxia, elevated CO_2
Normocytic, normochromic anemia

Potential complications

Angina, dysrhythmias
Heart failure
Myocardial infarction
Intestinal obstruction
Pleural/pericardial effusions
Stupor
Coma

Medical Management

IV fluids
IV albumin
High-protein, high-fiber, low-calorie, low-sodium diet
Restrict fluids
Thyroid hormone replacement with synthetic L-thyroxine
Glucocorticoids if myxedema develops
Diuretics
Stool softeners

Nursing diagnoses/interventions/evaluation

■ **NDX:** Fluid volume excess, extravascular, related to increased capillary permeability

Monitor intake and output q8h and prn
Monitor IV fluids, if administered, to prevent overhydration
Weigh patient daily and report significant gain to physician (significant gain is greater than 0.5 kg daily)
Monitor for signs and symptoms of excess extra-vascular volume
  Periorbital edema
  Jugular vein distention
  Increasing abdominal girth
  Presence of abdominal fluid wave
  Dependent edema of extremities
  Pulmonary edema: dyspnea, orthopnea, and/or crackles in lungs; monitor chest x-ray results
Monitor serum albumin levels, electrolytes, creatinine
Maintain high-protein diet to increase serum protein levels
Restrict fluids as determined by collaboration with physician
Monitor vital signs q4h and observe for
  Increased pulse
  Labored respirations
  Development of S_3 gallop
Be cautious in administering sedatives, especially barbiturates, because of increased sensitivity
Notify physician of development or worsening of any of the above signs or symptoms

Position patient on bed rest to alleviate dyspnea and support edematous areas

Expected outcome/evaluation

Vital signs are stable; electrolytes are within normal range; weight is returning to normal range for patient; intake and output are balanced; edema is resolving

■ **NDX:**   Altered thought processes related to altered metabolic processes

Assess level of orientation q4h and reorient patient as necessary; explain procedures clearly and slowly; repeat as necessary; break down tasks into easy-to-accomplish segments
Help patient to focus on tasks and reach self-care goals
Provide a stable, calm, and nonstressful environment
  Be consistent in timing and performance of activities and procedures
  Restrict visitors as necessary
  Avoid frequent changing of personnel
  Prevent emotionally upsetting or confusing situations
  Allow sufficient time for performance of procedures and activities
Plan care with patient
Allow sufficient time for patient to express needs and feelings
Assist patient to make choices and decisions
Provide diversional activities and materials
Assist significant other in acceptance of patient's slowness

Expected outcome/evaluation

Oriented to time, person, and place
Accomplishes planned self-care activities
Makes choices known to others
Discusses feelings and responses with significant other

■ **NDX:**   Potential for trauma related to risk of changes in sensory perception and coordination

Assess for development or worsening of perception/coordination defects q8h
Assess muscle strength and mobility daily
Explain necessary safety precautions
Assist patient with ambulation as necessary; provide aids to ambulation (walker, cane) as needed
Monitor pulse rate, complaints of dyspnea or chest pain during activity
Balance periods of activity and rest
Place articles patient may wish to use frequently within easy reach
Arrange environment simply; avoid unnecessary clutter
Remove potentially hazardous objects from patient's environment
Place bed in low position
Face patient when speaking

Speak slowly and clearly
Serve foods at tepid temperature to avoid thermal injury
Assist with bathing, shaving, and toileting as necessary
Use safety measures (e.g., jacket restraint; avoid wrist restraints) as necessary
Instruct patient to call for assistance when getting out of bed
Keep call light within easy reach at all times
Provide nighttime lighting
Keep side rails up at all times

Expected outcome/evaluation

Patient sustains no injuries

■ **NDX:**   Constipation related to decreased metabolic rate and/or decreased intestinal peristalsis, and decreased dietary bulk and fluids

Maintain low-calorie diet that includes high-fiber foods
Administer fluids to tolerance; remind patient to drink fluids hourly if not restricted
Monitor bowel pattern, consistency of color, odor of stool, and associated symptoms daily
Assess usual methods used to avoid constipation
Provide privacy
Assess effectiveness of stool softener, laxatives, administered
Encourage exercise as tolerated
Teach patient to respond promptly to urge to defecate; avoid straining
Assist patient with recognizing activities that stimulate urge to defecate (drinking warm liquids)
Encourage patient to atttempt defecation at same time each day to establish a routine
Monitor daily bowel pattern

Expected outcome/evaluation

Stool is normal in color, consistency, odor, and frequency

■ **NDX:**   Impaired skin integrity related to edema, dry, scaly skin, and immobility

Assess for redness or breakdown q24h; if patient is on bed rest, assess q8h
Administer skin care to pressure points four times daily and as necessary
Use superfatted soap for bathing; apply lotion after each bath or handwashing
Use elbow and heel protectors
Place patient on decubitus-prevention mattress or bed
Elevate edematous extremities with pillows
Assist and encourage patient to make small position changes q½ to 1h; turn q2h
Encourage ambulation when able; avoid sitting for long periods
Maintain optimal nutritional status

Conserve body temperature by use of blankets, warm clothing, etc.

Expected outcome/evaluation

Skin turgor is good; skin is intact; patient uses preventative measures

■ **NDX:** Knowledge deficit related to lack of exposure to information regarding disease process, treatment, and self-care

Explain basic concepts of the disease process and complications to report to physician
Explain reasons for physical and emotional changes
Teach name of medication, dosage, time and method of administration, purpose, side effects, and toxic effects
Emphasize that medication must not be discontinued without consulting physician
Emphasize importance of telling all health care personnel about disease and wearing medic alert band
Explain need to avoid taking over-the-counter medications without consulting physician
Explain that condition is potentially reversible if treatment regimen is followed
Emphasize importance of
　Ongoing outpatient follow-up
　Understanding of slowness and dullness
　Increasing self-care
　Avoiding very cold environments and stressful situations
　Adequate periods of rest alternating with increasing activity/exercise
　Maintaining balanced diet and adequate fluid intake
　Avoiding constipation
Discuss symptoms of infection to report to physician
　Temperature above patient's normal
　"Cold" or "flu" symptoms
　Redness or swelling around lesions
　Frequency of or burning on urination

Expected outcome/evaluation

Patient and/or significant other verbalizes understanding of disease process and principles of home and follow-up care

HYPERTHYROIDISM: THYROID CRISIS (STORM, THYROTOXIC CRISIS)

hyperthyroidism *Characterized by excessive production of thyroid hormone; causes may be classified as autoimmune (Graves' disease), viral, hyperplastic, genetic, or neoplastic, or it may be secondary to an acute systemic illness (excess thyroid hormone results in increased sympathetic tone, which is responsible for many of the assessment findings listed below)*

Graves' disease *Most prevalent form of hyperthyroidism; most commonly seen in women during the third and fourth decades of life*
thyroid crisis *A medical emergency caused by acute exacerbation of the symptoms of hyperthyroidism; usually precipitated by a stressful event such as surgery, infection, trauma, or acute cardiovascular disease*

Assessment
Observations/findings

Neurological
　Hyperthyroidism
　　Irritability/nervousness
　　Tremors
　　Insomnia
　　Emotional lability
　　Diplopia
　　Headache
　　Brisk deep tendon reflexes
　　Muscle weakness or atrophy
　Thyroid crisis
　　Extreme restlessness
　　Confusion or disorientation
　　Frank psychosis
　　Apathy
　　Stupor or delirium
　　Coma
　Eyes
　　Large, protruding eyes
　　Periorbital edema
　　Tremor of eyelids
　　Weakness or paralysis of extraocular muscles
Cardiovascular
　Hyperthyroidism
　　Palpitations
　　Rapid, bounding pulses
　　Wide pulse pressure
　　Irregular pulse/dysrhythmias
　　Systolic cardiac murmur
　　Edema
　Thyroid crisis
　　Profuse diaphoresis
　　Tachycardia disproportionate to change in BP
　　Atrial fibrillation
　　Weak pulses
　　Hypotension
Respiratory
　Hyperthyroidism
　　Dyspnea
　　Increased depth and rate of respiration
　Thyroid crisis: pulmonary edema
Gastrointestinal
　Hyperthyroidism
　　Weight loss
　　Increased thirst and/or appetite
　　Diarrhea

Nausea, abdominal pain
Hyperactive bowel sounds
Thyroid crisis
  Anorexia
  Protracted vomiting
  Severe abdominal pain
  Hepatomegaly
  Jaundice
Metabolic
  Profuse sweating
  Sensitivity to heat
  Increased tolerance to cold
  Enlarged thyroid gland
  Bruit over neck
Integumentary
  Skin: soft, warm, moist, shiny
  Reddened, hyperpigmented palms
  Hair: thinning, fine, straight (silky)
  Oily scalp
  Separation of nails from nail beds
Sexual/reproductive
  Oligomenorrhea
  Amenorrhea
  Diminished libido
  Decreased fertility
  Gynecomastia in males

Laboratory/diagnostic studies

Elevated total and free T_3 and T_4
TSH response to thyrotropin-releasing hormone
  (TRH) is flat
Thyroid radioiodide uptake test (RAIU)
  Low uptake in thyroiditis or excess thyroid hormone
    medication
  High uptake in Graves' disease
TSH decreased
Decreased T_3 resin uptake
Basal metabolism rate (BMR) increased

Potential complications

Fever over 106° F
Marked elevation in P and BP
Dangerous dysrhythmias
Congestive heart failure
Pulmonary edema
Widespread tremors
Circulatory collapse
Shock
Death

Medical Management

Antithyroid medications
Beta-blockers (Propranolol) for control of symptoms of
  excessive sympathetic stimulation
Radioactive ^{131}I therapy

Subtotal thyroidectomy
Eye lubricants
High-calorie, high-protein, high-carbohydrate, high-
  vitamin B diet; fluids to 3 to 4 L
Cooling measures, i.e., hyperthermia blanket
Acetaminophen
Thyroid crisis
  Reserpine/guanethidine to deplete tissue catechol-
    amines
  Hyperthermia control (aspirin is contraindicated)
  Cooling measures
  Volume expanders and/or vasopressors for hypotension
  Total parenteral nutrition
  Glucocorticoids
  Digoxin and/or diuretics for congestive heart failure

Nursing diagnoses/interventions/evaluation

■ **NDX:** Altered thought processes related to increased
stimulation of the sympathetic nervous system
by high levels of thyroid hormone

Assess level of consciousness, orientation, affect, and per-
  ception q4h to 8h; report negative changes
Discuss feelings and responses to situations and people;
  reinforce those that are appropriate
Provide a stable, calm, nonstressful, and nonstimulating
  environment
  Control extraneous noise
  Be consistent in timing and performing of activities and
    procedures
  Restrict visitors as necessary
  Avoid frequent changing of personnel
  Prevent emotionally upsetting situations when possible
Plan care with patient; give clear, concise explanations
Anticipate needs to prevent hyperactive reactions
Inform patient that activities may be restricted
Teach stress-reduction techniques and assess use by pa-
  tient
Provide diversional activities and materials that decrease
  stimulation; avoid those requiring fine motor manipu-
  lation
Reorient patient to environment as needed and provide
  orienting cues (e.g., clock, calendar, familiar pictures,
  etc.)
Monitor for adverse reactions to medications

Expected outcome/evaluation

Patient is oriented
Responds appropriately to situations and people
Uses stress-reduction techniques

■ **NDX:** Activity intolerance related to imbalance between oxygen supply and demand due to increased resting metabolic rate and intolerance
of heat

Assess baseline vital signs and prior activity level

Restrict activity to patient's level of tolerance by assessing physiological response to activity (i.e., assess vital signs during activity and compare to baseline)

Allow patient to set priorities for care within limits

Space procedures to allow adequate rest periods

Provide needed equipment, supplies to prevent expenditure of energy by patient before activity

Discontinue activity at onset of signs of intolerance: dyspnea, tachycardia, fatigue

Assist patient with those activities patient is unable to perform because of weakness or tremors

Plan daily activity and rest pattern that will facilitate increasing tolerance for self-care

Expected outcome/evaluation

Completes planned activities without evidence of intolerance

Asks for assistance only when needed

■ **NDX:** Sleep pattern disturbance related to an *increased* metabolic rate

Assess past and present sleep and activity patterns

Determine factors/techniques to induce sleep previously used by patient

Provide sleep aids requested by patient: warm drink, back rub, quiet music

Discuss other sleep aids, such as relaxation techniques

Discourage frequent daytime sleeping; provide nap times sufficient in length to produce REM sleep

Avoid intake of stimulants in diet

Assist patient with establishing a regular pattern of physical activity; reduce stimulating activities before sleep

Provide environment conducive to sleep: reduce lighting; close door to room; maintain quiet; maintain privacy

Avoid disturbing patient unnecessarily during the night for procedures

Schedule treatments and medications for daytime and evening hours when possible

Assess effectiveness of sleep-promoting activities daily

Expected outcome/evaluation

Sleep pattern is normal for patient

Patient expresses feeling rested, alert with energy to accomplish daily tasks

■ **NDX:** Altered nutrition: less than body requirements related to diarrhea, nausea, abdominal pain, and/or elevated BMR

Monitor intake of high-calorie, high-protein, high-carbohydrate, high-vitamin B diet

Offer frequent small meals and between-meal supplements

Consult patient as to food preferences

Avoid stimulants: coffee, tea, colas, or other beverages with caffeine or theobromine that increase feeling of fullness or peristalsis

Avoid foods with large amounts of fiber or highly seasoned foods

Encourage fluid intake to 2 to 3 L daily; avoid juices that may cause diarrhea

Provide environment with congenial visitors if patient desires

Weigh patient daily, same time, scale, clothing

Monitor intake and output q8h

Assess effectiveness of medication for nausea and abdominal pain

Expected outcome/evaluation

Weight is increasing to that which is normal for patient; takes prescribed diet without abdominal discomfort; has no diarrhea; intake and output are balanced

■ **NDX:** Potential for altered tissue integrity (eyes) related to compromised protective mechanisms

Assess for eye changes; excessive tearing, feeling of foreign object, inability to close eyes, signs of infection, irritation, or abrasions q4h to 8h

Provide sunglasses during the day prn

Administer lubricants as ordered

Patch or tape eyes during sleep to protect exposed cornea

Avoid getting foreign bodies in eyes (dirt, dust)

Assist and teach patient to perform eye motion exercises

Discuss feelings and techniques related to improving appearance

Ensure that patient understands that surgical intervention may be needed

Expected outcome/evaluation

Eyes remain moist without evidence of abrasions or infection

Patient uses methods to protect eyes and discusses feelings about appearance

■ **NDX:** Hyperthermia related to hypermetabolic state

Provide tepid sponge baths as necessary

Use light clothing and bed linens

Maintain cool environment

Assess effectiveness of hypothermia blanket when in use

Use measures to prevent skin breakdown

Administer acetaminophen as ordered (aspirin is contraindicated)

Increase fluid intake to 2500 ml/day

Monitor vital signs, level of consciousness, urinary output q2h to 4h

Collaborate with physician in using additional cooling measures when condition indicates

Expected outcome/evaluation

Patient is alert and responsive
Vital signs and urinary output are normal

 NDX: Potential for trauma related to risk of altered mental status

Use safety measures as necessary
  Pad side rails
    Avoid use of extremity restraints (may increase restlessness)
  Remove potentially hazardous objects from patient's environment and arrange furniture to prevent bumps or falls, e.g., bed in low position
  Provide fluids for drinking and bathing that will not burn if spilled or used immediately
Assess muscle strength, mobility, and mental status q4h to 8h
Provide information about need to follow safety precautions
Assist patient with ambulating as needed
Instruct patient to call for assistance when getting out of bed; keep side rails up
Keep call light within easy reach of patient
Keep personal articles patient may wish to use frequently within easy reach
  Encourage use of nonskid slippers
  Provide night light

Expected outcome/evaluation

Patient is not physically injured
  Understands safety precautions
  Calls for assistance when needed

NDX: Knowledge deficit related to lack of exposure to accurate information about disease process, treatment, and self-care

Explain basic concepts of the disease process, signs and symptoms of recurrence, and complications to report to physician
Explain that symptoms of disease *may be* reversible if medical regimen is followed
Explain that nervous symptoms are part of the disease process and will decrease with treatment
Provide reasons for physical and emotional changes
Stress importance of discussing feelings about changes
Teach name of medication, dosage, time and method of administration, purpose, side effects, and toxic effects
Explain need to avoid taking over-the-counter medications without checking with physician
Emphasize importance of ongoing outpatient care
Instruct patient to inform all health care givers of presence of disease, (physician, dentist) and wear medic alert bracelet

Emphasize importance of planned rest periods of adequate duration
Emphasize importance of avoiding stressful situations and using stress-reducing techniques
Emphasize that high-calorie, high-protein, high-carbohydrate, and high–vitamin B diet with increased fluids must be maintained until discontinued by physician
Discuss maintaining eye integrity: sunglasses, lubricants, protective coverings, and prescribed exercises

Expected outcome/evaluation

Patient and/or significant other verbalizes understanding of disease process and principles of home and follow-up care

HYPOPARATHYROIDISM

Rare condition characterized by a deficiency of parathyroid hormone; may be due to removal of or damage to parathyroid glands (e.g., during thyroid or other neck surgery or radiation treatment)

Assessment
Observations/findings

Neurological
  Paresthesias; lips, tongue, fingers, feet
  Tingling
  Tremor
  Hyperreflexia
  Positive Chvostek's and/or Trousseau's signs
  Papilledema
  Emotional lability
  Irritability
  Anxiety
  Depression
  Delirium
  Delusions
  Changes in level of consciousness
  Tetany
  Seizures
Musculoskeletal
  Stiffness
  Painful cramping, twitching spasms
  Weakness
  Fatigue
Cardiovascular
  Cyanosis
  Palpitations
  Cardiac dysrhythmias
  ECG changes: prolonged QT interval, peaked or inverted T waves, heart block
Respiratory
  Hoarseness

Laryngeal stridor/edema
Gastrointestinal
    Nausea, vomiting
    Abdominal pain
Renal: calculi formation
Integumentary
    Dystrophic, dry, scaly skin and nails
    Cutaneous pigmentation
    Thinning hair
    Alopecia
    Horizontal ridges on nails
    Brittle nails

Laboratory/diagnostic studies

Decreased serum calcium
Increased serum phosphorus
Decreased serum bicarbonate
Decreased or absent serum parathyroid hormone
Hypocalciuria
Hypophosphaturia

Medical Management

High-calcium, high-vitamin D, low-phosphorus diet and
    supplements
Phosphate binders (aluminum hydroxide)
Parenteral fluids
Calcium medications
If acute tetany, IV calcium administration

Nursing diagnoses/interventions/evaluation

■ **NDX:** Potential for injury related to risk of seizures or
    tetany resulting from hypocalcemia

Monitor vital signs and reflexes q2h to 4h
Monitor cardiac function continuously if ECG abnor-
    malities are present
Collaborate with physician in managing early symptoms
    of tetany by administering and monitoring effectiveness
    of parenteral fluids and calcium
Administer calcium cautiously as hypotensive thrombo-
    phlebitis can occur
Administer vitamin D and calcium supplements as ordered
Do not administer phosphate binders within 1 to 2 hr
    before or after calcium supplements or other medica-
    tions
Monitor serum levels of calcium and phosphorus q8h
When patient is on bed rest, pad rails and keep bed in
    low position
If seizure activity occurs when patient is out of bed:
    Assist patient to floor
    Remove potentially harmful objects
Assess patient for injury after seizure
Inform patient of seizure and reorient if necessary

Expected outcome/evaluation

Patient has no injuries; reflexes are normal; vital signs
    are stable; takes diet and medications as pre-
    scribed

■ **NDX:** Potential for ineffective airway clearance re-
    lated to laryngeal edema or seizure activity

Keep suction equipment and oral airway at bedside at all
    times
Have tracheostomy tray, oxygen, and manual resuscita-
    tion equipment readily available at all times

Laryngeal edema

Assess respiratory efforts and voice quality q2h and prn
Auscultate for subtle laryngeal stridor q4h
Report early symptoms to physician and collaborate to
    maintain open airway
Instruct patient to inform nurse or physician at first sign
    of tightness in throat or shortness of breath
Position patient to optimize airway clearance: keep head
    in neutral position, midline

Seizure

If seizure occurs
    Maintain airway
    Suction oropharynx as indicated prn
    Administer oxygen if ordered
    Monitor BP, P, R, and neurological signs
        Check after seizure and prn
    Note frequency, time, level of consciousness, body parts
        involved, and length of seizure activity
Be prepared to collaborate with physician in treating status
    epilepticus, e.g., intubation, medications
Continue preseizure care as indicated

Expected outcome/evaluation

Respiratory rate, rhythm, and depth are normal for patient
Lungs are clear on auscultation

■ **NDX:** Activity intolerance related to muscular weak-
    ness and/or fatigue

Assess past activity patterns
Assess for changes in musculoskeletal symptoms q8h
Assess response to activity
    Note changes in BP, P, R
    Stop activity when changes occur
    Increase participation in small increments as tolerance
        increases
    Teach patient to monitor response to activity and to
        alter, stop, or ask for assistance when changes occur
Plan care with patient to determine activities patient de-
    sires to accomplish; schedule assistance with others

Balance activity with rest

Keep articles and needed supplies within easy reach to decrease energy expenditure

Expected outcome/evaluation

Activity level is increasing daily without dyspnea, tachycardia, or elevated BP

Performs ADLs without effort

Additional nursing diagnoses to consider

Potential fluid volume deficit related to diarrhea, nausea, or vomiting

Altered thought processes related to neurological changes as evidenced by emotional lability, delirium, delusions

Potential for altered skin integrity related to dry scaly skin and immobility

■ **NDX:** Knowledge deficit related to lack of exposure to information regarding treatment and self-care

Explain basic concepts of the disease process

Discuss reasons for physical and emotional changes

Teach patient to check for and report early signs of tetany
  Tingling sensations
  Tremors
  Positive Chvostek's and/or Trousseau's sign
  Change in respiratory effort

Teach significant other to recognize patient's seizure activity and determine course of action to take
  Avoid restraining or interrupting behavior
  Observe and record behaviors exhibited before and during seizure
  Notify physician immediately

Stress importance of daily activity and exercise to tolerance and to report increasing muscle weakness or fatigue

Discuss importance of maintaining safe home environment

Teach name of medication, dosage, time and method of administration, purpose, side and toxic effects, that medication needs to be taken for life

Explain need to avoid taking over-the-counter medications without consulting physician

Emphasize importance of ongoing follow-up care

Instruct patient to maintain high-calcium, high-vitamin D, low-phosphorus diet and increased fluid intake

Expected outcome/evaluation

Patient and/or significant other verbalizes understanding of disease process and principles of home and follow-up care and demonstrates method to check for Chvostek's and Trousseau's sign

HYPERPARATHYROIDISM

Hyperparathyroidism may be due to either primary or secondary causes; in primary hyperparathyroidism hypertrophy of the gland is most commonly due to a benign adenoma but may be caused by other endocrine disorders; secondary hyperparathyroidism is due to excessive compensatory production of PTH that develops as a result of conditions that cause a decrease in calcium levels, such as renal disease

Assessment
Observations/findings

Neurological
  Easy fatigability
  Apathy
  Slow mentation
  Drowsiness
Musculoskeletal
  Muscular weakness
  Bone pain with weight bearing
  Arthralgia
  Bone deformities, shortened stature
  Hyporeflexia
Cardiovascular
  Hypertension
  ECG changes: broad T wave, short or prolonged QT interval, bradycardia
Gastrointestinal/nutritional
  Anorexia
  Nausea
  Weight loss
  Constipation
Renal
  Polyuria
  Dysuria
  Dehydration
  Renal colic
  Uremia

Laboratory/diagnostic studies

Hypercalcemia
Hypophosphatemia
Hyperchloremia
Low serum HCO_3
Increased urine phosphate and urine calcium
Anemia
Elevated parathyroid hormone (PTH) radioimmunoassay
X-ray examination: subperiosteal bone resorption
Ultrasound: enlarged parathyroid gland

Potential complications

Renal failure
Pathological bone fractures
Gastric ulcers

Pancreatitis
Stupor
Coma

Medical Management

Parenteral hydration: usually with normal saline
Avoidance of thiazide diuretics
Medications
    Sodium sulfate, sodium phosphate
    Glucocorticoids
    Calcitonin
    Mithramycin
Treatment of choice: surgical removal of the gland(s)

Nursing diagnoses/interventions/evaluation

■ **NDX:** Potential for fluid volume deficit (1) related to hypercalcemia

Monitor IV and oral fluid intake
    1000 ml/hr for short period may be given initially IV, then oral fluids to 3000 ml/day
Monitor vital signs, central venous pressure (CVP), and breath sounds q4h
Monitor intake, output, and electrolyte values q4h
Monitor cardiac rhythm for changes in T waves or QT intervals indicative of hypercalcemia
Assess muscle strength and mobility q4h
Assess reflexes q4h
Administer medications as ordered and observe for adverse reactions: hypotension with IV phosphates, extravasation with IV mithramycin
Weigh daily: same time, clothes, scale
Assess skin condition and turgor q8h
Maintain low-calcium, high-phosphorus diet
Collaborate with physician if any changes in physical condition are detected

Expected outcome/evaluation

Vital signs are stable; intake and output are balanced; electrolytes are within normal range; skin is warm and moist with good turgor

■ **NDX:** Potential for trauma related to risk of pathological fracture

Assess for pain; may be indicative of fracture
Maintain correct body alignment as indicated to prevent fractures
Assist patient with ambulation as needed
Provide aids to ambulation: walker, cane
Place articles within easy reach that patient may require frequently
Arrange environment simply; avoid unnecessary clutter
Provide night-light
Place call bell within easy reach at all times

Instruct patient to call for assistance before getting out of bed
Keep bed in low position with side rails up when in bed
Assist with personal hygiene as needed
Use safety measures (e.g., jacket restraint) as necessary if patient is confused
Remove potentially hazardous objects from patient's environment

Expected outcome/evaluation

No physical injury occurs; verbalizes no pain or increasing discomfort

■ **NDX:** Altered thought processes related to slow mentation, depression, and/or drowsiness

Assess level of consciousness and orientation q4h
Provide a stable, calm, and nonstressful environment
    Be consistent in timing and performance of activities and procedures
    Restrict patient's visitors as necessary
    Avoid frequent changing of personnel
    Prevent emotionally upsetting or confusing situations
Plan care with patient as appropriate
Anticipate needs
Reorient patient to environment as necessary
Explain procedures slowly and clearly; repeat as necessary
Encourage patient to take active role in care
Avoid administration of narcotics or sedatives if possible

Expected outcome/evaluation

Patient is alert, oriented and accomplishes self-care as planned

■ **NDX:** Knowledge deficit related to lack of information regarding disease process, treatment, and self-care

Explain basic concepts of the disease
Discuss reasons for physical and emotional changes
Teach name of medication, dosage, time and method of administration, purpose, side effects, and toxic effects
Explain need to avoid taking over-the-counter medications without consulting physician
Emphasize importance of ongoing outpatient follow-up
Instruct patient to maintain low-calcium, high-phosphorus diet
Instruct patient to maintain increased fluid intake
Emphasize importance of maintaining safe environment, need to report signs of fractures to physician

Expected outcome/evaluation

Patient and/or significant other verbalizes understanding of disease process and principles of home and follow-up care

ADRENOCORTICAL INSUFFICIENCY

Hypofunction of the adrenal cortex; primary adrenocortical insufficiency, Addison's disease, results in a deficiency of mineralocorticoids and glucocorticoids; secondary insufficiency results in a deficiency of only glucocorticoids; primary insufficiency is usually due to idiopathic atrophy of the cortex, most likely an autoimmune response, whereas secondary insufficiency may be due to pituitary tumor, postpartum pituitary necrosis, tumor of the third ventricle, head trauma, or optic gliomas

Assessment

Observations/findings

Neurological
  Mental fatigue
  Apathy
Musculoskeletal
  Weakness
  Fatigue
Cardiovascular
  Postural hypotension with reflex tachycardia
  Decreased tolerance of cold or stress
  Hypovolemia
Gastrointestinal
  Weight loss
  Anorexia
  Nausea, vomiting
  Abdominal pain
  Salt craving
  Diarrhea
Integumentary
  Hyperpigmentation; bronze coloration
  Decreased body hair
Sexual/reproductive
  Loss of secondary sex characteristics (especially in females)
  Amenorrhea
  Decreased libido

Diagnostic/laboratory studies

Increased serum ADH
Increased serum ACTH in primary; decreased in secondary
Hyponatremia
Hyperkalemia
Increased BUN
Metabolic acidosis
Increased plasma renin levels
Decreased plasma cortisol, no response to administration of ACTH in primary; gradual increase over several days in secondary
Decreased plasma aldosterone
Subnormal excretion in urine of 17-hydroxycorticoids and aldosterone-18-glucuronide
X-ray examination: small heart, adrenal calcification

Potential complications

Adrenal (Addisonian) crisis: medical emergency involving intensification of symptoms of adrenal insufficiency; usually precipitated by acute infection, trauma, surgery, or excessive loss of body salts
Observations/findings in adrenal crisis include
  Profound weakness, fatigue
  Severe hypotension
  Nausea, vomiting
  Dehydration
  Severe pain: back, abdomen, extremities
  Severe headache
  Hypopyrexia
  Hyperthermia in acute infection
  Shock
  Cardiac arrest
  Renal failure
  Azotemia
  Death

Medical Management

IV hydration and sodium replacement
Glucocorticoids: corticosteroids
Mineralocorticoids: fludrocortisone
In crisis: vasopressors, plasma expanders, supportive therapy (e.g., oxygen)
Antibiotics if infection is cause of episode
Diet and activity

Nursing diagnoses/interventions/evaluation

■ **NDX:** Potential for injury related to risk of adrenal crisis

Assess vital signs q4h and prn; report abnormal findings to physician immediately as severe hypotension can lead to vascular collapse
Monitor cardiac rhythm continuously if dysrhythmias occur: for hyperkalemia initially, then hypokalemia
Monitor intake and output q4h and prn; report output greater than intake
Monitor neurological status q4h; report increasing headache and confusion
Position patient to promote cardiovascular and respiratory function
Collaborate with physician, if adrenal crisis develops, to administer IV fluids, vasopressors, corticosteroids, and oxygen

Expected outcome/evaluation

Vital signs are stable and within normal limits; alert, oriented; intake and output are balanced

■ **NDX:** Potential for injury related to risk of inability to tolerate environmental stresses

Select quiet, nonstimulating room with noninfectious roommate

Avoid exposure to cold: provide extra blankets; have patient wear bed socks and use warm robe when out of bed

Administer steroid therapy as ordered

Consider need for increased doses of steroids during periods of stress (consult physician)

Always administer steroid therapy on time; do not alter hours of administration or dose abruptly

Medicate for pain or nausea as required

Encourage regular rest periods alternating with activity

Anticipate stressful situations and defuse if possible

Avoid discussing stress-producing topics; inform visitors

Monitor and restrict visitors if patient desires

Plan daily schedule with patient and avoid unexpected events

Expected outcome/evaluation

Begins to tolerate environmental stresses as evidenced by increased interest and participation in daily schedule and desire for visitors

Discusses disease process and asks questions

■ **NDX:** Potential for infection related to inability of adrenal cortex to produce steroids in times of stress

Monitor for signs and symptoms of infection; report if detected (URI, UTI, wounds, IV, or infection sites)

Have patient turn, cough, and deep breathe q2h while on bed rest

Avoid unnecessary invasive procedures (urinary catheterization)

Maintain sterile technique when caring for any skin lesions, tubes, drains, or IV lines

Culture suspicious wounds or secretions

Maintain optimal nutritional and fluid status

Avoid placing patient in room with other potentially infectious patients

Avoid having nursing personnel with infections care for patient

Screen visitors and restrict those with potential infections or instruct to wear mask and wash hands before visiting

Expected outcome/evaluation

Temperature is within normal range; no other signs of infection (respiratory, renal, or skin) present

■ **NDX:** Activity intolerance related to fatigue and weakness

Assess present activity level

Allow patient to move at own pace

Assist with active or perform passive ROM exercises while patient is on bed rest

Assist with ambulation and bed mobility as needed

Provide patient with assistive devices: walker, cane, over-the-bed trapeze, side rails

Anticipate need for help with daily activities (grooming, feeding, toileting)

Restrict patient's activities to level of tolerance

Discontinue activity at first signs of intolerance: tachycardia, fatigue, dyspnea, cardiac dysrhythmias, drop in blood pressure, complaints of vertigo

Expected outcome/evaluation

Performs ADLs without evidence of fatigue or weakness; vital signs remain within normal limits during ROM exercises, ambulation, and ADLs

■ **NDX:** Pain related to headache, back, extremity, abdomen

Identify, with help of patient, location, severity of pain, and factors that increase or decrease pain

Assess need for and administer pain medication as ordered

Explore with patient measures to reduce or relieve pain: positioning, use of pillows for support, warm or cold compresses, manipulation or massage of body part or area

Monitor effectiveness of interventions at routine intervals

Provide distraction from pain (conversation, visitors, reading materials, quiet music)

Assist patient with developing pain management techniques, such as progressive relaxation or guided imagery

Expected outcome/evaluation

Reports absence of pain

Exhibits relaxed body position and facial expression

Begins using relaxation techniques

■ **NDX:** Fluid volume deficit (1) related to inability of renal tubules to retain sodium and water

Monitor serum sodium levels q8h

Measure intake and output q8h and prn; report intake less than output

Weigh patient daily same time, scale, and clothing; observe for weight loss

Encourage fluid intake to 2500 ml/day or as ordered

Administer IV fluids and sodium replacement as ordered

Assess for signs and symptoms of hypovolemia or dehydration: poor skin turgor, weak pulses, tachycardia, thirst, low blood pressure, cool skin, increased body temperature, dry mucous membranes, change in mental status

Report occurrence of any of these signs or symptoms to physician without delay

Administer antiemetics as ordered

Provide diet high in sodium

Expected outcome/evaluation

Intake and output are balanced

Skin is moist with good turgor

Mucous membranes and tongue are moist
Weight is stable within ideal range for body build and height

■ **NDX:** Knowledge deficit related to lack of information regarding disease process, treatment, and self-care

Explain basic concepts of the disease process and symptoms of recurrence requiring medication dosage adjustment
Explain reasons for physical and emotional changes
Teach name of medication, dosage, time and method of administration, and toxic and side effects
Explain that hormone therapy must be continued throughout lifetime
Instruct that emergency IM medication must be carried at all times for use in times of stress
　Demonstrate method of administering IM injections to patient and significant other
Explain need to avoid taking over-the-counter medications without consulting physician
Emphasize importance of regular exercise alternating with rest periods and avoiding strenuous exercise
Teach patient to practice relaxation techniques daily
Explain need to avoid persons with infectious diseases (especially URIs)
Teach stress risk factors to report
　Infection
　Fever, persistent cough, flu, or cold
　Burning on urination
　Wounds that are red and swollen
　Injury
　Surgery
　Routine dental care
　Profuse sweating in hot weather or strenuous exercise
　Emotionally charged situations
　Positive or negative changes in lifestyle or relationships
Instruct patient to wear medical alert band and inform all health care providers of disease
Explain need for high-sodium, low-potassium diet with plenty of fluids

Expected outcome/evaluation

Verbalizes understanding of disease process
Continues medication therapy
States symptoms of recurrence and infection to report
Discusses plans to carry emergency medication
Wears medical alert bracelet
Discusses methods to incorporate diet, exercise, and rest periods into lifestyle
Demonstrates IM injection technique and relaxation technique

CUSHING'S SYNDROME AND CUSHING'S DISEASE

Cushing's syndrome arises from either ectopic ACTH-secreting tumors of the adrenals or from iatrogenic causes, such as excessive doses of cortisol or ACTH; Cushing's disease results from pathology of the pituitary gland in which the negative-feedback loop is faulty and the pituitary continues to secrete ACTH in the face of high levels of plasma cortisol; the effects on protein, carbohydrate, and lipid metabolism in both syndrome and disease are due to prolonged exposure to high levels of glucocorticoid hormone

Assessment
Observations/findings

Neurological
　Lability of mood: depression to mania
Musculoskeletal
　Buffalo hump
　Truncal obesity with thin extremities
　Supraclavicular fat pads
　Backache
　Muscle weakness or wasting
　Osteoporosis
Cardiovascular
　Hypertension
　Fluid retention with pitting edema
Gastrointestinal
　Polydipsia
　Weight gain
Renal
　Polyuria
Metabolic
　Impaired wound healing
　Increased susceptibility to infection
　Carbohydrate intolerance
Integumentary
　Moon face
　Thin, transparent skin
　Increased pigmentation
　Easily bruised
Sexual/reproductive
　Female masculinization
　Menstrual disorders
　Male feminization
　Impotence
　Decreased libido

Laboratory/diagnostic studies

Hyperglycemia
Metabolic alkalosis
Hypokalemia
Elevated plasma ACTH when tested throughout day
Elevated serum sodium and plasma cortisol

Plasma cortisol not suppressed with dexamethasone
White blood cell count (WBC) elevated
Hyperactive response to 8-hr ACTH stimulation test
Increased 24-hr urine cortisol and 17-hydroxycortico-
  steroids
Increased response to metapyrone

Potential complications

Pathological fractures
Congestive heart failure
Peptic ulcers

Medical Management

Transphenoid hypophysectomy (p. 349) or irradiation of
  pituitary adenoma if present (most common cause)
Diet: decreased calories and carbohydrates; low sodium
  and high potassium
Medications
  Mitotane
  Aminoglutethimide
  Metapyrone
  Cyproheptadine
  Correct electrolyte imbalance
Adrenalectomy (p. 347)

Nursing diagnoses/interventions/evaluation

■ **NDX:** Body image disturbance related to musculoskeletal, integumentary, and sexual/reproduc-
  tive changes

Maintain environment conducive to discussing body im-
  age changes
Discuss feelings related to changes with patient
Assist patient with identifying and developing personal
  strengths and coping mechanisms for dealing with phys-
  ical changes
Provide information about reversibility of symptoms with
  treatment
Assist with grooming to enhance appearance; personal
  hygiene, hair removal measures, attractive clothing
Respect patient's wishes for privacy
Be sensitive to needs
Set aside time each shift for active listening and emotional
  support
Consult mental health nursing specialist

Expected outcome/evaluation

Discusses feelings about changes in appearance
Verbalizes knowledge that reversal of symptoms will occur
  with treatment
Performs daily hygiene
Enhances appearance through judicious use of cosmetics
  and clothing if appropriate

■ **NDX:** Potential for infection related to impaired immune responses

Monitor temperature and for other signs or symptoms of
  infection q4h
Have patient turn, cough, and deep breathe q2h while
  on bed rest
Avoid unnecessary invasive procedures (urinary catheterization)
Use sterile technique when caring for any skin lesions,
  tubes, drains, or IV sites
Culture suspicious wound sites or secretions
Maintain optimal nutritional status
Avoid placing patient in room with other potentially infectious patient
Avoid having personnel with URI or other infections care
  for patient; monitor visitors for signs of infection and
  restrict as needed or teach handwashing and wearing
  mask before visit

Expected outcome/evaluation

Temperature within normal limits; no evidence of infection in integumentary, respiratory, and renal systems

■ **NDX:** Potential for impaired skin integrity related to
  fragile capillaries and/or thinning of skin

Assess for redness or skin breakdown q8h; if patient is on
  bed rest, assess q4h
Administer skin care to pressure points q4h and as needed
Use oil or lotion in bathwater; rinse and dry well
Avoid use of harsh soaps or rough towels
Use elbow and heel protectors and pull sheets
Place patient on decubitus-prevention mattress or bed
Assist and encourage patient to change positions fre-
  quently; teach and assist with ROM; ambulate as soon
  as possible; have patient avoid sitting position for longer
  than 1 hour
Maintain optimal nutritional status

Expected outcome/evaluation

Skin is intact and without evidence of redness

■ **NDX:** Activity intolerance related to musculoskeletal
  weakness due to increased protein catabolism

Allow patient to move at own pace: use side rails and
  overhead trapeze
Alternate activity with rest periods to aid in increasing
  tolerance
Assist with and provide aids to ambulation (walker, cane)
  as necessary
Anticipate need for help with daily activities; grooming,

toileting, feeding; provide needed supplies within reach to reduce energy expenditure

Restrict activities to patient's level of tolerance

Discontinue activity at first signs of intolerance: tachycardia, dyspnea, fatigue

Encourage patient to increase activity as tolerance increases, but to seek assistance with appearance of symptoms of intolerance

Expected outcome/evaluation

Increases participation in self-care and activities daily
Reports decreased feelings of weakness and fatigue

■ **NDX:** Altered thought processes related to excessive cortisol secretion

Evaluate past and present coping methods

Encourage discussion of feelings of loss of control

Discuss reactions that are out of proportion to event and methods for future coping

Explain that these mood swings will abate with treatment

Teach and assist with relaxation techniques

Provide a stable, calm, and nonstressful environment
Be consistent in timing and performance of activities and procedures
Restrict visitors as necessary
Avoid frequent changing of personnel
Prevent emotionally upsetting situations

Plan care with patient and anticipate needs

Provide diversional activities and materials of preference

Reorient patient to environment as needed
Explain procedures slowly and clearly; repeat as necessary

Expected outcome/evaluation

Patient is alert and oriented

Discusses feelings easily

Acknowledges inappropriate responses to situations and discusses plan for managing response

Practices relaxation techniques

■ **NDX:** Fluid volume excess related to excessive secretion of cortisol causing sodium and water retention

Monitor electrolyte values q4h to 8h and report abnormal findings to physician

Monitor intake and output q4h

Weigh patient daily: same time, scale, and clothing; report increasing weight

Avoid excessive fluid intake when patient is hypernatremic

Monitor ECG for abnormalities associated with electrolyte imbalances, usually hypernatremia and hypokalemia

Monitor blood pressure, pulse, and breath sounds q4h and report significant changes from patient's baseline

Assess dependent areas for edema
Provide support and skin care for edematous areas; turn and reposition q2h

Maintain high-protein, high-potassium, low-sodium, decreased-calorie diet

Expected outcome/evaluation

Vital signs and electrolytes are within normal range for patient; intake and output are balanced; weight is stabilized and within patient's normal limits; no evidence of edema present

Additional nursing diagnoses to consider

Altered nutrition: less than body requirements related to altered CHO metabolism and hyperglycemia (see Diabetes Mellitus, p. 332)

Potential for trauma related to risk of pathological fractures

Potential for injury related to risk of hypertension

■ **NDX:** Knowledge deficit related to lack of information regarding disease process, treatment, and self-care

Explain basic concepts of the disease

Discuss reasons for physical and emotional changes

Discuss and give written information about diet: low sodium, decreased CHO, and increased potassium

Explain importance of maintaining a safe environment and balancing activity with rest

Teach name of medication, dosage, time and method of administration, purpose, side effects, and toxic effects

Explain that medication must not be discontinued without consulting physician

Explain need to avoid taking over-the-counter medications without consulting physician

Emphasize importance of ongoing outpatient care

Prepare for adrenalectomy (p. 347) or radiotherapy of pituitary as indicated

Expected outcome/evaluation

Patient and/or significant other verbalizes understanding of disease process, principles of home and follow-up care, and plans for surgery or radiation therapy

PRIMARY ALDOSTERONISM

Overproduction of mineralocorticoids by the adrenal cortex caused by benign adenoma, or less commonly, by carcinoma or hyperplasia of the adrenal cortex

Assessment
Observations/findings

Neurological
  Muscle weakness
  Fatigue
  Paresthesia
  Paralysis of arms and legs
  Positive Chvostek's sign
  Tetany
  Autonomic dysfunction
Cardiovascular
  Hypertension
  Postural hypotension without reflex tachycardia
  Increased pulse when squatting
  Cardiomegaly
  Decreased conduction through myocardium
Renal
  Polyuria, especially nocturnal
  Polydipsia
  Azotemia

Laboratory/diagnostic studies

Elevated plasma aldosterone
Suppressed/nonstimulatable plasma renin activity
Failure to suppress aldosterone with usual maneuvers
Hypernatremia
Hypokalemia
Hypervolemia
Metabolic alkalosis
Urine excretion (24 hr) of 18-glucuronide
ECG
  Depressed ST segments and T waves; appearance of U
    waves
  Premature ventricular contractions
Iodocholesterol scan
CT scan of adrenal glands to localize an adenoma or to
  differentiate hyperplasia from adenoma
Adrenal venous catheterization

Potential complications

Renal failure
Heart failure

Medical Management

Adrenalectomy (p. 347)
  Unilateral for adenoma
  Bilateral for hyperplasia
Spironolactone
Low-sodium, high-potassium diet

Nursing diagnoses/interventions/evaluation

■ **NDX:** Fluid volume excess related to hypernatremia

Weigh patient daily same time, scale, and clothing; report
  to physician if gain of over 0.5 kg occurs

Measures intake and output q8h
Maintain low-sodium diet
Monitor serum sodium levels q8h
Monitor for signs and symptoms of fluid overload: pul-
  monary edema (dyspnea, orthopnea, crackles in lung
  fields)
Monitor chest x-ray examination results
Monitor vital signs q4h and prn; observe for increased
  pulse, development of S_3 gallop, and labored respira-
  tions
Notify physician of development or worsening of any of
  the preceding signs or symptoms
Monitor pedal pulses q4h
Monitor effectiveness and side effects of diuretics

Expected outcome/evaluation

Vital signs and breath sounds are within normal limits for
  patient
Intake and output are balanced

■ **NDX:** Potential for altered tissue perfusion; cardiopulmonary related to dysrhythmias due to hypokalemia

Maintain high-potassium diet: avocado, apricots, ba-
  nanas, meat, poultry, potatoes, milk
Administer potassium supplements as ordered
Monitor serum potassium levels q8h and prn
Monitor for signs and symptoms of hypokalemia
  ECG changes (ectopic beats, decreased T wave ampli-
    tude, increased U wave amplitude)
  Muscular weakness
  Neurological impairments
Collaborate with physician to alter development of any
  of the preceding signs or symptoms
Anticipate need for assistance with ADLs
Assist with active ROM exercises q8h if patient is on bed
  rest

Expected outcome/evaluation

Plasma potassium levels are within normal range
ECG exhibits normal sinus rhythm
Exhibits no signs of muscle weakness or paresthesia

■ **NDX:** Potential for injury related to risk of muscle
  weakness, paresthesia, autonomic dysfunction,
  and/or tetany

Assess neuromuscular function q4h to 8h; report changes
  indicative of potential tetany; increasing weakness or
  paresthesia
Allow patient to move at own pace; encourage use of side
  rails and trapeze for assistance
Assist with and encourage ambulation if patient is able;
  instruct patient to call before getting out of bed

Keep call bell within reach at all times

Provide aids to ambulation such as a walker or cane

Anticipate postural hypotension when patient gets out of bed or chair; if it occurs, have patient sit or lie down with head lower than heart

Keep bed in low position and side rails up

Use safety measures (padded side rails for tetany; oral airway) as needed

Remove potentially hazardous materials and objects from patient's environment

Expected outcome/evaluation

Patient sustains no physical injury

■ **NDX:** Knowledge deficit related to lack of information about disease process, treatment, and self-care

Explain basic concepts of the disease; signs and symptoms of hypokalemia, hypernatremia, and hypocalcemia to report to physician

Teach name of medication, dosage, time and method of administration, purpose, side effects, and toxic effects; if on spironolactone teach signs of hyperkalemia to report

Discuss importance of not discontinuing medication without checking with physician

Explain need to avoid taking over-the-counter medications without consulting physician

Discuss and prepare for adrenalectomy if planned

Emphasize importance of ongoing outpatient care

Emphasize importance of regular exercise alternating with rest periods

Discuss and provide information about therapeutic low-sodium, high-potassium diet

Emphasize importance of obtaining and wearing medical alert bracelet

Expected outcome/evaluation

Patient and/or significant other verbalizes understanding of disease process and principles of home and follow-up care

PHEOCHROMOCYTOMA

A chromaffin cell tumor of the adrenal medulla that secretes an excess of the catecholamines, epinephrine and norepinephrine; the increased catecholamines cause severe hypertension, increased metabolism, and hyperglycemia

Assessment
Observations/findings

Episodic; occurring every 2 months to 25 times each day

Neurological

Anxiety/nervousness

Feelings of impending doom

Headache

Insomnia

Paresthesia

Cardiovascular

Persistent or paroxysmal hypertension

Excessive diaphoresis

Tachycardia

Palpitations

Flushing

Respiratory

Tachypnea

Gastrointestinal/nutritional

Hyperglycemia

Nausea, vomiting

Weight loss, occasionally gain

Renal: decreased urine output

Precipitating risk factors

Postural change

Exercise

Laughing

Smoking

Urination

Change in body or environmental temperature

Vasovagal stimulus

Any event that increases pressure on tumor (pregnancy)

Laboratory/diagnostic studies

Elevated serum catecholamines

Elevated urine metanephrines and vanillylmandelic acid

Failure of serum catecholamines to respond by suppression after administration of clonidine

Hyperglycemia

Abdominal CT scan showing tumor location

Potential complications

Heart failure

Renal failure

Cerebrovascular accident (CVA)

Myocarditis

Dysrhythmias

Surgical morbidity or mortality

Medical Management

Surgical removal of the tumor(s)

Medications

α- and β-Adrenergic blockers

α-Methylparatyrosine

Nursing diagnoses/interventions/evaluation

■ **NDX:** Altered tissue perfusion, cardiopulmonary and renal, related to hypertensive episodes

Remain with patient during episodes of hypertension

Monitor blood pressure and pulse electronically q10min to 15min

Be prepared to administer antihypertensive medications

Position patient with head elevated 30 degrees to minimize effects on ICP

Perform neurological checks; auscultate chest for heart sounds, rate, and rhythm

Monitor breath sounds; observe for dyspnea

Measure urinary output qh; report if <30 ml/hr

Provide a calm, low-stimulus atmosphere

Monitor orthostatic vital signs; report if difference >10 mm Hg

Monitor intake and output q8h

Review events occurring before episode to determine etiology; discuss methods of avoiding precipitating events, if present, with patient

Keep bed dry and wrinkle-free if patient is diaphoretic

Provide quiet environment for adequate periods of rest

Expected outcome/evaluation

Orthostatic vital signs are within normal limits; intake and output are with output >30 ml/hr; verbalizes no palpitation, nervousness, or headache

■ **NDX:** Sleep pattern disturbance related to increased levels of circulating catecholamines

Assess usual sleep pattern and use of any aids

Provide sleep aids requested by patient: quiet music, warm drink

Discourage frequent daytime sleeping

Avoid intake of stimulants in diet

Assist patient with establishing a regular pattern of activity

Provide environment conducive to sleep: reduce lighting; close door to room; maintain quiet and privacy

Avoid disturbing patient at night for unnecessary procedures

Schedule treatments, procedures, and medications for daytime and evening hours when possible

Expected outcome/evaluation

Reports feeling well rested after sleep

Maintains energy throughout day without need for naps

■ **NDX:** Altered nutrition: less than body requirements related to increased metabolism and/or nausea

Assess nutritional status and food preferences

Assist patient to select daily menus and incorporate basic food groups

Provide several small meals if patient prefers

Ask patient's family to bring favorite foods from home, within limits of therapeutic diet

Assist patient with arranging meal tray and with feeding if necessary

Provide dietary consultation to reduce tyramine-containing foods in diet

Monitor blood glucose; report if elevated

Monitor food intake daily

Weigh patient daily; same time, scale, and clothing

Expected outcome/evaluation

Weight is increasing toward level required for body build and height

■ **NDX:** Knowledge deficit related to lack of information regarding disease process, treatment, and self care

Explain basic concepts of the disease process and potential risk factors

Discuss methods for avoiding hypertensive episodes

Provide written information about diet and reduction of tyramine-containing foods

Teach name of medication, dosage, time and method of administration, purpose, side effects, and toxic effects

Explain need to avoid taking over-the-counter medications without consulting physician

Emphasize importance of ongoing outpatient care

Provide information for obtaining medical alert bracelet and card

Refer to Adrenalectomy (p. 347) for preoperative patient teaching

Expected outcome/evaluation

Patient and/or significant other verbalizes understanding of disease process and principles of home and follow-up care

HYPOPITUITARISM

Decreased or absent secretion of one or more of the anterior pituitary gland hormones; causes are varied and may include malignancies, other tumors, infection, vascular changes, or physical injury such as head trauma; hypopituitarism may be a disorder of the pituitary gland itself or may be caused by insufficient pituitary stimulation by the hypothalamus

Assessment
Observations/findings*

General
    Wrinkled, waxy skin
    Hypothermia
    Low blood pressure
    Low serum glucose
Gonadotropin deficiency
    Regression of secondary sex characteristics
    Decreased libido
    Impotence, infertility

---

*Findings depend on which hormonal deficiencies are present.

Loss of muscle tone
Thyrotropin deficiency: see Hypothyroidism (p. 312); symptoms will be less severe
ACTH deficiency
    See Adrenocortical Insufficiency (p. 322)
    No hyperpigmentation
    No sodium depletion
Growth hormone deficiency
    Mental retardation in children
    Dwarfism/short stature
    Lack of development of secondary sex characteristics
    High-pitched voice
Prolactin deficiency: absence of lactation in postpartum women

Laboratory/diagnostic studies

Deficiency of serum cortisol, thyroxine, testosterone, and/or estrogen
Lack of compensatory increased levels of serum ACTH, TSH, FSH, and LH

Potential complications

Deficiencies are usually not severe (see specific disease entities)

Medical Management

Hormone replacement
    Glucocorticoids
    Thyroxine
    Gonadal steroids
    Growth hormone in children
    GnRH therapy in women to restore fertility

Nursing diagnoses/interventions/evaluation*

■ **NDX:** Body image disturbance related to changes in physical characteristics and capabilities

Encourage verbalization by patient of feelings related to physical changes
Assist patient with developing coping mechanisms to deal with changes
Reinforce patient's qualities that have positive effect on self-image
Answer questions and clarify misunderstandings regarding diagnosis and permanence or regression of changes
Assist patient with developing a plan to incorporate any permanent changes into lifestyle
Demonstrate acceptance of patient and encourage others to do the same
Reinforce behaviors that demonstrate acceptance of changes

---

*For further interventions refer to specific disease entity.

Expected outcome/evaluation

Verbalizes feelings about physical changes to others
Discusses strengths and sets realistic goals

■ **NDX:** Altered sexuality patterns related to hormonal deficiencies

Maintain privacy and confidentiality
Explore with patient and/or significant other usual patterns of sexuality and how current diagnosis may affect these patterns
Encourage patient and/or significant other to explore alternatives to usual patterns that consider limitations of the disease
Initiate referral to appropriate personnel if patient desires
Explore with patient and/or significant other alternatives to becoming parents if appropriate

Expected outcome/evaluation

Begins to discuss feelings about sexuality with partner
Verbalizes understanding of effect of diagnosis on sexual patterns
Accepts referral for counseling

■ **NDX:** Knowledge deficit related to lack of information regarding disease process, treatment, and self-care

Provide and discuss information about*:
    Basic concepts of the disease process
    Name of medication, dosage, time and method of administration, purpose, side effects, and toxic effects
    Importance of regular outpatient follow-up
    Need to avoid taking over-the-counter medications without consulting physician
    Importance of discussing feelings regarding body changes with significant other
    Signs and symptoms to report to physician (see specific disease)
    Provide referral for sexual counseling when appropriate

Expected outcome/evaluation

Patient demonstrates beginning of acceptance of change in physical characteristics and capabilities
Discusses alternatives to usual sexual patterns
Verbalizes understanding of disease process and home and follow-up care

CENTRAL DIABETES INSIPIDUS

Disorder of hypothalamus or posterior pituitary that results in insufficient synthesis or secretion of antidiuretic hormone; consequently, the renal mechanism for

concentration of urine is impaired and large amounts of dilute urine are excreted; causes may include head injury, neurological surgery, and hypothalamic tumors

Assessment
Observations/findings

Gastrointestinal
  Polydipsia
  Weight loss
  Dehydration
Renal
  Polyuria to 10 L daily
  Frequency
  Nocturia
Integumentary
  Dry skin and mucous membranes
  Poor turgor

Laboratory/diagnostic studies

Increased serum osmolality, >300 mosm/kg
Urine specific gravity of less than 1.007
Urine osmolality of less than 50 to 200 mosm/kg; increases
  with administration of pitressin
Electrolyte imbalances
Water deprivation studies
Hypertonic saline test

Potential complications

Severe dehydration
Hypotension
Shock

Medical Management

Parenteral fluids
ADH replacement therapy
  Pitressin tannate in oil
  Aqueous pitressin
  Lypressin nasal solution
Synthetic vasopressin: DDAVP
Chlorpropamide

Nursing diagnosis/interventions/evaluation

■ **NDX:** Fluid volume deficit (1) related to inability of renal tubules to concentrate urine in absence of ADH

Provide sufficient fluid of patient's preference to maintain
  equal intake and output per 24 hr
Supplement oral intake with IV fluids as ordered
Monitor intake and output q2h and notify physician if
  output is greater than 100 ml over intake or if output
  is greater than 200 ml/hr
Weigh patient daily, observing for weight loss or gain
With each voiding check urine for specific gravity; send
  urine for osmolality daily; report specific gravity <1.007
Assess for signs and symptoms of hypovolemia: tachycardia, poor skin tugor, weak pulses, low blood pressure,
  cool skin, increased body temperature, dry mucous
  membranes, changes in mental status
Report occurrence of any of preceding signs or symptoms
  to physician and initiate medical orders without delay
Administer ADH replacement therapy as ordered and
  monitor effectiveness
  Observe for side effects: hypertension, chest pain, uter-
    ine cramps, and increased peristalsis
  Monitor for overhydration: headache, changes in LOC,
    confusion
  Report abnormal findings
Monitor for hypoglycemia if taking chlorpropamide; give
  rapid-acting carbohydrates if symptoms present; report
  to physician

Expected outcome/evaluation

Intake and output are balanced
Intake is ≤2500 ml/day
Output is ≤100 ml/hr
Urine specific gravity is within normal limits
Skin is moist with good turgor
Weight is within patient's ideal limits
Vital signs are within normal limits

 NDX: Knowledge deficit related to lack of information regarding disease process, treatment and self-care

Explain basic concepts of disease process
Teach name of medication, purpose, time and method of
  administration, dosage, and toxic and side effects
  Explain need to monitor for side effects and report if
    present
  Teach to monitor urine specific gravity and measure
    intake and output (medication dosage may be based
    on appearance of symptoms)
  Instruct to weigh daily; report loss or gain as these are
    symptoms of recurrence or fluid retention, indicating
    change needed in medication dosage
  Demonstrate injection method if medication to be
    taken IM
Emphasize importance of maintaining fluid intake equal
  to output
Explain need to avoid liquids that may cause a diuretic
  effect: coffee, alcohol, tea
Emphasize importance of regular outpatient follow-up
Explain need to avoid taking over-the-counter medica-
  tions without consulting physician
Provide information to obtain medical alert bracelet and
  card

Expected outcome/evaluation

Verbalizes understanding of disease process, medication
  directions, symptoms to report, and need to obtain medical alert bracelet

Demonstrates measuring intake and output and urine specific gravity

Performs IM injection

DIABETES MELLITUS

A chronic disorder characterized by disturbances in carbohydrate, protein, and fat metabolism resulting from a complete or relative lack of insulin; two major classifications are type 1: insulin-dependent diabetes mellitus (IDDM) and type II: non-insulin–dependent diabetes mellitus (NIDDM) (Table 6-2); other classifications not discussed here are gestational diabetes, secondary diabetes, and impaired glucose tolerance diabetes.

Assessment

See Table 6-2 (p. 333)

Medical Management

See Table 6-2 (p. 333)

Nursing diagnoses/interventions/evaluation

■ **NDX:** Fluid volume deficit (1) related to absent or deficient insulin function

Assess vital signs q4h to 8h

Monitor intake and output q8h; check urine for ketones

Assess skin turgor; moisture and condition of mucous membranes q4h to 8h

Assess mental status

Monitor blood glucose before administration of insulin or oral hypoglycemics and meals, and/or according to a predetermined schedule, usually q4h initially

Begin teaching self-blood glucose monitoring (p. 338)

Monitor effectiveness of administration of insulin

Usually rapid-acting ordered initially, then intermediate-acting in split doses with or without addition of rapid-acting (type 1); may need to use 70/30 insulin if patient has difficulty mixing the two different types of insulin

Monitor effectiveness of oral hypoglycemics if ordered for NIDDM

Assess for continuing signs of hyperglycemia (see Assessment, p. 333)

Assess for signs of hypoglycemia; blood glucose ≤ 60 mg/dl, dizziness, lightheadedness, tachycardia, sweating, shakiness, or altered level of consciousness

Provide noncaloric fluids as well as those allowed on ADA diet to 2500 ml/day

Monitor electrolyte and CO_2 lab values

Assess for disturbances in electrolyes and CO_2 (Table 1-3, pp. 38-51)

Be aware of potassium shift as fluid volume deficit improves

Assist with ADLs when patient unable to complete because of weakness or malaise

Encourage self-care as condition improves

Expected outcome/evaluation

Vital signs are stable and within normal limits for patient; intake and output are balanced; ketones are not present in urine; skin is moist with good turgor; blood sugar, electrolytes, and CO_2 are within normal range; patient completes ADLs without expression of fatigue or weakness

■ **NDX:** Altered nutrition: less than body requirements related to diabetes mellitus (generally IDDM)

Assess dietary intake pattern and nutritional status

Provide dietary consultation for instruction about ordered ADA diet for patient and significant other

Assist patient to select daily menu based on ADA program prescribed; reinforce correct choices

Monitor daily food intake; assist at mealtimes when necessary because of fatigue, etc.

Provide exchanges for foods not taken at mealtimes

Provide relaxing environment and allow ample time for meals; visiting by support person may be helpful

Stress importance of regular meal and snack times, eating all foods and snacks provided or exchanging; remind not to save exchanges for another meal

Collaborate with physician to determine exercise program to meet patient's needs and lifestyle

Begin first phase of program

Assist patient to check need for additional carbohydrates before exercise through use of self-blood glucose monitoring (see Table 6-3)

Weigh daily; same time, scale, and clothing

Expected outcome/evaluation

Maintains stable weight or increases weight to that predetermined for body build

Selects menus based on ordered ADA diet and eats meals and snacks as scheduled

Monitors blood glucose

Determines type of snack and takes snack only if needed before exercise

■ **NDX:** Altered nutrition: more than body requirements related to diabetes mellitus, usually NIDDM

Assess baseline nutritional status; height, weight, activity level, eating patterns and preferences

Teach relationship of obesity to diabetes

TABLE 6-2. Two Major Classifications of Diabetes Mellitus

	Insulin-dependent diabetes mellitus (IDDM)	Non-insulin–dependent diabetes mellitus (NIDDM)
DEFINITION		
Onset	<30 yr	>40 yr
Etiology	Postulated that beta cell destruction occurs resulting from infection (usually viral) and/or autoimmune response in genetically disposed persons	Interaction between heredity and environmental factors such as obesity, diet, and lifestyle is postulated
Insulin	Early: present but deficient; late: usually absent	Normal to above normal quantity
ASSESSMENT		
Observation/findings	Polyuria Polydipsia Polyphagia Weakness Fatigue Malaise Weight loss Irritability Late symptoms: see Diabetic Ketoacidosis (DKA) (p. 340)	Fatigue Polyuria Polydipsia Vision changes Tingling, numbness of extremities Slow healing of cuts Skin infections or pruritis Drowsiness Late symptoms: see Hyperosmolar Hyperglycemic Nonketotic Coma (HHNC) (p. 343)
DIAGNOSTIC LABORATORY STUDIES		
FBS	>140 mg/dl	>140 mg/dl
Oral glucose tolerance (first 2 hr)	>200 mg/dl	>200 mg/dl
Blood insulin level	Trace to absent	Normal to high
Serum osmolality	300 mosm/kg	300 mosm/kg
Ketonuria	Usually present	Usually absent
Plasma pro-insulin	Not applicable	Normal to high
Plasma C-peptide	Absent	Normal to high
COMPLICATIONS		
Acute	Diabetic ketoacidosis (DKA) Hypoglycemia	Hyperosmolar hyperglycemic nonketotic coma (HHNC) Hypoglycemia Diabetic ketoacidosis (DKA)

Long-term	Microangiopathies
	  Retinopathy
	  Nephropathy
	  Neuropathy
	
	Macroangiopathies
	  Cardiovascular
	  Cerebrovascular
	  Peripheral vascular
		Microangiopathies
		  Retinopathy
		  Nephropathy
		  Neuropathy
		
		Macroangiopathies
		  Cardiovascular
		  Cerebrovascular
		  Peripheral vascular

MEDICAL MANAGEMENT		
	Insulin preparations: rapid-acting, intermediate-acting, usually in split doses Diet, usually ADA exchange (usually three balanced meals and three snacks) Regular exercise program Self-blood glucose monitoring Treatment of existing complications	Diet, usually ADA exchange with decreased calories (usually three balanced meals and one high-protein snack) Oral hypoglycemics may be ordered and/or insulin as well Regular exercise program Self-blood glucose monitoring Treatment of existing complications

Provide dietary consultation for calculation of caloric requirements and instruction of ordered ADA diet

Assist to select daily menu based on low-calorie, low-fat, ADA diet; reinforce correct choices

Encourage patient to include foods high in complex carbohydrates (may assist in weight reduction)

Assess daily food intake; replace foods not eaten

Weigh QOD same time, scale, and clothing; give positive reinforcement for any weight reduction

Monitor blood glucose before meals and at bedtime or before bedtime snack

Collaborate with physician to determine exercise program to meet patient's needs and lifestyle; begin first phase of program

Discuss need to monitor dietary intake and exercise level using a diary

Explore with patient ways to increase activity in daily routine and to add exercise program

Refer to diabetic and/or weight reduction support group

Expected outcome/evaluation

Verbalizes understanding of relationship of obesity to diabetes

Selects meals and snacks based on ADA and/or decreased caloric guidelines

Takes all foods at mealtimes and snacks

Monitors blood glucose as scheduled

Keeps diary of dietary intake and exercise level

Identifies persons to use for support in making lifestyle changes

Additional nursing diagnoses to consider

Altered tissue perfusion; peripheral, cardiopulmonary, cerebral, or renal related to microangiopathy or macroangiopathy

Sensory perceptual alterations: visual related to retinopathy

Sexual dysfunction related to neuropathy

Potential for infection related to hyperglycemia

Noncompliance with therapeutic plan, related to difficulty of integration of therapy into lifestyle

Altered patterns of urinary elimination related to nephropathy

■ **NDX:** Knowledge deficit related to lack of accurate information about disease, acute and long-term complications, diet, exercise, medications, blood glucose monitoring, hygiene-personal care, sick day rules, and travel guidelines

Disease

Explain diabetes mellitus specific to patient's type

Discuss control of disease through managing interrelationship among diet, maintenance of ideal weight, exercise program, medication if ordered, and blood sugar changes

Complications

Acute

Hypoglycemia (p. 343)

Diabetic ketoacidosis (DKA) (p. 340)

Long-term

Microangiopathies, macroangiopathies

Stress that maintaining control of blood glucose may decrease the risk of or minimize these complications

Discuss need to

Have regular medical follow-ups to check for early symptoms of complications; cardiovascular, peripheral, renal, neural, or visual

Visit ophthalmologist, dentist, and podiatrist regularly

Maintain control of blood pressure and cholesterol

Stop smoking and/or drinking alcoholic beverages

Follow prescribed diet, exercise program, take medications, follow personal hygiene guidelines, and consult physician at first appearance of symptoms

Teach symptoms of long-term complications to report to physician

Diet therapy

Reinforce explanation of prescribed ADA and/or calorie-reduction diet

Assist with setting realistic goals for weight reduction

Have patient and/or significant other calculate dietary needs and choose a sample diet, cutting down on foods with high cholesterol, saturated fats, salt, sugar, and alcohol

Discuss need to eat meals and snacks at regularly scheduled times every day

Stress need to determine additional food requirements before exercise by use of self-blood glucose monitoring; give samples to calculate snacks required

Stress that diet may be the only means of control for patients with NIDDM

Provide written material, names of personnel, and telephone numbers for questions and assistance with meal planning

Exercise

Discuss need for exercise program

Positive effect on blood glucose control increases optimal functioning of body

Collaborate with physician and patient to plan program of progressive exercise based on patient's interest and physical condition

Give details specifying exercise type, intensity, frequency, duration, warm-up and cool-down time

Teach pulse-taking to monitor target heart rate during exercise

Explain need to exercise 1 to 2 hours after meal and how to adjust dietary intake as required

Avoid exercise at peak insulin times

Check blood glucose before and 30 minutes after exercise

Medications

INSULIN

Provide information to patient and/or significant other about insulin

Action of the type(s) of insulin to be used

Time of day patient may expect to have reaction (peak action time; Table 6-4)

Factors that precipitate hypoglycemia reaction

Incorrect, increased dosage of insulin

Altered routine in mealtimes or exercise without planning

Stress

Other disease processes

Cold

Flu

Nausea, vomiting

Infection, etc.

Dosage may be adjusted according to blood test results as ordered by physician

Provide information about care of insulin and equipment

Keep opened insulin vial currently in use at room temperature and away from sunlight; keep no longer than 2 months or expiration date

Have at least one unopened vial stored in refrigerator, not in freezer

Observe expiration date

Be sure units marked on syringe are understood; ½ cc or ³⁄₁₀ cc syringes are in increments of 1 unit/line; 1 cc syringes are in increments of 2 units per line, 2 cc syringes in increments of 5 units/line

Handle syringe and needles carefully to avoid self-puncture

Maintain sterility of needle and syringe during procedure

Dispose of syringe and needle in safe container after use

Discuss use of special equipment for patients with vision problems or other handicaps

Provide instructions for preparing injection

Mix insulin by gently rolling bottle between hands; do not shake vigorously

Clean bottle top with alcohol

Read label and check expiration date

Insert air and withdraw exact dose

Withdraw rapid-acting insulin first if mixing two types of insulin (avoids contaminating rapid-acting with longer-acting insulin)

Read label again and check dosage

Discuss information about injection site with patient and significant other

Most rapid absorption occurs in abdomen, arms, and thighs

Importance of rotating site of injection with each dose of insulin to prevent atrophy, fibrosis, lipodystrophy, and decreased insulin absorption

Rotation within one body area, e.g., abdomen may be recommended to ensure same length of absorption time

Need to avoid injection into extremities just before exercise

Need to use each site only once each month (Fig. 6-2)

Need to record site used for each injection by location and number

Have patient and/or significant other demonstrate injection technique

Select site for injection

Clean skin with alcohol

Allow to air dry to prevent irritation

Hold syringe filled with correct insulin dosage as one would hold a pencil or a dart

TABLE 6-3. Before Exercise Snacks

Exercise	Blood sugar levels	Snack
SHORT WORKOUT		
Easy pace Examples: 15 min slow walk easy swim stretching	less than 100	1 fruit or 1 bread or 4 oz milk
	more than 100	no food needed
MODERATE WORKOUT		
Moderate pace Examples: 25-40 min brisk walk	less than 100	1 meat, 1 bread, and 1 fruit
stationary bike heavy housework	100-160	1 milk or 1 fruit or 1 bread
aerobics class	161-300	no food needed
LONG WORKOUT		
Hard pace Examples: 1 hour shoveling snow skiing	less than 100	1 meat, 2 breads, and 1 milk or 1 fruit
	100-160	1 meat, 1 bread, and 1 milk or 1 fruit
	161-225	1 milk and 1 bread
	226-300	1 milk or 1 bread

More food may need to be added than is given here if patient works out 2 to 4 hours after taking short-acting insulin. In 2 to 4 hours this type of insulin peaks, and blood sugar can drop very fast. Always carry carbohydrate snacks during exercise.

TABLE 6-4. Action of Insulin

Type	Company, product	Species source	Onset of action (hours)	Peak of action (hours)	Duration of action (hours)
CONVENTIONAL INSULINS					
Regular	Lilly (Iletin I)	B-P*	½	2-4	6-8
	Nordisk Nova	Pork	½	2½-5	6-8
Semilente	Lilly (Iletin I)	B-P	1-2	3-8	10-16
	Nordisk Nova	Beef	½-1	5-10	12-16
NPH (Isophane)	Lilly (Iletin I)	B-P	1-2	6-12	18-26
	Nordisk Nova	Beef	1-1½	4-12	24
Lente	Lilly (Iletin I)	B-P	1-3	6-12	18-26
	Nordisk Nova	Beef	1-1½	7-15	24
Protamine zinc	Lilly (Iletin I)	B-P	4-6	12-24	26-36
	Nordisk Nova	Beef	4-8	14-20	36
Ultralente	Lilly (Iletin I)	B-P	4-6	14-24	28-36
	Nordisk Nova	Beef	4-8	10-30	36
PURIFIED INSULINS†					
Regular	Lilly (Iletin II)	Beef or pork	½	2-4	6-8
	Nordisk Nova (Velosulin)	Pork	½	1-3	8
	Nordisk Nova (Actrapid)	Pork	½	2½-5	8
Semilente	Nordisk Nova (Semitard)	Pork	½-1	5-10	16
NPH (Isophane)	Lilly (Iletin II)	Beef or pork	1-2	6-12	18-26
			1-3	6-12	24-28
	Nordisk Nova (Insulatard)	Pork	1½	4-12	24
	Nordisk Nova (Prota-phane)	Pork	1½	4-12	24
Lente	Lilly (Iletin II)	Beef or pork	1-3	6-12	18-26
	Nordisk Nova (Monotard)	Pork	2½	7-15	22
	Nordisk Nova (Lentard)	B-P	2½	7-15	24
Protamine zinc	Lilly (Iletin II)	Beef or pork	4-6	14-24	26-36
Ultralente	Nordisk Nova (Ultratard)	Beef	4	10-30	36
Biphasic (30% regular, 70% NPH)	Nordisk Nova (Mixtard)	Pork	½	4-8	24
HUMAN INSULINS					
Regular	Lilly (Humulin-R)	Bacteria	½	2-4	6-8
	Nordisk/Nova (Novolin-R)	Semisynthetic	½	2½-5	6-8
NPH (Isophane)	Lilly (Humulin-N)	Bacteria	1-2	6-12	18-24
	Nordisk/Nova (Novolin-N)	Semisynthetic	1½	4-12	24
Lente	Lilly (Humulin-L) Nordisk/Nova (Novolin-L)	Semisynthetic	2½	7-15	24
Biphasic (30% regular, 70% NPH)	Nordisk/Nova 70/30	Semisynthetic	½	6-12	24

* B-P, mixed beef and pork insulin.
† The Food and Drug Administration recommends that purified insulins be used for all patients and human insulins be considered for new patients.

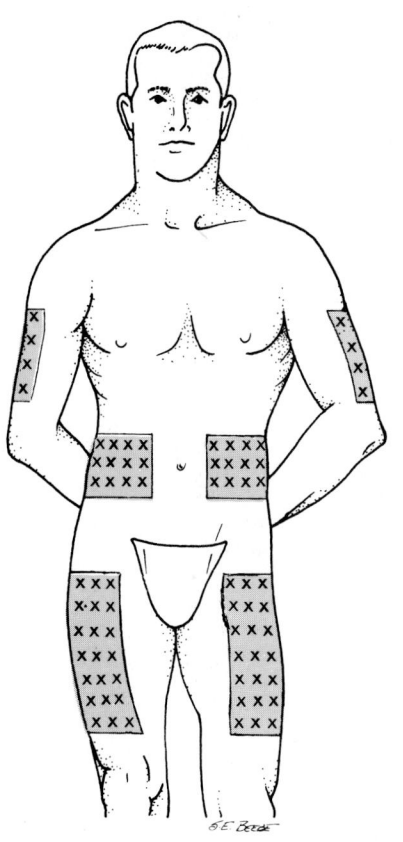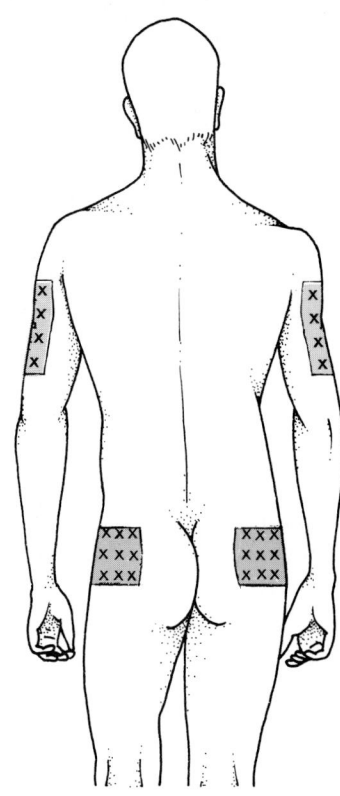

FIGURE 6-2. Rotation of insulin injection sites.

TABLE 6-5. Oral Hypoglycemics

Drug	Dosage range (mg/day)	Onset (hr)	Duration (hr)	Serum half-life (hr)
Tolazamide	100-1,000	4-6	10-18	7
Tolbutamide	250-3,000	1	6-12	4-5
Acetohexamide	250-1,500	1	8-24	6-8
Chlorpropamide	100-500	1	24-72	36
Glyburide	1.25-20	24	16-24	7-10
Glipizide	2.5-40	1-1.5	6-24	2-7

Insert needle at 90-degree angle (45-degree if little sub-cutaneous tissue) and quickly push into tissue up to hub of needle

Withdraw plunger to check for entry into blood vessel; if blood returns, withdraw syringe and start procedure over

Inject medication

Withdraw needle and hold alcohol swab on area for a few seconds; do not rub

Record date and time given, type of insulin, dosage, and site of injection in diary

ORAL HYPOGLYCEMICS

Provide information about medications when ordered
 Action and dosage (Table 6-5)

Monitor blood glucose level at specific times; usually four times/day until effective dosage achieved; then two to three times/wk with a complete profile one to two times/mo (before and after meals, at bedtime, and once during night)

Take exact dosage before meal(s)

Observe for hypoglycemic reactions (p. 343)
 Take 10 g carbohydrate (CHO) (p. 344) at first sign of

reaction to raise blood glucose level in 10 to 15 min; then take longer-acting CHO to offset recurrence

Discuss other side or toxic effects to report to physician or nurse if they last longer than 24 to 48 hrs

GI upset

Weakness

Paresthesia

Headache

Tinnitus

Skin rash

Jaundice

Photosensitivity

Intolerance to alcohol

Prolonged action of sedatives and hypnotics

Discuss planning for pregnancy with physician; notify immediately if pregnancy is suspected; oral hypoglycemic agents need to be stopped before pregnancy occurs and another regimen instituted in collaboration with physician

Self-blood glucose monitoring and urine testing

Give reasons for testing blood glucose

Maintain control of blood sugar

Reduce risk of complications

Instruct about blood glucose test

Frequency of testing

Usually before meals and exercise, 30 minutes after exercise, and to monitor any symptoms of hypoglycemia or hyperglycemia

Need to rotate sites of finger punctures

Use only sides of fingertips; produces less discomfort

Use at least six sites on each finger (Figure 6-3)

Advise that thumb and ring finger may have better blood flow

Methods to increase blood flow

Place hand in warm water a few minutes

Hold hand below heart level and "milk" finger (Figure 6-4)

Not using alcohol or povidone-iodine to clean finger as these products interfere with test results

Need to wash, rinse, and dry hands well before beginning procedure

Procedure for using lancet and finger puncture device

Procedure to use and read reagent strips or to use automated equipment

Care and storage of supplies and equipment

Disposal of lancets in safe container

Teach about urine testing

Urine testing for sugar does not indicate amount of sugar in the blood but does indicate that excess sugar from blood is spilling into urine; ketones

Test urine before meals and bedtime

Follow directions on container

Test urine for ketones when experiencing symptoms of hyperglycemia

Report presence to physician or follow predetermined plan

Store urine testing supplies in dry, cool, dark area away from oral medications and children

Record test results in diary

Note any medications taken as some give false readings; e.g., salicylates or ascorbic acid give false-positive readings

Explain changes to make in diet, exercise, or medication as a result of blood glucose or urine test as determined through collaboration with physician

Discuss need to maintain diary to record

Blood glucose/urine test

Medication and dosage

Exercise level

Symptoms and interventions taken

Missed meals or unusual situations

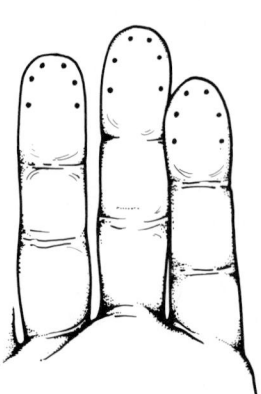

FIGURE 6-3. Finger puncture sites.

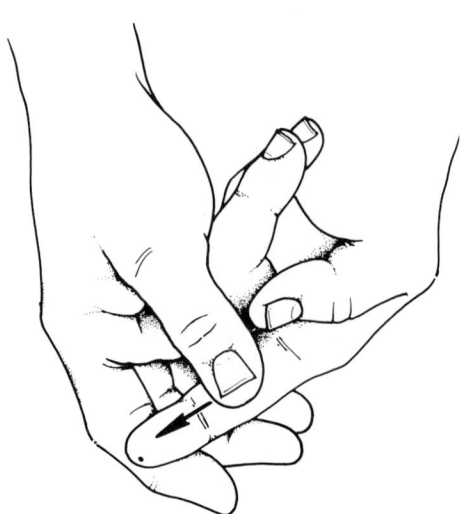

FIGURE 6-4. Milking finger to obtain blood sample.

Personal care and hygiene

SKIN, FOOT, AND LEG CARE

Provide information about daily care

Bathe daily using tepid water; check water temperature with thermometer, especially when bathing feet

Rinse and dry gently but thoroughly

Apply lubricating lotion; do not leave skin wet

Inspect body, especially feet, legs, and groin area daily; use mirror if unable to see any body part, e.g., bottom of feet

Check for cuts, cracks, blisters, corns, boils, calluses, or ingrown toenails; if found, wash with mild soap and water, dry well, and cover with dry, sterile dressing; notify physician if healing does not begin in 24 hours

Have podiatrist treat corns and calluses; do not use home remedies or devices

Keep feet dry; wear clean stockings, preferably with cotton feet, daily

Avoid tight-fitting stockings with elastic

Wear well-fitting shoes; break in new shoes gradually; alternate two pairs of shoes; do not go barefoot

Exercise feet throughout the day; curl toes, rotate ankles, bend and stretch knees and hips; avoid one position for long periods of time; walk in place if standing, stand and walk if sitting

Do not use hot water bottles or heating pads on extremities

Wear protective clothing for warmth or sunshielding

Use sunscreen, at least SPF 15, daily

Use gloves when exposed to harsh soaps, gardening, using an oven, or handling heavy, rough objects

Be cautious when using machinery, tools, and equipment

CARE OF TEETH

Brush teeth or clean dentures after sleep and meals and before bedtime

Floss at least daily

Examine mouth for irritated gums, bleeding, or ulcers

Report those that do not begin to heal in 24 hr

Schedule periodic dental examinations (usually every 6 months)

Tell dentist about condition and check with primary physician before scheduling extensive dental care or surgery

CARE OF EYES

Explain that eye changes (vision) may be temporary if blood sugar is high

Schedule yearly examinations with an ophthalmologist; more often if vision changes are noted

URINARY AND GENITAL CARE

Drink six to eight glasses of water/day

Avoid urinary tract or vaginal infections

Avoid fluids with caffeine or alcohol

Urinate as soon as urge is felt

Wash and dry genital area daily

Inspect for irritation and discharge

Shower rather than take tub baths

Wear underwear and/or panty hose with cotton crotch

Avoid douching except as ordered by physician

Report to physician if following symptoms occur

Urinary tract

Difficulty in voiding

Burning or pain on voiding

Incontinence

Vagina

Heavy discharge

Itching

Sick day rules

Explain that any illness, injury, or change in body functioning causes an increased need for glucose, which the body will automatically produce

Advise that a change in medication and food usually is required during these periods

Discuss signs and symptoms of illness, injury, or functional change that *may* require changes in medication or food

Injuries

Infections, including cold or flu

Nausea, vomiting

Diarrhea

Burns

Dental care

Surgery

Pregnancy

Emotional stress

Unaccustomed physical activities; periodic jogging, swimming, tennis

Instruct to increase testing of blood glucose and urine ketones to every 4 hr or at least four times/day during this period

Explain importance of notifying physician when

Blood glucose is 300 mg/dl or urine test results are 1% with or without ketones two successive times

Experiencing an inability to take oral food/fluids

Experiencing unusual thirst, increased urination, weakness, warm/flushed skin, blurred vision, or nausea and vomiting

Explain need to have blood or urine glucose and urine ketone record sheet nearby to report to physician when experiencing symptoms of high blood glucose

Instruct about action to take

Drink a cup or more of broth, tea, nondietetic carbonated drinks, gelatin, or fluids with electrolytes

Take insulin based on test results or discussion with physician

Travel tips

Discuss need to prepare for travel
Inform physician
Obtain immunizations well before trip when needed
Have generic prescriptions in duplicate for
Diabetic medications
Syringes and needles
Other medications needed
Have letter describing condition and treatment (in language of country visiting if possible)
Buy and "break-in" new shoes well in advance
Obtain identification bracelet or necklace if patient normally carries a card
Arrange for special meals while enroute
Importance of carrying supply of insulin and syringes in hand luggage to prevent exposure to extreme temperature and to prevent loss
Need to take supply of emergency medication to prevent or treat possible travel complications
Importance of carrying emergency carbohydrates and a meal
Method to alter meal, medication, and activity needs when traveling to other time zones
Where to obtain emergency assistance and how to express needs in language of country visited*
Importance of traveling with a companion when possible

DIABETIC KETOACIDOSIS (DKA)

Acute complication of diabetes mellitus, characterized by hyperglycemia, metabolic acidosis, increased plasma ketones, and severe dehydration

Assessment

See Table 6-6.

Medical Management

Regular insulin IV bolus or continuous drip (5 to 10 units/hr)
Rapid IV hydration: 1 L/hr (approximately 6 L)
Normal saline initially, then as serum glucose decreases, glucose is added to infusion
IV potassium replacement as indicated
$NaHCO_3$ replacement for pH less than 7.1
Central venous pressure (CVP)
ABG
Monitor ECG
Insulin subcutaneously
Treatment of infection if underlying cause

*International Association for Medical Assistance to Travellers Directory of English Speaking Physicians Throughout the World, 736 Center St., Lewiston, NY 14092; (716) 754-4883.

Nursing diagnoses/interventions/evaluation

■ **NDX:** Fluid volume deficit (1) related to osmotic diuresis

Monitor IV fluids; maintain large-bore IV for rapid infusion
Administer plasma expanders as ordered
Monitor BP, P, T, R q15min to ½h until stable for 1 hour than q½h until reactive and blood glucose controlled; then q4h to 8h
Assess for signs and symptoms of hypovolemic shock continuously: tachycardia, low blood pressure, weak, thready pulses, cool skin, increased body temperature, change in level of consciousness
Administer insulin; usually given IV initially
Rinse container and tubing with insulin per hospital policy before adding prescribed dose as insulin adheres to equipment and correct dosage may not be given
Note that smaller doses are required for HHNC than for DKA
Assess effectiveness; report glucose level that continues to rise, that falls too rapidly, or that is 120 mg/dl or lower
Measure capillary blood glucose qh
Measure urine ketones qh in DKA
Monitor ECG for changes; report signs of hyperkalemia or hypokalemia
Monitor electrolyte and ABG levels
Report changes and collaborate with physician to adjust fluids, electrolytes, and HCO_3
Monitor CVP if inserted
Insert nasogastric tube as indicated; monitor gastric drainage
Insert indwelling urinary catheter to straight drainage for exact assessment of output
Monitor intake and output qh and report output <30 ml/hr
Assess skin temperature, turgor, and capillary refill q2h

Expected outcome/evaluation

Vital signs are stable
Intake and output are balanced
Skin turgor is good
Electrolytes are within normal range
Blood glucose is within patient's normal range

■ **NDX:** Potential for injury related to confusion or seizures

Assess for presence of neurological/sensory deficits and respiratory status q4h
Maintain oral airway at bedside
Keep bed in low position with padded side rails in up position when patient is on bed rest

TABLE 6-6. Comparison of Diabetic Ketoacidosis (DKA), Hyperosmolar Hyperglycemic Nonketotic Coma (HHNC), and Hypoglycemia

Assessment	Observations/findings		
	DKA	HHNC	Hypoglycemia
Diabetes type	Usually IDDM	Usually NIDDM	IDDM or NIDDM
Onset	Hours to days	Hours to days	Minutes to 1 hr
Renal	Polyuria; osmotic diuresis Dehydration	Polyuria; osmotic diuresis Dehydration	
Neurological	Lethargy, drowsiness Paresthesia Slowed reflexes Confusion, disorientation	Unconsciousness (50%) Drowsiness Confusion, disorientation	Inability to concentrate Lack of coordination Numbness, tingling; lips, tongue Yawning, slurred speech Hyperreflexia, seizure activity Nighttime: nightmares, sleepwalking; restlessness
Respiratory	Tachypnea, Kussmaul's respiration Sweet, fruity breath	Tachypnea with shallow respiration	
Cardiovascular	Hypotension Tachycardia Weak pulses Warm to hot, dry, flushed skin Decreased turgor	Tachycardia Weak pulses Orthostatic hypotension Warm to hot, dry, flushed skin Decreased turgor	Tachycardia Cool, clammy skin
GI	Polydypsia Nausea, vomiting	Polydypsia	Hunger Nausea
Risk factors	Undiagnosed IDDM Insufficient insulin dosage Stressors: surgery, injury, infection Sudden decrease in exercise program Pregnancy	Undiagnosed NIDDM Insufficient oral hypoglycemic agent Stressors: surgery, injury, infections Sudden decrease in exercise program High-protein, high-calorie enteral or parenteral feedings Drug toxicities Dialysis Alcohol intake Pregnancy	Excessive insulin dosage, missed meal(s) Unplanned increase in exercise program Vomiting Alcohol intake Drug interactions Pregnancy

Laboratory/diagnostic studies

Assessment	DKA	HHNC	Hypoglycemia
Serum glucose	200-800 mg/dl	800-2000 ml/dl	<60 mg/dl
Serum ketones	Elevated	Normal to slightly elevated	
Urine acetone	Positive	Negative	Negative
Serum osmolality	300-350 mosm/L	>350 mosm/L	
PH	<7.38	7.30-7.42	
Sodium	<137	Elevated, normal, or low	
BUN	Elevated	Elevated	
Potassium	Normal or elevated then decreased	Normal or <3.5 mEq/L	

Potential complications

Assessment	DKA	HHNC	Hypoglycemia
	Shock Renal failure Death occurs if untreated	Thromboembolism Shock Seizures Coma Death occurs if untreated	Seizure Shock Coma Permanent brain damage Death occurs if untreated

Remove potentially hazardous materials from patient's immediate environment

Place articles frequently required within easy reach

Instruct patient to call for assistance before getting out of bed

Keep call light within patient's reach at all times

Be aware that patient's vision may be affected; assist with feeding, personal hygiene, and ambulation as needed

Maintain orientation to environment: assess level of consciousness and orientation q4h and prn

Provide stimulation in the environment that will assist in maintaining orientation: pictures from home, calendar, clock, radio, television

Address patient by name; review day, date, time, and current events with patient as necessary

Expected outcome/evaluation

Patient sustains no physical injuries
Remains alert and oriented to time, place, and person

■ **NDX:** Potential for infection related to increased susceptibility caused by hyperglycemia and protein depletion

Monitor for signs of infection q4h to 8h
Sites of invasive lines
Skin
Respiratory and urinary systems

Maintain sterility of invasive sites, e.g., IV, catheters, etc.
Provide meticulous, sterile daily care and rotate sites according to policy

Culture suspicious drainage

Teach and assist patient to turn, cough, and deep breathe q2h

Provide oral fluids to 2000 ml/day when allowed

Provide oral care q4h to 6h

Use aids to promote circulation and prevent skin breakdown when on bed rest

Expected outcome/evaluation

Temperature is within normal range
Cultures show no evidence of infection
Lungs and urine are clear
Skin is dry and clear with good turgor

■ **NDX:** Altered nutrition: less than body requirements related to deficiency of effective insulin

Assess diet and fluid intake before DKA

Provide ADA diet and fluids as prescribed

Maintain food diary when necessary to assist patient in determining intake

Weigh patient daily; same time, scale, and clothing

Administer insulin; assess effectiveness by monitoring blood glucose; collaborate with physician to adjust medication dosage as necessary

Determine possible factors leading to DKA episode
Not taking insulin
Not observing diet
Reduction in level of exercise
Infection, stress, injury, etc.

Expected outcome/evaluation

Weight is stable or increasing toward predetermined level for patient's build

Blood glucose level is within normal limits

■ **NDX:** Knowledge deficit related to lack of information about risk factors and prevention of DKA

Explain factors that predispose to ketoacidosis: increased food intake, omitted doses of insulin, failure to respond to increased need for insulin resulting from infectious process, decreased activity/exercise, stress, or pregnancy

Discuss early signs of DKA
Blood glucose 300 mg/dl or more
Ketones in urine
Unusual thirst
Increased urination
Hot, dry, flushed skin
Elevated temperature
Drowsiness
Nausea, vomiting, abdominal pain, diarrhea

Teach action to take when early signs noted

Continue diet and fluids
Take broth or tea if unable to tolerate food

Increase frequency of blood glucose testing

Have patient take insulin as scheduled or change dosage as indicated by tests, with physician approval, using algorithms

Test urine for presence of ketones

Notify physician if no improvement

Assess knowledge of diabetes mellitus and management through patient's maintenance of ADA diet, exercise program, diabetic medication schedule, and blood glucose monitoring

See Diabetes Mellitus (p. 332)

Expected outcome/evaluation

Verbalizes early signs of DKA and action to take when symptoms occur

Understands risk factors, and need to avoid these when possible

Verbalizes and demonstrates management of diabetes

HYPEROSMOLAR HYPERGYLCEMIC NONKETOTIC COMA (HHNC)

Metabolic disorder in which the blood sugar level is extremely elevated, increasing the serum osmolality and resulting in hypertonic dehydration; serum ketosis is usually not present

Assessment

See Table 6-6 (p. 341)

Medical Management

IV insulin administration
IV fluid administration, plasma expanders as needed
Electrolyte replacement as needed
    Electrolyte, blood glucose, and bicarbonate levels
    ABG
    Monitor ECG
    CVP
    Insulin subcutaneously and/or oral hypoglycemics

Nursing diagnoses/interventions/evaluation

See Diabetic ketoacidosis for the following diagnoses:
Fluid volume deficit (1) related to osmotic diuresis (p. 340)
Potential for injury related to confusion and/or seizures (p. 340)
Potential for infection related to increased susceptibility resulting from hyperglycemia and protein depletion (p. 340)
Altered nutrition: less than body requirements related to deficiency of effective insulin (p. 342)
See Diabetes Mellitus for altered nutrition: more than body requirements related to diabetes mellitus usually NIDDM (p. 332)

■ **NDX:** Potential for altered tissue perfusion; peripheral, cerebral, cardiopulmonary; related to risk of thromboembolism

Assess peripheral pulses q2h to 4h; report decreased amplitude or absence
Assess for thrombosis in extremities: vein—pain, swelling, tenderness, or Homan's sign; artery—mottling, cyanosis, coolness with delayed capillary refill
Teach active ROM exercises for extremities
    Assist with passive ROM if patient unable to perform
Apply thromboembolic or pneumatic alternating-pressure stockings to lower extremities
    Remove daily, check condition of legs, then reapply
Assess vital signs, heart and breath sounds, and neurological status q2h to 4h
    Assist patient to assume position to enhance cardiopulmonary effort
    Instruct patient to report sudden headache, chest pain, numbness in extremities

Expected outcome/evaluation

Vital signs are stable and within normal limits; patient reports no headache, chest pain, numbness, or pain in extremities and is alert and oriented

■ **NDX:** Knowledge deficit related to lack of information about risk factors and prevention of HHNC

Explain factors that predispose to HHNC
    Not taking oral hypoglycemic or insulin dosage
    Sudden decrease in exercise program
    Stressors: surgery, dental care, infections
    Increase in food intake
    Pregnancy
Review symptoms of HHNC
    See Assessment, Table 6-6
Teach action to take when signs of HHNC are noticed
    Continue diet and fluids
        Take broth or tea if unable to tolerate food
    Increase frequency of blood glucose monitoring
    Take oral hypoglycemic as scheduled or change dosage as indicated by tests with physician approval using algorithm
    Explain that insulin may be required during these situations
    Notify physician if no improvement
Assess knowledge of diabetes mellitus management including patient maintenance of ADA diet, adherence to exercise program, monitoring blood glucose, and taking of medications; see Diabetes Mellitus (p. 332)

Expected outcome/evaluation

Verbalizes signs of HHNC and action to take
Understands risk factors and need to avoid
Verbalizes and demonstrates diabetic management

HYPOGLYCEMIA

An abnormally low serum glucose level usually 60 mg/dl or less

Assessment

See Table 6-6 (p. 341)

Medical Management

10 g fast-acting oral CHO
50% glucose IV bolus
IV fluids $D_{10}W$

Nursing diagnoses/interventions/evaluation

■ **NDX:** Potential for injury related to insufficient glucose to meet metabolic needs

Hypoglycemia *requires immediate intervention* to prevent brain damage and death

Obtain blood glucose stat and be prepared to administer 50% glucose IV if patient is a diabetic and is comatose; then initiate IV of $D_{10}W$ if prescribed *or*

Obtain capillary blood glucose and give 10 g of fast-acting CHO if patient is exhibiting early signs of hypoglycemia

Continue to monitor blood glucose q15min to 30 min; slow-acting CHO may be needed to prevent recurrence of symptoms

Determine predisposing factor if possible
Decreased food intake
Increased exercise
Wrong medication, dosage, etc.

Consult physician, if no predisposing factor determined, for adjustment of insulin or oral hypoglycemic dosage

Monitor neurological and cardiovascular status q30min until fully reactive

Expected outcome/evaluation

Blood glucose within normal limits after ingestion of CHO or IV glucose; vital signs are stable; patient is alert and oriented

■ **NDX:** Potential for trauma related to rapid onset of altered level of consciousness (LOC) and seizure activity resulting from hypoglycemia

Keep oral airway and suction equipment at bedside
Pad side rails if patient is on bed rest
Assist to floor if patient is out of bed and remove hazardous objects
Note time, frequency, level of consciousness, body parts involved, and length of seizure activity
Obtain stat blood glucose and administer IV glucose as ordered
Notify physician of seizure
Suction oropharynx as needed
Assess for injury
Check pulse and pupils
Reorient as necessary
Determine predisposing factor for hypoglycemia

Expected outcome/evaluation

Patient is free of injury

■ **NDX:** Knowledge deficit related to lack of information about predisposing factors of hypoglycemia and prevention

Involve significant other and/or peers from work setting in teaching, as patient may not be able to intervene
Teach factors that may precipitate hypoglycemia; too much insulin or oral hypoglycemic medication, increased length of time between meals, omission of a meal or snack, unplanned exercise, extremely stressful situation, etc.

Discuss symptoms of hypoglycemia:
Mild: shaky, sweaty, cool feeling, irritable, weak, headache, nervous, drowsy, or personality changes
Moderate: nausea, faintness, disorientation, confusion
Severe: coma, seizure

Explain that hypoglycemic reactions may be different for each person
Any unusual feeling or symptom must be considered
Each patient must become familiar with initial reactions

Identify the time reactions will most likely occur; relate to type of insulin prescribed (see Table 6-4)

Teach action to take immediately: take 10 g of quick-acting carbohydrate
The following foods contain 10 g of quick-acting carbohydrate (CHO):

Orange juice	4 oz
Apple juice	4 oz
Grape juice	2 oz
Coca-Cola	3 oz
Ginger ale	4 oz
7-up	3 oz
Corn syrup	2 tsp
Honey	2 tsp
Granulated sugar	2½ tsp
Grape jam	2 tsp
Animal crackers	4
Space Food Stix	1
Gumdrops	10 small
Jelly beans	6
Hard candy such as Life Savers	5 or 6
Dextrose wafers or tablets as labeled	
Glucose paste, amount indicated on label	

Emphasize importance of always carrying fast-acting sugar in same pocket, and keeping juice or other drink in same container in same place in refrigerator for easy, quick accessibility

Check blood glucose 15 min after taking quick-acting CHO; then take slowly digested carbohydrate, such as milk, cottage cheese, bread, or peanut butter after response to fast-acting carbohydrate to offset a secondary reaction, if needed

Demonstrate method for glucagon administration to significant other; discuss action and dosage
Use if patient clamps mouth shut, is unable to swallow, or is unconscious; patient should respond in 5 to 15 min
Have patient eat slowly digested carbohydrate after responding
Follow physician's orders if no response
Telephone physician if further orders are not indicated
Give another injection of glucagon if ordered

Telephone for emergency help or take patient to emergency room of hospital

Demonstrate alternate method of glucagon therapy: oral glucose in tube; squeeze directly between cheek and gum area

Explain need to observe closely for further reaction for 1 to 1½ hr; avoid strenuous activity during this time

Determine predisposing factor after reaction is controlled

Emphasize importance of reporting frequent reactions to physician as directed

Give time of onset and duration until response to care

Discuss predisposing factor if known

Discuss prevention and early care

Always carry some form of quick-acting carbohydrate (see list, at left); take when first symptoms appear

Eat correct diet regularly; remember between-meal nourishment when included in diet

Test blood regularly for glucose (p. 337); anticipate probable reactions

Be aware of greater-than-normal activity or emotional stress; follow physician's directions to either notify physician, increase food intake, or decrease dosage of insulin

Discuss prevention of dosage errors

Check dosage of insulin or oral hypoglycemic with another person when possible

Record medication when it is taken to prevent duplication

Always wear medical alert band or chain and carry diabetic identification card

Determine ability to manage diabetes mellitus (p. 332)

Expected outcome/evaluation

Patient and/or significant other verbalize risk factors for hypoglycemia and action to take; demonstrate IM injection technique

Surgical Interventions

THYROIDECTOMY

Surgical removal of part (subtotal thyroidectomy) or all of the thyroid gland; usually reserved for patient who does not respond to medical treatment with antithyroid drugs; treatment of choice to remove very large goiters or those compressing surrounding structures; may also be performed for men and women of child-bearing age for whom radiation exposure is unwanted, patients allergic to antithyroid medications, and pregnant women

Preoperative Assessment and Care

Assess baseline vital signs

Assess voice quality and ability to swallow

Teach patient to support neck with towel to prevent strain on sutures, incision

Explain importance of not speaking postoperatively to prevent edema

Obtain pad and pencil for communicating postoperatively

Teach patient to turn and deep breathe; include use of incentive spirometer

Explain that hoarseness will subside after 4 to 5 days

Discuss pain management; use of pain rating scale

Reinforce physician's explanation of procedure; clarify any misconceptions, allow time for questions

Postoperative Assessment
Observations/findings

Increasing hoarseness

Change in tone or pitch of voice

Weak voice, inability to speak

Hypocalcemia

Numbness

Tingling

Twitching

Spasm, tetany

Positive Chvostek's or Trousseau's sign

Incision site

Color (redness)

Pain, guarding of site, intensity, location

Swelling

Drainage, bleeding

Airway

Choking sensation

Dysphagia

Complaints of heaviness or fullness in throat

Complaints of tight dressing

Stridorous respirations

Retraction of neck muscles

Cyanosis

Laboratory/diagnostic studies

Serum: total and free T_3 and T_4; calcium levels

Potential complications

Airway obstruction

Hemorrhage

Paralysis of recurrent laryngeal nerves

Hypothyroidism

Hypocalcemia

Tetany

Medical Management

IV fluids progressing to po diet

Treatment of complications

Pain management including throat spray or lozenges

Incentive spirometer

Nursing diagnoses/interventions/evaluation

■ <u>**NDX:**</u> Potential for ineffective airway clearance related to bleeding and/or laryngeal edema

Position patient on back with head elevated 30 degrees to 45 degrees

Teach and assist patient to turn, cough, and deep breathe q2h and prn

Keep suction equipment at bedside; gently suction oropharynx only when necessary

Have tracheostomy tray and oxygen immediately available

Monitor for signs of respiratory distress or obstructed airway qh: stridor, wheezing, coarse airway crackles, dyspnea, cyanosis, labored respirations

Check dressing for bleeding qh for first 24 hr

Notify physician if dressing requires reinforcement more than one time

Expected outcome/evaluation

Respirations and breath sounds are within patient's normal limits, no bleeding is present at surgical site

■ **NDX:** Potential for injury (tetany) related to hypocalcemia

Evaluate reflexes q4h to 8h; report neuromuscular irritability

Monitor calcium levels

Maintain quiet environment with bed in low position and side rail padded

Collaborate with physician in treating symptoms of tetany: parenteral fluids and medications

Expected outcome/evaluation

Patient exhibits normal reflexes

■ **NDX:** Potential for infection related to invasive surgical procedure

Monitor vital signs and breath sounds q4h to 8h

Change dressing daily and prn when wet; observe for signs and symptoms of infection or impaired healing: redness, swelling, foul drainage, fever

Promote incision healing: prevent stress on suture line, cleanse site daily as ordered, and apply dry, sterile dressing

Use only necessary dressing and tape; remove tape toward incision

Expected outcome/evaluation

Incision is dry and clean
Vital signs are stable
Lungs are clear

■ **NDX:** Potential for impaired verbal communication related to damage and/or manipulation of laryngeal nerves

Monitor voice quality q2h

Monitor for edema at surgical incision and glottis

Discourage talking for first 48 hr

Reassure patient that voice should return to normal after a few days

Provide alternate means of communication (e.g., pad and pencil)

Keep call bell within reach at all times

Report increasing hoarseness to physician

Anticipate patient's needs

Expected outcome/evaluation

Uses alternate communication methods for 48 hr postoperatively

Communicates verbally without voice change

Has no edema at incision

■ **NDX:** Pain related to surgical incision

Assess patient for verbal and nonverbal signs of pain

Have patient use pain rating scale to indicate intensity of pain

Discuss with patient factors that increase or relieve pain

Assist patient with finding physical position of comfort

Prevent tension on suture line
Use pillows to maintain head alignment; use sandbags if pillows insufficient

Prevent flexion or extension of head and neck

Teach patient to keep head in a neutral position

Instruct patient to use hands to support head during movement

Assist patient with using distraction as means of pain control: guided imagery, progressive relaxation, soft music, reading, visitors

Monitor effectiveness of pain medications

Administer analgesic throat spray or lozenges as ordered and as patient desires

Expected outcome/evaluation

Expresses feeling of well-being and comfort; posture and face are relaxed

■ **NDX:** Knowledge deficit related to lack of exposure to accurate information regarding home and follow-up care

Teach care of surgical incision

Emphasize importance of supporting incision until healed

Teach prescribed head and neck exercises: flexion, lateral movement, and hyperextension

Discuss symptoms of recurrent hyperthyroidism, hypothyroidism, or hypocalcemia to report to physician

Discuss symptoms of wound infection to report to physician

Emphasize importance of
Rest and relaxation

Managing stressful situations and emotional outbursts with stress management techniques

Proper nutrition and fluid intake

Ongoing outpatient care

Teach name of medication, purpose, time and method of administration, dosage, side effects, and toxic effects

Explain need to avoid taking over-the-counter medications without consulting physician

Expected outcome/evaluation

Patient and/or significant other verbalizes understanding of home and follow-up care

PARATHYROIDECTOMY

Surgical removal of the parathyroid glands; if surgery is performed for adenoma, total removal of all involved glands is done; if the cause of hyperparathyroidism is hyperplasia, three total glands are removed and three fourths of the fourth gland is removed, leaving sufficient gland to prevent hypocalcemia in most patients

Postoperative Assessment
Observations/findings

Signs and symptoms of hypocalcemia
  Paresthesia
  Tingling
  Stiffness
  Cramping
  Tremor
  Tetany
Respiratory
  Hoarseness
  Laryngeal stridor
  Cyanosis
Incision site
  Redness
  Pain; location, intensity
  Swelling
  Drainage
  Bleeding
  Choking sensation
  Complaints of heaviness or fullness in throat
  Dysphagia

Laboratory/diagnostic studies

Serum calcium levels
Serum phosphorus levels

Potential complications

Hemorrhage
Hypocalcemia: seizures, tetany
Respiratory arrest

Medical Management

IV fluids, progressing to diet as tolerated

Treatment of complications
Pain management

Nursing diagnoses/interventions/evaluation

See Thyroidectomy (p. 345)

ADRENALECTOMY

Surgical removal of the adrenal gland(s); unilateral removal may be performed for benign adenomas, whereas bilateral removal is done for malignant ACTH-producing tumors; other diseases of the adrenal glands, such as Cushing's diseases or pheochromocytoma, a catecholamine-secreting tumor, may also require removal

Preoperative Assessment and Care

Assess baseline vital signs to determine control of predisposing disease factors, e.g., hypertension in pheochromocytoma or primary aldosteronism

If scheduled for bilateral removal explain that patient must take cortisone preparation throughout life; if unilateral for only 6 mo to 2 yr

Monitor blood glucose for control of hyperglycemia

Teach patient to turn, cough, and deep breathe

Encourage questions and discussion of fears and anxiety

Administer preoperative steroid

Postoperative Assessment
Observations/findings

Signs of adrenal crisis (p. 322)
  Falling blood pressure
  Tachycardia; weak, thready pulses
  Elevated temperature
  Restlessness
  Profound weakness
  Lethargy
  Hypoglycemia
  Electrolyte imbalance
  Seizures
Dehydration
Flatulence
Site of incision
  Redness
  Pain
  Swelling
  Drainage, bleeding
  Impaired healing
Respiratory distress
  Decreased breath sounds
  Tachypnea, bradypnea

Laboratory/diagnostic studies

Decreased serum aldosterone levels
Decreased serum steroid levels

Hyperglycemia
Hyperkalemia

Potential complications

Renal dysfunction
Atelectasis
Adrenal crisis
Coma
Cardiac arrest

Medical Management

IV fluids progressing to po diet when the bowel sounds return
Incentive spirometer
Treatment of complications
Pain management

Nursing diagnoses/interventions/evaluation

■ **NDX:** Potential for injury related to risk of adrenal crisis

Monitor cardiovascular, neurological, respiratory, and renal function q4h
  Assess vital signs q4h and prn; report abnormal findings to physician
  Monitor neurological status q4h; report increasing headache and confusion
  Monitor cardiac rhythm continuously if dysrhythmias occur because of electrolyte imbalances
  Monitor intake and output q4h and prn; report output that is greater than intake
Position patient to promote cardiovascular and respiratory function
Collaborate with physician to administer IV fluids, vasopressors, corticosteroids; assess effectiveness

Expected outcome/evaluation

Vital signs are stable and within patient's normal range; intake and output are balanced; patient is alert and oriented when reactive

■ **NDX:** Pain related to surgery

Assess for verbal and nonverbal signs of pain; use pain rating scale
Administer pain medications and assess effectiveness
Discuss with patient factors that increase or decrease pain
Assist patient with finding position of comfort
Assist patient with using distraction as means of pain control: guided imagery, progressive relaxation, soft music, visitors
Maintain support of surgical incision during movement or ambulation
Increase ambulation as tolerated

Expected outcome/evaluation

Appears calm/relaxed
States pain is at tolerable level or absent
Uses learned pain control techniques

■ **NDX:** Potential for infection related to surgical incision and abnormal cortisol levels

Change dressing daily and when wet; observe for signs of infection, impaired healing, dehiscence, redness, swelling, foul drainage, fever
Culture suspicious drainage
Promote incisional healing
  Prevent stress on suture line
  Remove sutures when ordered
  Use dry, sterile dressing when changing
  Use only necessary amount of tape and remove in direction of incision
  Cleanse site daily
  Instruct patient to avoid touching incision site
Avoid unnecessary invasive procedures
Assist patient to turn, cough, and deep breathe q2h
Monitor for signs of URI and UTI
Screen personnel and visitors for infections; restrict if present

Expected outcome/evaluation

Temperature is within normal range
Breath sounds are clear
Incision is healing
Urine is clear

■ **NDX:** Potential fluid volume deficit related to unstable levels of circulating steroids

Maintain IV fluids to 2500 ml/day
Monitor serum electrolytes q8h and prn
Calculate intake and output q4h to 8h; report intake less than output
Weigh patient daily; observe for weight loss
Administer sodium replacement as ordered in diet or IV fluids if NPO
Assess for signs and symptoms of fluid/electrolyte imbalance: poor skin turgor, weak pulses, tachycardia, thirst, low blood pressure, cool skin, cardiac dysrhythmias, increased body temperature, change in mental status
Report any of the preceding signs or symptoms to physician without delay and carry out medical orders received
Check blood sugar via fingerstick q8h

Expected outcome/evaluation

Intake and output are balanced
Weight is stable
Skin is warm and moist with good turgor

Vital signs are stable
Blood glucose is within normal levels

■ **NDX:** Knowledge deficit related to lack of information about home and follow-up care

Discuss symptoms of adrenal crisis to report
Emphasize importance of reporting risk factors to physician immediately for medication adjustment
  Infection: fever, cold, flu, persistent cough, burning on urination, wounds that do not heal
  Injury, surgery, dental care
  Profuse sweating
  Strenuous, unusual activity
  Emotionally charged events
  Infections, no matter how minor
Explain need to avoid persons with infections, especially URIs
Teach name of medications, dosage, time and method of administration, side and/or toxic effects
Demonstrate IM injection method to patient and significant other
Emphasize importance of carrying injectable cortisol for administration in emergency
Explain that if bilateral adrenalectomy was performed, steroid therapy will be needed for remainder of life
Teach care of incision and to report signs of infection
Emphasize importance of
  Adequate rest
  Moderate exercise
  Good nutrition
  Ongoing outpatient care, being certain to inform all physicians, dentists, other health care providers of surgery and prescribed medications
Explain that if surgery was for Cushing's syndrome, these symptoms will slowly recede
Emphasize importance of wearing medical alert band or chain and carrying identification card

Expected outcome/evaluation

Patient and/or significant other verbalizes understanding of symptoms and risk factors to report, general home care instruction, need for continued medication; demonstrates IM injection techniques

HYPOPHYSECTOMY

Surgical removal of pituitary gland to remove adenomas, to slow growth of endocrine-dependent tumors, to correct Cushing's disease, and as palliative therapy in certain types of breast and prostate cancer; usually performed via transphenoid approach

Preoperative Assessment and Teaching

Assess for upper airway infection, report if present (surgery will be delayed)

Discuss and teach postoperative care and rationale
  Presence of nasal packing
  Graft site, usually thigh
  Need for mouth breathing
  No toothbrushing
  Avoid coughing, sneezing, or noseblowing
  Decreased smell and taste
Encourage questions
  Reinforce physician's explanation of procedure
  Allow time for discussion of fears and anxiety

Postoperative Assessment
Observations/findings

Signs and symptoms of increased intracranial pressure (ICP)
  Increasing restlessness
  Decreasing level of consciousness
  Unequal pupils
  Visual changes
  Widened pulse pressure
  Bradycardia
  Respiratory arrest
Gum line incision
  Pain; location, intensity
  Redness
  Swelling
  Edema
  Drainage or bleeding
Nasal packing
  Intact
  CSF drainage (may be postnasal drip): frequent swallowing, coughing
  Bleeding
  Patent airway
Thigh, graft site
  Redness
  Swelling
  Drainage

Laboratory/diagnostic studies

Hormone levels
Electrolyte levels
Blood sugar levels

Potential complications

Cerebrospinal rhinorrhea
Meningitis
Hemorrhage
Diabetes insipidus (p. 330)
Adrenal crisis (p. 322)
Severe hypoglycemia (p. 343)
Decreased levels of sex hormones

Medical Management

Indwelling catheter
Incentive spirometer

IV fluids progressing to po diet
Treatment of complications
Pain management

Nursing diagnoses/interventions/evaluation

■ **NDX:** Potential for injury related to risk of increased intracranial pressure

Assess for signs and symptoms of increased ICP qh for first 24 hr, then q4h; check neurological and vital signs
Notify physician at once if onset of restlessness or if pupillary or vital signs change
Maintain head of bed elevated 30 degrees
Avoid turning, extending, and flexing head for first 24 hr
Avoid having patient cough vigorously or use other valsalva maneuvers for any reason; use stool softeners if needed
Maintain calm, dimly lit environment
Pace care to avoid excessive stimulation; allow adequate undisturbed rest periods

Expected outcome/evaluation

Vital signs are within normal limits
Remains alert, oriented with reactive pupils
Has no cough

■ **NDX:** Potential for ineffective airway clearance related to nasal packing, postnasal drip, and/or dry oropharynx

Assess for intactness of nasal packing q2h; determine if packing is slipping posteriorly
Patient must maintain mouth breathing; maintain oral mucous membranes in moist condition
Provide oral care with saline solution or diluted mouthwash q2h and prn
Supply humidity to room or via face mask if necessary
Keep suction at bedside; gently suction oropharynx only when absolutely necessary
Remind patient to deep breathe and turn q2h, to avoid forceful coughing
Monitor for signs of respiratory distress: stridor, wheezing, labored respirations, cyanosis
Check dressing and oropharynx for bleeding or CSF leakage q2h to 4h prn

Expected outcome/evaluation

Breath sounds, respiratory rate and rhythm are within normal limits
Nasal packing is intact without bleeding or postnasal drip
Mucous membranes are moist
Color is good

■ **NDX:** Potential for infection related to disruption in dura mater

Monitor incision for signs and symptoms of infection q4h
Evaluate drainage for CSF leakage (positive glucose reagent strip); report immediately
Assess for early signs of meningitis; chills, fever, malaise, headache, vomiting, nuchal rigidity; report immediately
Do not use toothbrush until incision is healed
Avoid foods that would irritate incision
Instruct patient not to touch dressing or packing; use sterile technique to change mustache pad each time it becomes damp

Expected outcome/evaluation

Temperature is within normal limits
Nasal packing negative for CSF
Incision is clean without signs of infection

■ **NDX:** Potential fluid volume deficit related to risk of surgically induced diabetes insipidus

Assess for signs of diabetes insipidus
Monitor intake and output q8h
Measure output qh; report if >200 ml/hr
Report intake >3000 to 4000 ml/24 hr
Monitor urine specific gravity; report if <1.010
Collaborate with physician to correct condition if condition is present
Monitor vital signs, skin turgor, and mucous membranes q4h to 8h
Weigh patient daily, same time, clothing, and scale; monitor for weight loss

Expected outcome/evaluation

Vital signs are stable
Intake is <2500 ml/24 hr
Urine output is <150 ml/hr and specific gravity is within normal range
Weight is stable
Skin turgor is good

■ **NDX:** Pain at surgical site or headache

Assess patient for verbal and nonverbal signs of pain
Be aware that severe headache may be a sign of increased ICP
Discuss with patient factors that relieve pain; facilitate use of these if possible
Assist patient with finding position of comfort, maintaining neutral head position with head elevated 30 degrees
Teach relaxation techniques
Provide means of distraction from pain: guided imagery, soft music, visitors as tolerated
Administer pain medications as ordered; be aware that they may mask signs of increased ICP

Expected outcome/evaluation

Verbalizes increasing comfort and no headache
Face and body are relaxed
Uses relaxation techniques

■ **NDX:**   Knowledge deficit related to lack of information regarding home and follow-up care

Explain that decrease in taste and smell for several months is expected

Explain need to avoid persons with infections, especially upper respiratory infections (URIs)

Discuss symptoms of incisional or systemic infection to report to physician

Emphasize importance of avoiding vigorous coughing, straining, and nose-blowing

Emphasize importance of ongoing patient care

Discuss signs and symptoms of hormonal imbalances to report to physician (see specific disease relating to hormone deficiency)

Teach name of medication(s), dosage, time and method of administration, side effects, and toxic effects

    Emphasize that hormone therapy will continue throughout lifetime

Explain need to notify care giver about unusual stress so medication dosages can be changed if needed

Provide information for obtaining medical alert bracelet and card

Expected outcome/evaluation

Patient and/or significant other verbalizes understanding of home and follow-up care

BIBLIOGRAPHY

American Diabetes Association: *Foot care for the diabetic*, Los Angeles, 1989, Southern California Affiliate, Inc, American Diabetes Association.

Butts D: Fluid and electrolyte disorders associated with diabetic ketoacidosis and hyperglycemic hyperosmolar nonketotic coma, *Nurs Clin North Am* 22(4):827, 1987.

Bybee D: Saving lives in parathyroid crises, *Emerg Med* 19(5):62, 1987.

Bybee D: Saving lives in thyroid crises, *Emerg Med* 19(6):20, 1987.

Diabetic teaching manual, Los Angeles, 1987, Southern California Kaiser Permanente Medical Center.

Gavin JR III: Diabetes and exercise, *Am J Nurs* 88(2):178, Feb, 1988.

Germain CP, Nemchik RM: Diabetes self-management and hospitalization, *Image J Nurs Scholar* 20(2):74, 1988.

Green Hernandez CM: Surgery and diabetes: minimizing the risks, *Am J Nurs* 87(6):788, June, 1987.

Gulanick M et al: *Nursing care plans: nursing diagnosis and treatment*, ed 2, St Louis, 1990, Mosby–Year Book.

Hurxthal K: Quick: Teach this patient about insulin, *Am J Nurs* 88(8):1097, August, 1988.

Ihde JK, Jacobsen WK, and Briggs BA: *Principles of critical care*, Philadelphia, 1987, WB Saunders.

Kim MJ, McFarland GK, and McLane AM: *Pocket guide to nursing diagnosis*, ed 4, St Louis, 1990, Mosby–Year Book.

Knight-Macheca MK: Educating the Hospitalized diabetic: a nurse's responsibility, *Curr Con Nurs* 2(4):11, 1988.

Mampalam T et al: Transphenoid microsurgery for Cushing disease: a report of 216 cases, *Ann Intern Med* 109(6):487, 1988.

Melby J: Therapy of Cushing disease: a consensus for pituitary microsurgery, *Ann Intern Med* 109(6):445, 1988.

Nath C, Murray S, and Ponte C: Lessons in living with type II diabetes mellitus, *Nurs 88* p. 45, August, 1988.

Pagana KD, Pagana TJ: *Diagnostic testing and nursing implications*, ed 3, St Louis, 1990, Mosby–Year Book.

Ramsey PW: Hyperglycemia at dawn, *Am J Nurs* 87(11):1424, November, 1987.

Sarsany S: Thyroid storm, *RN* 51(7):46, 1988.

Thompson JM et al: *Mosby's manual of clinical nursing*, ed 2, St Louis, 1989, CV Mosby.

Ulrich C, Canale S, and Wendell, S: *Nursing care planning guides: a nursing diagnosis approach*, ed 2, Philadelphia, 1990, WB Saunders.

Utiger RD: *The thyroid: physiology, hyperthyroidism, hypothyroidism and the painful thyroid—endocrine and metabolism*, ed 2, New York, 1987, McGraw-Hill.

Williams RH: *Textbook of endocrinology*, Philadelphia, 1985, WB Saunders.

7

Musculoskeletal System

MUSCULOSKELETAL ASSESSMENT

Subjective Data

Pain and/or edema in muscles, joints, or bones with or without movement
Weakness in extremities
Limited activity and movement
Sensory changes
Anorexia; loss of weight
Insomnia
Tires easily
Unsteady gait or stance
Frustration, anger at self

Objective Data

General appearance
Age, weight
Vital signs: BP, T, P, and R
Joint(s) inflamed, edematous, and/or warm to touch
Impaired neurovascular status of extremity(ies)
Deformities
Paralysis
Contractures
Posture
Abnormal body alignment
Limited ability or inability to move in bed
Abnormal gait; needs assistance
Decreased handgrip and range of motion (ROM)
Internal and external rotation of extremities
Ability to perform ROM exercises
Contusions, lacerations, scars
Wounds: amount and type of drainage
Facial and body gestures indicating pain
Loss of extremity
Pressure ulcers
Skin rashes
Allergies
Tenseness
Presence of casts, braces, prostheses, crutches, traction, cane, or walker
Nutritional history

Ability to use trapeze in bed, to sit up, and to turn
Ability to perform activities of daily living (ADLs)
Constipation
Dependence, independence, and interdependence

Pertinent Background Information

CONCURRENT DISEASES AND/OR CONDITIONS

Spinal cord injury, nerve impairment
Cerebrovascular accident (CVA)
Rheumatoid arthritis
Arthritis
Bursitis
Polyneuritis
Multiple sclerosis
Muscular dystrophy
Myasthenia gravis
Fracture
Ruptured disc
Meniere's disease
Labyrinthitis
Osteoporosis
Congenital conditions
Low back pain
Lupus erythematosus
Gout
Blood dyscrasias

PREVIOUS SURGERY AND/OR ILLNESS

Poliomyelitis
Hemiplegia, paraplegia
Cerebral palsy
Orthopedic surgery
Spinal surgery
Parkinson's disease
Ataxia
Alcoholism
Syphilis
Impaired vision and/or hearing
CVA
Hyperparathyroidism
Osteoporosis

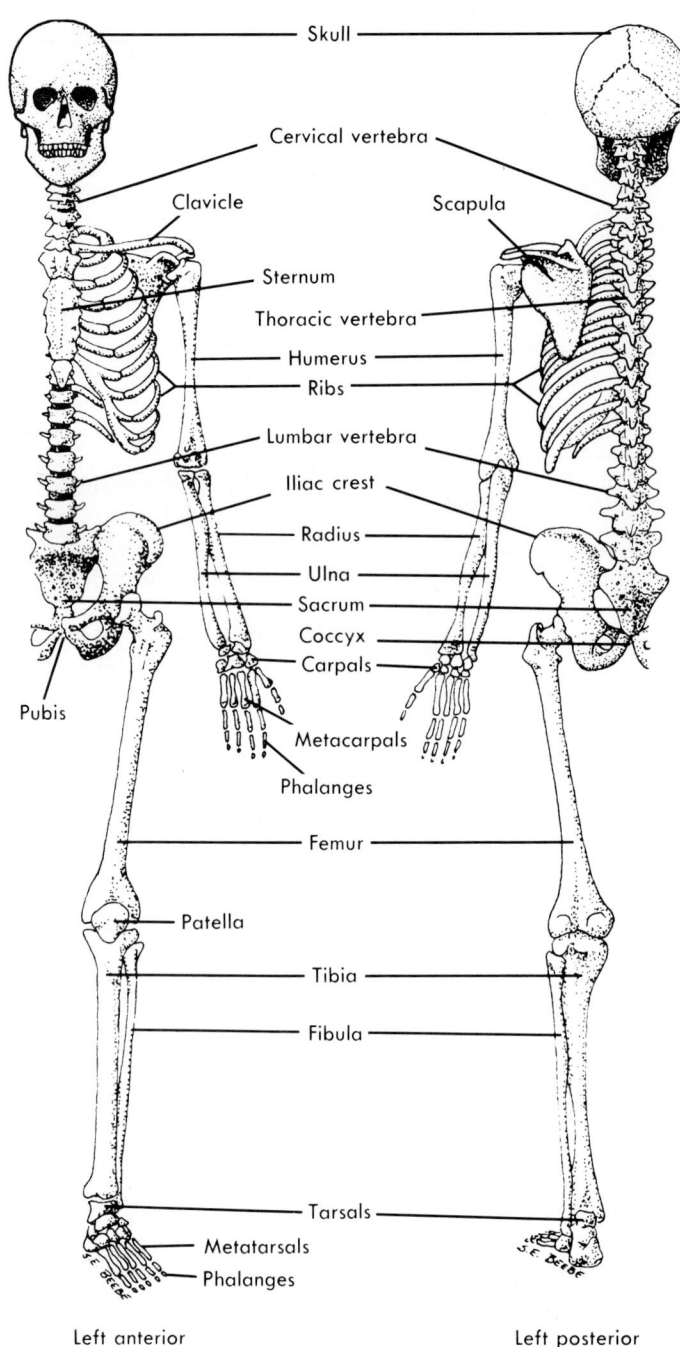

Left anterior   Left posterior

FIGURE 7-1. Musculoskeletal system.

Rickets, osteomalacia
Tuberculosis

FAMILY HISTORY

Carcinoma
Diabetes
Tuberculosis

SOCIAL HISTORY

Hazardous job or recreation (e.g., construction work or
    contact sports)

Safety measures used
Accident proneness
Alcohol, chemical substance, tobacco use

MEDICATION HISTORY

Antiinflammatory agents: steroid and nonsteroid
Sedatives
Tranquilizers
Analgesics
Acetylsalicylic acid
Antimalarials

Antiemetics
Anticoagulants
Antidepressants
Insulin
Oral hypoglycemics
Psychotherapeutic agents
Antibiotics
Antihypertensive agents

Diagnostic Aids

LABORATORY STUDIES

Serum
    Calcium
    Phosphorus
    Alkaline phosphatase
    Erythrocyte sedimentation rate (ESR)
    Creatinine clearance
    BUN
    Uric acid
    SGOT, SGPT, creatinine phosphokinase (CPK)
Urine
    Calcium
    Phosphorus
    Creatinine, uric acid

PROCEDURES

X-ray examination of bones
Arthrogram
Arthroscopy
Myelograms
Fluoroscopy
Arteriograms
Venograms
Bone marrow aspiration
Bone or muscle biopsy
Incision and drainage of joint
Aspiration of joint
Electromyogram (EMG): muscle and nerve conduction studies
Bone scan
Computed tomography (CT scan)
Thermography
Magnetic resonance imaging (MRI)

ORTHOPEDIC SEPSIS: ACUTE PYOGENIC ARTHRITIS, ACUTE OSTEOMYELITIS

acute pyogenic arthritis Acute bacterial infection affecting one or more joints caused by trauma or a penetrating wound; highest incidence is in children

acute osteomyelitis Infection of the long bones caused by acute local infection or bone trauma, usually caused by Escherichia coli, Staphylococcus aureus, or Streptococcus pyogenes

Assessment

Observations/findings

Pain, redness, and swelling in affected joint; increases with motion
Chills
Rapid elevation of temperature
Diaphoresis
Muscular spasms around affected joint
Tachycardia
Headache
Restlessness
Irritability
Weakness

Laboratory/diagnostic studies

CBC, blood cultures
Joint radiological study
Culture of joint aspirate

Potential complications

Limited motion, contractures
Ankylosing of joint
Degenerative joint changes
Chronic osteomyelitis

Medical Management

Parenteral fluids with antibiotics
Antibiotics, analgesics
Irrigant solution
Immobilization of joint
Compresses; warm, moist, or alternate warm and cold
Diet, activity
Excision, aspiration, drainage, irrigation of joint

Nursing diagnoses/interventions/evaluation

■ **NDX:** Impaired physical mobility related to pain and swelling

Maintain bed rest; handle affected extremity gently
Immobilize joint/extremity with use of cast, splint, and/or pillows to maintain alignment; elevate to reduce edema
Assist with and teach active or perform passive ROM exercises to unaffected extremities q4h and deep breathe q½h
Involve in planning care and encourage self-care participation
Increase socialization
Monitor for signs of deep vein thrombosis (DVT): calf pain, Homan's sign (calf pain or dorsiflexion of foot), edema
Administer skin care prn
Increase activity after fever and swelling subside or drainage decreases
Initiate ROM exercise of affected joint/extremity

Monitor tolerance before increasing activity
Provide resistive exercises
Protect affected joint/extremity from trauma
Assist patient to chair; elevate affected extremity
Ambulate with crutches; advance to walker or cane as tolerated
Provide a safe environment
Instruct patient in weight bearing
Provide encouragement and support for each accomplishment

Expected outcome/evaluation

Patient's
Mobility and joint use are improving
Participation in own care is increasing
Edema is diminishing

■ **NDX:** Potential for infection related to progression of bacterial invasion

Draw blood cultures immediately; monitor results
Maintain parenteral fluids with antibiotics
Monitor vital signs q4h; institute cooling measures as needed
Apply warm, moist compresses or alternate warm and cold compresses
Collaborate with physician and prepare patient for excision and drainage if infected lesion presents
Take cultures of aspirated fluid
Irrigate lesion if irrigating catheter is in place; continuous irrigation with antibiotics may be ordered
Monitor intake and output of irrigant
Do not allow irrigating bottle to run dry
Keep patient warm and dry
Observe for skin breakdown.
Monitor incision for bleeding
Change dressing prn; maintain rigid aseptic technique
Provide high-calorie, high-protein diet as tolerated to promote healing; assist with meals as needed
Encourage fluids to upper limits for age and weight
Remove splints daily if ordered and monitor skin condition

Expected outcome/evaluation

Patient's
Vital signs are stable
Incision is healing without evidence of extension of infection

■ **NDX:** Pain related to inflammation, incision, and drainage

Assess location, intensity, and type of pain
Provide analgesics as indicated; assess effectiveness of pain relief measures
Assist patient with changing position frequently; support affected extremity; administer back rubs

Provide diversional activities
Discuss and promote alternate pain relief measures

Expected outcome/evaluation

Patient
Reports that level of pain is tolerable
Appears more relaxed, comfortable
Balances periods of activity with rest

■ **NDX:** Knowledge deficit related to lack of information about home care management

Provide and discuss information on prescribed rehabilitation program: physical therapy and home instructions
Demonstrate incision care and stress importance of aseptic technique and a daily shower
Provide information about disease process and complications
Discuss signs and symptoms to report to physician
Tenderness, pain, discomfort
Fever, malaise
Drainage from incision
Provide medication schedule, including name, dosage, purpose, and side effects: instruct patient to take all prescribed medications
Stress importance of nourishing diet and increased fluid intake
Promote regular visits with physician

Expected outcome/evaluation

Patient
Demonstrates ability to perform incision care
Verbalizes understanding of disease process, potential complications, and rehabilitation program
Expresses understanding of medication schedule

PROGRESSIVE SYSTEMIC SCLEROSIS (SCLERODERMA)

A chronic inflammatory disease of the connective tissue (collagen) affecting many organs and their connective tissue in its later stages

Assessment
Observations/findings

Joints/skin
Edema
Muscle weakness
Tough, hard skin, progressing to taut and shiny
Tenderness, pain in joints, fingers, and toes
Skin rash (hands, feet)
Altered self-concept
History of
Pulmonary fibrosis, dyspnea
Myocardial sclerosis, dysrhythmia
Renal incompetence

Esophageal lesions, paralytic ileus, malabsorption syndrome

Raynaud's phenomenon

Laboratory/diagnostic studies

Skin biopsies, angiography

Elevated ESR, rheumatoid factor

Positive antinuclear antibody studies

Renal, GI, and pulmonary studies

Potential complications

Bowel obstruction

Congestive heart failure

Nephrosclerosis

Esophageal thickening

Lung fibrosis

Atrophic changes in skin

Medical Management

Analgesics, antipyretics, antibiotics

Corticosteroids, potassium (Potaba), antihypertensives

Cholinergics for dysphagia

Diet, activity, rest

Physical therapy

Surgical intervention: joint arthroplasty

Nursing diagnoses/interventions/evaluation

■ **NDX:** Impaired physical mobility related to pain and edema of joints

Promote and perform prescribed exercise program

Perform passive or assist with and teach active ROM exercises

Maintain correct body alignment

Allow time to complete self-care

Provide mobilization devices prn; ensure correct use

Encourage use of affected joints to maintain function

Keep joints warm and protected

Ambulate with assistance as tolerated

Encourage use of shoes with good support; avoid slippers

Expected outcome/evaluation

Patient

Participates actively in treatment program

Uses mobilization devices correctly

States discomfort is less intense

■ **NDX:** Potential alteration in tissue perfusion; renal, cardiopulmonary, peripheral, related to risk of altered blood flow

Assess renal function

Measure intake and output q8h

Monitor for hypertension; administer antihypertensives as indicated

Encourage fluid intake of 2500 ml/24 hr if not contraindicated

Monitor output, color, consistency, frequency, and for retention

Assess cardiopulmonary function

Monitor vital signs for dysrhythmias

Assess ECG, pulmonary function studies, and arterial blood gases as indicated

Assess breath sound in all lobes q4h to 8h; monitor for diminished sounds, dullness, friction rub

Monitor respirations, observe for dyspnea, cough, shortness of breath, pain

Assist with deep breathing exercises as needed; encourage incentive spirometer if appropriate

Administer corticosteroids if indicated

Assess peripheral function

Monitor peripheral pulses q4h; assess digits for sensation and temperature

Observe hands, feet for blanching, cyanosis, redness (Raynaud's phenomenon)

Assess for parasthesia, numbness, tingling of extremities

Expected outcome/evaluation

Patient's

Vital signs are normal within parameters of disease

Intake and output are balanced

Arterial blood gases are within normal limits

Peripheral pulses are present

■ **NDX:** Potential for altered nutrition related to the risk of digestive dysfunction resulting from other organ involvement

Assess GI function

Monitor nutrition and fluid intake; observe for dysphasia, reflux, and esophageal stricture

Administer potassium amino benzoate (Potaba) and anticholinergic as indicated; assess effectiveness/side effects

Provide well-balanced, high-fiber diet, fluids

Encourage small, frequent meals

Measure intake

Assess ability to chew foods well

Auscultate abdomen for bowel sounds; observe stools for fat

Measure abdominal girth as baseline

Monitor for distention, pain, tenderness

Weigh patient daily, same clothes, scale, and time

Expected outcome/evaluation

Patient

Ingests intake adequate to maintain weight

Evidences normal skin turgor

Tolerates well-balanced diet without discomfort

■ **NDX:** Potential for impaired skin integrity related to altered skin turgor

Assess skin integrity and observe for rashes, excoriation, breaks, or ulcers

Change position frequently to reduce pressure and promote comfort

Elevate legs to prevent edema; avoid long periods of chair sitting; avoid use of donuts and rings

Provide skin care frequently, keeping skin well lubricated with lotions; do not massage reddened areas

Encourage fluid intake to 2500 ml/day if not contraindicated

Ambulate as soon as able

Expected outcome/evaluation

Patient

Exhibits warm, dry and intact skin

Verbalizes and demonstrates ability to perform skin care within parameters of disease process

■ **NDX:** Body image disturbance related to altered body structure/function

Encourage and allow time for patient to discuss feelings about body image change

Allow time to discuss anger and denial

Assess present coping styles and provide support for strengths that assisted in the past

Encourage communication with significant other

Promote independence and provide positive feedback for tasks accomplished

Encourage social interaction with family and friends

Expected outcome/evaluation

Patient

Seeks out others to help maintain self-esteem

Actively participates in own care

Uses positive coping skills in dealing with altered body image

■ **NDX:** Knowledge deficit related to lack of information about home care management and disease process

Reinforce physician's explanation of progression of disease, treatment, and prognosis; clarify any misconceptions

Promote independence in ADLs to lessen complications

Explain signs and symptoms of specific organ involvement to report to physician

Discuss medications: name, purpose, schedule, dosage, and side effects; explain need to avoid medications not ordered by physician

Stress importance of nutritious high-fiber diet, prescribed exercise schedule, and planned rest periods

Promote follow-up visits with physician

Expected outcome/evaluation

Patient

Verbalizes understanding of disease process, symptoms

to report to physician, and medication schedule

Performs ADLs within limited activity ability

Understands importance of physician visits

GOUTY ARTHRITIS

Acute and/or chronic arthritis of the joints caused by impaired uric acid production

Assessment
Observations/findings

Affected joint (usually metatarsophalangeal joint of great toe)

Excruciating pain

Tenderness

Redness

Increased heat

Swelling

Shiny

Vein distention

Deformity

Anorexia

Headache

Elevated temperature

Chills

Constipation

Subcutaneous tophi: ears, joints, knuckles

Laboratory/diagnostic studies

Serum and uric acid elevated, WBC, ESR

Microscopic examination of joint aspirate

X-ray examination of affected area

Potential complications

Decreased urine output

Hypertension

Renal calculi

Medical Management

Antigout agents: probenecid (Benemid), colchicine (Colsalide)

Nonsteroid antiinflammatory agents: phenylbutazone (Butazolidin), indomethacin (Indocin), ibuprofen (Motrin)

Analgesics, antipyretics, allopurinol

Cold packs

Low-purine diet

Nursing diagnoses/interventions/evaluation

■ **NDX:** Pain related to gout and edema

Assess intensity, location, and type of pain; use pain rating scale

Maintain patient in position of comfort with affected joint, initially foot, supported and in alignment; place cradle over foot; no weight bearing

Elevate affected area to reduce edema and promote venous
    return
Administer analgesics and antigout and antiinflammatory
    agents; observe for side effects
    Colchicine: nausea, vomiting, bloody diarrhea, oli-
        guria, hematuria
    Phenylbutazone: nausea, vomiting, diarrhea, rash,
        edema, hypertension, leukopenia
Encourage fluids to 2500 ml/day
Monitor serum uric acid levels

Expected outcome/evaluation

Patient
    Reports pain is at a tolerable level
    Appears calm and relaxed
    Exhibits lessening or absent edema

■ **NDX:**   Impaired physical mobility related to joint pain
                and immobility

Increase activity as pain and swelling subside
Ambulate with assistance; use walker or cane
Perform ROM exercise carefully to affected joint
Promote return to normal activities

Expected outcome/evaluation

Patient
    Performs ROM adequately in affected joint
    Ambulates with walker or cane without discomfort

■ **NDX:**   Knowledge deficit related to lack of information
                about medications and home care management

Provide medication schedule, including name, dosage,
    purpose, and side effects, and explain necessity of taking
    colchicine hourly at onset of acute attacks
Report side effects of medications immediately; avoid sa-
    licylates if taking probenecid
Discuss importance of diet (avoiding foods high in purine
    and alcohol), exercise, and rest program
Explain importance of high fluid intake (2500 ml/day)
Encourage follow-up visits with physician

Expected outcome/evaluation

Patient
    Accurately verbalizes understanding of diet, activity,
        and exercise regimen
    Expresses awareness and knowledge of medication
        schedule/side effects

FRACTURES

A break in bone continuity; there are many types of frac-
tures—a few major ones are as follows
compound or open fracture *A break with bone protrud-*
ing through the skin

simple or closed fracture *A break with the skin left in-*
tact
complete fracture *A break through the entire bone; bone*
may be displaced
incomplete fracture *A break through only part of the*
bone

Assessment
Observations/findings

Fracture site
    Pain, tenderness, edema
    Skin open or intact
    Color and temperature of surrounding tissues
    Presence of pulse distal from break
    Numbness, tingling
    Bleeding, hematoma
    Restricted, limited mobility
    Abnormal position of extremity
Signs of shock: hypotension, tachycardia

Laboratory/diagnostic studies

Radiological films of fracture
CBC, electrolytes
Arthroscopic aspirate studies

Potential complications

Malunion, delayed union, or nonunion of fracture
Thrombophlebitis
Fat embolism
Compartment syndrome (knee, elbow)
Infection
Nerve compression

Medical Management

Open or closed reduction of fracture
Joint arthroplasty or total replacement
Analgesics, narcotics, sedatives, antibiotics, muscle re-
    laxants
Application of cast, traction, splint, and/or sling
Ice application
Antiembolic stockings
Bed rest in specific position
Diet, activity, rest, mobility restrictions
Physical therapy

Nursing diagnoses/interventions/evaluation

■ **NDX:**   Impaired physical mobility related to fracture
                and injury to surrounding tissues

Maintain bed rest in prescribed position to facilitate heal-
    ing.
Elevate affected extremity and apply ice bags indicated
Support affected extremity above and below fracture when
    moving, turning, and lifting
Monitor cast, traction, and sling q1h initially, then q4h;

observe for cast integrity and position of traction weights and sling

Assist with and teach use of trapeze and other methods of moving and turning

Perform passive or assist with and teach active ROM exercises to unaffected joints

Explain restrictions and limitations in activity

Encourage patient to perform ADLs within scope of limitations; provide supplies; assist as necessary

Assist with and teach patient use of urinal or bedpan for elimination; administer perineal care as needed

Expected outcome/evaluation

Patient
  Regains mobility to optimal level
  Participates actively in treatment plan
  Seeks assistance as needed
  Verbalizes needed restrictions and understands rationale

■ **NDX:** Potential for altered tissue perfusion; peripheral, related to location of fracture and risk of arteriovenous flow alteration

Monitor pulses distal from fracture qlh and 2h and observe for color, temperature, and sensation

Assess capillary refill; report normal findings; compare with opposite extremity

Maintain body alignment and prescribed position

Observe for signs of compartment syndrome (p. 382)

Apply antiembolic stockings: remove daily to inspect for pressure, pain, and redness

Expected outcome/evaluation

Patient's
  Pulses distal to fracture are present
  Skin is warm
  Capillary refill is normal (2 to 4 sec)

■ **NDX:** Potential for altered tissue perfusion: cerebral and/or cardiopulmonary related to risk of fat embolus

Assess cardiopulmonary status
  Monitor vital signs q2h to 4h; take apical pulse
  Auscultate chest for breath sounds q4h; observe for diminished sounds and dyspnea

Assist and teach patient to turn and cough q2h and deep breathe qlh

Assess level of consciousness (LOC) and mental status q4h to 8h

Monitor ABGs

Instruct patient to report headache or chest pain immediately

Expected outcome/evaluation

Patient
  Presents normal vital signs

Exhibits clear breath sounds
Presents laboratory values within normal limits
Remains alert, oriented
Reports no headache or chest pain

■ **NDX:** Potential for impaired tissue integrity related to surgical reduction, puncture wounds

Assess wound integrity and observe for signs of infection or drainage especially at pin sites
  Administer antibiotics and assess effectiveness/side effects
  Monitor and change dressings prn
  Monitor temperature
Monitor traction/casts for pressure points
  Provide frequent skin care to bony prominences and around cast/traction openings
  Turn patient frequently; maintain body alignment
  Maintain dry, wrinkle-free bed linen
Provide foam, air, or water mattress as needed
  Use bed cradle to prevent pressure

Expected outcome/evaluation

Patient's
  Tissue integrity is maintained

■ **NDX:** Pain related to fracture and/or trauma

Assess location, intensity, and type of pain; use pain rating scale

Administer narcotics, analgesics, and muscle relaxants; avoid allowing pain to become severe; assess effectiveness of pain relief measures

Provide quiet environment initially and encourage diversional activities

Assist with and teach alternate pain management methods

Change position frequently and administer back rubs and massages

Encourage ambulation with assistance when tolerated

Involve physical therapy department in instructions in use of crutches, walker, or cane

Expected outcome/evaluation

Patient
  Reports a reduction in pain
  Presents a relaxed manner
  Participates in diversional activities

■ **NDX:** Anxiety related to altered health status/situational crisis

Monitor patient's level of anxiety (p. 13)
Reinforce physician's explanation of treatment and expected outcome; clarify misconceptions
Encourage and allow time for verbalization of feelings

Teach and assist with stress management techniques

Assess present coping behaviors and encourage use of behaviors that were successful in managing past experiences

Encourage interaction with significant other and with friends and relatives

Explain all procedures and treatments; involve patient in plan of care; provide options; encourage safe decision-making

Expected outcome/evaluation

Patient

Demonstrates relaxation techniques correctly

Verbalizes a feeling of less tension, apprehension

Appears calm and relaxed

Participates in activities appropriately

■ **NDX:** Knowledge deficit related to lack of information about home care management

Stress importance of prescribed rehabilitation plan of activity, rest, and exercise

Provide and review diet instructions regarding type and amount; need to avoid weight gain if applicable

Discuss medications: name, purpose, schedule, dosage, and side effects

Discuss signs and symptoms to report to physician: severe pain, changes in temperature, color, or sensation in extremity, foul odor or drainage from wound

Explain cast, splint, sling care as indicated

Encourage follow-up visits with physician

Expected outcome/evaluation

Patient

Verbalizes understanding of prognosis, treatment, and rehabilitation programs

Demonstrates ability to care for immobilizing devices

Expresses knowledge of symptoms, potential complications

MAXILLOMANDIBULAR FIXATION

Surgical procedure to reduce and repair jaw fractures or deformities

Preoperative Assessment and Care

Assess respiratory status; observe for signs of upper respiratory infection (URI)

Explain purpose of wires after surgery and provide method of communication: pad and pencil, Magic Slate, etc.

Assist with and teach patient method for pushing secretions through clamped jaw (if possible) and demonstrate use of oral suction catheter

Discuss importance of oral hygiene and oral suctioning, and teach procedure

Demonstrate feeding procedure using straw or syringe

Explain possibility of nasopharyngeal airway and/or nasogastric tube and aspiration postoperatively

Perform facial scrub and oral hygiene preoperatively

Administer prescribed antibiotics

Answer all questions and allow time for verbalization of fears and anxieties

Postoperative Assessment
Observations/findings

Edema of
Face
Base of tongue
Front of neck
Nose

Pain

Nausea, vomiting; aspiration of emesis

Dyspnea

Elevated temperature

Apprehension

Drainage from mouth

Location of wire cutters or scissors

Laboratory/diagnostic studies

CBC, electrolytes

Radiological examinations for alignment of fracture

Potential complications

Respiratory distress

Aspiration pneumonia

Hemorrhage, shock

Medical Management

Analgesics, sedatives, antibiotics

Parenteral fluids

Nasogastric aspiration, NPO

Oxygen therapy

Ice packs

Wire and band cutting procedure

Diet, activity, rest

Nursing diagnoses/interventions/evaluation

■ **NDX:** Potential for aspiration related to wired jaws

Tape wire cutters or scissors to head of bed; if aspiration is imminent, cut wires as needed

Maintain bed rest with head elevated when reactive

Assess patient's ability to swallow

Perform oral suctioning prn; assist and teach patient to clear airway and perform suctioning

Provide and maintain suction apparatus at all times; observe for edema, drainage, and bleeding

Teach patient techniques to avoid vomiting; deep breathing, swallowing

Control with antiemetics as needed

Monitor nasogastric tube and low, intermittent suction apparatus if applicable; maintain patency with normal saline irrigations prn

Apply ice bags to reduce swelling

Monitor vital signs q4h to 8h

Auscultate chest for breath sounds q4h to 8h

Instruct patient to report immediately inability to manage self-suctioning or feeling of nausea

Maintain parenteral fluids and decrease amount as fluid intake increases

Provide clear liquid to full high-calorie liquid diet as tolerated after nasogastric tube had been removed

    Assist and teach patient to use straw or feed with syringe; give small amount and wait for swallowing before continuing

    Follow each feeding with water and mouth care

    Provide small, frequent meals

    Consult dietitian regarding alternatives in food selections (i.e., commercially prepared formulas)

Measure intake and output q8h

Expected outcome/evaluation

Patient

    Performs self-suctioning to remove secretions

    Ingests liquid diet without nausea

    Presents clear breath sounds

    Presents stable vital signs

■ **NDX:** Pain related to surgical procedure

Assess type, intensity, and location of pain; administer prescribed analgesics; use pain rating scale; assess effectiveness of pain relief measures

Assist patient with changing position frequently while in bed

Maintain quiet environment

Administer back rubs to promote comfort

Offer diversional activities

Administer frequent oral hygiene; use water jet, if available, or mouth swabs; keep lips well lubricated

Ambulate patient with assistance as needed

Assist with and teach alternate pain management techniques

Apply ice bags to reduce discomfort

Expected outcome/evaluation

Patient

    Reports a tolerable level of pain

    Appears calm, relaxed

    Balances sleep with activities adequately

■ **NDX:** Impaired verbal communication related to jaw wiring

Maintain call light within easy reach

Provide means of communications; pad and pencil, Magic Slate

Allow time for patient to write out thoughts and questions

Encourage patient to express fears and anxieties

Maintain equipment for communication and place within easy reach

Expected outcome/evaluation

Patient

    Demonstrates ability to use alternate methods of communication

    Appears comfortable with method selected

■ **NDX:** Knowledge deficit related to lack of information about home care management

Provide and review diet instruction for full liquid diet and foods allowed: blended junior foods, eggnogs, and milk shakes; demonstrate use of straw or syringe

Discuss importance and purpose of small, frequent meals

Stress and teach oral hygiene; demonstrate use of Water Pic and dental wax to keep lips moist

Demonstrate method for cutting wires and under what circumstances to cut (wires will remain for 6 to 8 weeks)

Explain signs and symptoms to report to physician: fever, increased pain, edema, foul odor from mouth

Discuss obtaining all medications in liquid form

Promote follow-up visits with physician

Expected outcome/evaluation

Patient

    Demonstrates ability to feel self adequately and maintain correct oral hygiene

    Verbalizes signs/symptoms of potential complications

    Expresses understanding of emergency wire-cutting procedure

SPINAL SURGERY

Surgery performed to relieve pressure on the spinal nerves and/or cord caused by a herniated disc, trauma, displaced fracture, incomplete vertebral dislocation from rheumatoid arthritis, osteoporosis, or insertion of rods to correct scoliosis; incision may be anterior or posterior in cervical, thoracic, or lumbar areas

laminectomy *Removal of part of the disc lamina*

discectomy *Removal of part of the disc*

spinal fusion *Solidification of several vertebrae by grafting bone from the iliac crest of the tibia*

microsurgical dorsal root rhizotomy *Severing of the sensory nerve root to the painful area; provides symptomatic relief and causes loss of sensation and possible motor damage; performed when other treatments have been unsuccessful*

Facet joint rhizotomy *Needle insertion into the facet joint with destruction of the nerve by microwave current; provides symptomatic relief*

Harrington rod internal fixation for scoliosis Surgical correction of scoliosis by insertion and implantation of a rod or rods along the posterior vertebral spine to correct the existing concavity or convexity; a posterior spinal fusion is performed concurrently

Preoperative Assessment and Teaching

Assess patient's neurovascular and respiratory status, and location, intensity, and duration of pain

Discuss with and teach patient postoperative care and rationale

    Definition and importance of prescribed postoperative position and body alignment

    Methods for turning, coughing, and deep breathing

    Use of trapeze and method for getting in and out of bed

    Necessary movement limitations and activities allowed

        ROM and isometric exercises

        Gluteal contractions, quadriceps setting

Provide firm mattress and bedboard if spinal fusion is to be performed

Harrington rod internal fixation patients may have halo traction brace or Risser cast in place preoperatively

Cervical fusion or fracture patients may have head immobilized before surgery with head collar, brace, halo cast, or traction (Crutchfield tongs); these devices will accompany patient to operating room

Explain that body brace, cast, or mold will be in place after surgery for thoracic and lumbar fusion; these devices are made ready for patient before surgery

Explain that a Hemovac or a Jackson-Pratt drain will be in place, and drainage may be profuse

Explain that there will be a second incision from bone graft site for spinal fusion

Discuss possibility of nasogastric aspiration and urinary drainage catheter; for thoracoabdominal approach, chest tubes may be in place

Explain that pain may be less with laminectomy, discectomy, or rhizotomy, but more with spinal fusion; discuss pain management

Encourage patient to ask questions; provide emotional support

    Reinforce physician's explanation of surgical procedure

    Allow time for and discuss patient's fears and anxieties

Postoperative Assessment
Observations/findings

Decreased sensation and motor activity of extremities

Circulatory status of extremities: change in color, temperature, or pulse

Respiratory status (especially in cervical surgery)

    Difficulty in breathing

    Cyanosis

    Tachypnea

    Diminished cough

Body alignment: presence of immobilization devices

Location and character of pain

Character and amount of

    Wound drainage

    Hemovac drainage if present

    Urinary output

Laboratory/diagnostic studies

CBC, electrolytes

Spinal radiological examinations

Urine for culture/sensitivity

Potential complications

Neurovascular damage

Hemorrhage

Shock

Urinary retention, infection

Abdominal distention

Paralytic ileus

Atelectasis, hypostatic pneumonia

Pulmonary embolus

Wound infection

Nonunion

Medical Management

Analgesics, antibiotics, antiemetics, stool softeners

Parenteral fluids with electrolytes

Urinary drainage catheter

Hemovac drainage, dressing change

Oxygen therapy, incentive spirometer

Transcutaneous electrical nerve stimulation (TENS) unit (p. 60), patient controlled analgesia (PCA) (p. 59)

Immobilization devices: brace, cast, corset

Diet, activity, rest

Antiembolic stockings

Nursing diagnoses/interventions/evaluation

■ **NDX:** Ineffective breathing pattern related to anesthesia, surgical incision, and pain

Assess respiratory status q2h

    Assist and teach patient to deep breathe q1h

    For cervical surgery

        Check respirations q½h for rate, rhythm, quality, and distress signs

        Maintain bed rest with head of bed elevated 30 to 45 degrees

        Observe for diminished cough reflex

        Assess face and neck for edema qh

Maintain comfort with analgesics to improve respiration

Auscultate chest for breath sounds q2h

Monitor vital signs q2h for 8 hr, then q4h

Provide incentive spirometer q1h to 2h

Expected outcome/evaluation

Patient's

    Breath sounds are normal

Respiratory rate and rhythm are regular
Face and neck edema is absent

■ NDX: Potential fluid volume deficit related to NPO status and/or abnormal fluid loss

Maintain NPO
Administer parenteral fluids with electrolytes as ordered
Connect nasogastric tube and low intermittent suction apparatus, if applicable; irrigate with measured amounts of normal saline to maintain patency
Connect indwelling urethral catheter and closed gravity drainage system
 Monitor output qh; if output is less than 20 to 30 ml/hr, notify physician
 Measure intake and output q8h
Monitor dressing(s) for drainage q2h for 24 hr, than q4h
 Patient may be in supine position for extended period; assessment must be made by feeling dressing
 Check Hemovac drainage and graft incision qlh to 2h
 Change dressing prn with initial change by physician
Monitor Hgb, Hct, and electrolytes
Administer naso-oral hygiene q2h; keep areas moist
Monitor vital signs q4h
Auscultate abdomen for bowel sounds q8h; report return to physician; observe for distention
 Provide diet as tolerated when bowel sounds return or nasogastric tube is clamped or removed
 Initiate clear liquids and increase to soft or regular diet
 Measure intake and output until adequate for patient
Remove indwelling urethral catheter as ordered
 Obtain specimen for culture
 Institute voiding measures as needed
Administer stool softeners as ordered

Expected outcome/evaluation

Patient's
 Vital signs are stable
 Intake and output are balanced
 Skin turgor is normal

■ NDX: Potential for infection; related to invasive procedure and reduced primary defenses

Monitor vital signs q4h
Monitor Hgb, Hct, WBC
Monitor dressing(s) for drainage q2h for 24 hr, then q4h
Change dressings prn; physician may wish to do initial dressing
Report excess drainage, bleeding to physician
Culture suspicious drainage

Expected outcome/evaluation

Patient's
 Incision remains clean, dry, and intact

Temperature is normal
Laboratory values are within normal limits

■ NDX: Impaired physical mobility related to musculoskeletal impairment and pain

Maintain bed rest, usually in supine or prone position
Maintain immobilization of spine
 Placement of immobilization devices
Maintain body alignment throughout all procedures
 No knee flexion
 For cervical surgery, sandbags on both sides of head may be ordered if no immobilization device is present
 Do not flex head forward
 Elevate head of bed 40 to 60 degrees
Assess motor activity, sensation, color, pulse, and temperature of lower extremities q2h
 Report changes to physician
 For cervical surgery; assess upper extremities for color, pulse, and temperature q2h; report changes to physician
Turn patient only as prescribed
 Administer pain medication 30 min before turning when possible
 Use logrolling method
 Turn q2h from back to side to side
 While turning
  Support patient's legs with pillow between knees
  Support head with small pillow
  Roll in one continuous motion
  Support back with pillows
 Administer skin care with each turn; assess pressure points
Remove immobilization device as ordered and check for altered skin integrity
Balance rest periods with activity
Increase activity as prescribed
 Initiate quadriceps setting and gluteal contractions
 Assist with and teach active or perform passive ROM exercises q4h as indicated according to surgical procedure
 Avoid sudden movements or twisting of extremities or neck
 Involve physical therapist if available
Ambulate with assistance when tolerated
 Maintain patient in immobilization device or apply immobilization device as indicated; Harrington rod patients will have body cast or two-piece plastic shell (turtle shells)
 Assist with and reinforce teaching of method for sitting up and getting out of bed
 Have patient wear supportive shoes
 Apply antiembolic hose; remove daily, inspect skin for rash, broken areas
 Assist patient in walking

Observe for vertigo, nausea, and hypotension
Observe gait
Avoid shuffling feet
Place patient in straight-back chair with feet on floor
Increase ambulation to tolerance; have patient avoid standing, sudden movements, and twisting
Encourage self-care as tolerated; assist with and teach modified ADLs as needed

Expected outcome/evaluation

Patient
Regains mobility to optimal level
Demonstrates ability to use mobilizing devices
Maintains proper body alignment
Participates in rehabilitation plan

■ **NDX:** Pain related to surgical intervention

Assess location, type, and intensity of pain; use pain rating scale and medicate as needed for continuous comfort
Administer analgesics; avoid morphine for cervical surgery patients; monitor for effectiveness/side effects
Assist patient with changing position frequently, maintaining correct body alignment to promote comfort
Provide and teach use of TENS unit if applicable
Discuss and teach alternate pain relief measures
Instruct patient in use of PCA
Encourage diversional activities

Expected outcome/evaluation

Patient
Reports that pain is at tolerable level
Appears relaxed and comfortable
Cooperates and attempts use of alternate pain management techniques

■ **NDX:** Knowledge deficit related to lack of information about home care management

Stress importance of prescribed activity, exercises, and restrictions
Degree of activity and self-care allowed; ways to avoid overdependence
Need to maintain good body alignment
No heavy lifting or strenuous exercise, automobile driving or riding, stooping, or bending
Methods of knee bending
Need to avoid fatigue; to exercise to tolerance with frequent rest periods
ROM exercises as allowed
Straight-backed chair for sitting
Convalescent period (may be an extended length of time: 2 to 9 months)
Need to wear immobilization device as ordered; method of application, care, and removal of device; observ-

ance of device for areas that may cause skin irritation or breakdown
Firm mattress with bedboard (essential)
Provide and review instructions on diet and fluid intake; explain ways to avoid weight gain and constipation
Discuss and demonstrate incisional care
Signs and symptoms of wound infection
Need to shower daily with mild soap and to observe skin for signs of irritation; apply lotion as needed
For tibial graft incision site: need to wear elastic bandage for edema and rewrap qid
Discuss signs and symptoms to report to physician
Decreased motor activity and/or sensation in extremities
Increased pain in surgical area
Elevated temperature
Discuss medications: name, schedule, purpose, dosage, and side effects
Promote follow-up visits with physician

Expected outcome/evaluation

Patient
Verbalizes understanding of rehabilitation program, symptoms to report to physician, and medication schedule
Demonstrates ability to perform ADLs and care for incision
Verbalizes understanding of use of immobilization device

FRACTURE OR DISLOCATION OF CERVICAL SPINE

A condition of the cervical spine in which one or more vertebrae are fractured or dislocated; either condition may cause pressure on the spinal cord, resulting in neurovascular dysfunction

Assessment
Observations/findings

Neck pain, headache
Signs of spinal cord compression
Loss of mobility and sensation below compression
Urinary retention
Paroxysmal hypertension
Bradycardia
Dyspnea

Laboratory/diagnostic studies

Radiological examination of cervical spine
Baseline CBC, urinalysis, electrolytes

Potential complications

Respiratory distress
Abdominal distention, paralytic ileus
Decreased bowel and urine function
Complete paralysis of all extremities and trunk

Medical Management

Immobilization devices: Halo traction, Crutchfield tongs, skeletal traction

Analgesics, muscle relaxants, stool softeners

Parenteral fluids with electrolytes

Diet, activity, rest

Nursing diagnoses/interventions/evaluation

■ **NDX:** Impaired physical mobility related to musculoskeletal impairment and bed rest

Maintain bed rest in correct body alignment; have patient avoid lifting or twisting head; use sandbags until immobilization device is applied

Maintain and monitor immobilization device, Halo traction, cervical head halter, skeletal traction, Stryker frame, or Circolectric bed; maintain cervical spine in extension

Assess neurovascular status q2h; monitor pulses, color, temperature, sensation, and mobility of all extremities

Perform passive or assist with and teach active ROM exercises for all extremities q2h

Promote isometric exercises q2h to 4h

Apply antiembolic hose; remove daily and monitor skin integrity

Encourage lower leg movement to promote venous return

As fracture heals, traction is replaced with casts (Halo, Minerva) or neck brace; it is worn continuously; monitor for comfort and correct fit

Ambulate with assistance; monitor for vertigo and weakness; progress slowly

Expected outcome/evaluation

Patient

Participates in rehabilitation plan and activity schedule

Regains mobility to optimal level

Performs ROM and isometric exercises accurately

■ **NDX:** Potential for impaired skin integrity related to pressure resulting from physical immobilization

Provide alternating pressure, gel, foam, air mattress to maintain skin integrity

Administer skin care q2h without turning if necessary

Change positions in small ways q1h to 2h to decrease amount of pressure

Apply lotions and provide massage and back rubs; do not massage reddened areas

Maintain wrinkle-free bottom sheets

Monitor bilateral skull dessings and tong placement of skeletal traction; observe amount of drainage and cleanse areas q4h with half-strength hydrogen peroxide or normal saline; allow to dry and apply antibiotic ointment; redress

Monitor weights for correct amount and placement; *never release traction, and keep weights off floor*

Expected outcome/evaluation

Patient

Maintains skin integrity around insertion sites

Moves about in bed frequently and maintains body alignment

Verbalizes understanding of needed immobilizing device

■ **NDX:** Potential for self-care deficit: feeding, bathing, toileting related to restricted positioning and trauma

Assess level of dependency

Plan care to meet needs as identified; e.g.: provide total care only for those areas of self-care in which patient cannot participate

FEEDING

Maintain parenteral fluids with electrolytes until oral intake is adequate for patient

Collaborate with physician and provide well-balanced diet when tolerated

Initiate clear-to-full liquids and progress to soft or regular diet

Provide foods easily chewed and swallowed

Assist with feeding or feed as needed

Observe for signs of dysphagia

Encourage patient to make food selections

Serve food attractively arranged

Provide oral hygiene before and after meals

BATHING

Discuss and plan daily care and routines with patient

Encourage self-care; instruct to avoid overexertion or fatigue

Provide needed equipment for patient comfort and ADLs

Assist as needed or perform total care if patient is dependent

Promote increasing self-care as tolerated by patient

TOILETING

Measure intake and output; monitor for urine retention

Offer bedpan regularly or keep close at hand

Encourage fluid intake of 2500 ml/day if not contraindicated

Provide privacy and perform perineal care as needed

Monitor bowel sounds; observe for decreased sounds, distention (paralytic ileus)

Avoid constipation with stool softeners, natural laxatives, high-fiber diet

Expected outcome/evaluation

Patient

Regains independence as activity and mobility increase

Participates in self-care to optimal level

Maintains weight normal for age, height

■ **NDX:** Pain related to fracture, trauma, edema

Assess location, type, and intensity of pain; use pain rating scale

Administer analgesics and muscle relaxants; avoid morphine; assess effectiveness of pain relief measures

Administer back rubs and massages to promote comfort

Encourage patient to change position slightly at frequent intervals; reinforce correct body alignment

Provide diversional activities

Discuss and teach alternate pain relief measures

Expected outcome/evaluation

Patient

Reports reduced level of discomfort

Seems relaxed; rest and sleep are adequate

Participates in diversional activities

Additional nursing diagnoses to consider

Ineffective breathing pattern related to location of fracture and frank spinal cord injury (see Spinal Cord Injury, p. 426)

Self-care deficit related to frank injury

■ **NDX:** Knowledge deficit related to lack of information about home care management

Stress importance of prescribed activity and immobilization device

Avoiding fatigue with planned rest periods

Signs and care of pressure points from device

Length of time device is to be worn

Demonstrate application and care of immobilization device

Explain importance of well-balanced diet; avoid weight gain

Avoid constipation with use of stool softeners; discuss importance of activity, exercise, and fluids

Discuss maintaining a safe environment to prevent accidents and falls

Encourage diversional activities

Promote follow-up visits with physician

Expected outcome/evaluation

Patient

Demonstrates understanding of activity program and use of immobilization device

Seeks assistance appropriately

Demonstrates ability to apply and care for immobilization device

ANKYLOSING SPONDYLITIS

A progressive inflammatory disease of the vertebral column and surrounding tissues that begins in the low back and eventually causes ankylosing and deformity of the entire spinal column; etiology is unknown

Assessment

Observations/findings

Vertebral pain and stiffness on arising; may radiate to buttocks

Limited mobility

Fatigue, malaise, chest discomfort

Anorexia, weight loss

Conjunctivitis, urethritis, polyarthritis

Kyphosis

Laboratory/diagnostic studies

Radiological examination of spine

Histocompatability antigen HLA B27 (positive)

ESR (elevated)

Potential complications

Neurological damage

Respiratory dysfunction, depending on stage of progression

Thrombophlebitis

Fractured vertebrae

Polyarthritis

Medical Management

Analgesics, antipyretics, nonsteroid antiinflammatory agents, stool softeners

Exercise program, physical therapy

Bedboard, firm mattress, small pillow

Back brace, corset

Surgical intervention: cervical spinal fusion, osteotomy

Nursing diagnoses/interventions/evaluation

■ **NDX:** Impaired physical mobility related to musculoskeletal impairment and pain

Assess present mobility and observe for increased impairment

Assist with and reinforce prescribed exercise program

ROM exercises, ambulation, self-care, and ADLs as tolerated

Discuss importance of making rest periods infrequent since they are not beneficial

Provide diversional activities

Prepare bed with bedboard, firm mattress, and small pillow; administer frequent back rubs and massages

Monitor vital signs q4h

Assess neurovascular status; monitor peripheral pulses and check extremities for color, warmth, sensation, edema, and weakness q4h

Assist with and teach deep breathing exercises to promote respiratory and peripheral-vascular function

Monitor skin and mucous membranes for irritation, rashes, or breaks

Administer antiinflammatory agents; observe for side effects; gastric discomfort, diarrhea, constipation

Maintain elimination patterns

Encourage fluid intake of 2500 ml/day if not contraindicated

Promote ambulation; assist as needed

Expected outcome/evaluation

Patient

Participates in exercise program

Seeks assistance as needed

Maintains coordination and mobility at optimal level

■ **NDX:** Pain related to inflammation/edema

Assess location, intensity, and type of pain; observe for
progression of pain to new areas

Administer analgesics; assess effectiveness of pain relief
measures

Maintain back brace or corset

Encourage frequent small position changes to increase
comfort

Promote diversional activities

Teach and assist with alternate pain management techniques

Expected outcome/evaluation

Patient

Reports a reduction in discomfort

Presents a more relaxed behavior

Demonstrates learned pain-reducing skills with increasing success

■ **NDX:** Body image disturbance related to altered body
structure/function disturbance

Allow time for and encourage verbalization of feelings and
concerns

Reinforce physician's explanation of disease process, treatment, and expected outcome; clarify misconceptions

Provide a supportive environment and assist patient with
identifying positive coping styles

Provide realistic hope and set short-term goals to be attained; praise patient for each task accomplished or
attempted

Encourage communication with significant other and socialization with family and friends

Encourage self-care as tolerated

Promote adherence to treatment plan to postpone further
development of deformities

Expected outcome/evaluation

Patient

Verbalizes feelings/concerns and uses adaptive coping
skills in dealing with altered image

Participates in treatment regimen and seeks assistance
appropriately

Performs ADLs at optimal level

Additional Nursing Diagnosis to Consider

Self-care deficit related to increasing musculoskeletal impairment

■ **NDX:** Knowledge deficit related to lack of information
about home care management

Stress importance and benefits of maintaining prescribed
exercise program; including swimming and other non–
weight-bearing exercises as tolerated

Discuss medications: name, schedule, purpose, dosage,
and side effects

Promote physical therapy activities; ROM, deep breathing; avoid excessive rest

Demonstrate application and care of brace or corset

Encourage nutritious diet and adequate fluid intake

Stress importance of safe environment to prevent fractures

Discuss signs and symptoms of disease progression: increased pain and immobility

Promote follow-up visits with physician

Refer to social worker if job change required; arrange help
at home if necessary

Expected outcome/evaluation

Patient

Verbalizes understanding of disease process, treatment
plan, and symptoms of disease progression

Demonstrates application and care of brace or corset

Expresses understanding of medication schedule

HIP SURGERY

internal fixation *Surgical repair of hip fractures using
an internal fixation device, such as a nail, pin, screw,
or plate, or a combination thereof*

cup arthroplasty *Surgical repair of a diseased acetabu-
lum; the head of the femur is covered with a metal cup
or mold and is placed into the reconstructed acetabu-
lum; the cup prevents the two surfaces from fusing and
reestablishes joint function*

Preoperative Assessment and Care

Assess respiratory, neurovascular, nutritional, and integumentary status

Assess hearing, visual status, and presence of other diseases

Monitor traction (Buck's or Russell)

Discuss with and teach patient

Method of coughing and deep beathing or use of incentive spirometer

ROM exercises to unaffected extremities

Postoperative position to be maintained

Gluteal and abdominal contractions and quadriceps setting

Dorsiflexion and plantar flexion of foot

Importance of leg abduction postoperatively; avoidance of adduction

Use of trapeze, abduction brace, and pillow

Method of bladder and bowel elimination

Method of pain management

Teach and discuss use of patient controlled anesthesia (PCA) (p. 59)

Discuss and assist patient in dealing with fears and anxieties

Reinforce physician's explanation of surgical procedure and follow-up care

Encourage communication with significant other

Elderly patients may need instructions repeated with each task or procedure

Provide praise or encouragement for tasks attempted and completed

Postoperative Assessment
Observations/findings

Correct placement of affected leg

Location and character of pain

Neurovascular status of affected extremity

Urinary output, vital signs

Color and amount of wound drainage

Mental alertness

Respiratory status

Laboratory/diagnostic studies

CBC, electrolytes, blood gases

Radiological examination of hip

Potential complications

Hemorrhage

Shock

Urinary retention, infection

Confusion, if elderly

Decubitus ulcers

Atelectasis

Thrombophlebitis

Wound infection

Pin or prosthesis slippage
    Extreme internal or external rotation
    Severe pain
    Localized edema of hip

Malunion of fracture
    Severe pain
    Elevated temperature
    Severe muscle spasms

Fat embolus
    Difficulty in breathing
    Cough   .
    Chest petechiae
    Tachycardia

Medical Management

Position to be maintained

Analgesics, muscle relaxants, antibiotics

Parenteral therapy with electrolytes, urinary catheter

Oxygen therapy, incentive spirometer

Diet, activity, rest

Nursing diagnoses/interventions/evaluation

■ **NDX:**   Impaired physical mobility related to surgical incision and temporary inability to bear weight

Maintain bed rest in prescribed position with firm mattress and trapeze

Monitor vital signs and urine output q4h

Perform neurovascular assessment q2h to 4h

Assist and teach patient to cough and deep breathe qh
    Auscultate chest for breath sounds q8h
    Provide incentive spirometer
    Observe for dyspnea and chest pain

Turn patient on unaffected side q2h; maintain body alignment with pillow between knees and at back; turn on affected side if ordered

Ambulate with assistance (cup arthroplasty patients are bedfast longer); assist patient with dangling at bedside, then with standing and pivoting on unaffected leg into chair (no weight bearing); involve physical therapy department if available

Assist with and teach ROM exercises to unaffected extremities q4h, and with ROM exercises to knee, foot, and ankle of affected leg; passive continuous ROM machine may be ordered (p. 389)

Encourage and teach use of walker and increase ambulation and weight bearing as tolerated

Assist with ADLs as needed

Promote self-care as soon as patient able

Monitor intake/output

Monitor elimination patterns

Balance rest periods with activity

Expected outcome/evaluation

Patient
    Regains mobility and weight bearing to optimal level
    Participates in rehabilitation plan
    Progressively participates in own care

■ **NDX:**   Potential for infection related to invasive procedure and lowered primary defenses

Assess incision for Hemovac placement; observe for increased drainage

Monitor incision for drainage q2h to 4h

Change dressings as needed; report bleeding, increased drainage to physician

Observe for signs of infection; culture suspicious drainage

Monitor vital signs q4h

Provide well-balanced diet to promote healing

Expected outcome/evaluation

Patient's
  Vital signs are normal
  Incision is healing
  Surrounding tissue is clean, dry, and intact

■ **NDX:**   Pain related to surgical procedure and impaired mobility

Assess location, intensity, and character of pain
Assess neurovascular status; especially for calf pain (thrombophlebitis)
Administer analgesics; assess effectiveness of pain relief measures
Be alert for severe increase in pain caused by prosthetic slippage or malunion of fracture; report immediately
Provide frequent skin care and back rubs; change position slightly to prevent skin breakdown
Monitor dosage of analgesics for the elderly patient since confusion and disorientation may result with normal dosage
Encourage and increase self-care activities as tolerated
Provide diversional activities
Teach and assist with alternate pain relief measures

Expected outcome/evaluation

Patient
  Reports a reduction in pain level
  Appears more relaxed and calm
  Participates in self-care with less discomfort

Additional nursing diagnoses to consider

Altered tissue perfusion: cardiopulmonary, cerebral related to fat embolus
Impaired skin integrity related to mechanical factors and/or physical immobilization

■ **NDX:**   Knowledge deficit related to lack of information about home care management

Stress importance of following prescribed rehabilitation plan: amount of weight bearing, activities allowed, and correct body alignment
Discuss need for nutritious diet and fluids to facilitate bone union and to maintain circulation and elimination
Prevent constipation with natural laxative/stool softeners
Discuss signs and symptoms to report to physician: increased incision or leg pain, fever, decreased urinary output, signs of wound infection
Demonstrate incision care
Promote increasing self-care and ADLs as tolerated
Encourage follow-up visits with physician and physical therapist

Expected outcome/evaluation

Patient
  Demonstrates understanding of rehabilitation and exercise plan
  Demonstrates incision care accurately
  Verbalizes understanding of symptoms to report to physician and importance of follow-up care
  Shows ability to perform ADLs independently to optimal level

TOTAL JOINT ARTHROPLASTY: HIP, KNEE, ANKLE, SHOULDER, ELBOW, WRIST, FINGER

Replacement of a total joint with a prosthesis to provide stability and motion; performed on diseased or traumatized joints

Preoperative Assessment and Care

Assess respiratory, neurovascular, nutritional, and integumentary status
Assess hearing and visual status and presence of other diseases (diabetes, arthritis)
Discuss with and teach patient
  Method of coughing and deep breathing
  ROM exercises to unaffected extremities
  Postoperative restrictions or limitations; these may differ according to physician preference
  Total hip arthroplasty (Figure 7-2, A)
    Gluteal and abdominal contractions and quadriceps setting
    Dorsiflexion and plantar flexion of foot
    Hip hiking, isometric exercises
    Use of trapeze and continuous passive motion device
    Importance of leg abduction or adduction postoperatively, depending on surgical approach
  Total knee arthroplasty (Figure 7-2, B)
    Quadriceps setting, gluteal contractions, and flexion-extension exercises
    Straight leg lifts
    Use of continuous epidural analgesia
  Total shoulder arthroplasty
    Presence of sling to support affected arm; no side elevation of arm
    Prescribed exercises of fingers, wrist, and elbow
  Total elbow arthroplasty
    Presence of abduction humerus splint to prevent rotation
    Elbow will be immobilized at 90 degrees of flexion
    Prescribed wrist and finger exercises
  Total wrist arthroplasty (Figure 7-2, C)
    Presence of volnar splint to prevent wrist flexion
    Prescribed finger and arm exercises
  Total thumb replacement
    Presence of immobilizing splint or brace to provide

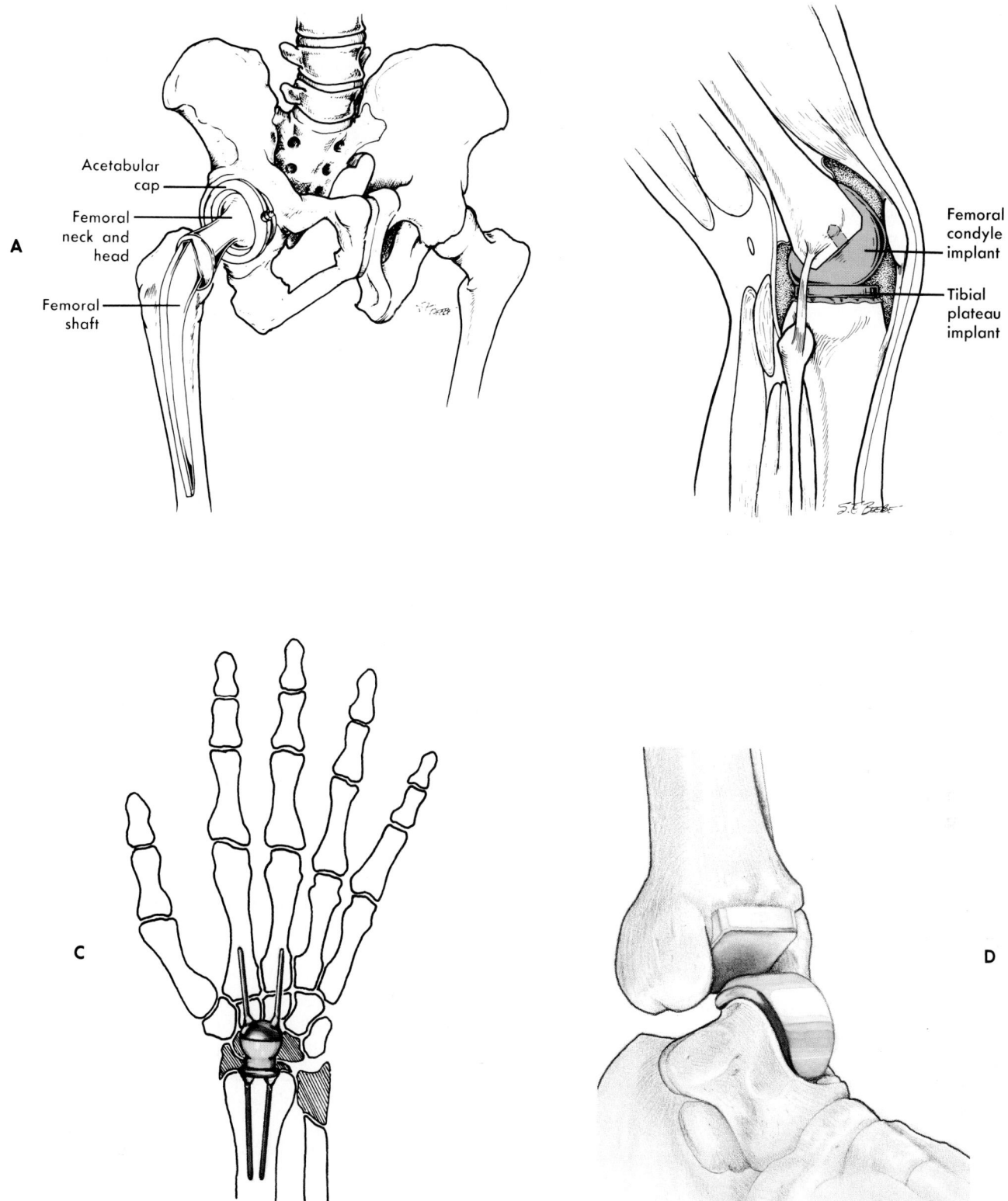

FIGURE 7-2. A, Oblique view of total hip arthroplasty. **B,** Total knee arthroplasty. **C,** Total wrist arthroplasty. **D,** Total ankle arthroplasty.

wrist and thumb support but allowing for movement of fingers

Prescribed finger and arm exercises

Total finger arthroplasty

    Presence of immobilizing splint or brace that provides involved finger support but allows movement of other fingers

    Prescribed exercises for arm and unaffected fingers

Total ankle arthroplasty (Figure 7-2, D)

    Presence of posterior plaster cast and Hemovac suction apparatus

    Method of crutch walking

    Prescribed exercises for toes and knee

Involvement of physical therapy department in planning rehabilitation goals

Methods of bladder and bowel elimination

Methods of pain management; patient controlled analgesia (PCA) (p. 59)/continuous epidural analgesia (p. 59)

Administer antibiotics and anticoagulants

Measure for antiembolic stockings

Discuss sequential compression devices

Administer surgical scrub bid

Discuss and assist patient in dealing with fears and anxieties

    Reinforce physician's explanation of surgical procedure and follow-up care

    Encourage communication with significant other

    Repeat instructions as needed with each procedure or task for elderly patients

    Provide praise and encouragement for tasks attempted and/or completed

Postoperative Assessment
Observations/findings

Neurovascular status of involved extremity

    Peripheral pulse, pallor, cyanosis, edema

    Sensation, temperature, mobility

Site of incision

    Wound drains

        Hemovac

        Excessive bleeding or drainage

Location and character of pain

Respiratory status

Position of affected joint and extremity

Mental alertness

Laboratory/diagnostic studies

Electrolytes, CBC, prothrombin time (PT)

Joint radiological study

Potential complications

Disorientation (elderly patient)

Tachycardia

Tachypnea

Chest pain

Atelectasis

Pneumonia

Thrombophlebitis

Pulmonary embolus

Hemorrhage

Shock

Fat embolus

Wound infection

Compartment syndrome (knee, elbow)

Medical Management

Postoperative position of involved extremity

Parenteral fluids with electrolytes initially; then diet as tolerated

Incision and draining apparatus care

Cast splint, brace, sling: device depends on joint replaced

Analgesics, antibiotics, sedatives, antipyretics, anticoagulants, stool softeners, laxatives, antiinflammatory agents

PCA device, TENS unit

Oxygen therapy, incentive spirometer

Antiembolic stockings, sequential compression device

Diet, rest

Physical therapy: exercise depends on joint replaced

Nursing diagnoses/interventions/evaluation

■ **NDX:** Impaired physical mobility related to surgical procedure of joint involved and pain

Maintain bed rest with affected joint in prescribed position

    Provide firm mattress, trapeze, and overhead frame

    Maintain support of joint through use of splint, brace, sling, or cast

Perform passive or assist with and teach active ROM exercises to unaffected joints

Reinforce restrictions and limitations on affected joint to prevent dislocation

Maintain elimination patterns with increased fluid intake, high-fiber diet

Assist with ADLs as needed

Turn patient as ordered; support joint to maintain immobilization and body alignment

Monitor skin for reddened areas; massage bony prominences prn

Maintain wrinkle-free linens

Promote quadriceps, gluteal muscle sets and isometric exercises as indicated

Ambulate patient with assistance (duration of bed rest depends on joint replaced)

    Provide ambulatory aids as needed

    Observe weight-bearing restrictions

    Monitor for vertigo, weakness, and nausea

Continuous passive ROM machine may be ordered for affected extremity of hip and knee arthroplasty patients

Expected outcome/evaluation

Patient
    Maintains proper body alignment in bed and while ambulating
    Increases weight bearing as prescribed
    Expresses understanding of and participates in rehabilitation regimen
    Progressing toward self-care

■ **NDX:**   Potential alteration in tissue perfusion: peripheral related to risk of reduced blood flow, tissue edema

Monitor vital signs q2h to 4h and prn
Assess neurovascular status of affected extremity q1h for 12 hr, then q4h; observe color, temperature, pulse, sensation, and mobility; observe for signs of thrombophlebitis (p. 70) and compartment syndrome (p. 382)
Monitor antiembolic stocking or sequential compression device
Encourage foot flexion q2h to 4h to promote venous return if applicable
Apply ice bags to affected joint
Monitor CBC, electrolytes, and PT
Maintain parenteral fluids; monitor intake and output; observe for urinary retention
Administer anticoagulants; assess effectiveness and for side effects

Expected outcome/evaluation

Patient's
    Vital signs are stable
    Laboratory values are within normal limits
    Extremities are warm, pink and pulses are palpable

■ **NDX:**   Potential for infection (wound, pneumonia) related to surgical intervention and immobility

Monitor incision and dressings for drainage and presence of drain or Hemovac
    Attach drain or Hemovac to prescribed apparatus; monitor output for color and amount q4h
    Reinforce and change dressings prn; observe for signs of healing process or wound infection
    Administer wound irrigation with antibiotics as indicated
Assess respiratory status q4h; observe for pain, dyspnea, and tachypnea
Auscultate chest for breath sounds q4h; observe for diminished breath sounds
Initiate use of incentive spirometer q1h to 2h

Expected outcome/evaluation

Patient's
    Incision is clean, dry, intact

    Temperature is normal
    Respiratory rate/rhythm are regular
    Breath sounds are normal

■ **NDX:**   Pain related to surgical intervention and impaired mobility

Assess location, intensity, and character of pain
Administer analgesics, sedatives, and/or antiinflammatory agents; assess effectiveness of pain relief measures, monitor dosage for elderly patients, since prescribed dose may cause disorientation
Apply and monitor TENS unit (p. 60)
Monitor patient controlled or continuous epidural analgesic as indicated
Change position frequently to prevent fatigue and pressure on bony prominences; administer back rubs or massage as indicated
Provide diversional activities
Discuss and teach alternate pain relief techniques
Promote self-care activities as tolerated
Monitor for severe chest or affected joint pain; may indicate emboli or displacement of joint

Expected outcome/evaluation

Patient
    Displays more relaxed affect
    States pain is at tolerable level
    Participates in diversional activities

■ **NDX:**   Knowledge deficit related to lack of information about rehabilitation plan and home care management

Stress importance of and provide written instructions for prescribed rehabilitation program: daily exercises and/or ROM for affected joint, activity allowed, physical therapy involvement
Discuss and demonstrate incision care
Provide medication schedule, including name, purpose, dosage, and side effects; if patient is taking anticoagulants, explain need to have PT checked regularly, to observe for bleeding, to avoid aspirin use
Explain need to use soft toothbrush, electric razor while on anticoagulant
Discuss need to take prophylactic antibiotics before invasive procedure, including dental cleaning or procedure
Explain importance of high-protein, high-fiber diet and increased fluid intake to facilitate healing and prevent constipation
Discuss need for a safe environment
Discuss signs and symptoms of wound infection, dislodgment to report to physician: fever, inflammation, pain, immobility
Promote follow-up visits with physician

Expected outcome/evaluation

Patient

Verbalizes understanding of rehabilitation plan, medication, and laboratory schedule

Demonstrates incision care accurately

Expresses knowledge of precautions to follow and symptoms of potential complications

AMPUTATION OF LEG: ABOVE OR BELOW KNEE

Surgical removal of part of the leg because of trauma, disease, tumors, or congenital anomalies; a skin flap is generally constructed to facilitate healing and use of prosthetic equipment

Preoperative Assessment and Care

Monitor neurovascular status, both extremities

Observe affected extremity for open, draining sites

Obtain baseline vital signs

Administer skin preparation as ordered

Encourage and allow time for verbalization of fears and anxieties

Reinforce physician's explanation of operative procedure and phantom limb sensation

Begin to deal with body image change, loss, and grief; listen carefully and support positive coping behaviors; assist patient with expressing feelings to significant other

Explain process of and preparation for rehabilitation

Strengthen muscles of upper extremities for crutch walking

Push-ups from prone position

Alteration of flexing and extending arms holding weights

Sit-ups from seated position

Practice crutch walking

Practice quadriceps setting exercises, gluteal contraction exercises, and leg lift of affected extremity unless contraindicated

Practice use of overhead trapeze attached to frame

Explain types of prostheses available if appropriate

Immediate postsurgical fitting (IPSF) and immediate postoperative prosthesis (IPOP); used for immediate or early ambulation and weight bearing; cast is applied to stump and prosthesis is attached to cast

Delayed: dressing and elastic bandage are applied to stump; prosthesis is not made for 2 to 3 months

Postoperative Assessment
Observations/findings

Location, intensity, and type of pain

Type of dressing or rigid plaster cast

Position of stump

Stump dressing, amount and color of drainage, presence of drains, Hemovac

Respiratory status, vital signs

Laboratory/diagnostic studies

CBC, fasting blood sugar (FBS; for diabetics)

Potential complications

Hemorrhage, dehiscence

Wound infection

Phantom pain

Contractures

Abduction deformity

Medical Management

Position of stump postoperatively

Type of dressing and/or postsurgical fitting applied

Analgesics, antibiotics, antipyretics, sedatives

Exercises, physical therapy

Diet, activity, rest

Nursing diagnoses/interventions/evaluation

■ **NDX:** Impaired physical mobility related to pain and musculoskeletal impairment

Maintain bed rest in prescribed position

Elevate stump, usually for 24 hr; avoid pillow unless it is removed for 30 min q2h to prevent contractures; avoid outward rotation

Elevate head no more than 30 degrees

Turn from side to back to abdomen (after 24 hr) q2h

Assist with and teach active or perform passive ROM exercises q4h to unaffected extremities

Assist with and teach adduction and extension exercises to affected extremity q4h

Assist with ambulation

Without prosthesis

Avoid long periods of chair-sitting

Provide ambulation devices: crutches, walker

Encourage use of good walking shoes and maintain stump in normal position—relaxed and in downward position; involve physical therapy department

With prosthesis

Assist with measuring for prosthesis

Provide ambulation device: crutches, walker

Increase ambulation with prescribed amount of weight bearing; involve physical therapy department

Assist with and reiterate postoperative conditioning exercises: trunk flexion, sit-ups, hopping in place, hopping with walker

Expected outcome/evaluation

Patient

Expresses understanding of treatment and exercise plan

Cooperates/participates in needed activities
Maintains correct body alignment
Exhibits no contractures

■ **NDX:** Potential fluid volume deficit related to increased drainage or bleeding at surgical site

Administer parenteral fluids and anticoagulants as indicated
Monitor vital signs and LOC q2h and 4h
Monitor intake and output 8h
Monitor dressings and incision for color and amount of drainage and for presence of drains or Hemovac; observe for bleeding; outline bleeding area on dressing with pen and write date and time
Maintain tourniquet at bedside in case of hemorrhage
Monitor Hgb, Hct, PT, and electrolytes
Monitor postsurgical cast for bleeding and mark area as discussed previously; observe for cast slippage and report to physician

Expected outcome/evaluation

Patient's
  Vital signs are within normal limits
  Alert and oriented
  Wound is healing
  Skin is warm/dry

■ **NDX:** Potential for infection related to surgical procedure and lowered primary defenses

Change stump dressing and elastic bandage to produce shrinkage and prepare for prosthesis
  Wash and dry area, expose it to air before reapplying dressing
  Perform at least bid
  Observe for signs of infection and increasing edema
  Begin stump strengthening and conditioning; push against pillow and increase to firmer surface as tolerated
Change postsurgical cast dressing; wash and dry area; allow it to air dry bid
  Apply properly fitting stump sock prn
  Observe incision and surrounding area for increasing edema and signs of wound infection
  Massage stump toward suture line as ordered: usually 1 week postoperatively
  Reapply postsurgical cast
Maintain dry dressing; cover with plastic while using bed pan or if incontinent
Begin teaching dressing change procedure
Monitor temperature q4h
Provide high-protein diet and encourage fluids to upper limits for age and weight to promote healing
Administer antibiotics and/or antipyretics; monitor for effectiveness/side effects

Expected outcome/evaluation

Patient
  Participates in maintaining aseptic techniques
  Remains afebrile with adequate wound healing

■ **NDX:** Pain related to surgical intervention and immobility

Assess character, intensity, and location of pain; observe for compartment syndrome in below-the-knee amputation (p. 382)
Administer analgesics and sedative; assess effectiveness of pain relief measures
Assist patient with changing position slightly at frequent intervals to reduce fatigue and pressure; provide back rubs
Provide diversional activities
Teach and assist with alternate pain relief measures
Monitor use of TENS unit or patient controlled anesthesia (PCA)
Discuss and explain phantom pain and that it is normal and usually temporary
Coordinate care to provide rest periods

Expected outcome/evaluation

Patient
  States that pain is at a tolerable level
  Appears calm, relaxed; is able to sleep and rest adequately
  Understands phantom pain theory

■ **NDX:** Body image disturbance related to loss of body part

Encourage and allow time for patient to express feelings of loss and grief
Assist in identifying positive coping behaviors and provide encouragement and praise for strengths observed
Provide praise for attempted and/or completed tasks
Encourage patient to discuss and view stump
Encourage patient to perform self-care activities and involve patient in stump care as soon as tolerated; promote independence
Promote communication with significant other
Explain all procedures and treatments
Provide a supportive environment
Encourage socialization with another amputee

Expected outcome/evaluation

Patient
  Begins using positive coping skills in dealing with loss of body part
  Begins expressing feelings of acceptance of altered self
  Participates in self-care activities (ADLs) and stump care

■ **NDX:** Knowledge deficit related to lack of information about rehabilitation program and home care management

Stress importance of and review rehabilitation program; involve physical therapy department in daily exercises and stump strengthening and conditioning

Demonstrate dressing changes, incision care, skin care, and technique for massage of stump

Discuss and demonstrate care of IPSF/IPOP as indicated; consult physical therapy department or provide referral for permanent prosthesis

Promote safe home environment; instruct patient to wear rubber-soled shoe as indicated

Discuss signs and symptoms to report to physician: fever, inflammation of incision, prolonged phantom pain, increasing edema of stump

Discuss importance of well-balanced diet; avoiding weight gain

Refer to support group

Encourage follow-up visits with physician/physical therapist

Expected outcome/evaluation

Patient
  Demonstrates ability to care for incision/cast
  Verbalizes understanding of prescribed rehabilitation regimen
  Expresses knowledge of symptoms to report to physician and needed safety precautions

ARTHROSCOPIC SURGERY OF KNEE

Management of various knee disorders, using an arthroscope; small surgical instruments are introduced via a trocar and scope into the knee joint, and needed surgical procedures are performed; this technique allows for early rehabilitation and return to work, as well as decreased patient discomfort and confinement

Preoperative Assessment and Care

Determine presence of both pedal pulses
Discuss with and teach patient
  ROM exercises to unaffected extremities
  Restrictions and limitations postoperatively
    These will vary with physicians and according to extent of surgery
    Usually patient is out of bed on evening of surgery, but with no weight bearing
  Method of crutch walking
  Methods of pain management
Administer antiseptic scrub to affected knee
Reinforce physician's explanation of procedure
Explain that local anesthetic is usually used

Postoperative Assessment
Observations/findings

Position of knee and degree of elevation
Character and amount of drainage
Type of immobilization device (rarely used)
Neurovascular status of affected leg: pulse, color, temperature, sensation, mobility
Location and character of pain

Potential complications

Edema
Hemorrhage
Thrombophlebitis (p. 70)
Postoperative arthrosis
Compartment syndrome (p. 382)

Medical Management

Analgesics, antibiotics, sedatives
Position of knee postoperatively, exercises, ambulation
Ice bag to knee
Diet, activity, rest

Nursing diagnoses/interventions/evaluation

■ **NDX:** Potential for altered tissue perfusion: peripheral, related to arthroscopy and risk of altered arteriovenous flow

Elevate leg to promote venous return
Monitor neurovascular status of affected extremity q1hfor 4 hr, then q4h; check pulse, color, temperature, sensation, and mobility
Monitor vital signs q4h
Apply ice pack to knee to reduce swelling

Expected outcome/evaluation

Patient's
  Affected leg is warm, dry, mobile
  Vital signs are stable
  Pedal pulses are palpable

■ **NDX:** Impaired physical mobility related to discomfort and prescribed immobilization

Maintain bed rest in position of comfort with involved knee elevated in slight flexion
Encourage ROM exercises of unaffected extremities q2h
Ambulate with assistance, usually on evening of surgery
  Assist patient with getting out of bed, keeping affected leg elevated until standing; no weight bearing until ordered
  Assist patient with use of crutches
  Increase ambulation as tolerated
  Provide rest periods between ambulations
Initiate and assist with prescribed exercises; these depend on physician preference and extent of surgery
  Involve physical therapy department if applicable

Teach dorsiflexion and plantar flexion of foot and increasing flexion of knee

Expected outcome/evaluation

Patient
Demonstrates increasing mobility
Participates in exercise program
Ambulates correctly with crutches

■ **NDX:** Pain related to invasive procedure

Assess location, intensity, and type of pain; severe unrelenting pain and edema may indicate compartment syndrome
Administer analgesics and/or sedatives; assess effectiveness and for side effects
Provide diversional activities

Expected outcome/evaluation

Patient
Reports a reduced level of discomfort
Exhibits relaxed facial expressions
Sleeps for longer periods at night

■ **NDX:** Knowledge deficit related to lack of information about home care management and rehabilitation program

Stress importance and goals of pescribed rehabilitation program
Amount of weight bearing and knee flexion allowed
Elevation of leg while sitting
Avoiding twisting knee
Dorsiflexion and plantar flexion exercises of feet
Planned rest periods between exercises
Ambulation with crutches
Dates and times of physical therapy visits
Swimming should be encouraged
Discuss signs of wound infection to report to physician
Promote follow-up care with physician

Expected outcome/evaluation

Patient
Correctly repeats purpose and goals of prescribed rehabilitation plan
Reviews symptoms to report to physician

EXTERNAL FIXATION FOR COMPLICATED FRACTURES

A surgical procedure to immobilize and reduce complicated fractures; stabilizing pins or wires are inserted into and/or through the bone and attached to an external metal frame (Figure 7-3); may be applied to jaw, arm, leg, ribs, pelvis, fingers, or toes; another type of fixator is the Ilizarov external fixator (Figure 7-4)

Preoperative Assessment and Teaching

Preoperative teaching may be limited, depending on urgency of needed treatment
Assess neurovascular and respiratory status
Discuss with and teach patient
Methods of coughing and deep breathing and/or use of incentive spirometer
Necessary ROM exercises, quadriceps setting, and gluteal contractions according to location of fracture
Use of trapeze
Necessary movement limitations and activities allowed
Importance of external fixator
Reinforce physician's explanation of procedure

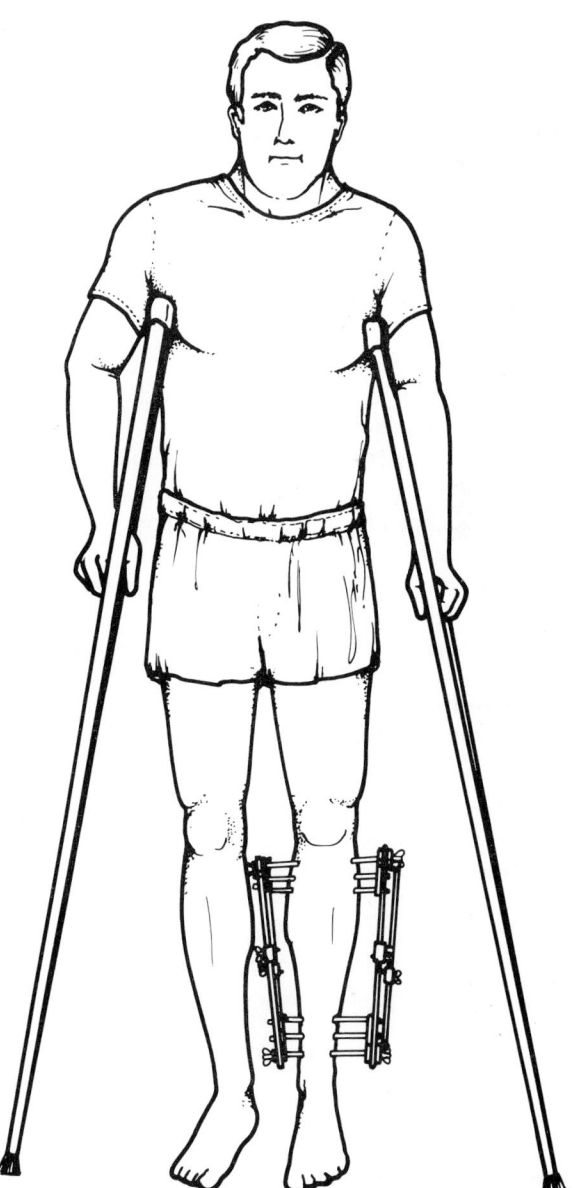

FIGURE 7-3. External fixation for complicated fractures.

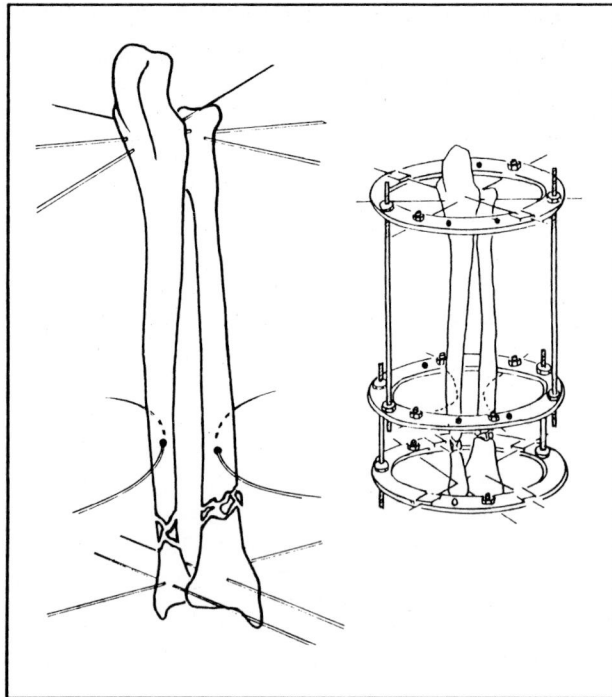

FIGURE 7-4. Treatment of fracture of the ulna with dislocation of the head of the radius using Ilizarov external fixator. (From Ilizarov external fixator general surgical technique brochure, Richards Medical Co, Memphis, Tenn, 1990.)

Fixator usually causes little pain or discomfort, and allows for early ambulation

Device is unsightly, but long-range results are primary goal

Explain that extremity will be elevated postoperatively to reduce edema

Involve physical theray department, if available, for crutch walking and exercises

Administer prescribed antibiotics and skin prep

Postoperative Assessment
Observations/findings

Elevation and position of extremity
Edema of extremity at operative site and below
Presence of supportive dressings
Character and amount of drainage from wound and pin sites
Neurovascular status of affected extremity; color, sensation, mobility, peripheral pulse, temperature
Location, intensity, and character of pain

Laboratory/diagnostic studies

CBC
Radiological examination of affected bone

Potential complications

Hemorrhage
Shock

ILIZAROV EXTERNAL FIXATOR

An external fixator, developed by Gauril Ilizarov, that allows control over a variety of bone disorders, including rotation, angulation, translation, lengthening, and shortening. It preserves limb function and blood supply and promotes healing. Also known as a compression-distraction apparatus, it can be assembled in more than 600 different ways and, therefore, is very versatile (Figure 7-4).
Indications:
  Open, closed fractures
  Nonunion, pseudoarthrosis of long bones
  Limb lengthening, shortening
  Correction of deformities, defects of bony or soft tissue
Postoperative care is essentially the same as for the external fixator on p. 377.

Wound or pin site infection
Nonunion, malunion
Neuromuscular dysfunction
Compartment syndrome

Medical Mangaement

Position of affected extremity
Analgesics, antibiotics, antipyretics, sedatives, antibacterial cream
Ice bag to area
Diet, activity, ambulation, rest

Nursing diagnoses/interventions/evaluation

■ **NDX:** Impaired physical mobility related to musculoskeletal impairment and pain

Maintain bed rest in position of comfort with extremity elevated
Assist with and teach active ROM exercises to unaffected extremities q2h to 4h; initiate quadriceps setting, gluteal contractions, or palmar or dorsal flexion as needed
Assist and teach patient to cough and deep breathe qh
Monitor neurovascular status of affected extremity q1h for 24 hr, then q4h
Monitor vital signs q4h
Ambulate when edema of soft tissues has decreased
  Holding fixator with both hands, assist patient to sitting position on bed side; observe for vertigo and nausea
  Always support fixator, not extremity
  Assist patient to ambulate with crutches or sling as indicated
Do not change or adjust fixator bars (can cause misalignment)
  No weight bearing until ordered

Physical therapy department should be involved where available

Elevate extremity while sitting up

Expected outcome/evaluation

Patient

Demonstrates mobility returning to optimal level

Cooperates with, participates in exercise program

Uses supporting devices correctly

■ **NDX:** Potential for infection related to pins and fixator insertion

Monitor pin sites, incision, and supportive dressing q1h to 2h for drainage and edema

Initiate pin site and incision care bid

Assess for pain, tenderness, redness, and tension around each pin site

Culture drainage suggestive of infection

Cleanse around each pin site with hydrogen peroxide; rinse with normal saline

Apply antibacterial agent around each pin

Allow to air dry

Cover each pin head with cork or rubber tip to prevent injury

Cleanse fixator with sterile water

Assist with and teach patient wound, pin site, and fixator care as soon as patient is physically and emotionally able

Change incision dressings bid prn; observe for wound healing

Apply ice bags to areas to reduce edema

Expected outcome/evaluation

Patient's

Tissue around pin sites remains clean and dry

Incision and surrounding area are healing

Demonstration of incision and pin care is adequate

■ **NDX:** Pain related to surgical intervention and immobility

Assess location, intensity, and character of pain; observe proximal joint for compartment syndrome signs; unrelenting pain, edema (p. 382)

Administer analgesics and sedatives; assess effectiveness of pain relief measures

Assist patient with changing position frequently while in bed to prevent fatigue and pressure

Provide diversional activities

Discuss and teach alternate pain management techniques

Expected outcome/evaluation

Patient

States pain is at a tolerable level

Appears more relaxed and calm

Reports ability to sleep and rest for increasing length of time

■ **NDX:** Body image disturbance related to external fixator

Provide supportive environment

Promote and allow time for expression of feelings; encourage communication with significant other

Assist in identifying positive coping patterns; acknowledge strengths

Promote self-care activities and praise tasks attempted or completed

Stress that fixator is temporary and promote its positive aspects

Reinforce purpose of fixator

Expected outcome/evaluation

Patient

Attempts to express concerns/feelings

Begins to use positive coping skills in dealing with altered self-image

Seeks assistance appropriately

■ **NDX:** Knowledge deficit related to lack of information about rehabilitation program, care of external device, and home management

Provide and review written goals, restrictions, and activities of rehabilitation program as outlined by physician

Demonstrate care of pins, fixator, and incision

Observe return demonstration

Stress importance of not tampering with fixator since it may alter alignment of fracture

Explain that showering is permitted but that patient needs to avoid swimming since chlorine and salt corrode metal

Stress importance of diet and elimination

Discuss signs and symptoms of wound infection to report to physician

Encourage follow-up visit with physician/physical therapy department

Expected outcome/evaluation

Patient

Verbalizes understanding of rehabilitation and exercise plan

Demonstrates ability to perform fixator, pin, incision care correctly

Verbalizes signs of potential complications

DIGITAL REPLANTATION

Surgical reconnection of severed digit(s) after trauma by a sharp object, crushing blow, or avulsion; general criteria for replantation include thumb replacement, multiple digit replacement, or replacement if patient is a child or if patient's occupation requires manual skills; surgery must be performed within 24 hr

Preoperative Assessment and Care

Preservation of digit(s)
  Wrap digit(s) in gauze soaked with normal saline
  Place in plastic bag
  Place bag in ice
  Never place digit directly on ice
  Care of amputated stump: apply sterile pressure dressing and elevate hand as ordered
Administer parenteral fluids with antibiotics as ordered
Administer anticoagulant and tetanus toxoid as ordered
Assess respiratory, cardiovascular, and neurological status
Determine presence or absence of further trauma or injury
Assess medication and medical history; diseases such as diabetes, chronic obstructive pulmonary disease (COPD), vascular disease, rheumatoid arthritis, osteoarthritis, and bleeding tendencies inhibit replantation success
Determine dominant hand
Assess emotional status where possible
  Be alert for maladaptive behavior since functional return depends on patient's motivation, emotional acceptance, and willingness to adapt to alterations in body image and lifestyle
    Reinforce physician's explanation of surgical procedure
    Discuss and deal with fears and anxieties
    Encourage communication with significant other
Discuss with and assist patient to understand that nicotine and caffeine are potent vasoconstrictors and therefore are prohibited

Postoperative Assessment
Observations/findings

Neurovascular status of digit
  Sensation, color, temperature
  Capillary refill, skin turgor
  Edema
Anatomic position of digit, wrist, and elbow, and elevation of each
Presence or absence of skin graft and graft site
Character and amount of drainage from incision
Location and character of pain

Laboratory/diagnostic studies

CBC, PT
Radiological examination of replantation

Potential complications

Hemorrhage
Shock
Vascular thrombosis or occlusion
Wound infection
Inappropriate or maladaptive behavior
Nonunion or malunion of digit(s)

Medical Management

Position and immobilization of wrist, hand, and digits
Analgesic, antibiotics, anticoagulants
Physical therapy department involvement
Leech therapy (see box)
Fluorometry
Diet, activity, rest

Nursing diagnoses/interventions/evaluation

■ **NDX:** Potential for altered tissue perfusion: peripheral, related to risk of interruption of arteriovenous flow

Maintain bed rest in position of comfort within confines of prescribed position of affected arm
Maintain warm environment to prevent vasoconstriction; avoid topical pressure on affected limb
Apply heat to promote vasodilation
Elevate affected arm on pillow above heart level
  Wrist and hand elevated 30 degrees
  Forearm in prone position
  Elbow flexion of no more than 10 to 15 degrees since further flexion may impair venous return
Maintain prescribed position of affected arm during repositioning
Assess neurovascular status of digit(s) qh
  Check sensation, temperature, color, pulse, skin turgor, and capillary refill
  Digit is pinker and capillary refill is faster immediately after surgery; accurate assessment and recording are imperative
  Report alterations in color to physician immediately
    Pink to white or mottled: arterial occlusion
    Pink to dusky purple: venous congestion
    Leech therapy is used for venous congestion
    Initiate fluorometry readings as indicated
    Both nurses should assess status at change of shift
Monitor vital signs q4h for 24 hr, then qid; monitor BP on unaffected arm
Check dressing qh for drainage; report excess bleeding to physician; change dressing as indicated
Monitor Hgb, Hct, and PT
Maintain parenteral fluids with antibiotics and anticoagulants; assess effectiveness and monitor for side effects of medications
Observe for occult bleeding; gums and injection sites if patient is on anticoagulants
Measure intake and output

Expected outcome/evaluation

Patient's
  Arteriovenous flow is maintained

LEECH THERAPY

After microsurgery for digital replantation, leeches are introduced to the digit where venous congestion is present to drain the engorgement and restore normal venous circulation.

PRETHERAPY ASSESSMENT OF DIGIT

Venous congestion
  Skin color: pink, dusky purple
  Capillary refill: brisk
  Skin turgor: swollen, distended
  Temperature: cool

PRETHERAPY PREPARATION

Cleanse area with warm water
Explain procedure
Warn patient not to touch leech after it is applied
Place gauze or towels around site to prevent leech from escaping
Physician will apply leech to skin

INTRATHERAPY ASSESSMENT/CARE

After application of leech, monitor continually until leech is fully distended (10 to 15 min)
Leech will usually drop off once this occurs
If leech does not drop off, gently stroke it with an alcohol sponge
Never grasp leech with forceps as regurgitation might occur, resulting in a wound infection

POSTTHERAPY ASSESSMENT/CARE

Once the leech has dropped off the digit, gently pick it up and place it in alcohol-filled container and send it for disposal
Cleanse site and apply dressing as site will continue to drain and ooze for 24 to 48 hours
Assess digit for improved color, turgor, temperature

Digit is warm and pink
Capillary refill, skin turgor, and sensation are within normal limits
Vital signs are normal
Laboratory values are within normal limits

■ **NDX:**   Potential for disuse syndrome related to surgical procedure with prescribed immobilization of hand

Teach active ROM exercises q4h to unaffected extremities while patient is in bed
Ambulate with assistance
  Maintain forearm and hand in sling
  Observe for vertigo and nausea
Involve patient and physical and occupational therapy

departments in establishing rehabilitation goals according to physician's order
Individualize goals according to
  Healing process and progress
  Patient's motivation to master manual skills
  Patient's willingness to use replanted digit
  Patient's acceptance of replanted digit into body image
Assist patient with and teach modified ADLs according to prescribed limitations dictated by surgery and if affected arm is dominant
Begin exercise program as planned
Encourage use of nondominant hand if appropriate
Allow time for completion of tasks
Provide a supportive environment
Promote diversional activities
Encourage visitation

Expected outcome/evaluation

Patient
  Undertakes using nondominant hand
  Participates in activities, ADLs, rehabilitation program
  Sets realistic goals for self and strives to complete tasks

■ **NDX:**   Pain related to trauma and surgical procedure

Assess location, intensity, and character of pain; use pain rating scale
Administer analgesic; assess effectiveness of pain relief measures
Assist patient with changing position frequently to prevent pressure and fatigue; maintain elbow flexion at prescribed amount
Discuss and teach alternate pain relief measures if applicable
Provide diversional activities

Expected outcome/evaluation

Patient
  Reports a tolerable level of pain
  Presents a calm, relaxed facial affect
  Sleeps/rests for longer periods

■ **NDX:**   Body image disturbance related to replanted digit

Assess degree of acceptance of replanted finger
Provide time for and assist patient in expressing feelings, encourage communication with significant other
Explain all procedures and treatments
Assess present and past coping behaviors and reinforce positive coping patterns that helped in the past
Stress positive aspects of replantation
Reinforce physician's explanation of expected outcome of surgical procedure; clarify misconceptions
Involve patient in self-care as soon as physically and emotionally able

Expected outcome/evaluation

Patient
  Begins to incorporate replanted digit into body image
  Verbalizes concerns/feelings and begins to understand
    expected outcome
  Participates appropriately in self-care

■ **NDX:** Knowledge deficit related to lack of information
            about home care management

Stress and review importance of prescribed rehabilitation
  program
  Degree of movement of digit allowed and duration and
    times of exercise
  Exercises for wrist, elbow, and arm
  Position of arm, elbow, and hand during rest and am-
    bulation
Stress that using and wanting to use the digit are the most
  important factors in function return
Paresthesia may last 4 to 6 months, whereas return of
  function may take a year
Replanted digit(s) may be shorter than opposing digits(s)
Demonstrate incision care and discuss signs of wound in-
  fection
Stress importance of well-balanced diet, fluid intake, rest,
  and daily exercise
Explain symptoms to report to physician
  Changes in color and temperature of digit
  Increased incision pain and/or edema
  Wound infection
Discuss importance of physical therapy and follow-up visits
  with physician

Expected outcome/evaluation

Patient
  Verbalizes understanding of prescribed rehabilitation
    program, performs beginning exercises
  States understanding of symptoms of potential compli-
    cations
  Demonstrates incision care correctly

COMPARTMENT SYNDROME

*Increased pressure in compartments of the forearm or
  lower leg after trauma; within compartments are muscles, blood vessels, and nerves, and any internal pressure (trauma, surgery, edema, bleeding) or external
  pressure (tight casts or dressings, IV infiltrations) can
  cause impaired circulation, nerve damage, and muscle
  weakness; if left unchecked, necrosis with loss of extremity and renal failure, acidosis, and shock (crush
  syndrome) can occur*

Assessment
Observations/findings

Pain in compartment area: increasing, unrelenting, and
  unrelieved by narcotics

Swelling and localized redness
Pain with passive motion of fingers or toes
Paresthesia of hand or foot
Absent pulse below compartment
Progressive loss of motor function

Laboratory/diagnostic studies

Deep vein thrombosis (DVT) studies
Ankle or brachial index
Vascular occlusion studies
CBC, PT

Potential complications

Neurovascular dysfunction of extremity
Muscle weakness
Necrosis, amputation
Renal failure, acidosis
Shock

Medical Management

Analgesics, antibiotics
Dressing and cast removal; cast window made
Neurovascular check q½h
Tissue pressure monitoring, fasciotomy

Nursing diagnoses/interventions/evaluation

■ **NDX:** Altered tissue perfusion: peripheral, related to
            interruption of arteriovenous flow, edema,
            trauma

Monitor and assess pain q½h if syndrome is suspected
Notify physician immediately if pain in extremity is
  Increasing
  Unrelenting
  Unrelieved by narcotics
  Occurring during passive motion of fingers or toes
  Be aware that this type of pain is primary indicator of
    compartment syndrome; other symptoms may take
    longer to appear
Remove dressing or have windows cut in cast immediately
  as ordered
Assess neurovascular status of foot or hand bilaterally
  q15min to 30min
Measure forearm or calf bilaterally for presence of or in-
  crease in edema q1h to 2h
If no improvement is noted, prepare for and assist with
  tissue pressure monitoring (p. 383), a means to measure
  fascial pressure (normal fascial pressure is about 0 to 30
  mm Hg, and when this pressure nears 30 mm Hg capillaries and arteries will close, causing occlusion)
Needle may be removed or left in place for continuous
  monitoring, depending on technique used
Prepare for fasciotomy as ordered (longitudinal incision
  into fascia surrounding compartment to release pressure)

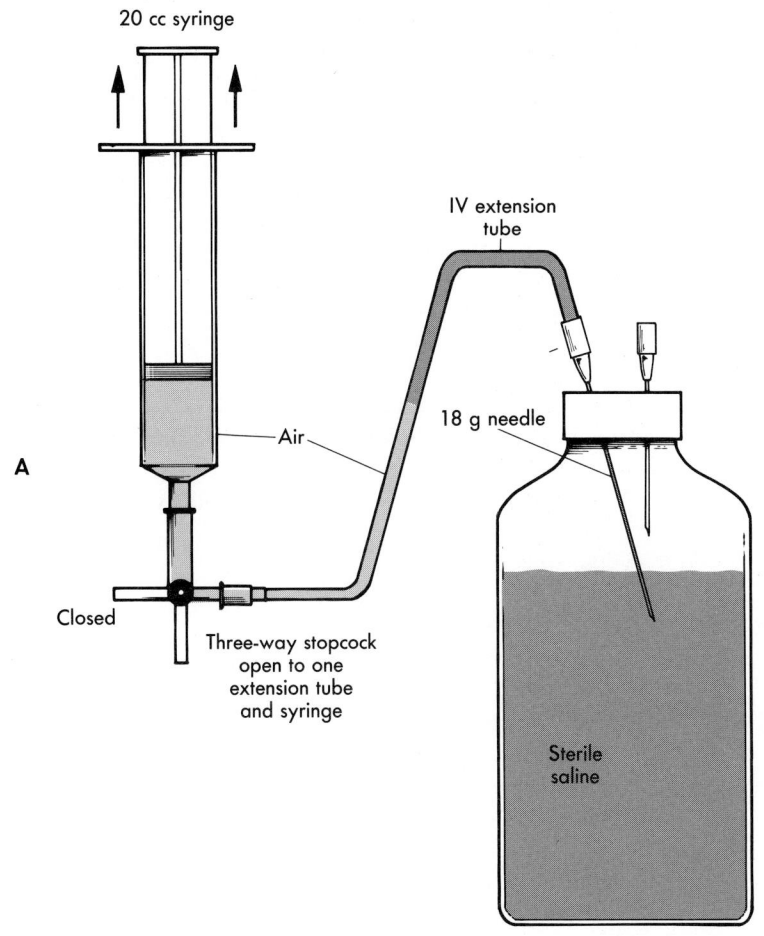

A

20 cc syringe

IV extension tube

Air

18 g needle

Closed

Three-way stopcock open to one extension tube and syringe

Sterile saline

FIGURE 7-5. Whiteside technique for measuring tissue pressure. **A,** Initial setup showing air and saline in extension tube. **B,** Connection of second extension tube from closed stopcock to manometer. When stopcock control is in down position, a closed system between manometer and fascia is established.

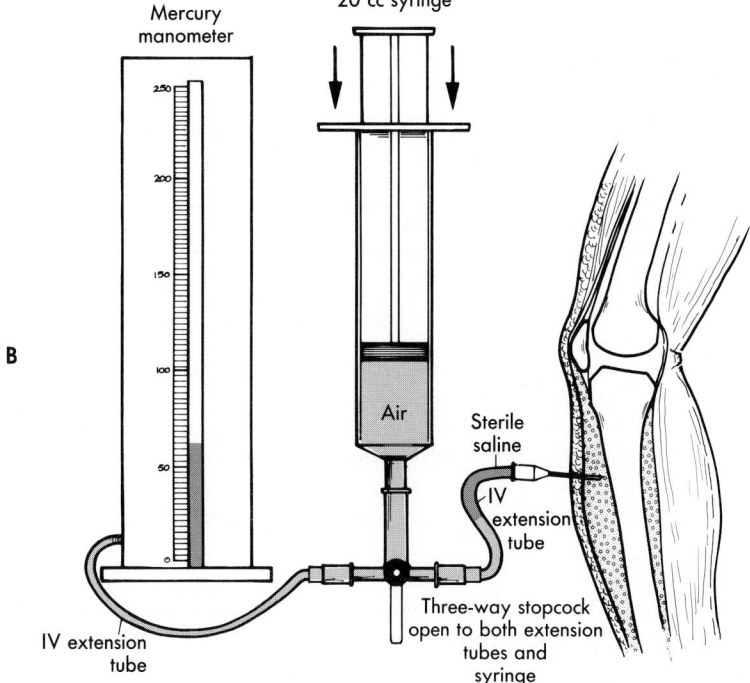

B

Mercury manometer

20 cc syringe

Air

Sterile saline

IV extension tube

IV extension tube

Three-way stopcock open to both extension tubes and syringe

Postoperatively, extremity will be immobilized in posterior cast or splint

Be aware that wound may be left open, with future grafting required, and that it may be a long, painful procedure

Change dressings as needed; observe for altered alignment of extremity

Continue neurovascular monitoring qh; observe for return of color, temperature, and capillary refill

Assess pain and monitor effectiveness after analgesic administration

Expected outcome/evaluation

Patient's

Compartment pressure is reduced as evidenced by palpable peripheral pulses, reduced muscle edema, minimal discomfort

Extremity is warm and dry, capillary refill is normal

Mobility is intact

■ **NDX:** Anxiety/fear related to lack of knowledge of the syndrome and situational crisis

Reinforce physician's explanation of syndrome, procedure, outcome, and rehabilitation plan

Allow time for verbalization of fears and explain all treatments as much as possible

After procedure assist patient in identifying coping strengths and discuss ways of dealing with wound and possible skin grafting

Encourage communication with significant other

Promote self-care activities

Provide diversional activities

Expected outcome/evaluation

Patient

Begins to observe wound and discuss feelings about it

Participates in own care

Verbalizes understanding of treatment and rehabilitation plan

TISSUE PRESSURE MONITORING

A procedure for measuring fascial tissue pressure to diagnose compartment syndrome; two techniques are available

Whiteside technique A one-time insertion of a needle into the fascia for measuring pressure (Figure 7-5)

Infusion technique A transducer monitoring system using essentially the same equipment as the Whiteside technique but can also be used for continuous monitoring, this technique is more accurate (not shown)

Preprocedure Assessment and Care

Explain procedure to patient (patient will have severe forearm or lower leg pain)

Check baseline BP

Equipment needed

Local anesthetic, needle, and syringe

Vial of bacteriostatic normal saline

Three-way stopcock

Mercury manometer

20 ml sterile syringe

Two 18-gauge needles

Two IV extension tubes

Prepare muscle site for injection and equipment as shown in Figure 7-5

Position patient as comfortably as possible

Interventions

Prepare site with antiseptic

Assist physician with anesthetizing exposed muscle site

Following diagram A (see Figure 7-5)

Withdraw enough saline with syringe to fill IV tube half full

Close stopcock

Following diagram B (see Figure 7-5)

Assist physician with needle insertion into fascia

Connect second IV tube to manometer and close stopcock

Move stopcock control to down position opposite syringe; this provides closed system

Gently depress syringe barrel to increase pressure in system; manometer will begin to register

When closed system pressure exceeds fascial pressure, some saline will enter fascia; amount of saline in IV tubing will decrease

Observe manometer at this point; this is tissue pressure reading

Assist with second fascial injection to verify initial reading

Normal fascial tissue pressure is 0 to 30 mm Hg; readings of 30 mm Hg or more are usually diagnostic of compartment syndrome, but this may vary according to physician

Monitor bilateral peripheral pulses and measure calf, forearm, thigh, or arm for edema

Assist patient with assuming position of comfort and prepare for fasciotomy if ordered

BUNIONECTOMY (KELLER OR MAYO ARTHROPLASTY)

Surgical correction of hereditary or acquired hallux valgus: acute angulation of the first metatarsophalangeal joint

Preoperative Assessment/Teaching

Assess mobility and neurovascular status of toes

Discuss with and teach patient

Crutch walking

Use of walker

Toe flexing

Quadriceps setting

ROM exercises

Postoperative Assessment
Observations/findings

Neurovascular status of affected toes: color, temperature, sensation, edema
Location and character of pain
Site of incision for drainage and bleeding
Placement of plaster toe cap or splint

Potential complications

Fever
Wound infection
Recurrence of hallux valgus

Medical Management

Analgesics, antipyretics
Type of immobilization device
Ambulation, weight bearing
Diet, activity, rest
Ice bags to affected site

Nursing diagnoses/interventions/evaluation

■ **NDX:** Altered physical mobility related to musculoskeletal impairment

Maintain bed rest until fully reactive
  Elevate foot of bed
  Place bed cradle over feet
  Monitor immobilization device for pressure areas and circulatory constriction
Ambulate with assistance, usually 24 to 48 hr postoperatively
Monitor vital signs q4h and affected foot for color, temperature, sensation, and edema q2h for 24 hr, then qid
Assist patient with performing ROM exercises q4h while in bed
Assist and teach patient to turn and deep breathe q2h to 3h while in bed; hold affected foot during turn and place on pillow after turn has been completed
Apply plaster walking boot if ordered
Initiate flexing exercises of toes five times qh when edema subsides and as ordered

Expected outcome/evaluation

Patient
  Performs rehabilitation exercises correctly
  Participates in self-care activities
  Presents normal peripheral pulse, color, temperature, sensation, mobility of affected foot

■ **NDX:** Pain related to surgical intervention

Assess location, intensity, and character of pain; use pain rating scale
Administer analgesics; assess effectiveness of pain relief measures and monitor for side effects

Apply ice bag to area to promote comfort
Assist patient with changing position frequently while on bed rest
Provide diversional activities

Expected outcome/evaluation

Patient
  States that pain is at tolerable level
  Appears relaxed and calm
  Sleeps for increasing number of hours

■ **NDX:** Knowledge deficit related to lack of information about home care management

Stress importance of and review foot and incision care and prescribed exercises
  Demonstrate dressing change
  Explain need for foot soaks in warm, soapy water after sutures are removed; need to dry feet well
  Discuss care of plaster boot if applicable
  Demonstrate toe and foot ROM exercises
  Explain importance of proper footwear
Discuss activities allowed; encourage self-care and ADLs
Discuss signs of wound infection to report to physician: fever, pain, edema
Encourage follow-up care with physician

Expected outcome/evaluation

Patient
  Verbalizes understanding of rehabilitation and treatment plan
  Participates in ADLs adequately
  Expresses understanding of signs of wound infection
  Performs incision care accurately

TRACTION MANAGEMENT

Method of providing a pulling effect to an extremity or body part while also maintaining a countertraction (pull in opposite direction) (see Table 7-1 and Figures 7-6 through 7-9)

CAST MANAGEMENT

Casts are applied to immobilize musculoskeletal tissues after trauma; they are made of plaster, fiberglass, plastic, or cast tape

Assessment
Observations/findings

Type of cast applied, moistness
Neurovascular status of affected extremity
Location, intensity, and character of pain
Integumentary status at edges and under cast
GI, renal, and/or respiratory dysfunction (body or cervical cast)

TABLE 7-1. Traction Management

Type	Balanced suspension	Skin	Skeletal
Definition	Skeletal or skin traction applied to a lower extremity while weights and a splint simultaneously provide countertraction to and suspension of that extremity	Light or temporary traction applied directly to the skin to align fracture and reduce muscle spasm	Insertion of a pin or wire directly into the bone to provide continuous traction

General interventions (same for all types of traction listed in this table)	Maintain constant pull in line with deformity
	Assess and maintain ropes and pulleys
	  Taut
	  Riding freely over pulleys
	  Free of bedding
	  Knots secure
	  Adequate space between pulley and traction
	Monitor and maintain weights
	  Hanging free
	  Off floor
	  Away from bed
	  NOTE: *Never remove weights; never lift weights*
	Monitor and maintain countertraction
	  Elevation of bed under part to which traction is applied
	  Pull exerted against fixed point
	  Pull exerted against traction in opposite direction		

Interventions for specific type of traction	Maintain anatomical position of extremity
	Maintain 20-degree angle between thigh and bed
	Have heel clear of sling under calf
	Maintain abduction of extremity
	Monitor femoral and popliteal pulses
		Observe carefully for slippage and bunching up of bandage
		Replace bandage prn
		Observe for pressure areas at distal end of bandage (wrist or heel), especially if weight is greater than 7 pounds
		Check neurovascular status q2h to 4h
			Cover ends of pin with cork
			Observe site of insertion
			  Redness
			  Swelling
			  Discharge
			  Odor
			  Bleeding
			Clean skin around puncture sites as ordered; do not remove crusts around pin sites
			Monitor neurovascular status q2h to 4h

Pelvic	Side arm	Cervical	Bryant's	Halo
Traction provided to lower back to reduce low back pain	Skin traction to the humerus to maintain alignment after open reduction procedure	Application of cervical halter with traction to relieve neck pain or when a cervical fracture is suspected	Treatment of fractures of femur shaft in young children	Metal brace attached to the skull and iliac crest or femur with pins; provides spinal support after spinal fusion or for preoperative treatment of scoliosis
Ensure that pelvic girdle is proper size for patient and that pelvic girdle fits snugly over iliac crests and pelvis Inspect skin areas over iliac crests for pressure points q4h Pelvic straps must be equal in length and unrestricted	Maintain position as directed by physician Check neurovascular status of affected arm q2h to 4h Notify physician immediately if any change is noted Apply chest restraint sheet for countertraction prn	Position without pillows Monitor so weight and pulley are free of wall Observe for pressure areas Jaws, chin, and ears Side of head Back of head Pad as necessary for comfort	Raise buttocks slightly from mattress Observe bandages carefully for slippage and bunching over heel cords Observe for skin sloughing on both legs Check feet for color, pulses, temperature, and sensation q2h to 4h Use harness restraint to prevent turning over Avoid thick, wide diapers between legs	Cover ends of pins with cork Observe pin insertion sites Redness Swelling Drainage Odor Bleeding Clean skin around pin sites as ordered; do not remove crusts Monitor straps for areas of constriction Pad pressure points as necessary for comfort Do not alter amount of traction applied

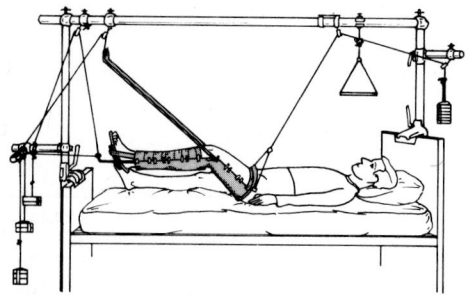

FIGURE 7-6. Balanced suspension with Thomas' splint and Pearson's attachment.

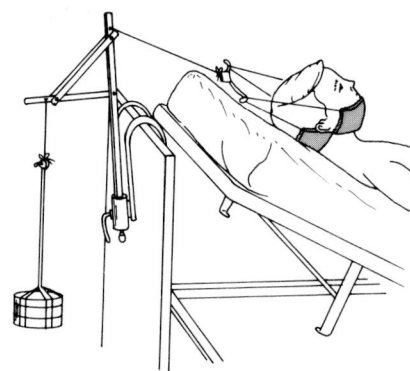

FIGURE 7-8. Cervical traction.

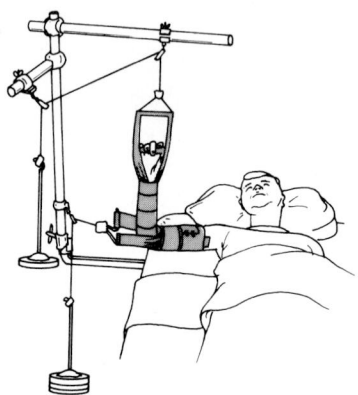

FIGURE 7-7. Traction of humerus.

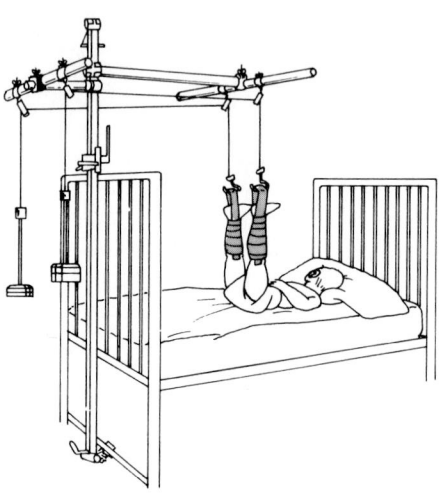

FIGURE 7-9. Bryant's traction.

Potential complications

Neurovascular impairment
Fever
Skin impairment
Infection
Compartment syndrome (see p. 382)

Interventions
General

Maintain correct body alignment
Inspect skin under edges of cast for irritation q2h to 4h
  Apply lotion to reachable areas (no powder)
  Massage areas gently until lotion absorbed
  Keep cast dry
  Apply moleskin tape to cast edges to prevent irritation
Monitor pulses, skin color, warmth, sensation, and capillary refill (if appropriate) distal to cast

Casts on extremities

Maintain bed rest in prescribed position, usually until cast dries; patients with plastic or fiberglass casts may ambulate as ordered
Expose cast to air until dry
Elevate cast on firm pillow(s)

Explain that skin will feel warm under cast until cast dries
Elevate each joint higher than preceding joint (e.g., hand higher than elbow); avoid restriction of brachial artery
If blood or drainage appears on cast
  Mark spot with circle
  Note date and time
  NOTE: Use china or permanent marker on plastic or fiberglass cast
  Observe for further drainage q2h; if present report to physician

Body, hip spica, cervical casts

Maintain bed rest in prescribed position until cast dries
  Use bedboard and firm mattress
  Provide trapeze on bed
  Support feet with footboard
Expose cast to air until dry unless quick-drying plaster is used
  Cover uncasted areas only; maintain warmth
  Protect privacy by covering perineal area with towel (hip spica); protect edge with plastic to prevent soiling

Use palms of hands only when handling wet cast; handle cast as little as possible until dry (approximately 8 hr)

When turning

Use enough personnel to maintain alignment

Turn patient to prescribed side

Place side rails up

Support chest and cast with pillows

Turn entire body at one time

Avoid twisting body beneath cast

Do not use abduction crossbar (hip spica) to lift or turn

On discharge

Provide information on and stress importance of prescribed activities and rehabilitation exercises

Demonstrate turning procedure for patient in spica cast and reiterate crutch-walking procedure where appropriate

Discuss need to keep cast out of water; use plastic bag for showering

Notify physician immediately if cast becomes wet

Suggest clothing that can be put on easily

Discuss measures to ensure warmth of affected digits

Demonstrate neurovascular monitoring of affected extremity(ies) as needed

Discuss signs and symptoms to report to physician

Fever; foul odor from cast

Increasing pain or decreased sensation

Demonstrate skin care around cast

CONTINUOUS PASSIVE MOTION DEVICE

A patient-guided machine that provides passive exercise to the hip and knee after surgery or trauma, similar devices are available for ankle, shoulder, wrist, and fingers

Purpose

Facilitates early movement and increased flexion of joint

Prevents stiffness of joint and contractures of tissue

Enhances circulation and healing

Reduces pain of or psychological resistance to flexion and edema

Assessment/Procedure

Physician's order to include

Initial degree of flexion; number of degrees to increase flexion/hour and number of hours/day to use

Restrictions or special instructions for use

Assess patient's ability to operate and manage device

Explain purpose of machine and its advantages

Remove any splints before applying device

After machine is set up by physical therapist or cast or traction technician

Place extremity on device and check the following

Lower buttock is against femur support

Knee is directly over center of frame

Foot if firmly against foot plate

Apply Velcro safety straps to extremity; check that they do not interfere with gear assembly

Set automatic flexion and/or extension motion as ordered by physician (usually at 10)

Increase flexion 1 to 5 degrees qh as ordered

Assess patient's tolerance before increasing flexion

Adjust speed as prescribed (maximum speed to flex joint from 0 to 110 degrees is about 1 min, 40 sec; minimum speed is approximately 12 min; slow speeds are used initially and at night to facilitate sleep)

Set ROM limits as ordered by physician

Instruct patient in use of controls

Control has three settings: flexion, stop, and extension

Once device is operating, patient can control movement, stop, or reverse at any point within preset range limits

Each time machine is applied, reduce flexion 5 degrees for about 15 min and then increase to original setting

Encourage patient to use machine as much as possible and as tolerated

BIBLIOGRAPHY

Barker E: Action stat! spinal cord injury, *Nursing '90* 20(11):33, 1990.

Berg EE: *Progress in orthopaedic surgery: the 1980s in review*, Orthop Nurs 9(3):29, 1990.

Carpentino LJ: *Handbook of nursing diagnosis*, Philadelphia, 1990, JB Lippincott.

Ceccio CM: Teaching the elderly amputee to meet the world, *RN* 51(9):70, 1988.

Ceccio CM: Understanding therapeutic beds, Orthop Nurs 9(3):57, 1990.

Ceron GE, Rakowski-Reinhardt AC: Action stat! autonomic dysreflexia, *Nursing '91* 21(2):33, 1991.

Cmiel PA, Cavanaugh CE: Digital replantation in children, *Am J Nurs* 89(9):1158, 1989.

Doenges ME et al: *Nursing care plans: guidelines for planning patient care*, ed 2, Philadelphia, 1989, FA Davis.

Dunajcik LM: The hip: when the joint must be replaced, *RN* 52(4):62, 1989.

Gamron RB: Taking the pressure out of compartment syndrome, *Am J Nurs* 88(8):1076, 1988.

Gulanick M et al: *Nursing care plans*, ed 2, St Louis, 1990, Mosby–Year Book.

Guzzetta CE et al: *Clinical assessment tools for use with nursing diagnoses*, St Louis 1989, CV Mosby.

Kim MJ et al: *Pocket guide to nursing diagnoses*, ed 3, St Louis, 1989, CV Mosby.

Krug BM: The hip: nursing fracture patients to full recovery, *RN* 52(4):56, 1989.

Lavin RJ: The high-pressure demands of compartment syndrome, *RN* 52(2):22, 1989.

Lovell HW, Anderson CL: Put your patient on the right bed, *RN* 53(5):66, 1990.

Mather MLS: The secret to life in a spica, *Am J Nurs* 87(1):56, 1987.

McFarland GK, McFarlane EA: *Nursing diagnosis and intervention*, St Louis, 1989, CV Mosby.

Miller RA, Evans WE: Immediate postop prosthesis, *Am J Nurs* 87(3):310, 1987.

Miller RA, Evans WE: Nurse and patient: allies preventing amputation, *RN* 51(7):38, 1988.

Morris L et al: Nursing the patient in traction, *RN* 51(1):26, 1988.

Morris L et al: Special care for skeletal traction, *RN* 51(2):24, 1988.

Nelson L et al: Improving pain management for hip fractured elderly, *Orthop Nurs* 9(3):79, 1990.

O'Hara MM: Leeching: a modern use for an ancient remedy, *Am J Nurs* 88(12):1656, 1988.

Peters VJ, Fox JM: Knee surgery clears a hurdle, *RN* 51(7):20, 1988.

Redheffer GM, Bailey M: Assessing and splinting fractures, *Nursing '89* 19(6):51, 1989.

Romeo JH: The critical minutes after spinal cord injury, *RN* 51(4):61, 1988.

Smith JE: Applying the continuous passive motion device, *Orthop Nurs* 9(3):54, 1990.

Southern JP: How to access an epidural implanted port, *Nursing '90* 20(7):48, 1990.

Thelan LA et al: *Textbook of critical care nursing,* St Louis, 1990, Mosby–Year Book.

Thompson JM et al: *Mosby's manual of clinical practice,* ed 2, St Louis, 1989, CV Mosby.

Willey T: High-tech beds and mattress overlays: a decision guide, *Am J Nurs* 89(9):1142, 1989.

8
CHAPTER

Neurological System

NEUROLOGICAL ASSESSMENT

Subjective Data

Dizziness
Vertigo
Weakness (bilateral or unilateral)
Paralysis
Headaches
Numbness
Bowel and/or bladder dysfunction
Pain
   Onset
   Duration and severity
   Location and radiation
   Character: throbbing, dull, prickling, tight
Memory loss, lapses
Tremors, tics
Nervousness
Syncope
Seizures
Irritability
Drowsiness
Hallucination
Confusion
Disturbances in
   Smell
   Taste
   Vision

Objective Data

Mental status
Level of consciousness
   See Glasgow Coma Scale (GSC)
   Awake, alert, and oriented; able to maintain conversation
   Responds to verbal and/or painful stimuli
   Drowsy, lethargic, sleeplike
   Able to follow commands
   Disoriented and stuporous
   Unable to respond to verbal or painful stimulus
   Comatose
Behavior
   General appearance
   Personal grooming
   Verbal expression

   Facial expression
   Ability to concentrate, express ideas
Intellectual or cognitive function
   Memory: immediate, recent, and past
   Abstract reasoning; insight
Emotional status
   Affect
   Mood

GLASGOW COMA SCALE (GCS)

Assessment scale designed to quickly and quantitatively evaluate level of consciousness in relation to eye opening, motor response, and verbal responses

Scores of 9 or greater (15: normal) not indicative of coma and may be assigned to responses indicating increased arousal states; scores of 7 or less qualify as coma; lowest score of 3 is compatible with but not indicative of brain death

EYE OPENING

Open spontaneously	4
Open to voice	3
Open to pain or noxious stimuli	2
No response; unable to open eyes because of bandages or edema	1

MOTOR RESPONSE

Obeying simple commands	6
Localizing pain	5
Flexion withdrawal (pain)	4
Abnormal flexion (pain); decorticate rigidity	3
Abnormal extension (pain); decerebrate rigidity	2
No motor response	0

VERBAL RESPONSE

Oriented	5
Confused	4
Verbalizes; inappropriate words	3
Vocalizes; incomprehensible words, sounds	2
No verbal response	1

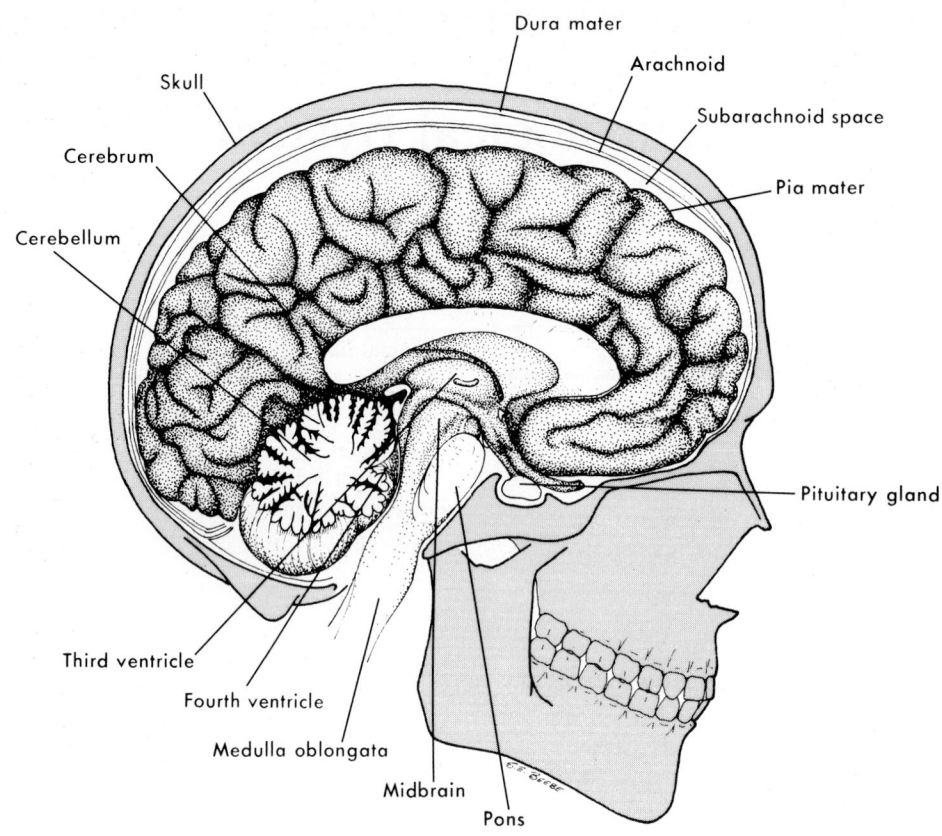

FIGURE 8-1. Nervous system.

Level of dependence vs. independence in activities of daily living (ADLs)
Sensory dysfunctions
 Visual agnosia
 Tactile agnosia
Dysarthria
Language dysfunction
 Motor, expressive aphasia: Broca's aphasia
 Aphemia (pure word mutism)
 Sensory, receptive aphasia (Wernicke's aphasia)
 Auditory verbal agnosia (pure word deafness)
Apraxia
Meningeal signs
 Brudzinski's sign: to assess meningeal irritation—patient in supine position bends knees to avoid pain when neck is flexed
 Kernig's sign: to assess meningeal irritation—patient in supine position with hips flexed is unable to extend knees without pain
 Nuchal rigidity: stiff neck
 High-pitched cry
 Severe retraction of head
 Arm and leg extension
Abnormal findings of particular gaits and postures
General appearance
 Skin

  Temperature
  Color, discolored areas
  Turgor
  Rashes
  Angiomatous lesions
  Moles
Vital signs
 BP
  Both arms, standing, sitting
  Increased
  Decreased
  Widening pulse pressure
 Arterial pulses
 Respirations (Table 8-1)
  Rate
  Rhythm
  Quality
  Type of breathing pattern
  Chest movements
  Breath sounds
Eyes (Figure 8-3)
 Pupils
  Equality
  Size
   Pinpoint

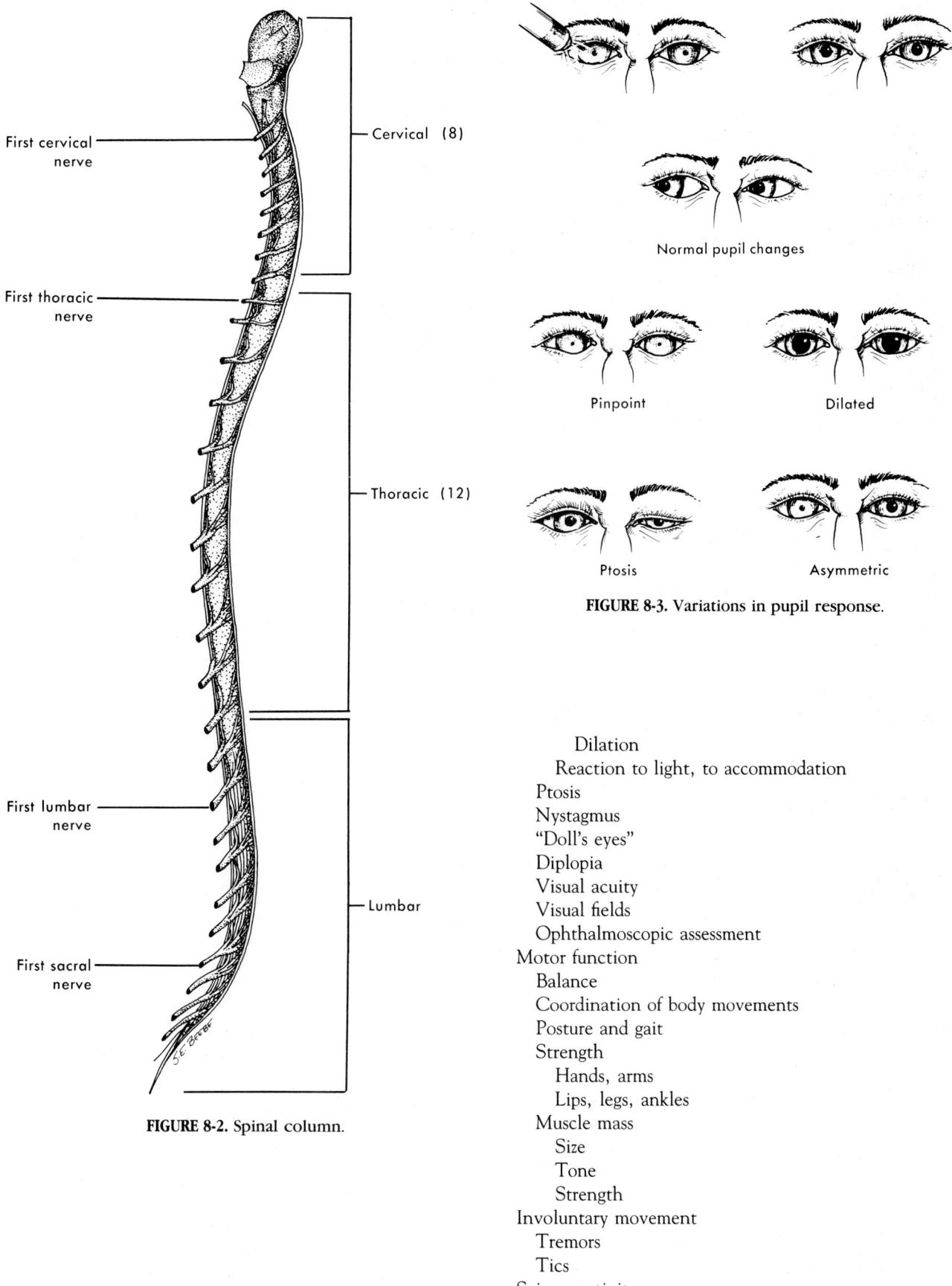

First cervical
nerve

First thoracic
nerve

First lumbar
nerve

First sacral
nerve

Cervical (8)

Thoracic (12)

Lumbar

FIGURE 8-2. Spinal column.

Normal pupil changes

Pinpoint   Dilated

Ptosis   Asymmetric

FIGURE 8-3. Variations in pupil response.

      Dilation
        Reaction to light, to accommodation
    Ptosis
    Nystagmus
    "Doll's eyes"
    Diplopia
    Visual acuity
    Visual fields
    Ophthalmoscopic assessment
Motor function
    Balance
    Coordination of body movements
    Posture and gait
    Strength
        Hands, arms
        Lips, legs, ankles
    Muscle mass
        Size
        Tone
        Strength
Involuntary movement
    Tremors
    Tics
Seizure activity

TABLE 8-1. Patterns of Respiration in Neurological Dysfunction

Terms	Description	Selected neurological causes
Eupnea	Normal breathing	
Cheyne-Stokes respirations	Breathing characterized by regular, alternating periods of hyperpnea and apnea; breathing builds from respiration to respiration in a smooth crescendo and, as peak is reached, declines in an equally smooth decrescendo; ordinarily, hyperpneic phase endures longer than apneic phase	Deep bilateral diencephalic lesions, hypertensive encephalopathy, uremia, anoxia, or imminent transtentorial herniation
Central neurogenic hyperventilation	Sustained regular, rapid hypocapnic hyperpnea	Midbrain lesions
Biot's respirations	Regular periods of hyperventilation and irregular periods of apnea	
Apneustic respirations	Ataxic, gasping, shallow breathing	Infarction at midpontine or caudal pontine level, usually as a result of basilar artery occlusion
Posthyperventilation apnea	Respirations interrupted for up to 30 seconds after five voluntary breaths in wakeful patients	Diffuse metabolic or structural forebrain disease
Cluster breathing	Breaths follow each other in disorderly sequence with irregular pauses between them	Low pons or high medulla lesion; may be result of expanding lesion in posterior fossa (cerebellar hemorrhage)
Ataxic breathing	Completely chaotic pattern with deep and shallow breaths occurring randomly; progressively leads to apnea	Dorsomedial medulla dysfunction; may appear in relation to meningitis or acute parainfectious demyelination

From Barber JM, Stokes LG, and Billings DM: *Adult and child care: a client approach to nursing,* ed 2, St Louis, 1977, CV Mosby.

TABLE 8-2. Reflexes

Reflexes	Associated nerve function
SUPERFICIAL	
Upper abdominal	T-8, T-9
Lower abdominal	T-10, T-11, T-12
Cremasteric	T-12, L-1
Gluteal	L-4 to S-3
DEEP TENDON	
Biceps	C-5, C-6
Triceps	C-6, C-7, C-8
Finger flexion	C-7 to T1
Brachioradialis	C-5, C-6
Patellar	L-2, L-3, L-4
Achilles	S-1, S-2
PATHOLOGICAL FINDINGS	
Babinski's sign (plantar)	L-4, L-5, S-1, S-2
Chaddock's sign	L-4, L-5, S-1, S-2
Clonus	

Reflex responses (Table 8-2)

Classification		Description
0	(0)	Absent
1	(+)	Sluggish or diminished
2	(++)	Active or normal
3	(+++)	Slightly hyperactive or increased response
4	(++++)	Brisk with intermittent or transient clonus
5	(+++++)	Very brisk with sustained clonus

Autonomic functions
  Bowel and/or bladder dysfunctions
  Sexual dysfunction
Cranial nerve abnormalities (Table 8-3)
Nutritional assessment
  Weight, height
  Anthropometric measurements
    Triceps skinfold (TSF)
    Arm muscle circumference (AMC)
    Mid-upper arm circumference (MUAC)

INFANTS

Fontanel evaluation
  Bulging
  Flat
  Pulsating
Cry quality: high pitched
Reflexes

TABLE 8-3. Cranial Nerve Function

Nerve	Findings
I. Olfactory	Smell
II. Optic	Visual acuity, visual fields; examination of fundi
III. Oculomotor	Pupillary reflex, external ocular muscles inducing upward, downward, and medial movements; involvement will cause ptosis, dilation of pupils
IV. Trochlear	Ocular movements; involvement will cause inability to look downward and laterally; nystagmus
V. Trigeminal	Sensory function: corneal reflex, skin of face and forehead, mucosa of nose and mouth; motor function; maxillary "jaw" reflex
VI. Abducens	Ocular movements; involvement will cause inability to look downward and laterally; nystagmus
VII. Facial	Motor function of upper and lower face; involvement will cause asymmetry of face and paresis; sensory function is tested by taste
VIII. Acoustic	Cochlear nerve test: hearing, lateralization, air and bone conduction; involvement will cause tinnitus, decreased hearing, or deafness
IX. Glossopharyngeal X. Vagus	Motor function: pharyngeal gag reflex, swallowing; vocal cord assessment: speak clearly without hoarseness
XI. Accessory	Strength of trapezius and sternocleidomastoid muscle; involvement will cause inability to elevate shoulder
XII. Hypoglossal	Motor function of tongue; involvement will cause lateral deviation, atrophy, tremor, inability to extend or move tongue from side to side

Moro's
Grasping
Rooting
Sucking
Muscle tone
Jitteriness
Tremors
Seizures

Pertinent Background Information

HISTORY OF PRESENT ILLNESS

Description of past or concurrent neurological or muscular
  disorders
Recent operations or hospitalization
Epilepsy
Loss of consciousness
Headaches
Hypertension
Cancer
Coronary artery disease
Hyperlipidemia
Pernicious anemia
Diabetes
Coarctation of aorta
Allergies
Seizure disorders
Infections
Motor and/or sensory disturbances
Behavioral or emotional changes
Head trauma/spinal trauma
Drug abuse
Dietary restrictions
Pregnancies

FAMILY HISTORY

Hypertension
Seizure disorders

Neurological disorders
Cancer
Strokes
Mental retardation
Mental illness
Sudden unexplained death

SOCIAL HISTORY

Sleep patterns
Exercise and activity level
Occupation; work patterns, exposure to toxic substances
Travel history, recent
Leisure activities
Dietary preferences
Smoking
Alcohol consumption
Psychosocial patterns
  Personality changes
  Relationships with family and friends
Social support system
School history; learning disorders

MEDICATION HISTORY

Prescription medications
Over-the-counter medications
Use of controlled substances

Diagnostic Aids

LABORATORY STUDIES

Cerebrospinal fluid (CSF) analysis
Complete blood cell count (CBC)
Erythrocyte sedimentation rate (ESR)
Gastric analysis with histamine
Blood chemistries
Arterial blood gases and pH
Blood glucose

Fluid and electrolyte levels
Enzyme studies

DIAGNOSTIC PROCEDURES

Skull films
Spinal films
Electroencephalogram (EEG)
Myelogram
Lumbar puncture
Cisternal puncture
Ventricular puncture
Electromyogram (EMG)
Tomogram
Echoencephalogram (EEG)
Pneumoencephalogram (PEG)
Ventriculography
Brain scan
Computed tomography (CT) scan
Positron emission tomography (PET) scan
Magnetic resonance imaging (MRI)
Cerebral angiography
Doppler scan: carotid and transcranial
Cerebral blood flow (CBF)
Biopsy
   Brain
   Nerve
   Muscle
Nerve conduction velocity determination
Caloric
Pulmonary function
   Vital capacity (VC)
   Minute ventilation
   Tidal volume

SURGICAL PROCEDURES

Craniotomy; burr holes
Cranioplasty
Craniectomy
Cordotomy
Sympathectomy
Laminectomy
Ventriculostomy
Ablative procedures
Vascular surgery

DIAGNOSTIC PROCEDURES

Numerous procedures, both invasive and noninvasive, performed for neurological diagnostics; general guidelines for preprocedure preparation and postprocedure observations/interventions are listed

Preprocedure Preparation

For all tests or procedures patient and family or significant others should be fully informed of the nature of the procedure, its rationale, and risks involved

Reinforce physician's explanation
Explain procedure and any sensations or discomforts that will be experienced during and after procedure
Reinforce importance of cooperation and immobility of patient for appropriate procedures
Determine patient's allergies to iodine or procaine, or kidney function when indicated
Whenever possible, be present to provide physical and emotional support during procedure
Obtain signed informed consent as indicated

Postprocedure Observations/Interventions

Changes in level of consciousness or orientation
Changes in any neurological functions: speech, range of motion (ROM), visual acuity, sensory function
For vascular procedures: observe for hemorrhage, bleeding, and stability in vital signs
Maintain positioning postprocedurally as indicated
Restrict fluids and/or foods as ordered
Maintain bed rest as ordered
Measure intake and output
Control pain as indicated

CARE OF PATIENT WITH ALTERED CONSCIOUSNESS

altered consciousness (lowered) The state in which alteration in the interaction of the cerebral hemisphere and the reticular activating system (RAS) results in an inability of the individual to relate to himself and his environment

Assessment
Observations/findings

Level of consciousness: Glasgow Coma Scale (see box on p. 391)
   Eye opening
   Motor response
   Verbal response
   Eye movements (see Level of Consciousness under Neurological Assessment, p. 393)
   Agitation
Motor function assessment
Motor function abnormalities
   Flaccidity
   Contractures
   Spasticity
   Abnormal posturing: decortication, decerebration
Respiratory function
   Airway patency
   Secretions
   Respirations
      Rate
      Patterns
         Cheynes-Stokes
         Apneustic

Cluster
 Ataxic
 Breath sounds: equal or decreased
 Dullness
 Crackles
Cardiovascular function
 Heart rate, rhythm, quality
 Carotid, peripheral pulses
 BP
Temperature
 Hypothermia
 Hyperthermia
Skin
 Color
 Turgor
Nutritional assessment
 Dietary intake
 Weight loss
 Decreases in anthropometric measurements

Laboratory/diagnostic studies

Electrolytes, chemistry profile
 Fasting blood sugar (FBS)
 Sodium
 Chloride
 Potassium
 Calcium
 Phosphorus
 Magnesium
Serum ETOH (alcohol)
CSF
Arterial blood gas (ABG) studies
Urine
 Toxicology screening
 Creatinine clearance
Intracranial pressure (ICP) may be elevated
Skull x-ray examination
CT scan
EEG

Potential complications

Respiratory
 Aspiration, atelectasis
 Pneumonia
 Neurogenic pulmonary edema
 Adult respiratory distress syndrome (ARDS)
Decubitus, constipation, contractures, malnutrition
Corneal ulceration
Dysrhythmias
Disseminated intravascular coagulation (DIC)
Urinary tract infection (UTI)

Medical Management

Oxygen/ventilatory support
Respiratory therapy
Fluids and electrolytes

ICP monitoring
Nutritional support
Medications
 ICP drugs
 Diuretics
 Antiarrhythmics
 Antihypertensives
 Antibiotics

Nursing diagnoses/interventions/evaluation

■ **NDX:** Potential for ineffective breathing pattern related to neurological impairment

Assess and monitor respirations: rate, depth, and pattern; assess ventilation effort
Maintain patent airway; maintain neck in midline position; avoid flexion of neck
Administer oxygen and humidification as indicated
Administer assisted ventilation as indicated
Assess for signs and symptoms of respiratory distress
Auscultate lung sounds q4h to 8h or as indicated
Insert oral nasopharyngeal airway as indicated for managing secretions; suction naso-oropharynx prn
Monitor arterial blood gases
Monitor tidal volume
Elevate head of bed to 30 degrees if possible to
 Maximize breathing potential
 Maintain in prone or semiprone position
 Turn side to side and prone q2h to optimize alveolar expansion

Expected outcome/evaluation

Patient demonstrates patent airway
 Respirations: normal rate, rhythm, and pattern of breathing

■ **NDX:** Self-care deficit: nutrition, hygiene/bathing, toileting, mobility, related to alteration in level of consciousness

Assess nutritional status; establish baseline weight
Maintain nutritional balance
 Assess daily caloric and fluid requirements
 Administer high-calorie, high-protein tube feedings q2h to 3h as ordered; check tube placement to prevent aspiration
 Initiate hyperalimentation or intralipid therapy as indicated
Comb hair daily; shampoo every week as indicated
Keep nails clipped and clean
Administer oral hygiene q2h to 4h and prn
 Remove dentures
 Brush teeth three times a day
 Clean mucous membranes with water and/or alkaline mouthwash

Keep lips moist with cold creams or glycerin-type lip-sticks

Initiate oral lavages as indicated

Inspect tongue daily for cuts or crusting

Perform eye inspection and care q4h

Observe for signs of corneal ulcerations, keratitis, in-flammation, or irritation

Remove any formed crusts

Cleanse with lubricating eye drops

Close eyes and apply eye shield as necessary

Apply topical ointments as indicated

Avoid positioning patient on side with eyes open

Administer nose care q4h to 5h

Remove any formed crusts

Apply ointment to nares

Change nasal tube q72h as ordered; alternate nares

Inspect ears q4h to 6h for signs of dry or fresh drainage

Report any fresh drainage to physician

Remove crusts as ordered

Ensure elimination

Connect indwelling catheter to closed gravity drainage as ordered

Monitor urinary output; assess for clarity, sedimentation

Use external catheters as ordered

Care for catheter q8h and prn

Monitor daily bowel movement; if none, check for im-paction q2d to 3d

Initiate bowel program

Give stool softeners daily

Give mild cathartics q2d to 3d

Give enemas as ordered

Expected outcome/evaluation

Patient's needs for hygiene, nutrition, elimination, and toileting are met

■ **NDX:**   Potential for impaired skin integrity

Assess and monitor skin integrity q4h to 8h

Inspect ears, elbows, heels, and all pressure points care-fully

Administer skin care q2h

Use air mattress or egg crate mattress

Apply heel and elbow guards

Massage back and pressure points with lanolin-based lotions

Use cottonseed oil over feet and hands to prevent loss of cutaneous oil

Keep bed linen taut, dry, and wrinkle-free

Turn and reposition q2h

Remove and clean skin around any tubes (nasogastric or endotracheal) daily

Expected outcome/evaluation

Patient's skin integrity is maintained

■ **NDX:**   Impaired physical mobility related to neurolog-ical impairment

Assess muscle mass and joint motion daily

Monitor for signs of joint contractures

Perform passive ROM exercise to all extremities q2h to 4h and prn; involve large (arms, legs) and small (fingers, toes) muscle groups

Maintain body in proper alignment; reposition q2h; use rolls, pillows as necessary

Apply splints as necessary

Expected outcome/evaluation

Patient remains free of joint contractures; muscle is main-tained

Demonstrates full ROM and joint mobility

Level of physical mobility is appropriate for physical status

■ **NDX:**   Potential for injury related to neurological im-pairment

Assess mental and physical status to determine potential for injury

Initiate strategies to prevent injury that are appropriate for physiological status

Maintain bed in low position, with side rails up if patient is unattended

Pad side rails if patient is restless or agitated

Provide hand mittens as indicated; remove q8h for hand care

Provide soft restraints; contraindicated if seizures occur

Speak softly to patient, reassuring and explaining proce-dures and activities

Expected outcome/evaluation

Patient is free of injury

■ **NDX:**   Sensory-perceptual alteration related to neu-rological disease or trauma

Assess level of consciousness q8h; monitor and record level of mental awareness

Speak to patient; orient to day, hour, and location

Explain all activities and procedures

Encourage family, friends to talk to patient and to touch patient

Assess environmental stimuli; eliminate as much as pos-sible noises that are excessive or disturbing

Keep environment appropriate to time of day; open shades during day, turn out lights at night

Structure routine activities

Provide items around bed that will increase meaningful stimuli: clocks, calendars, personal favorite objects

Expected outcome/evaluation

Patient demonstrates stabilization of emotions and/or absence of signs of agitation or distress

■ **NDX:**   Ineffective family coping related to situational crisis and/or prolonged disability that exhausts supportive capacity

Provide correct and updated information

Assist family to have a realistic perception of patient's condition and prognosis

Assist family members to identify potential role changes necessary to maintain family integrity

Provide emotional support for family or significant other (e.g., allow to express feelings of loss, anger)

Encourage verbalization of feelings of death, dying, and loss

Permit and encourage participation in patient care as desired

Allow family to do small tasks for patient: combing hair, applying lotion, ROM exercises, etc.

Encourage use of resources to help in adjusting to situation (e.g., clergy, counseling)

Expected outcome/evaluation

Family (member)
   Demonstrates ability to deal with situation
   Verbalizes feelings
   Seeks information to understand situation
   Displays decreased anxiety regarding being with patient

Additional nursing diagnoses to consider

Ineffective airway clearance
Impaired gas exchange
Potential for infection: urinary, respiratory

SEIZURE DISORDER (CONVULSIONS, EPILEPSY)

Sudden and violent involuntary motor movements of a group of skeletal muscles; generally are transitory and often involve disturbances in consciousness as well as motor-sensory and/or autonomic function (see box)

Assessment
Observations/findings

Assess patient for characteristics before, during, and after seizure activity

Document time, length, and body parts involved

Loss of consciousness or alteration in consciousness

Motor activity
   Tonic, clonic
   Jerking, patting, rubbing movements
   Sudden, brief contractions of muscle groups
   Fluttering of eyelids
   Facial jerking
   Lip smacking

Movements may be confined to one area or may spread from one side to the other

Head and eyes deviate to the side

Respiratory function
   Tachypnea
   Apnea
   Difficulty in breathing
   Occluded airway

Laboratory/diagnostic studies

EEG
Echoencephalogram
CT scan/magnetic resonance imaging (MRI)
Urine screening
Serum chemistries
   Hypoglycemia
   Increased BUN
Serum ETOH

Potential complications

Physical trauma, self-inflicted injury
Aspiration pneumonia
Respiratory impairment
Status epilepticus

Medical Management

Medications (Table 8-4)
   Anticonvulsants
   Sedatives
   Barbiturates
Diet
   Regular
   Ketogenic
Surgery
   Resection of irritable focus

GENERALLY RECOGNIZED SEIZURE CLASSIFICATIONS

GENERALIZED

Tonic-clonic (grand mal)
Absence (petit mal)
Myoclonic
Akinetic
Atonic

PARTIAL

Motor: focal motor (Jacksonian), simple partial
Sensory: focal sensory (e.g., sensory, visual, auditory, gustatory)
Psychomotor: temporal lobe, complex partial

TABLE 8-4. Drugs Used in Seizure Disorders

Drug	Plasma therapeutic levels	Average daily dose	Side and toxic effects
Acetazolamide (Diamox)		1-3 g 750 mg	Drowsiness; aplastic anemia; headache; paresthesia
Carbamazepine (Tegretol)	4-10 μg/ml	450-700 mg (maximum dose 1200 mg); children: 20-30 mg/kg	Skin rash; blurred vision; ataxia; bone marrow depression
Clonazepam (Clonopin)	40-100 μg/ml	1.5-20 mg; children: 100-200 μg/kg/day	Drowsiness; ataxia; anorexia; behavior changes
Diazepam (Valium)		8-30 mg	Drowsiness; ataxia
Ethosuximide (Zarontin)	40-90 μg/ml	500-1500 mg; children: 20-40 mg/kg	Drowsiness; aplastic anemia; headache; lethargy
Mephenytoin (Mesantoin)		200-600 mg; children: 100-400 mg	Nystagmus; ataxia; skin rashes; serious toxicity common; pancytopenia
Methsuximide (Celontin)		300-600 mg	Drowsiness; ataxia; anorexia; aplastic anemia
Paramethadione (Paradione)		300-900 mg	Nephrotoxicity; neutropenia
Phenobarbital (Luminal)	20-40 μg/ml	80-120 mg; adults: 60-250 mg; children: 3-6 mg/kg	Drowsiness; ataxia; nystagmus
Phenytoin, sodium diphenylhydantoin (Dilantin)	10-20 μg/ml	300 mg or 4-7 mg/kg/day	Drowsiness; ataxia; nausea; rash; gingival hyperplasia; nystagmus; anemia
Primidone (Mysoline)	7-15 μg/ml	750-1500 mg; children: 10-25 mg/kg	Drowsiness; ataxia
Trimethadione (Tridione)		900-1200 mg/day; children: 900 mg/day	Bone marrow depression; dermatitis; photophobia; irritability
Valproic acid (Depakene)	50-100 μg/ml	1000-3000 mg; children: 15-60 mg/kg	Nausea; hepatotoxicity

Nursing diagnoses/interventions/evaluation

■ **NDX:** Potential for injury: trauma related to rapid onset of altered state of consciousness and seizure activity

Preconvulsive care
  Pad side rails
  Maintain bed in low position
  When patient is on bed rest, raise padded side rails
  Assist patient to identify auras
Convulsive care
  If out of bed during seizure activity, ease patient to floor and remove objects of potential harm; loosen constrictive clothing
  Turn head to side
  Note frequency, time, level of consciousness, body parts involved, and length of seizure activity
  Provide privacy
  Administer medications as ordered (see Table 8-4)
Postconvulsive care
  Assess and monitor patient carefully after seizure
  Maintain effective patent airway
  Assess patient for injury carefully, inspecting oral cavity
  Check BP, P, and R and do neurological check immediately after seizure and prn
  Assess for

  Altered level of consciousness
  Malaise
  Nausea, vomiting
  Muscular soreness, backache, or back weakness
  Aspiration
    Choking, difficulty in breathing, cyanosis
    Decreased or absent breath sounds
    Tachycardia
    Tachypnea
Provide emotional support
Inform patient of seizure and reorient if necessary
Resume routine activity

Expected outcome/evaluation

Patient is free of injury

■ **NDX:** Potential for ineffective breathing pattern related to neurogenic impairment

Preconvulsive care
  Keep oral airway at bedside
  Have suction equipment readily available
  Administer oxygen as ordered
Postconvulsive care
  Maintain patent airway

Suction oropharynx as indicated prn
Administer oxygen as ordered

Expected outcome/evaluation

Patient
Demonstrates patent airway
Lungs are clear
Respiration rate and depth are clear

■ **NDX:** Social isolation related to lack of friends, groups because of stigmatization associated with seizure (epilepsy) disorders

Assess past experiences with social contacts, the degree and amount of discrimination, ostracism of patient by family, friends, classmates, co-workers
Establish trust
Discuss feelings of loneliness; validate normality of feelings
Assist patient to identify barriers, actual or perceived, in establishing meaningful relationships
Offer support and encouragement to engage in social activities
Assist in identifying diversional activities that will decrease loneliness
Refer to and encourage participation in support groups

Expected outcome/evaluation

Patient
Verbalizes feelings of isolation
Identifies barriers to interaction with others
Seeks participation in social groups
Speaks to others

■ **NDX:** Knowledge deficit related to lack of information about disease process and home care management

Assist patient and family to recognize auras, type of seizure activity involved, and course of action to take
Discuss importance of not restraining or interrupting behavior
Observe and record behaviors exhibited during preictal and convulsive phases
Instruct patient and family about the nature of disorder and need to attempt to adopt positive attitude toward patient's life and treatment
Dispel and clarify common fears and myths about convulsive disorders
Epilepsy is not a form of insanity
It does not get progressively worse
Emphasize importance of communication between patient and family regarding feelings of shame and humiliation associated with epilepsy
Explain importance of identifying aura and course of action to take
Explain need to identify and avoid stimuli that can stimulate onset of seizure activity

Flickering lights
Certain sounds
Certain types of food
Full bladder
Discuss medications: name, dosage, frequency of administration, purpose, and toxic or side effects
Stress importance of taking medication as ordered, of not skipping dose
Explain need to avoid taking over-the-counter medications without checking with physician
Explain importance of maintaining regularity of diet, exercise and all activity
Explain importance of well-balanced diet; avoid excessive use of alcohol
Discuss importance of avoiding overexertion
Explain to family
Need to encourage patient to continue with normal routines, such as work, recreation, and other outside interests
Need to avoid being overprotective; assure patient and family that activity often inhibits seizure occurrence
Discuss need to avoid excessive physical and emotional excitement or stress; need to avoid stimulants and alcohol
Instruct patient to wear or carry medical alert band or card
Discuss available agencies for use as references, such as Epilepsy Foundation of America*
Educate patient regarding possible limitations or restrictions of driving privileges

Children

Discuss child's needs with parents
To have an understanding about condition
To participate actively in care and treatment
To avoid rigid restrictions and overprotection
Emphasize importance of allowing child to attend regular school and engage in normal activities with other children
Stress need to inform school nurse and/or teacher of
Patient's epileptic status
Child's understanding of the disorder
Treatment to implement should seizure occur while child is at school

Expected outcome/evaluation

Patient and/or significant other demonstrates knowledge and understanding of home care and disease management

Other nursing diagnoses to consider

Disturbance in self-esteem related to repeated negative interpersonal experiences

---

*Epilepsy Foundation of America, 4351 Garden City Dr., Landover, Md., 20785.

Ineffective coping: individual, related to inadequate support systems

CEREBROVASCULAR DISRUPTIONS

Alterations in cerebrovascular circulation; may be classified as ischemic or hemorrhagic

ischemic disruption Disruption of cerebral blood flow caused by thrombosis, embolus, or hemorrhage

subarachnoid hemorrhage (SAH) Bleeding into the subarachnoid space caused by ruptured cerebral aneurysm, hypertensive hemorrhage, ruptured arteriovenous malformation

intracerebral hemorrhage Bleeding into cerebral tissue; caused by hypertensive rupture of cerebral vessel

Assessment
Observations/findings
ISCHEMIC

Altered level of consciousness
  Vertigo
  Drowsiness
  Stupor
  Mental confusion
  Disorientation
  Irritability
  Coma
Visual disturbances
  Diplopia
  Ptosis
  Monocular blindness
  Photophobia
Sensory disturbances
  Tingling
  Numbness
  Tinnitus
Motor disturbances
  Paresis
  Weakened reflexes
  Hemiplegia
Dysphasia
Aphasia
Nausea, vomiting
Elevated T and BP
Tachycardia
Tachypnea
Positive Kernig's and Brudzinski's signs

HEMORRHAGIC

Subarachnoid hemorrhage (SAH)
  Symptoms generally abrupt in onset
  Increasing intracranial pressure
  Altered level of consciousness

  Headaches (may be severe)
  Vertigo
  Mental confusion
  Stupor
  Coma
  Ocular disturbances
  Hemiparesis or hemiplegia
  Nausea, vomiting
  Sweating and/or chills
  Meningeal irritation
    Nuchal rigidity
    Positive Kernig's or Brudzinski's signs
    Photophobia
    Blurred vision
    Irritability, restlessness
    Elevated temperature
Intracerebral hemorrhage
  Altered level of consciousness
    Mental confusion
    Stupor
    Coma
  Severe hypertension
  Respiratory distress
Arteriovenous malformation
  Headaches
  Seizure activity
  Motor/sensory deficits
  Aphasia
  Dizziness
  Fainting

Laboratory/diagnostic studies

CT scan or MRI
Lumbar puncture and CSF evaluation (may not be performed because of elevated ICP)
  Elevated pressure
  Xanthochromic to grossly bloody
  Elevated protein (80 mg to 130 mg/100 ml)
  Elevated WBC
  Decreased glucose
Clotting studies
Cerebral angiography
Skull x-ray examinations
Brain scan
Regional cerebral blood flow studies (CBF)
Carotid Doppler flow studies

Potential complications

Cerebral vasospasm
  Focal neurological deterioration
  Cerebral ischemia
  Cerebral infarction
Hydrocephalus
Rebleeding

Medical Management

ISCHEMIC

Parenteral therapy
Medications
  Anticonvulsants
  Antiplatelet aggregation
  Antihypertensives
  Corticosteroids
  Diuretics
  Antihistamines
  Narcotic analgesic
Ventilatory support when indicated
Cardiac monitoring
Seizure precautions
Intracranial pressure monitoring
Nutritional support

HEMORRHAGIC

Ventilator/oxygen support
Arterial blood gases
Complete activity restriction
Intracranial pressure (ICP) monitoring
Parenteral therapy
Medications
  Antihypertensives
  Corticosteroids (dexamethasone)
  Antifibrinolytics (aminocaproic acid)
  Stool softeners
  Antipyretics
  Analgesics (codeine)
Hyperventilation
Surgery
  Aneurysm: clipping, ligation
  Arteriovenous malformation (AVM): embolization,
    surgical excision of AVM
Treatment of vasospasm
  Hypervolemic-hypertensive therapy
    Fluid and volume expanders
  Medications
    Serotonin antagonists (reserpine)
    Kanamycin sulfate
    Calcium-blocking agents (nifedipine, verapamil)
    Barbiturates
  Hemodynamic monitoring

Nursing diagnoses/interventions/evaluation

■ **NDX:** Alteration in cerebral tissue perfusion related
to vasospasm secondary to hemorrhagic injury

Assess neurological status q15min to 30min or as indicated
Monitor for changes or signs of cerebral vasospasm
Maintain bed rest with head of bed elevated 15 to 60
  degrees
Check BP, P, and R q15min to 30min

```
SUBARACHNOID PRECAUTIONS

Provide private room with dim artificial lighting
Ensure complete bed rest
Maintain quiet environment
Reduce environmental stimuli
Limit visitors
Provide all nursing care
Administer stool softeners
```

Report any sudden changes in BP, pupillary, or neuro-
  logical status immediately
Assess and monitor respirations and ventiliation; provide
  oxygen as indicated
Monitor ABGs as ordered
Check rectal temperature q2h to 4h; hypothermia or cool-
  ing measures may be indicated
Initiate subarachnoid precautions (see box above)
Maintain intake and output
Initiate treatment for vasospasm as ordered
  Auscultate lung sounds q4h to 8h
  Maintain head of bed in flat position
  Monitor PCWP, PAD, SVR, and BP to achieve and
    maintain within prescribed parameters

Expected outcome/evaluation

Patient demonstrates effective cerebral perfusion
  Is oriented to time, person, place
  No alteration in consciousness
  Vital signs within normal limits

■ **NDX:** Alteration in cerebral tissue perfusion related
to increased intracranial pressure secondary to
hemorrhagic injury

Assess neurological status q15min to 30min or as indicated
Check BP, P, and R q15min to 30min
Monitor for signs and symptoms of increasing ICP (p.
  439); report any changes in BP, P, or neurological status
  immediately
Maintain head of bed elevated 30 to 45 degrees
Maintain head and neck in midline position
Monitor intake and output
Report an increase in systolic BP of > 20 mm Hg with
  widened pulse pressure
Initiate monitoring of ICP as ordered; report an increase
  of > 15 mm Hg lasting 15 to 30 min
Administer medications as ordered

Expected outcome/evaluation

Patient demonstrates effective cerebral perfusion

Is oriented to time, person, place
No alteration in consciousness
ICP ≤ 15 mm Hg
No clinical signs of increased ICP

■ **NDX:** Pain (headache, nuchal rigidity) related to irritation of meninges secondary to subarachnoid
hemorrhage

Assess type, location and severity of pain
Monitor for signs of increasing pain or discomfort; report
any changes in character of pain
Administer medications as ordered: analgesics
Maintain quiet environment; remove or modify any stim-
uli that may heighten pain or discomfort; dim lights
Explain all procedures and treatments
Organize care to maximize periods of quiet and rest
Move or reposition patient gently; avoid excessive
movement

Expected outcome/evaluation

Patient reports pain relief
Achieves comfort level
Appears comfortable; sleeps and rests quietly

■ **NDX:** Knowledge deficit related to lack of information
about disease process and home care manage-
ment

Provide explanation of primary clinical disorder, causes,
and treatment as indicated
Encourage questions; correct any misconceptions
Discuss medications: name, dosage, frequency of admin-
istration, purpose, and toxic or side effects
Explain need to avoid taking over-the-counter medica-
tions without checking with physician
Explain need to increase activities as ordered
Explain importance of physical activity as tolerated
Explain need for planned rest periods
Discuss symptoms of progression of condition to report to
physician
Explain importance of ongoing outpatient care
NOTE: for stroke victims (see p. 408)

Expected outcome/evaluation

Patient
Demonstrates knowledge and understanding of home
care management
Verbalizes understanding of limitations and allowances
regarding activities and exercise
Repeats all relevant information regarding medications,
time of dose, side effects, and purpose

Additional nursing diagnoses to consider

Anxiety related to perceived and actual biological threat
Ineffective breathing related to neurological impairment

Unilateral neglect related to cerebrovascular accident

CEREBROVASCULAR ACCIDENT (CVA) (STROKE)

*Onset of neurological deficits related to decreased cere-
bral blood flow caused by occlusion or stenosis of
blood vessels from embolism, thrombosis, or hemorrhage, resulting in ischemia of the brain, (NOTE: Symptoms depend on location and size of lesion)*

Assessment
Observations/findings

Symptoms may be rapid in onset or may take several min-
utes or hours to complete
Altered level of consciousness
Loss of sensation and reflexes
Usually unilateral
May be temporary or permanent
Generalized weakness
Flaccid or spastic muscle tone
Pupil inequality
Ptosis of eyelid
Visual deficits
Blurred vision
Partial loss of vision
Drooping mouth
Elevated BP
Paralysis: may be unilateral or bilateral
Communication dysfunction
Motor and sensory aphasia
Apraxia
Agnosia
Dysphagia
Bladder and bowel incontinence
Nausea and vomiting
Bruits: carotid, femoral, iliac arteries or abdominal aorta

Laboratory/diagnostic studies

Lumbar puncture and CSF
Normal or elevated pressure
Elevated protein level
CT scan
MRI
Cerebral arteriography
EEG
Brain scan
B-mode ultrasound
Skull x-ray examination
Echoencephalography
Doppler ultrasonography

Potential complications

Increased ICP
Herniation

Aspiration, atelectasis
Respiratory failure
Seizure activity
Cardiac dysrhythmias
Malnutrition
Contractures, ankylosis

Medical Management

Airway patency support
  Oxygen-assisted ventilation
  Tracheostomy
Bed rest
Nutritional and fluid management
Medications
  Antihypertensives
  Antifibrinolytics
  Antispasmodics
  Anticonvulsants
  Anticoagulants
  Antipyretics
  Corticosteriods
Electrocardiogram (ECG) and cardiac monitoring
Hypothermia
ICP monitor
Indwelling catheter
Neurological rehabilitation

Nursing diagnoses/interventions/evaluation

■ **NDX:** Ineffective airway clearance related to impaired cough and inability to handle secretions

Assess and monitor respirations, cough reflex, and secretions
Position body and head to avoid obstruction of airway and provide optimal secretion removal
Suction secretions prn
Insert oral or nasopharyngeal airway to maintain airway patency
Auscultate chest for breath sounds q2h to 4h
See Care of Patient with Altered Consciousness (p. 396)
Administer oxygen/humidification as ordered
Provide mechanical ventilation as ordered
Monitor arterial blood gases and hemoglobin as indicated

Expected outcome/evaluation

Patient demonstrates patent airway
  Chest expansion is symmetrical
  Breath sounds are clear to auscultation
  ABGs and vital signs are within normal limits
  No signs of respiratory distress

■ **NDX:** Impaired mobility: physical, related to impaired neurophysiological function

Assess functional ability and extent of impairment; record and monitor changes and improvements

Maintain body alignment; use bedboard, air mattress, or footboard as indicated (Figure 8-4)
Turn and reposition q2h
Elevate affected limbs on pillow
Use pull sheet when indicated
When patient is on side, support with pillows; may use hand rolls and arm splints to maintain patient in functional position (see Figure 8-4)
Perform active and/or passive ROM exercise to all extremities q2h to 4h and prn (Figures 8-5 and 8-6)
Assist and encourage patient to perform quadriceps setting and gluteal exercises q4h
Encourage hand, finger, and foot exercises
  Have patient squeeze rubber sponge ball
  Perform extension and flexion
  Perform extension of fingers, legs, and feet
Assist patient with using supportive devices as indicated: overhead trapeze, braces, wheelchair, canes, walker
Apply antiembolic stockings
Encourage use of involved side when possible
Instruct patient to use good extremity to support weaker side (e.g., lift involved left leg with good right leg or lift involved left arm with good right arm)
Encourage patient to perform basic ADLs as soon as possible using unaffected side
  Bathing
  Brushing teeth
  Combing hair
  Eating
Begin progressive ambulation as ordered; assist to balanced sitting position; begin with transfer procedure from bed to chair to regain position sense
Consult with physical and occupational therapy departments regarding activity program

Expected outcome/evaluation

Patient
  Demonstrates optimal physical mobility and function within physiological limitations
  Demonstrates behaviors and skills necessary for resumption of activities

■ **NDX:** Unilateral neglect related to right/left cerebral hemisphere lesions secondary to neurological illness and trauma

Assess degree of neurological deficit and patient's perception and awareness of deficit
Orient patient to environment on regular basis
Provide realistic feedback
Provide a safe environment
  Remove unnecessary furniture and equipment
  Place call bell, bedside stand, and personal items on unaffected side within reach
  Keep side rail up on affected side
  Observe and anticipate needs

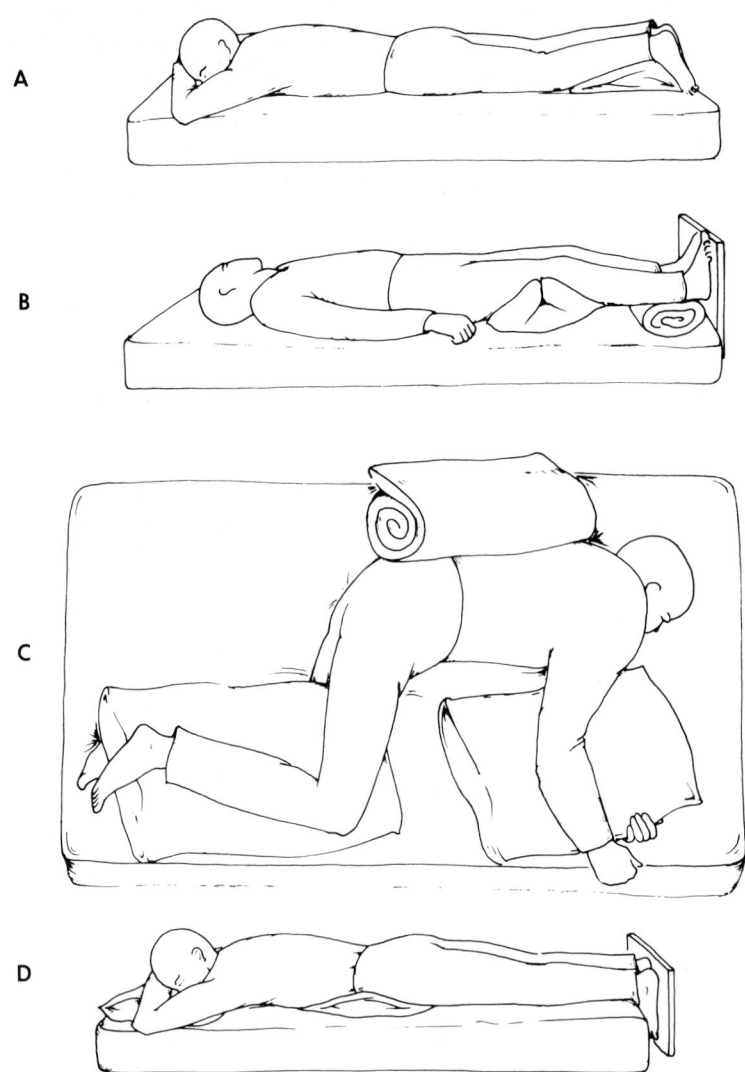

FIGURE 8-4. Various body positions to maintain correct alignment. **A,** Prone position. **B,** Supine position. **C,** Side-lying position. **D,** Prone position with support of feet.

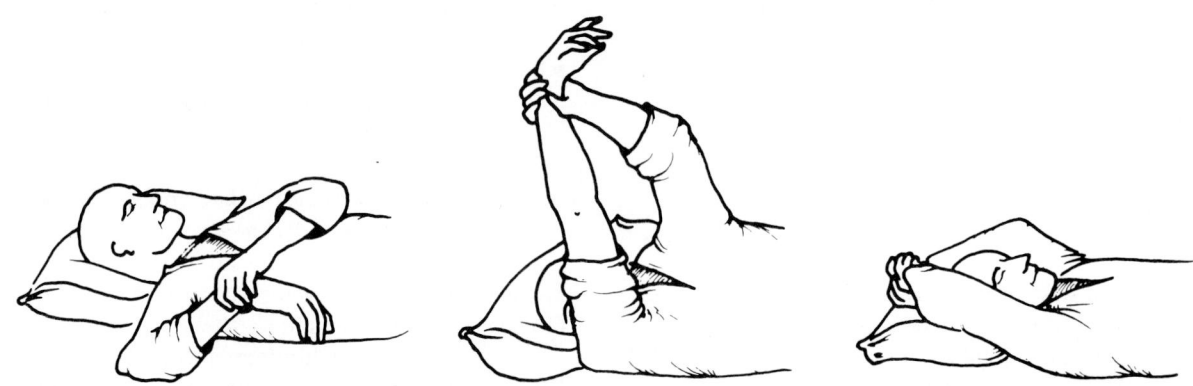

FIGURE 8-5. Range of motion of affected shoulder and elbow.

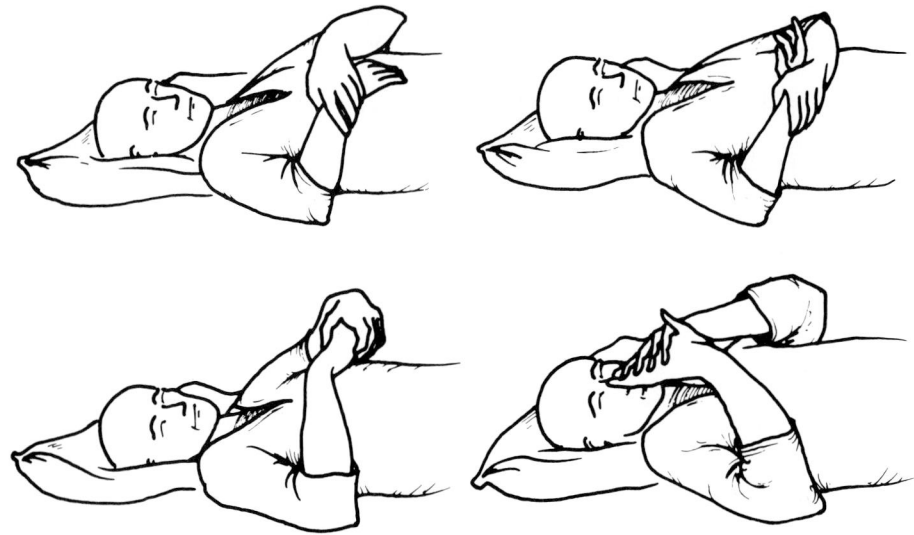

FIGURE 8-6. Range of motion of affected wrist and hand.

Approach and speak to patient from unaffected side

Assist patient to recognize and deal with perceptual deficit

Initially: arrange environment within perceptual field

After initial stress: promote increased attention to neglected side

Encourage patient to look at affected side

Stay with patient, touching or stroking affected side; encourage patient to handle affected limbs

Instruct and remind patient to include affected limbs when performing simple tasks

Use tactile stimulation to reintroduce patient to affected limbs; use scented lotions or different texture materials to stimulate different sensations

Consult with rehabilitation team to design a rehabilitation program

Encourage patient to participate in ADLs; begin by teaching individual components of an activity, then later integrate components into total activity

Encourage activities that will force patient to look at or involve affected side (e.g., place food closer toward affected limb)

Expected outcome/evaluation

Patient

Demonstrates a realistic perception of deficit

Is free of injury

■ **NDX:** Self-care deficit: hygiene, feeding, and/or toileting, related to impaired physical mobility and alteration in cognitive process

Assess degree of disability in performing self-care activities (bathing, feeding, toileting)

Administer skin care q4h to 5h

Use oil-based lotions

Inspect area over bony prominences daily for any breakdown

Provide for total physical hygiene as indicated

Comb hair daily; shampoo qwk as indicated

Keep nails clipped and clean

Administer oral hygiene q4h to 8h; brush teeth; clean mucous membranes with water and/or alkaline mouthwash

Assess and monitor nutritional status

Administer tube feedings as ordered; check tube placement to prevent aspiration

Initiate oral feedings as indicated

Progress from clear liquids

Assist with feedings as necessary

Observe for difficulty in swallowing

Position on side with head of bed elevated if feeding patient in bed

Encourage fluid intake to 2000 ml/day unless contraindicated

Ensure regular elimination

Connect indwelling catheter to closed gravity drainage system as ordered; provide catheter care q8h and prn

Use external catheters as ordered

Offer bedpan/urinal q2h to 4h if catheter is not used

Monitor daily bowel movement; if none check for impaction q2d to 3d

Give stool softener or enemas as ordered

Expected outcome/evaluation

Patient's needs for hygiene, nutrition, elimination, and toileting are met

---

COMMUNICATION DEFICIT

Expressive aphasia (Broca's aphasia): inability to express oneself verbally

Receptive aphasia (Wernicke's aphasia): inability to understand the spoken word

Global aphasia: combination of expressive and receptive aphasia

---

■ **NDX:** Impaired communication related to injury to cerebral speech center

Assess type of communication deficit (see box above)

Assess patient's ability to speak, comprehend, read, or write

Stand within patient's line of vision; when speaking allow patient to observe lips and hands

Speak in normal voice, do not shout or speak loudly

Speak slowly using simple sentences and common vocabulary; use vocabulary patient understands

Ask questions that can be answered with a yes or no response

Allow time for patient to respond to questions

Be supportive and accepting of behavior as patient shows signs of frustration

Offer assurance that speech will begin to improve over time

Provide flash cards with pictures or words of common objects that patient can point to

Consult with speech therapist to identify an appropriate means of communication

Expected outcome/evaluation

Patient is able to communicate basic needs

■ **NDX:** Knowledge deficit related to lack of information about disease process

Assess level of understanding of an adjustment to disability

Explain to family

  Need to encourage as many independent activities as possible; be alert to limitations

  Need to set realistic, achievable goals

  Need to avoid being overprotective

  Need to praise any tasks accomplished

  Importance of dealing with body image changes and behavioral changes

  Need to allow patient to be expressive

Encourage diversional activities

  Reading to patient

  Watching television

  Listening to radio

Plan regular rest periods; avoid fatigue

Encourage verbalization and communication between patient and family

Be sympathetic to emotional upsets but be firm in carrying out regimen

Reinforce physician's explanation of medical management

Stress importance of ongoing outpatient care and follow-up visits

Stress importance of continuation of rehabilitation program

Instruct patient and significant other in proper dietary and fluid needs

Stress importance of safety measures: side rails, ramps, flat shoes, removal of scatter rugs

Expected outcome/evaluation

Patient and/or significant other demonstrates knowledge and understanding of home care management

  Demonstrates passive and/or active ROM exercises

  States all relevant information regarding medications, time of dose, side effects, and purpose

  Identifies high-calorie, high-protein food and states understanding of need for maintenance of diet

  States understanding of fluid intake maintenance to avoid infection risk and constipation

Other nursing diagnoses to consider

Potential for impaired skin integrity

Self-concept disturbance: body image, self-esteem

Powerlessness

BRAIN TUMORS

Abnormal growths of primary, metastatic, or developmental origin occurring within the brain or supporting structures

Assessment
Observations/findings

Headache: localized or general; may increase with activity

Dizziness occurring with position change; vertigo

Altered level of consciousness

Decreased response to verbal and painful stimuli

Inability to follow commands

Mental or personality changes

  Irritability

  Forgetfulness

  Loss of memory

  Impaired judgment

  Depression

Pupils: unequal response to light

Papilledema

Diplopia

Blurring or decreased vision

Ptosis

Tinnitus
Loss of hearing
Weakness or paralysis of face and/or extremities
Discoordination of extremities
Paresthesia
Gait
  Staggering
  Uncoordinated
  Wide-based walking
Difficulty in chewing with dysphagia
Vomiting with or without nausea
Aphasia
Agraphia (inability to express oneself in writing)
Obesity

ACCORDING TO LOCATION

FRONTAL LOBE

Inappropriate affective responses; forgetfulness
Lack of concern; loss of social graces
Facetiousness
Poor judgment
Impaired sphincter control
Focal motor seizures
Headaches

TEMPORAL LOBE

Recent memory loss
Visual phenomenon: "déjà vu"
Auditory disturbances: "auditory agnosia"
Psychomotor seizure
Olfactory or gustatory hallucinations
Sensory aphasia

OCCIPITAL LOBE

Visual disturbances
  Central blindness
  Cortical blindness and anosognosia
  Visual hallucinations

CEREBELLUM

Uncoordination: ataxia
Loss of equilibrium
Nausea, vomiting
Vertigo

PARIETAL LOBE

Sensory loss/agnosia
Apraxia
Body perceptional disorders

ACCORDING TO TYPE

GLIOMAS (ASTROCYTOMAS)

Occurring in cerebral hemispheres
Headache

Vomiting
Personality changes; irritable, apathetic

ACOUSTIC NEUROMAS

Vertigo
Ataxia
Parasthesia and weakness of face (cranial nerves V, VII)
Loss of corneal reflex
Decreased sensitivity to touch or pain (cranial nerves V, XI)
Unilateral hearing loss

MENINGIOMAS

Seizures
Unilateral exophthalmos
Extraocular muscle palsy
Visual disturbances
Olfactory disturbances
Paresis

PITUITARY ADENOMAS

Acromegaly
Hypopituitarism: decreased thyroid, pancreatic, and gonadal function
Cushing's syndrome
Female: amenorrhea, sterilization
Male: loss of libido, impotence
Visual disturbances
Diabetes mellitus
Hypothyroidism
Hypoadrenalism
Diabetes insipidus
Inappropriate antidiuretic hormone (IADH)

Laboratory/diagnostic studies

Physical and neurological examination
Visual fields examination
MRI
Skull x-ray examination
Lumbar puncture
  CSF: elevated protein
EEG
Echoencephalography
CT scan
Cerebral angiography
Serum glucose, prolactin levels

Potential complications

Herniation
Elevated BP
Seizure activity
Neurological deficit: mild to severe
Increased ICP
Alteration in respiratory function

Alteration in consciousness
Personality change

Medical Management

Surgical excision
  Microsurgery
  Laser surgery
Medications
  Corticosteroids
  Anticonvulsants
  Antacids
  Laxatives
Radiation therapy
Chemotherapy
Fluid/electrolyte therapy
Oxygenation/ventilatory support
ICP monitoring
Neurological rehabilitation

Nursing diagnoses/interventions/evaluation

■ **NDX:** Alteration in cerebral tissue perfusion related to increased intracranial pressure secondary to tumor

Obtain and record baseline history of signs and symptoms, monitor for signs of progression
Assess level of consciousness q4h to 5h and prn
Use Glasgow Coma Scale for rapid assessment (p. 391)
Assess quality and strength of facial muscles and extremities q4h to 5h
Monitor BP, P, and R, and do neurological check q2h to 4h and prn
Monitor for and intervene at signs of increasing intracranial pressure (p. 439)
Maintain seizure precautions
Maintain safe environment
  Use side rails with padding
  Use soft restraints
Maintain quiet environment
Check rectal temperature q2h to 4h; hypothermia or cooling measures may be indicated
Administer medications as ordered
Monitor for signs of mental and personality changes

Expected outcome/evaluation

Patient demonstrates improved or normal cerebral tissue perfusion
  Neurological signs are within acceptable limits
  Is alert and oriented
  No signs of ICP

■ **NDX:** Potential for self-care deficit: hygiene, feeding, toileting, and/or mobility related to perceptual, cognitive, and/or neurological impairment

Assess for degree of disability in performing ADLs: bathing, feeding, toileting, and mobility
Monitor for signs of progressive disability
Assist with daily physical hygiene care as indicated
  Administer oral hygiene prn
  Administer skin care
Familiarize patient with surroundings if eyesight and/or visual fields are impaired
Ensure elimination
  Use external or indwelling catheter as indicated
  Initiate voiding measures as necessary
  Have patient avoid constipation and straining through use of stool softeners or mild laxatives
Maintain diet as ordered
Feed and assist with nutritional intake as needed
Ambulate as tolerated; assist as necessary with wheelchair, walker, or cane
If patient is unable to ambulate, assist and teach patient to turn, cough, and deep breathe q2h and prn
Elevate head of bed to 30 to 45 degrees
Perform active and passive ROM exercises to all extremities q4h to 5h

Expected outcome/evaluation

Patient's self-care needs are met

■ **NDX:** Anxiety related to actual or perceived biological or psychological threat

Assess for signs and symptoms of fear and anxiety, noting verbal and nonverbal expressions
Explore feelings, encouraging patient to discuss fears and concerns regarding diagnosis and prescribed therapies
Provide emotional support
Offer simple explanations to questions
Assist patient to deal with anxiety, providing alternate methods for dealing with stress (e.g., guided imagery, relaxation techniques)

Expected outcome/evaluation

Anxiety level is reduced
Patient appears calm and is able to verbalize feelings and concerns

■ **NDX:** Knowledge deficit related to lack of information about disease process and home care management

Assess level of understanding regarding disease process and prescribed treatments
Reinforce physician's explanation of the disease and its causes, symptoms, and treatment
Encourage questions; assess for any misconceptions
Discuss medications: name, dosage, frequency of administration, purpose, and toxic or side effects

Explain need to avoid taking over-the-counter medications without checking with physician

Explain need for well-balanced diet

Explain need for ongoing rehabilitation therapy as ordered

Expected outcome/evaluation

Patient and/or significant other verbalizes knowledge and understanding of home care management, disease process, and prescribed treatment

Additional nursing diagnoses to consider

Altered comfort: pain (headache)

Potential alteration in communication, verbal

Potential for injury secondary to seizure activity

CRANIOCEREBRAL TRAUMA

Any sudden impact or blow to the head with or without loss of consciousness; the following are types of head injuries

linear fracture A break in the continuity of bone without displacing bone tissue

comminuted fracture Multiple breaks leading to fragmentation of bone

depressed fracture Bone fragments displaced below the surface of the skull

compound fracture A fracture complicated by laceration of surrounding scalp or membranes

concussion Shock to brain soft tissue without bruising or lacerations; accompanied by temporary memory loss and amnesia lasting approximately 48 hr

contusion Shock to brain soft tissue with bruising and laceration; accompanied by loss of consciousness and amnesia; patient may exhibit varying degrees of consciousness: stupor, agitation, disorientation, coma

coup-contracoup phenomenon Brain injury resulting from acceleration type of injury causing contusion and laceration in areas remote or opposite from the site of impact

subdural hematoma An accumulation of blood between the arachnoid and dura mater resulting from contusion or laceration of subdural blood vessels; symptoms (headaches, increasing drowsiness, seizures, unilateral pupil dilation) may not occur for weeks or months

epidural hematoma Bleeding in the epidural space between the skull and dura mater; usually involves a temporoparietal fracture, which results in a lacerated middle meningeal artery; transient loss of consciousness occurs and is followed by lucid periods; patient then lapses into unconsciousness again with signs of rapidly developing increased ICP; this is usually a surgical emergency

Assessment
Observations/findings

Altered level of consciousness; periods of consciousness followed by unconsciousness

Headache

Dizziness, vertigo

Posturing
  Decorticate rigidity
  Decerebrate rigidity
  Motor and/or sensory movement of extremities: unilateral, bilateral
  Weakness, paresis, paralysis, stimulus, response

Mental changes
  Irritability
  Restlessness
  Confusion
  Delirium
  Stupor
  Coma

Pupillary response
  Size, equality, response to light
  Corneal reflex

Brainstem integrity
  EOM (extraocular movement), gag or swallow reflex

Airway patency
  Rate and rhythm of respirations
  Breathing pattern
  Secretion management

Unequal pupils and uncoordinated eye movement

Periocular edema, ecchymosis

Seizure activity

Hematemesis

Projectile vomiting

Lacerations and abrasions around head and face

Drainage from ears and nose

Elevated temperature

Elevated or decreased BP

Increased weakness

Paresis or paralysis

Facial asymmetry

Aphasia

Nuchal rigidity

Dehydration

Polyuria

Bruit over carotid artery

Laboratory/diagnostic studies

Skull x-ray examinations

Cervical x-ray examinations

CT scan

MRI

Lumbar puncture; CSF sampling (may be contraindicated)

Pneumoencephalogram

Cisternogram

ABGs

Serum electrolytes, osmolality

CBC

EEG

Echoencephalogram

Potential complications

Increased ICP
Hemorrhage
Brain herniation
Respiratory failure
Neurological deficit: mild to severe
    Paresis
    Paralysis
Extracranial dissection

Medical Management

Respiratory management
Oxygenation/mechanical ventilation with volume ventilation
Surgical repair
    Craniotomy
    Ventriculostomy
    Cranioplasty
    Shunting procedures
    Tracheostomy
Medications
    Anticonvulsants
    Diuretics
    Corticosteroids
    Analgesics
    Barbiturates
ICP monitoring
Cardiac monitoring
Fluid and electrolyte management
Nutritional support
Physical therapy
Rehabilitation

Nursing diagnoses/interventions/evaluation

■ **NDX:** Potential alteration in tissue perfusion: cerebral, related to increased intracranial pressure secondary to acute head injury

Assess neurological status q15min to 30min as indicated; establish baseline parameters
Monitor and record signs of improvement or deterioration
Assess for signs of increased ICP (p. 439)
Check BP, P, and R q15min to 30min decreasing frequency as condition stabilizes
Initiate ICP monitoring as ordered; report increase of > 15 mm Hg lasting 15 to 30 min
Elevate head of bed 30 degrees; maintain head in midline position
Maintain quiet environment
Avoid or minimize activities known to precipitate valsalva maneuvers (e.g., prolonged suctioning)
Administer medications as ordered

Expected outcome/evaluation

Patient demonstrates no signs of increased intracranial pressure

Is oriented to time, place, situation
No alteration in level of consciousness
ICP of ≤ 15 mm Hg
No clinical signs of increased ICP

■ **NDX:** Ineffective airway clearance related to impaired neurological function

Assess and monitor respiratory function and secretions
Maintain patent airway: endotracheal tube or tracheostomy as ordered; suction prn
Position head to avoid obstruction of airway and provide optimal secretion removal
Administer oxygen, humidification, or mechanical ventilation as ordered
Auscultate lungs q4h to 8h
Obtain and monitor ABGs; maintain $PaCO_2$ as ordered to prevent hypoxia and hypercapnia
Assist in coughing and deep breathing when patient is conscious
Maintain head of bed elevated to 30 degrees if patient is unconscious, unless contraindicated, to maximize airway patency and control secretions
Check BP, P, R, and Glasgow Coma Scale (p. 391) q15min to 30min; report any pupillary or mental changes immediately since changes may signal respiratory embarrassment

Expected outcome/evaluation

Patient demonstrates effective breathing pattern
Clear breath sounds
ABGs and vital signs within normal limits
No signs of respiratory distress

■ **NDX:** Alteration in sensory/perceptual, cognitive, visual, auditory, kinesthetic, related to neurological trauma

Assess level of consciousness, orientation, mood/affect, and thought process; monitor and record changes
Assess for any sensory deficits: responses to pain, touch; changes in vision: blurred vision, changes in visual field, depth and perception
Assess and monitor motor coordination; ability to locate body parts
Orient to reality: environment, situation, individuals interacting with patient
Interpret sights, sounds, smells in environment
Speak in calm voice with normal tone
Maintain eye contact
Provide meaningful stimuli: clocks, calendars
    Place patient near window to differentiate day and night
Structure daily activities and routines
Place common and familiar object within field of vision

Maintain safety precautions
  Bed in low position, side rail up
  Assist with ambulation
  Remove potentially dangerous objects
Encourage decision-making, exploration of environment

Expected outcome/evaluation

Patient demonstrates improved level of consciousness, appropriate perceptual functioning

■ **NDX:** Potential for alteration in self-concept/body image related to perceived changes in physical and personal self-image

Assess perception of body image and relate to degree of disability
Provide emotional support; allow patient to verbalize needs and to participate in planning care
Encourage verbalization of feelings about body image and functional changes
Acknowledge and praise attempts to improve body image (e.g., wearing make-up, selecting clothing)
Assist patient to accept physical disability; assist patient to identify other physical characteristics that remain unchanged
Offer supportive counseling
Encourage participation in counseling and/or self-help group

Expected outcome/evaluation

Patient verbalizes positive expression of body image
  Demonstrates signs of decreasing body image disturbance

■ **NDX:** Knowledge deficit related to lack of information about disease process and home care management

Discuss nature of disorder, treatment, and procedures; explain as they occur
Explain to family need to encourage verbalization about any body image change or limitations
Explain need to ambulate as tolerated
Explain importance of planned rest periods

Discuss possible residual effects such as dizziness, headache, and memory loss, which may persist for 3 to 4 months after trauma
Discuss medications: name, dosage, frequency of administration, purpose, and toxic or side effects
Explain need to avoid taking over-the-counter medications without checking with physician
Discuss symptoms of progression of condition to report to physician
Explain importance of ongoing outpatient care
  Physician's visits
  Physical therapy
Explain importance of diet as ordered; need to chew and swallow slowly
Discuss care of abrasions or lacerations as indicated

Expected outcome/evaluation

Patient and/or significant other demonstrates knowledge and ability needed for self-care and home care management

Additional nursing diagnoses to consider

Impaired mobility: physical, related to neurophysiological function (see Cerebrovascular Accident, p. 405)
Potential unilateral neglect related to right cerebral hemisphere lesions secondary to neurological trauma (see Cerebrovascular Accident, p. 405)

SPINAL CORD INJURIES

cord injuries *Injuries in which the spinal cord is compressed by fractured or displaced vertebrae, bleeding, or edema*
cervical cord injuries *Level of injury is located in the cervical spine C-2 to C-6*
thoracic cord injuries *Level of injury is located in the thoracic spine T-1 to T-12*
lumbar cord injuries *Level of injury is located in the lumbar spine L-1 to L-2*
NOTE: Clinical descriptions of spinal cord injuries generally refer to deficits in terms of upper motor neuron (UMN) and lower motor neuron (LMN): UMN injuries involve the corticobulbar or corticospinal tract and result in muscle spasticity and increased tendon reflexes;

TABLE 8-5. Clinical Manifestations of Upper and Lower Motor Neuron Lesions

Upper motor neuron	Lower motor neuron
Muscle spasticity, possible contractures	Muscle flaccidity
Little or no muscle atrophy	Muscle atrophy
Hyperreflexia	Loss of muscle tone
	Hyporeflexia or areflexia
	Fasciculations
Damage above level of brainstem will affect opposite side of the body	Muscle changes will be in muscles supplied by that nerve—usually muscle on same side as lesion

From Rudy EB: *Advanced neurological and neurosurgical nursing*, St Louis, 1984, CV Mosby.

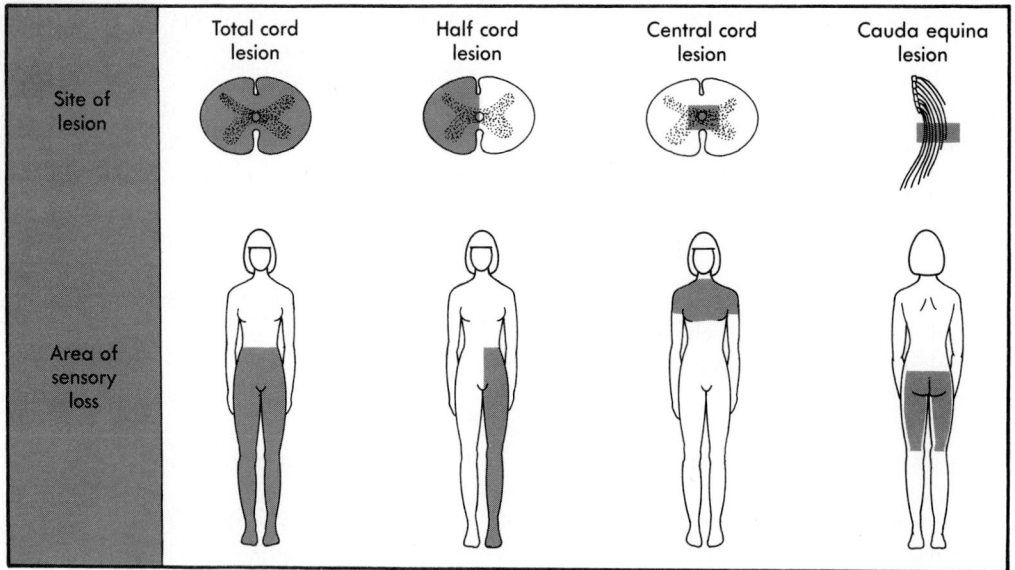

	Total cord lesion	Half cord lesion	Central cord lesion	Cauda equina lesion
Site of lesion				
Area of sensory loss				

FIGURE 8-7. Common patterns of sensory abnormality. *Upper diagrams,* site of lesion; *lower diagrams,* distribution of corresponding sensory loss. (From Thelan LA, Davie JK, and Urden LD: *Textbook of critical care nursing: diagnosis and management,* St Louis, 1990, Mosby—Year Book.)

LMN injuries involve anterior horn cells or nerve fibers after their exit from the spinal cord and result in muscle flaccidity, loss of reflexes, loss of tone, and muscle atrophy (Table 8-5) (Figure 8-7)

Assessment
Observations/findings
CORD INJURIES

Loss of power, movement, and sensation of extremities below level of injury
Pain at level of injury
Urinary retention
Priapism
Absence of vasomotor tone and perspiration in cervical and upper thoracic cord injuries

CERVICAL CORD INJURIES

Paralysis of all extremities and trunk
Respiratory failure: hypoxemia
Bladder and bowel disturbances
  Bladder retention, spasticity
  Bowel incontinence
Autonomic dysreflexia
  Bradycardia
  Sweating
  Elevated temperature
  Paroxysmal hypertension
  Headache
  Neurogenic shock

THORACIC CORD INJURIES

Paralysis of lower extremities; initially muscles are flaccid—later become spastic
Paralysis of bladder, bowel, and sphincters
Pain to chest or back
Abdominal distention
Loss of sexual function

LUMBAR CORD INJURIES

Paralysis of lower extremities, bladder, and rectum
  Flaccid muscles during spinal shock phase
  Spastic muscular activity
Loss of sexual function

Laboratory/diagnostic studies

X-ray examination: vertebral fractures
CT scan
MRI
Arterial blood gases
CBC with differential
Electrolytes

Potential complications

Respiratory arrest
Spinal shock
  Complete transection
    Flaccid paralysis below level of injury
    Loss of reflexes below level of injury
    Loss or proprioception, sensations of touch, temperature, and pressure below level of injury

Loss of somatic and visceral sensations
Loss of ability to perspire below level of injury
Decreased BP
Urinary retention
Paralytic ileus
Bowel dysfunction
Possible priapism
Bladder dysfunction
Urinary tract infection
Autonomic dysreflexia
Sexual dysfunction
Malnutrition: acute or chronic
Decubitus
Contractures, ankylosis
Spasms
Foot-drop, wrist-drop
Behavioral changes
    Anxiety
    Grief reaction
    Acute depression

Medical Management

Surgical
    Decompression: laminectomy
    Stabilization: spinal fusion
    Skull tongs (Crutchfield, Vinke, Cone, Gardner-Wells)
    Halo traction
Ventilatory support; tidal volume measurements
Medication
    Muscle relaxants
    Tranquilizers
    Anticoagulants
    Laxatives
    Antacids
    Steroids
Stryker or Foster frame or kinetic treatment table
Splints, braces
Cardiac monitoring
Fluid/electrolyte management
Intake and output
Urinary catheterization
Neurological rehabilitation

Nursing diagnoses/interventions/evaluation

■ **NDX:**   Ineffective breathing pattern related to neurogenic or traumatic injury

Maintain patent airway; avoid flexion of the neck
Assess respiratory function, noting rate, quality, and depth of respirations
Assess ability and quality of cough
Assess motor-sensory function to ensure adequate rhythm or pattern of respiration
Auscultate breath sounds
Administer assisted ventilation and oxygenation as ordered; measure vital capacity and minute ventilation to ensure adequate ventilation
Be aware that tracheostomy may be indicated
Provide nasal or oropharyngeal airway and suction as needed
Monitor vital signs with neurological check q1h to 2h as indicators of impaired ventilatory status
Obtain and monitor ABGs

Expected outcome/evaluation

Patient demonstrates effective breathing pattern
    Chest expansion is symmetrical
    Breath sounds are clear to auscultation
    ABGs and vital signs are within normal limits
    No sign of respiratory distress

■ **NDX:**   Self-care deficit: hygiene, feeding, toileting, and/or mobility related to neurophysiological impairment

Assess level of injury and related disability in performing self-care needs
Maintain NPO until chewing, swallowing, and gastrointestinal (GI) function is established
Provide nutritional support as ordered; consult with dietician to establish nutritional needs
Assist with feedings as necessary
Encourage fluid intake to 2000 ml/day unless contraindicated
Connect indwelling catheter to closed gravity drainage system as ordered
Check urine for presence of calculi
Administer catheter care bid
Give colon lavage or enemas q3d as ordered
Perform passive ROM exercises to extremities; check with physician before starting exercises
Assist and teach muscle-building exercises as indicated
    Squeeze toys
    Rubber balls
    Clay
Use trapezes and pulleys
Apply antiembolic stockings
Administer oral hygiene q2h to 4h; brush teeth
Administer skin care q2h to 4h
    Give back rubs
    Use sheepskin
    Use footboard
    Use heel and/or elbow guards
Provide for total physical hygiene as indicated
    Comb hair daily; shampoo weekly as indicated
Explain importance of skin care

Expected outcome/evaluation

Patient's self-care needs are met

Fluid and nutritional needs are met
Elimination needs are met
Skin, oral, and eye hygiene needs are met
Passive or active range of motion exercise is performed

■ **NDX:** Grieving dysfunction related to loss of physio-psychosocial well-being

Assess and monitor patient's perceptions of medical conditions and prognosis response from staff, significant others, social network
Assess stage of grieving that patient is experiencing
Shock and disbelief
Provide simple but honest explanation to questions regarding diagnosis, treatments, and prognoses, identify and correct misconceptions
Permit and encourage expressions of emotions
Allow use of denial; avoid confronting patients when experiencing distorted perceptions
Point out reality in nonthreatening manner
Refrain from judgmental responses
Avoid reinforcement of denial
Provide encouragement and supportive counseling
Anger
Accept expressions of emotion; avoid arguing
Identify manipulative and disruptive behavior; set limits on acting-out when necessary

Expected outcome/evaluation

Patient demonstrates beginning of resolution of feelings
Participates in prescribed treatment
Is able to express thoughts and feelings related to loss

■ **NDX:** Knowledge deficit related to lack of information about diagnosis and potential home care management

Ensure that patient and significant other are informed about disease and prognosis
Prepare for chronicity and duration of rehabilitative process
Discuss medications: name, dosage, route, side effects, and purpose
Refer to appropriate rehabilitative and counseling resources

Expected outcome/evaluation

Patient and/or significant other demonstrates knowledge and understanding of home care management
Demonstrates passive or active ROM exercises
States all relevant information regarding medications, time of dose, side effects, and purpose
Identifies high-calorie, high-protein foods and states understanding of need for maintenance of diet
States understanding of fluid intake maintenance to avoid infection risk and constipation

Additional nursing diagnoses to consider

Impaired mobility: physical alteration in sensory perception
Powerlessness
Alteration in skin integrity
Incontinence, reflex
Altered bowel elimination: constipation

SURGICAL INTERVENTION OF CENTRAL NERVOUS SYSTEM

Surgical repair of conditions involving the brain, spinal cord, cranial nerves, and cerebral vasculature
craniotomy Surgical revision, resection, or removal of growths or abnormalities within the cranium; consists of removing and replacing bones of the skull to provide access to intracranial structures
craniectomy Removal of a portion of the skull; includes burr hole performance

Assessment
Postoperative observations/findings

Level of consciousness
See Glasgow Coma Scale for rapid assessment (p. 391)
Pupillary response; ocular movement
Visual disturbances
Periocular edema
Focal neurological deficits
Pain: headache
Personality changes
Respirations
Rate
Pattern
Motor-sensory function
Paresthesia
Paralysis

Laboratory/diagnostic studies

CBC
Serum chemistries: BUN, FBS, creatinine

Potential complications

Seizure activity
Increased ICP
Diabetes insipidus
Hemorrhage
Infection of bone graft
Cardiac dysrhythmias
Meningitis
Thrombophlebitis
Adult respiratory distress syndrome (ARDS)

Medical Management

Oxygenation/ventilatory support
Medications
Corticosteroids

Anticonvulsants
Antiemetics
Antipyretics
Analgesics
Diuretics
Antibiotics
Antacids
Histamine-blocking agents
Stool softeners
Parenteral therapy
Diet
ICP monitoring
Cardiac monitoring
Physical therapy
Neurological rehabilitation

Nursing diagnoses/interventions/evaluation

■ **NDX:** Potential for ineffective breathing pattern related to postanesthesia recovery and possible neurological depression

Assess spontaneous respiratory function: monitor rate, quality, and depth of respirations
See Care of Patient in Recovery Room (p. 28)
Maintain patent airway
Maintain neck in neutral position
Position on side with head of bed elevated to 30 degrees
Report any change in vital signs, level of consciousness, or restlessness immediately
Administer oxygen with assisted ventilation as ordered
Monitor arterial blood gases
Maintain parenteral therapy as indicated
Assess ventilatory status
Auscultate chest for breath sounds q1h to 2h and prn
Maintain optimal positioning to promote ventilatory status
Assist and teach patient to turn and deep breathe q2h

Expected outcome/evaluation

Patient demonstrates effective breathing pattern
Chest expansion is symmetrical
Breath sounds are clear to auscultation
ABGs and vital signs are within normal limits
No signs of respiratory distress

■ **NDX:** Alteration in cerebral/peripheral tissue perfusion related to interruption of arterial flow

Maintain bed rest with head of bed elevated 15 to 30 degrees or as ordered
Check BP, P, and R and do neurological check q15min to 30min
Monitor ICP and report sustained elevations or trends to elevation immediately

Report immediately any sudden changes in BP, pupillary or neurological status, numbness, tingling, weakness, or loss of pulses
Assess for restlessness and seizure activity
Check rectal temperature q2h to 4h; hypothermia or cooling measures may be indicated
Maintain parenteral fluids as ordered
Maintain bed rest; use firm mattress or bedboard
Provide cervical collar or cervical traction as ordered
Keep head in neutral or slightly flexed position

Expected outcome/evaluation

Patient maintains adequate tissue perfusion
Is alert and oriented
Cognitive processes are intact
Evidences sensory-motor integrity

■ **NDX:** Self-care deficit: feeding, hygiene, toileting, and/or mobility, related to physical postoperative limitations

Assess degree of functional disability
Maintain proper positioning as indicated by surgical restrictions
Limit activities and perform nursing functions as indicated
Maintain quiet environment
Administer skin care q4h to 5h
Give back rubs
Use air mattress (for patient in traction)
Use sheepskin
Check for redness, irritation, and pressure areas q2h to 4h when patient is in traction
Provide additional padding and pressure reduction if indicated
Keep skin dry
Meet all physical hygiene needs as indicated
Provide passive or active ROM to nonoperative extremities
Maintain patient NPO until otherwise ordered
Provide fluid and/or diet within restrictions as ordered; assess for swallowing and chewing ability
Maintain adequate elimination
Initiate voiding measures as appropriate
Monitor time and amount

Expected outcome/evaluation

Patient's self-care needs are met
Medications are administered as ordered
Fluid and nutritional needs are met
Elimination needs are met
Skin, oral, and eye hygiene needs are met
Passive or active ROM exercises are performed
Planned rest periods are maintained

■ **NDX:** Knowledge deficit related to lack of information about disease process and potential home management

Assess cognitive and motor skills; assess level of understanding regarding diagnosis and prescribed treatment

Explain nature of disorder, symptoms, and importance of maintaining traction, corset, or braces at home

Explain to family need to encourage verbalization; to deal with body image changes and anxieties over disability and loss of work

Teach principles of body mechanics

Avoid bending from waist: keep back straight, bend knees, and lower body to pick up objects

Use straight, flat chairs; avoid soft-cushioned chairs

Avoid crossing knees

Avoid lifting while back is flexed or twisted

Explain need to avoid constipation through use of stool softeners, mild laxatives, and/or fruit juices and roughage in diet

Explain need to avoid extremes of hot and cold to lower extremities because of possible sensory nerve loss

Explain need to avoid hyperextension of spine while sleeping; to avoid sleeping in prone position or straight supine position

Explain need to sleep on side with knees and hips in flexion

Explain need to wear corset or brace support as ordered

Explain need for exercise as ordered; instruct patient to stop exercises if pain is unrelieved or worsens

Explain importance of maintaining diet as ordered

Discuss medications: name, dosage, time of administration, purpose, and side effects

Explain need to avoid taking over-the-counter medications without checking with physician

Explain importance of ongoing outpatient care

Physician's visits

Physical therapy

Ensure that patient and/or significant other demonstrates proper use and maintenance of traction and corsets

Expected outcome/evaluation

Patient and/or significant other demonstrates knowledge and understanding of home care management

Demonstrates passive or active ROM exercises

States all relevant information regarding medications, time of dose, side effects, and purpose

Identifies high-calorie, high-protein food and states understanding of need for maintenance of diet

States understanding of fluid intake maintenance to avoid infection risk and constipation

ALZHEIMER'S DISEASE

Progressive deterioration of intellect, memory, personality, and self-care, leading to severe dementia from degeneration of nerve cells in the cerebral cortex

Assessment
Observations/findings
EARLY

Memory loss

Loss of orientation to time and location

Inability to recognize family and friends

Lack of recent memories but able to recall early life events

Personality changes

Apathy, loss of initiative

Anxiety, fear, belligerence, stubbornness

Suspicion progressing to paranoia

Loss of sense of humor

Insensitivity to others

Intellectual changes

Difficulty in making decisions or plans

Inability to calculate (e.g., money transactions)

Loss of train of thought during conversations

Requiring repetitive directions

Inattentiveness

Conversation changes: slow speech, loss of words, use of cliches

Fatigues easily

Mood

Reactive depression

Crying spells

Lethargy

Neglect of self-care

Nocturnal wandering

ADVANCED

Apathetic, mute

Inability to recall recent or remote events

Disorientation/confusion

Inability to perform ADLs

Incontinence

Potential complications

Physical and/or psychological dependence

Social isolation

Injury

Dehydration/malnutrition

Medical Management

Supportive management

Physiological and psychological support measures for patient and family to enhance coping with progressive deterioration

*Nursing diagnoses/interventions/evaluation**

■ **NDX:** Potential for injury related to deterioration of physiological and cognitive function

Maintain safety precautions

---

*Care and teaching are combined to provide nurse and family with consistent approach.

Have attendant with patient during any treatment or procedure
Remove or disconnect door locks
Avoid having patient use razors without assistance
Avoid potentially dangerous tasks (e.g., smoking, cooking)
Assist with ADLs

Expected outcome/evaluation

Patient is free of injury
Demonstrates no signs of physical injuries

■ **NDX:** Alteration in thought processes related to loss of memory

Explain to patient and family the nature of this disorder; that it is progressive
Assist with reality orientation
Introduce all care givers by name each time; repeat on regular basis
Writing instructions and directions may be helpful
Provide large-face clock and current calendar
Orient patient to day, hour, and location frequently
Speak in quiet tones
Maintain calm atmosphere; avoid rushing
Use consistency and repetition with patient
Give singular, simple instructions

Expected outcome/evaluation

Patient demonstrates enhanced interpretation of reality
Oriented to environment, self, time
Makes wants and needs known

■ **NDX:** Self-care deficit: hygiene, nutrition, and/or toileting related to physiological and/or psychological dependence

Assess degree of self-care needs
Provide for physical hygiene needs: bathing, shampooing, skin and oral care
Provide properly balanced diet
Administer diet as ordered; present one course at a time (e.g., salad first, then entree)
Assist patient in cutting food as needed
Establish regular bowel habits
Determine patient's normal patterns
Instruct patient to go to bathroom at scheduled times
Recognize signs of impaction
No formed stool for 3 days
Semiliquid stools
Restlessness
Discuss treatment for impaction: laxative, suppository, enema
Establish routine voiding measures
Remind patient to go to bathroom q2h
Avoid giving fluids before bedtime
Use disposable diapers prn
Administer medications as ordered

Expected outcome/evaluation

Patient's self-care needs are met
Nutritional intake is adequate
Elimination needs are met

■ **NDX:** Potential for ineffective family coping related to long-term deteriorating effects of disease process

Provide emotional support
Refer family to support groups
Refer to social services for financial concerns and potential placement
Refer to home care services for potential in-home assistance for home maintenance and management problems
Ensure that family and/or significant others are informed about disease process and physician's instructions for supportive care

Expected outcome/evaluation

Family and/or significant others are coping effectively with home management and proper resources are being used for patient care needs, counseling, and financial assistance

PARKINSON'S DISEASE

A progressive, degenerative disease of the brain's dopamine neuronal system, most commonly idiopathic in nature

Assessment
Observations/findings

Rigidity of limbs: arms lose natural swing and remain at side of body
Tremors
Exaggerated by stress and anxiety
Most severe when limb is resting; absent during sleep
Fingers: pill-rolling movement
Head: to-and-fro tremor
Movements
Voluntary body movements become slower (bradykinesia)
Starting activities become difficult (akinesia)
Posture
Bent forward
Walking with slow, short, shuffling steps
Breaking into run if pushed
Uncoordinated and/or loss of muscular activity: impaired writing (micrographia)
Restlessness (motor restlessness, akathisia)
Stiffness and diffuse pain in legs and shoulders
Blank facial expression (masked facies)
Wide-eyed
Infrequent blinking of eyes
Speech
Slowed, soft, monotonous

Dysarthric
Slurred
Soft spoken, decreased volume
Dysphagia
Excessive salivation and drooling
Emotional changes
Depression
Nervousness
Mood swings
Hallucinations
Paranoia
Dementia
Side effects of drugs

Laboratory/diagnostic studies

CSF
Usually within normal limits
May show slight increase in protein level
CT scan
Normal results or may show cerebral atrophy
Mild microcytic anemia
GI studies
Hypomotility
Delayed emptying of stomach
Varying degrees of bowel distention
EEG
Normal with minimal slowing
Marked or moderate slowing and/or disorganization (with marked dementia or bradykinesia)

Medical Management

Surgical stereotactic thalamotomy to relieve contralateral tremor and rigidity
Medications
Levodopa
Carbidopa (Sinemet)
Anticholinergics
Benztropine mesylate (Cogentin)
Trihexyphenidyl (Artane)
Antiparkinsonian and antihistamine
Orphenadrine hydrochloride (Disipal)
Diphenhydramine hydrochloride (Benadryl)
Amantadine hydrochloride (Symmetrel)
Ethopropazine hydrochloride (Parsidol)
Nutritional therapy
Physical therapy
Occupational therapy
Speech therapy
Surgery
Stereotactic thalamotomy

Nursing diagnoses/interventions/evaluation

■ **NDX:** Impaired mobility: physical, related to neurological degenerative disorder

Assess level of disability
Encourage ambulation to tolerance
Assist to chair
Perform active or passive ROM exercises q4h to all extremities
Neck
Hands and fingers
Wrists
Elbows
Knees
Evaluate effectiveness of drug therapy
Initiate gait-retraining program; consult with physical therapy department
Provide physical therapy as ordered: massage and stretching exercises
Have patient practice lifting legs while walking rather than shuffling; try to maintain erect position
Maintain planned rest periods
Conduct occupational therapy as indicated by amount of tremors
Assist patient with turning q2h to 4h if unable to move self

Expected outcome/evaluation

Patient demonstrates optimal level of mobility appropriate for physical disability

■ **NDX:** Alteration in self-care ability; feeding, hygiene

Assess functional disability related to self-care needs
Assess nutritional needs; consult with dietitian
Maintain well-balanced soft diet
Avoid foods and medications that contain pyridoxine HCl (vitamin B_6)
Maintain frequent small feedings as indicated
Maintain fluid intake to 2000 ml/day unless contraindicated
Maintain supplemental high-calorie fluids such as eggnog, milk shakes, and malts
Use bibs and straws as indicated; place food and drinks within easy reach of patient
Initiate voiding measures as necessary
Institute bladder control program as indicated
Have patient avoid constipation through use of high-residue foods, stool softeners, and/or enemas
Provide or assist with general hygiene as indicated
Administer oral hygiene q4h to 6h and prn
Encourage self-care as tolerated: bathing, mouth care

Expected outcome/evaluation

Patient's self-care needs are met
Demonstrates optimal nutritional intake
Demonstrates skin integrity

■ **NDX:** Potential for alteration in self-concept related to actual or perceived changes in physical and personal self-image

Provide emotional support; allow patient to verbalize needs and to participate in planning care

Encourage verbalization of feelings about body image and functional changes

Acknowledge and support attempts to improve appearance

Permit expression of emotions

Encourage use of support groups

Expected outcome/evaluation

Patient experiences self-respect and self-confidence
   Achieves goals that reflect awareness of abilities and limitations
   Acknowledges and supports attempts to improve appearance
   Permits expression of emotions
   Uses support groups

■ **NDX:** Knowledge deficit related to lack of information about diagnosis and home care maintenance

Assess level of understanding regarding disease and treatments prescribed

Reinforce physician's explanation of disease and its causes, symptoms, and treatment

Discuss importance of verbalization about loss of body function, self-esteem, and sexuality

Explain that behavioral changes may be part of disease process or may be due to medications

Emphasize need to discuss feelings about symptoms
   Tremors
   Drooling
   Slurred speech

Explain to family
   Need to provide psychological support
   Need to emphasize capabilities rather than limitations
   Need to encourage active participation in family activities
   Need to encourage socialization
   Need to encourage independence; avoid overprotection
   Need to permit patient to do things for himself
      Self-care
      Feedings
      Dressing
      Ambulation
      That although patient may be physically disabled, he is intellectually normal

Discuss need for family to show security, love, a need for patient, and patience with and understanding of patient's slowness and clumsiness

Explain that frustration over tremors and dependence may be source of patient's irritability and loss of self-interest

Discuss agencies available for use as resources, such as the American Parkinson Disease Association[*]

Explain importance of daily exercise to delay progression of disease

Explain importance of performing any physical task that is difficult 5 to 10 times a day

Explain importance of ongoing outpatient care
   Physician's visits
   Physical therapy

Discuss medications: name, dosage, frequency of administration, purpose, and toxic or side effects

Explain need to avoid taking over-the-counter medications without checking with physician

Explain need for well-balanced, soft diet; limit high-protein foods, which may block effects of drugs
   Cut foods for patient
   Place all utensils within easy reach
   Use blender for thick foods
   Use braces for severe tremors occurring during meals
   Maintain fluid intake to 2000 ml/day unless contraindicated
   Serve frequent, small feedings
   Serve supplemental high-calorie fluids such as eggnog and milk shakes
   Use straws and bibs for excessive drooling
   Avoid food high in vitamin B_6 (reverses effects of levodopa)
   Instruct patient to swallow slowly and to take small bites of food

Explain need for activity
   Plan rest periods
   Perform passive or active ROM exercises to all extremities
   Encourage family or significant other to participate in physical therapy exercise of stretching and massaging muscles
   Give warm baths
   Encourage daily ambulation outdoors but have patient avoid extremely hot or cold weather
   Encourage patient to practice lifting feet while walking, using heel-toe gait, and swinging arms deliberately while walking
   Place head of bed or back of chair on blocks to facilitate getting out of bed or chair; use pulleys such as sheets tied to end of bed
   Have patient avoid sitting for long periods of time
   Encourage patient to dress daily
      Avoid clothing with buttons; use zippers instead
      Avoid shoes with laces or snaps
   Provide diversional activities depending on extent of tremors and disability

---

[*]American Parkinson Disease Association, 116 John St., New York, N.Y., 10038; National Parkinson's Foundation Hotline: 1-800-327-4545.

Reading
Watching television
Listening to radio
Engaging in hobbies
Painting

Prevent falls and injuries by clearing walkways of furniture and scatter rugs; build side rails on stairs and in tub or shower

Provide supports as indicated when patient is ambulating with walker or cane

Provide speech therapy
Instruct patient to speak slowly and practice reading aloud slowly in an exaggerated manner
Provide electronic amplifiers as ordered for weak voice

Explain need for oral hygiene q2h to 4h and prn; need to control drooling
Have tissues easily accessible to patient (e.g., in pockets)
Have patient use bib while eating
Clean corners of mouth after eating and prn
Apply ointment if necessary

Explain importance of proper elimination
Conduct voiding measures as necessary
Conduct bladder control program as necessary
Provide raised toilet seat with side rails in home to facilitate sitting and standing

Expected outcome/evaluation

Patient and/or significant other demonstrates optimal knowledge concerning Parkinson's disease and related home maintenance

Additional nursing diagnoses to consider

Impaired communication: verbal
Potential for injury
Social isolation

MULTIPLE SCLEROSIS (DISSEMINATED SCLEROSIS)

A chronic, progressive disease characterized by scattering of demyelinating lesions in the central nervous system (CNS), which affect the white matter of the brain and spinal cord

Assessment
Observations/findings

Fatigue; may be increased by heat (e.g., hot bath or shower)
Sensory impairment
Numbness
Tingling
Loss of position sense: staggering gait
Weakness of extremities
Facial palsy

Hyperactive reflexes
Poor coordination
Ataxia
Spasticity of extremities
Tremors
Staggering gait
Dizziness, vertigo
Visual disturbances
Diplopia
Blurred vision
Dilation of affected pupil when light is shone into eye (Marcus Gunn phenomenon)
Nystagmus
Optic neuritis
Speech impairment: scanning speech
Muscular spasms
Positive Babinski's sign
Weakness of throat muscles: difficulty in chewing and swallowing
Impotence
Fecal and/or urinary incontinence or retention
Mental changes
Mood swings
Depression
Euphoria
Irritability
Apathy
Inattention
Lack of judgment
Memory deficits

Laboratory/diagnostic studies

CSF
Usually normal
Normal with low protein
Increased white blood cell count (WBC)
Increased gamma globulin level
MRI
Myleography
CT scan

Potential complications

Neurological deficit; paralysis, quadriplegia
Sexual dysfunction
Spastic bladder, urinary retention
Respiratory failure

Medical Management

Medications
Antiinflammatory agents
ACTH
Corticosteroids
Muscle relaxants
Immunosuppressive agents
Vitamin B

Antidepressants
Antianxiety drugs/tranquilizers
Beta-adrenergic blocking agents
Physical therapy
Occupational therapy
Rehabilitation
Psychotherapy/counseling
Nutritional therapy

Nursing diagnoses/interventions/evaluation

■ **NDX:**   Impaired mobility: physical, related to neuro-muscular impairment

Assess and monitor degree of physical disability
NOTE: Limit activity level when patient is unduly tired, during periods of exacerbation
Maintain quiet, relaxing, and cool environment
Institute activity
   Massage and stretch muscles
   Perform resistive exercises to all extremities and joints
   Perform active or passive ROM exercises q4h to 5h and prn
   Instruct patient to avoid exercising when tired and on hot days
   Encourage ambulation to tolerance
   Encourage self-care activities
   Avoid use of heating pad; measure bathwater temperature (heat reduces muscle strength)
   Plan all activities to avoid fatigue
   Plan rest periods
   Encourage diversional activities during periods of exacerbation
      Reading
      Watching television
      Listening to radio and/or talking books
If patient is confined to bed rest
   Position comfortably
   Turn q2h to 4h and prn
   Perform active or passive ROM exercises q2h to 4h
   Perform dorsiflexion of ankles and quadriceps q2h to 4h
   Help patient out of bed and into chair two or three times daily
   Feed as necessary; hand braces may be indicated

Expected outcome/evaluation

Patient
   Demonstrates improved or minimal degree of physical immobility
   Participates in activities that promote improved function
   Verbalizes understanding of conditions that may exacerbate symptoms

■ **NDX:**   Alteration in elimination: bowel and bladder, related to neuromuscular impairment

Assess degree of functional disability
Initiate bladder program as indicated
   Assess bladder function and voiding pattern (urgency, frequency, incontinence, nocturia)
   Measure intake and output
   Catheterize intermittently as indicated
   Teach self-catheterization whenever possible
   Plan bladder dysfunction program as appropriate for spasticity or flaccidity
Institute bowel control program
   Establish regular bowel routines
   Avoid constipation
Maintain high-fiber diet
Encourage fluids to 3000 ml/day unless contraindicated

Expected outcome/evaluation

Patient
   Maintains bladder and bowel elimination
   Has stable intake and output
   Evidences no bladder distention
   Has regular bowel evacuation pattern
   Does not experience fecal impaction

■ **NDX:**   Activity intolerance related to generalized weakness secondary to neuromuscular disease

Assess energy level and ability to carry out activities
Assess sleep and rest patterns; determine when patient feels strongest
Schedule nursing care, procedures, and tests to permit maximum periods of rest
Plan periods of uninterrupted rest
Assist patient to plan activities at level of ability
Instruct patient to avoid activities when tired or on days that are hot

Expected outcome/evaluation

Patient demonstrates improved activity tolerance
   Verbalizes understanding of activity allowance and limitations
   Verbalizes understanding of need to balance activities and periods of rest

■ **NDX:**   Potential for disturbance in self-concept: body image and self-esteem, related to altered perception of self

Assess patient's perception of illness and physical disabilities
Encourage questions and verbalization of feelings
Provide accurate explanation of disease process
Acknowledge and permit discussion related to actual and perceived changes
Acknowledge concerns about body image

Be supportive of patient's emotional changes and needs for improving image and esteem

Permit expression of emotion

Expected outcome/evaluation

Patient experiences self-confidence and demonstrates beginning of adaptation to physical changes

■ **NDX:** Potential for ineffective airway clearance related to motor weakness and/or immobility

Assess respiration: rate, depth, and pattern; assess degree of respiratory effort and cough reflex

Suction oral pharynx as needed

Assist and teach patient to cough and deep breathe q2h to 4h and prn

Maintain patent airway and avoid flexion of patient's neck if immobile

Auscultate breath sounds q2h to 4h and prn

Position patient for maximal respiratory expansion and control of respiratory secretions

Expected outcome/evaluation

Patient demonstrates effective breathing pattern
  Chest expansion is symmetrical
  Breath sounds are clear to auscultation
  ABGs and vital signs are within normal limits
  No signs of respiratory distress

■ **NDX:** Knowledge deficit related to lack of information about disease process

Assess level of understanding regarding disease process

Explain nature of disease, emphasizing that this is not a hereditary disease

Explain that warm weather and hot baths may increase weakness

Explain importance of avoiding fatigue and becoming overworked or emotionally stressed, since these may be precipitating factors in exacerbation

Explain importance of exercising regularly; need to maintain rest periods

Explain need to do muscle stretching exercises daily

Explain need for ROM exercises for patient with spasticity

Explain importance of daily routines for activities and rest periods

Discuss need for patient support when ambulating with walker, cane, or braces as indicated

Instruct patient to walk with a wide base, keeping feet apart

Emphasize importance of speech therapy; instruct patient to speak slowly and practice reading aloud

Emphasize need for diversional activities
  Reading
  Watching television
  Listening to radio
  Knitting
  Playing quiet games

Explain importance of decubitus care if patient is confined to bed rest or wheelchair

Explain importance of regulating bathwater temperature; need to avoid extremes of hot and cold because of loss of temperature change sense

Discuss symptoms of disease progression to report to physician

Explain importance of avoiding persons with infections, especially URIs

Discuss symptoms of cold or flu to report to physician
  Elevated temperature
  Chills
  Cough
  Extreme fatigue

Encourage activity as long as patient is able
  Recreational activities
  Work
  Household chores

Encourage verbalization

Allow time for patient to complete all activities and deal with any body image changes and loss of self-esteem

Encourage socialization with friends and family

Encourage independence and self-care to point of tolerance

Expected outcome/evaluation

Patient and/or significant other demonstrates knowledge necessary for home maintenance management

Additional nursing diagnoses to consider

Potential alterations in sensory perceptions: visual
Role performance: altered
Coping: ineffective individual

MYASTHENIA GRAVIS

A neuromuscular disorder characterized by muscular weakness and fatigue resulting from a defect in transmission of motor impulses at the neuromuscular junction; probably a result of an autoimmune response

Assessment
Observations/findings

Fatigue
Expressionless facies/facial droop
Generalized weakness
  Increased with exercise
  May be confined to one area
  Weakness of face, jaw, neck, arms, hands, and/or legs
Difficulty in raising arms above head or extending fingers outward
Dysphagia/drooling

Difficulty in chewing
Weak, high-pitched, soft voice
Ptosis of one or both eyelids
Ocular palsy
Diplopia
Inability to walk on heels; may walk on toes
Strength decreases as day progresses
Stress incontinence
Anal sphincter weakness
Respirations
  Shallow
  Decreased vital capacity (VC)
  Use of accessory muscles
  Muffled cough

Laboratory/diagnostic studies

CT scan of chest or chest x-ray examination indicating
  thymoma
Tensilon test
Single-fiber electromyogram
Nerve conduction studies
Anti-acetylcholine receptor (ACLR) antibody test

Potential complications

Myasthenia crisis
Cholinergic crisis
Neuromuscular deficit: mild to severe
Pneumonia
Aspiration, atelectasis
Respiratory failure

Medical Management

Surgery
Plasmapheresis
  Thymectomy
  Tracheostomy
Mechanical ventilation/oxygen therapy
Physical therapy
Occupational therapy
Medications
  Anticholinesterase
  Corticosteroids
  Pituitary hormones
Nutritional support

Nursing diagnoses/interventions/evaluation

■ **NDX:** Impaired communication: verbal related to
  neuromuscular disease

Assess degree of speech impairment
Avoid rushing patient: provide sufficient time to respond
Provide for alternative communication methods if vocal-
  ization is impaired

Magic Slate
Pencil and pad
Provide handkerchief or tissues
Stand close to patient; listen carefully

Expected outcome/evaluation

Accepted method of communication is established
  Verbalizes understanding of alternative methods of
  communicating need

■ **NDX:** Self-care deficit: feeding, hygiene, related to
  decreased motor function

Assess severity of deficits
Initiate a self-care plan that permits patient maximum
  participation
Maintain regular diet as tolerated; with persistent dys-
  phagia, tube feeding may be indicated; small, frequent
  feedings may be indicated
Administer oral hygiene q2h to 4h, after meals, and prn
Meet physical hygiene needs as indicated
Administer skin care q4h to 6h
  Turn patient q2h to 4h if patient is unable to ambulate
  Apply sheepskin
  Rub back
Administer eye care q4h to 5h
  Remove any formed crusts
  Place eye patch over affected eye
  Administer eye drops as ordered

Expected outcome/evaluation

Patient's self-care needs are met as evidenced by optimal
  nutritional status and skin integrity

■ **NDX:** Alteration in mobility related to neuromuscular
  weakness

Assess degree of physical limitations
Assess medications, check dosage, times taken
Work with patient to determine time of day patient is
  weakest
Increase activity to tolerance; plan treatments and major
  activities early in day or 30 min after medication is
  taken
Perform passive or active ROM exercises q4h to 5h and
  prn
Maintain planned rest periods
Administer medication as ordered
  Anticholinesterase: to be given 20 to 30 min before
    meals; note increase in muscular strength within 30
    min of taking medication
  Medication should always be taken at scheduled time;
    never miss a dose (rationale: anticholinesterase max-
    imizes physical mobility)

Expected outcome/evaluation

Patient experiences optimal mobility

■ **NDX:** Potential for alteration in self-concept: body image, related to actual or perceived changes in physical and personal self-image

Assess patient's understanding and feelings about disease and the effect it has had on physical appearance

Provide emotional support; allow patient to verbalize needs and to participate in planning care

Encourage verbalization of feelings about body image and function changes

Expected outcome/evaluation

Patient demonstrates positive strategies to deal with body image and functional changes

■ **NDX:** Knowledge deficit related to lack of information about disease process and home care management

Assess level of understanding regarding disease process
Explain to family
   Need to encourage patient to deal with body image changes and fears of permanent disability, dying, or loss of body function
   Need to encourage verbalization
   Need to encourage independence and continued socialization
Discuss medications: name, dosage, time of administration, purpose, and side effects
   Anticholinesterase
      Importance of dosage
         Take at scheduled times
         Do not miss doses
         Take with milk, crackers, or bread
         Avoid taking with coffee, or fruit or tomato juice
         Avoid taking with sedatives or tranquilizers
      Toxic side effects: muscular weakness, abdominal cramps, diarrhea
Discuss symptoms and first signs of drug toxicity to report to physician
Explain need to avoid taking over-the-counter medications without checking with physician
Explain need to wear medical alert band
Discuss symptoms of recurrence or progression of disease or of any complications, such as respiratory failure, to report to physician
Explain importance of avoiding persons with infections, especially URIs
Discuss symptoms of URI to report to physician
   Increased weakness
   Low-grade fever
   Chills
   Cough

Explain need to avoid use of tobacco and alcohol and prolonged exposure to hot or cold weather
Explain importance of ongoing outpatient care
Explain need to maintain regular diet according to patient's status
   Serve soft or solid food as tolerated
   Arrange foods and utensils so as to be easily managed by patient
   Instruct patient to chew small pieces of food well and to eat slowly
Explain need for exercise to tolerance; to avoid strenuous activity
   Plan activities when maximum effect of medication is seen; patient will usually exhibit most strength in morning or after nap
   Assist in planning ADLs in a manner in which patient will accomplish tasks without too many motions
Explain need for active or passive ROM exercises to all extremities
Explain need for planned rest periods and at least 8 hr of sleep at night
Emphasize need for diversional activities
   Reading
   Watching television
   Listening to radio
   Knitting
   Working puzzles
Emphasize importance of avoiding physical and emotional stress
Discuss need for speech therapy; instruct patient to speak slowly and practice reading aloud
Explain need to use eye patch over affected eye or frosted lens to increase clear vision if diplopia persists
Explain importance of avoiding constipation; may need to use stool softeners or mild laxatives
Explain need for adequate fluid intake: up to 2000 ml/day unless contraindicated
Discuss available agencies for use as references, such as Myasthenia Gravis Foundation[*]
Refer patient and/or significant other to Visiting Nurses Association or social service worker for obtaining any necessary equipment for home use, such as suctioning equipment

Expected outcome/evaluation

Patient and/or significant other demonstrates knowledge of the disease process and home management needs

MYASTHENIA GRAVIS CRISIS, CHOLINERGIC CRISIS

myasthenia gravis crisis Acute exacerbation of myasthenic process resulting in increased signs of weakness;

---

[*]Myasthenia Gravis Foundation, 53 W. Jackson Blvd., Suite 1352, Chicago, Ill., 60604.

usually a result of infection, surgery, or emotional upset

cholinergic crisis *Acute exacerbation of muscle paralysis resulting from an overdose of anticholinesterase*

Assessment
Observations/findings
MYASTHENIA GRAVIS CRISIS

Respiratory distress progressing to periods of apnea and respiratory failure
Tachypnea
Extreme muscular weakness
Extreme fatigue
Restlessness
Anxiety
Irritability
Difficulty in handling secretions
Dysphagia
Inability to chew or move jaws
Facial weakness
Speech impairment
Elevated temperature
Ptosis of one or both eyelids

CHOLINERGIC CRISIS

Respiratory distress progressing to periods of apnea and respiratory failure
Dyspnea and wheezing
Vertigo
Blurred vision
Lacrimation
Salivation
Anorexia
Abdominal cramping
Nausea and vomiting
Dysarthria
Dysphagia
Muscular cramps and spasms (fasciculations)
Extreme weakness
Toxic effects of anticholinesterase
    Anorexia
    Abdominal cramps
    Nausea, vomiting
    Excessive salivation
    Sweating
    Diarrhea

Potential complications

Aspiration
Respiratory failure
Respiratory arrest

Medical Management

Oxygen-assisted ventilation
Tracheostomy
Intake and output

Medication therapy; reduce or withdraw anticholinergic drugs
NPO as indicated

Nursing diagnoses/interventions/evaluation

■ **NDX:** Ineffective breathing pattern related to neuromuscular (respiratory) impairment

Assess respirations: rate, depth, pattern, and respiratory effort
Maintain patent airway
Administer oxgyen with assisted ventilation as ordered
Inspect and auscultate chest frequently to monitor adequate ventilation
Monitor VC q2h to 4h as ordered
Assist and teach patient to turn, cough, and deep breathe q2h as possible
Suction q1h to 2h and prn
Monitor consciousness until breathing pattern is stabilized
Check rectal temperature q2h to 4h; cooling measures may be ordered to decrease work of breathing
Maintain bed rest to maximize effective breathing
    Elevate head of bed 30 degrees as tolerated
    Maintain body alignment
Administer medication to optimize ventilatory muscular activity
    Reduce or withdraw anticholinergic drugs as ordered; may be given to differentiate type of crisis
        Myasthenia gravis crisis: patient worsens
        Cholinergic crisis: patient improves
    Keep atropine at bedside; *avoid use of morphine*
Maintain ventilatory support until crisis is resolved, then resume noncrisis management

Expected outcome/evaluation

Patient demonstrates effective breathing pattern without ventilatory support
Respiratory rate, rhythm, and pattern are within normal limits without mechanical support

AMYOTROPHIC LATERAL SCLEROSIS (ALS)

A progressive lower motor neuron disorder of unknown etiology that results in muscular wasting and atrophy; commonly known as "Lou Gehrig's disease"

Assessment
Observations/findings

Irregular muscular fasciculations
Cramping
Incoordination of movement of hands and fingers
Muscle stiffness and wasting involving hands, arms, and shoulders
Spastic gait
Progressive weakness, flaccidity, and atrophy of legs
Dysarthria

Dysphagia
Dyspnea
Excessive drooling
Loss of reflexes

Laboratory/diagnostic studies

Elevated creatinine phosphokinase (CPK)
CSF: elevated protein
Myelography
CT scan: cerebral atrophy
Muscle biopsy
Electromyelogram
Nerve conduction studies

Potential complications

Neuromuscular deficit: mild to severe
Respiratory infection
Aspiration, atelectasis
Injury
Respiratory failure

Medical Management

Cricopharyngeal myotomy to alleviate dysphagia
Cervical esophagostomy
Transtympanic neuroectomy
Medications
   Anticholinesterase
   Steroids
   Antibiotics
   Muscle relaxants
Oxygenation/ventilatory support
Cardiac monitoring
Parenteral fluids/nutritional support
Physical therapy
Occupational, speech therapy

Nursing diagnoses/interventions/evaluation

■ **NDX:** Ineffective airway clearance related to progressive neuromuscular impairment

Assess respiratory function and ability to handle secretions
Assess ability to swallow; maintain NPO if reflexes are weak
Maintain patent airway through
   Proper body and head positioning
   Suctioning q2h to 4h as indicated
   Encouraging coughing and deep breathing as patient's condition permits
Observe for alterations in respiratory rate and pattern
Auscultate chest for breath sounds q6h to 8h
Administer oxygen, humidification, and ventilatory support as ordered
Perform chest percussion and vibration to loosen secretions
Test muscular strength for respiratory effort by monitoring tidal volume and VC

Expected outcome/evaluation

Patient demonstrates effective breathing pattern
   Chest expansion is symmetrical
   Breath sounds are clear to auscultation
   ABGs and vital signs are within normal limits
   No signs of respiratory distress

■ **NDX:** Self-care deficit: feeding, bathing, and/or toileting related to progressive neuromuscular deterioration

Assess degree of self-care deficit
Encourage self-care as long as possible
   Bathing
   Feeding
Direct nursing care to promote self-care and prevention of complications according to severity of symptoms
Administer oral hygiene q4h to 5h
Provide physical hygiene as indicated
Check gag reflex
Modify eating patterns as gag reflex diminishes
Maintain high-calorie, high-protein soft diet as tolerated
Initiate tube feedings as indicated
Administer skin care q4h and prn
   Use air mattress
   Use sheepskin
   Use footboard
   Rub back
Anticipate and manage elimination needs
Have patient avoid constipation
   Encourage drinking fluids
   Use daily suppositories or stool softeners

Expected outcome/evaluation

Patient's
   Self-care needs are met
   Fluid and nutritional needs are met
   Elimination needs are met
   Skin, oral, and eye hygiene needs are met

■ **NDX:** Alteration in physical mobility related to muscle weakness and wasting secondary to neuromuscular deterioration

Assess and document level of motor function
Consult with physiotherapist to outline an appropriate exercise program
Perform active or passive ROM exercises q4h to all extremities
Apply necessary braces or splints to support ankles and hands
Turn q2h to 4h if patient is confined to bed
Encourage ambulation to tolerance
Avoid strenuous exercise
Administer or supervise physical therapy as ordered: massage and stretching exercises

Maintain planned rest periods

Test muscular strength of extremities q4h and prn

Expected outcome/evaluation

Patient maintains full ROM to affected limbs
  Motor function is maintained
  Demonstrates use of support devices

■ **NDX:** Powerlessness related to perceived and/or actual lack of control over body function

Assess feelings and perceptions of physical deterioration

Assess expressions of dissatisfaction and frustration over inability to perform tasks

Provide emotional support; be aware that there is no cure
  Focus and support use of motor functions that still exist
  Encourage expression of feelings

Assist family and patient with accepting reality of progressive loss of bodily functions

Be supportive; encourage active listening and expression of feelings by patient and family members

Permit patient to participate in care as long as possible

Expected outcome/evaluation

Patient
  Experiences an increased sense of control over life situation and prescribed activities
  Verbalizes feelings of increased control
  Participates in decisions regarding physical care and activities

■ **NDX:** Knowledge deficit related to lack of information about disease process and home management

Assess level of understanding regarding disease

Reinforce physician's explanation of disease, symptoms, progression, and management

Emphasize that although activity is impaired, cognitive processes are not affected

Emphasize importance of verbalization of feelings about progressive muscular wasting and weakness

Emphasize need to discuss feelings about
  Excessive salivation
  Weakening voice, hoarseness
  Dysphagia

Emphasize need for family to encourage active participation in family activities

Demonstrate use of electrolarynx to facilitate vocalization as tolerated

Discuss need to develop alternative methods of communication when voice becomes nonfunctional: use of eyes and eyelid blinking

Explain importance of ongoing outpatient care and physician's visits

Explain need for high-calorie, high-protein soft diet as tolerated

Assist patient with dealing with problems of swallowing
  Place pureed foods on posterior aspect of tongue
  Cut foods for patient
  Use wrist and hand braces
  May need to consider nasogastric or gastrostomy feedings

Explain need for oral suctioning as disease progresses

Instruct patient to swallow slowly to avoid danger of aspiration

Explain need for oral hygiene q2h to 4h and prn
  Have tissues easily accessible to patient
  Have patient use bib while eating
  Clean corners of mouth after eating and prn

Discuss use of braces, splints, and/or cervical collars for support of hands, ankles, and neck

Explain need to avoid strenuous exercise/activity

Explain need to perform ROM activities as tolerated

Discuss agencies available for use as resources

Explain need to provide skin care frequently, turning patient q2h to 4h to alternate potential pressure areas

Explain need to provide for and anticipate elimination needs

Expected outcome/evaluation

Patient and/or significant other demonstrates knowledge and understanding of home care management
  Demonstrates passive or active ROM exercises
  States all relevant information regarding medications, time of dose, side effects, and purpose
  Identifies high-calorie, high-protein foods and states understanding of need for maintenance of diet
  Demonstrates understanding of use of supportive devices to maintain physical mobility

Additional nursing diagnoses to consider

Ineffective breathing pattern related to neuromuscular degeneration

Impaired verbal communication

Potential for injury: trauma

GUILLAIN-BARRÉ SYNDROME (ACUTE INFECTIOUS POLYNEURITIS; POLYRADICULITIS)

A neurological syndrome of acute ascending paralysis; etiology is unknown, but syndrome generally follows a recent infection; onset is rapid, and symptoms are generally reversible

Assessment
Observations/findings

Symmetrical muscular weakness of lower extremities, progressive to arms, trunk, head, and face

Ascending paresthesia, pain
Paralysis of upper extremities may be partial, or complete quadriplegia may develop
Absent or diminished deep tendon reflexes
Unstable BP: Hypertension (during acute phase), hypotension
Sinus tachycardia, bradycardia
Choking, difficulty in breathing, tachypnea
Decreased or absent breath sounds
Dysphagia, difficulty in swallowing
Speech impairment
Low-grade fever
Urinary retention or infection

Laboratory/diagnostic studies

Lumbar puncture
 CSF
  Increased protein
  Normal WBC
Electromyography
Nerve conduction studies

Potential complications

Autonomic dysfunction
 Postural hypotension
 ECG changes: dysrhythmias
 Urinary, rectal incontinence
Aspiration, atelectasis
Respiratory failure
 Decreased tidal volume
 Hypercapnia
Respiratory arrest
Neuromuscular deficit
 Atrophy
 Contractures

Medical Management

Endotracheal intubation; tracheostomy
Oxygen/mechanical ventilation
Arterial blood gases
Chest physiotherapy
Physical and/or occupational therapy
Medications
 Antibiotics
 Analgesics (not opiates)
 Steroids
 Pituitary hormones
Bed rest; monitoring of muscular strength
Parenteral therapy
Enteral or oral nutrition with high-protein, high-calorie diet
Cardiac monitoring
Plasmapheresis

Nursing diagnoses/interventions/evaluation

 NDX: Potential for ineffective breathing pattern related to neuromuscular impairment (ascending paralysis)

Assess respiratory function, noting rate, depth, and pattern 1qh to 2h and prn
Maintain patent airway
Administer oxygen, humidification, and assisted ventilation as ordered
Assess and monitor tidal volume and vital capacity
Provide tracheostomy care if indicated (p. 232)
Monitor closely for signs of impending respiratory failure; do not leave patient unattended during periods of respiratory distress
Auscultate chest q2h to 4h
Elevate head of bed 30 degrees
Maintain body alignment and position
Monitor vital signs with neurological signs q1h to 2h and prn for change
Test muscular strength q4h to 8h
Suction prn
Assist and teach coughing and deep breathing as appropriate
Keep intubation equipment and mechanical ventilator on standby in acute phase

Expected outcome/evaluation

Patient demonstrates effective breathing pattern
 Chest expansion is symmetrical
 Breath sounds are clear to auscultation
 ABGs and vital signs are within normal limits
 No signs of respiratory distress

 NDX: Alteration of sensory perception related to neuromuscular paralysis: tactile, communication, visual

Assess and monitor signs of sensory alterations (e.g., inability to differentiate hot and cold, dull and sharp)
Record changes/improvement daily
Establish and maintain means of communication
 Call bell within reach
 Magic Slate, pad and pencil, or word board at bedside
Administer eye care q2h to 4h; remove crusts, apply eye shields, and administer artificial tears
Administer analgesics as indicated
Assist patient to differentiate tactile sensations (e.g., what is hot or cold)
Protect from injury
 Test bath water and foods for appropriate temperature
 Keep all sharp objects out of reach
 Assist patient to turn q2h; observe for pressure points
Keep call bell within reach

Expected outcome/evaluation

Patient demonstrates increase in sensory stimulation
   Sustains no injuries
   Is able to communicate needs

■ **NDX:**   Impaired physical mobility related to progressive weakness and paresthesia secondary to neuromuscular disease

Assess and document degree of functional ability
Maintain bed rest; position patient to level of comfort
Support extremities with pillows and footboards
Change position q2h to 4h; administer skin care q2h to 4h as indicated
Perform passive ROM to all extremities
Increase frequency of nursing functions as patient's condition requires
Encourage ambulation as tolerated
   Begin by having patient sit on bedside with support, progressing to chair two to three times daily
   Later have patient walk in room or hall for 15 min four times daily
Administer analgesics as indicated
Consult with physical therapy department for structured exercise program
Maintain planned rest periods

Expected outcome/evaluation

Patient experiences optimal level of mobility
   Performs passive and active ROM
   There are no complications related to immobility (e.g., contractures, decubiti)

■ **NDX:**   Alteration in nutrition: less than body requirements, related to neuromuscular weakness

Assess and record ability to chew, swallow, and cough on daily basis
Monitor daily caloric intake
Consult with dietitian as indicated
Weigh daily
Administer diet as tolerated; progress from soft to solid foods as tolerated
Supplement feedings with high-calorie, high-protein fluids such as eggnog and milk shakes
Administer enteral feedings as indicated
Encourage fluids to 2000 ml/day unless contraindicated
Maintain parenteral fluids as indicated and ordered

Expected outcome/evaluation

Patient's nutritional and fluid needs are met
   Weight is maintained or increased

■ **NDX:**   Potential for powerlessness related to perceived/actual loss of body function imposed by progressive physical deterioration

Assess feelings of frustration, anxiety, and fear over loss of body function
Provide emotional support, thorough explanations, and reassurance
Be alert to emotional changes and mood swings
Encourage patient's participation and expression of needs and feelings
Encourage participation in self-care activities
Support and focus on existing body function (eating, dressing, shaving) as indicated
Consult and provide physical, occupational, and psychosocial support

Expected outcome/evaluation

Patient
   Feels in control of or participates in as many routine activities as possible
   Participates in decision-making and activities related to care
   Identifies need areas
   Participates in self-care
   Participates in diversional activities
   Optimal communication is established

■ **NDX:**   Knowledge deficit related to lack of information about disease process

Ensure that patient and/or significant other understands that recovery may take up to 1 year or more
Stress importance of dealing with body image changes and fears of permanent disability, loss of function, and dying
Explain to family
   Need to encourage verbalization
   Need to encourage independence and socialization
   Need to encourage self-care as a strategy for health maintenance
   Importance of allowing patient to take meals with family
Discuss medications: name, dosage, frequency of administration, purpose, and side effects
Explain need to avoid over-the-counter medications without checking with physician
Stress need to avoid individuals with infections, especially URIs
Encourage diversional activities: TV, reading, radio
Stress importance of high-calorie, high-protein diet
Reinforce need to arrange utensils and foods for easy patient management
Stress need to maintain fluid intake of 2000 ml/day
Teach patient to avoid constipation by drinking fluids

Explain importance of ongoing outpatient care, including physical and/or occupational therapy

Encourage need to exercise to tolerance

Explain use of warm baths to alleviate stiffness and pain

Ensure that patient and/or significant other demonstrates

    Active and passive ROM exercise with massage to all extremities

    Strengthening and mobility exercises to fingers

    Exercises that increase mobility and strength of fingers; use of rubber squeeze toys, balls, or clay

Expected outcome/evaluation

Patient and/or significant other demonstrates knowledge and understanding of home care management

    Demonstrates passive/active ROM exercises

    States all relevant information regarding medications, time of dose, side effects, and purpose

    Identifies high-calorie, high-protein foods and states understanding of need for maintenance of diet

    States understanding of fluid intake maintenance to avoid infection risk and constipation

    Demonstrates abilities in physical hygiene care

    States principles important in maintaining skin integrity

Additional nursing diagnoses to consider

Potential alteration in bowel elimination: incontinence

Potential alteration in patterns of urinary elimination

Anxiety

Pain

NEUROLOGICAL INFECTIONS

Those conditions in which a microorganism has gained entry into the body, producing a reaction, brain abscess, or meningitis

brain abscess *Secondary to systemic infections or may be introduced through trauma; results in space-occupying lesions causing a potential for increased ICP*

meningitis *Infection of the meninges, causing inflammatory reaction in the pia-arachnoid membrane; may be caused by bacteria or virus (acute aseptic meningitis)*

encephalitis *Infection of the brain parenchyma*

Assessment
Observations/findings
GENERAL

(NOTE: See box below for specific findings)

History of recent URI, sinus or ear infection, penetrating trauma, or basal skull fracture

Headache

Elevated temperature

Meningeal irritation

    Nuchal ridgidity

    Positive Kernig's and Brudzinski's signs

    Photophobia

Altered level of consciousness: irritability, disorientation to coma

---

SPECIFIC FINDINGS ASSOCIATED WITH BACTERIAL MENINGITIS, VIRAL ENCEPHALITIS, BRAIN ABSCESS

Bacterial meningitis	Viral encephalitis	Brain abscess
Elevated temperature (101° F - 103° F/38° C to 39.5° C)	Altered LOC	**ACUTE**
Altered LOC: memory loss, disorientation to delirium to coma	Aphasia	Chills and fever
	Hemiparesis	Confusion
Meningeal irritation	Ataxia	Drowsiness
Oligenia	Nystagmus	Seizures: local or generalized
Muscle hepatoma, flaccid paralysis	Ocular paralysis	Motor or sensory deficits
Deafness	Facial weakness	
Petechial hemorrhage		**SECOND STAGE**
Increased ICP		Headache, recurrent and severe
		Confusion to stupor
		Increased ICP

LABORATORY/DIAGNOSTIC STUDIES

CSF	CSF	CSF
Turbid	Increased WBC with mononuclear cells	Increased WBC (lymphocytes)
Increased WBC	Increased (slightly) protein	Increased (high) protein
Increased protein	Normal glucose	Normal glucose
Decreased glucose		Elevated CSF pressure (200-300 mm H$_2$O)
Elevated CFS pressure (>180 mm H$_2$O)		

Cranial nerve dysfunction (III, IV, VI, VII, VIII)
    Ocular palsies
    Facial paresis
    Deafness
    Vertigo
Diplopia
Seizures: focal, generalized
Malaise
Anorexia

Laboratory/diagnostic studies

Lumbar puncture
CSF
    Protein level and pressure
    Glucose level
Serum blood cultures
EEG
CT brain scan
X-ray examination
    Chest
    Skull
    Sinus

Potential complications

Increased ICP
Neurological deficit
    Paresis
Herniation
Pneumonia
Respiratory failure

Medical Management

Institutional protocol for isolation or infection control as
    indicated by organism (identified)
Medications
    Antibiotic therapy
    Analgesics
    Anticonvulsants
    Antipyretics
Ventilatory/oxygenation support
Hypothermia
ICP monitoring
Fluid/electrolyte therapy

Nursing diagnoses/interventions/evaluation

■ **NDX:** Ineffective thermoregulation related to infectious process

Monitor temperature q4h to 8h or as indicated
Administer antipyretic medications as ordered
Maintain room temperature to 68° F or 20° C
Initiate cooling measures as indicated
    Give tepid sponge bath
    Remove excess bedclothes
    Use hypothermia blanket
Encourage fluid intake

Expected outcome/evaluation

Patient is normothermic; temperature is 98.6° F or 37° C

■ **NDX:** Pain: headache related to cerebral tissue irritation

Maintain quiet environment; darken room if photophobia
    occurs
Maintain bed rest; assist patient in assuming position of
    comfort
Administer analgesics as ordered
Administer comfort measures
    Elevate head to 30 degrees
    Put cool cloth over eyes
    Apply ice cap to head

Expected outcome/evaluation

Patient
    Verbalizes absence of or improved headache
    Appears to be resting quietly

■ **NDX:** Potential for ineffective breathing related to increased ICP and depressed cerebral functioning

Assess and monitor respirations: rate, depth, and breathing pattern
Assess respiratory status q1h to 2h as indicated
Auscultate breath sounds
Monitor ABGs as ordered
Administer oxygen/ventilatory support as ordered
Position patient for optimal ventilation
Assist and instruct patient to turn and deep breathe q2h
    to 4h
Suction prn
Check BP, P, R, and level of consciousness prn as indications of neurological and respiratory stability

Expected outcome/evaluation

Patient demonstrates effective breathing pattern
    Chest expansion is symmetrical
    Breath sounds are clear to auscultation
    ABGs and vital signs are within normal limits
    No signs of respiratory distress

■ **NDX:** Knowledge deficit related to lack of information about disease process and eventual home management

Discuss medications: name, dosage, frequency of administration, purpose, and toxic or side effects
Explain need to avoid taking over-the-counter medications without checking with physician
Explain to family need to encourage verbalization; help
    patient understand nature of disorder
Explain need to increase activities as ordered
Explain importance of physical activity as tolerated
Explain need for planned rest periods

Discuss symptoms of progression of condition to report to
physician
Explain importance of ongoing outpatient care

Expected outcome/evaluation

Patient and/or significant other demonstrates knowledge
and understanding of home care management
States all relevant information regarding medications,
time of dose, side effects, and purpose

SUBSTANCE ABUSE (DRUG ABUSE AND INTOXICATION)

NOTE: Care of the intoxicated patient will depend on the
amount and type of drug ingested; for severe drug overdose or intoxication refer to Care of Patient with Altered Consciousness, Shock Syndrome, Respiratory
Failure, and Seizures.

Alcohol Intoxication
Assessment
Observations/findings

Acute intoxication
  Confusion
  Slurred speech
  Ataxia
  Depressed deep tendon reflexes

DRUGS COMMONLY ABUSED

NARCOTICS
Opium
Heroin (horse, smack)
Oxycodone
Codeine
Methadone
Hydromorphone (Di-
  laudid)
Meperidine (Demerol)

HALLUCINOGENS
LSD (acid)
Mescaline
DMT
Scopolamine
Atropine
Phencyclidine: PCP
  (angel dust, crystal,
  dust mist, peace
  pill, superweed)
Psilocybin

ORGANIC SOLVENTS
Glue
Cleaning fluid

DEPRESSANTS
Alcohol
Barbiturates
Meprobamate
Chloral hydrate
Glutethimide (Doriden)

STIMULANTS
Cocaine (coke)
Amphetamines
Methylphenidate (Ritalin)

CANNABIS
Marijuana (grass, weed,
  joints)
Hashish (weed oil, hash)

Nystagmus
Anxiety, restlessness
Dilated pupils
Stupor
Coma
Gastric irritation: vomiting
Withdrawal
  Anxiety
  Tremors
  Diaphoresis
  Nausea, vomiting
  Anorexia
  Confusion
  Moroseness
  Confabulation
  Delirium tremens
  Seizure activity
  Uncontrolled rage
  Hallucination
  Toxic psychosis
Chronic intoxication
  Mental confusion
  Cerebellar degeneration
    Ataxic gait
    Nystagmus
    Dysarthric speech
  Nutritional deficiencies
  Myopathy
  Hepatic coma
  Seizure disorders
  Marchiafava-Bignami syndrome (progressive organic
    dementia)
  Wernicke's syndrome
    Ophthalmoplegia
    Apathy, apprehension
    Confusion
    Coma
  Korsakoff's syndrome
    Disorientation to time and place
    Peripheral neuropathy
    Confabulation

Laboratory/diagnostic studies

Serum ETOH (Table 8-6)
Serum chemistries

Potential complications

Aspiration
Hypertension
Severe stages
  Hypoventilation
  Hypotension
  Hypothermia
  GI hemorrhage
  Myocardial infarction (MI)

Medical Management

Acute

Ventilatory support and management: oxygenation/ventilatory

Fluid/electrolyte therapy

Medications during withdrawal

Phenothiazines

Tranquilizers

Barbiturates

Anticonvulsants

Thiamin

Nursing diagnoses/interventions/evaluation

■ **NDX:** Potential for ineffective breathing pattern

Maintain patent airway: assisted ventilation as indicated

See Care of Patient with Altered Consciousness (p. 396) and Respiratory Failure (p. 223)

Position to optimize respiratory excursion, airway patency, and secretion removal

Monitor BP, P, and R q2h to 4h and prn

Provide oral or nasopharyngeal airway as indicated

Suction prn

Auscultate breath sounds prn

Provide oxygenation/respiratory therapy

Monitor ABGs as indicated

Avoid use of sedatives; may potentiate effects of alcohol

Provide soft restraints as indicated

    Keep restraints loose

    Position patient on side or stomach

Expected outcome/evaluation

Patient demonstrates effective breathing pattern

    Chest expansion is symmetrical

    Breath sounds are clear to auscultation

    ABGs and vital signs are within normal limits

    No signs of respiratory distress

■ **NDX:** Ineffective individual coping related to inadequate coping methods

TABLE 8-6. Serum Alcohol Levels

Serum alcohol levels	Effects
Mild: 0.5 to 1.5 mg/ml	Muscular incoordination, personality changes; talkative, morose, noisy
Moderate: 1.5 to 3 mg/ml	Marked ataxia, mental impairment, incoordination, prolonged reaction time, nausea, vomiting, diplopia
Severe: 3 to 5 mg/ml	Dysarthria, amnesia, hypothermia, hypoventilation, coma

Maintain quiet, supportive environment; avoid punitive approach

Maintain safety precautions for anxious and restless patients

Provide supportive counseling services to patient when receptive

Ensure that patient and/or significant other is knowledgeable about effects of alcohol abuse

Expected outcome/evaluation

Patient

    Demonstrates effective coping strategies

    Discusses effects of alcohol abuse

    Attends counseling/educational support groups

Chemical Substance Abuse

Intermittent or chronic use of stimulants or depressants resulting in alterations in mental and physiological function

Assessment

Observations/findings

DEPRESSANTS: NARCOTICS, OPIATES*

Level of consciousness

    Apathy

    Withdrawal

    Euphoria

    Coma

Airway obstruction

Stridor

Decreased BP

Tachycardia or bradycardia

Pupillary changes

    Pinpoint (opiates)

    Dilated (barbiturates)

Depressed gag and swallow reflexes

Respiratory distress, respiratory rate < 8/min or > 30/min

Seizure activity

Hypothermia

Method of administration

    Oral

    Subcutaneous: "skin popping"

    Nasal insufflation: "snorting"

    Intravenous

    Signs of withdrawal

        Abdominal and muscular pain

        Severe cramping

*Refers to all drugs that possess some morphinelike activity.

HALLUCINOGENS, STIMULANTS
GENERAL

Anxiety progressing to pain
Paranoid reaction
Combativeness progressing to violence
Insomnia
Hallucinations
  Auditory
  Visual
Confusion
Ataxia
Depression: mild to severe
Suicidal tendencies
Anorexia
Nausea
Headache
Elevated BP
Elevated temperature
Tachycardia palpitations
Hypertension progressing to crisis
Pupillary changes: dilated
Photophobia
Diplopia
Horizontal and vertical nystagmus
Hot flashes
ECG changes
  Dysrhythmias
    ST-T wave changes
Decreased urine output

LSD, MESCALINE

Hyperactivity
Pupil dilation
Increased vital signs
Low doses: euphoria
High doses: hallucinatory psychosis

PCP: "ANGEL DUST"

Low-to-moderate doses: effect begins within 5 min and
  peaks within 30 to 60 min
  Elevated systolic and diastolic pressures
  Tachycardia
  Increased deep tendon reflexes
  Small pupils
  Nystagmus: horizontal and vertical (persists for 4 days)
  Tremors, clonus
  Euphoria
  Amnesia
  Agitation
  Image distortion
  Increased urine output
High doses
  Slurred speech
  Drowsiness
  Depressed deep tendon reflexes

Seizures
Opisthotonos
Bradypnea
Decreased BP
Disordered thought processes, hallucinations

Laboratory/diagnostic studies

Serum chemical screening
Urinalysis
Arterial blood gases

Potential complications

Aspiration
Respiratory failure
MI
Shock
Acute psychosis

Medical Management
Depressants

Respiratory support with oxygenation or ventilation
Fluid/electrolyte therapy
Emetics
Gastric lavage
Activated charcoal for ingested opiates
Naloxone for opioid overdose
Peritoneal dialysis

Stimulants

Decreased external stimuli
Medications
  General
    Barbiturates, phenothiazines
    Sedatives, anticonvulsants
  For LSD, mescaline
    Diazepam (oral)
    Avoid phenothiazine; may potentiate psychotic re-
      action
  For PCP
    Haloperidol
    Diazepam
    Activated charcoal (high doses)
  Parenteral fluids
  Gastric suction for PCP
  Psychiatric liaison

Nursing diagnoses/interventions/evaluation

■ **NDX:**   Potential for ineffective breathing pattern

Refer to p. 396 if patient arrives in coma or in respiratory
  failure
Assess respirations q2h to 4h, noting rate, quality, and
  depth
Assess level of consciousness and monitor q2h to 4h
Report any changes in consciousness or vital signs to physician

Administer parenteral fluids as ordered

Understand that peritoneal dialysis may be indicated for long-acting barbiturates

Obtain accurate and detailed history regarding drug ingested: type, amount, time of ingestion, method of administration

Administer emetics as ordered; contraindicated in presence of depressed gag reflex, seizures, or coma

Administer gastric lavage as ordered (within 2 hr of ingestion); endotracheal tube is usually inserted before lavage in comatose patient

Keep patient physically active and stimulated

Provide patient with positive reassurance about condition; avoid punitive approach

Be firm, patient, and understanding

Administer medication as ordered: naloxone (Narcan) for opiate overdose; effects can be noted within 1 to 2 min for IV

Give activated charcoal orally for ingested opiates

Check BP and P on admission and q4h as indicated by condition

Monitor cardiac status for dysrhythmias

Meet self-care needs as indicated

Expected outcome/evaluation

Patient demonstrates effective breathing pattern
    Chest expansion is symmetrical
    Breath sounds are clear to auscultation
    ABGs and vital signs are within normal limits

■ NDX: Potential for violence

Admit to private room when possible

Decrease external stimuli
    Use low lighting
    Avoid loud voices and rapid movements

NOTE: Administration of the following care may heighten patient's paranoid state and cause increased agitation; approach patient quietly, using friend to assist if required

Allow friend or family member to remain in room during all procedures to assist in "talking down"

Provide patient with support, reassurance, and reality-defining information

Instruct patient to avoid trying to differentiate between real perceptions and effects of drug; remind patient that effects of drug will end

Avoid mechanical restraints

Approach cautiously; avoid whispering to others

Explain all procedures; allow same person to care for patient at all times

Administer medications as ordered

Avoid phenothiazine (may potentiate effect or produce anticholinergic crisis)

Administer parenteral fluids as ordered

Monitor BP, P, and R q2h to 4h or as indicated by level of consciousness

Expected outcome/evaluation

Patient demonstrates calm and nondestructive behavior

■ NDX: Knowledge deficit related to lack of information about potential side effects of drug abuse and dependence

Explore patient's willingness to participate in self-help and support group experiences

Provide supportive, nonjudgmental approach to patient

Provide opportunity for participation in counseling and group support

Expected outcome/evaluation

Patient understands effects of drug abuse and dependence

LUMBAR PUNCTURE (SPINAL TAP)

Puncture usually made at the junction of the third and fourth lumbar vertebrae to obtain CSF for purposes of measuring CSF pressure and laboratory examination

Preprocedure Preparation

Explain procedure

Have patient empty bowel and bladder

Position patient on side with spine close to edge of bed; support soft mattress with bedboards

Maintain aseptic technique throughout procedure
    Handle specimen with care
    Ensure specimen delivery to laboratory within 30 min to ensure diagnostic accuracy

Explain to patient that procedure may be uncomfortable

Explain importance of immobilization during procedure

Instruct patient to breathe normally; not to hold breath

Provide patient with physical and emotional support during procedure

Postprocedure Assessment
Observations/findings

Altered level of consciousness

Headache: mild to severe

Nuchal rigidity

Hypotension

Tachycardia

Tachypnea

Bleeding from site of puncture

Elevated temperature

Laboratory/diagnostic studies

Normal adult CSF
    Pressure: 70 to 200 mm of water
    Color: colorless, clear

Glucose level: 45 to 75 mg/100 ml
Protein level (total): 20 to 45 mg/100 ml
Red blood cells: none
White blood cells: 0 to 5 cells/mm^3
Microorganisms: none
Normal child CSF (above 6 months)
Pressure: 70 to 200 mm of water
Color: colorless, clear
Glucose level: > 40 mg/100 ml
Protein level (total): < 40 mg/100 ml
Red blood cells: none
White blood cells: 0 to 4/mm^3
Microorganisms: none

Potential complications

Headache
Infection

Immediate Postprocedure Care

Maintain bed rest; place patient in supine position, keeping head of bed flat for 4 to 8 hr as ordered; if headache occurs, elevate feet 10 to 15 degrees above bed
Assist and teach patient to turn and deep breathe q2h to 4h
Check BP, P, and R q15min for four times, then qh for four times, then as ordered
Control pain as ordered
Observe site of puncture for redness, swelling, or drainage and report any symptoms to physician
Maintain diet as ordered
Force fluids unless contraindicated
Explain importance of keeping head and body position flat in bed

Ongoing Care

Resume activities as ordered
Ambulate to tolerance

HYPOTHERMIA: CARE OF PATIENT

Controlled reduction and maintenance of body temperature to decrease the metabolic rate

Assessment
Observations/findings
PATIENT

Shivering
Decreased BP
Bradycardia
Bradypnea
Altered level of consciousness
Medication reactions
Pupil inequality

EQUIPMENT

Cooling solution; amount in unit
Patency of connections
Pads

Potential complications

Dysrhythmias
Increased ICP
Respiratory failure
Decreased urinary output
Intestinal ileus
Frostbite and burns

Immediate Care

Take and record temperature before starting treatment and q5min until desired temperature is reached, then q15min
Check BP, P, and R and do neurological check q5min to 10min while temperature is stabilizing
Observe for any change in skin color or for presence of edema and induration; report any changes to physician immediately
Assist and teach patient to turn, cough, and deep breathe q1h to 2h
Measure intake and output; measure output qh; report output less than 30 ml/hr to physician; specific gravity test may be ordered
Connect indwelling catheter to closed gravity drainage as ordered
Auscultate chest for breath sounds q1h to 2h
Administer medication for shivering as ordered
Test gag reflex before administering any oral fluids or food to patients with temperatures of less than 90° F (32.2° C)
Perform naso-oral suction as indicated
Administer skin care q1h to 2h
   Lubricate skin before and during procedure with oil or lotion
   Place bath blankets over thermal blankets
Maintain good body alignment
Perform passive or active ROM exercises q4h
Administer oral hygiene q1h to 2h; keep lips well lubricated
Administer nose care q1h to 2h
Provide emotional support
   Remain with patient when anxious
   Anticipate needs

Ongoing Care
Patient

Check BP, T, P, and R and do neurological check q30min for four times, then q4h for 24 hr, then as ordered
Check any dressing and all skin surfaces q1h to 2h until patient's temperature is stable
Measure intake and output

Assist and teach patient to turn, cough, and deep breathe
q2h

Resume care of disease as ordered

Equipment

Check for leaks or punctures in pads before applying to
patient

INCREASED INTRACRANIAL PRESSURE (ICP)

*Slow or sudden elevation in CSF pressure caused by
edema, hemorrhage, or trauma; caused by increase in
CSF or obstruction to outflow*

Assessment
Observations/findings

Deterioration in level of consciousness
  Restlessness
  Instability
  Anxiety
  Confusion
  Lethargy
Motor weakness
  Paresis
Progressive weakness or paralysis of extremities
Headache: location, duration, severity
Pupil dysfunction (ipsilateral to edema or lesion)
Visual disturbances
  Diplopia
  Blurring
  Decreased acuity
Papilledema
Decreasing respiratory rate progressing to periods of apnea;
  Biot's or Cheyne-Stokes respirations
Elevated BP (systolic); widened pulse pressure
Pulse rate decreased to 50 beats/min or below
Vomiting (projectile), nausea
Elevated temperature
Seizure activity
After cranial surgery
  Swelling around surgical site
  Elevation of bone flap

Laboratory/diagnostic studies

Lumbar puncture
Continuous ICP monitoring
Cerebral perfusion pressure
ABGs

Potential complications

Deterioration of neurological function
Respiratory failure
Herniation

Medical Management

Management of ventilatory status
  Oxygenation
  Ventilatory support
  Hyperventilation
Medications
  Osmotic diuretics
  Fluid restriction
  Steroids
  Anticonvulsants
  Barbiturate coma
  Antiinfectives
  Antacids
Fluid restriction
Cardiac monitoring
Surgical intervention
Ventricular drainage

Nursing diagnoses/interventions/evaluation

■ **NDX:** Alteration in tissue perfusion: cerebral, related
to sustained elevations in intracranial pressure

Assess and monitor level of consciousness, reporting any
changes immediately
Maintain patent airway
Elevate head of bed to 30 degrees
Maintain bed rest
  Avoid semiprone or prone position
  Avoid flexion of neck
  Avoid compression of neck veins
  Avoid extreme hip flexion
Monitor BP, P, and R q30min; if possible take BP on
same arm each time
Perform neurological check q30min using Glasgow Coma
Scale (p. 391); report scores of 8 or less or any significant
changes
Check rectal temperature q2h to 4h and prn; perform
cooling measures as needed
Monitor ABGs q4h to 8h as indicated
Maintain parenteral fluids as ordered; hypertonic solutions
may be ordered
Monitor intake and output
Initiate specific medical management as indicated
Avoid valsalva-type maneuvers: vomiting, retching,
straining; initiate measures to avoid constipation as in-
dicated
Avoid isometric muscular contractions; instruct patient
to avoid pushing feet against bedboard
Perform passive ROM activities as ordered
Avoid stress-producing procedures during rapid eye move-
ment (REM) stages of sleep
Explain and prepare for diagnostic tests and/or return to
surgery as ordered
See standard of care for primary condition

Expected outcome/evaluation

Patient
    Remains free of injury
    Demonstrates appropriate orientation and level of consciousness
    Demonstrates vital signs within normal limits
    Demonstrates an effective breathing pattern
    Demonstrates normal intracranial pressure
    Demonstrates normal ROM

INTRACRANIAL PRESSURE (ICP) MONITORING

Insertion of a catheter for purposes of monitoring ICP and/or removing CSF

intraventricular (ventriculostomy) Placement of catheter into lateral ventricle; CSF may be removed for control of ICP or diagnostic evaluation

subarachnoid method Screw or commercial bolt with stopcock that can be rapidly passed into subarachnoid space

epidural method Placement of sensor through a burr hole between the skull and dura

Assessment
Observations/findings
PATIENT

Normal levels: 1 to 15 mm Hg
Moderate elevation: 15 to 40 mm Hg
High levels: >40 mm Hg
Cerebral perfusion pressure (CPP): 50 to 85 mm Hg
    Calculation of formula:

$$CPP = MABP \text{ (mean arterial blood pressure)} - ICP$$

    CPP < 50 mm Hg: ischemia
    CPP < 20 to 30 mm Hg: irreversible ischemia
Wave forms
    A waves: large plateau formations characterized by varying increases and decreases of ICP ranging from 50 to 90 mm Hg and lasting 5 to 20 min; related to cerebral dysfunction
    B waves: occur more regularly—1½ to 1/min, ranging from 10 to 50 mm Hg
    C waves: rapid rhythmic oscillations at amplitudes to 20 mm Hg
Hemodynamic measurements
    Intraarterial pressure
    Pulmonary capillary wedge pressure (PCWP)
    Pulmonary artery diastolic pressure
    Cardiac output (CO)
Level of consciousness
Decreased BP
Increased ICP: changes determined by baseline pressure
CSF
    Clear
    Cloudy
    Blood tinged
    Xanthochromic
Elevated temperature

EQUIPMENT

Flush solution
    Ringer's lactated injection
    Normal saline solution
Pressure line tubing
Transducer
Pressure monitor

Potential complications

Meningitis
Hemorrhage: catheter insertion site
Infection
    Swelling
    Inflammation
    Redness
    Leaking of CSF

Preparation
PATIENT

Reinforce physician's explanation of procedure, duration, and equipment that will be used
Record baseline observations of patient and ICP at time of insertion

EQUIPMENT

Calibrate all equipment before insertion
    Transducer
    Recording display unit
Position transducer to eye of patient for ventriculostomy or at level of both for subarachnoid screw
Be aware that insertion must be done under sterile conditions

Ongoing Care
PATIENT

Maintain head of bed elevated at 30 degrees with patient in supine position; avoid neck flexion, prone position, or extreme hip flexion
Assess pressures qh, prn, and after changes in body position or condition
Notify physician if plateau wave forms begin to increase steadily
Calculate CPP qh
Assess and report any changes in level of consciousness or pressures to physician
Check BP, P, and R and do neurological check q1h to 2h
Check rectal temperature q2h to 4h
Check dressing q1h to 2h
Change dressing qd
Never flush or irrigate ventricular cannula

Administer stool softeners as ordered; have patient avoid straining

See Increased Intracranial Pressure (ICP) (p. 49)

NOTE: The following items may change pressure readings
  Obstructed airway
  Suctioning
  Body position
  Valsalva maneuver

Report any changes in patient's condition to physician

Observe monitor during removal of CSF for precipitous drop in pressure

Remove CSF slowly and by gravity; never aspirate

EQUIPMENT

Level transducer to eye of patient for ventriculostomy; to bolt for subarachnoid screw

Flush pressure tubings with 10 ml of fluid at a time

Check patency of pressure lines q4h; remove air bubbles

Prevent kinking, compression, or tension on tubing

Calibrate transducer q4h to 6h or as indicated by manufacturer; never apply direct pressure to diaphragm of transducer

Change pressure tubing q24h

BOWEL TRAINING

Method of bowel evacuation by reflex conditioning

Assessment
Observations/findings

Impaction

Diarrhea

Bowel incontinence

Dehydration

Autonomic hyperreflexia (dysreflexia)
  Restlessness
  Chills
  Hypertension
  Diaphoresis
  Headache
  Elevated temperature
  Bradycardia
  Flushing

Patient Teaching/Discharge Planning

Explain purpose and necessity of developing bowel regulation

Encourage patient's participation in developing a program

Assess previous bowel habits

Establish regular bowel habits
  Time of day that will be convenient for patient once discharged: after breakfast
  Development of program to have bowel evacuation at same time each day or q3d

Administer medications as indicated
  Stool softeners
  Mild laxatives

Teach exercises that will help develop abdominal muscles and tone
  Pushing up
  Bearing down
  Contracting abdominal muscles

Ensure privacy

Provide bedside commode rather than bedpan when possible; encourage sitting position rather than lying

Keep equipment easily available at bedside

Teach patient to recognize signals or "cues" that may indicate full bowel
  Goose pimples
  Perspiration
  Raising of hair on arms or legs
  Sense of fullness

Instruct patient to eat diet high in fiber

SKULL TONGS AND HALO TRACTION

Methods of immobilizing the neck and stabilizing the spine

Assessment
Observations/findings

Site of insertion of tongs
  Redness
  Swelling
  Drainage

Skin condition: decubiti of scapula, coccyx, and heels

Alignment of head, pulleys, and weights: avoid patient's head touching head of bed

Weights
  Pounds ordered
  Off floor, hanging freely

Position of bed

Ongoing Care

Inspect and clean site of insertion q1h to 2h; remove *any* formed crusts with hydrogen peroxide q6h to 8h and prn

Administer skin and scalp care q2h to 4h
  Use air mattress
  Use sheepskin
  Give back rubs
  Keep bed linen dry and wrinkle-free
  Avoid powders

Perform passive ROM exercises to all extremities q4h

Check alignment of pulleys and weights q4h to 6h; sandbags may be indicated for restlessness as ordered

Turn patient q2h as ordered

Assist and teach patient to deep breathe q2h

Establish means of communication and keep within easy reach of patient: call bell

Assist with ambulation as indicated for patient with halo traction

Patient Teaching

Explain purpose of tongs
Explain methods of turning when possible
Explain importance of keeping head straight

CARE OF PATIENT ON A CIRCLE BED

Assessment
Observations/findings
PATIENT

Body alignment
Pressure areas
Numbness of any area
Dizziness or nausea related to turning
Foot-drop
Anxiety

BED

Position, condition, and proper functioning of
  Canvas supports
  Anterior and posterior frame
  Locks
  Side rails
  Armrests
  Wheel brakes
  Footboard
  Electrical outlets

Ongoing Care

Check position, condition, and proper functioning of bed parts before use and daily; report breakage, missing parts, or malfunction to appropriate person
Turn and reposition patient as ordered
  Free drainage tubing and call light before patient turning and reaffix after turning
  Maintain any traction during turning
Turn slowly; inform patient of frequency of turns; reassure patient when turning
Use footboard at all times
Place armrests in desired position
Provide some method to increase patient's field of vision when possible

STRYKER FRAME

Metal frame bed used to facilitate administration of nursing care to patient with spinal cord injuries

Assessment
Observations/findings
PATIENT

Body position
  Straight body alignment

  Place in center of frame
  Body parts not resting on metal frame
Skin
  Temperature
  Color
Pressure areas
Pulse
Respirations
Lightheadedness
Numbness

EQUIPMENT

Canvas supports
Arm and foot supports
Locks
Frame
  Anterior
  Posterior

Preparation of Unit

Check unit for security of bolts, locks, and frame before placing patient on Stryker frame
Prepare bed with linens, foam mattress, arm rests, and footboards before receiving patient

Ongoing Care

Turn patient q2h during day
Turn patient q4h during night
Check P and R before and after turning
Free all excess tubing before turning
Secure all bolts tightly before turning
Reassure patient when turning
Administer skin care q2h and 4h and prn
Inspect pressure points q2h to 4h

GENERAL REHABILITATIVE CARE OF NEUROLOGICAL PATIENT

May involve minimal to long-term chronic rehabilitative care; specialized settings have programs designed to meet special need areas; the following discussion describes general guidelines for observation and intervention in the care of the neurologically impaired patient

Conditions Requiring Rehabilitative Approach

Cognitive impairment
  Alteration in memory
  Alteration in speech, auditory, or visual function
Sensory-perceptual impairment
Impaired physical mobility
Paralysis
Behavioral changes
Spinal cord injuries
Alteration in elimination function
Self-care deficit

Ineffective individual coping
Chronic pain

Rehabilitative Approach

Reinforce physician's explanation of disorder and its limitations and allowances
Deal with behavioral response
    Allow patient to go through stages of grief over loss of body function
    Be supportive but firm in dealing with patient
Encourage verbalization of feelings and fears
Use positive and reassuring approach to patient
Encourage independence when possible; be alert to limitations
Involve family or significant other in care and instructions
Establish program for ADLs
Encourage patient's participation in developing a program
Establish daily routines of activity and rest periods
    Sample

7:00 to 7:30	Morning care
7:30 to 8:30	Breakfast
9:00 to 9:30	Commode (bowel training)
9:30 to 10:30	Bath
10:30 to 11:00	Chair, stretcher
11:00 to 12:00	Bed rest; turn and position
12:00 to 12:30	Lunch
12:30 to 2:30	Bed rest; turn and position
2:30 to 3:00	Exercises
3:00 to 5:00	Bed rest
5:00 to 6:00	Chair, stretcher, Dinner
6:00 to 9:00	Bed rest
9:00 to 9:30	Exercises
9:30 to 10:00	Evening care
10:00 PM to 7:00 AM	Bed rest

Turn and reposition to
    Right side
    Left side
    Prone position
    Supine position
Attempt to avoid sensory deprivation by providing
    Calendars
    Clocks
    Pictures
    Include schedule for favorite television or radio programs, hobbies, and visiting hours
Explain all treatments and procedures as they occur
Alert staff to patient's emotional changes and mood swings
Allow patient time to express needs
Refer to social service, Visiting Nurses Association, and/or local rehabilitation centers as ordered
Report symptoms of urinary tract infection to physician
    Foul odor of urine
    Sedimentation, pus, or blood in urine
    Decreased output
    Low-grade fever
    Chills

Encourage participation in bowel and bladder training
Avoid constipation
Cleanse perineal region; wipe from front to back after urination
Cleanse perineal region with soap and water after each bowel movement
Give high-calorie, high-protein diet as ordered; avoid high-calcium foods

Activities

Explain importance of exercise programs
Exercise to tolerance; avoid fatigue
Assist and instruct patient to use assistive devices as ordered
Plan rest periods
Encourage patient to participate in self-care as indicated

Nutrition

Assess daily caloric needs
Maintain high-calorie, high-protein, low-residue diet as ordered
Limit high-calcium and gas-producing foods

Elimination

Encourage fluids to 3000 ml/day unless contraindicated
Have patient avoid constipation through use of stool softeners, mild cathartics, suppositories, and/or enemas
Check for bowel movement q3d
Institute bowel and bladder programs
Avoid overdistention of bladder and bowel
Initiate intermittent catheterization as indicated

Patient Teaching

Ensure that patient and/or significant other knows and understands
    Importance of exercise programs
    Need to exercise to tolerance; to avoid fatigue
    Importance of fluid intake; measure intake and output
    Importance of turning q2h to 4h while in bed
    Need to inspect skin and bony prominences for detection of breakdown
    Importance of skin care q2h to 4h while in bed
    Need to avoid constrictive clothing below level of lesion (e.g., garters, belts)
    Need to avoid urinary tract infections
    Need to avoid overdistention of bladder; empty on regular basis
    Need for fluid to 3000 ml/day
Need to ensure daily bowel evacuation to avoid fecal impaction; encourage participation in bowel training (p. 441)
Need for ongoing support and counseling services
    Sexual counseling: patients can engage in some form of satisfying sexual activity
        Limitations depend on site of injury; incomplete in-

juries and high cord injuries allow for varying amounts of sensation and sexual function—even if spinal reflexes are absent, sensation of genital organs may endure

Female reproductive system usually remains intact; patient can bear children—refer for family planning counseling

Refer to appropriate support services
  Vocational rehabilitation
  Recreational rehabilitation
  Home care

PARAPLEGIA

Paralysis of the lower extremities resulting from injury to the spinal cord

Assessment
Observations/findings

Atrophy of nonfunctioning body parts
See Musculoskeletal Assessment (p. 353)
Bladder distention
Dysuria
Bowel incontinence, impaction

Rehabilitation

Give praise for tasks completed
Avoid tasks that patient cannot complete
Provide diversional activities as indicated
  Reading
  Watching television
  Listening to radio
  Working puzzles
  Listening to tape cassettes
Establish means of communication
  Call bell within reach
  Calling out to nurse

Bed activities

Perform weight-bearing exercises
  Begin elevating head of bed, progressing to high-Fowler's position as tolerated when condition stabilizes
  Use tilt or circle bed as ordered
    Begin elevating patient's head at 10 degrees for 10 to 15 min three times daily, progressing to 15 degrees for 1 hr two or three times daily
    Keep legs wrapped with elastic stockings as ordered
    Take BP before tilting patient and q5min at 10 degrees; in absence of hypotension or dizziness, progress to 15 degrees as tolerated
    Gradually progress to 90-degree elevation as tolerated
Change position qh: maintain body alignment
  Prone position
  Supine position
  Rolling to side
  Sitting up

Moving forward and backward
Check placement of lower extremities with each movement
Administer skin care q2h to 4h
  Use air mattresses
  Use sheepskin
  Give back rubs with lanolin-based lotions
  Put foam rubber pads on chairs
  Keep bed linen dry and wrinkle-free
  Place rubber sheet under bath blanket
  Use body corset as ordered
Perform muscle-building exercises
  Active ROM exercise to support extremities
  Dumbbells: extending and flexing of arms
  Overhead trapezes
  Push-ups
  Sit-ups
  Hand-finger exercises
    Rubber sponge balls
    Extension and flexion
Teach method of turning self and pulling up in bed

Wheelchair activities

Get patient out of bed two or three times daily
Demonstrate method of transferring from bed to wheelchair, and from wheelchair to toilet or shower
Demonstrate management of wheelchair: moving forward, backward, turning, stopping, and locking

Self-care activities

Encourage self-care as tolerated
  Bathing
  Dressing
  Combing hair
  Shaving
  Oral hygiene
Encourage patient to wear own clothing: pajamas, slippers, or shoes

Motion activities

Use long leg braces as ordered
Perform physical therapy as ordered
  Weight-bearing exercises
  Parallel bar exercises
  Balancing exercises
  Crutch-walking exercises
To relieve spasticity
  Perform active or passive ROM exercises
  Wear long leg braces
  Give medications as ordered

Elimination

Perform urinalysis weekly as indicated
Check urine output for sedimentation or presence of renal calculi

Perform intermittent catheterization as ordered
Initiate bowel and bladder programs
Teach self-catheterization when appropriate

QUADRIPLEGIA

Paralysis of the upper and lower extremities resulting from injury to the spinal cord (thoracic and cervical regions)

Assessment
Observations/findings

Loss of sweating reflex
Bladder distention and incontinence
Mass reflex of bladder
    Muscular spasms
    Diaphoresis
    Elevated BP
    Headache

Rehabilitation

Encourage staff to allow time for patient care; do not rush patient
Provide diversional activities as indicated
    Reading
    Socializing with nursing staff
Provide means of communication
    Calling out to nurse
    Whistling

Bed activities

Maintain good body alignment
Use circle bed as indicated
Turn and position patient q1h to 2h
    Use supports: sandbags and pillows
    Avoid external rotation of lower extremities
    Position patient: supine, prone, and on side
Cough and deep breathe q1h to 2h
Administer skin care q1h to 2h
    Use air mattress
    Use footboard
    Use sheepskin
    Keep bed linen dry and wrinkle-free
    Rub back and heels with lanolin-based lotions
    Change bed clothing prn
    Place rubber sheet under bath blanket to be used as draw sheet
    Assist with or provide perineal care after each voiding or bowel movement
    Begin elevating head of bed as condition stabilizes, progressing to high-Fowler's position as tolerated
Tilt table or circle bed as ordered
    Begin raising head to 10 degrees for 10 to 15 min three times daily, progressing to 20 degrees for 1 hr two or three times daily, on to 90 degrees for 1 hr two or three times daily, on to 90 degrees as tolerated

Take BP before tilting patient and at 5 to 10 min intervals as head is being raised; in absence of hypotension or dizziness progress to 90 degrees
Apply elastic bandages or stockings as ordered

Wheelchair activities

Use three or four persons to transfer patient to stretcher chair or stretcher for 15 to 30 min two to three times daily as ordered
Encourage wheelchair activity as ordered as condition stabilizes
Provide braces, splints, and other supports as ordered
Take safety measures
    Soft jacket restraints
    Soft abdominal binders
    Side rails when indicated

Self-care activities

Encourage patient to wear clothing from home and to make selections

Motion activities

To relieve spasticity
    Perform gentle passive ROM exercises
    Have patient wear braces
    Give medications as ordered
    Prepare for rhizotomy or chordotomy as ordered

Nutrition

Give tube feedings as indicated
Position patient with head of bed at 30 to 45 degrees
Feed patient
    Allow 30 to 45 min for feeding time
    Give small bites of food
Perform oral hygiene q4h and after meals
    Clean with hydrogen peroxide and water
    Gargle and mouthwash
    Brush teeth

Elimination

Provide indwelling or external catheter to closed gravity drainage as ordered
Instruct patient to develop exercise or signals that may help to stimulate urge to defecate
    Smoking
    Pressure on inner thigh
    Stroking anus
    Digital rectal stimulation
    Drinking coffee
    Massaging abdomen downward or right to left
Instruct patient to respond to "cues" promptly
Discuss importance of established well-balanced diet that includes bulk and roughage
Discuss foods to avoid
    Bananas
    Beans

Cabbage

Foods that have been previously constipating

Encourage fluids to 3000 ml/day unless contraindicated

Include prune and orange juice and coffee in daily diet as preferred

Discuss possible programs to develop

Instruct patient to take 8 to 10 oz of prune juice 12 hr before time set for defecating; insert glycerin suppository high in rectum 15 to 20 min before set time, then place patient on bedpan, toilet, or commode

Insert lubricated glycerin suppository 2 hr before set time and position patient in sitting position or transfer to bedpan or commode

Instruct patient to drink 4 to 8 oz of prune juice each night

Instruct patient to drink a warm drink 30 min before set time

Water

Coffee

Milk

Insert laxative suppository for 2 to 4 days, then glycerin suppository for 2 to 4 days; note length of time between insertion and defecation; place patient on bedside commode at appropriate time; if no bowel movement, give small tap water enema

Instruct patient to recognize signs of impaction

No formed stool for 3 days

Semiliquid stools

Restlessness and increased feeling of discomfort

Discuss treatment for impaction

Laxative suppository

Tap water or oil-retention enemas

Manual clearing of bowel followed by enema

BIBLIOGRAPHY

Adams HP: Current status of antifibrinolytic therapy for treatment of patients with aneurysmal subarachnoid hemorrhage, *Curr Concepts Cerebrovasc Dis* 16(5):23, 1981.

Aita JF: Why patients with Parkinson's disease fall, *JAMA* 247(4):515, 1982.

Alter M: Amyotrophic lateral sclerosis, *Med Times* 110(10):42, 1982.

Barry K, Texerian S: The role of the nurse in the diagnostic classification and management of epileptic seizures, *J Neurosurg Nurs* 15(4):243, 1983.

Blount M, Kinney AB, Stove M: Plasma exchange in management of myasthenia gravis, *Nurs Clin North Am* 14(1):173, 1979.

Budassi S, Barber J: *Mosby's manual of emergency care: practices and procedures*, ed 2, 1984, CV Mosby.

Campbell VG: Neurological system. In Thompson JM et al: *Mosby's manual of clinical nursing*, ed 2, St Louis, 1989, Mosby–Year Book.

Campion HR et al: Trauma scare, *Crit Care Med* 9(9):672, 1981.

Conway BL: *Carini and Owens' neurological and neurosurgical nursing*, ed 8, St Louis, 1982, CV Mosby.

Cuddy PG: Management of acute opioid intoxication, *CCQ* 4:65, 1982.

Dau PC et al: Plasmapheresis and immunosuppressive drug therapy in myasthenia gravis, *N Engl J Med* 297(21):1134, 1977.

Davis J, Niason C: *Neurologic critical care*, New York, 1979, Van Nostrand Reinhold.

Department of Health, Education and Welfare: *Guidelines for stroke care*. Washington, DC, 1976, US Government Printing Office.

Essentials of the neurological examination, Philadelphia, 1974, Smith Kline & French.

Glanze WD et al: *Mosby's medical nursing and allied health dictionary*, ed 3, St Louis, 1990, Mosby–Year Book.

Goodman G: *The pharmacological basis of therapeutics*, ed 7, 1985, MacMillan Publishing.

Hart RG, Sherman DG: The diagnosis of multiple sclerosis, *JAMA* 247(4):498, 1982.

Hickey F: *The clinical practice of neurological and neurosurgical nursing*, ed 2, Philadelphia, 1986, JB Lippincott.

Johanson BC et al: *Standards for critical care*, ed 3, St Louis, 1988, Mosby–Year Book.

Knoben JE, Anderson PO, and Watanabe AS: *Handbook of clinical drug data*, ed 4, Hamilton, Ill, Drug Intelligence Publication.

Krenzel JR, Rohrer LM: *Handbook of care of paraplegic and quadriplegic individuals*, Chicago, 1972, National Association of Paraplegia and Quadriplegia.

Krenzelok EP: Phencyclidine—a contemporary drug of abuse, *CCQ* 4:55, 1982.

Lewis SM, Collier IC: *Medical surgical nursing: assessment and management of clinical problems*, New York, 1983, McGraw-Hill.

Mauss N, Mitchel P: Increased intracranial pressure, an update, *Heart Lung* 5:919, 1976.

Myasthenia gravis: a manual for physicians, New York, 1971, Myasthenia Gravis Foundation.

Nikas D, Konkoly L: Nursing responsibilities in arterial and intracranial pressure monitoring, *J Neurosurg Nurs* 7:116, 1975.

Nursing the multiple sclerosis patient, Chicago, 1969, National Multiple Sclerosis Society.

Phipps WJ, Long BC, and Woods NF: *Medical-surgical nursing: concepts and clinical practice*, ed 4, St Louis, 1990, Mosby–Year Book.

Purchase G: *Neuromedical, neurosurgical nursing*, London, 1977, Ballière Tindall.

Redelman K, ed: Neurological injuries, *CCQ* 2(1), 1979.

Ricci M: *Educational core curriculum for neuroscience nursing*, vol 2, ed 2, Park Ridge, Ill, 1984, American Association of Neuroscience Nurses.

Richmond TS, ed: Neurotrauma, *Nurs Clin North Am* 21(4):549, 1986.

Rimel R, John J, and Edlich RF: Assessment of recovery following head trauma. In Redelman K, ed: Neurological injuries, *CCQ* 2(1):97, 1979.

Snyder M: A guide to neurological and neurosurgical nursing, New York, 1983, John Wiley & Sons.

Taylor J, Ballenger S: *Neurological dysfunction and nursing intervention*, New York, 1980, McGraw-Hill.

Teasdale G, Jennett B: Assessment of coma and impaired consciousness: a practical scale, *Lancet* 2:81, 1974.

Tongs TG: "The alcohols" in poisonings and overdose, *CCQ* 1(4), 1982.

Turner M: Intracranial hypertension. In Redelman K, ed: Neurological injuries, *CCQ* 2(1):67, 1979.

Tyson GW et al: Acute care of the spinal cord injured patient. In Redelman K, ed: Neurological injuries, *CCQ* 2(1):45, 1979.

Vogt G, Miller M, Esluer M: *Mosby's manual of neurological care*, St Louis, 1985, CV Mosby.

Walton Sir JN: *Brain diseases of the nervous system*, ed 9, New York, 1985, Oxford University Press.

William A: Classification and diagnosis of epilepsy, *Nurs Clin North Am* 9:747, 1974.

Wing S: Cervical spine injuries: treatment and related nursing care, *J Neurosurg Nurs* 9:138, 1977.

Genitourinary System

GENITOURINARY ASSESSMENT

Subjective Data

Frequency of urination
Urgency
Strangury (painful urination, a drop at a time)
Burning on urination
Dribbling
Incontinence
    Functional
    Reflex
    Stress
    Total
    Urge
Hesitancy
Poor force of urinary stream
Nocturia
Enuresis
Hematuria
Pneumaturia
Complaints of pain
    Back
    Flank
    Costovertebral angle
    Abdominal
    Bladder spasms
    Urethral
    Genital
    Scrotal
    Testicular
    Perineal
    Rectal
Nausea, vomiting
Anorexia
Diarrhea
Constipation
Painful intercourse
Impotence

Objective Data

Physical examination
    Kidney (abdominal mass, flank mass, costovertebral angle tenderness)
    Bladder (presence of distention, pain)
    Urethra (drainage, discharge)
    Vagina (drainage, discharge, redness, inflammation)
    External genitalia (redness, sores, ulcers/lesions, rash, inflammation, pain)
    Testes/scrotum (enlargement, mass, tenderness)
    Prostate via rectum (size, consistency, induration)
Urine
    Color
    Odor
    Amount
        Polyuria
        Oliguria
        Anuria
    Specific gravity
    Voiding patterns (voiding diary)
    Presence of catheter
Pain (location, type, duration, precipitating and alleviating factors)
BP, T, P, and R
Weight
Fluid and electrolyte balance
Dehydration
Edema
Skin (dry, scaly, pale, or yellow-tan)
Uremia
Anemia
Congestive heart failure (CHF)
Pericarditis

Pertinent Background Information

CONCURRENT DISEASES AND/OR CONDITIONS

Hypertension
Diabetes
Tuberculosis
Allergies
    Shellfish
    Iodine
    Isotope dyes
    Penicillin
    Nonsteroidal antiinflammatory agents
Hormonal imbalance
Anemia
Systemic lupus erythematosus
Multiple myeloma
Vascular disease: polyarteritis
Sickle cell disease
Amyloidosis
Leukemia

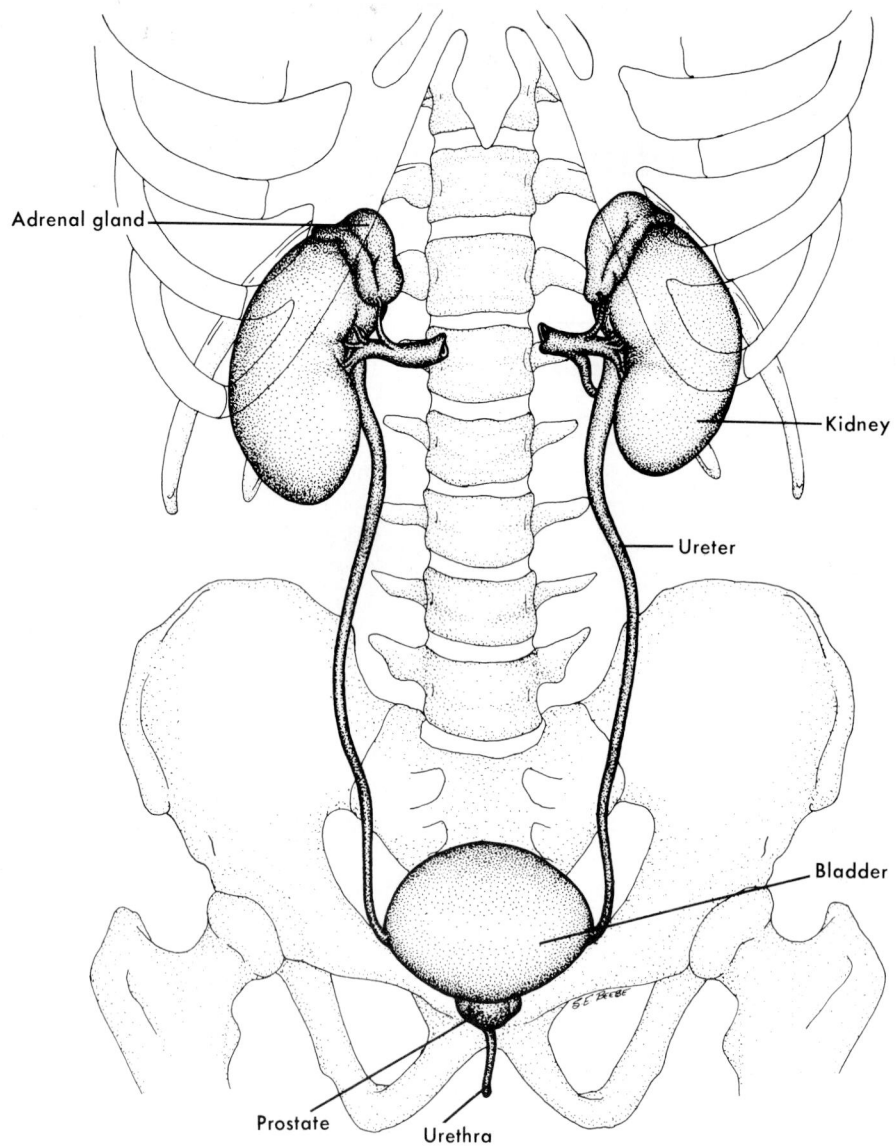

FIGURE 9-1. Genitourinary system.

Gout
Hyperparathyroidism
CVA
Brain tumor
Traumatic brain injury
Alzheimer's disease
Spinal cord injury
Transverse myelitis
Guillain-Barré syndrome
AIDS
Chemotherapy
Trauma
Presence of continuous, indwelling catheter
Frequent intermittent catheterization
Renal radiological procedures

Exposure to sexually transmitted diseases
Forceps delivery
Date of last menstrual period

PREVIOUS SURGERY OR ILLNESS

Genitourinary (GU) trauma/injury
Urological and/or renal surgery
Congenital anomalies
Urinary tract infections
Hereditary and/or noninherited renal disease
Kidney transplant
Kidney and/or bladder stones
Tuberculosis
Recent blood transfusion
Sexually transmitted disease
Multiple births

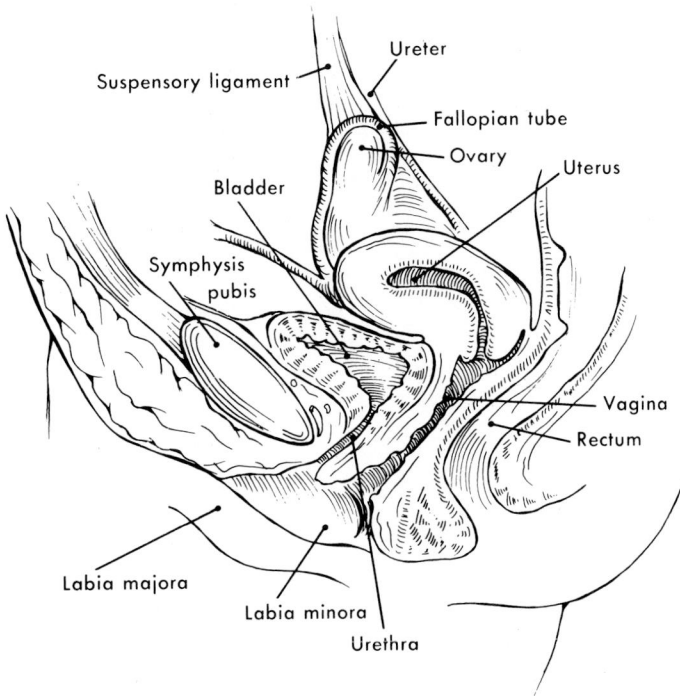

FIGURE 9-2. Female genitourinary and reproductive system. (From Meeker MH, Rothrock JC: *Alexander's care of the patient in surgery,* ed 9, St Louis, 1991, Mosby–Year Book; modified from Keuhnelian J, Sanders V: *Urologic nursing,* New York, 1970, Macmillan Publishing.)

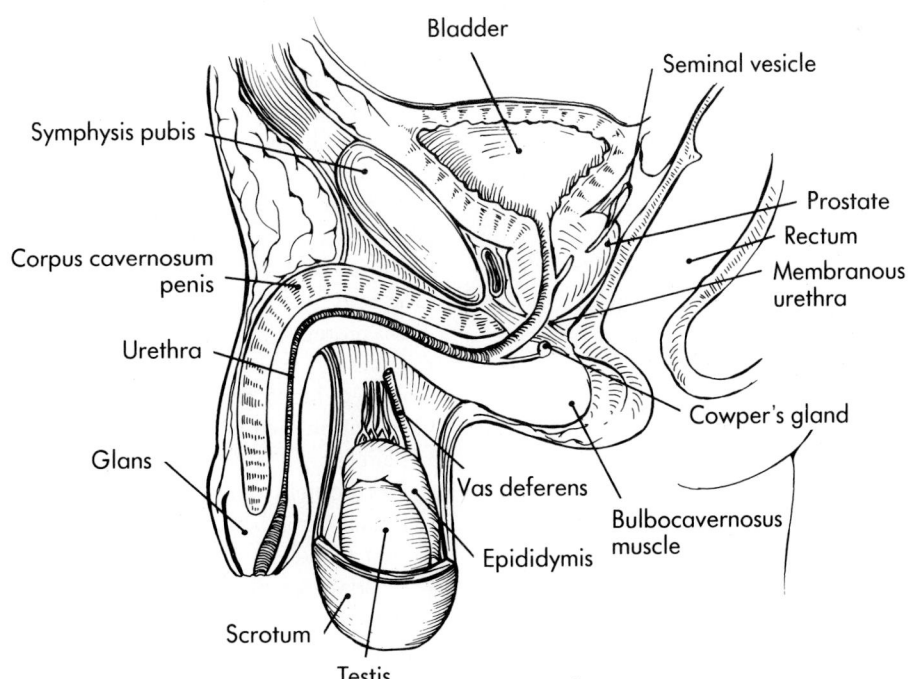

FIGURE 9-3. Male genitourinary and reproductive system. (From Meeker MH, Rothrock JC: *Alexander's care of the patient in surgery,* ed 9, St Louis, 1991, Mosby–Year Book; modified from Keuhnelian J, Sanders V: *Urologic nursing,* New York, 1970, Macmillan Publishing.)

FAMILY HISTORY

Hereditary and/or noninherited renal disease
Hypertension
Diabetes
Congenital anomalies
Cancer

SOCIAL HISTORY

Drinking of coffee, tea, cola, or alcoholic beverages
Smoking
Sexual activity
Occupation (e.g., contact with chemicals, plastic, pitch,
  tar, or rubber)
Use of feminine hygiene sprays
Use of perfumed soaps
Tub baths

MEDICATION HISTORY

Penicillin and/or other antibiotics
Hormones
Anticoagulants
Nonsteroidal antiinflammatory agents
Analgesics
Alpha-adrenergics
Alpha-adrenergic agonists
Alpha-blockers
Beta-adrenergics
Diuretics
Decongestants
Antipsychotropics
Antidepressants
Antiparkinsonian agents
Papaverine

Laboratory Tests

Urinalysis
  Color
  Clarity
  Odor
  pH
  Specific gravity
  Osmolality
  Sediment
  Red blood cells
  Pus
  Bacteria
  White blood cells
  Casts
  Crystals/calculi
  Blood
  Protein
  Glucose
  Creatinine
  Urea
  Uric acid

Electrolytes
  Sodium
  Potassium
  Chloride
  Calcium
  Phosphorus
  Magnesium
Urine culture and sensitivity
Urine collection (24 hr)
  Aldosterone
  17-Hydroxycorticosteroids
  17-Ketosteroids
  Catecholamines
    Norepinephrine
    Epinephrine
    Dopamine
  Stones
    Oxalate
    Cystine
  VMA
  Calcium
  Phosphorus
  Uric acid
Urine clearance tests
  Inulin
  Creatinine
  Phenosulfonphthalein (PSP)
Serum analysis
  Osmolality
  Electrolytes
    Sodium
    Potassium
    Chloride
    Calcium
    Phosphorus
    Magnesium
    Alkaline phosphatase
Blood urea nitrogen (BUN)
Creatinine
Uric acid
Total protein
Albumin
Complete blood cell count (CBC)
Coagulation factors
  Platelets
  Prothrombin time (PT)
  Partial thromboplastin time (PTT)
Tumor markers
  Prostatic specific antigen
  AFP
  HCG

Diagnostic Tests

Radiographic studies
  Kidney, ureter, bladder (KUB) x-ray examination

Excretory urogram
Nephrotomogram
Retrograde pyelogram
Retrograde cystogram, voiding cystourethrogram
Retrograde urethrogram
Renal angiogram (renogram)
    Renal arteriogram
    Renal venogram
Renal computed tomography (CT) scan
Renal and prostate ultrasonography
Radionuclide imaging
Endoscopic studies
    Cystoscopy
    Cystourethroscopy
    Ureteroscopy
    Percutaneous renal endoscopy (nephroscopy)
Renal biopsy
Urodynamic studies
    Cystometrogram
    Uroflowmetry
    Pressure flow study
    Urethral pressure profile
    Electromyography and electromyogram
Dynamic infusion cavernosometry and cavernosography
Magnetic resonance imaging

URINARY TRACT INFECTION (UTI)

An infection in any part of the urinary tract, caused by bacteria, primarily Escherichia coli; *risk and severity are enhanced by conditions such as vesicoureteral reflux, urinary tract obstruction, urinary stasis, recent urethral instrumentation, and septicemia*
lower urinary tract infections
urethritis An infection of the urethra
cystitis An infection localized in the bladder
prostatitis An infection of the prostate gland
upper urinary tract infection
pyelonephritis An infection causing inflammation of the renal parenchymal tissue and renal pelvis, caused by a systemic infection but usually resulting from an ascending infection of the lower urinary tract.

Assessment
Observations/findings
LOWER UTI

Suprapubic discomfort
Low back pain
Bladder spasms
Dysuria
Urinary frequency
Urinary hesitancy
Urinary urgency
Nocturia
Hematuria
Pyuria
Malodorous urine

UPPER UTI*

Flank pain
Tender, enlarged kidney
Costovertebral tenderness
Abdominal rigidity
Fever
Chills
Malaise
Anorexia
Nausea, vomiting
Decreased urine output
Elevated temperature

Laboratory/diagnostic studies

Urinalysis
    Cloudy
    Bacteria
    Pyuria
    White blood cells
    Red blood cells may be present
Positive urine culture and sensitivity
Radiography
    KUB
    Excretory urography
    Cystoscopy

Potential complications

Progression of UTI upward to kidney, resulting in
    Sepsis
    Nausea, vomiting, dehydration
    Parenchymal scarring
    Renal abscess
    Perinephric abscess
Recurrence (20% to 50% chance)
Formation of urinary calculi

Medical Management

Antibiotic therapy determined by urine culture and sensitivity
Fluids
Analgesics
Cystoscopy
IVP
Bed rest with gradual return to activities as tolerated
Surgical intervention if obstruction is present

Nursing diagnoses/interventions/evaluation

■ **NDX:** Infection related to presence of bacteria in the urinary tract

Assess temperature q4h and report if greater than 101°F (38.5°C)
Note character of urine; report if cloudy and malodorous

---

*Findings are in addition to those for lower UTI.

Collect midstream and/or clean-voided urine for culture and sensitivity when output is suspicious

Encourage high oral fluid intake, up to 2500 ml/day, to flush out bacteria, unless contraindicated

Monitor repeat urine specimens for culture and sensitivity to determine response to therapy

Instruct patient to void when urge is felt, before and after intercourse, and q3h to 4h except during sleep

Instruct patient to take time to empty bladder completely with each voiding

Teach patient to shower daily with antibacterial soap

Teach female patient to avoid tub baths

Provide good perineal hygiene; keep area clean and dry

Teach female patient to administer perianal care after each bowel movement and to wipe from front to back

Expected outcome/evaluation

Exhibits no signs of UTI, as evidenced by absence of flank pain, suprapubic tenderness, voiding symptoms, fever, chills, and/or malaise

Urine culture is negative for bacteria

■ **NDX:** Altered patterns of urinary elimination (dysuria, urgency, frequency, and/or nocturia) related to UTI

Measure and document urine output with each voiding; maintain voiding diary

Encourage voiding every 2 to 3 hr

Palpate bladder q4h for distention

Provide easy access to bathroom, bedpan, or urinal

Help patient assume a comfortable position for urination

Provide well-lighted area for patients with nocturia

Instruct patient to avoid drinking fluid for 2 to 3 hr before bedtime and to void before bedtime to achieve maximal sleep

Instruct patient to avoid coffee, tea, cola, and alcoholic beverages, which exacerbate irritative symptoms

Explain all diagnostic procedures used to further evaluate UTI

Expected outcome/evaluation

Patient voids with pattern of urinary elimination as near normal as possible, as evidenced by absence of dysuria, urgency, frequency, nocturia, and with balanced intake and output.

■ **NDX:** Pain related to UTI

Assess nature, intensity, location, duration, and precipitating and alleviating factors of pain

Provide bed rest; increase activities as ordered and tolerated

Provide nonpharmacological comfort measures: assist pa-

tient with assuming comfortable position, provide sitz baths and warm perineal soaks, teach relaxation techniques and guided imagery, and/or provide diversional activity

Encourage high oral fluid intake to dilute urine

Monitor and document pain relief and any undesirable side effects

Notify physician of unrelieved or increasing pain

Expected outcome/evaluation

Reports a decrease in pain and a decrease in burning on urination

Shows a relaxed facial expression and body position

■ **NDX:** Knowledge deficit related to lack of exposure to information about disease process, methods of prevention, and home care and follow-up instructions

Instruct patient to drink 2000 to 2500 ml of fluid/day unless contraindicated

Instruct patient to avoid coffee, tea, cola, and alcoholic beverages

Teach methods of preventing recurrence of UTI
  Empty bladder q4h; avoid prolonged bladder distention
  Women
    Keep perineal region clean and dry; wipe from front to back after each bowel movement
    Empty bladder before and after intercourse
    Shower with antibacterial soap; avoid perfumed soaps
    Avoid tub baths, especially bubble baths
    Report and treat vaginal discharge promptly
    Avoid use of feminine hygiene sprays and douches
    Wear cotton underpants; avoid nylon underpants
    Wear loose, nonrestrictive clothing

Teach symptoms of recurrence of UTI and instruct patient to report their presence to physician

Instruct patient to complete prescribed course of antibiotics

Teach method and importance of obtaining midstream urine specimen for culture and sensitivity after course of antibiotic therapy

Teach method of self-monitoring urine test for bacteria (Microstix)

Teach name of medication, dosage, schedule, purpose, and side effects

Instruct patient to avoid taking over-the-counter medications without checking with physician

Emphasize importance of ongoing outpatient care because of high incidence of recurrent infection

Expected outcome/evaluation

Patient and/or significant other verbalizes understanding of disease process, methods of prevention, and home care and follow-up instructions; is able to state symptoms of recurrence of UTI to report to physician; and return-demonstrates self-monitoring urine test for bacteria (Microstix) and midstream urine collection technique

URINARY INCONTINENCE

An involuntary loss of urine, classified into five types: functional, stress, reflex, urge, and total

General Assessment (All Types)
Observations/findings

Existing diseases/conditions
Pregnancy history
Sexual history
Fluid intake
Age and physical condition
Current medications
Change in urinary patterns
    Use voiding diary noting
        Time and amount voided; continent/incontinent
        Strength of urge/stream
        Activity before incontinence
        Voiding interval
        Fluid amount in relation to voiding time

Laboratory/diagnostic studies

Voiding cystourethrogram
Urodynamic testing
IVP
Retrograde urethrogram
Cystoscopy
Urethroscopy
Urinalysis and culture
Bladder biopsy

Functional Incontinence

The involuntary loss of urine, which is unpredictable and occurs when continent people are unable or unwilling to get to the bathroom on time; there is no impairment of the urinary system; associated with emotional illness, head injury, joint and muscle abnormalities, and pain

Assessment and Medical Management

See Table 9-1, comparison of five types of incontinence (p. 454)

Nursing diagnoses interventions/evaluation

■ **NDX:** Functional incontinence related to sensory, cognitive, or motor deficits, or altered environment

Assess usual pattern of voiding through use of voiding diary; maintain diary to assess effectiveness of planned program

In collaboration with physician assess effect of medications and determine possible changes in drug, dosage, or schedule to decrease risk of incontinence
Monitor intake and output; adjust intake so that largest amounts are taken at time of day patient is best able to remain continent; ensure a fluid intake of 2000 ml/day unless restricted

Cognitive deficit

Assess cognitive deficit and tailor voiding program as needed
Determine usual interval between voidings
Plan a fixed voiding schedule to eliminate incontinence, such as q2h, and then assist patient
    Discuss schedule with patient and have patient void at specified times or assist patient at scheduled times
Prompt voiding by questioning patient at scheduled times; assist as necessary
Provide positive reinforcement for continent behavior

Motor/sensory deficits

Assess for sensory or motor deficits that inhibit patient from reaching bathroom or receptacle in time to void without incontinence
Determine optimal interval to avoid incontinence
Plan fixed voiding schedule initially then increase interval in small increments of time to q3h to 4h
Assist with voiding as necessary
    Provide equipment to enable patient to toilet alone; bedpan or urinal within reach; trapeze or walkers for easy movement; bedside commode, elevated toilet seats; bars in bathrooms, etc.
Assess pain and comfort level; administer ordered medications or assist with alternate pain relief measures before timed voiding
Assess bowel elimination qd; remove impactions if present; institute bowel training program when appropriate

Altered environment

Orient patient to location of bathroom and/or placement of equipment
Assess environment to determine obstacles that may inhibit patient's reaching toileting facilities on time
Modify identified obstacles or hazards
Maintain privacy for voiding
Place call light and needed equipment within reach
Answer call light *promptly* to assist patient
Suggest use of bed clothes and robes that permit easy removal for voiding
Place furniture to permit easy access to bathroom
Keep bed in low position with rails down if safety factors allow
Use night light or keep bathroom door ajar with light on

Expected outcome/evaluation

    Remains continent

TABLE 9-1. Incontinence Assessment and Medical Management*

Factors	Functional incontinence	Stress incontinence	Reflex incontinence	Urge incontinence	Total incontinence
SPECIFIC ASSESSMENT					
Character of voiding urge	Usually strong	Sudden, associated with increased abdominal pressure	None	Very strong with inability to delay voiding	None
Amount voided	Moderate to large	Small, usually < 50 ml	Moderate	Small to large	Constant leakage
Nocturia (more than two times)	May be present	Not usual	Always	Common	Always
Frequency of urination (more than q2h)	Variable	Increased	Regular intervals related to volume	Increased	Constant, unpredictable
Awareness of incontinence	Aware	Aware	Unaware; however, sympathetic response may be present: diaphoresis, flushing of skin, "gooseflesh," nausea	Aware	Unaware
Precipitating factors	Inability to read receptacle Environmental problems, e.g., lack of privacy, side rails up on bed	Increased intra-abdominal pressure Obesity Laughing Coughing Sneezing Lifting Exercise	Full bladder Bladder contraction or spasm	Sensation of full bladder and inability to reach receptacle on time, Catheter use Increased fluids Increased urine concentration Alcohol, caffeine use	Unpredictable
MEDICAL MANAGEMENT					
	Evaluate medication regimen and change as necessary and possible Behavioral therapy	Surgery Vesicourethral suspension Artificial urinary sphincter Periurethral injection Alpha-adrenergics Estrogen therapy Anticholinergics Skin care management	Intermittent catheterization External catheter drainage Surgery; continent diversion Indwelling catheter (last resort) Skin care management	Medications Anticholinergics Antispasmodics Treatment of infections Evaluate diuretic therapy and change when possible; e.g., schedule Reduced-calorie diet Skin care management	Surgery Repair fistulas Correct congenital defect Artificial sphincter Urinary diversion External collecting devices Skin care management

* Adapted from McFarland GK, McFarlane EA: *Nursing diagnosis and intervention*, St Louis, 1989, CV Mosby.

Through change in medication, dosage, or schedule
Using a fixed or prompted schedule
By habit training
Through environmental alterations (list)
Intake and output are balanced with at least 2000 ml of fluid intake/day

■ **NDX:** Potential for impaired skin integrity related to incontinence

Assess perineal area for redness, irritation, swelling, or breaks
Cleanse skin with mild soap and water or no-rinse cleaners and dry well after each incontinent episode
Apply skin barrier, protective spray, or sealant
Keep bed linen dry and wrinkle-free
Use absorbent products, briefs, shields, or underpads if incontinent episodes are frequent
  Be certain plastic does not touch skin, causing maceration from increased perspiration

Expected outcome/evaluation

Patient's perineal skin is intact

■ **NDX:** Body image disturbance related to incontinence

Provide an accepting and supportive atmosphere
Determine how incontinence has affected patient's daily activities and sex life
Encourage expression of feelings of anxiety, fear, embarrassment, anger, frustration, and/or helplessness
Promote feelings of self-worth by stressing positive features in patient's life
Be nonjudgmental when cleaning patient after an episode of incontinence
Suggest methods to control odor: good perineal hygiene; change clothing as needed; avoid foods that cause a strong odor in urine
Provide suggestions to help maintain a satisfactory level of sexual expression; alternate positions, empty bladder before intercourse, etc.
Encourage communication with significant other
Provide assistance from other professionals to help deal with emotional changes (psychiatrist, sexual counselor)
Encourage participation in support group

Expected outcome/evaluation

Discusses feelings of anxiety, embarrassment; changes in lifestyle with care giver or significant other
Expresses feeling less anxious and more able to manage changes
Participates in ADL
Makes arrangements to meet with support group
Seeks assistance from other professionals when needed

■ **NDX:** Knowledge deficit related to lack of exposure to information about controlling incontinence

Review need for maintaining voiding schedule
Discuss importance of maintaining fluid intake at 2000 to 2500 ml/day, increasing amounts at times when patient has better control of voiding
Discuss methods for preventing and handling unexpected incontinence
  Void before social activities, trips, etc.
  Plan sexual activity for times when bladder is empty
  Carry a change of clothing for use in unexpected episodes of incontinence
  Discuss availability of undergarments or shields with absorbent materials
Teach signs and symptoms of UTI to report
Stress need to evaluate episodes of incontinence for precipitating factors and to make changes as necessary; report continued incontinence
Provide facts about incontinence and numbers of people affected
Reinforce need to continue communication with significant other; use of support groups and other health professionals
Discuss need to perform activities of daily living and resume self-care within capabilities
Teach name of medication, dosage, side and toxic effects to report, and need to take as scheduled
Emphasize need to keep regular laboratory and follow-up appointments

Expected outcome/evaluation

Patient and/or significant other verbalizes understanding of need to maintain voiding schedule, take fluids to 2000 ml/day, take measures to prevent or manage unexpected incontinence, report symptoms of UTI, keep follow-up appointments, alter environment to avoid risk of incontinence

Stress Incontinence

The involuntary loss of less than 50 ml of urine occurring with increased intraabdominal pressure; this type of incontinence is associated with decreased tone of the pelvic floor muscles or damage to the internal sphincter or bladder neck caused by surgery, trauma, radiation, decreased estrogen levels, or UTI

Assessment and Medical Management

See Table 9-1, comparison of five types of incontinence

Nursing diagnoses/interventions/evaluation

■ **NDX:** Stress incontinence related to weak pelvis and structure supports, overdistention between voidings, or high intraabdominal pressure

Assess usual pattern of voiding through use of voiding diary; maintain voiding diary to assess effectiveness of interventions

Observe urinary meatus to check for leakage when patient has a full bladder

Instruct patient to cough while in lithotomy position; if no leakage, repeat with patient at 45-degree angle; continue with patient standing if no previous leakage

Monitor intake and output; adjust intake so that largest amounts are taken at time of day patient is best able to remain continent; ensure a fluid intake of 2000 ml/day unless restricted

Teach patient that decreased fluid intake does not decrease incontinent episodes

In collaboration with physician assess effect of medications and determine possible changes in drug, dosage, or schedule to decrease frequency of incontinence

Weak pelvic and structural supports

Teach techniques to strengthen pelvic muscles (pubococcygeus)

Kegel exercises

Identify pelvic muscles by

Tightening muscles around anus while sitting or standing

Starting and stopping urine flow while voiding

Keeping buttocks, thigh, and abdominal muscles relaxed

Perform quick Kegel exercises

Tighten and relax pelvic muscles as rapidly as possible

Perform slow Kegel exercises

Tighten muscle group and hold for a count of 10, then relax

Pull in-push out exercises

Use pelvic and abdominal muscles to pull up pelvic floor as though trying to suck water

Push out or bear down to push imaginary water out

Daily schedule

Week 1: do 10 of each exercise: quick and slow Kegel exercises and pull in-push out exercises, four times a day

Each succeeding week increase each exercise by five, completing four sets a day

Results should be seen in about 3 months

Instruct patient to tighten pelvic muscles before coughing, laughing, or any activity that increases abdominal pressure, to attempt to prevent leakage

Overdistention

Assess factors leading to overdistention; increased fluid intake, use of diuretics, or decreased frequency of urination resulting from immobility, unwillingness to ask for assistance, etc.

Assess abdomen for bladder distention immediately after an episode of incontinence

Discuss reasons for avoiding overdistention of bladder

Institute habit training during early period of muscle strengthening

Plan a fixed voiding schedule

Set interval shorter than that in which incontinence occurs such as q2h

Discuss schedule with patient and have patient void at specified times, or assist patient with toileting at scheduled times

Prompt voiding by questioning patient at scheduled times; assist as necessary

Begin bowel training to increase interval very gradually over weeks or months as pelvic muscles strengthen

Alter other factors that cause patient to delay toileting

Provide positive reinforcement for continent behavior

High intraabdominal pressure

Discuss with patient fact that weight reduction may decrease incidence of incontinence

Provide dietary consultation to plan weight-reduction diet, incorporating preferences with preexisting medical conditions

Have patient make daily menu selections

Praise efforts taken to reduce weight

Weigh weekly to determine effectiveness

Institute exercise program to tone body and assist with weight reduction; ensure that program is appropriate for age, existing medical or surgical condition

Expected outcome/evaluation

Performs pelvic muscle exercises daily; incontinent episodes are decreasing or patient voids on a regular schedule and does not have a distended bladder or episodes of incontinence; weight is decreasing and patient begins exercise program; intake and output are balanced with at least 2000 to 2500 ml/day intake of nonirritating type fluids

■ **NDX:**   Potential for impaired skin integrity related to incontinence

Assess perineal area for redness, irritation, swelling, or breaks

Cleanse skin with mild soap and water or no-rinse cleaners and dry well after each incontinent episode

Apply skin barrier protective spray or sealant

Keep bed linen dry and wrinkle-free

Use absorbent products, briefs, shields, or underpads, if incontinent episodes are frequent

Be certain plastic does not touch skin, causing maceration from increased perspiration

Expected outcome/evaluation

Patient's perineal skin is intact

■ NDX: Body image disturbance related to incontinence

Provide an accepting and supportive atmosphere

Determine how incontinence has affected patient's daily activities and sex life

Encourage expression of feelings of anxiety, fear, embarrassment, anger, frustration, and/or helplessness

Promote feelings of self-worth by stressing positive features in patient's life

Be nonjudgmental when cleaning patient after an episode of incontinence

Suggest methods to control odor: good perineal hygiene; change clothing as needed; avoid foods that cause a strong odor in urine

Provide suggestions to help maintain a satisfactory level of sexual expression; empty bladder before intercourse, use alternate positions, etc.

Encourage communication with significant other

Provide assistance from other professionals to help deal with emotional changes (psychiatrist, sexual counselor)

Encourage participation in support group

Expected outcome/evaluation

Discusses feelings of anxiety, embarrassment; changes in lifestyle with care giver or significant other

Expresses feeling less anxious and more able to manage changes

Participates in ADLs

Makes arrangements to meet with a support group

Seeks assistance from other professionals when needed

■ NDX: Knowledge deficit related to lack of exposure to information about management of incontinence

Discuss need to do pelvic muscle exercises daily; to reduce weight to that determined for age, body type, and height, to void routinely to avoid bladder distention

Discuss importance of maintaining fluid intake at 2000 to 2500 ml/day, increasing amounts at times throughout the day when patient has better control of incontinence

Review techniques to control odor of urine

Discuss availability of absorbent shields, briefs, or undergarments

Teach signs of skin impairment; early action to take and signs to report

Teach signs and symptoms of UTI to report

Provide facts about incontinence and numbers of people affected

Reinforce need to continue communication with significant other; use of support groups and other health professionals

Discuss need to perform activities of daily living and resume self-care within capabilities

Teach name of medication, dosage, side and toxic effects to report, and need to take as scheduled

Emphasize need to keep regular laboratory and follow-up appointments

Expected outcome/evaluation

Patient and/or significant other verbalizes understanding of need to perform daily pelvic muscle exercises, void routinely to prevent bladder distention, reduce weight to decrease intraabdominal pressure, change wet garments and/or bed linens routinely, maintain intake of nonirritating liquids to 2000 ml/day, resume self-care activities, keep follow-up appointments, take measures to prevent skin breakdown, report symptoms of UTI and skin impairment and demonstrates pelvic muscle exercises

Reflex Incontinence

The involuntary loss of urine at fairly predictable intervals; the detrusor contraction is stimulated by a full bladder; the bladder empties but a large residual usually remains; this type of incontinence is associated with spinal cord lesions above S-2 to S-4, traumatic injuries, tumors, multiple sclerosis, other demyelinating diseases, and some cerebral lesions

Assessment and Medical Management

See Table 9-1, comparison of five types of incontinence (p. 454)

Nursing diagnoses/interventions/evaluation

■ NDX: Reflex incontinence related to neurological impairment

Assess usual pattern of urinary elimination; use voiding diary

Assess for signs patient may experience before incontinence; diaphoresis, flushing, pilomotor response (gooseflesh), or nausea

Instruct patient to call for assistance with voiding when first sign is experienced

In collaboration with physician determine acceptable residual urine volume (usually 50 to 75 ml)

Continue checking for residual volume until desired level is obtained

Explore mechanisms that may trigger bladder emptying; stroking inner thigh, tapping or stroking lower abdomen, anal stimulation, or stroking vulva or glans penis

Determine usual voiding interval

Before next expected voiding, place patient in optimal voiding position, if possible, to practice these mechanisms

Perform sterile catheterization to determine residual amount

Continue use of triggering mechanisms if successful and checking of residual volume until desired residual volume level is obtained

Discuss inability to use mechanisms or residual volume that is more than desired amount with physician to determine need for intermittent catheterization

Assess fluid intake and urine output volume to determine optimal interval for intermittent catheterization to prevent overdistention of bladder with sequelae; usually q3h initially

Continue to adjust fluid intake to lengthen interval to 5 to 6 hr while ensuring an intake of 2000 to 2500 ml/day

Assess for autonomic dysreflexia (hyperreflexia); pounding headache, blurred vision, hypertension to 300 mm Hg, profuse diaphoresis and flushing above level of spinal injury; severe pilomotor response and pale skin appearing below injury level; nausea, restlessness, and nasal congestion that may be present.

Immediately elevate head of bed, empty bladder, and notify physician

Expected outcome/evaluation

Intake and output are balanced; with at least 2000 ml intake/day; symptoms of UTI are absent; patient uses triggering mechanism to initiate voiding and empties bladder with residual volume within acceptable limits, or is unable to use triggering mechanisms and bladder is emptied by intermittent catheterization at increasing intervals with a volume of no more than 300 ml

■ **NDX:** Potential for impaired skin integrity related to incontinence

Assess perineal area for redness, irritation, swelling, or breaks

Cleanse skin with mild soap and water or no-rinse cleaners and dry well after each incontinent episode

Apply skin barrier protective spray or sealant

Keep bed linen dry and wrinkle-free

Use absorbent products, briefs, shields, or underpads if incontinent episodes are frequent

Be certain plastic does not touch skin, causing maceration from increased perspiration

Apply external collection device if incontinence continues and skin shows signs of breakdown

Expected outcome/evaluation

Patient's perineal skin is intact

■ **NDX:** Body image disturbance related to incontinence

Provide an accepting and supportive atmosphere

Determine how incontinence has affected patient's daily activities and sex life

Encourage expression of feelings of anxiety, fear, embarrassment, anger, frustration, and/or helplessness

Promote feelings of self-worth by stressing positive features in patient's life

Be nonjudgmental when cleaning patient after an episode of incontinence

Suggest methods to control odor; good perineal hygiene, change clothing as needed, avoid foods that cause a strong odor in urine

Provide suggestions to help maintain a satisfactory level of sexual expression; alternate positions, empty bladder before intercourse

Encourage communication with significant other

Provide assistance from other professionals to help deal with emotional changes (psychiatrist, sexual counselor)

Encourage participation in support group

Expected outcome/evaluation

Discusses feelings of anxiety, embarrassment; changes in lifestyle with care giver or significant other

Expresses feeling less anxious and more able to manage changes

Participates in ADLs

Makes arrangements to meet with a support group

Seeks assistance from other professionals when needed

■ **NDX:** Knowledge deficit related to lack of exposure to information about controlling incontinence

Discuss importance of maintaining fluid intake at 2000 to 2500 ml/day and coordinating intake with output to keep output volume to 300 ml or less with each voiding

Teach patient using self-stimulation to initiate voiding and to check for residual urine on a regular basis as determined in consultation with physician

Teach intermittent self-catheterization (p. 463) to patient and/or significant other

Discuss need to maintain regular schedule for self-catheterization

Discuss and provide written information about signs of autonomic dysreflexia and action to take

Discuss methods for preventing and handling unexpected incontinence

Be aware of activities that stimulate voiding (stroking, scratching legs or genitalia, etc.) and to avoid if possible

Initiate voiding or perform self-catherization before social activities, trips, etc.

Plan sexual activity for times when bladder is empty

Carry self-catheterization equipment for use when unplanned delays may occur

Carry a change of clothing for use in unexpected episodes of incontinence

Discuss availability of undergarments or shields with absorbent materials

Teach signs of skin impairment; early action to take and signs to report

Teach signs and symptoms of UTI to report

Provide facts about incontinence and numbers of people affected

Reinforce need to continue communication with significant other; use of support groups and other health professionals

Discuss need to perform activities of daily living and resume self-care within capabilities

Emphasize need to keep regular laboratory and follow-up appointments

Expected outcome/evaluation

Patient and/or significant other verbalizes understanding of need to maintain fluid intake to 2000 ml/day; need to empty bladder at intervals so that no more than 300 ml is obtained; measures to take to prevent or manage unexpected incontinence; symptoms of and action to take at first sign of autonomic hyperreflexia; measures to take to prevent skin breakdown; symptoms of UTI and skin impairment to report; to resume self-care activities, and keep follow-up appointments. Demonstrates self-catheterization procedure and checking for residual urine

Urge Incontinence

The involuntary loss of urine occurring after a strong urge is felt but when the patient is unable to hold the urine long enough to reach the bathroom or receptacle; this type of incontinence is associated with: detrusor instability caused by disorders of the central nervous system, such as CVA, Parkinson's disease, Alzheimer's disease, brain tumors, or trauma; reduced bladder capacity resulting from long-term indwelling catheter, abdominal surgery, trauma, or tumors; bladder irritation resulting from infection or ingestion of irritating fluids; or overdistention of the bladder resulting from increased fluid intake or decreased intervals between voidings

Assessment and Medical Management

See Table 9-1, comparison of five types of urinary incontinence (p. 454)

Nursing diagnoses/interventions/evaluation

■ **NDX:** Urge incontinence related to decreased bladder capacity, bladder irritability, overdistention of the bladder, or neurological deficits

Assess usual pattern of voiding through use of voiding diary; maintain diary to assess effectiveness of planned program

In collaboration with physician assess effect of medications and determine possible changes in drug, dosage, or schedule to decrease risk of incontinence

Assess for sensory or motor deficits that inhibit patient from reaching bathroom or receptacle in time to void without incontinence

Provide equipment to enable patient to toilet alone; bedpan or urinal within reach; trapeze or walkers for easy movement; bedside commode, elevated toilet seats; bars in bathrooms, etc.

Assess pain and comfort level; administer ordered medications or assist with alternate pain relief measures before timed voiding

Monitor intake and output; adjust intake so that largest amounts are taken at time of day patient is best able to remain continent; ensure a fluid intake of 2000 ml/day unless restricted

Overdistention

Assess factors leading to overdistention; increased fluid intake, use of diuretics, or decreased frequency of urination resulting from immobility, unwillingness to ask for assistance, etc.

Assess abdomen for bladder distention after incontinent episode

Discuss reasons for avoiding overdistended bladder

Determine usual interval between voidings

Plan a fixed voiding schedule

Set interval shorter than that in which incontinence occurs, such as q2h

Discuss schedule with patient and have patient void at specified times, or assist patient with toileting at scheduled times

Prompt voiding by questioning patient at scheduled times; assist as necessary

Alter other factors that cause patient to delay toileting

Provide positive reinforcement for continent behavior

Decreased bladder size/neurological deficit

Determine optimal interval to avoid incontinence

Plan fixed voiding schedule initially

Set interval shorter than that in which incontinence occurs

Increase interval in small increments of time until bladder capacity increases to about 200 to 250 ml q4h without incontinence

Maintain fixed or prompted schedule if incontinence continues to occur when interval is increased in several trials

Assist with voiding as necessary

Provide equipment to enable patient to toilet alone; bedpan or urinal within reach; trapeze or walkers for eacy movement; bedside commode, elevated toilet seats; bars in bathrooms, etc.

Irritable bladder

Assess for UTI and report if present

Discuss need to maintain fluid intake to at least 2500 ml/day

Disabuse patient of idea that a decreased fluid intake will decrease risk of incontinence

Explain that increased fluids will dilute urine, thereby decreasing irritable symptoms

Discuss need to avoid irritating fluids, such as drinks with caffeine or alcohol

Expected outcome/evaluation

Remains continent while increasing interval between voidings or remains continent on a fixed schedule; is not able to increase intervals between voidings without incontinence. Intake and output are balanced with at least 2000 to 2500 ml/day of nonirritating fluids

■ **NDX:** Potential for impaired skin integrity related to incontinence

Assess perineal area for redness, irritation, swelling, or breaks

Cleanse skin with mild soap and water or no-rinse cleaners and dry well after each incontinent episode

Apply skin barrier, protective spray, or sealant

Keep bed linen dry and wrinkle-free

Use absorbent products, briefs, shields, or underpads if incontinent episodes are frequent

Be certain plastic does not touch skin, causing maceration from increased perspiration

Expected outcome/evaluation

Patient's perineal skin is intact

■ **NDX:** Body image disturbance related to incontinence

Provide an accepting and supportive atmosphere

Determine how incontinence has affected patient's daily activities and sex life

Encourage expression of feelings of anxiety, fear, embarrassment, anger, frustration, and/or helplessness

Promote feelings of self-worth by stressing positive features in patient's life

Be nonjudgmental when cleaning patient after an episode of incontinence

Suggest methods to control odor; good perineal hygiene, change clothing as needed, avoid foods that cause a strong odor in urine

Provide suggestions to help maintain a satisfactory level of sexual expression; alternate positions, empty bladder before intercourse

Encourage communication with significant other

Provide assistance from other professionals to help deal with emotional changes (psychiatrist, sexual counselor)

Encourage participation in support group

Expected outcome/evaluation

Discusses feelings of anxiety, embarrassment; changes in lifestyle with care giver or significant other

Expresses feeling less anxious and more able to manage changes

Participates in ADLs

Makes arrangements to meet with a support group

Seeks assistance from other professionals when needed

■ **NDX:** Knowledge deficit related to lack of exposure to information about controlling incontinence

Discuss voiding schedule and how patient will incorporate into daily activities, e.g., use of reminder such as a timer

Discuss use of a voiding diary

Discuss need to increase intervals between voidings when appropriate

Discuss importance of maintaining fluid intake at 2000 to 2500 ml/day, increasing amounts at times of day when patient has better control of voiding; discuss type of fluids to take

Discuss methods for preventing and handling unexpected incontinence

Void before social activities, trips, etc.

Plan sexual activity for times when bladder is empty

Carry a change of clothing for use in unexpected episodes of incontinence

Discuss availability of undergarments or shields with absorbent materials

Stress need to evaluate episodes of incontinence for precipitating factors and to make changes as necessary; report continued incontinence

Teach signs and symptoms of UTI to report

Teach signs of skin impairment; early action to take and signs to report

Provide facts about incontinence and numbers of people affected

Reinforce need to continue communication with significant other; use of support groups and other health professionals

Discuss need to perform activities of daily living and resume self-care within capabilities

Emphasize need to keep regular laboratory and follow-up appointments

Expected outcome/evaluation

Patient and/or significant other verbalizes understanding of need to maintain voiding schedule, increasing intervals as established; to maintain intake of nonirritating liquids to 2000 ml/day; to resume self-care activities; to keep follow-up appointments; and to alter environment to avoid risk of incontinent episodes, repeats measures to take to prevent or manage unexpected incontinence; measures to take to prevent skin breakdown; symptoms of UTI and skin impairment to report

Total Incontinence

The involuntary, unpredictable or continuous loss of urine; this type of incontinence is associated with neurological diseases or conditions, anatomical deficits, such as fistulae, or damage from surgery, trauma, or radiation

Assessment and Medical Management

See Table 9-1, comparison of five types of urinary incontinence (p. 454)

Nursing diagnoses/interventions/evaluation

■ **NDX:** Total incontinence related to neurological dysfunction, independent contraction of detrusor reflex caused by surgery, trauma, or radiation, or anatomical problems such as fistulae

Assess type of incontinence in collaboration with physician using voiding diary and checking for residual to rule out other types

In collaboration with physician assess effect of medications and determine possible changes in drug, dosage, or schedule to decrease frequency of incontinence

Provide absorbent briefs, undergarments, and underpads; plan schedule for routine changes q1h to 2h during period when most fluids are being taken, then q2h to 3h during sleep periods

Provide call light within reach and have patient who can communicate call when wet; stress importance of not staying wet for long periods of time

Provide absorbent briefs, undergarments, and underpads for self-care when patient can manage without assistance

Expected outcome/evaluation

Patient changes wet garments routinely without assistance, or wet absorbent garments, underpads and bed linen are changed routinely

■ **NDX:** Potential for impaired skin integrity related to incontinence

Assess perineal area for redness, irritation, swelling, or breaks

Cleanse skin with mild soap and water or no-rinse cleaners and dry well after each incontinent episode

Apply skin barrier protective spray or sealant

Keep bed linen dry and wrinkle-free

Use external collection devices if skin shows any signs of breakdown

  Males

    Condom catheter with drainage bag

      Check penis regularly for excoriation or constriction and condom for twisting and pooling of urine

    Retracted penis pouch with drainage bag

      Clip hair and apply skin protective barrier film before applying

      Check regularly for excoriation

  Females

    Prepare skin and apply external device

    Check regularly for excoriation

  Connect external devices to collection system

  Coil tubing to prevent dependent loops

  Keep drainage bag below bladder at all times

  Be certain plastic does not touch skin, causing maceration from increased perspiration

Expected outcome/evaluation

Patient's perineal skin is intact; external collection device drains urine and patient remains dry without pooling of urine in device

■ **NDX:** Body image disturbance related to incontinence

Provide an accepting and supportive atmosphere

Determine how incontinence has affected patient's daily activities and sex life

Encourage expression of feelings of anxiety, fear, embarrassment, anger, frustration, and/or helplessness

Promote feelings of self-worth by stressing positive features in patient's life

Be nonjudgmental when cleaning patient after an episode of incontinence

Suggest methods to control odor; good perineal hygiene, change clothing as needed, avoid foods that cause a strong odor in urine

Provide suggestions to help maintain a satisfactory level of sexual expression

Encourage communication with significant other

Provide assistance from other professionals to help deal with emotional changes (psychiatrist, sexual counselor)

Encourage participation in support group

Expected outcome/evaluation

Discusses feelings of anxiety, embarrassment; changes in lifestyle with care giver or significant other

Reports feeling less anxious and more able to manage changes

Participates in ADLs

Makes arrangements to meet with a support group

Seeks assistance from other professionals when needed

■ **NDX:** Knowledge deficit related to lack of exposure to information about management of incontinence

Discuss importance of maintaining fluid intake at 2000 to 2500 m/day, increasing amounts at times when patient has better control of wetness

Review techniques to control odor of urine

Discuss availability of absorbent briefs, undergarments, or underpads

Review procedure for applying external collecting device; have patient or significant other apply device; coach as needed

Teach signs of skin impairment; early action to take and signs to report

Teach signs and symptoms of UTI to report

PATIENT CARE STANDARDS

Provide facts about incontinence and numbers of people
affected

Reinforce need to continue communication with significant other; use of support groups and other health
professionals

Discuss need to perform activities of daily living and resume self-care within capabilities

Teach name of medication, dosage, side and toxic effects
to report, and need to take as scheduled

Emphasize need to keep regular laboratory and follow-up
appointments

Expected outcome/evaluation

Patient and/or significant other verbalizes understanding
of need to change wet garments and/or bed linen routinely, to maintain intake of nonirritating liquids to
2000 ml/day, to resume self-care activities, to keep
follow-up appointments; repeats measures to take to
prevent skin breakdown, symptoms of UTI and skin
impairment to report

ACUTE URINARY RETENTION

*A condition in which the bladder becomes distended with
urine and the patient is unable to completely empty
the bladder; major cause is obstruction; other causes
include a neurogenic bladder, trauma, postoperative
complications, anxiety, muscle tension, and side effects
of medications*

Assessment
Observations/findings

Urinary pattern (voiding diary)
　Cessation of urination
　Decrease in volume
　Inability to start stream
　Decrease in force of stream
　Interruption of flow
　Frequency with small amounts
　Dribbling
　Dysuria
　Postvoiding residual > 100 ml
Output less than intake
Bladder distention
Bladder tenderness
Suprapubic pain
Restlessness
Anxiety
Diaphoresis
Cystitis
Administration of medications
　Anticholinergics
　Antihistamines
Fecal impaction

Laboratory/diagnostic studies

Urinalysis
Urine culture and sensitivity
Serum electrolytes
Serum creatinine
Serum BUN
Kidney, ureter, bladder (KUB) x-ray examination
IVP
Urodynamic studies

Potential complications

UTI
Electrolyte imbalance
Hemorrhage
Shock

Medical Management

Catheterization
Cholinergics to stimulate bladder contraction (Urecho-
line)
Analgesics to control pain
Antibiotics in presence of infection
IV hydration
Surgery to remove or bypass obstruction

Nursing diagnoses/interventions/evaluation

■ **NDX:** Urinary retention related to obstruction or neuromuscular dysfunction

Assess bladder for distention
Monitor intake and output q8h
Use voiding measures to facilitate bladder emptying
　Ensure privacy
　Place patient in comfortable position to urinate
　Run tap water near patient
　Flush toilet
　Place patient's hands in warm water
　Apply heat to suprapubic area as ordered
　Pour warm water over perineum
　Assist patient with using relaxation techniques
　Place a few drops of oil of peppermint in bedpan or on
　　cotton ball and hold briefly in front of urinary meatus
　Pull pubic hairs slightly
　Stroke inner aspect of thigh gently
　Stroke inner aspect of thigh with ice
Observe for and document desired effects and side effects
of medications
　Collaborate with physician to determine effect of pre-
　　scribed medications on retention and need to change
　　medications, schedule, or dosage
Apply ice to perineum if swelling present; e.g., postpartum
Medicate before voiding to decrease pain
Have patient double void to empty bladder more com-
pletely
Assess intake; initiate voiding schedule to correlate with
intake

Check postvoiding residual if voiding occurs; report if >
100 ml

Intermittent catheterization may be required if voiding
techniques fail

Catheterize patient as ordered

Avoid use of guide wire

Notify physician if unable to pass catheter; do not force

Notify physician if bright red urine occurs after decompression

Measure and record urinary output qh

Monitor for postobstructive diuresis; report urine output
greater than 200 ml/hr

If postobstructive diuresis occurs

Monitor vital signs, intake, and output to prevent dehydration qh

Monitor serum and urine electrolytes and osmolality

Monitor for signs and symptoms of electrolyte imbalance

Assist and teach patient technique of self-catheterization

Teach purpose of procedure; to completely empty bladder on a regular time schedule, usually q3h to 4h

Instruct patient to have necessary equipment available

Magnifying mirror (female)

Measuring container

Two No. 14 French catheters

Pan or toilet

Water-soluble lubricant

Soap and water

Clean washcloth

Clean towel

Instruct patient to perform good handwashing technique before and after self-catheterization

Teach self-catherization procedure

Women

Perform catheterization procedure in semi-Fowler's
position initially; later can sit or stand over toilet

Identify urinary meatus by looking in magnifying
mirror initially; later can sit on or stand over
toilet

Men

Perform catheterization procedure sitting on stool
or toilet

Both sexes

Clean meatus, labia, or glans with soap and water

Grasp catheter 3 to 4 inches from tip

Lubricate tip of catheter

Insert catheter in urethral meatus until urine flows
out

Women will insert catheter 3 to 5 cm

Men will insert catheter until urine flows

Allow urine to flow into pan or toilet until bladder
is empty

Remove catheter

Measure output

Wash catheter in soap and water

Rinse well

Dry catheter; roll in clean towel

Place catheter in clean plastic or paper bag for
storage

Expected outcome/evaluation

Reports normal voiding pattern; no evidence of bladder
distention; intake and output are balanced

■ **NDX:** Pain related to bladder fullness and inability to
void

Assess nature, intensity, location, duration, and precipitating and alleviating factors of pain

Provide bed rest; increase activities as ordered and tolerated

Provide nonpharmacological comfort measures: assist patient with assuming a comfortable position, provide sitz
baths and warm perineal soaks, teach relaxation techniques and guided imagery, and/or provide diversional
activity

Encourage high oral fluid intake

Administer other pain medication as ordered

Assess vital signs before and after administering pain medications

Monitor and document pain relief and any undesirable
side effects

Notify physician of unrelieved or increasing pain

Expected outcome/evaluation

Reports a decrease in pain and a decrease in burning
on urination

Shows a relaxed facial expression and body position

■ **NDX:** Potential for infection (UTI) related to urinary
obstruction and/or urine stasis

Assess temperature q4h and report if greater than 101° F
(38.5° C)

Note character of urine; report if cloudy and malodorous

Collect midstream and/or clean-voided urine for culture
and sensitivity as ordered

Encourage high oral fluid intake, up to 2500 ml/day, to
flush out bacteria unless contraindicated

Obtain repeat urine specimens for culture and sensitivity
as ordered, to determine response to therapy

Teach patient to shower daily with antibacterial soap

Teach female patient to avoid tub baths

Provide good perineal hygiene; keep area clean and dry

Teach female to administer perianal care after each bowel
movement and to wipe from front to back

Expected outcome/evaluation

Exhibits no signs of UTI; temperature is within normal
range; urine culture is negative

■ **NDX:** Knowledge deficit related to lack of information about disease process, and home care and follow-up instructions

Instruct patient to force fluids up to 2500 ml/day unless contraindicated

Instruct patient to avoid alcohol, coffee, tea, and cola beverages, which may cause irritation

Instruct patient to measure urine after each void and to note character of urine, time and force of stream (urinary diary if appropriate)

Teach voiding measures

Instruct patient to perform prescribed self-catheterization

Teach symptoms of recurrence and instruct patient to report these symptoms to physician

Teach symptoms of UTI and instruct patient to report these symptoms to physician

Teach name of medication, dosage, schedule, purpose, and side effects

Instruct patient to avoid over-the-counter medications without checking with physician

Teach importance of ongoing outpatient care

Expected outcome/evaluation

Patient and/or significant other verbalizes an understanding of acute urinary retention, and home care and follow-up instructions; states symptoms of recurrence and UTI to report to physician; and return-demonstrates self-catheterization technique

SURGERY FOR FEMALE URINARY INCONTINENCE

Marshall-Marchetti-Krantz operation A surgical procedure for correcting stress incontinence; the urethra and vesical neck of the bladder are suspended to restore the normal vesicourethral angle by suturing the paraurethral anterior vaginal wall to the periosteum of the symphysis pubis and to the lower rectal fascia via a suprapubic incision

Pereya procedure A surgical procedure performed vaginally to restore the normal vesicourethral angle, thus decreasing stress incontinence; the urethra and vesical neck are suspended by suturing the anterior vaginal wall to the rectal fascia

Other procedures include Pereya-Raz, Stame, and Buret

Assessment
Observations/findings

Urinary output
  Amount
  Color
  Character
UTI
Incision
  Redness
  Pain
  Swelling
  Drainage
Difficulty in voiding after removal of catheter

Laboratory/diagnostic studies

Urinalysis
Urine culture and sensitivity
Cystoscopy
Excretory urography
Urine flow rate measurement
Urethral pressure profile
Bonney-Read-Marshall test (vesical neck elevation test)

Potential complications

UTI
Postoperative complications
  Atelectasis
  Thrombophlebitis
  Pulmonary embolism
  Paralytic ileus
  Wound infection

Medical Management

NPO until bowel sounds are audible
Parenteral fluids until liquids or diet is tolerated
Intake and output
BP, T, P, and R per postoperative procedure
Analgesics
Stool softeners
Indwelling urethral catheter and/or suprapubic tube for 4 to 6 days postoperatively (Marshall-Marchetti-Krantz operation)
Indwelling urethral catheter for 2 days postoperatively (Pereya procedure)

Nursing diagnoses/interventions/evaluation

■ **NDX:** Pain related to surgical incision and manipulation of organs, and to periostitis

Assess nature, intensity, location, duration, and precipitating and alleviating factors of pain; use pain rating scale

Assess nonverbal signs of pain

Check urethral catheter and/or suprapubic tube for obstruction; secure so there is no tension; position to enhance drainage

Assess incision site for redness, tenderness, swelling, and drainage

Provide nonpharmacological comfort measures
  Assist patient with assuming a comfortable position
  Teach relaxation techniques
  Teach and assist with guided imagery techniques
  Provide diversional activity
  Provide a restful environment
Observe for desired effects and side effects of medications
Instruct patient to splint incision when turning, coughing, and deep breathing

Consult with physician if measures fail to provide adequate pain relief or if a dosage or interval change in pain medication is needed

Expected outcome/evaluation

Reports feeling a decrease in pain
Has a relaxed facial expression and body position

■ **NDX:** Altered patterns of urinary elimination related to presence of urethral catheter and/or suprapubic tube

Maintain patency of catheter
  Keep tubings below level of patient's bladder
  Keep urine draining freely, avoid clamping or kinks in tubing
  Anchor suprapubic tube to patient's abdomen
  Irrigate suprapubic tube only under direct order
Measure and document intake and urinary output q8h, or more frequently if necessary
Palpate bladder for distention if output is low
Explain to patient that presence of catheter may cause urge to urinate
Maintain integrity of closed gravity drainage system at all times
Clean periurethral area bid
  Protect patient's privacy
  Remove all crusts and mucus from catheter
Reduce swelling of urinary meatus if present
  Apply anesthetic ointment to urethral meatus if ordered
  Avoid placing tension on catheter
Follow clamping routine as ordered
Remove indwelling catheter as soon as possible when ordered
Use measures to facilitate voiding
  Ensure privacy
  Place patient in a comfortable position to urinate
  Run tap water near patient
  Flush toilet
  Place patient's hands in warm water
  Apply heat to suprapubic area if ordered
  Pour warm water over perineum
  Assist patient with using relaxation techniques
  Place a few drops of oil of peppermint in bedpan or on cotton ball and hold briefly in front of urinary meatus
  Pull pubic hairs slightly
  Stroke inner aspect of thigh gently
  Stroke inner aspect of thigh with ice
  Observe voiding pattern; use voiding diary
  Measure urinary output after each voiding
  Note character of urine; report any abnormalities to physician
  Report retention of urine with overflow to physician
  If residual urine is greater than 100 ml postvoid, a postvoid catheter program may be ordered

Perform intermittent catheterization as ordered
Instruct patient to avoid staying in sitting position for prolonged periods of time
Administer stool softeners and laxatives as ordered
Instruct patient to avoid straining during bowel elimination

Expected outcome/evaluation

Urethral catheter and suprapubic tube remain patent for their duration
Intake and output are balanced
Does not experience difficulty in voiding in 2 to 3 days after catheter removal
Exhibits no symptoms of retention

■ **NDX:** Potential for infection related to risk of UTI resulting from presence of indwelling urethral catheter and/or suprapubic tube

Monitor patient's temperature and report if greater than 101° F (38.5° C)
Maintain sterile technique when performing intermittent catheterization and if catheter irrigations are performed
Note character of urine; report if cloudy and malodorous
Monitor urine culture and sensitivity reports
Encourage high oral fluid intake, up to 2500 ml/day, to flush out bacteria, unless contraindicated
Teach patient to shower daily with antibacterial soap
Teach female patient to avoid tub baths
Provide good perineal hygiene; keep area clean and dry
Teach female to administer perianal care after each bowel movement, and to wipe from front to back

Expected outcome/evaluation

Temperature is within normal range for patient; urine is clear and culture report is negative

■ **NDX:** Potential for altered in tissue perfusion: peripheral, cardiopulmonary or gastrointestinal, related to risk of interrupted blood flow as evidenced by thrombophlebitis, pulmonary embolism, or paralytic ileus.

Thrombophlebitis

Monitor for and report signs of venous thrombosis (pain, tenderness, warmth, or redness in extremity, positive Homan's sign)
Apply antiembolic stockings as ordered
Assist and teach patient to perform passive ROM exercises to extremities q2h to 4h; avoid straight leg exercises
Avoid placing patient in a sitting position for prolonged periods of time
Avoid pressure or putting pillows under knees
Instruct patient not to cross legs
Administer anticoagulants as ordered

Pulmonary embolism

Monitor for and report signs and symptoms of pulmonary embolism (sudden chest or shoulder pain, cough, hemoptysis, dyspnea, tachycardia, hypertension, cyanosis, restlessness, decreased PO_2)

If symptoms of pulmonary embolism occur
  Place patient in semi- or high-Fowler's position
  Administer O_2 as ordered
  Monitor vital signs qh
  Maintain strict bed rest
  Administer anticoagulants as ordered
  Prepare patient for diagnostic tests (lung scan, venography, pulmonary angiography)

Paralytic ileus

Monitor for and report signs of paralytic ileus (absent or diminished bowel sounds, persistent or worsening abdominal pain and cramping, distended, firm abdomen, failure to pass flatus)

Maintain NPO until active bowel sounds are audible or passage of flatus is noted

Auscultate for bowel sounds q4h

Insert and maintain nasogastric tube as ordered

Encourage early ambulation

Instruct patient to avoid smoking and/or chewing gum in order to reduce air swallowing

Administer stool softeners, laxatives, or enemas as ordered

Expected outcome/evaluation

  Vital signs are stable
  Breath sounds are clear
  Reports no chest pain or difficulty breathing
  Bowel sounds are present without reports of abdominal pain
  Performs extremity ROM exercises without pain
  No evidence of redness or swelling in legs

■ **NDX:** Potential for wound infection related to surgical incision

Monitor for and report signs and symptoms of wound infection (fever, chills, redness, swelling, tenderness, purulent and/or malodorous wound drainage)

Check surgical incision q4h for redness, swelling, tenderness, and purulent drainage

Assess temperature q4h

Monitor WBC

Obtain wound culture of suspicious drainage

Use good handwashing technique and teach and encourage patient to do the same

Instruct patient to avoid touching incision, dressings, and drainage

Maintain sterile technique when changing dressings and performing wound care

Administer antibiotics as ordered

Expected outcome/evaluation

  Incision is clean and dry; temperature is within normal range

■ **NDX:** Knowledge deficit related to lack of exposure to information about postoperative routine, and home care and follow-up instructions

Teach postoperative routine; encourage patient to participate in care

Instruct patient to avoid persons with infections

Instruct patient to get plenty of rest; to exercise to tolerance and to plan frequent rest periods

Instruct patient to avoid heavy lifting and heavy housework for 6 weeks or as indicated by physician

Teach patient good body mechanics; instruct patient to bend knees to pick up items from the floor

Instruct patient to avoid standing or sitting for long periods of time.

Instruct patient to avoid constipation and to avoid straining when having a bowel movement

Instruct patient to avoid sexual activity for 6 weeks or as indicated by physician

Instruct patient to avoid tub baths and to shower daily

Teach self-catheterization procedure when required (see p. 463)

Instruct patient to report signs and symptoms of UTI and methods to avoid UTI

Teach patient to perform wound care and dressing change as indicated

Instruct patient to monitor for and report signs and symptoms of wound infection (fever, chills, redness, swelling, tenderness, and purulent and/or malodorous drainage from incision)

Teach name of medication, dosage, schedule, purpose, and side effects

Instruct patient to avoid taking over-the-counter medications without checking with physician

Teach importance of ongoing outpatient care

Expected outcome/evaluation

Patient and/or significant other verbalizes an understanding of postoperative routine, and home care and follow-up instructions; states signs and symptoms to report to physician; and return-demonstrates wound care, dressing change, and self-catheterization if required

ARTIFICIAL URINARY SPHINCTER (AUS)

A fluid-filled system with a silicone rubber cuff that surrounds the urethra and functions as a urinary sphincter, a pump is implanted in the labia of the female and in the scrotum of the male or may be external, and a balloon reservoir sits in the abdomen, when the pump is squeezed, the fluid leaves the cuff and flows into the balloon (reservoir), thus allowing the urethra to open and the patient to void (Figure 9-4)

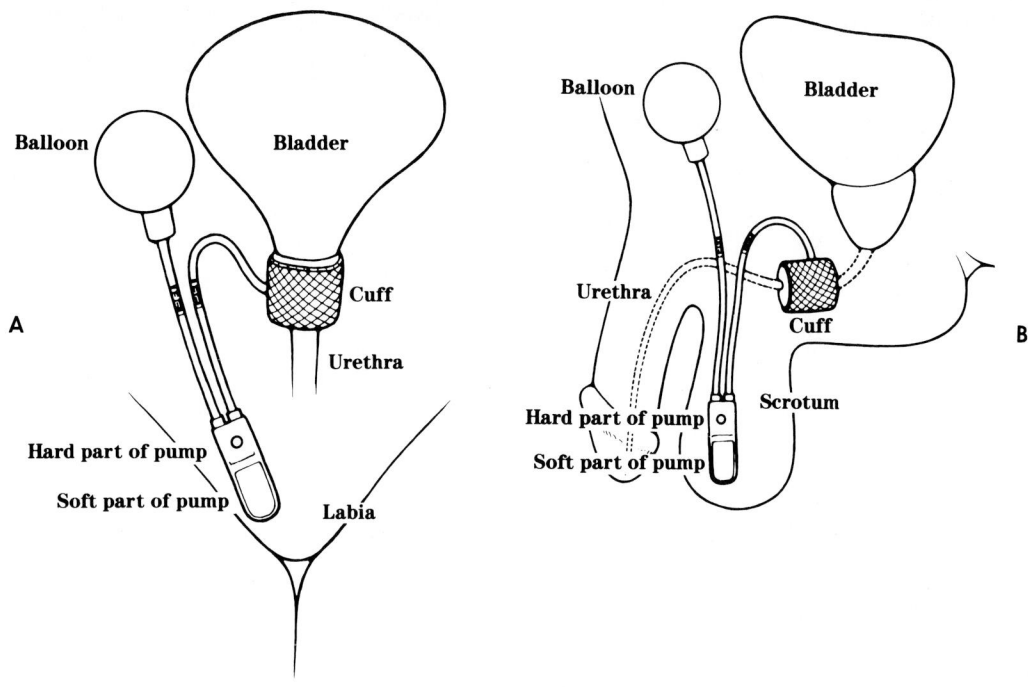

FIGURE 9-4. Artificial urinary sphincter. **A,** Bladder neck implantation, female. **B,** Bulbous urethra implantation, male. (From American Medical Systems Inc.: Publication 50715, 1985, Minnetonka, Minn. Illustrations by Michael Schenk.)

Assessment
Observations/findings

Urine
  Amount
  Character
Incontinence
Leakage of urine
Scrotal swelling
Labial swelling
Bladder spasms
Incision
  Pain
  Redness
  Swelling
  Tenderness
  Purulent and/or malodorous drainage
Elevated temperature

Laboratory/diagnostic studies

Urinalysis
Urine for culture and sensitivity
See Urinary Incontinence, (p. 453)

Potential complications

UTI
Infection
Rejection of artificial urinary sphincter
Malfunctioning artificial urinary sphincter

Medical Management

NPO until bowel sounds are audible
Parenteral fluids until liquids or diet is tolerated
Intake and output
BP, T, P, and R per postoperative routine
Analgesics
Stool softeners
Antibiotics

Nursing diagnoses/interventions/evaluation

■ **NDX:** Pain related to low, transverse, deep surgical incision and bladder spasm

Assess nature, intensity, location, duration, and precipitating and alleviating factors of pain, use pain rating scale
Assess nonverbal signs of pain
Monitor urine flow; check patency of urethral catheter
Report signs and symptoms of urinary retention to physician
Assess scrotum/labia for swelling
Provide nonpharmacological comfort measures
  Assist patient with assuming a comfortable position
  Teach relaxation techniques
  Teach and assist with guided imagery
  Provide diversional activity
  Provide a restful environment

Maintain Trendelenburg's position, if ordered, to decrease scrotal swelling

Apply ice bag to scrotum and/or perineal area for 12 to 48 hr or as indicated by physician

Monitor and document pain relief and side effects of medication

Consult with physician if measures fail to provide pain relief, or if a dosage or interval change in pain medication is needed

Expected outcome/evaluation

Reports a decrease in pain
Shows a relaxed facial expression and body position

■ **NDX:**   Altered patterns of urinary elimination related to presence of artificial urinary sphincter and bladder spasms

Measure and document urinary output qh

Note character of urine; report any abnormalities to physician

Maintain patency of uninflated urethral catheter for 1 to 5 days or as ordered by physician

Monitor and report signs and symptoms of urinary retention

Locate pump qh postoperatively and document

Notify physician immediately if unable to palpate pump (it may have traveled into inguinal canal; *this is an emergency*)

Remove urethral catheter as ordered when swelling goes down and patient can palpate artificial urinary sphincter

Once urethral catheter is removed, use an external collecting device to prevent contact of urine with skin

Begin activating pump when ordered

Pump bulb q2h during the day and once midway through the night

Deflate device while patient is asleep and connect patient to an external urine collecting device; may use pads for female, changing as necessary to maintain dryness

Teach patient to palpate and operate artificial urinary sphincter (AUS)

Provide privacy while palpating, teaching, or activating pump

Explain to patient that there may be some incontinence of urine at times

Report any leakage of urine to physician

Expected outcome/evaluation

No signs of urinary retention are present
Urethral catheter drains clear urine when present
Operates AUS successfully without leakage of urine

■ **NDX:**   Potential for infection; (UTI, wound infection), and rejection of artificial urinary sphincter related to implantation of foreign body surrounding urinary tract

Assess temperature q4h; report if greater than 101° F (38.5° C)

Assess site of incision for and report redness, swelling, tenderness, and purulent and/or malodorous drainage

Note character of urine; report abnormalities to physician

Monitor for and report signs and symptoms of UTI

Maintain a closed drainage system for duration of indwelling urethral catheter

Force fluids up to 2000 ml/day unless contraindicated

Maintain sterile technique when performing wound care and dressing changes

Monitor for and report signs and symptoms of rejection (erosion, increasing pain, abdominal tenderness, swelling, urinary retention)

Administer antibiotics as ordered

Expected outcome/evaluation

Temperature is within normal limits
Incision is clean and dry
No symptoms of rejection are present

■ **NDX:**   Knowledge deficit related to lack of exposure to information regarding activation of artificial urinary sphincter, and home care and follow-up instructions

Instruct patient to force fluids up to 2500 ml/day unless contraindicated

Instruct patient to avoid smoking, tea, coffee, and alcohol

Teach patient to palpate pump and to activate artificial urinary sphincter

Locate pump in labia or scrotum with thumb and forefinger of dominant hand

Locate and gently support tubing above pump with nondominant hand to prevent pump from slipping away

Using thumb and forefinger of dominant hand, squeeze pump until it reaches decompressed state (usually three times); this opens cuff, allowing urine to flow

Explain to patient that within 1 to 3 min, cuff will automatically refill and compress urethra, thus maintaining continence

If urine does not flow

Instruct patient to cough (this increases intraabdominal pressure and thus facilitates urine flow)

Instruct patient to move from supine to sitting or standing position

Instruct patient to use voiding measures (see nursing diagnosis of altered patterns of urinary elimination under Acute Urinary Retention, p. 462)

Explain that some patients may need to deflate pump twice to fully empty bladder

Instruct patient to pump bulb flat q2h during the day and once midway through the night for 3 weeks postoperatively or as ordered by physician; thereafter, patient may pump bulb to urinate only when sensation of bladder fullness occurs; instruct patients with no feeling of fullness to empty bladder q3h to 4h

Instruct patient not to leave device completely inflated while asleep; instruct patient to use smallest amount of fluid necessary for continence

Instruct patient to report leakage of urine to physician

Instruct patient to report if pump goes flat or if it requires more squeezes to inflate

Explain that some incontinence may occur, especially with activities such as cycling or horseback riding

Teach and instruct patient to report signs and symptoms of UTI to physician

Teach and instruct patient to report signs and symptoms of rejection and wound infection to physician

Instruct patient to wear a medical alert tag, so that if patient is ever unconscious, the pump may be activated and urine eliminated

Expected outcome/evaluation

Patient and/or significant other verbalizes function of artificial urinary sphincter, symptoms to report to physician, and home care and follow-up instructions; palpates pump; and operates artificial urinary sphincter

INDWELLING URETHRAL CATHETER MANAGEMENT

A catheter inserted through the urethra into the bladder to drain urine (Figure 9-5)

Assessment
Observations/findings

Distended bladder
Bladder spasms
UTI
  Cystitis
  Epididymitis
    Elevated temperature
    Chills
    Pyuria
Edema of urethral meatus: paraphimosis
Reflux of urine into bladder
After catheter removal
  Dysuria
  Frequency of urination
  Urinary retention with overflow
  Inability to urinate
  Urethral stricture
    Dribbling
    Difficulty in initiating urinary stream
    Small urinary stream

Incontinence
Hematuria

Laboratory/diagnostic studies

Urinalysis
Urine for culture and sensitivity

Potential complications

Progressive UTI
Septicemia
Urinary tract calculi
Difficulty in voiding after removal

Medical Management

Fluid intake 2500 ml/day unless contraindicated by primary conditions
Periodic catheter change
Antibiotics in presence of infection

Interventions

Encourage fluids to 2500 ml/day unless contraindicated
Measure and document urinary output q8h or more frequently if necessary
Note character of urine; report abnormalities
Palpate bladder for distention if output is low
Explain to patient that presence of catheter may cause urge to urinate
Maintain patency of catheter
  Avoid clamping or occluding catheter
  Avoid irrigating catheter unless ordered
  Keep catheter below level of bladder
Maintain integrity of closed gravity drainage system at all times
Maintain tension-free catheter
  Tape drainage tubing to inner aspect of lateral thigh (female)
  Tape catheter to abdomen or upper thigh (male)
Clean periurethral area bid
  Protect patient's privacy
  Remove all crusts and mucus from catheter
Reduce swelling of urinary meatus if present

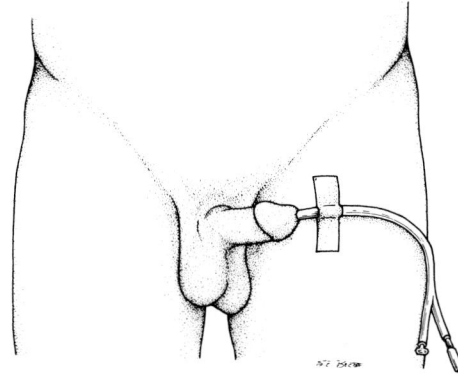

FIGURE 9-5. Indwelling urethral catheter.

Apply anesthetic ointment to urethral meatus if ordered

Maintain closed gravity drainage system; avoid contamination if catheter must be disconnected and reconnected

Collect urine specimens only by aspirating urine through catheter collection portal with sterile 10 ml syringe and 25-gauge needle

To remove catheter:

Use measures to facilitate voiding

Ensure privacy

Place patient in a comfortable position to urinate

Run tap water near patient

Flush toilet

Place patient's hands in warm water

Apply heat to suprapubic area if ordered

Pour warm water over perineum

Assist patient with using relaxation techniques

Place a few drops of oil of peppermint in bedpan or on cotton ball and hold briefly in front of urinary meatus

Pull pubic hairs slightly

Stroke inner aspect of thigh gently

Stroke inner aspect of thigh with ice

Measure urinary output for 24 hr after catheter removal

Note character of urine; report abnormalities to physician

Observe voiding pattern; report retention of urine with overflow to physician

Upon discharge

Instruct patient to avoid placing tension on catheter and to check for patency of catheter q4h

Instruct patient to avoid clamping or kinking tubing and to keep drainage system below level of bladder; may place drainage system in shopping bag when ambulating

Instruct patient to clean periurethral area bid

Teach patient care of collecting bags, leg bags, and tubing

Wash daily with soap and water

Soak for 15 min in a mild vinegar solution

Rinse with lukewarm water

Protect ends of catheter and tubing with clean gauze square when disconnecting or before reconnecting catheter to drainage system

Teach patient procedure for attaching catheter to leg bag and/or closed drainage system

Instruct patient to report absence of urine, persistent leakage around catheter, accidental removal of catheter, back pain, elevated temperature or cloudy urine

URINARY DIVERSION

Diversion of urinary flow, bypassing the bladder by transplanting the ureters into the skin, intestine, ascending colon, or an isolated section of intestine

Conduits

ureteroenterocutaneous diversion

The ureters are anastomosed to an isolated section of intestine, which provides a bridge for urine to pass quickly through an abdominal stoma to an external appliance

ileal conduit

Bricker procedure. The ureters are anastamosed into a prepared segment of the ileum, which is sutured closed at one end, forming a blind pouch; the other end is connected to an opening in the abdominal wall; remaining bowel is reanastomosed to provide normal gastrointestinal (GI) function (Figure 9-6)

jejunal conduit

A portion of the jejunum may be used if the ileum has been damaged, use of the jejunum predisposes patients to electrolyte imbalances

Continent Urinary Diversion

An internal reservoir for urine is constructed with an abdominal stoma, eliminating need for an external appliance

ileal reservoir

Kock pouch. The ureters are anastamosed into a prepared segment of the ileum, forming a pouch that contains two nipple valves: one nipple valve prevents reflux of urine, and the other nipple valve maintains continence; the pouch is then anchored to the abdominal wall (Figure 9-7)

ileocecal reservoir The ureters are implanted into the mucosa of the ascending colon by an antirefluxing method, the ileum with a nipple valve formation is implanted in the abdomen; the cecum and ascending colon form the reservoir

Cutaneous Ureterostomy

A surgical procedure in which one or both ureters are implanted into an opening in the abdominal wall (Figure 9-8)

Assessment
Observations/findings

Urine

Color; hematuria

Character

Amount; oliguria

Intestinal obstruction

Diarrhea

Stoma/ureteral buds

Placement

Type

Inverted

Flush with skin

Protruding

Color

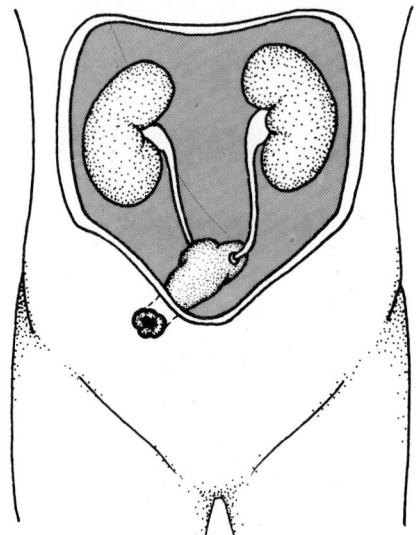

FIGURE 9-6. Ileal conduit.

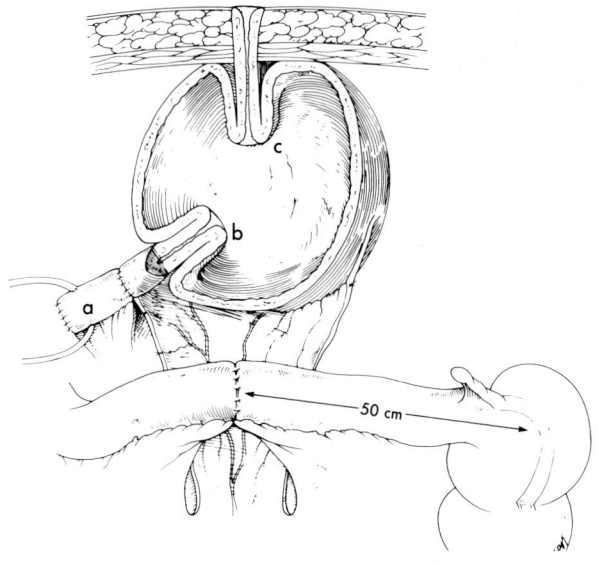

FIGURE 9-7. Kock continent ileal reservoir. *a,* Original ileal conduit with implanted ureters; *b,* reflux-preventing nipple valve; *c,* continence-maintaining nipple valve. (From Gerber A: J Enterostom Ther 12:15, 1985.)

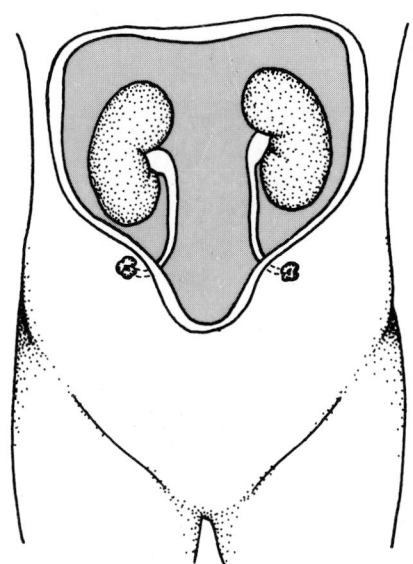
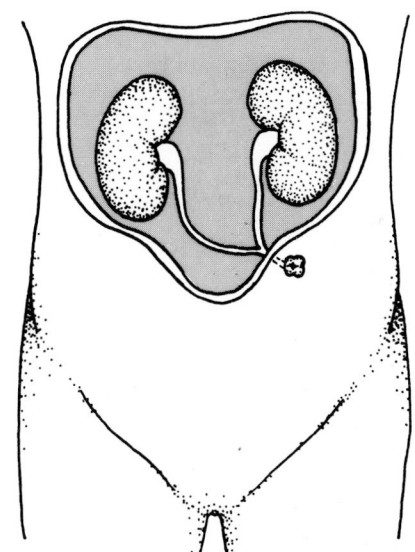

FIGURE 9-8. Cutaneous ureterostomies.

Cyanosis
Necrosis
Prolapse
Retraction
Edema
Stenosis
Skin excoriation
Pressure sores under faceplate of external appliance
Infection at stomal site/ureteral buds

Fungus
Yeast
Bacteria
Collection bag
Kinks
Compression
Leakage around bag
Offensive odor
Urinary fistula: urine from incision

Bowel fistula: feces from incision
Incision
   Redness
   Pain
   Swelling
   Drainage
   Dehiscence
   Evisceration
Elevated temperature
Back pain
Disturbance in self-concept: body image

Laboratory/diagnostic studies

Urinalysis
Urine culture and sensitivity
Serum BUN
Serum creatinine
Serum electrolytes

Potential complications

Hemorrhage
Shock
Atelectasis
Thrombophlebitis
Pulmonary embolism
Electrolyte imbalance
   Potassium loss
   Hyperchloremic acidosis
   Metabolic acidosis
Paralytic ileus
Peritonitis
UTI: pyelonephritis
Hydronephrosis
Renal failure

Preoperative Assessment and Care

Assess knowledge of surgery and change in body function
Allow ample time for discussion of fears and questions
Provide information about equipment, tubes, and drains to expect postoperatively depending on type of diversion
Discuss bowel preparation and patient's role; begin preparation routine
Arrange consultation with ET nurse to determine location of stoma in collaboration with patient and physician

Postoperative
Medical Management

Bowel preparation; enemas, medication, and diet
NPO until active bowel sounds are present
Connection of nasogastric tube to low, intermittent suction
BP, T, P, and R per postoperative routine
Serum electrolyte monitoring
Intake and output
Parenteral fluids with electrolytes as needed

Analgesics, antipyretics
Antibiotics
Stool softeners

Nursing diagnoses/intervention/evaluation

■ **NDX:** Pain related to surgical incision and/or urinary obstruction

Assess nature, intensity, location, duration, and precipitating and alleviating factors of pain
Assess nonverbal signs of pain
Check patency of catheters
Report signs and symptoms of urinary retention or absence of urinary drainage to physician
Assess incision and scrotum for swelling
Provide nonpharmacological comfort measures
   Assist patient with assuming a comfortable position
   Teach relaxation techniques
   Teach and assist with guided imagery
   Provide diversional activity
   Provide a restful environment
Monitor and document pain relief and side effects of medication
Consult with physician if measures fail to provide pain relief or if a dosage or interval change in pain medication is needed

Expected outcome/evaluation

Reports a decrease in pain
Exhibits a relaxed facial expression and body position

■ **NDX:** Altered patterns of urinary elimination related to urinary diversion

Monitor urine from all sources for color, clarity, and volume qh for first 24 hr then q4h to q8h; report output of < 30 ml/hr
   Conduit: stoma; may have ureteral stents and/or conduit catheter/stent
   Continent diversion: stoma and Kock-reservoir catheter; may have ureteral stents: ileocecal-ureteral stents from stoma may have reservoir catheter via stab wound
   Ureterostomy-stoma(s); may have ureteral stents
   Expect pink-colored urine first 24 hr; mucus from conduit and continent diversions is normal
   Label each collecting container and catheter/stent as to "right" or "left" and type
   Connect each catheter/stent to a separate closed gravity drainage system or pouch
   Keep separate, accurate output record for each source of drainage
Maintain patency of catheters/stents
   Prevent kinking of drainage tubing
   Keep drainage bag below level of patient's kidneys
   Position patient in bed so that flow of urine is not impeded

Keep ureteral catheters securely taped

Monitor function of drains if present; drainage may be pink for first 24 hr; expect decreasing drainage

Assess size, shape, color, type, and placement of stoma/ ureteral buds qh for 24 hr then q4h to 8h

Notify physician if color of stoma/ureteral buds is not red or pink or if shape of stoma/ureteral buds appears to be changing

Encourage fluid intake to 2500 ml/day; calculate intake q8h

Monitor urine output closely for 24 hr after removal of ureteral catheters

Avoid having patient sit in chair for long periods; ambulation and movement facilitate urine drainage from conduit

Expected outcome/evaluation

Urinary output is > 30 ml/hr

Intake and output are balanced

Urine is clear, yellow

Stoma/ureteral buds are pink and swelling is decreasing

■ **NDX:**   Potential for impaired skin integrity related to risk of skin contact with urine

Inspect skin around stoma and report signs of redness, breakdown, and/or excoriation

Check for leakage of urine around ostomy bag, dressing, drains, or catheters

Notify physician if leaks occur around ureteral catheter

Keep skin clean and dry

Change dressings when wet

Change temporary appliance as needed

Clean skin around stoma/ureteral buds with soap and water; remove mucus present on and around stoma; note that mucus is not an expected finding in ureterostomy

Rinse thoroughly with water; pat dry

Place rolled 4 × 4 inch gauze over stoma/bud opening; tampon can also be used

Apply skin barrier; allow to dry completely

Measure stoma/bud size; bag opening should be 1/16 to 1/8 inch wider than stoma/bud

Make a pattern and leave at bedside

Check correctness of pattern q2d

Remove 4 × 4 inch gauze or tampon

Apply temporary bag directly to skin barrier around stoma/bud

Avoid wrinkles or creases in bag

Angle bag to patient's side when in bed and toward feet when ambulating

Attach ostomy pouch to bedside drainage system at night

Reapply ostomy pouch prn if leakage or poor seal occurs

Assist and teach patient to empty appliance q2h

Fit patient with ostomy pouch; be aware that 3 to 6 weeks after operation, stoma will shrink to normal size

Arrange a visit by enterostomal therapist if available

Expected outcome/evaluation

Patient's skin around stoma is dry and intact

■ **NDX:**   Potential for body image disturbance related to loss of normal body function and presence of urinary stoma/bud on abdomen

Be aware that patients facing this type of surgery are under considerable emotional stress

Be sensitive to changes in patient's lifestyle

Encourage patient to express feelings

Actively listen

Explain to patient that feelings of grief are normal

Answer questions honestly

Be aware of coping mechanisms and expect that patient may exhibit irrational or inappropriate behaviors, irritability, and lack of motivation

Encourage adaptive coping behaviors

Set limits on maladaptive behaviors, especially if they are detrimental to patient's health

Instruct patient that there are no social limitations

Patient may participate in any sport except boxing, and sports requiring body contact (football, wrestling); or heavy weight lifting should also be avoided

Explain to patient that there are no clothing limitations except that girdles should not be worn

Explain to patient that there are no sexual limitations unless surgery includes cystectomy in male patient

Reassure patient that stoma will not smell bad; suggest methods to control odor

Encourage communication with significant other (one of the most common fears is that patient's family—especially patient's spouse—will not be able to accept stoma/bud)

Encourage patient to look at and touch stoma as soon as possible

Encourage patient to participate in emptying and changing appliance

Include spouse/significant other in teaching

Arrange for visit by an ostomate

Provide for psychiatric consultation if necessary

Expected outcome/evaluation

Verbalizes feelings related to change in body image to care giver and/or significant other

Looks at and cares for urinary diversion

Begins to resume ADLs

■ **NDX:**   Potential for infection related to surgical incision and risk of ascending bacteriuria or peritonitis

Monitor temperature q4h and report if greater than 101° F (38.5° C)

Monitor and report signs and symptoms of UTI (see Urinary Tract Infection [UTI], p. 451)

Maintain closed drainage systems

Encourage fluids up to 2500 ml/day unless contraindicated

Check surgical incision and stab wounds q4h

Monitor for and report signs and symptoms of wound infection (fever, chills, redness, swelling, tenderness, purulent and/or malodorous wound drainage)

Use good handwashing technique and teach and encourage patient to do the same

Instruct patient to avoid touching incision, dressings, or drainage

Maintain sterile technique when changing dressings and performing wound care; change dressing as soon as it becomes wet; be certain pouch over stoma does not overlap incision; trim pouch to avoid suture line

Obtain cultures of suspicious drainage

Monitor for and report signs and symptoms of peritonitis (abnormal drainage from wound or urethra, i.e., large quantities of cloudy, purulent fluid or stool in drainage; prolonged abdominal distention with rebound tenderness; prolonged absence of bowel sounds; sudden rise in temperature)

Monitor results of methylene blue test as ordered

Expected outcome/evaluation

Temperature is within normal range for patient

Surgical incision is clean, dry, and healing

Urine cultures are negative

Bowel sounds are present

Urethral drainage is clear mucus (if present)

■ **NDX:** Potential for ineffective breathing pattern related to pain, fatigue

Auscultate chest for and report diminished, absent, and adventitious breath sounds

Assess breathing pattern and respiratory effort; report use of accessory muscles, increased rate and changed rhythm

Assist patient with turning, coughing, and deep breathing q1h to 2h

Assist patient with incentive spirometer to maximize lung expansion as ordered

Note character and amount of sputum; report any abnormalities to physician

Monitor for and report signs and symptoms of impaired gas exchange (confusion, restlessness, irritability, cyanosis, diaphoresis, decreased PO_2, increased PCO_2)

Administer pain medication at proper intervals to manage pain and to help patient perform coughing and deep breathing exercises more effectively

Expected outcome/evaluation

Respiratory rate and rhythm are regular

Breath sounds are normal

Uses incentive spirometer and deep breathes as instructed

■ **NDX:** Potential fluid volume deficit related to risk of excessive losses and electrolyte imbalances

Monitor serum electrolytes

Measure and document intake and output

Inspect skin turgor

Monitor parenteral fluids with electrolytes

Monitor for and report signs and symptoms of

Hyperchloremic acidosis: nausea, vomiting, irregular pulse, muscle weakness, tachypnea, lethargy, diarrhea

Metabolic acidosis: apathy, disorientation, weakness, Kussmaul's respirations

Hyponatremia: apathy, twitching, seizures, nausea, vomiting, tachycardia, thready pulse

Reabsorption dehydration: thirst, headache, diuresis

Monitor for signs and symptoms of hypokalemia and hyponatremia, especially in patient with ileal conduits

Encourage early ambulation to prevent urinary stasis and thus decrease risk of electrolyte imbalance

Use dietary sources for replacement of electrolytes

If patient is confused or has symptoms of increased neuromuscular activity, keep bed in low position, elevate side rails, and institute other safety measures

Expected outcome/evaluation

Intake and output are balanced

Electrolytes are within normal limits

Skin is warm, dry with good turgor

Heart rate and rhythm are within normal limits for patient

Is alert and oriented

■ **NDX:** Knowledge deficit related to lack of information regarding postoperative routine, symptoms to report to physician, and home care and follow-up instructions

Teach postoperative routine for incision care

Instruct patient to maintain prescribed diet

Instruct patient to take fluids to 2500 ml/day

Teach patient effects of diuretic substances such as alcoholic beverages, tea, and coffee

Instruct patient to exercise to tolerance, to avoid heavy lifting, and to plan frequent rest periods

Instruct patient to shower daily

Instruct patient to empty appliance q2h to 3h; instruct patient not to allow more than 100 ml of urine to accumulate at one time

Explain importance to ureterostomy patients of not irrigating ureteral buds

Instruct patient to attach appliance to bedside closed gravity drainage system at night, keeping drainage apparatus lower than tube

Teach patient how to change appliance

  Instruct patient to change appliance early in morning, after fluids have been restricted for 2 to 3 hr, or prn if leakage occurs

  Have patient sit in front of mirror

  Have patient bend over to allow conduit to empty

  Moisten edge of faceplate with adhesive solvent and gently remove it

  Instruct patient not to smoke or be near an open flame when removing pouch (solvent is flammable)

  Keep skin free from direct contact with urine; place rolled 4 × 4 inch gauze over stoma/bud until pouch is applied; never leave in stoma

  Wash skin with soap and water and rinse well (patient may shower); pat dry or use hair dryer on low setting

  Inspect skin and stoma for signs of irritation

  Instruct patient to clip hairs; to never shave around stoma/buds

  Apply faceplate to skin; check size and shape to ensure that it is 1/16 to 1/8 inch around stoma

  Place appliance over stoma/bud

  Have appliance extend down, toward thigh

Teach methods of managing appliances

  Wash appliance with soap and lukewarm water

  Soak in distilled vinegar

  Rinse well with lukewarm water

  Air dry overnight

  Teach methods of controlling odor

    Avoid foods that give strong odor to urine

    Use deodorizing tablets or drops in pouch

Explain to patient where to purchase supplies

Provide written list of needed supplies, especially size and type of appliance

Instruct patient to avoid constipation

Teach importance of resuming normal sexual activity unless patient has cystectomy and is male (potential for impotence)

  Offer counseling if appropriate

Instruct patient to report the following symptoms to physician

  Absence of urine

  UTI

  Hematuria

  Pain in back or abdomen

  Elevated temperature

  Incision redness, pain, swelling, or drainage

  Severe skin excoriation

  Retraction of stoma

  Malaise

  Nausea, vomiting

  Abdominal distention; pain

Schedule follow-up care for patient with continent diversion for self-catheterization of reservoir

Expected outcome/evaluation

Patient and/or significant other verbalizes understanding of postoperative routine, symptoms to report to physician, and home care and follow-up instructions; and return-demonstrates wound and skin care, as well as emptying, changing, and caring for appliance

POLYCYSTIC KIDNEY DISEASE

A hereditary, incurable renal disease in which multiple outpouchings (cysts) of the nephrons occur in both kidneys; the cysts may be filled with urine, serous fluid, blood, or a combination; as the cysts enlarge, they distort and compress surrounding renal tissue and blood vessels, causing ischemia and necrosis; eventually, too few normal nephrons remain to support patient, and end-stage renal disease slowly develops

Assessment
Observations/findings

Family history of polycystic kidney disease
Abdominal fullness
Palpable abdominal mass
Pain
  Flank
  Abdominal
  Lumbar
Hypertension
Intracranial aneurysm in circle of Willis
Variable urine output
Proteinuria
Hematuria
Recurrent UTI
Progressive renal failure (see Renal Failure, p. 482)
Susceptibility to infections
Anemia
Other cystic organs
  Pancreas
  Lung
  Spleen
  Liver
Psychosocial problems
  Hopelessness
  Depression
  Anxiety
  Fear of death

Laboratory/diagnostic studies

Urinalysis
Urine culture and sensitivity
Serum electrolytes
Urine electrolytes
BUN
Serum creatinine

Urine creatinine clearance
CBC
KUB
Renal ultrasound
Renal biopsy
Infusion nephrotomogram

Potential complications

Ruptured cysts causing infection and hemorrhage
Intracranial bleeding
Renal calculi
End-stage renal disease

Medical Management*

Antihypertensive medications, diuretics
Antibiotics
Fluid restriction/parenteral fluids
Analgesics
Dietary restriction of protein and sodium
Dialysis and renal transplant if renal failure occurs (see Renal Failure, 482)
Genetic counseling

Nursing diagnoses/interventions/evaluation

■ **NDX:** Pain related to renal cysts

Assess nature, intensity, location, duration, and precipitating and alleviating factors of pain; use pain rating scale
Assess nonverbal signs of pain
Provide nonpharmacological comfort measures
    Assist patient with assuming a comfortable position
    Teach relaxation techniques
    Teach and assist with guided imagery technique
    Provide diversional activity
    Provide a restful environment
Observe for desired effects and side effects of medication
Consult with physician if measures fail to provide adequate pain relief or if a dosage or interval change for pain medication is needed

Expected outcome/evaluation

Reports a decrease in pain
Exhibits a relaxed facial expression and body position

■ **NDX:** Potential for fluid volume excess or deficit related to incompetence of kidney

Monitor for and report signs of fluid deficit (hypotension, poor skin turgor, decreased urinary output, thirst, dry mucous membranes, weight loss)
Monitor for and report signs of fluid excess (CHF, hy-

pertension, weight gain, edema, decreased urine output, S_3, S_4, distended neck veins)
Monitor serum and urine electrolytes and osmolality; report abnormal laboratory values to physician
Monitor for and report signs and symptoms of electrolyte imbalance
Measure and document intake and output q4h to 8h
Note character of urine
Measure urine specific gravity q8h
Weigh patient daily at same time with same clothing and scale
Avoid fluid dehydration; monitor administration of parenteral and oral fluids carefully
Avoid fluid excess; if fluids are restricted administer medications at mealtimes and space allowed fluids throughout day
Maintain dietary restrictions as ordered (low sodium, low protein)

Expected outcome/evaluation

Intake and output are balanced
Weight is stable and within normal range for patient
Vital signs are within patient's normal range
Urine is clear, yellow

■ **NDX:** Potential for infection (UTI, local, systemic) related to disease process, depressed immune system, and/or presence and rupture of fluid-filled cysts

Monitor for and report signs and symptoms of infection (elevated temperature; chills; flushed skin; sore throat; adventitious breath sounds; cough; thick, colored sputum; redness, swelling, tenderness, or drainage from wound)
Check temperature q4h and report if above 101° F (38.5° C)
Note character of urine; report if cloudy and malodorous
Avoid instrumentation and/or catheterization of urinary tract
If urethral catheter is present, maintain closed gravity drainage system
Monitor for and report signs and symptoms of UTI, and take measures to prevent UTI (see Urinary Tract Infection [UTI], p. 451)
Encourage coughing and deep breathing
Use good handwashing technique; teach and encourage patient to do the same
Instruct patient to avoid persons with infections
Take measures to prevent skin breakdown
Encourage early ambulation

Expected outcome/evaluation

Temperature is within normal range

---

*Medical management is preventive, supportive, and symptomatic in nature.

Breath sounds are clear
Urine is clear yellow to amber

■ **NDX:** Grieving related to loss of function of major organ system, changes in lifestyle, decision of having no children, and life-threatening prognosis

Be sensitive to changes and restrictions in patient's lifestyle
Encourage patient to express feelings of frustration, anger, fear, and uncertainty
Actively listen
Observe for behavioral and emotional signs of grieving (denial, anger, crying, withdrawal, noncompliance, dependency, etc.)
Be patient and empathetic as patient experiences emotional changes and develops coping mechanisms
Set limits on maladaptive coping mechanisms if they interfere with patient's well-being
Support adaptive behaviors that suggest a progression and resolution of grieving process
Support realistic hope; answer questions honestly, providing requested information
Provide assistance from other professionals to help patient with emotional changes (social worker, clergy, psychiatrist)
Teach and reteach about disease process and management
Involve family and significant others in teaching process
Encourage and provide genetic counseling

Expected outcome/evaluation

Begins progression through grieving process as evidenced by expression of feelings to care giver or significant other
Uses support system and adaptive coping mechanisms
Complies with treatment plan
Participates in self-care activities

■ **NDX:** Potential for altered tissue perfusion related to risk of hypertensive crisis

Monitor for and report signs and symptoms of hypertensive crisis q8h (hypertension, tachycardia or bradycardia, confusion, decreased level of consciousness, headache, tinnitus, nausea, vomiting, seizures, dysrhythmias, cerebrovascular accident [CVA])
Monitor BP and heart rate q4h; report systolic BP greater than 160 and diastolic BP greater than 90 to physician
Assess effectiveness of antihypertensive medication
Maintain bed in a low position with side rails elevated

Expected outcome/evaluation

Vital signs remain stable
Patient is alert and oriented with no signs of seizures or CVA

■ **NDX:** Knowledge deficit related to lack of exposure to information about disease process, and home care and follow-up instructions

Instruct patient to maintain dietary and fluid restrictions; provide written instructions
Instruct patient to observe character of urine after each voiding
Instruct patient to report hematuria to physician
Teach methods of preventing UTI
Instruct patient to exercise to tolerance, plan frequent rest periods, and sleep 6 to 8 hr per night
Instruct patient to keep warm and dry
Teach importance of genetic counseling before having children
Teach patient to report symptoms of disease progression
Teach name of medication, dosage, schedule, purpose, and side effects
Instruct patient to avoid taking over-the-counter medications without checking with physician
Teach importance of ongoing outpatient care

Expected outcome/evaluation

Patient complies with treatment plan and participates in self-care activities
Patient and/or significant other verbalizes symptoms to report to physician, and home care and follow-up instructions

GLOMERULONEPHRITIS

A group of diseases that result in an inflammatory reaction and/or necrotizing lesions within the glomeruli; usually caused by an immunological response

Assessment
Observations/findings

History of beta-hemolytic streptococcal infection
History of systemic lupus erythematosus or other autoimmune disease
Dull flank pain
Headache
Low-grade fever
Fatigue
Anorexia
Nausea
Elevated BP
Urine
  RBC
  Casts
  Nocturia
  Proteinuria
Azotemia
Edema
Facial in morning
Sacrum with bed rest

Ankles in evening
Retina (visual disturbances)
Circulatory overload
Sodium retention
Water retention
Dyspnea
On exertion
Supine position
Crackles, rales, pulmonary edema

Laboratory/diagnostic studies

Urinalysis
Urine protein excretion (24-hr)
IVP or retrograde pyelograms
BUN
Serum creatinine
Serum protein
Serum complement (decreased)
Antistreptolysin O titer (increased)
Renal biopsy
Throat and blood cultures
Hepatitis B antigen
Immunoelectrophoresis of serum and urine
Fibrin split products
Pulmonary function tests EKG and other cardiac function
tests

Potential complications

Infection
Renal failure (p. 482)
Anemia
Hypertensive encephalopathy
Cardiac failure, CHF

Medical Management

Bed rest
BP, T, P, and R q4h
BUN, creatinine, and urine protein monitoring
Intake and output
Fluid replacement according to fluid loss
Dietary sodium and fluid restriction: high-carbohydrate,
low-protein diet in presence of renal failure and/or low
potassium
Antibiotics in presence of infection
Corticosteroids and cytotoxic agent to decrease immune
system response and antibody formation
Antihypertensives to control BP
Diuretics to remove fluid
Plasmapheresis to remove antibodies

Nursing diagnoses/interventions/evaluation

■ **NDX:** Activity intolerance related to protein depletion and/or renal dysfunction

Monitor for excessive body depletion of protein (proteinuria, albuminemia)

Use dietary protein to replace protein loss
Provide high-calorie, high-carbohydrate diet
Enforce bed rest as ordered
Provide exercise within prescribed activity restriction
Plan activities with frequent rest periods
Plan a progressive regimen (as tolerated) to return to nor-
mal level of activity; evaluate BP and urine protein
excretion

Expected outcome/evaluation

Adheres to activity plan
BP remains within patient's normal limits without excessive protein excretion as activity is increased

■ **NDX:** Potential fluid volume excess related to sodium
and water retention and renal dysfunction

Monitor for and report signs and symptoms of fluid excess
(hypertension, CHF, weight gain, edema, S_3, S_4, neck
vein distention, and visual disturbances)
Measure and document intake and output q4h to 8h
Note amount and character of urine; report decreased
urine output to physician
Measure urine specific gravity q8h; report if elevated
Weigh patient daily at same time with same clothing and
scale
Arrange consultation with dietitian to teach sodium and
protein restricted diet; encourage patient to select menu
based on these principles
Replace fluids according to fluid loss
Provide ice chips to control thirst; include in intake cal-
culation
Monitor electrolytes and report abnormal laboratory val-
ues, and signs and symptoms of electrolyte imbalance
Hypokalemia: abdominal cramps, lethargy, arrythmias
Hyperkalemia: muscle cramps and weakness
Hypocalcemia: neuromuscular irritability
Hyperphosphatemia: hyperreflexia, paresthesias, mus-
cle cramps, itching, seizures
Uremia: confusion, lethargy, restlessness
Assess effectiveness of electrolytes administered parenter-
ally and orally
See nursing diagnosis of potential for fluid volume excess
under Renal Failure (p. 482)

Expected outcome/evaluation

Does not exhibit signs or symptoms of fluid excess, as
evidenced by stable weight, usual mental status, normal breath sounds, and absence of hypertension and
edema
Intake and output are balanced

■ **NDX:** Potential for infection (UTI, local, systemic)
related to depressed immune system

Assess effectiveness of administered immunosuppressive medications and cytotoxic agents

Monitor serum WBC, antibodies, and T cell values; report abnormal laboratory values to physician

Check temperature q4h and report if above 101° F (38.5° C)

Note character of urine; report if cloudy and malodorous

Avoid instrumentation and/or catheterization of urinary tract

If urethral catheter is present, maintain closed gravity drainage system

Monitor for and report signs and symptoms of UTI and take measures to prevent UTI (see Urinary Tract Infection [UTI], p. 451)

Auscultate chest for breath sounds q4h; report adventitious breath sounds to physician

Encourage coughing and deep breathing

Use good handwashing technique; teach and encourage patient to do the same

Instruct patient to avoid persons with infections

Take measures to prevent skin breakdown

Encourage early ambulation

Expected outcome/evaluation

Temperature and laboratory studies are within normal range

Breath sounds are clear

Urine is clear, yellow

Skin is dry and intact

■ **NDX:** Potential for altered tissue perfusion: cerebral/cardiopulmonary, related to risk of hypertensive crises

Monitor for and report signs and symptoms of hypertensive crisis (hypertension, tachycardia or bradycardia, confusion, decreased level of consciousness, headache, tinnitus, nausea, vomiting, seizures, dysrythmias, CVA)

Monitor BP and heart rate q4h; report systolic BP greater than 160 and diastolic BP greater than 90 to physician

Assess effectiveness of antihypertensive medication

Maintain bed in a low position with side rails elevated

Expected outcome/evaluation

Remains alert and oriented

BP and HR remain within patient's normal limits

■ **NDX:** Knowledge deficit related to lack of exposure to information about disease process, and home care and follow-up instructions

Discuss and provide written information about high-carbohydrate, low-protein, low-sodium diet

Instruct patient to:

Maintain fluid restriction as ordered

Weigh self daily at same time with same clothing and scale

Report weight gain to physician

Take and record temperature daily

Measure and record intake and output

Use good handwashing technique

Take BP daily at same time in same position and in same arm, and rest 5 min before taking BP

Teach patient to report symptoms of recurrence and progression of disease to physician

Rapid weight gain

Progressive edema: puffy eyes, swollen extremities

Elevated BP

Lethargy

Decreased urine output: less than 600 ml in 24 hr

Teach patient to avoid fatigue: to exercise only to tolerance, to plan frequent rest periods, and to sleep 6 to 8 hr per night

Teach patient to avoid persons with infections, especially upper respiratory infections, strep throat, and UTI; crowds

Instruct patient to report symptoms of infection to physician

Elevated temperature

Sore throat

Flu

Cough

Change in character of urine

Teach methods for preventing UTI

Instruct patient to:

Shower daily with antibacterial soap; women should avoid tub baths

Avoid pregnancy

Avoid overeating (appetite may be increased because of medications)

Avoid constipation

Teach medication name, dosage, schedule, purpose, and side effects

Instruct patient to avoid taking over-the-counter medications without checking with physician

Teach importance of ongoing outpatient care; teach need for long-term medical care, even though patient may feel well

Expected outcome/evaluation

Patient and/or significant other verbalizes understanding of disease process and progression, and home care and follow-up instructions; and return-demonstrates measuring and recording of intake and output, BP, weight, and using good handwashing technique

URINARY CALCULI (UROLITHIASIS)

Formation of stones in the kidney (pelvis or calyx) and their passage in the path of urine flow; renal calculi are classified according to their composition—they are usually composed of calcium, uric acid, cystine, phos-

phate, oxalate, or struvite; the stones may vary in size from a few millimeters up to a size that occupies the entire renal pelvis

Assessment
Observations/findings

Pain
  Back
  Flank
  Abdominal
  Groin
  Renal colic
  Ureteral colic
Distress
Anxiety
Nausea, vomiting
Urine
  Hematuria (microscopic or gross)
  Oliguria
UTI
  Elevated temperature
  Chills
  Dysuria
  Pyuria
  Frequency of urination
  Urgency of urination

Laboratory/diagnostic studies

Serum
  BUN
  Creatinine
  Calcium
  Phosphorus
  Uric acid
Urine
  Urinalysis
  Urine culture and sensitivity
  Urine collection (24-hr)
    Creatinine clearance
    Calcium excretion
    Phosphorus excretion
    Magnesium excretion
    Uric acid excretion
    Cystine excretion
    Oxalate excretion
Chemical analysis of stones passed or extracted
Radiological studies
  KUB
  Excretory urography with nephrotomogram
  Renal ultrasound
  Renal CT scan

Potential complications

UTI: pyelonephritis
Sepsis
Complete urinary obstruction
Hydronephrosis
Renal failure
Loss of a kidney: nephrectomy

Medical Management

Treatment according to chemical composition of stone
  Calcium stone
    Thiazide diuretics
    Low-calcium diet
    Oral phosphates
  Uric acid stone
    Allopurinol
    Sodium bicarbonate to alkalinize urine
    Sodium citrate
    Potassium phosphate
    Low-purine diet
  Cystine stone
    D-Penicillamine
    Sodium bicarbonate to alkalinize urine
    Low–animal protein diet
  Struvite stone
    Penicillin
    Drugs to acidify urine
Analgesics and antispasmodics for pain management
Antiemetics for nausea and vomiting
Antibiotics in presence of infection
Intake and output
Fluid intake up to 3000 ml/day unless contraindicated
Catheterization
Urine culture
Straining of all urine for stones and analysis
Evaluation of parathyroid function
Evaluation for absorptive hypercalcuric state

Surgical Interventions

Stone destruction

extracorporeal shock wave lithotripsy (ESWL) *A noninvasive procedure in which the patient is anesthetized and is placed on a pillow of water through which an electric spark is passed, causing high energy shock waves, which shatter the stone; patient then passes the stone through the urine*
Stone basket and ureteroscopy using ultrasonic fragmentation
laser lithotripsy *An endoscopy tube is threaded up the ureter to the stone and laser energy is passed through a fine wire into the stone, breaking it into fine pieces*

Percutaneous nephrostomy/nephrolithotripsy

Insertion of a tube into the renal calyx and through the parenchyma to the other side of the kidney
endoscopic removal of stone *After percutaneous nephrostomy, an endoscope is passed and the stone is extracted*
percutaneous stone dissolution *Lithotriptic agents that*

dissolve the stone are injected into nephrostomy tube

percutaneous ultrasonic lithotripsy (PUL) *A procedure using local anesthesia in which an ultrasonic probe is inserted into the renal pelvis via a nephrostomy tube and is positioned against the stone; pulses of ultrasound are administered and disintegrate the stone, which is then suctioned or irrigated out through the nephrostomy tube*

Surgical stone extraction

pyelolithotomy *Removal of stone through an incision into the renal pelvis*

nephrolithotomy *Removal of stone through a longitudinal incision across the middle two thirds of the kidney, requiring a parenchymal incision*

ureterolithotomy *Removal of stone by incision into the ureter*

cystolithotomy *Removal of stone by incision into the bladder*

nephrectomy *Removal of a kidney*

Nursing diagnoses/interventions/evaluation

▪ **NDX:** Pain related to passage of renal stone and/or surgical incision

Assess nature, intensity, location, duration, and precipitating and alleviating factors of pain; use pain rating scale

Monitor for syncopal episodes associated with renal colic (intense pain)

Assess for nonverbal signs of pain (restlessness, wrinkled brow, clenched fists, elevated BP and heart rate)

Monitor urine flow; check patency of catheters

Report signs and symptoms of urinary retention to physician

Assess incision site for redness, swelling, tenderness, and drainage

Provide nonpharmacological comfort measures

    Assist patient with assuming a comfortable position

    Teach relaxation techniques

    Teach and assist with guided imagery

    Provide diversional activity

    Provide a restful environment

    Encourage forcing fluids to dilute urine and flush stone

    Assist patient with ambulation, if tolerated, to promote movement of stone

Monitor and document pain relief and side effects of medications

Consult with physician if measures fail to provide adequate pain relief or if a dosage or interval change in pain medication is needed

Expected outcome/evaluation

Reports a decrease in pain

Presents a relaxed facial expression and body position

▪ **NDX:** Potential fluid volume deficit related to nausea and vomiting

Assess factors that contribute to nausea

Remove noxious sights and smells from room

Perform measures to relieve pain and anxiety

Provide a quiet, restful environment

Administer antiemetics as ordered

Monitor and document effects of medication

Instruct patient to change positions slowly

If emesis occurs, assess and document character and amount

Provide oral hygiene with each emesis

Provide small, frequent meals

Encourage patient to eat dry foods (toast, crackers)

Encourage patient to eat slowly

Expected outcome/evaluation

Patient reports a decrease in nausea and absence of vomiting

▪ **NDX:** Altered patterns of urinary elimination related to presence of stone in path of urine flow

Assess patient's "normal" voiding pattern; use voiding diary

Monitor and document complaints of dysuria, frequent urination, urgent urination, and hematuria

Measure urine output qh or with each voiding

Measure and record output from all catheters, drains, and tubes separately, if present

Be aware that a double J ureteral stent may be in place; assess for presence of suture from urinary meatus attached to stents to be used for removal

Monitor and report signs of urinary retention

Assess bladder for distention q4h

Insert Foley catheter if ordered

Maintain patency of all catheters; avoid kinks, loops, or tension in catheters or tubing

Instruct patient to avoid Fowler's position and to move about carefully to avoid dislodging catheters

Ensure that all collecting systems are below level of patient's bladder

Care of tubes and catheters

    Tape securely but allow for patient movement

    Label type and "right" or "left" to avoid errors

    Secure connection sites

    Use sterile technique when disconnecting and reconnecting

Maintain nephrostomy tube

    Tape to patient's flank

    Never clamp

    Irrigate only with a physician's direct order; be aware that irrigating may cause bleeding, infection, or mechanical damage to kidney

    Have a similar tube available at bedside

    Notify physician immediately if nephrostomy tube becomes dislodged

Maintain ureteral catheter
Tape to urethral catheter or patient's flank
Never clamp
Irrigate only with a physician's direct order; aspirate with sterile syringe to ensure patency of catheter then irrigate gently with a second sterile syringe using no more than 5 ml of sterile normal saline
Note character of urine; report abnormalities
Strain all urine and send for crystallographic analysis
Describe and report passage of stone
Force fluids up to 2500 ml/day unless contraindicated
Instruct patient to collect urine for stones, urinalysis, culture and sensitivity, and 24-hr urine collection
Explain and prepare patient for diagnostic tests

Expected outcome/evaluation

Patient resumes normal voiding pattern
Intake and output are balanced
Stone is passed

■ **NDX:** Potential for altered skin integrity related to wound drainage

Monitor surgical dressings for drainage; change dressings when wet
Note and document wound drainage, odor, color, and consistency; keep skin clean and dry
Inspect skin around catheters and tubes and report redness, breakdown, and excoriation
Apply an ostomy pouch and skin barrier around wounds where there is prolonged or copious drainage
Maintain patency of catheters; avoid kinks in drainage appliances

Expected outcome/evaluation

Patient shows no signs or symptoms of skin redness, breakdown, or excoriation

■ **NDX:** Knowledge deficit related to lack of exposure to information about disease process, postoperative routine, symptoms to report to physician, and home care and follow-up instructions

Instruct patient to force fluids to 2500 ml/day
Instruct patient to maintain diet as ordered
Teach patient to measure and strain urine
Instruct patient to save stone and report passage of stone to physician
Instruct patient to observe character of urine and to report abnormalities to physician
Teach patient methods to avoid UTI (see Urinary Tract Infection [UTI], p. 451)
Instruct patient to avoid persons with infections
Teach patient to use good handwashing technique
Instruct patient to exercise to tolerance, to take frequent rest periods, and to sleep 6 to 8 hr/day

Instruct patient to monitor and report
Elevated temperature
UTI
Incision redness, swelling, tenderness, or drainage
Hematuria
Symptoms of recurrence
Teach care of incision and dressing change
Teach medication name, dosage, schedule, purpose, and side effects
Instruct patient to avoid taking over-the-counter medications without checking with physician
Teach importance of ongoing outpatient care

Expected outcome/evaluation

Patient and/or significant other verbalizes understanding of disease process, postoperative routine, and home care and follow-up instructions; and return-demonstrates wound care, dressing change, measuring and recording of urine output, and straining of all urine

RENAL FAILURE

acute renal failure *A sudden decrease in renal function; causes are classified into three major categories: (1) prerenal hypoperfusion (decreased cardiac output, shock, vascular disorders), (2) intrarenal syndrome (acute tubular necrosis [ATN], acute allergic interstitial nephritis, glomerulonephritis), and (3) postrenal syndrome (obstruction of urine flow); acute renal failure can be divided into three phases (1) oliguric, (2) diuretic, and (3) recovery; with proper management acute renal failure may be reversible, but it has a high mortality rate (40% to 60%)*

chronic renal failure *An irreversible disease of the kidney, characterized by a progressive loss of renal function, leading to end-stage renal disease and death; most common causes of chronic renal failure include glomerulonephritis, pyelonephritis, congenital hypoplasia, polycystic kidney disease, diabetes, hypertension, systemic lupus, Alport's syndrome, and amyloidosis*

Assessment
Observations/findings

Neurological
Headache
Blurred vision
Nystagmus
Personality changes
Irritability
Malaise
Peripheral neuropathy
Paresthesias
Motor weakness
Decreased level of consciousness
Drowsiness
Confusion

Stupor
Coma
Seizure activity
Respiratory
Shortness of breath
Hyperventilation
Pulmonary edema
Pneumonia
Cheyne-Stokes respirations
Ammonia breath
Uremic lung
Cardiovascular
Hypertension
Tachycardia
CHF
Dysrhythmias
Myocardiopathy
Pericarditis
Cardiac tamponade
Fluid and electrolytes
Oliguria
Anuria
Edema: weight gain
Dehydration: weight loss
Hyperkalemia
Hyperphosphatemia
Hypermagnesemia
Hypocalcemia
Hypoproteinemia
Hyperlipidemia
Metabolic acidosis
Gastrointestinal
Bitter, metallic taste in mouth
Oral ulcerations
Anorexia
Malnutrition
Nausea, vomiting
Diarrhea
Constipation
Pancreatitis
Hemorrhage
Integumentary
Dry, scaly skin
Pale, sallow, yellow, or bronze color
Brittle, pale nail beds
Petechiae
Pruritis
Bruising
Uremic frost
Hematological
Anemia
Coagulopathy
Platelet deficiency
Musculoskeletal
Osteomalacia
Osteitis fibrosis

Osteosclerosis
Loss of muscle mass
Endocrine
Amenorrhea
Sexual dysfunction
Infertility
Hyperparathyroidism
Glucose intolerance
Immunological
Elevated temperature
Elevated WBC
Infection
Septicemia
Drug toxicity
Psychosocial
Anxiety
Fear
Powerlessness
Grieving
Denial
Noncompliance
Depression
Alteration in relationship with significant others

Laboratory/diagnostic studies

Serum BUN
Serum creatinine
Serum electrolytes
Urinalysis
Urine osmolality
Urine electrolytes
Creatinine clearance
Uric acid serum and urine
KUB
Renal ultrasound
Renal CT scan
IVP
Renal biopsy

Potential complications

Progressive loss of renal function
Fluid and electrolyte imbalance
Infection/sepsis
Hemorrhage
Cardiovascular failure
Respiratory failure

Medical Management

Maintenance of fluid and electrolyte balance
Fluid restriction
Daily weights
Medications*

---

*Dosages of medications may need to be altered depending on whether they are excreted primarily by the kidney, are nephrotoxic, or are dialyzed out.

Diuretics
Antihypertensives
Aluminum hydroxide antacids
Kayexalate
Vitamin D
Multivitamins
Ferrous sulfate
Calcium
Sodium bicarbonate
Diphrenhydramine
Dietary management
  High carbohydrate
  Low protein
  Low potassium
  Low sodium
  Total parenteral nutrition (TPN)
Blood transfusion
Peritoneal dialysis
Hemodialysis
Renal transplant
Treatment of complications

Nursing diagnoses/interventions/evaluation

■ **NDX:**   Fluid volume excess related to decreased ability of kidney to extract water and to retain sodium

Monitor and document intake and output accurately qh
Weigh patient daily at the same time with same clothing and scale
Monitor for elevated BP
Monitor serum electrolytes; report abnormal laboratory values or signs and symptoms of electrolyte imbalance
Hyperkalemia—irritability, nausea, diarrhea, intestinal colic, arrythmias, and peaked T wave on electrocardiogram (ECG)
  Restrict dietary potassium as ordered
  Administer polystyrene sulfonate (Kayexalate) as ordered
  Avoid administration of whole blood; use washed packed cells
Hyperphosphatemia—hyperreflexia, paresthesias, muscle cramps, and seizures
  Administer aluminum hydroxide antacids as ordered
  Restrict dietary phosphorus (peanuts, poultry, milk, cheese, corn, peas)
Hypermagnesemia—hypoactive deep tendon reflexes, decreasing level of consciousness, hypotension, decreased respirations, bradycardia, flushed skin, nausea, and vomiting
  Restrict dietary magnesium (nuts, whole-grain breads and cereals, meat, milk, and legumes)
  Avoid use of laxatives and antacids containing magnesium
Hypocalcemia—abdominal cramps; muscle cramps; carpopedal spasm; tingling of fingertips, toes, and circumoral area; positive Chvostek's and Trousseau's signs;

tetany; change in mental status; seizures; and dysrythmias
Provide sources of dietary calcium (e.g., dairy products)
Assess for signs of tetany
Assess level of consciousness; note changes in mental status
Assess heart sounds for presence of S₃ and/or S₄ and breath sounds for rales
Assess for peripheral edema and distended neck veins
Restrict fluids as ordered; give medications with meals when possible: divide fluids over remainder of day
Provide ice chips to control thirst and include amount in intake
Hard candies as well as frequent mouth care may help control thirst

Expected outcome/evaluation

Intake and output are balanced
Weight is stable
Breath and heart sounds are normal
No edema is present
Electrolytes are within normal limits for patient

■ **NDX:**   Potential fluid volume deficit related to risk of diuretic phase of disease process and/or bleeding (acute)

Monitor intake and output q4h to 8h; include insensible loss
Assess skin turgor, capillary refill, BP, HR, and weight for signs of dehydration
Encourage fluids to limit allowed
Monitor serum sodium
Assess patient for and report signs of unusual bleeding (petechiae, prolonged bleeding with venipuncture, bleeding gums, increased abdominal girth, significant drop in BP)
Guiac all GI tract fluids; report positive results
Monitor coagulation times (PT, PTT, platelets), Hgb, and Hct
Use smallest-gauge needle possible for all venipunctures and injections
Apply pressure to site after injections, and venous and arterial punctures, until bleeding stops
Caution patient to avoid activities that increase potential for trauma and bleeding

Expected outcome/evaluation

Capillary refill is 1 to 2 sec
Skin turgor is good
Intake balances output
Exhibits no evidence of bleeding

■ **NDX:**   Altered nutrition: less than body requirements, related to anorexia, nausea and vomiting, dietary restrictions, and oral ulcerations

Assess nutritional status

Monitor patient's weight daily

Consult with dietitian to plan menus incorporating dietary restrictions, calorie requirements, and patient's preferences

Encourage patient to control menu planning as much as possible

Encourage patient to express feelings about dietary restrictions

Encourage meals from home as long as they follow dietary restrictions

Be empathetic and reexplain purpose of dietary restrictions

Provide oral hygiene before and after meals and prn

Provide smaller, more frequent meals if patient is nauseated or experiences early satiety

Administer antiemetics on a timely basis before meals

Provide a pleasant environment during meals

Monitor percentage of meals eaten

    Offer replacements when necessary

Expected outcome/evaluation

Patient maintains adequate nutritional status as evidenced by weight within normal range for height, age, and body type, and by normal levels of serum albumin, total protein, iron, Hgb, and Hct

 NDX: Altered skin integrity related to immobility, uremia, capillary fragility, and edema

Assess patient's skin for redness, bruising or breakdown, turgor, and temperature

Keep skin clean and dry

Assist patient with cleansing and drying perineal area after bowel elimination

Administer skin care with lotion to avoid dryness

Avoid use of harsh soaps on patient's skin

Instruct patient not to scratch pruritic areas

Apply emollient lotion or cream to pruritic areas

Assess effectiveness of medications used to relieve pruritis

Encourage ambulation as tolerated

Assist patient with turning and changing position q2h if on bed rest

Keep bed linen wrinkle-free

Use an egg-crate mattress or sheepskin to decrease skin irritation

Apply protectors to heels and elbows

Remove any clothes, jewelry, etc. that may compromise skin circulation

Handle edematous areas carefully

Instruct and assist patient with ROM exercises

Administer IM injections with caution to minimize bruising

Provide direct pressure to venipuncture sites for 5 min or longer to prevent bleeding or bruising

Maintain adequate nutrition

Expected outcome/evaluation

Skin is warm, dry, and intact with good turgor

Verbalizes absence of pruritis

 NDX: Activity intolerance related to inadequate tissue oxygenation, anemia, inadequate nutrition, and difficulty in resting and sleeping

Identify factors that reduce patient's activity tolerance

Assess patient's present daily schedule

Adjust patient's schedule to provide rest periods between activities and adequate nocturnal sleep

Limit visitors or length of stay as necessary

Allow patient to set daily activity goals

Encourage gradual progression of activities as tolerated

Encourage self-care activities; assist as needed

Provide praise for all attempts to increase activity

Assess patient's response to increase in activity

Maintain adequate nutrition

Expected outcome/evaluation

Patient demonstrates an increase in activity tolerance as evidenced by verbalization of feeling less fatigued and getting adequate rest and by as near-normal resumption of ADLs as possible

■ NDX: Potential for infection related to depressed immune system, inadequate nutrition, and hospitalization

Monitor for and report signs and symptoms of infection (fever, chills, elevated WBC, increased heart rate, adventitious breath sounds, colored or increased sputum, cloudy and foul-smelling urine, redness, swelling, or drainage where there is skin breakdown, vaginal or urethral drainage, or ulceration of oral mucosa)

Monitor T, P, R, and BP every shift or more often if necessary

Monitor culture specimens obtained

Use excellent handwashing technique and teach patient the same

Maintain sterile technique with all invasive procedures and when caring for catheters, tubes, lines, dressings, and dialysis accesses

Maintain skin and mucosal integrity by providing good skin care and oral hygiene

Instruct patient to perform good perineal care

Avoid invasive procedures and indwelling catheters if possible

Maintain adequate nutrition

Discourage contact with persons having an infection

Maintain a clean environment

Encourage activity (ambulation if possible)

Encourage patient to take deep breaths and cough

Expected outcome/evaluation

Patient remains free of local or systemic infection as evidenced by absence of fever or leukocytosis; negative urine, sputum, and blood cultures; and absence of inflammation or drainage where there is a break in skin integrity or in oral mucosa

■ **NDX:** Grieving related to loss of function of major organ systems, changes in lifestyle, and life-threatening prognosis

Be sensitive to changes and restrictions in patient's lifestyle

Encourage patient to express feelings of frustration, anger, fear, and uncertainty

Actively listen

Observe for behavioral and emotional signs of grieving (denial, anger, crying, withdrawal, noncompliance, dependency, etc.)

Be patient and empathetic as patient experiences emotional changes and develops coping mechanisms

Set limits on maladaptive coping mechanisms if they interfere with patient's well-being

Support adaptive behaviors that suggest a progression and resolution of grieving process

Support realistic hope; answer questions honestly, providing requested information

Provide assistance from other professionals to help patient with emotional changes (social worker, clergy, psychiatrist)

Teach and reteach about disease process and management

Involve family and significant others in teaching process

Expected outcome/evaluation

Patient begins progression through the grieving process as evidenced by expression of feelings to care giver or significant other, use of support system, and effective coping mechanisms, and by compliance with treatment plan and participation in self-care activities

■ **NDX:** Knowledge deficit related to lack of exposure to information about disease process of renal failure, home care, and follow-up instructions

Instruct patient to eat high-carbohydrate, low-protein, low-sodium diet as ordered and avoid salt substitutes

Teach amount of daily fluid allowed in diet and that thirst is not a reliable indicator of fluid needs

Teach importance of and instruct patient to measure and note character of all output (urine, stools, and emesis)

Instruct patient to report decreasing ability to urinate to physician

Instruct patient to weigh self daily at same time with same clothing and scale and to accurately record weight

Instruct patient to take BP daily at same time in same

arm and in same position, and to rest briefly before taking it

Teach signs and symptoms of infection and instruct patient to notify physician of their occurrence

Instruct patient to avoid persons with infections, to avoid crowds, and to use good handwashing technique

Instruct patient to maintain good skin care

Shower daily

Avoid detergent soaps

Apply lanolin-based lotion or cream to skin

Avoid scratching skin

Teach and instruct patient to report symptoms of disease progression (rapid weight gain, lethargy, decreased urine output, absence of urine output for 24 hr, elevated BP, presence of edema)

Instruct patient to avoid fatigue: to exercise to tolerance, to plan frequent rest periods, and to sleep 6 to 8 hr per night

Teach name of medication, dosage, schedule, purpose, and side effects

Emphasize need to avoid taking over-the-counter medications without checking with physician

Teach importance of ongoing outpatient care

Expected outcome/evaluation

Patient and/or significant other is able to verbalize understanding of renal failure, fluid and dietary restrictions, and plan of follow-up care; identify ways to decrease the risk of further kidney damage, infection, and bleeding; state signs and symptoms to report to physician; and demonstrate ability to weigh self, measure intake and output, and take BP accurately

PERITONEAL DIALYSIS

A treatment indicated in renal failure, using the peritoneum as the dialyzing membrane to correct electrolyte and fluid imbalances and to remove toxic waste or drugs normally excreted by the kidneys; a catheter is inserted into the peritoneal cavity, and a hypertonic, warmed solution (dialysate) is infused by gravity into the peritoneal cavity and allowed to dwell; during the dwell time, osmosis occurs, moving water from the blood into the dialysate, and diffusion occurs, moving toxins and waste across the peritoneal membrane into the dialysate; after the appropriate dwell time, the dialysate and excess fluid are drained from the peritoneal cavity (Figure 9-9)

intermittent peritoneal dialysis (IPD) Can be performed manually or with a cycler; patient is dialyzed for 6 to 10 hr periods, four to five times a week, using a predetermined amount of dialysate with a set dwell time

continuous ambulatory peritoneal dialysis (CAPD) Used to treat chronic renal failure and performed by the patient; dialysis changes are done continuously (24 hr a day, 7 days a week); dialysate dwells in peritoneal cavity for 4 hr during the day and 8 hr during the night

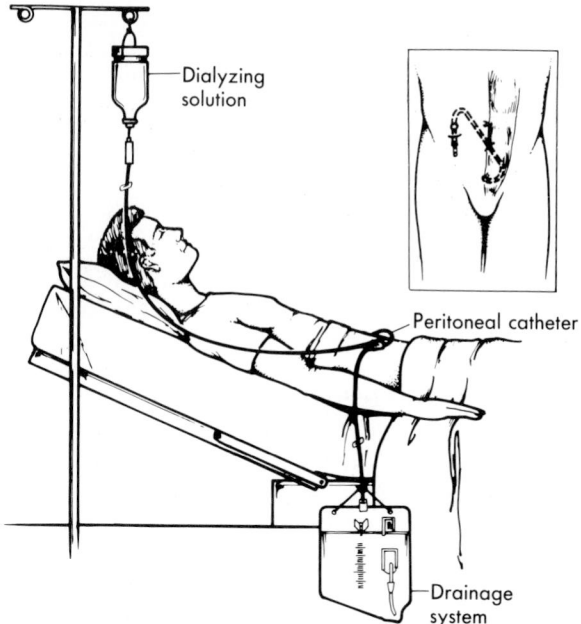

FIGURE 9-9. Acute peritoneal dialysis. *Insert,* Indwelling peritoneal catheter.

continuous cycling peritoneal dialysis (CCPD) *A combination of IPD and CAPD; a cycler performs three dialysate exchanges at night; during the day, dialysate is instilled and allowed to dwell in the peritoneal cavity the entire day and is drained at the end of the day*

Assessment
Observations/findings

Fluid imbalance
    Overhydration
       Rapid weight gain
       Edema
    Dehydration
       Rapid weight loss
       Hypovolemia
Respiratory system
    Tachypnea
    Rales
    Pulmonary edema
    Pneumonia
Cardiovascular system
    Tachycardia
    Bradycardia
    Cardiac dysrhythmias
    Shock
    Pericardial friction rub
    Congestive heart failure (CHF)
GI system
    Abdominal pain
    Nausea, vomiting
    Diarrhea
Neurological system

Confusion
    Decreased level of consciousness
    Seizure activity
Metabolism: hyperglycemia
Hypothermia
Catheter insertion site
    Redness
    Pain
    Swelling
    Drainage
    Drainage of dialysate around catheter
    Bleeding
Retention of dialysate
Dialysate
    Cloudy
    Bright red
    Fecal colored
    Foul smelling
Psychological
    Anxiety
    Disturbance in self-concept
    Fear of death

Laboratory/diagnostic studies

Serum electrolytes
Serum creatinine
Serum BUN
Serum protein
Urine glucose
See Renal Failure (p. 482)

Potential complications

Hyperosmolar coma
See Renal Failure (p. 482)
Perforated bladder
Perforated bowel
Infection
Peritonitis
Hemorrhage

Medical Management

Maintenance of fluid and electrolyte balance
    Restriction of fluids
    Daily weights
Medications*
    Diuretics
    Antihypertensives
    Aluminum hydroxide antacids
    Polystyrene sulfonate (Kayexalate)
    Vitamin D
    Multivitamins
    Ferrous sulfate

---

*Dosages of medications may need to be altered depending on whether they are excreted primarily by the kidney, are nephrotoxic, or are dialyzed out.

Calcium
Sodium bicarbonate
Diphenhydramine
Dietary management
  High carbohydrate
  Low protein
  Low potassium
  Low sodium
  TPN

Nursing diagnoses/interventions/evaluation

■ **NDX:**   Potential for infection related to presence of peritoneal catheter

Maintain sterile technique when connecting and disconnecting peritoneal catheter from dialysis system and when adding medication to dialysate

Maintain closed drainage system; use distal emptying valve to empty collecting unit

Wear clean masks, goggles, and sterile gowns and gloves when catheter is manipulated; have patient wear mask

Use povidone-iodine to clean connection site between catheter and dialysis tubing

Disconnect dialysis tubing from catheter and insert a sterile male Luer-Lok cap into open end of dialysis catheter

Apply antibacterial ointment to catheter insertion site

Be certain catheter is securely anchored; avoid tension

Apply sterile dressing to insertion site

Change dressing q24h or whenever wet or soiled

Monitor and report catheter site redness, swelling, or drainage

Monitor and report leakage of dialysate around catheter site

Report and culture turbid, cloudy, malodorous, bloody, or feces-stained outflow dialysate; this indicates perforated bowel, peritonitis, or hemorrhage

Check temperature q4h and report if above 101° F (38.5° C)

Auscultate chest for breath sounds q4h; report adventitious breath sounds to physician

Encourage coughing and deep breathing

Use good handwashing technique; teach and encourage patient to do the same

Instruct patient to avoid persons with infections

Take measures to prevent skin breakdown

Encourage early ambulation

Prevent UTI (see Urinary Tract Infection [UTI], p. 451)

Avoid use of indwelling urethral catheter; use intermittent catheterization as required

Expected outcome/evaluation

Outflow dialysate remains clear and is without odor
Insertion site is clean and dry
Temperature is within normal limits
Breath sounds are clear
Urine is clear, yellow

■ **NDX:**   Potential for altered fluid volume; excess, related to fluid retention, or deficit, related to abnormal loss caused by hypertonicity of dialysate or inadequate fluid replacement

Monitor baseline vital signs at beginning of each dialysis treatment, q15min during first exchange, and q1h thereafter

Report elevated or decreased BP, bounding pulse, tachycardia, or dyspnea to physician

Measure abdominal girth before initial treatment and then daily; obtain baseline weight, then weigh daily when peritoneal cavity is drained; report increasing weight or abdominal girth, a sign of retention of dialysate

Monitor intake and output

Maintain dialysis record
  Amount of solution instilled
  Amount of solution returned; notify physician if patient retains 500 ml or more
  Time of beginning and end of dialysis cycle
  Fluid balance
  Number of exchanges
  Medication used in dialyzing solution
  Patient's weight

Replace or restrict IV or oral fluid according to previous day's output plus 400 to 600 ml to replace insensible loss as ordered

Monitor serum electrolytes; report abnormal laboratory values or signs and symptoms of electrolyte imbalance
  Hyperkalemia—irritability, nausea, diarrhea, intestinal colic, dysrhythmias, and peaked T wave on ECG
  Hyperphosphatemia—Hyperreflexia, paresthesias, muscle cramps, and seizures
  Hypermagnesemia—hypoactive deep tendon reflexes, decreasing level of consciousness, hypotension, decreased respirations, bradycardia, flushed skin, nausea, and vomiting
  Hypocalcemia—abdominal cramps, muscle cramps, carpopedal spasm, tingling of fingertips, toes, and circumoral area, positive Chvostek's and Trousseau's signs, tetany, change in mental status, seizures, and dysrythmias

Assess for fluid overload and report hypertension, distended neck veins, bounding pulse, or peripheral edema

Assess for rales and dyspnea; if present drain dialysate, elevate head of bed, and notify physician

Evaluate outflow for obstruction, tubing kinks, or drainage around catheter

Assess for signs of constipation, which can cause outflow problem; assess effectiveness of stool softeners or laxatives

Assess for fluid volume deficit: hypotension, tachycardia, poor skin turgor, weight loss; report symptoms if present and collaborate with physician to adjust dialysate or dwell time

Expected outcome/evaluation

Weight remains stable
Abdominal girth is unchanged
BP, HR, and breath sounds are within normal limits
for patient
Skin turgor is good without presence of edema

■ **NDX:** Activity intolerance: related to inadequate tissue oxygenation, anemia, inadequate nutrition, and/or difficulty in resting and sleeping

Identify factors that reduce patient's activity tolerance
Assess patient's present daily schedule
Adjust patient's schedule to provide rest periods between activities and adequate nocturnal sleep
Limit visitors or length of stay as necessary
Maintain activity restrictions as ordered
Allow patient to set daily activity goals
Encourage gradual progression of activities as tolerated by patient
Encourage self-care activities; assist as needed
Provide praise for all attempts to increase activity
Assess patient's response to increases in activity
Maintain adequate nutrition

Expected outcome/evaluation

Verbalizes feeling rested
Resumes ADLs
Vital signs remain within patient's normal limits during activity

■ **NDX:** Pain related to cold or acidic dialysate, rapid infusion, or peritoneal infection

Assist patient with assuming a comfortable position during dialysis; change positions prn to promote comfort
Warm dialysate solution before infusion
Prevent air from entering peritoneal cavity during infusion of dialyzing solution; keep drip chamber three-fourths full
Monitor for pain radiating to shoulder, which may result from air accumulation under diaphragm
Monitor for signs of peritonitis and report
Monitor for rectal pain (may indicate improper catheter placement)
Instill no more than 2000 ml of dialyzing solution at one time
If pain occurs during infusion, slow infusion rate
Maintain tension-free patent drainage system
When administering CAPD, leave some dialyzing solution in peritoneal cavity (this prevents dialysis catheter from becoming plugged, thus facilitating infusion and drainage)

Expected outcome/evaluation

Reports a decrease in pain
Exhibits a relaxed facial expression and body position

■ **NDX:** Anxiety related to life-threatening complications of disease process and peritoneal dialysis

Teach patient about renal failure
Orient patient to environment
Announce any changes in routine; explain delays
Explain all procedures of peritoneal dialysis (i.e., implantation of catheter, exchanges, etc.)
Stress simplicity of peritoneal dialysis
Reinforce physician's explanation of procedure
Stress advantages to patient: more liberal diet and fluid intake usually
Teach relaxation techniques, such as music therapy or use of imagery
Encourage patient to verbalize feelings
Actively listen
Support adaptive coping mechanisms
Encourage communication with significant other
Encourage sharing common problems with others (group experiencing dialysis)

Expected outcome/evaluation

Verbalizes feelings of anxiety and uncertainty to care giver or significant other
Identifies adaptive coping mechanisms
Verbalizes feeling of increased psychological comfort
Begins to use relaxation techniques

■ **NDX:** Body image disturbance related to presence of peritoneal catheter

Be aware that patient is under considerable emotional stress
Be sensitive to changes in patient's lifestyle
Encourage patient to express feelings
Actively listen
Answer questions honestly
Be aware of coping mechanisms and expect that patient may exhibit irrational or inappropriate behaviors, irritability, and lack of motivation
Encourage adaptive coping behaviors
Set limits on maladaptive behaviors, especially if they are detrimental to patient's health
Instruct patient that there are no social limitations; patient may participate in any sport except boxing or sports requiring body contact (football, wrestling); heavy weight lifting should also be avoided
Explain to patient that there are no clothing limitations except that bikinis or girdles should not be worn

Explain to patient that there are no sexual limitations
Encourage communication with significant other
Encourage patient to look at and care for catheter as soon as possible
Include spouse/significant other in teaching
Provide for a psychiatric consultation if necessary

Expected outcome/evaluation

Verbalizes feelings related to body image change to care giver or significant other
Looks at and begins to care for peritoneal catheter

■ **NDX:** Knowledge deficit related to lack of exposure to information about renal failure, peritoneal dialysis procedure, and home care and follow-up instructions

Teach about disease process and progression of renal failure (see Renal Failure, p. 482)
Teach need and procedure for peritoneal dialysis
Discuss and provide written information about diet and fluids
Instruct patient to monitor and maintain daily records for
  Dialysis record
  Intake and output
  Weight (using same scale, clothing, and empty peritoneal cavity)
  BP, T, and P
Instruct patient to take measures to prevent UTI
Instruct patient to report the following symptoms to physician
  Elevated temperature
  Elevated or decreased BP
  Abdominal pain
  Abdominal distention
  Nausea, vomiting
  Vertigo
  Rapid weight gain
  Edema
  Catheter insertion site
    Redness
    Pain
    Swelling
    Drainage
  Dialysate Outflow Solution
    Turbid
    Cloudy
    Malodorous
    Bloody
    Feces stained
  Symptoms of progression of renal failure
Teach skin and peritoneal catheter care
  Protect catheter from damage
  Keep sterile cap and dressing in place

Wash catheter insertion site gently with soap and water, rinse well, and pat dry
Apply antibacterial ointment to catheter site daily
Cover site with sterile dressing
Teach name of medication, dosage, purpose, schedule, and side effects
Instruct patient to avoid taking over-the-counter medications without checking with physician
Instruct patient to have blood drawn for laboratory analysis as ordered by physician
Teach importance of ongoing outpatient care

Expected outcome/evaluation

Patient and/or significant other verbalizes understanding of renal failure, peritoneal dialysis procedure, symptoms to report to physician, home care, and follow-up instructions; return-demonstrates care of peritoneal catheter and dialysis procedure

CARE OF PATIENT AFTER HEMODIALYSIS

A treatment used in renal failure to remove toxic wastes, excess water, and fluid, and to correct electrolyte imbalance, by the principles of filtration, osmosis, and diffusion, using an external dialyzing system; three types of vascular access may be used: shunt—temporary, external connection between an artery and vein (Figure 9-10); fistula—permanent, internal connection or a graft between an artery and vein in the arm or thigh (Figure 9-11); subclavian or femoral lines—temporary, external catheter in a large vein

Assessment
Observations/findings

Patency of vascular access (shunt or fistula)
  Bruits
  Thrills
  Color of blood in shunt
  Unrelieved pain, numbness, tingling, change in color or temperature of extremity
  Poor capillary refill in extremity
Vascular access site
  Pain
  Redness
  Swelling
  Drainage
Fluid overload
Dehydration

Laboratory/diagnostic studies

Coagulation studies
  PT
  PTT
  Platelets
Serum BUN
Serum creatinine
Serum electrolytes

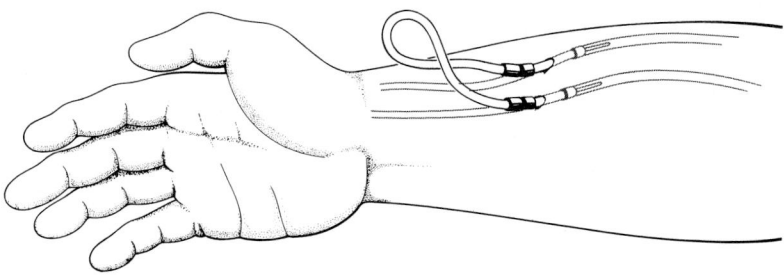

FIGURE 9-10. External arteriovenous shunt. (From Beare PG, Myers JL: *Principles and practice of adult health nursing,* St Louis, 1990, Mosby—Year Book.)

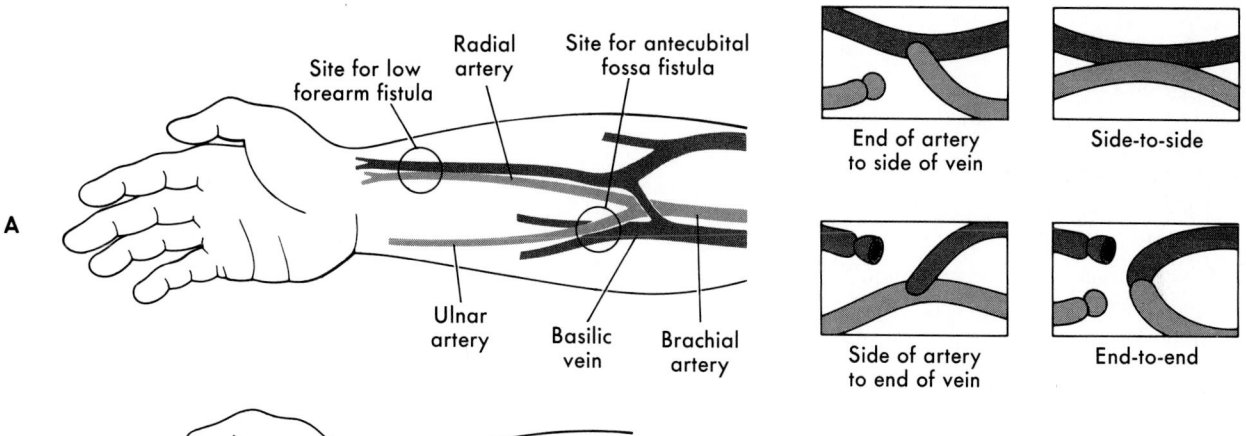

FIGURE 9-11. Internal arteriovenous fistula. **A,** Types of fistula construction. **B,** Appearance of arm with fistulas. (From Beare PG, Myers JL: *Principles and practice of adult health nursing,* St Louis, 1990, Mosby—Year Book.)

Urinalysis
Urine osmolality
Urine electrolytes
Creatinine clearance
Uric acid serum and urine

Potential complications

Hemorrhage
Air embolism
   Cyanosis
   Hypotension
   Weak, rapid pulse
Severe hypotension
Hepatitis
Septicemia

Medical Management

Maintenance of fluid and electrolyte balance
   Restriction of fluids
   Daily weights

Medications*
   Diuretics
   Antihypertensives
   Aluminum hydroxide antacids
   Polystyrene sulfonate (Kayexalate)
   Vitamin D
   Multivitamins
   Ferrous sulfate
   Calcium
   Sodium bicarbonate
   Diphenhydramine
Dietary management
   High carbohydrate
   Low protein
   Low potassium

---

*Dosages of medications may need to be altered depending on whether they are excreted primarily by the kidney, are nephrotoxic, or are dialyzed out.

Low sodium
TPN
Blood transfusion
Treatment of complications

Nursing diagnoses/interventions/evaluation

 NDX: Potential alteration in tissue perfusion, peripheral, related to risk of vascular access clotting, disconnection, or infection

Assess for and document patency of venous access q8h
    Auscultate for bruits
    Palpate for thrills and blood temperature
    Observe color of blood and condition of surrounding skin
For shunt, subclavian or femoral line
    Monitor access for leakage
    Maintain smooth rubber-tipped clamps and tourniquet at bedside in case of line disconnection
    Wrap shunt securely with gauze, exposing only a portion of loop to evaluate patency
    Never cut off dressings at access site or puncture tubing
    If disconnection occurs, clamp tubing and notify physician immediately
    If tubing is pulled out, apply pressure at site; notify physician STAT; apply tourniquet above site if needed
For fistula
    Inspect needle puncture sites after dialysis for bleeding
    Apply pressure to stop bleeding if present and hold for 5 min; recheck for bleeding q5min thereafter until no bleeding occurs for 15 to 20 min
Monitor for and report signs and symptoms of clotting of venous access (dark or separated blood within shunt, site cool to touch, absence of bruits and/or thrills)
Monitor for and report signs and symptoms of inadequate peripheral perfusion (sudden, unrelieved pain, numbness, tingling, decreased capillary refill time, or change in color and temperature of extremity distal to access site)
Keep subclavian or femoral lines patent with heparin solution by infusion or priming
Never kink tubing
Never take BP, start IV lines, or draw blood from shunt arm
Avoid tight clothing, jewelry, and name bands on extremity of access site
Monitor for and report signs of infection (redness, swelling, increased temperature or drainage)
Use sterile technique to perform dressing changes

Expected outcome/evaluation

Vascular access is intact as evidenced by presence of bruits and thrills, warm red blood circulating
Site of access and distal extremity are warm with capillary refill time at 1 to 2 sec

 NDX: Altered fluid volume: excess, related to kidney's inability to regulate fluid balance and/or retention of dialysate, or deficit, (1) related to inadequate fluid replacement, excessive fluid removal during dialysis, and/or bleeding caused by heparinization

Assess for fluid overload; hypertension, distended neck veins, bounding pulse, edema, rales, and dyspnea; report
Monitor intake and output q2h to 4h
Weigh patient daily, same time, scale, and clothing
Monitor vital signs q1h to 2h
Assess for fluid volume deficit; hypotension, tachycardia, poor skin turgor; dry mucous membranes, weight loss
Assess and measure baseline abdominal girth
Provide and encourage fluids to allowed limit; usually amount equal to output plus allowance for insensible loss
Monitor for electrolyte inbalances
    Hyperkalemia—irritability, nausea, diarrhea, intestinal colic, arrythmias, and peaked T wave on ECG
    Hyperphosphatemia—hyperreflexia, paresthesias, muscle cramps, and seizures
    Hypermagnesemia—hypoactive deep tendon reflexes, decreasing level of consciousness, hypotension, decreased respirations, bradycardia, flushed skin, nausea, and vomiting
    Hypocalcemia—abdominal cramps, muscle cramps, carpopedal spasm, tingling of fingertips, toes, and circumoral area, positive Chvostek's and Trousseau's signs, tetany, change in mental status, seizures, and dysrythmias
Assess patient for and report signs of unusual bleeding (petechiae, prolonged bleeding with venipuncture, bleeding gums, increased abdominal girth, significant drop in BP)
Guiac all GI tract fluids; report positive results
Monitor coagulation times (PT, PTT, platelets) and Hgb and Hct
Use smallest-gauge needle possible for all venipunctures and injections
Apply pressure to site after injections and venous and arterial punctures until bleeding stops
Caution patient to avoid activities that increase potential for trauma and bleeding

Expected outcome/evaluation

Vital signs are stable
Intake and output are balanced
Weight is stable
Abdominal girth is unchanged
Skin turgor is good
Mucous membranes are moist
Breath sounds are clear
No bleeding is noted

■ NDX: Grieving related to loss of kidney function, changes and restrictions in lifestyle, and life-threatening prognosis

Be sensitive to changes and restrictions in patient's lifestyle

Encourage patient to express feelings of frustration, anger, fear, and uncertainty

Actively listen

Observe for behavioral and emotional signs of grieving (denial, anger, crying, withdrawal, noncompliance, dependency, etc.)

Be patient and empathetic as patient experiences emotional changes and develops coping mechanisms

Set limits on maladaptive coping mechanisms if they interfere with patient's well-being

Support adaptive behaviors that suggest a progression and resolution of the grieving process

Support realistic hope; answer questions honestly, providing requested information

Provide assistance from other professionals to help patient with emotional changes (social worker, clergy, psychiatrist)

Teach and reteach about disease process and management

Involve family and significant others in teaching process

Expected outcome/evaluation

Patient shows signs of progression through the grieving process as evidenced by expression of feelings to care giver or significant other, utilization of support system and coping mechanisms, and compliance with treatment plan

■ NDX: Knowledge deficit related to lack of information about hemodialysis procedure, home care and follow-up instructions, and care of access site

Teach about disease process and progression of renal failure

Discuss need and procedure for hemodialysis

Discuss and provide written instructions about care of vascular access

Palpate for thrills qd

Report clotting of access

Absence of thrills

Dark or separated blood (shunt)

Pain, numbness, tingling, change in color and temperature of extremity

Procedure for managing disconnection (shunt)

Always carry rubber-tipped clamp

Report signs of infection at site

Never have BP taken, IV started, or blood drawn in extremity with access

Avoid wearing tight clothing or jewelry on access site extremity

Protect site from injury

Keep sterile dressing on site

Teach patient to measure and record intake and output and to weigh daily; report decreasing or no urine output and increasing weight

Discuss fluid and diet restrictions; provide consultation with dietician to plan meals

Provide access to professionals to assist in grieving process as necessary

Teach symptoms of progression of renal failure (see Renal Failure, p. 482)

Teach name of medication, dosage, purpose, schedule, and side effects

Instruct patient to have blood drawn for laboratory analysis as ordered by physician

Teach importance of ongoing outpatient care

Expected outcome/evaluation

Patient and/or significant other verbalizes understanding of vascular access care, symptoms to report to physician, and home care and follow-up instructions; return-demonstrates care of access site

NEPHRECTOMY: TOTAL/PARTIAL

Total or partial surgical removal of a kidney, via a flank, transabdominal, or thoracoabdominal incision; indicated in the treatment of renal malignancy, chronic pyelonephritis, trauma, polycystic kidney disease, renal vascular disease, congenital deformity, or renal calculi, or for the purpose of donation

Assessment
Observations/findings

Urine output
  Character
  Amount
  Color
    Hematuria
    Pyuria
    Oliguria
    Sediment
Status of other kidney
  Present
  Functional
Tension-free catheters
Patent drainage system, below level of kidney
  Ureteral catheter
  Stents
  Nephrostomy tube
  Drains
Hemorrhage
Shock
Site of incision
  Redness
  Pain
  Swelling
  Drainage

Elevated temperature
Grieving

Laboratory/diagnostic studies

BUN
Serum creatinine
Serum electrolytes
CBC
Coagulation studies
Blood typing and cross matching
Tissue compatability testing
   Human leukocyte antigen (HLA)
   Mixed lymphocyte culture (MLC)
Urinalysis
Urine culture and sensitivity
Urine creatinine clearance (24-hr)
IVP
Radionuclide studies
Renal perfusion scan
Renal ultrasound
Renal arteriography
Chest x-ray examination

Potential complications

Pneumonia
Pneumothorax
   Tachypnea
   Absent breath sounds
   Adventitious breath sounds
Atelectasis
Hemorrhage/shock
Paralytic ileus
Infection

Medical Management

T, P, and R per postoperative routine
NPO until bowel sounds are audible
Nasogastric tube to low, intermittent suction
Chest x-ray examination
Incentive spirometry
Parenteral fluids until liquids and/or diet is tolerated
Monitoring of fluid and electrolyte balance
Intake and output
Wound management
Urethral and ureteral catheters
Nephrostomy tube
Stents
Antibiotics
Analgesics
Stool softeners, laxatives

Nursing diagnoses/interventions/evaluation

■ **NDX:** Potential fluid volume deficit related to hemorrhage or hypovolemia

Assess surgical dressing, tubes, stents, and catheters for

bleeding qh and report presence to physician
Instruct patient to take caution not to dislodge tubes or catheters when turning and repositioning
Monitor intake and output q4h to 8h; report imbalances
Assess vital signs and skin turgor, temperature, and mental status q4h to 8h
Provide fluids as soon as tolerated

Expected outcome/evaluation

Vital signs are stable
Skin is warm and dry
Incision is beginning to heal
No evidence of bleeding via tubes, catheters, or stents
Intake and output are balanced

■ **NDX:** Potential for ineffective breathing pattern related to depressant effects of anesthetics and pain medications, or to reluctance of patient to breathe deeply because of incision pain

Position patient for optimal chest excursion
Assist patient with turning, coughing, and deep breathing q2h and prn
Assist patient with incentive spirometer to maximize lung expansion as ordered
Assess BP, heart rate and rhythm q2h
Assess breath sounds q4h
Report diminished or absent breath sounds to physician
Assess skin for signs of cyanosis and diaphoresis
Monitor for and report symptoms of impaired gas exchange (confusion, restlessness, irritability, decreased PO_2, increased PCO_2)
Administer analgesics at proper intervals to manage pain and to help patient perform coughing and deep breathing exercises more effectively
Administer O_2 as ordered
Assist in insertion of chest tubes if necessary
Secure connections and collection device for chest tubes
Maintain patency and integrity of chest tubes if present

Expected outcome/evaluation

Patient maintains an effective breathing pattern as evidenced by unlabored respirations, full chest expansion, absence of diminished or adventitious breath sounds, ability to clear secretions, and normal arterial blood gas values (ABGs)

■ **NDX:** Pain related to surgical incision

Assess nature, intensity, location, duration, and precipitating and alleviating factors of pain
Assess nonverbal signs of pain
Check catheters and/or drainage tubes for obstruction
Assess incision site for redness, tenderness, swelling, and drainage

Provide nonpharmacological comfort measures
  Assist patient with assuming a comfortable position
  Teach relaxation techniques
  Teach and assist with guided imagery techniques
  Provide diversional activity
  Provide a restful environment
Observe for desired effects and side effects of medications
Instruct patient to splint incision when turning, coughing, and deep breathing
Consult with physician if measures fail to provide adequate pain relief or if dosage or interval change for pain medication is needed

Expected outcome/evaluation

Reports increasing comfort
Moves easily
Exhibits relaxed facial expression and body position

■ **NDX:** Altered patterns of urinary elimination related to temporary urinary diversion or urinary retention related to nephrostomy tube, ureteral catheter, and surgical intervention

Assess patient's "normal" voiding pattern
Monitor for and document complaints of dysuria, frequent urination, urgent urination, and hematuria
Measure urine output qh or with each voiding
Measure and record output from all catheters, drains, and tubes separately, if present
Monitor for and report signs of urinary retention
  Assess bladder for distention q4h
  Insert Foley catheter if ordered
Maintain patency of all catheters; avoid kinks, tension, or loops in catheters or tubing
Instruct patient to avoid Fowler's position and to move about carefully to avoid dislodging catheters
Care for tubes and catheters
  Tape securely; never clamp
  Secure connection sites
  Use sterile technique when disconnecting or reconnecting
  Ensure that all collecting systems are below level of patient's bladder
Maintain nephrostomy tube, if present
  Tape securely
  Never clamp
  Irrigate only with a physician's direct order; be aware that irrigating may cause bleeding, infection, or mechanical damage to kidney
  Have a similar tube available at bedside
  Notify physician immediately if nephrostomy tube becomes dislodged
Maintain ureteral catheter, if present
  Tape to urethral catheter or patient's thigh
  Never clamp

Irrigate only with a physician's direct order
  Irrigate gently with no more than 5 ml of sterile normal saline, using a sterile syringe as ordered
Encourage fluids up to 2500 ml/day unless contraindicated
Use voiding measures if necessary after catheter removal
  Ensure privacy
  Place patient in a comfortable position to urinate
  Run tap water near patient
  Flush toilet
  Place patient's hands in warm water
  Apply heat to suprapubic area if ordered
  Pour warm water over perineum
  Assist patient with using relaxation techniques
  Place a few drops of oil of peppermint in bedpan or on cotton ball and hold briefly in front of urinary meatus
  Pull pubic hairs slightly
  Stroke inner aspect of thigh gently
  Stroke inner aspect of thigh with ice
Assess voiding stream force; volume, character of urine, and frequency; report abnormalities

Expected outcome/evaluation

Tubes and catheters remain patent that drain clear urine while in place
Patient voids with good force, clear, yellow urine when catheters and tubes are removed
Volume remains at > 30 ml/hr

■ **NDX:** Potential for altered tissue perfusion: peripheral, cardiopulmonary, and GI, related to risk of thrombophlebitis, pulmonary embolism, or paralytic ileus

Monitor for and report signs of venous thrombosis (pain, tenderness, warmth, or redness in extremity; positive Homan's sign, absent pedal pulses)
Apply antiembolic stockings as ordered; remove daily and assess skin integrity
Assist and teach patient to perform passive ROM exercises to extremities q2h to 4h; avoid straight leg exercises
Avoid placing patient in a sitting position for prolonged periods of time
Avoid pressure or putting pillows under knees
Instruct patient not to cross legs
Monitor for and report signs and symptoms of pulmonary embolism (sudden chest or shoulder pain, cough, hemoptysis, dyspnea, tachycardia, hypertension, cyanosis, restlessness, decreased PO_2)
If symptoms of pulmonary embolism occur
  Place patient in semi-Fowler's or high-Fowler's position
  Administer O_2 as ordered
  Monitor vital signs qh
  Maintain strict bed rest
  Prepare patient for diagnostic tests (lung scan, venography, pulmonary angiography)

Monitor for and report signs of paralytic ileus (absent or diminished bowel sounds, persistent or worsening abdominal pain and cramping, distended, firm abdomen, failure to pass flatus)

Maintain NPO until active bowel sounds are audible or passage of flatus is noted

Auscultate for bowel sounds q4h

Insert and/or maintain nasogastric tube as ordered

Encourage early ambulation

Instruct patient to avoid smoking and/or chewing gum to reduce air swallowing

Expected outcome/evaluation

Verbalizes no leg, chest, or abdominal pain

Pedal pulses are present

Negative Homan's sign

Respiratory rate and rhythm are within normal range

Breath sounds are clear

Bowel sounds are present

Passes gas and stool

■ **NDX:** Potential for infection related to surgical incision, presence of tubes and catheters

Monitor for and report signs and symptoms of wound infection q4h (fever, chills, redness, swelling, tenderness, purulent and/or malodorous wound drainage)

Assess temperature q4h

Obtain wound culture of suspicious drainage

Use good handwashing technique and teach and encourage patient to do the same

Instruct patient to avoid touching incision, dressings, and drainage

Maintain sterile technique when changing dressings and performing wound care

Assess tube and catheters for cloudy, malodorous drainage; report if present; increase fluids to 2500 ml/day

Use sterile technique when manipulating drainage tubes, catheters, and tubes

Expected outcome/evaluation

Incision is dry and healing is beginning

Drainage from tubes and catheters is clear yellow and without odor

■ **NDX:** Grieving related to loss of major body organ; fear that recipient may reject kidney, if for donation

Assess patient's perception of effect of loss of a kidney

Explain that remaining kidney will take over

If kidney is being used for transplantation

Explore concerns with donor and family that kidney may be rejected

Provide emotional support to donor and donor's family

Prepare donor and family for possibility that donated kidney may be rejected and explain that this does not mean donated kidney was inadequate

Refer donor and family for counseling if needed

Be sensitive to changes and restrictions in patient's lifestyle

Encourage patient to express feelings of frustration, anger, fear, and uncertainty

Actively listen

Observe for behavioral and emotional signs of grieving (denial, anger, crying, withdrawal, noncompliance, dependency, etc.)

Be patient and empathetic as patient experiences emotional changes and develops coping mechanisms

Set limits on maladaptive coping mechanisms if they interfere with patient's well-being

Support adaptive behaviors that suggest a progression and resolution of grieving process

Support realistic hope; answer questions honestly, providing requested information

Provide assistance from other professionals to help patient with emotional changes (social worker, clergy, psychiatrist)

Teach and reteach about disease process and management

Involve family and significant others in teaching process

Expected outcome/evaluation

Begins progression through the grieving process as evidenced by expression of feelings to care giver or significant other

Uses support system and effective coping mechanisms;

Complies with treatment plan

Participates in self-care activities

Discusses possibility of rejection of kidney by recipient

■ **NDX:** Knowledge deficit related to lack of exposure to information about postoperative routine, symptoms to report to physician, and home care and follow-up instructions

Instruct patient to take measures to prevent UTI

Instruct patient to force fluids up to 2500 ml/day unless contraindicated

Instruct patient to avoid activities that may endanger remaining kidney, e.g., contact sports such as football

Instruct patient to exercise to tolerance, to plan frequent rest periods, and to avoid heavy lifting for at least 1 year

Teach care of incision and surgical dressing change

Teach care of nephrostomy tube or ureteral catheter if present

Discuss symptoms and instruct patient to report

UTI

Elevated temperature

Incision and nephrostomy/ureteral catheter site redness, swelling, pain, or drainage

Teach medication name, dosage, schedule, purpose, and side effects

Instruct patient to avoid taking over-the-counter medications without checking with physician

Teach importance of ongoing outpatient care

Instruct patient to inform health care providers of presence of nephrostomy or ureteral catheter and history of nephrectomy

Expected outcome/evaluation

Patient and/or significant other verbalizes understanding of postoperative routine, symptoms to report to physician, and home care and follow-up instructions; and return-demonstrates care of incision, nephrostomy, and ureteral catheter

RENAL TRANSPLANT: CARE OF RECIPIENT*

A functioning kidney is removed from a living donor or a human cadaver and is transplanted into the right or left iliac fossa of the recipient; the renal blood vessels of the donor organ are anastomosed to the recipient's iliac artery and vein, and the ureter is transplanted into the bladder or anastomosed to the recipient's ureter, to establish urinary tract continuity (Figure 9-12)

Assessment
Observations/findings

Rejection of kidney (Table 9-2)
    Transplant site: redness, swelling, tenderness
    Elevated temperature
    Elevated WBC
    Decreased urinary output
    Hematuria

*See Nephrectomy (p. 493) for care of donor.

Increased proteinuria
Sudden weight gain of over 2 lb (0.9 kg) in 24 hr
Acute onset of hypertension
Restlessness
Irritability
Lethargy
Increased serum BUN
Increased serum creatinine
Atelectasis: diminished or absent breath sounds
Tachycardia
Tachypnea
Pulmonary edema
Cardiac dysrythmias

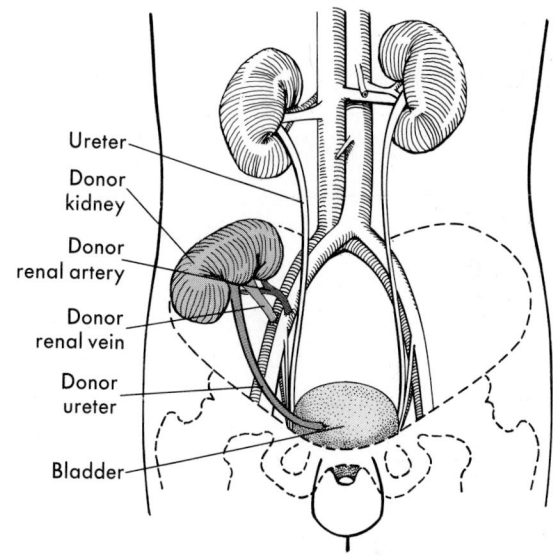

FIGURE 9-12. Location of transplanted kidney showing anastomosis of renal artery, renal vein, and ureter. (From Phipps WJ, Long BC, Woods NF et al: *Medical-surgical nursing: Concepts and clinical practice*, ed 4, St Louis, 1991, Mosby–Year Book.)

TABLE 9-2. Classification of Rejection

Hyperacute	Acute	Chronic
Rejection occurs as soon as new kidney is implanted	Rejection occurs 1 week to 3 months after kidneys has been implanted	Rejection occurs at any time after surgery
Rejection is caused by presence of antibodies in recipient that cause polymorphonuclear leukocytes to clot, thus blocking glomerular and peritubular capillaries	Immune response leukocytes and red blood cells invade vascular endothelium and intertubular vasculature; renal blood flow is decreased; therefore necrosis of renal tubules occurs	There is gradual decline in kidney function; glomerular filtration is decreased, and serum creatinine and serum urea nitrogen are elevated; proteinuria occurs, and sodium is decreased in urine
Rejection is usually irreversible	Rejection may be reversible	Early detection and treatment may decrease decline in kidney function
Transplanted kidney is removed immediately	Attempt is made to save new kidney	Attempt is made to save kidney
Patient resumes hemodialysis	Patient may need to resume dialysis treatments	Patient may need to resume dialysis treatments

Thrombophlebitis
Pulmonary embolism
Hemorrhage
Infection (UTI, local, systemic)
  Incision
    Redness
    Pain
    Swelling
    Drainage
    Dehiscence
Character and amount of urine output
  Oliguria to anuria
  Large quantities of dilute urine
Location and patency of arteriovenous (AV) shunt
  Bruits
  Thrills
Cataracts
Psychosocial problems
  Grieving
  Disturbance in self-concept
  Anxiety
  Depression
Sensory deprivation
Sensory overload

Laboratory/diagnostic studies

See Renal Failure, p. 482
Blood typing and cross matching
Tissue compatibility testing
Chest x-ray examination
ECG

Potential complications

Rejection
Renal artery stenosis, thrombosis, aneurysm
Shock
Paralytic ileus
Side effects of immunosuppressive drugs
Diabetes
Cushing's syndrome
GI bleeding
Glaucoma

Medical Management

BP, T, P, and R per postoperative routine
Intake and output
Monitoring of BUN, creatinine, and electrolytes
Parenteral fluids with electrolytes
NPO until bowel sounds are audible
Chest x-ray examination
Incentive spirometry
Reverse isolation
Hemodialysis
Immunosuppressive medications
Analgesics
Stool softeners, laxatives

Nursing diagnoses/interventions/evaluation

■ **NDX:** Pain related to surgical incision

Assess nature, intensity, location, duration, and precipitating and alleviating factors of pain
Assess nonverbal signs of pain
Check urethral catheter, if present, for obstruction; secure to avoid tension
Assess incision site for redness, tenderness, swelling, and drainage
Provide nonpharmacological comfort measures
  Assist patient with assuming a comfortable position
  Teach relaxation techniques
  Teach and assist with guided imagery techniques
  Provide diversional activity
  Provide a restful environment
Observe for desired effects and side effects of medications
Instruct patient to splint incision when turning, coughing, and deep breathing
Consult with physician if measures fail to provide adequate pain relief or if a dosage or interval change in pain medication is needed

Expected outcome/evaluation

Verbalizes feeling a decrease in pain
Exhibits a relaxed facial expression and body position

■ **NDX:** Potential for altered fluid volume: excess or deficit related to kidney's inability to regulate fluid balance immediately after transplant and/or inadequate fluid replacement

Monitor vital signs q2h to 4h
Weigh patient daily, same time, clothing or bed clothing, scale
Monitor intake and output q4h
  Measure urine output qh
Auscultate lungs for breath sounds q2h to 4h
Monitor skin turgor, condition of mucous membranes, and mental status q4h
Monitor CVP to assess volume changes
Maintain patency of drainage catheters
Monitor for and report excessive drainage at surgical site
Monitor serum electrolytes; report abnormal values or signs and symptoms of electrolyte imbalance
Administer fluids equal to output/hr plus designated amount for insensible losses (may be 20 to 30 ml/hr)
  Expect that some patients will have 200 to 500 ml output/hr; report <30 ml/hr output
Fluids may need to be restricted with low or no output
Maintain integrity of vascular access line (see Hemodialysis, p. 490)

Expected outcome/evaluation

Vital signs and weight remain stable

Intake and output are balanced with output of >50 ml/hr

Skin turgor is good

Mucous membranes are moist and pink

Lungs are clear

■ **NDX:** Potential for infection related to immunosuppression

Maintain reverse isolation if ordered

Assess temperature q4h and report if greater than 101° F (38.5° C) (temperature may not be elevated with infection because of immunosuppressive therapy)

Inspect incision daily for signs of redness, swelling, or drainage

Use strict sterile technique with dressing change and manipulation of incision line and catheters

Note character of urine; report if cloudy and malodorous

Avoid instrumentation/catheterization of urinary tract

If urethral catheter is present, maintain closed gravity drainage system

Monitor for and report signs and symptoms of UTI and take measures to prevent

Encourage high oral fluid intake, up to 2500 to 3000 ml/day, to flush out bacteria unless contraindicated

Auscultate chest for breath sounds q4h; report adventitious breath sounds to physician

Encourage coughing and deep breathing q1h to 2h; assist with incentive spirometer

Use good handwashing technique; teach and encourage patient to do the same

Instruct patient to avoid persons with infections

Take measures to prevent skin breakdown

Encourage and assist with early ambulation

Obtain specimens of suspicious drainage for culture and sensitivity

Expected outcome/evaluation

Patient is afebrile

Incision is dry and beginning to heal

Urine is clear, yellow without sediment

Lungs are clear

Skin has no breaks

Sites of IVs are healing

■ **NDX:** Potential for altered patterns of elimination related to changes in bladder structure, blockage of indwelling catheter, and/or leakage of ureter anastomoses

Assess preoperative voiding history

If oliguric, bladder may be reduced in size or atrophied

Assess urine for color, character, presence of sediments or clots qh immediately postoperatively; then q2h to 4h

Assess abdomen/bladder for distention q1h to 2h

Maintain closed catheter drainage system

Arrange tubing to prevent kinks and backflow of urine

Secure catheters to prevent tension

Observe urine; expect blood tinged in immediate postoperative period; flow obstructed by blood clots may require irrigation; use caution if irrigating ureteral and urethral catheters so anastomosis is not disturbed

Instruct patient to void q1h to 2h after removal of catheters to avoid distending bladder and increasing tension on anastomosis; and to report changes in color, character of urine, or presence of bleeding or clots

Expected outcome/evaluation

Catheters remain patent that drain urine free of sediment and clots while in place

Voids q2h and states urine remains clear, yellow without clots

Bladder is not distended on palpation

■ **NDX:** Potential for diversional activity deficit related to reverse isolation

Monitor for signs of diversional activity deficit (boredom, apathy, frequent napping during the day, etc.)

Explain rationale for reverse isolation

Familiarize patient with environment

Suggest and provide appropriate diversional activities (puzzles, books, model kits, handicrafts, cards, etc.)

Encourage patient to become involved in self-care activities to provide a sense of accomplishment (i.e., leg exercises, coughing and deep breathing, measuring and recording intake and output)

Encourage patient to verbalize feelings

Spend extra time with patient

Allow patient some control over scheduling of activities, treatments, and visitation

Encourage significant others to stagger visits throughout the day

Suggest that significant other bring radio, tape player, or other favorite items from home

Request consultation from psychiatric department or pastoral care if necessary

Expected outcome/evaluation

Verbalizes decreased feelings of isolation and boredom

Identifies and participates in diversional and self-care activities

■ **NDX:** Potential for altered protection related to risk of rejection of transplant and medication side effects

Monitor for and immediately report signs and symptoms of rejection (redness, swelling, and tenderness over transplant site; elevated temperature; elevated WBC;

decreased urine output; increased proteinuria; sudden weight gain; simultaneously increased BUN and serum creatinine; acute onset of hypertension; symptoms of sodium retention; edema)

Measure and document intake and output qh

Measure BP qh

Measure temperature q2h and report if greater than 101°F (38.5°C)

Monitor for and report side effects of immunosuppresive medications

Symptoms of bone marrow suppression, leukopenia, anemia, and thrombocytopenia azathioprine (Imuran), cyclophosphamide (Cytoxan)

Nausea and vomiting (azathioprine, cyclophosphamide); if nausea and vomiting occur, administer antiemetics as ordered

Symptoms of hepatotoxicity (azathioprine, cyclosporine); monitor bilirubin and CBC; report abnormal laboratory values

Symptoms of nephrotoxicity; gingival hyperplasia, tremors, and hirsutism (cyclosporine)

Signs of adrenal insufficiency; depressive and/or psychotic episodes, and GI bleeding (steroids)

Prepare patient for surgery to remove rejected kidney if hyperacute reaction occurs

Support patient and family

Expected outcome/evaluation

No signs or symptoms of rejection are present

Laboratory values are within normal limits for patient

Immunosuppressants as tolerated without presence of side effects

■ **NDX:** Potential for ineffective coping related to prolonged hospitalization, stages of transplant organ acceptance, and possibility of rejection

Assess patient's present coping mechanisms and what has worked in patient's past

Support adaptive coping mechanisms

Set limits on maladaptive coping mechanisms if they interfere with patient's health and well-being

Monitor for progression through stages of acceptance of transplant organ

Foreign body stage: kidney feels strange; patient feels that kidney is sticking out of body

Partial internalization stage: patient moves about cautiously; overemphasizes kidney's fragility

Complete internalization: patient accepts kidney and focuses on it only during direct conversation related to kidney

Recognize that patient may regress to previous stage(s)

Encourage patient to express feelings

Encourage family support and involvement

Consult with clergy, social service, and psychiatrist if necessary

Expected outcome/evaluation

Shows signs of progression through the stages of transplant organ acceptance

Identifies and uses adaptive coping mechanisms and support system

■ **NDX:** Knowledge deficit related to lack of information about postoperative routine, symptoms to report to physician, home care, and follow-up instructions

Instruct patient to prevent infections

Limit visitors and avoid large groups of people

Avoid persons with infections

Teach methods to prevent UTI (p. 451)

Demonstrate good handwashing technique

Demonstrate wound care and dressing change

Instruct patient to take temperature at same time twice a day

Teach and instruct patient to report to physician

Hematuria

Temperature over 101° F (38.5° C)

Increased pulse rate

Weight gain of over 2 lb (0.9 kg) in 1 day or 4 lb (1.8 kg) in 1 week

Lethargy

Decreased urine output: <600 ml in 24 hr

Tenderness over new kidney

Respiratory distress

Restlessness or irritability

Sudden change in BP

Edema

Symptoms of rejection

Instruct patient to:

Weigh self daily at same time with same clothing and scale

Take BP daily at same time in same position and in same arm, and to rest 5 min before taking it

Maintain prescribed dietary and fluid restrictions

Avoid overeating (appetite may increase because of medications)

Measure and record intake and output

Instruct patient to:

Exercise to tolerance, avoid strenuous exercise, plan frequent rest periods, and avoid heavy lifting and excessive bending

Wait 2 weeks before driving a car and avoid use of seat belts that may press on new kidney

Avoid drinking alcoholic beverages until allowed to do so by physician

Avoid sexual activity for 6 weeks or as indicated by physician

Avoid pregnancy until indicated by physician

Explain that symptoms of original disease may develop in new kidney

Explain that there is an increased risk of developing a malignancy—especially lymphomas, skin and lip cancers—and signs to report

Discuss name of medication, dosage, schedule, purpose, and side effects

Instruct patient to:

Never stop taking immunosuppressive drugs without a physician's order

Avoid taking over-the-counter medications without checking with physician

Teach importance of ongoing outpatient care

Have blood drawn for laboratory tests at regular intervals as ordered by physician

Have eye examinations q6 months for glaucoma and cataracts

Notify physician before going to dentist

Wear a medical alert bracelet

Expected outcome/evaluation

Patient and/or significant other verbalizes an understanding of postoperative routine, symptoms to report to physician, and home care and follow-up instructions; and return-demonstrates handwashing technique, care of incision, taking and recording of BP, T, and weight, and measuring and recording of intake and output

PROSTATIC HYPERTROPHY

Enlargement of glandular and cellular tissue of the prostate gland related to endocrine changes associated with aging; the prostate gland surrounds the neck of the bladder and urethra; therefore, prostatic hypertrophy frequently prevents the bladder from emptying

Assessment
Observations/findings

Hesitancy in starting flow of urine

Stream of urine reduced

Force

Size

Incomplete emptying of bladder: residual urine

Urgency of urination

Frequency of urination

Nocturia: three times or more

Dysuria

Hematuria

Bladder neck obstruction: acute retention of urine

UTI: cystitis

Enlargement and tenderness of prostate

Laboratory/diagnostic studies

Urinalysis

Urine culture and sensitivity

Serum creatinine

Serum BUN

Acid phosphatase

WBC

Cystoscopy

Excretory urography/IVP

Retrograde studies

Potential complications

Pyelonephritis

Hydronephrosis

Azotemia

Uremia

Medical Management

Catheterization

Antibiotics

Intake and output

Surgery

Transurethral resection of prostate (TURP)

Suprapubic prostatectomy

Retropubic prostatectomy

Radical retropubic prostatectomy

Cystostomy drainage of bladder

Nursing diagnoses/interventions/evaluation

■ **NDX:** Urinary retention related to enlarged prostate

Assess intake and output q4h to 8h

Assess force of urinary stream, frequency, and time required to initiate stream; use voiding diary

Encourage patient to void q2h to 4h and to obey impulse to void

Take caution when administering medications that may cause urinary retention

Restrict dietary alcohol, coffee, tea, and cola

Catheterize patient after each voiding as ordered to determine amount of residual urine; report if greater than 100 ml

Use voiding measures

Monitor serum BUN and creatinine

Expected outcome/evaluation

Voids in adequate amounts with no evidence of bladder distention

Residual volume measures less than 75 to 100 ml

■ **NDX:** Potential for infection related to use of urinary catheter and/or urinary retention

Check temperature q4h and report if above 101° F (38.5° C)

Note character of urine; report if cloudy and malodorous

If urethral catheter is present, maintain closed gravity drainage system

Use sterile technique for intermittent catheterization while hospitalized

Monitor abdomen/bladder for distention

Monitor for and report signs and symptoms of UTI; take measures to prevent UTI (see Urinary Tract Infection [UTI], p. 451)

Use good handwashing technique; teach and encourage patient to do the same

Expected outcome/evaluation

Temperature is within normal range
Urine is clear, yellow, and without odor
Bladder distention is not evident

■ **NDX:** Pain related to acute urinary retention

Assess nature, intensity, location, duration, and precipitating and alleviating factors of pain

Provide nonpharmacological comfort measures: assist patient to comfortable position, provide sitz baths and warm perineal soaks, teach relaxation techniques and guided imagery, and/or provide diversional activity

Monitor and document pain relief and any undesirable side effects

Notify physician of unrelieved or increasing pain

Expected outcome/evaluation

Reports a decrease in pain
Shows a relaxed facial expression and body position

■ **NDX:** Knowledge deficit related to lack of information about disease process, symptoms to report to physician, and home care and follow-up instructions

Instruct patient to force fluids up to 1500 to 2000 ml/day unless contraindicated

Teach patient to measure urine output after each voiding; to note increased hesitancy, decreased force of stream, increasing frequency; to report these findings as well as maintaining a voiding diary

Instruct patient not to allow bladder to become too full
Instruct patient to urinate q2h to 4h
Teach self-catheterization if required
Teach patient symptoms to report to physician
Inability to void
UTI
Instruct patient to remain as active and mobile as possible
Instruct patient to avoid long automobile, bus, or train rides unless voiding is possible at any time
Teach medication name, dosage, schedule, purpose, and side effects
Instruct patient to avoid taking over-the-counter medications without checking with physician
Teach importance of ongoing outpatient care

Expected outcome/evaluation

Patient and/or significant other verbalizes understanding of disease process, symptoms to report to physician, and home care and follow-up instructions; and return-demonstrates measuring urine output and self-catheterization if required

PROSTATECTOMY

Removal of part or all of the prostate gland

__transurethral resection of prostate (TURP)__ Removal of part or all of the prostate gland via a cystoscope or resectoscope inserted through the urethra

__suprapubic prostatectomy__ Removal of the prostate gland through an incision made in the bladder (Figure 9-13)

__retropubic prostatectomy__ Removal of the prostate gland via an incision in the lower abdomen through the anterior prostatic fossa without entering the bladder (Figure 9-14)

__perineal prostatectomy__ Radical removal of prostate gland through an incision between the scrotum and rectum

__radical retropubic prostatectomy__ Removal of the prostate gland, including the capsule, seminal vesicles, and adjacent tissue through an incision in the lower abdomen; the urethra is anastomosed to the bladder neck for prostatic cancer (Figure 9-15)

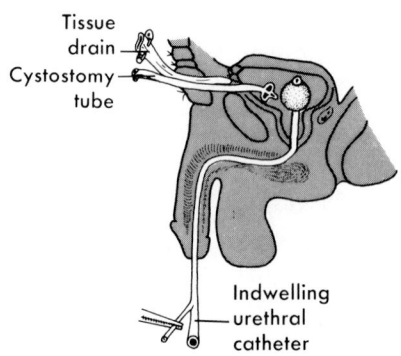

FIGURE 9-13. Suprapubic prostatectomy.

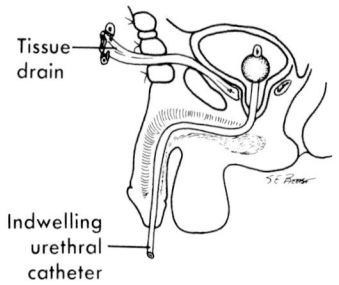

FIGURE 9-14. Retropubic prostatectomy.

Assessment
Observations/findings

Urinary output
 Character
 Amount
Hermorrhage: bright red drainage and clots from catheter
Shock
Bladder spasms
Distended bladder
 Suprapubic pain
 Elevated BP
 Tachycardia
 Diaphoresis
 Restlessness
Dilutional hypernatremia
 Elevated BP
 Headache
 Disorientation
 Pulmonary edema
Dilutional hyponatremia
 Muscular weakness
 Apprehension
 Nausea, vomiting
 Hyperpnea
 Hypotension
Extravasation of urine into abdominal cavity
 Tense, rigid abdomen
 Elevated temperature
 Renal failure
Patent, tension-free catheters
 Kinking
  Mucous plugs
  Blood clots
 Closed gravity drainage system
 Continuous bladder irrigation
 Leakage of urine around suprapubic catheter
Removal of indwelling catheter
 Incontinence
 Dysuria

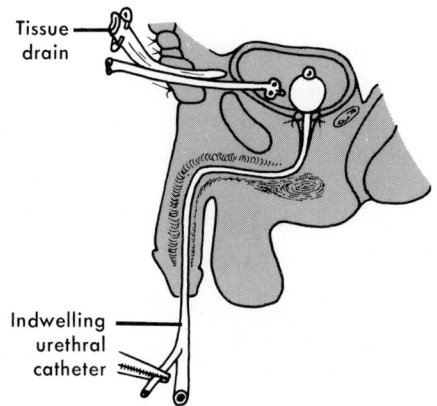

FIGURE 9-15. Radical retropubic prostatectomy.

Hematuria
Bladder neck contracture
 Dribbling
 Frequent urination
 Difficulty in initiating urinary stream
 Small urinary stream
Urinary retention with overflow
Urinary fistula
Inability to urinate
Incisional redness, swelling, pain, drainage

Laboratory/diagnostic studies

Urinalysis
Urine culture and sensitivity
Serum creatinine
Serum BUN
Acid phosphatase
WBC
Cystoscopy
IVP/excretory urography
Retrograde studies
Hgb, Hct
Serum electrolytes

Potential complications

Dilutional hyponatremia (TURP)
Infection
Circulatory complication involving testicle
Hydrocele
Shock
Acute urinary retention
Paralytic ileus
Pelvic abscess
 Elevated temperature
 Pain on walking

Medical Management

BP, T, P, and R per postoperative routine
Analgesics
Antispasmodics
Continuous bladder irrigation
Intermittent bladder irrigation
Parenteral IV therapy
Intake and output
NPO until bowel sounds are audible

Nursing diagnoses/interventions/evaluation

■ **NDX:** Pain related to surgical incision, bladder spasms, and urinary retention

Assess nature, intensity, location, duration, and precipitating and relieving factors of pain
Assess for nonverbal signs of pain (restlessness, wrinkled brow, clenched fists, elevated BP and HR)
Provide alternate comfort measures

Assist patient to assume comfortable position

Teach relaxation technique and assist with guided imagery

Observe and document desired and side effects of medications

Intermittently irrigate urethral/suprapubic catheters as ordered; use sterile normal saline and sterile syringe

Instill solution gently; never force

Continue irrigation until urine is clear of clots

If measures fail to provide relief, consult with physician for dosage or interval change

Expected outcome/evaluation

Reports a decrease in pain

Shows a relaxed facial expression and body position

■ **NDX:** Altered patterns of urinary elimination related to surgical resection and bladder irrigation

Assess urethral and/or suprapubic catheters for patency

Observe color, character, and flow of urine and presence of clots through catheters q2h

Record amount of irrigant and urine output; subtract irrigant from output; report retention and urine output of <30 ml/hr

Notify physician if complete occlusion of catheter occurs

Irrigate catheters to remove clots

Maintain continuous bladder irrigation (CBI) as ordered

  Use sterile normal saline as ordered for irrigation

  Maintain sterile technique

  Instill irrigating solution through smallest lumen of catheter

  Regulate flow of solution at 40 to 60 drops/min or to maintain clear urine

Frequently assess outflow lumen for patency

Encourage 2000 to 2500 ml of oral fluids/day unless contraindicated

After catheter removal

  Measure urine after each voiding; observe force of stream

  Assess bladder for retention

  Use voiding measures

    Provide privacy

    Have patient stand

    Institute voiding schedule

  Perform intermittent catheterization to check for residual urine as ordered; report if greater than 100 ml

  Avoid bladder distention

Expected outcome/evaluation

Catheters remain patent while in place

Clots irrigated out of bladder and do not obstruct blood flow through catheter

Irrigant is returned through outflow with no retention

Urine output exceeds 30 ml/hr

Voids without overflow or retention when catheter is removed

■ **NDX:** Potential for infection related to presence of catheters in bladder and presence of surgical incision

Check temperature q4h and report if above 101° F (38.5° C)

Note character of urine; report if cloudy and malodorous

Assess incision for pain, redness, swelling, or leakage of urine q4h

Change dressing using sterile technique

Maintain closed gravity drainage system

Monitor for and report signs and symptoms of UTI

Use good handwashing technique; teach and encourage patient to do the same

Remove catheters as soon as possible

Monitor for and report redness, swelling, pain, or leakage around suprapubic catheter

Expected outcome/evaluation

Temperature is within patient's normal limits

Incision is dry without evidence of infection

Voids clear urine without difficulty

■ **NDX:** Potential fluid volume excess related to absorption of irrigation fluid (TURP)

Monitor for and report signs and symptoms of dilutional hyponatremia (low serum sodium, change in mental status, confusion, restlessness, muscles twitching, convulsions, nausea, vomiting, SOB, elevated BP)

Monitor intake and output q4h to 8h

Carefully calculate irrigant instilled and amount returned; report decreased return

Stop irrigation at first signs of fluid excess; notify physician

Use syringe to irrigate catheter to remove clots if ordered

Expected outcome/evaluation

Intake and output (minus irrigant) are balanced

Irrigant is totally returned

Alert, oriented, and shows no abnormal motor function

■ **NDX:** Potential fluid deficit related to excessive blood loss

Monitor for and report signs and symptoms of hemorrhage (hypotension, tachycardia, dyspnea, cool, clammy skin, syncope, hematuria)

Monitor abdominal/suprapubic dressing q2h for bleeding

Monitor urethral and suprapubic catheters q2h for excessive bleeding (drainage that does not change to pinkish-red after irrigation but remains thick and bright red or dark red)

Report excessive bleeding and/or gross hematuria to physician

Maintain traction on catheter if instituted; usually 4 to 8 hr postoperatively

Do not manipulate rectum, e.g., no rectal temperatures

Be alert for signs of DIC

Monitor Hct and Hgb as ordered

If hemorrhage occurs

Place patient flat in bed

Notify physician

Expected outcome/evaluation

Vital signs remain stable

Incision exhibits no signs of redness, swelling, or increased temperature

Catheter drainage remains pink-tinged for 48 hr then clear, yellow

Skin is warm and dry

■ **NDX:** Potential for ineffective breathing pattern related to anesthetics

Assist patient with incentive spirometer to maximize lung expansion as ordered

Teach and assist patient to turn, cough, and deep breathe q2h

Assess breath sounds q4h

Report diminished or absent breath sounds to physician

Assess skin for signs of cyanosis and diaphoresis

Monitor for and report symptoms of impaired gas exchange (confusion, restlessness, irritability, decreased PO_2, increased PCO_2)

Administer pain medication at proper intervals to manage pain and to help patient perform coughing and deep breathing exercises more effectively

Expected outcome/evaluation

Lungs clear on auscultation; respiratory rate and rhythm are within normal limits

Performs coughing and deep breathing exercises without difficulty

■ **NDX:** Sexual dysfunction related to impotence (radical prostatectomy) and/or altered sexuality patterns related to retrograde ejaculation (suprapubic surgeries)

Provide opportunities for discussion of sexuality between patient and significant other

Provide information about expectation of return of sexual functioning

Impotence occurs in radical procedures (penile prosthesis may be recommended by physician)

Retrograde ejaculation occurs with suprapubic approach

Sexual function may be restored in 6 to 8 weeks but patient remains infertile

Provide information about sexual counseling

Provide reassurance that as surgical site heals, good urinary control will return

Teach and encourage patient to practice perineal exercises to promote muscular control of incontinence and sexual function

Expected outcome/evaluation

Patient discusses feelings about sexuality with significant other

Seeks counseling when needed

■ **NDX:** Knowledge deficit related to lack of information about postoperative routine, symptoms to report to physician, and home care and follow-up instructions

Instruct patient to

Avoid sitting for long periods of time, such as with long automobile trips

Perform perineal exercises 10 to 20 times qh after urethral catheter has been removed

Tense perineal muscles by contracting rectal sphincter

Hold position, then relax

Start and stop stream while voiding to increase muscle tone

Maintain diet prescribed and avoid coffee, tea, and cola; avoid alcohol for 1 month or as indicated by physician

Exercise to tolerance, avoid strenuous exercise, and plan frequent rest periods

Shower daily

Avoid sexual activity for 1 month or as indicated by physician; reinforce physician's explanation of retrograde ejaculation

Teach and instruct patient to report symptoms to physician

Heavy bleeding (intermittent hematuria is expected for 2 to 4 weeks)

Difficulty in voiding

Incision redness, swelling, pain, drainage

Elevated temperature

Pain on walking

Instruct patient to avoid constipation

Teach care of incision and dressing change

Discuss name of medication, dosage, schedule, purpose, and side effects

Instruct patient to avoid taking over-the-counter medications without checking with physician

Teach importance of ongoing outpatient care

Expected outcome/evaluation

Patient and/or significant other verbalizes understanding of postoperative routine, symptoms to report to physician, and home care and follow-up instructions; and return-demonstrates perineal exercises and care of incision

PENILE IMPLANT

Surgical implantation of a prosthesis in the penis for the treatment of impotence; three types of prostheses are used; a silicone rubber prosthesis, which leaves the penis in a constant state of semierection; an inflatable penile prosthesis that contains two cylinders in the corpora cavernosa (penile shaft), a balloon reservoir in the extraperitoneal space beside the bladder, and a pump in a subcutaneous pouch in the lower scrotum; and an inflatable self-contained prosthesis (see Figures 9-16 and 9-17)

Assessment
Observations/findings

Scrotal edema
Scrotal discoloration
Incisional
    Pain
    Redness
    Swelling
    Drainage
Elevated temperature
Mechanical failure of prosthesis
Urinary retention
Hematuria
Incontinence
Psychosocial problems
    Anxiety
    Fear that prosthesis will fail

Laboratory/diagnostic studies

Nocturnal penile tumescence test
    Snap gauge test
Doppler ultrasound flow meter for penile blood flow
Penile arteriogram
Sacral evoked response
Bulbocavernous reflex/artery time
Dynamic infusion cavernosometry
Dynamic infusion cavernosography

Potential complications

Rejection of prosthesis
Mechanical failure of prosthesis
Extravasation of fluid of prosthesis reservoir into surrounding tissue
Urethral or glans erosion
Persistent penile pain

Medical Management

Counseling therapy
Hormonal therapy
Revascularization

Penile prosthesis implantation
    Semirigid penile prosthesis
    Inflatable penile prosthesis
Postoperative care
    NPO until bowel sounds are audible
    Parenteral IV until liquids and/or diet is tolerated
    Monitoring of BP, T, P, and R per postoperative routine
    Analgesics
    Ice to scrotum
    Antibiotics
    Stool softeners, laxatives

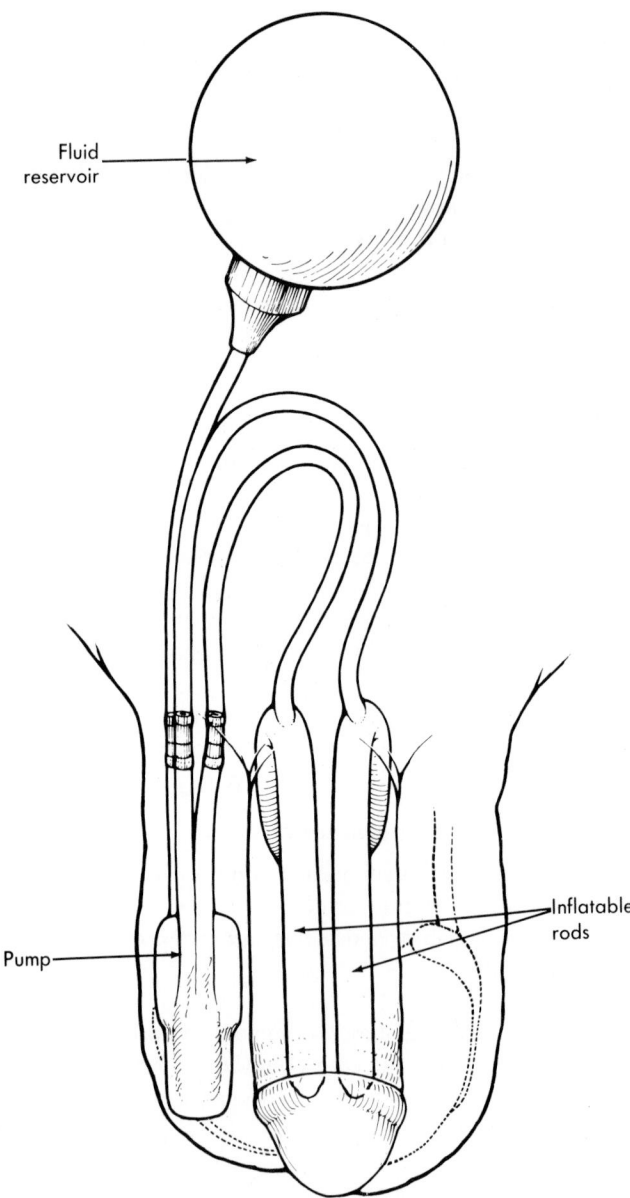

FIGURE 9-16. Implantation of penile prosthesis. Inflatable penile prosthesis, frontal view. (From Lerner J, Khan Z: *Mosby's manual of urologic nursing,* St Louis, 1982, CV Mosby; courtesy American Medical Systems, Inc, Minneapolis, Minn.)

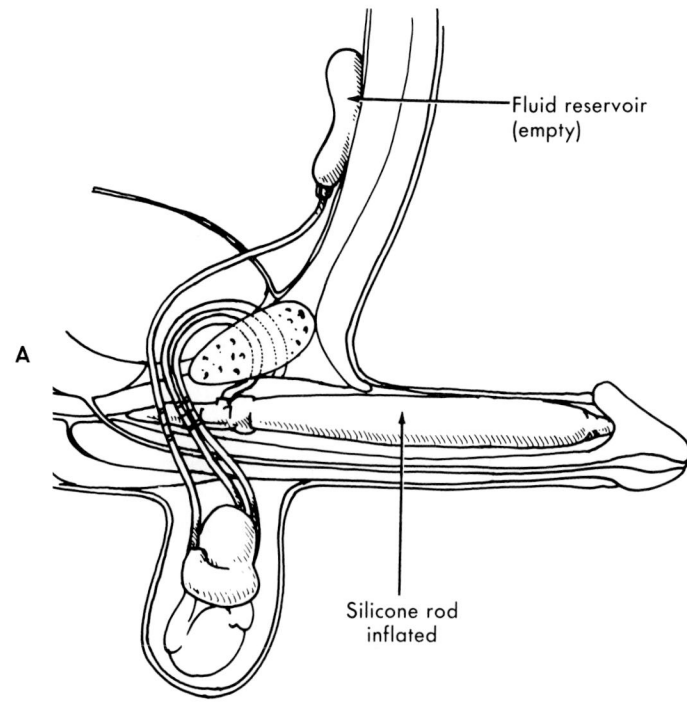

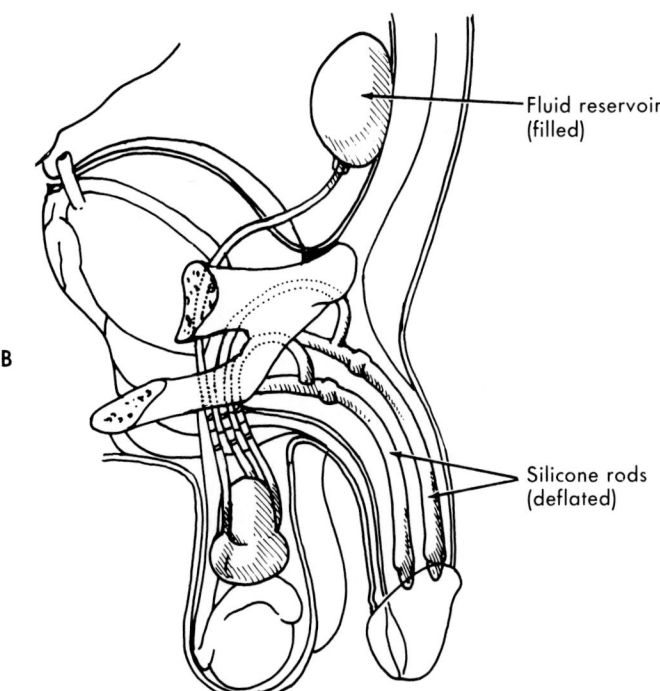

FIGURE 9-17. Inflatable prosthesis, sagittal view. **A,** Penis in erect position. **B,** Penis in flaccid position. (From Lerner J, Khan Z: *Mosby's manual of urologic nursing,* St Louis, 1982, CV Mosby; courtesy American Medical Systems, Inc, Minneapolis, Minn.)

Nursing diagnoses/interventions/evaluation

■ **NDX:** Pain related to surgical incision

Assess nature, intensity, location, duration, and precipitating and alleviating factors of pain

Assess nonverbal signs of pain; be aware that patient may not verbalize need for pain medication because of embarrassment

Elevate scrotum as ordered

Pack scrotum in ice as ordered: check that weight does not increase discomfort

Use bedcradle to elevate bed linen

Explain to patient that some scrotal swelling and discoloration is normal and may last for 7 to 10 days

For inflatable implants, keep patient in Trendelenburg's position for 24 hr to prevent scrotal edema

Check urethral catheter for obstruction

Provide nonpharmacological comfort measures

Assist patient with assuming a comfortable position

Teach relaxation techniques

Teach and assist with guided imagery techniques

Provide diversional activity

Provide a restful environment

Observe for desired effects and side effects of medications

Consult with physician if measures fail to provide adequate pain relief or if dosage or interval change in pain medication is needed

Expected outcome/evaluation

Reports a decrease in pain

Shows a relaxed facial expression and body position

■ **NDX:** Potential for infection and/or rejection related to surgical incision and implantation of a foreign object

Monitor for and report signs and symptoms of rejection (elevated temperature, elevated WBC, pain, redness, and swelling; pallid, stretched skin; appearance of device outline and pain over implant site, urinary retention); report if present

Assess incision for redness, swelling, drainage, or increasing pain

Use sterile technique for dressing changes

Pull pump down into most dependent part of scrotum beginning second postoperative day to prevent inguinal migration

Teach and assist with perineal care after bowel movement

Expected outcome/evaluation

Temperature is within normal range

Incision is dry without evidence of redness or swelling

Outline of implant is not visible over penis

■ **NDX:** Body image disturbance related to penile prosthesis, fear that implant will fail, and/or previous experiences with impotence

Assess feelings regarding prosthesis and function

Maintain a calm, accepting attitude when discussing impotence or implant

Encourage patient to verbalize feelings of embarrassment or anxiety, and fears and concerns

Encourage patient to look at and participate in care of dressings and location of pump, etc.

Assure patient that participation in sports and other activities will not be restricted after healing occurs

Explain that looser-type clothing will disguise appearance of semirigid implants

Assure that mechanical failure of pump can usually be corrected under local anesthetic if this is a concern

Provide privacy when teaching or activating prosthesis

Include significant other in teaching

Encourage communication with significant other

Refer for sexual counseling when appropriate

Expected outcome / evaluation

Discusses feelings about implant with significant other

Participates in care

■ **NDX:** Knowledge deficit related to lack of information about inflation of prosthesis, symptoms to report to physician, and home care and follow-up instructions

Teach name and type of prosthesis

Teach patient to inflate prosthesis

Use model or picture

Instruct patient to locate pump in scrotum between thumb and forefinger

Instruct patient to inflate prosthesis by squeezing bulb 10 to 15 times between thumb and index finger

To deflate pump, press release valve on side of pump between thumb and forefinger

Explain to patient that prosthesis need not be deflated all the way; do not squeeze penis to completely empty cylinders

Inflation schedule

First week: qd

Second week: bid

Third week: qd plus firmly inflate and leave inflated for 30 min qd

Fourth week: qd plus firmly inflate and leave inflated for 30 min bid

Explain to patient that prosthesis restores erectile capability but has no effect on ejaculation, fertility, or orgasm; these remain as before implant; e.g., if sperm production is normal, he may father a child

Explain to patient that implant erection will probably not be exactly the same as that achieved naturally before onset of impotence

Instruct patient to avoid intercourse for 6 weeks, or until incision heals, or as indicated by physician

Instruct patient to avoid tight, restrictive underclothing for 2 to 3 weeks postoperatively

Instruct patient that he may shower

Instruct patient to avoid strenuous activity, heavy lifting, jogging, or sports for about 3 weeks

Instruct patient to report symptoms to physician

Incision redness, pain, swelling, drainage

Elevated temperature

Inability to urinate

Penile pain

Teach medication name, dosage, schedule, purpose, and side effects

Instruct patient to avoid taking over-the-counter medications without checking with physician

Teach importance of ongoing outpatient care

Expected outcome / evaluation

Patient and/or significant other verbalizes an understanding of penile prosthesis, symptoms to report to physician, and home care and follow-up instructions; and return-demonstrates inflation and deflation of penile prosthesis

BIBLIOGRAPHY

Abels L: *Critical care nursing: a physiologic approach*, St Louis, 1986, CV Mosby.

Allen A, Gorman S, eds: *The post anesthesia review for certification*, Richmond, Va, 1985, American Society of Post Anesthesia Nurses.

Birdsall C, Brassil D: How do you use renal irrigations? *Am J Nurs*, July, 87(7):909, 1987.

Briggs BA, Acute renal failure. In: Ihde JK, Jacobsen WK, and Briggs BA: *Principles of critical care*, Philadelphia, 1987, WB Saunders.

Bristoll S, et al: The mythical danger of rapid urinary drainage, *Am J Nurs* March, 89(3):344, 1989.

Colling J: Educating nurses to care for the incontinent patient, *Nurs Clin North Am* 23(1);279, 1988.

Collste L, Lindskog M: Phenylpropanolamine in the treatment of female urinary incontinence, *Urology*, October, (4):398, 1987.

Conti MT, Eutropius L: Preventing UTIs: what works? *Am J Nurs* March, 87(3):307, 1987.

Corriere JN Jr: *Essentials of urology*, New York, 1986, Churchill-Livingstone.

Gerber A: The Kock continent ileal reservoir: an alternate to the conventional urostomy, *J Enterostom Ther* 12(1):15, 1985.

Gruendemann B, Huth-Meeker M: *Alexander's care of the patient in surgery*, ed 8, St Louis, 1987, CV Mosby.

Gulanick M et al: *Nursing care plans: nursing diagnosis and treatment*, ed 2, St Louis, 1990, CV Mosby.

Hanno PM, Wein AJ: *A clinical manual of urology*, Norwalk, Conn, 1987, Appleton-Century-Crofts.

Howe SM, Bates P: The cranberry juice cure: fact or fiction? *AUAA Journal* 8(1), 1987.

Kim MJ, McFarland GK, McLane AM: *Pocket guide to nursing diagnosis*, ed 4, St Louis, 1990, CV Mosby.

Lawrence RM: Current therapy of urinary tract infections and pyelonephritis, *Semin Nephrol* 6(3):241, 1986.

Mackett MCT: Organ transplantation. In: Ihde JK, Jacobsen WK, and Briggs BA, eds: *Principles of critical care,* Philadelphia, 1987, WB Saunders.

McFarland GK, McFarlane EA: *Nursing diagnosis and intervention: planning for patient care,* St Louis, 1989, CV Mosby.

Pagana KD, Pagana TJ: *Diagnostic testing and nursing implications,* ed 3, St Louis, 1990, CV Mosby.

Palmer M: Incontinence: the magnitude of the problem, *Nurs Clin North Am* 23:139, 1988.

Petillo M: The patient with a urinary stoma: nursing management and patient education, *Nurs Clin North Am,* 22(2):263, 1987.

Pieper B, et al: Inventing urine incontinence devices for women, *Image: J Nurs Scholar* 21(4):205, 1989.

Reznichek CG, Reznichek R: The problem most men won't talk about, *RN,* March, 53(3):28, 1990.

Richard C: *Comprehensive nephrology nursing,* Boston, 1986, Little, Brown.

Stewart C: Nephrolithiasis, *Emergency Clin North Am,* 6(3):617, 1988.

Wein AJ: *Voiding function and dysfunction: a logical approach,* New York, 1988, Year Book Medical Publishers.

Wyngaarden J, Smith L, eds: *Cecil textbook of medicine,* ed 17, Philadelphia, 1985, WB Saunders.

Female Reproductive System

FEMALE REPRODUCTIVE SYSTEM ASSESSMENT

Subjective Data

Lower abdominal pain
Cramps
Vaginal bleeding; color and amount
Vaginal discharge
  Mucoid
  Thick white
  Frothy, watery, yellow-green
  Thick, yellow-green or brown, and bloody
  Yellow
  Odoriferous
  Duration
Itching
Swelling
Redness
Painful intercourse
Urination
  Stress incontinence
  Burning on urination
  Pain, urgency, or frequency
Breasts
  Tenderness

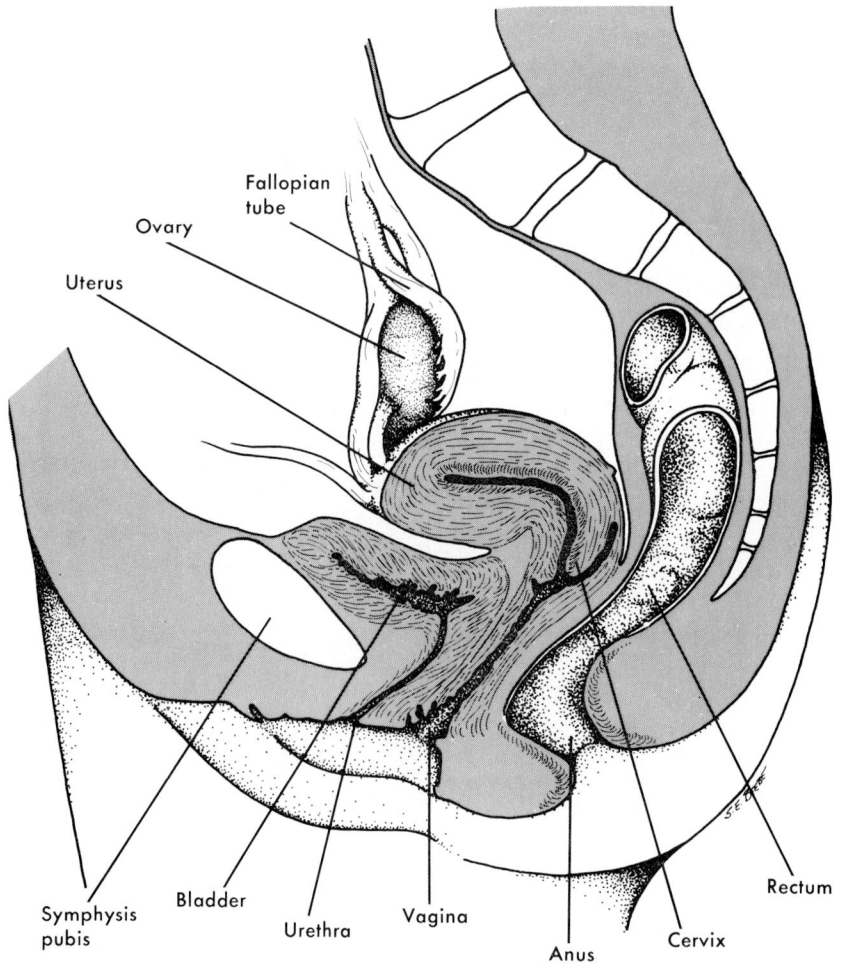

FIGURE 10-1. Female reproductive system.

Pain
Stinging sensation
Burning
Nipple discharge

Objective Data

General appearance
Vital signs, weight
Breasts
  Size
  Symmetry
  Contour
  Lumps, bumps
  "Orange peel" texture
  Venous pattern
  Moles, nevi
  Dimpling
  Erythema
Nipples
  Color
  Discharge (serous, bloody, purulent)
Abdomen
  Contour

Lesions
Scars
Stretch marks
Symmetry
Visible pulsations
Visible peristaltic waves
Presence of bowel sounds in each quadrant
External genitalia
  Labia majora
    Edema
    Redness
    Lumps
    Lesions
    Symmetry
    Pigmentation (nevi)
  Clitoris
    Edema
    Redness
  Urethral orifice
    Size
    Redness
    Discharge
  Discharge

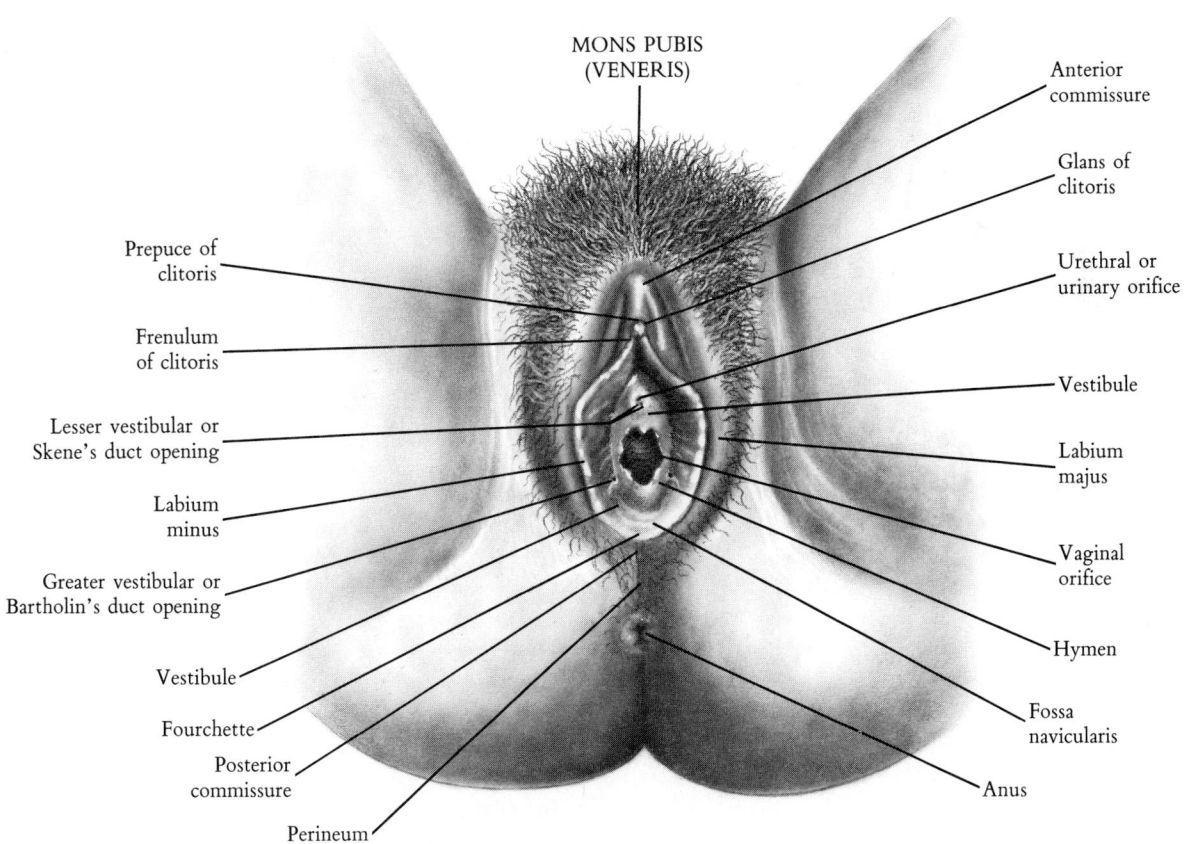

FIGURE 10-2. External female genitalia. (From Seidel HM, Boll JW, Dains JE et al: *Mosby's guide to physical examination,* ed 2, St Louis, 1991, Mosby–Year Book; originally from Bohah, Jensen, and Zalar, 1989.)

Bloody
Purulent
Odoriferous
Introitus
  Presence or absence of hymenal ring
  Hymenal tags
  Edema
  Redness
  Drainage
    Mucoid (normal)
    Thick, white, cheesy (typical of moniliasis)
    Purulent
    Frothy, watery, yellow-green (typical of tricho-
      moniasis)
    Thick, yellow-green or brown, and bloody (typical
      of upper genital tract infection)
    Bloody
    Yellow; thin with odor
Perineum
  Scars
  Redness
  Edema
  Excoriation

Pertinent Background Information

CONCURRENT DISEASES OR CONDITIONS

Menstrual cycle
  Age at onset
  Length of cycles (duration)
  Interval between cycles
  Regularity of cycles
  Amount and type of flow
    Number of tampons or napkins used
    Date of most recent douching
    Type of contraceptive used
  Date of last menstrual period (LMP)
  Associated symptoms (pain, menorrhagia, metror-
    rhagia, etc.)
Pregnancy
  Number of pregnancies and outcome of each
  Complications of pregnancy and delivery and/or abor-
    tion
Menopause
  When occurred
  Related symptoms
    Hot flashes; night sweats
    Dry vaginal mucosa
    Insomnia
Gastrointestinal (GI) system
  Constipation
  Hemorrhoids
Endocrine system
  Hypothyroidism
  Hyperthyroidism
  Stein-Leventhal syndrome

Blood dyscrasias
Hypertension
AIDS
Sexually transmitted diseases

PREVIOUS SURGERY OR ILLNESS

Gynecological surgery
Other major surgery or illness (of abdomen, endocrine
  system, etc.)

FAMILY HISTORY

Cancer
Sickle cell disease
Thyroid disorder
Diabetes
Other diseases
Death resulting from gynecological-related conditions
Maternal diethylstilbestrol (DES) usage

SOCIAL HISTORY

Sexual activity; abnormal lesions or discharge in sexual
  partner
Contraception
Patterns of tobacco, alcohol, and prescription/nonpre-
  scription drug use

MEDICATION HISTORY

Oral contraceptives
Estrogen therapy
Intrauterine contraceptive device (IUD)
Phenothiazines
Digitalis
Diuretics

Diagnostic Aids

Bimanual examination
Basal body temperature
Papanicolaou (Pap) test
Wet mount
Culture
Punch biopsy
Endobiopsy
Dilation and curettage (D & C)
Cold-knife conization
Colposcopy
Hysteroscopy
Culdoscopy
Culpotomy
Laparoscopy
Ultrasound
Insufflation
Mammography
Thermography
Radionuclide imaging
Galactography
Hysterosalpingography

LABORATORY STUDIES

Human chorionic gonadotropin (HCG) level

Serum luteinizing hormone (LH) and follicle-stimulating hormone level (FSH)

Thyroid function studies

    Basal metabolic rate (BMR)

    Protein-bound iodine (PBI) level

Adrenal function

    17-Ketosteroids

    Corticosteroids

Venereal disease research laboratory (VDRL) test

PELVIC INFLAMMATORY DISEASE (PID)

An infectious process of the pelvic cavity that may include the fallopian tubes, ovaries, pelvic peritoneum, veins, and pelvic connective tissue (Figures 10-3 and 10-4)

Assessment
Observations/findings

Abdominal and pelvic pain

Low back pain

Dyspareunia

Fever

Malodorous, purulent vaginal discharge

Malaise, general aching

Nausea, vomiting

Pruritus or maceration of vulva

Diarrhea

Bloating

Laboratory/diagnostic studies

Elevated white blood cell count (WBC)

Elevated erythrocyte sedimentation rate

Culture of purulent secretions positive for organisms

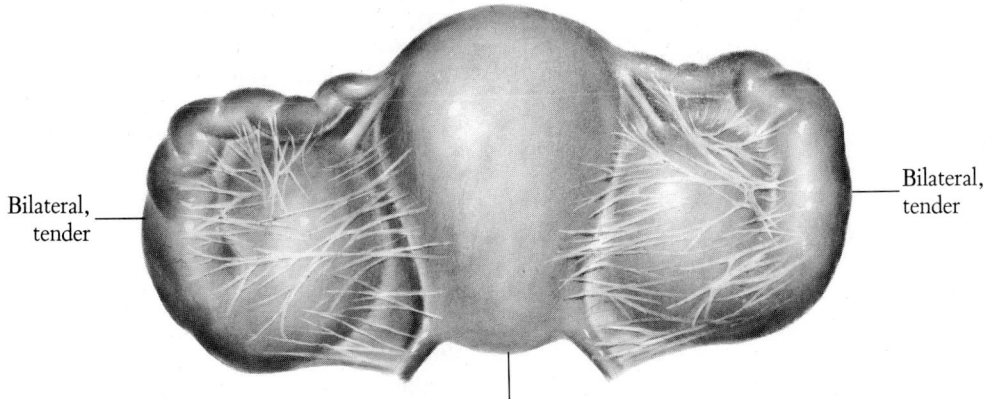

Bilateral, tender

Bilateral, tender

Movement of cervix painful

FIGURE 10-3. Pelvic inflammatory disease. (From Seidel HM, Boll JW, Dains JE et al: *Mosby's guide to physical examination,* ed 2, St Louis, 1991, Mosby–Year Book.)

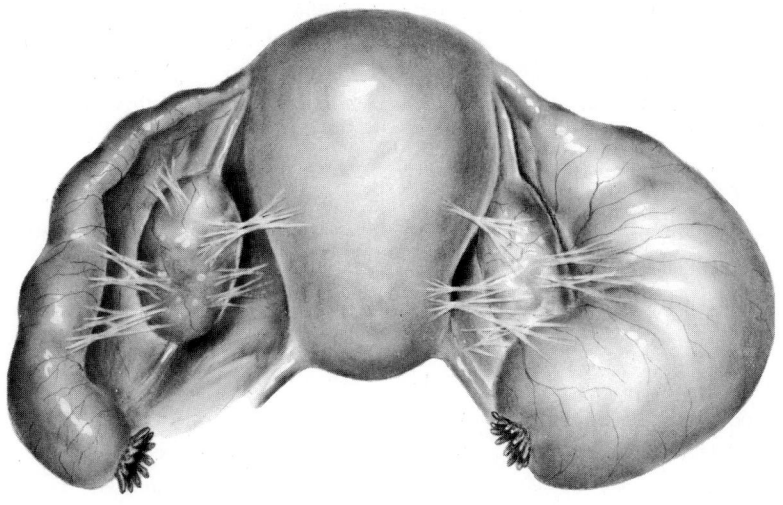

Advanced

Pyosalpinx

FIGURE 10-4. Salpingitis. (From Seidel HM, Boll JW, Dains JE et al: *Mosby's guide to physical examination,* ed 2, St Louis, 1991, Mosby–Year Book.)

Laparoscopic visualization of pelvic inflammation
Ultrasound of tubo-ovarian abscess, if present
Needle culdocentesis for WBCs or nonclotting blood

Potential complications

Urinary tract infection
Peritonitis
Tubo-ovarian abscess
Infertility
Paralytic ileus

Medical Management

Antibiotics as determined by sensitivity
Bed rest in semi-Fowler's position or position of comfort
Parenteral fluids
Nasogastric suctioning if ileus is present
Removal of intrauterine device if present
Removal of tampon if present
Analgesics

Nursing diagnoses/interventions/evaluation

■ **NDX:** Pain related to pelvic inflammation and protective guarding

Maintain complete bed rest in semi-Fowler's position or position of comfort
Administer analgesics as needed
Increase activity as tolerated

Expected outcome/evaluation

Patient states that pain is relieved

■ **NDX:** Potential for impaired skin integrity secondary to vaginal drainage

Assist and teach patient to perform gentle perineal care q3h to 4h and prn; blot skin dry (avoid rubbing)
Teach patient to wipe from front to back after elimination
Ensure that bed covers do not result in excessive warmth of perineal area

Expected outcome/evaluation

Patient's skin integrity is maintained as evidenced by absence of excoriation of perineal area

■ **NDX:** Knowledge deficit related to lack of information about disease process

Explain importance of handwashing both before and after contact with perineum
Explain need to use perineal pads, to change them as needed, and to wrap and properly dispose of them; avoid use of tampons
Explain that a shower is preferred to a tub bath
Promote good nutrition with diet as tolerated

Teach measures to prevent disease if condition is caused by gonococcus or chlamydia
Emphasize need for sexual partner to be examined or treated
Discuss alternative methods of conception control if condition is related to an intrauterine device
Explain importance of avoiding douching, intercourse, or use of tampons for 1 week after antibiotic therapy or as directed by physician
Discuss symptoms of recurrence that should be reported to physician

Expected outcome/evaluation

Patient
   Demonstrates understanding of instructions
   Verbalizes intent to comply with temporary restrictions

TOXIC SHOCK SYNDROME (TSS)

An acute bacterial infection caused by penicillinase-resistant Staphylococcus aureus; most often associated with continuous use of super-absorbent tampons during menses

Assessment
Observations/findings

Sudden onset of high fever
Myalgia
Vomiting
Watery diarrhea
Sore throat
Headache
Profound fatigue
Macular erythematous rash (sunburn-like) on palms and soles
Eventual desquamation within 1 to 2 weeks after rash appears
Impaired joint mobility
Decreased circulation of fingers and toes
Alterations in level of consciousness: disorientation, confusion
Vaginal, oropharyngeal, or conjunctival hyperemia
Severe peripheral edema
Diminished urine output
Hypotension

Laboratory/diagnostic studies

Elevated
   WBC and differential
   Blood urea nitrogen (BUN)
   Creatinine
   Bilirubin
   Serum glutamic-oxaloacetic transaminase (SGOT)
   Creatinine phosphokinase (CPK)

Decreased
  Platelets

Potential complications

Pulmonary edema
Adult respiratory distress syndrome (ARDS)
Sudden hypotension progressing to shock
Disseminated intravascular coagulation (DIC)

Medical Management

Antibiotics
Vital signs monitoring
Parenteral fluids to 3000 ml daily unless contraindicated
Septic shock management as indicated

Nursing diagnoses/interventions/evaluation

■ **NDX:** Alteration in tissue perfusion related to exchange problems associated with septic shock and/or ARDS

For specific desired outcome and interventions, see Shock Syndrome (p. 105) and Adult Respiratory Distress Syndrome (ARDS) (p. 225)

■ **NDX:** Knowledge deficit related to lack of information about home care needs

Explain need to avoid use of tampons until vaginal cultures are negative
Instruct patient to thoroughly wash hands before tampon insertion
Instruct patient to use tampons made of cotton, avoiding the super-absorbent, noncotton type
Explain need to change tampons frequently and need to rotate using tampons and sanitary napkins (consider wearing napkins at night)
Emphasize importance of avoiding tampons altogether if there is a concurrent skin infection such as a boil caused by *Staphylococcus aureus*
If the following symptoms occur, instruct patient to discontinue use of tampons immediately and report symptoms to physician
  Nausea
  Vomiting
  Diarrhea
  Fever

Expected outcome/evaluation

Patient demonstrates understanding of home care and follow-up instructions

HYDATIDIFORM MOLE

Tumor mass of chorionic cells in the uterus that mimics pregnancy; about 10% become malignant

Assessment
Observations/findings

Vaginal bleeding
Uterine cramping
Enlarged uterus (larger than pregnant uterus for same date)
Absence of fetal heart tones
Absence of fetal movement
Vaginal expulsion of vesicular tissue
Hypertension
Hyperthyroidism
Nausea, vomiting
Excessive weight loss

Laboratory/diagnostic studies

Elevated HCG titer
Ultrasonography

Medical Management

Evacuation of mole by suction curettage
Routine preprocedural and postprocedural care

Nursing diagnoses/interventions/evaluation

■ **NDX:** Anxiety related to situational crisis associated with pseudocyesis

Encourage verbalization about outcome of diagnosis and treatment
Use active listening skills and assist patient and family with use of adaptive coping strategies to reduce anxiety about pseudocyesis
Involve bereavement counselor as appropriate
Involve spouse/significant other in dealing with loss/grief

Expected outcome/evaluation

Patient demonstrates a reduction in anxiety and exhibits appropriate coping behaviors

■ **NDX:** Knowledge deficit related to lack of information about preprocedural and postprocedural care and risk of choriocarcinoma

Explain preoperative and postoperative vital sign and care routines
Reinforce physician's explanation of current condition, risk factors, avoidance of pregnancy (usually for 1 year), need for periodic HCG titers and chest x-ray examinations, and follow-up outpatient care

Expected outcome/evaluation

Patient and/or significant other demonstrates understanding of home care and follow-up instructions

DILATION AND CURETTAGE (D & C)

Expansion of the cervix and scraping of the endometrial lining of the uterus for diagnostic and/or therapeutic purposes

Assessment
Observations/findings

Excessive vaginal bleeding
Pelvic and low back pain
Hematuria
Foul odor of vaginal drainage
Elevated temperature

Potential complications

Endometritis
Sepsis
Uterine rupture
Hemorrhage

Medical Management

T, P, R, and BP monitoring
Pad count as indicated
Intake and output for 2 to 4 hr; notation of amount and
color of first-voided urine after procedure
Analgesics as indicated

Nursing diagnoses/interventions/evaluation

■ **NDX:** Pain related to uterine cramping

Administer analgesics as ordered
Maintain bed rest immediately after procedure, progressing to activity as tolerated

Expected outcome/evaluation

Patient experiences minimal discomfort

■ **NDX:** Potential for infection related to traumatized
intrauterine tissue secondary to intrauterine curettage

Administer perineal care after elimination as necessary
Monitor temperature and pulse
Explain importance of wiping from front to back after
elimination
Explain that shower is preferred to tub bath for 3 to 4
days
Note amount, color, and odor of vaginal drainage and
change perineal pads as necessary q2h and prn
Understand that vaginal packing, if used, is usually re-
moved by physician

Expected outcome/evaluation

Patient does not develop endometritis or vaginitis as evidenced by euthermia and normal drainage

■ **NDX:** Knowledge deficit related to lack of information
about home care, self-care management

Explain that vaginal bleeding or spotting may continue
for a week and that mild cramps may continue for 2 to
3 days

Explain that minimal activity is recommended for 2 to 3
days
Explain that coitus, douching, and use of tampons should
be delayed for 1 to 2 weeks or as indicated by physician
Discuss symptoms that should be reported to physician
Excessive bleeding, heavier than a menstrual period
Foul odor of vaginal drainage
Temperature over 100° F (37.8° C)
Severe lower abdominal cramps or pain

Expected outcome/evaluation

Patient verbalizes understanding of home care and follow-
up instructions

TUBAL PREGNANCY AND SALPINGECTOMY

tubal pregnancy *Implantation of the fertilized ovum in
the fallopian tube is the most common type of ectopic
pregnancy; often related to pelvic inflammatory disease resulting in tubal stricture after salpingitis*
salpingectomy *Removal of the fallopian tube*

Assessment
Preoperative observations/findings
UNRUPTURED TUBE

Low abdominal pain and tenderness: unilateral or gen-
eralized
Vaginal bleeding: usually scanty and dark brown; inter-
mittent or continuous
Signs of pregnancy
Amenorrhea
Nausea, vomiting
Urinary frequency
Breast changes

RUPTURED TUBE (Figure 10-5)

Severe lower abdominal pain: may be sudden and stabbing
Vaginal bleeding may or may not be present
Dizziness
Fainting
Pallor
Progressive supine hypotension
Referred supraclavicular pain

Laboratory/diagnostic studies

Culdocentesis (positive for free blood)
Laparoscopy
Ultrasonography
Complete blood cell count (CBC), electrolytes, type and
screen/cross
Urinalysis

Postoperative observations/findings

Site of incision
Redness
Pain

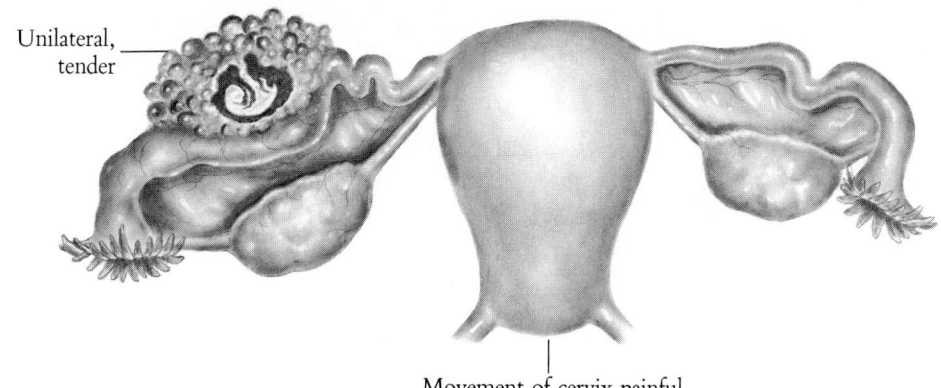

Unilateral, tender

Movement of cervix painful

FIGURE 10-5. Ruptured tubal pregnancy. (From Seidel HM, Boll JW, Dains JE et al: *Mosby's guide to physical examination,* ed 2, St Louis, 1991, Mosby–Year Book.)

Swelling
Drainage
Elevated temperature
Feelings of loss and grief

Potential complications

Paralytic ileus
Pneumonia
Hemorrhage, anemia
Shock

Medical Management

Parenteral fluids
Analgesics
Antiflatulant medications
Indwelling catheter to closed gravity drainage
Vital signs
Intake and output
Anti-Rh globulin
Progression of postoperative diet from clear liquids to full meal after return of bowel sounds

Nursing diagnoses/interventions/evaluation

■ **NDX:** Pain related to incision and abdominal distention

Assist patient with assuming position of comfort
Administer analgesics as ordered
Auscultate abdomen for bowel sounds; insert rectal tube and/or give Harris flush as ordered for abdominal distention

Expected outcome/evaluation

Patient reports that discomfort is minimal

■ **NDX:** Anticipatory grieving related to loss of pregnancy

Encourage verbalization of feelings

Assist patient with working through grieving process by using supportive statements
Involve "grief"/bereavement counselor as appropriate
Involve spouse or significant other with loss and grief

Expected outcome/evaluation

Patient demonstrates successful progress through grieving process with absence of characteristics of dysfunctional grieving

■ **NDX:** Impaired physical mobility related to discomfort in the immediate postoperative period

Observe site of incision and reinforce and change dressing as necessary
Demonstrate same and assist patient with performing care
Encourage and assist patient as needed with early ambulation; increase activity to tolerance
Involve social service worker regarding placement of other children at home if necessary since emergency surgery of mother prohibits preoperative planning for their care

Expected outcome/evaluation

Patient
Performs self-care activities
Is fully ambulatory before discharge

■ **NDX:** Knowledge deficit related to lack of information about ectopic pregnancy

Discuss symptoms of wound infection to report to physician
Explain need for activity to tolerance
Explain importance of planned rest periods
Emphasize importance of prevention of pregnancy for 2 to 4 months or as indicated by physician
Explain that childbearing ability can be diminished, especially if tubal pregnancy was a result of PID or anomaly of the tube resulting in bilateral obstruction

Expected outcome/evaluation

Patient and/or significant other verbalizes understanding of home care and follow-up instructions

TOTAL ABDOMINAL HYSTERECTOMY AND BILATERAL SALPINGO-OOPHORECTOMY (TAH-BSO)

Surgical removal of the uterus, cervix, both fallopian tubes, and ovaries through an abdominal incision to treat malignant neoplastic disease, leiomyomas (Figure 10-6), and chronic endometriosis

Assessment
Observations/findings

Vaginal discharge other than serosanguineous and/or with foul odor
Redness, pain, swelling, or drainage at incision site
Fever
Difficulty in voiding
Diminished or absent bowel sounds
Maladaptive comments related to self-concept

Laboratory/diagnostic studies

Urine culture and sensitivity after catheter removal
Hemoglobin and hematocrit postsurgically

Potential complications

Infection: intraabdominal or incisional
Urinary tract infection
Paralytic ileus
Pneumonia

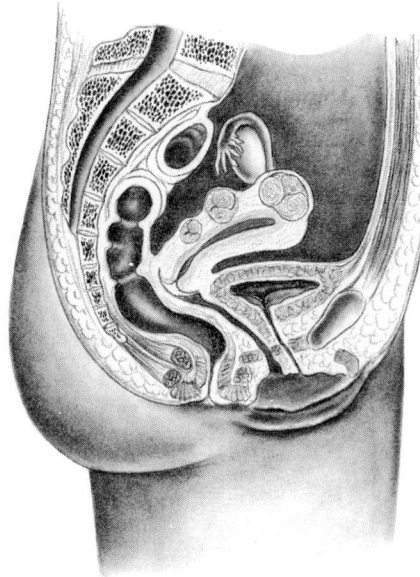

FIGURE 10-6. Myomas of the uterus (fibroids). (From Seidel HM, Boll JW, Dains JE et al: *Mosby's guide to physical examination,* ed 2, St Louis, 1991, Mosby—Year Book.)

Hemorrhage
Thrombophlebitis
Pulmonary embolus

Medical Management

NPO until bowel sounds are audible
Parenteral fluids until liquids or diet is tolerated
Indwelling catheter to low-gravity drainage system
Intake and output
BP, T, P, and R per postoperative procedure
Analgesics and stool softeners
Hormone replacement as indicated

Nursing diagnoses/interventions/evaluation

■ **NDX:** Altered peripheral tissue perfusion related to interruption in arterial and venous flow secondary to surgical intervention

Monitor vital signs as ordered
Avoid placing patient in high-Fowler's position and placing pressure under knees
Avoid sitting with knees bent and/or crossing legs
Apply antiembolic stockings as ordered
Auscultate bowel sounds q6h to 8h; maintain NPO status until bowel sounds are active
Assist with ambulation as needed
Encourage ambulation and/or leg exercises

Expected outcome/evaluation

Patient's
   Vital signs remain within normal presurgical limits
   Circulation remains normal without evidence of pelvic stasis or peripheral thrombophlebitis
   Bowel function is resuming

■ **NDX:** Pain related to surgical incision

Assist patient in assuming a position of comfort
Place pillow on abdomen for support when patient is coughing
Assist with bed bath on first postoperative day as necessary and until patient is able to bathe or shower

Expected outcome/evaluation

Patient
   Reports that she is comfortable
   Reports pain is reduced

■ **NDX:** Ineffective breathing pattern related to discomfort and postsurgical status

Assist with turning, coughing, and deep breathing q2h and prn, decreasing frequency as patient becomes more active

Assist and teach patient to use incentive spirometer as indicated

Auscultate chest for breath sounds q8h, then prn

Expected outcome/evaluation

Patient has normal breath sounds on auscultation, and inhalation/exhalation pattern enables adequate ventilation

■ **NDX:** Impaired skin integrity related to surgical incision

Observe incision for condition q4h or as indicated

Cleanse incision area as indicated; keep it clean and dry

Report signs of infection to physician, e.g., redness, swelling, or discharge

Change or reinforce dressing as necessary

Explain to patient importance of avoiding lifting or placing strain on abdominal muscles; avoid straining at stool

Expected outcome/evaluation

Patient's incision remains clean, dry, and intact without signs of infection

■ **NDX:** Potential for colonic constipation related to NPO status and manipulation of pelvic and abdominal structures during surgery

Progress to high-protein or high-residue diet as ordered

Encourage adequate fluid intake

Give Harris flush or insert rectal tube for gas as indicated

Assist patient with assuming lateral Sims position if this promotes expulsion of flatus

Encourage ambulation

Give stool softeners or mild laxatives as ordered

Expected outcome/evaluation

Patient has expelled flatus and defecated before discharge

■ **NDX:** Altered urinary elimination related to post-surgical sensory motor impairment

Connect indwelling catheter to closed gravity drainage bag

Give catheter care as indicated

Promote micturition at regular intervals when catheter is removed

Expected outcome/evaluation

Patient voids q.s. without difficulty

■ **NDX:** Potential disturbance in self-esteem related to body image change and value of reproductive organs

Encourage patient's comments and questions about surgery, progress, and prognosis

Reinforce correct information and provide factual information to correct any misconceptions; common misconceptions are that after a hysterectomy a woman grows fat and flabby, develops facial hair, becomes wrinkled, old, and masculine, loses her mind, or becomes depressed and nervous; normal concerns usually in need of discussion are fear of death, disfigurement, cancer, loss of femininity, pain, loss of childbearing ability, and changes in sexuality

Encourage verbalization of feelings with significant others

Discuss hormone replacement therapy if appropriate

Expected outcome/evaluation

Patient

    Demonstrates adaptive responses related to self-concept

    Asks appropriate questions

    Gives correct information related to procedures and prognosis

    Indicates that she has discussed concerns with partner

■ **NDX:** Knowledge deficit related to lack of information about home care needs

Explain need to avoid coitus, douching, tampons, or anything in vagina for 4 to 6 weeks or as indicated by physician

Instruct patient to ambulate at regular intervals and to avoid sitting for prolonged periods at home or when traveling

Instruct patient to care for incision with general cleanliness and daily bathing; to report signs of infection to physician, including redness, swelling, pain, discharge, increase in vaginal drainage, and foul odor

Explain need to avoid heavy lifting and vigorous activities for 6 weeks after surgery

Explain need to avoid constipation and straining at stool

Emphasize importance of maintaining regular outpatient gynecological examinations

Explain need to take estrogen-progesterone hormones as ordered (if surgical menopause is caused by removal of all ovarian tissue)

Expected outcome/evaluation

Patient and/or significant other demonstrates understanding of home care and follow-up instructions

BIBLIOGRAPHY

Anderson JR and Wilson MD: Caring for teenagers with salpingitis, *Contemp Ob/Gyn* 35(8):103, 1990.

Brown HP: Recognizing common STD's in adolescents, *Contemp Ob/Gyn* 33(3):47, 1989.

Cohen I: Chlamydia trachomatis in the perinatal period, *Contemp Ob/Gyn* 33(6):22, 1989.

Danforth DN, ed: *Obstetrics and gynecology*, Philadelphia, 1987, Harper & Row.

Gidwani GP: Treating endometriosis in the adolescent, *Contemp Ob/Gyn* 33(4):75, 1989.

Harger JH: Genital herpes infections, *Contemp Ob/Gyn* 35(5):83, 1990.

Iams JD, Zuspan FP, and Quilligan EJ, eds: *Manual of obstetrics and gynecology*, St Louis, 1990, Mosby–Year Book.

Nettina SM: When patients with genital herpes turn to you for answers, *Nursing 89* 19(8):69, 1989.

Scott J: Dangerous liaison, *Los Angeles Times Magazine*, March 11, 1990.

Witkin SS: Chronic recurrent vaginal candidiasis, *Contemp Ob/Gyn* 35(7):56, 1990.

11
CHAPTER

Integumentary System

INTEGUMENTARY SYSTEM ASSESSMENT

Subjective Data

Skin
  Itching
  Painful
  Rash
  Oily
  Dry
  Rough
  Bumpy
  Thin
  Peeling
  Puffy
  Blisters
  Hot
  Cold
  Changes in skin color
  Liver spots: aging spots
  Boils
  Use of Retin-A

Objective Data

Skin
  Color
    Cyanosis
      Lips
      Circumoral area
      Mucous membranes
      Earlobes
      Nail beds
    Jaundice: sclera
    Pallor: conjunctiva, nail beds
    Pigmentation distribution; freckling, moles
  Turgor
  Elasticity
  Intactness
  Rashes
  Moisture
  Temperature
  Cleanliness
  Odor
  Edema
  Needle marks
  Insect bites
  Scabies

Acne, calluses, corns
Exudate
Uremic frost: beard, eyebrows
Sclerema
Striae
Pressure areas over bony prominences
Decubitus ulcers
Nails
  Cleanliness
  Brittleness
  Condition of surrounding tissue
  Clubbing of fingers and toes
  Lines, pitting
  Ram's horn shape: turning under fingertip
  Spoon shape: concave
Hair
  Distribution and configuration
  Texture
  Color
  Quantity
  Parasites
  Alopecia
Lesions
  Macula (<5 mm)
    Flat
    Discolored
  Papule (<5 mm)
    Elevated
    Discolored
  Patch (>5 mm)
    Flat
    Discolored
    Scaly
  Exanthema
    Macular
    Papular
  Vesicle
    Blister
    Serous exudate
  Pustule
    Blister
    Purulent exudate
  Bulla
    Large blister
    Flaccid
    Tense

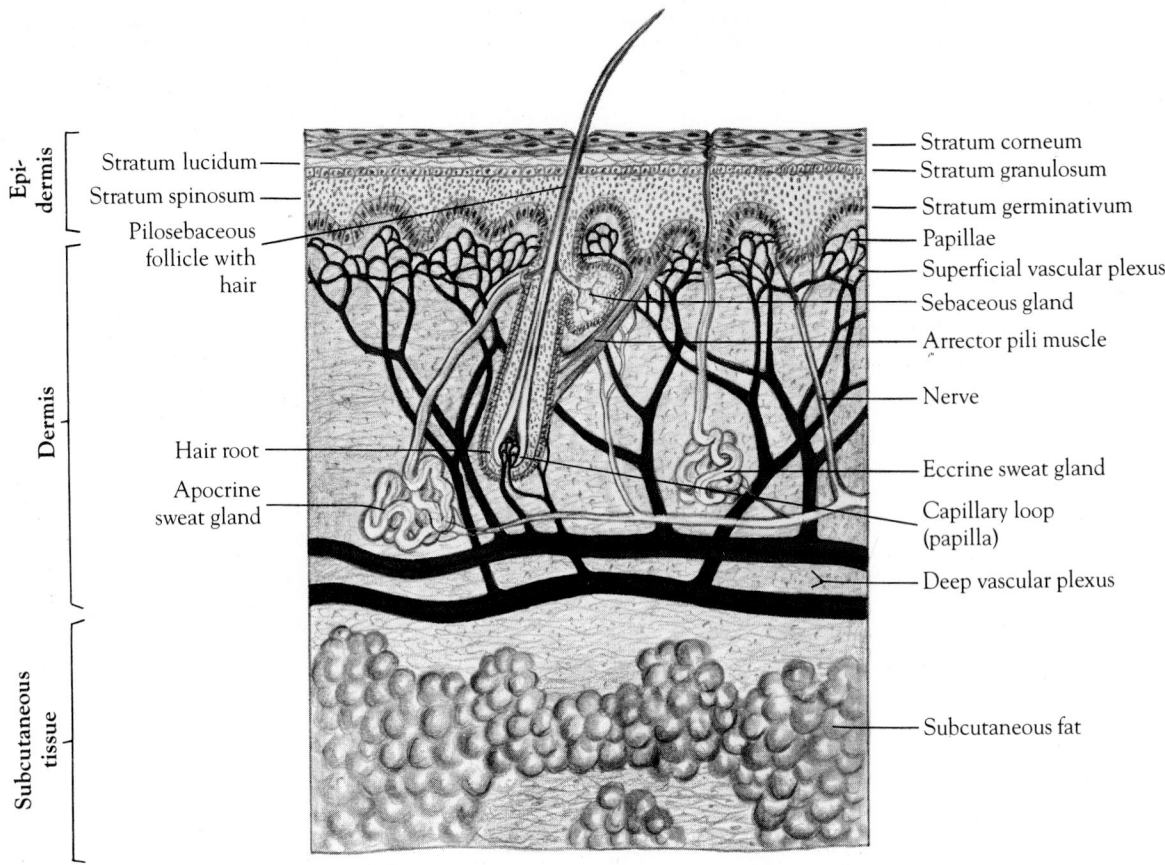

FIGURE 11-1. Structures of skin. (From Thompson JM, McFarland GK, Hirsch JE et al: *Mosby's manual of clinical nursing,* ed 2, St Louis, 1989, Mosby–Year Book.)

Plaque
  Thickened
  Coalesced papules
  Elevated
Tumor (>5 cm)
  Solid
  Movable
Cyst
  Semisolid
  Fluid filled
  Encapsulated
  Serous or purulent exudate
Crusts: dried exudate
Scales: flakes of dead epidermis
Hive (wheal)
  Swollen
  Hot
  Raised
  Itchy
  Transient
Wart
  Elevated
  Color

Mole
  Irregular vs. regular border
  Flat or raised
  Excessive/mixed pigment
Comedo: blackhead/whitehead
Chancre
  Small
  Hard or ulcerated
Excoriation: break
Ulcer: necrosis
Cicatrix: scar
Keloid: excessive tissue formation around lesion or scar
Petechia
  Small
  Bright red
  Flat
Lipoma: subcutaneous fatty lump
Nodule (5 mm to 5 cm)
Fissure
Telangiectasia
Erosion

Pertinent Background Information

FAMILY HISTORY AND CONCURRENT DISEASES

Allergies
Exposures to external allergens
  Cosmetics
  Soaps
  Medication
  Plants
  Chemicals
Exposures to internal allergens
  Drugs
  Food
Travel history
Exposure to parasites
Response to sun

MEDICATION PRESENTLY BEING TAKEN

Injectable medication
Prescription medication
Over-the-counter medication
Creams, lotions, ointments
Hygienic practices
Sexual practices

Diagnostic Aids

Diagnosis of causative disease
Skin and lesion cultures
Electron microscopy
Diascopy
Immunofluorescence (IF)
Lupus erythematosus prep
Punch biopsies, cytology
Allergy skin testing
Blood culture
Skin scraping
  Potassium hydroxide (KOH) testing for fungus

PRESSURE ULCER

An area of cellular necrosis, usually over a bony prominence, that results from tissue hypoxia caused by pressure

Assessment
Observations/findings

Location of pressure area
  Back of head
  Ear rims, cheeks
  Shoulder blades, acromion process
  Elbows, heels, toes
  Sacrum, buttocks, coccyx
  Hips, greater trochantar, ischial tuberosities
  Inner knee, cuter, inner ankle
  Medical and lateral condyles
  Breast (women), genitalia (men)

Stage of necrosis
  I. Erythema only, no break in skin
  II. Partial thickness; loss of skin involving epidermis, often into dermis
  III. Full thickness; involves epidermis, dermis into or exposing subcutaneous tissue
  IV. Deep tissue loss through subcutaneous tissue into fascia, muscle, bone
Immobility
Elevated temperature
Medical history (diabetes, carcinoma, anemia)
Pain, numbness
Nutritional status
Age, weight, mental acuity
Moisture, incontinence, perspiration
Hydration

Laboratory/diagnostic studies

Lesion culture
Complete blood cell count (CBC), electrolytes
Serum albumin

Potential complications

Infection
Further necrosis

Medical Management

Diet, vitamin, mineral supplements
Surgical and chemical debridement
Systemic and topical antibiotics

Nursing diagnoses/interventions/evaluation

■ **NDX:** Impaired tissue integrity related to immobility

Preventive measures
  Maintain skin integrity by keeping skin clean and dry
  Perform skin care daily and prn
  Bathe with mild soap and warm water; remove powder and ointments
  Rinse skin and pat dry thoroughly
  Apply lotion to feet, elbows, and back, and massage gently; remove excess
  Administer perineal care after elimination
Turn patient q2h: side, back, side
Assess and monitor pressure points qid and prn
Assist and teach patient to change position slightly every 15 to 30 min to avoid pressure and fatigue
Maintain clean, comfortable bed with wrinkle-free sheets
Administer back rubs and massage bony prominences with bland emollient; avoid alcohol
Prevent and eliminate pressure and friction by placing pillows between pressure areas (knees, ankles)
Prevent pressure with the following devices
  Alternating pressure mattress
  Foam or static air mattress overlay

Flotation mattress
Silicone pads
Heel and elbow guards to reduce friction
Assist with and teach active or perform passive range-of-motion (ROM) exercises to all extremities q4h
Increase activity as allowed: assist patient out of bed and into chair; avoid sitting for more than 30 min
Maintain head of bed at 45 degrees or less

Expected outcome/evaluation

Patient
Verbalizes understanding of procedures needed to prevent tissue breakdown
Participates in treatment/activities
Expresses sense of well-being

■ **NDX:** Impaired tissue integrity related to mechanical factors

Assess skin and identify stage of ulcer development
Involve enterostomal therapist if available
Eliminate causative factors
Initiate appropriate ulcer care for stages I and II
Cleanse skin at least q8h with mild soap and water and pat dry
Massage skin gently to increase circulation; avoid vigorous rubbing; bathe only as necessary
Do not massage reddened areas
Turn q1h to 2h; use turn sheet; avoid sliding
Maintain wrinkle-free sheets
Provide special pads, mattresses, beds as indicated
Position patient on unaffected areas
Protect skin surface and affected area with one of, or combination of, the following
Apply skin prep/gel
Cover area with moisture-permeable transparent dressing (Opsite) or hydrocolloid wafer barrier
Apply Granulex spray q8h according to manufacturer's directions
Continue one type of application, or combination, for 48 to 72 hr; if improvement is apparent, continue applications; if no improvement is noted, begin another type of treatment
Initiate appropriate ulcer care for stages III and IV
Assess ulcer for size, location, color, odor, and amount and type of drainage
Monitor temperature for elevation
Evaluate ulcer for infection and culture as needed
Administer wound care according to hospital standard of care
If healing is not evident, prepare for debridement as ordered
After debridement, change dressings as ordered; may range from gauze to hydrocolloids to absorbent gel-type dressing

Expected outcome/evaluation

Patient
Exhibits skin/tissue color, integrity, and temperature returning to normal
Demonstrates ability to perform exercises/activities to prevent tissue damage

■ **NDX:** Impaired tissue/skin integrity related to malnutrition

Assess patient's ability to chew and swallow food, determine dietary preferences, and provide appropriate type of diet; assist with feeding as needed
Explain diet rationale to patient and the need for high-protein, high-carbohydrate foods to promote healing; involve nutritionist and perform calorie count
Offer frequent small feedings on attractive trays; provide supplemental feedings
Promote involvement of significant other
Encourage involvement in food selection
Increase fluid intake to 2500 ml/day if not contraindicated
Weigh patient daily at same time with same clothing and scale; report 0.5 kg loss to physician
Monitor CBC, electrolytes, and serum albumin
Measure intake and output q8h; ensure intake equals output

Expected outcome/evaluation

Patient
Regains/maintains weight consistent with age/height
Participates in meal planning
Presents normal laboratory values

■ **NDX:** Knowledge deficit related to lack of information about home management and care

Provide written instructions for pressure ulcer care
Demonstrate cleansing procedure and application of medication and dressings as ordered; observe return demonstrations
Explain dietary regimen and provide written instructions
Stress importance of daily weights
Discuss signs and symptoms to report to physician
Weight loss; elevated temperature
Increased drainage from ulcer
Foul odor from dressing
Further necrosis around ulcer
Reddened areas at other pressure points
Explain importance of increasing activity as tolerated, of changing positions frequently while in bed, and of avoiding pressure on affected area
Promote follow-up visits with physician

Expected outcome/evaluation

Patient
Demonstrates ability to care for pressure ulcer at home

Verbalizes understanding of treatment, activity, and dietary regimen

Expresses understanding of symptoms to report to physician

CELLULITIS

An acute streptococcal, staphylococcal infection of the skin and subcutaneous tissue, usually caused by bacterial invasion through a broken area in the skin; however, it may occur with no site of entry evident; it usually occurs on the lower extremities

Assessment
Observations/findings

Localized pain, redness, swelling, tenderness of skin
Lymphangitic streaks
Skin resembling skin of orange (peau d'orange)
Presence of open wound
Amount, color, odor of drainage
Fever, chills, malaise
Headache, tachycardia
Hypotension

Laboratory/diagnostic studies

CBC: increased white blood cell count (WBC), eosinophils
Erythrocyte sedimentation rate (ESR) increased
Cultures: lesion and blood

Potential complications

Systemic infection
Ulceration

Medical Management

Antibiotics, analgesics, antipyretics
Position and immobilization of extremity
Alternate cool/warm compresses
Diet, activity

Nursing diagnoses/interventions/evaluation

■ **NDX:** Impaired skin integrity related to altered turgor, circulation, and edema

Assess impairment; size, depth, color, drainage q4h
Maintain bed rest with extremity elevated and immobilized for 2 or 3 days to decrease edema and promote circulation
Maintain aseptic techniques
Apply compresses and dressings
Monitor temperature q4h; report elevation to physician

Expected outcome/evaluation

Patient's
  Lesion begins to heal and area is free of further infection
  Skin is clean, dry and surrounding area is edema-free
  Temperature returns to normal

■ **NDX:** Pain related to tissue inflammation

Assess pain for intensity using pain rating scale
Maintain affected extremity in prescribed position
Explain need for immobilization for 48 to 72 hr
Administer analgesic as appropriate; assess effectiveness
Change position frequently, maintaining alignment, to prevent pressure and fatigue
Assist with and teach alternate pain relief measures; imagery, relaxation, etc.
Promote diversional activities

Expected outcome/evaluation

Patient
  Reports a reduction in pain and discomfort that is at a tolerable level
  Appears calm; has relaxed facial expression
  Alternates sleep with activity appropriately

■ **NDX:** Knowledge deficit related to lack of information about home care management

Demonstrate wound care and dressing-change procedure; stress importance of aseptic technique
Discuss maintaining prescribed elevation and immobilization of extremity
Encourage activity to tolerance utilizing supportive devices: sling, crutches
Explain signs and symptoms to report to physician
  Wound pain or increased drainage
  Fever, chills, headache
  Odor from dressings and wound
Discuss medication schedule, including name, purpose, dosage, and side effects
Stress importance of nutritional diet to promote wound healing
Promote follow-up visits with physician

Expected outcome/evaluation

Patient
  Performs wound care correctly using appropriate aseptic precautions
  Expresses understanding of expected progress, signs of infection, and medication schedule

BURN MANAGEMENT

Classification of Burns

Superficial: epidermis is red, with no blister formation
Partial thickness: epidermal and dermal layers are blistered, with subcutaneous edema and pain
Full thickness: all layers of skin are involved, and fat, muscle, nerves, blood supply, and bone may be affected

Assessment: Full-thickness Burns
Observations/findings

Percentage of body surface involved (Figure 11-2)
Classification
Anatomical location
Age of patient
Cause of burn
  Hot liquid: usually partial thickness
  Flame: some areas may be full thickness
  Explosion: may be full or partial thickness
  Chemical: difficult to evaluate
  Electrical: usually full thickness
History of preexisting illness
Other body trauma
  Fractures
  Deep tissue destruction

Respiratory tract trauma
Respiratory distress caused by toxic inhalation
Hypotension, tachycardia, shock
Presence of pain

Laboratory/diagnostic studies

CBC, electrolytes, serum albumin, oxyhemoglobin,
  BUN, creatinine, bilirubin, alkaline phosphatase
Arterial blood gases, glucose, carbooxyhemoglobin
Urinalysis for hemoglobin, myoglobin, albumin, glucose,
  acetone, specific gravity
Chest and body radiology, bronchoscopy, lung scan
Electrocardiogram (ECG)

Potential complications

Hyponatremia (first 48 hr)
Hypernatremia (after 48 hr)

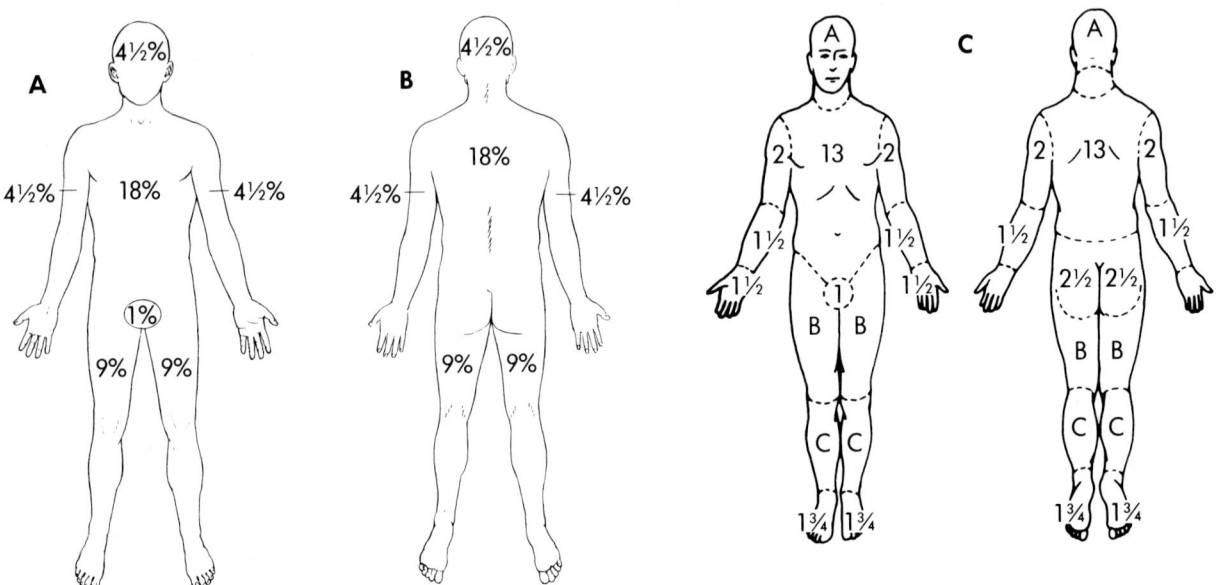

Relative percentages pf areas affected by growth
(age in years)

	0	1	5	10	15	Adult
A: half of head	9½	8½	6½	5½	4½	3½
B: half of thigh	2¾	3¼	4	4¼	4½	4¾
C: half of leg	2½	2½	2¾	3	3¼	3½

Second degree _____ and
Third degree _____ =
Total percent burned ___

FIGURE 11-2. Estimation of adult burn injury: rule of nines. **A,** Anterior view. **B,** Posterior view. **C,** Estimation of burn injury: Lund and Browder chart. Areas designated by letters *(A, B,* and *C)* represent percentages of body surface area that vary according to age. The accompanying table indicates the relative percentages of these areas at various stages in life. (From Sabiston DC Jr, editor, *Textbook of surgery: the biological basis of modern surgical practice,* ed 11, Philadelphia, 1977, WB Saunders Co.)

Hyperkalemia (first 48 hr)
Hypokalemia (after 48 hr)
Hypoproteinemia
Dehydration
Hypoxia
Circulatory collapse
Hematuria, oliguria
Anemia
Adult respiratory distress syndrome (ARDS)
Gastric atony
Septic shock
Curling's ulcer (as early as first week; as late as ninth week)
Fecal impaction
Emotional shock
Disseminated intravascular coagulation (DIC)

Medical Management

Narcotics, sedatives, analgesics, insulin, tetanus
Broncholytic agents, steroids, diuretics, antacids
Antibiotics, vasodilators
Oxygen therapy, postural drainage, tracheal aspiration
Mechanical ventilation, endotracheal tube
Parenteral fluids with electrolytes and vitamins
Hemodynamic monitoring, Swan-Ganz catheter
Transfusion/plasma
Nasogastric suction/indwelling urinary catheter
Diet, NPO, total parenteral nutrition (TPN), fluid-replacement formula, tube feedings
Burn care, hydrotherapy, physiotherapy
Escharotomy, fasciotomy
Skin graft

Nursing diagnoses/interventions/evaluation

■ **NDX:** Impaired gas exchange related to alveolar-capillary membrane and/or hypovolemia

Assess respiratory status
Monitor breath sounds qh; observe for decreased breath sounds, tachypnea, dyspnea, cough, pallor, and cyanosis
Monitor for signs of hypoxia: tachycardia, altered mental acuity
Monitor arterial blood gases and vital signs
Maintain patent airway; perform orotracheal suction as needed; position patient for optimal ventilation
Monitor mechanical ventilation and endotracheal tube for correct settings and function
Assist patient with turning q2h and deep breathing qh
Provide rest periods; avoid overexertion and assist with ADLs as needed
Administer oxygen therapy
Administer broncholytic agents

Expected outcome/evaluation

Patient's
    Respirations are slow, regular

Breath sounds are clear
Arterial blood gases are within normal limits

■ **NDX:** Fluid volume deficit (2) related to burns

Monitor for dehydration
Maintain NPO
Administer parenteral fluids with electrolytes
Monitor intake and output q4h
Monitor indwelling catheter and closed gravity drainage system
    Measure output qh; report less than 30 to 50 ml/hr in adults; 1 to 1.5 ml/kg/hr in children
    Observe for hematuria
Monitor BUN, creatinine, urine specific gravity
Weigh daily: same time, clothes, scale
Monitor mental acuity q8h

Expected outcome/evaluation

Patient's
    Intake is balanced with output
    Skin turgor is normal
    Mucous membranes are moist

■ **NDX:** Altered tissue perfusion; cardiopulmonary, gastrointestinal, peripheral, renal, cerebral, related to hypovolemia/edema

Cardiopulmonary

Assess for signs of dehydration
    Skin turgor if able
    Mucous membranes
    Decreased urine output
Monitor vital signs q1h to 2h (48 hr)
Monitor CVP, Swan-Ganz lines
Monitor for dysrhythmias
Administer blood replacement as prescribed
Monitor CBC, electrolytes, arterial gases
Encourage leg movement, if able, to promote venous return
Assess respiratory status; depth, rate, quality q2h to 4h

Gastrointestinal

Assess bowel sounds q4h; measure girth if sounds are absent
Observe for nausea/vomiting
Monitor nasogastric tube functioning
    Measure output q4h
    Maintain patency
    Observe for signs of bleeding
Maintain bowel function and stool
    Softeners, natural laxatives
    Observe for diarrhea, constipation
    Monitor for signs of bleeding

Peripheral

Monitor extremities for color, temperature, mobility, sensation
Assess pedal pulses q4h
Monitor antiembolic stockings if applicable
  Remove daily and observe skin for redness
Encourage ROM exercises to promote circulation
Provide warmth to extremities
Assess for compartment syndrome; unrelenting calf, thigh, arm pain, edema

Renal

Maintain NPO
Administer parenteral fluids with electrolytes as ordered
Monitor intake and output q4hr
Monitor indwelling catheter and closed gravity drainage system
Measure output qh; report less than 30 to 50 ml/hr in adults; 1 to 1.5 ml/kg/hr in children
  Observe for hematuria; monitor with Hemastix
  Monitor specific gravity
Assess skin turgor for dehydration
Monitor BUN, creatinine, urine specific gravity
Weigh daily; same time, clothes, scale

Cerebral

Assess mental acuity and level of consciousness q8h
Assess neurological status; document baseline assessment
Monitor blood gases; report decrease in PO_2 to physician

Expected outcome/evaluation

Patient's
  Tissue perfusion is adequate as evidenced by normal vital signs, balanced intake and output, normal laboratory results and arterial blood gases
  Respirations are slow, regular
  Peripheral pulses are present
  Available skin turgor, mucous membranes are normal

■ **NDX:** Potential for infection related to inadequate primary defenses; trauma

Maintain isolation precautions and aseptic technique; wear gown, mask, gloves as indicated
Monitor vital signs q2h to 4h
Monitor for signs of infection
Monitor invasive hemodynamic monitoring lines and indwelling urethral catheter for infection
  Culture as indicated
Assess laboratory values; CBC, urinalysis, electrolytes
Limit visitors to patient's significant others, especially exclude people with upper respiratory infections (URIs)
Administer tetanus toxoid as indicated
Administer topical/systemic antibiotics as indicated; assess effectiveness/side effects

Monitor for sepsis; fever, tachypnea, altered sensorium, decreased platelets, hyperglycemia
Initiate local burn therapy using the following principles; these are general considerations
  Culture burn areas as needed
  Cleanse burn and remove all pieces of detached epithelium; cleanse with saline or mild soap and tap water (hexachlorophene is not recommended)
  Debride, using sterile equipment
    Remove dirt and blood
    Shave surrounding area
  Prevent destruction of viable epithelium; prevent burned surfaces from touching viable skin or other burned surfaces
  Produce environment unfavorable to bacterial growth
  Aid separation of burn slough
  Apply skin coverage as soon as possible
Initiate one of the following topical burn agents as ordered
  Silver nitrate
    Antiinfective agent; penetrates burn slowly, is very painful; burn/dressings must be kept saturated; causes electrolyte imbalance and turns all surfaces black
  Povidone-iodine (Betadine)
    Broad spectrum antiinfective; is very painful and may cause increased iodine absorption
  Silver sulfadiazine 1% (Silvadene)
    Broad spectrum antibiotic; is slow to absorb but is relatively painless; may decrease WBC
    Monitor serum chloride and pH; WBC
  Mafenide acetate (Sulfamylon)
    Antiinfective agent; penetrates burn well but is painful; may cause rash, decreased $PaCO_2$

Expected outcome/evaluation

Patient's
  Burned areas begin to heal adequately
  Temperature is normal
  Laboratory values are within normal limits
  Surrounding tissue is clean, dry, and intact

■ **NDX:** Impaired tissue integrity related to trauma

Assess skin for signs of trauma, rashes, reddened areas
Maintain in prescribed position or position of comfort
Assess pressure areas; change position and support with pillows, padding as indicated
Provide bathing and oral care as needed
Monitor mucous membranes if nasogastric tube in place; keep nares moist
Administer lotions to unaffected areas to promote comfort and prevent breakdown
Assess size, depth, color of burned area; observe surrounding tissue for redness or necrosis
Maintain isolation procedures as indicated

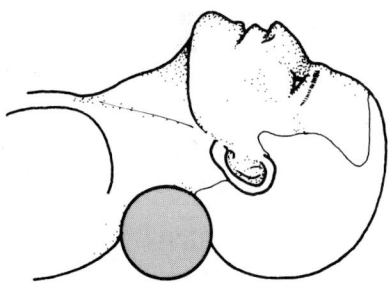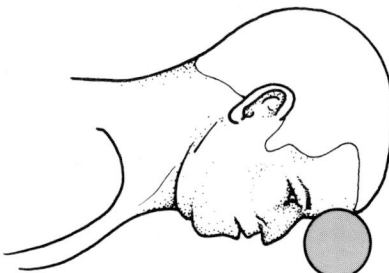

FIGURE 11-3. Positioning for head and neck burns to prevent contractures.

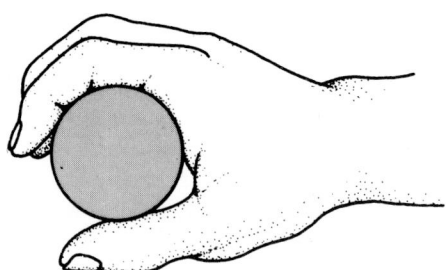

FIGURE 11-4. Positioning of hand burn to prevent contractures.

Monitor burn covering, dressing prn
   Opsite: thin, occlusive dressing for partial-thickness
      burns
   Biosynthetic: nylon fabric membrane for preautograft
      use
   Synthetic: hydroactive material for small burns
Monitor skin graft area
   Homograft: from deceased person
   Autograft: from unburned area of patient
   Heterograft: pigskin or synthetic
   Autologous: epithelium cells cultured into sheets
Maintain correct body alignment and elevate affected
   graft, dressing site if appropriate
Avoid pressure on site; use bed cradle prn
Monitor sites q4h for signs of healing
Maintain dressings/grafts as indicated
Apply pressure garment to prevent scarring as indicated

Expected outcome/evaluation

Patient's
   Healing is adequate
   Burn sites are regenerating new tissue
   Other tissue/skin areas are free from trauma

■ **NDX:**   Impaired physical mobility related to decreased
            strength and endurance

Maintain bed rest in prescribed position
Monitor neurovascular status q2h to 4h
Maintain body alignment within parameters of treatment

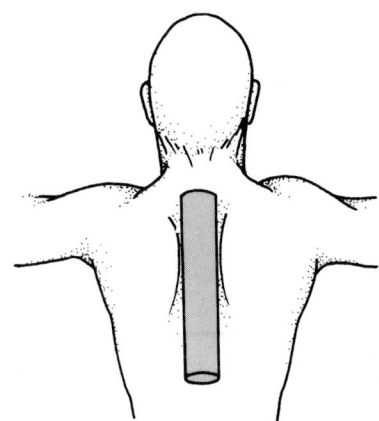

FIGURE 11-5. Placement of contracture roll for upper chest, axilla, and arm burns.

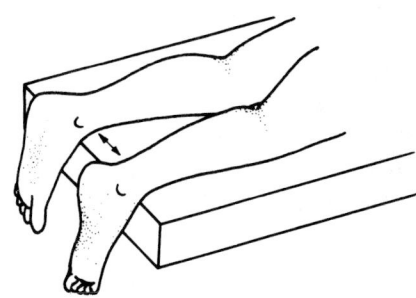

FIGURE 11-6. Correct foot and ankle positioning to prevent foot and ankle contractures.

Prevent contractures and/or hypertrophy
   Head and neck: do not use pillows (Figure 11-3)
   Hand (Figure 11-4)
   Upper chest, axilla, and arms (Figure 11-5): maintain
      arm at 90-degree angle, away from body and slightly
      above shoulder
   Ankles and feet (Figure 11-6): use footboard with pa-
      tient in supine position
   Legs: traction/splints may be used
Explain necessity of positions, since they can be uncom-
   fortable; position of comfort can be position for forming
   contractures

Assist with and teach active or perform passive ROM exercises on unaffected extremities

Coordinate care to allow for rest periods

Encourage patient to perform self-care activities

Change position frequently to prevent fatigue and pressure; CircOlectric bed may be required to promote position changes

Refer patient for physiotherapy and/or hydrotherapy as indicated

Ambulate as soon as possible

Expected outcome/evaluation

Patient

Participates in prescribed activities and therapy

Maintains correct body alignment

Demonstrates ability to balance rest with activities

■ **NDX:**   Alteration in nutrition: less than body requirements, related to thermal injury

Maintain adequate hydration, nutrition to replace lost fluids and promote healing

Provide TPN (p. 173), tube feedings (p. 166) if appropriate

Calculate and initiate fluid replacement formula as ordered (p. 841)

Provide high-protein, high-calorie diet as ordered and tolerated

Protein: 3 g/kg/day

Fat: 20% of calories

Carbohydrate: remainder of calories

Provide small, frequent meals; encourage oral fluids; milk, juice

Perform meticulous calorie count pc

Involve patient in food selection, likes, dislikes

Encourage family to provide home-cooked food

Perform oral hygiene before and after meals

Assist with feeding as needed; advance position to sitting in chair for meals when tolerated

Weigh daily; same time, clothes, scale

Expected outcome/evaluation

Patient

Regains lost weight to within 2% to 5% of normal

Participates in food selection and calorie count

Selects foods that increase healing potential

■ **NDX:**   Pain related to burn immobility

Cover burn to decrease discomfort if applicable

Maintain comfortable temperature/humidity

Assess location, type, and severity of pain; assess intensity with pain rating scale

Administer analgesics; assess effectiveness of pain relief measures; decrease narcotics as soon as possible

Perform dressing changes only after patient is medicated or as needed

Provide diversional activities

Encourage use of alternate pain relief measures

Encourage small shifts in position to promote comfort

Expected outcome/evaluation

Patient

Reports a tolerable pain level

Presents calm, relaxed facial affect

Expresses ability to sleep for increasing number of hours

■ **NDX:**   Body image disturbance related to disfigurement from burns

Assess feelings of loss, anxiety

Express acceptance of feelings

Encourage and allow time for verbalization of concerns/feelings; include significant others; provide privacy

Set realistic short-term goals and acknowledge tasks attempted and/or completed

Allow patient to progress through stages of grief at own pace

Maintain nonjudgmental attitude and avoid nonverbal rejection; discourage maladaptive behavior

Assess present coping attitudes and assist patient with identifying successful past behaviors

Promote self-care activities as soon as possible

Involve patient with unit routine and other burn patients

Refer to social service agencies for financial, family, and educational assistance

Expected outcome/evaluation

Patient

Begins to acknowledge altered image

Discusses feelings/anxieties with increasing confidence

Undertakes goal setting for future

Participates in self-care activities

■ **NDX:**   Knowledge deficit related to lack of information about home care management

Provide written dietary instructions; discuss importance of maintaining normal weight and adequate fluid intake

Explain rehabilitation plan and use of pressure garment if applicable

Discuss maintaining normal activity with planned rest periods; avoid boredom with diversional activities

Demonstrate burn care as necessary; avoid sunlight, detergents, and fabric softeners

Promote use of moisturizers, sunscreen to decrease irritation

Explain symptoms to report to physician

Fever, malaise

Bleeding, odor, and drainage from burn area

Discuss medication schedule, including name, purpose,

dosage, and side effects; caution patient to avoid over-the-counter medications unless approved by physician

Avoid contact with persons with infections, especially URIs

Expected outcome/evaluation

Patient

Verbalizes understanding of rehabilitation plan, potential complications, and medication schedule

Performs burn care accurately

Expresses understanding of need for diversional activities

Calculation of Fluid Replacement for Burns: Brooke Formula

NOTE: Many formulas are in use; Brooke formula is moderate and most frequently used

Calculation for Adults

First 24 hr (calculated from time of burn, not admission)

Colloids (albumin, dextran, or plasma): 0.5 ml/kg/percentage body surface burned

Lactated Ringer's solution: 1.5 ml/kg/percentage body surface burned

Five percent dextrose in water: 2000 ml; adjusted to keep urine output at 30 to 50 ml/hr

Half of each solution is to be given in the first 8 hr, a fourth in the second 8 hr, and a fourth in the third 8 hr

Second 24 hr

Colloids (albumin, dextran, or plasma): half the amount is given in the first 24 hr

Lactated Ringer's solution: half the amount is given in the first 24 hr

Five percent dextrose in water: 2000 ml

Calculation for Children

First 24 hr (calculated from time of burn, not admission)

Colloids (dextran or plasma; use albumin cautiously): 0.5 ml/kg/percentage body surface burned

Electrolyte solution (1:3 with 5% dextrose in water): 1.5 ml/kg/percentage body surface burned

Five percent dextrose in water

Up to 2 years of age: 150 ml/kg

2 to 5 years of age: 100 ml/kg

5 to 8 years of age: 75 ml/kg

8 to 12 years of age: 50 ml/kg

BIBLIOGRAPHY

Bayley EW, Smith GA: The three degrees of burn care, *Nursing '87* 17(3):34, 1987.

Carpentino LJ: *Handbook of nursing diagnosis,* Philadelphia, 1990, JB Lippincott.

Colburn L: Preventing pressure ulcers, *Nursing '90* 20(12):60, 1990.

Conforti C: Dressed for successful healing, *Nursing '89* 19(3):58, 1989.

Cuzzell JZ, Willey T: Pressure relief perennials, *Am J Nurs* 87(9):1157, 1987.

Doenges ME et al: *Nursing care plans: guidelines for planning patient care,* ed 2, Philadelphia, 1989, FA Davis.

Gulanick M et al: *Nursing care plans,* ed 2, St Louis, 1990, Mosby–Year Book.

Gurevich I: Counseling the patient with herpes, *RN* 53(2):22, 1990.

Guzzetta CE et al: *Clinical assessment tools for use with nursing diagnoses,* St Louis, 1989, CV Mosby.

Kim MJ et al: *Pocket guide to nursing diagnoses,* ed 3, St Louis, 1989, CV Mosby.

Martin LM: Nursing implications of today's burn care techniques, *RN* 52(5):26, 1989.

McFarland GK, McFarlane EA: *Nursing diagnosis and intervention,* St Louis, 1989, CV Mosby.

Moriarty MB: How color can clarify wound care, *RN* 51(9):49, 1988.

Murray SM, Thompson R: We've organized our approach to pressure sores, *RN* 54(1):42, 1991.

Nettina SM: When patients with genital herpes turn to you for answers, *Nursing '89* 19(8):61, 1989.

Smith GA, Savinski-Bozinko G: Giving emergency care for burns, *Nursing '89* 19(9):55, 1989.

Thelan LA et al: *Textbook of critical care nursing,* St Louis, 1990, Mosby–Year Book.

Ulrich SP, Canale SW, and Wendell SA: *Nursing care planning guides,* ed 2, Philadelphia, 1990, WB Saunders.

12
CHAPTER

Optic and Auditory Systems

ASSESSMENT

Subjective Data

Blurred or double vision
Light, flashes, rainbows, or halos seen
Decreased or absent vision
Decreased night or peripheral vision
Objects held too near or far
Collides with unfamiliar objects
Eye fatigue and strain
Tenderness or pain: sudden or gradual onset
Eyes water and itch
Dryness of eyes
Increased tearing
Trauma to head, face, or eyes
Inability to see in bright light
Headache
Squinting
Frequent falls
Clumsiness

Objective Data

General appearance
Age of patient
Vital signs: elevated BP, T, P, or R
Wears glasses, contact lenses, or eye patch
Position of reading material
Conjunctivitis
Drainage
  Amount
  Type
Hemorrhage
Rubbing eyes
Eyelid changes; edema, ptosis, redness, eversion, inversion
Amount of dependence or independence
Visual acuity
Exophthalmos
Ability to close eyelid(s)
Ability to blink
Abnormal eye movement
Opaqueness of eyeball
Increased tearing
Head tilts to improve vision
Squinting
Medication, eye drops used

Allergies
Strabismus
Nystagmus
Scleral edema, infection, jaundice
Chalazion
Foreign body
Laceration, contusion
Enucleation

Pertinent Background Information

CONCURRENT DISEASES OR CONDITIONS

Multiple sclerosis
Diabetes mellitus
Hypothyroidism
Hyperthyroidism
Sinus problems
Hypertension
Cerebral associated diseases, trauma, or tumors
Sexually transmitted diseases
Myasthenia gravis
Glaucoma
Cataract
Retinal detachment
Autoimmune diseases
Arthritis, rheumatism

PREVIOUS SURGERY OR ILLNESS

Eye surgery or treatments
Head or face trauma
Oxygen therapy as newborn
Coma
Hypertension
Substance abuse
Retinal degeneration

FAMILY HISTORY

Glaucoma
Diabetes mellitus
Cataracts
Retinitis pigmentosa

SOCIAL HISTORY

Hazardous job or recreation
Safety precautions taken
Alcohol or drug abuse
Sexually transmitted diseases

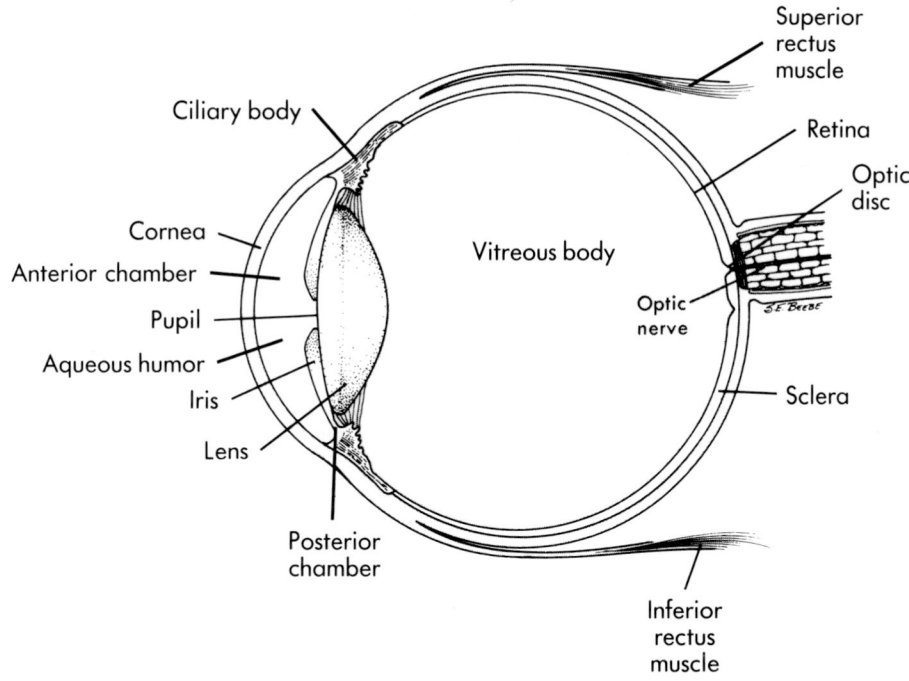

FIGURE 12-1. The eye.

MEDICATION HISTORY

Antibiotics
Antiemetics
Miotics
Acetazolamide
Mydriatics
Beta blockers
Epinephrine derivatives
Steroids (systemic, topical)
Antilipidemic agents
Hydroxychloroquine sulfate (Placquenil)

Diagnostic Aids

PROCEDURES

Visual fields and acuity
Biopsy and cultures
Magnetic resonance imaging (MRI)
Computed tomography
X-ray studies of orbit and skull
Ophthalmoscopic evaluation
Tonometry
Fluorescein angiography
Ultrasonography
Gonioscopy
Brain scan
Ultrasound
Electroretinogram (ERG)
Color vision test
Refraction
Microscopic procedures
Conjunctival scrapings

VISUALLY IMPAIRED PATIENT

Assessment
Observations/findings

Status of impairment
    Temporary (eye patch, shield)
    Permanent
Duration of impairment
Degree of visual loss
Degree of acceptance of impairment
Cause of visual impairment: diabetes, stroke, aneurysms, brain tumor, trauma, glaucoma, etc.
Condition of eyes: drainage, redness, pain, edema, squinting, abnormal eye movements, rubbing, opacities
Ability to perform ADLs

Nursing diagnoses/interventions/evaluation

■ **NDX:** Alteration in sensory perception related to visual impairment

Familiarize patient with surroundings
    Place all utensils and personal articles within easy reach and maintain consistent placement
    Use patient's sense of touch and smell during orientation
    Explain location of doors, windows, furniture, bathroom, and other patients
Establish effective lines of communication
    Always identify self when approaching or touching patient
    Call patient by name

Explain purpose of visit and visit often, especially at night

Use visual aids: magnifying glasses, large print

Encourage and assist with independence

Explain position of food on tray and prepare food as necessary; use clock sequence (e.g., plate at 6 o'clock, fruit at 10 o'clock, milk at 1 o'clock); assist only as needed

Initiate grooming procedures as tolerated

Explain position of articles and place in same position each time

Withdraw assistance gradually

Expected outcome/evaluation

Patient

Performs self-care within limits of impairment

Communicates effectively using learned skills

■ **NDX:** Potential for injury; trauma related to visual impairment

Maintain safe environment

Place side rails up while patient is in bed

Keep bed in locked, low position

Place call bell and needed articles within easy reach

Maintain environment as described (e.g., furniture, footstools, IV poles, wastebaskets)

Keep doors fully open or closed

Flag chart, indicating degree, type of visual impairment and eye affected

Encourage patient to call nurse before ambulating; assist by standing on affected side

Instruct to avoid use of sharp items such as razors, scissors, and glass without supervision

Expected outcome/evaluation

Patient

Demonstrates ability to perform activities in a safe manner

Verbalizes understanding of needed limitations

■ **NDX:** Anxiety related to degree of visual impairment

Assess level of anxiety and normal coping mechanisms

Encourage and allow time for verbalization of feelings

Explain daily plan of care and procedures

Allow as much independence as safety permits

Provide reassurance by being available and answering all questions

Provide time for use of relaxation measures

Encourage visitors and communication with significant others

Identify and reinforce use of adaptive coping mechanisms

Present a calm, caring attitude

Provide diversional activities

Expected outcome/evaluation

Patient

Identifies causative factors of anxiety

Accepts limitations and seeks ways to use remaining sight

Seeks assistance appropriately

■ **NDX:** Disturbance in body image related to visual impairment

Discuss with patient and significant others alternatives in managing ADLs

Assess past coping mechanisms that have been successful

Allow time for patient to verbalize feelings

Demonstrate acceptance of these feelings

Provide quiet, encouraging environment

Assist with and teach new skills as needed

Discuss small, realistic goals

Provide praise and encouragement

Promote support by significant other

Encourage involvement with others

Assist patient in discussing and accepting altered visual acuity

Encourage independence as tolerated

Encourage use of other senses: touch, smell, hearing

Expected outcome/evaluation

Patient

Demonstrates adaptive responses to altered body image

Expresses awareness of change and progresses toward acceptance

■ **NDX:** Knowledge deficit related to lack of information about self-care and home management

Reinforce safety precautions related to furniture placement, sharp objects and corners, scatter rugs, objects on floor, etc.

Reinforce physician's explanation of disease, disease process, and need to notify physician of any changes in condition

Assist patient and/or significant other in managing ADLs

Promote self-care within limits of visual impairment

Demonstrate procedure for instillation of eye drops

Refer to home health care agency and/or organizations* for the visually impaired

Maintain regular outpatient care visits with physician

Expected outcome/evaluation

Patient

Expresses knowledge of disease process and prognosis

Demonstrates procedure for eye drop instillation accurately

---

*American Foundation for the Blind, 15 West 16th St., New York, NY 10011.

Verbalizes understanding of availability and locations of outside resources

ACUTE GLAUCOMA: ADULT ONSET

acute (narrow-angle) glaucoma Disease characterized by suddenly impaired vision resulting from intraocular pressure caused by imbalance in production and excretion of aqueous humor

Assessment
Observations/findings

Rapid onset of severe pain in eye(s)
Blurred vision
Headache
Rainbows in artificial light
Halos around lights
Nausea, vomiting
Dilated pupil(s)

Laboratory/diagnostic studies

Tonometry
Gonioscopy
Visual fields
Visual acuity

Potential complications

Infection
Increased intraocular pressure (IOP)
Increased visual impairment
Blindness if untreated

Medical Management

Miotic beta blocker eye drops
Carbonic anhydrase inhibitors
Hyperosmotic agents
Antiemetics
Analgesics
Laser iridotomy
Iridectomy

Nursing diagnoses/interventions/evaluation

■ **NDX:** Pain related to increased intraocular pressure (IOP)

Assess type, intensity, and location of pain; be alert for signs of increased intraocular pressure
Use pain rating scale to determine analgesia dose
Maintain bed rest in quiet, darkened room with head elevated 30 degrees or in position of comfort
Administer analgesics and diuretics: assess for effectiveness/side effects
Avoid nausea and vomiting as these increase IOP: administer antiemetics as needed
Assess visual acuity

Administer back rubs, position changes to promote comfort

Expected outcome/evaluation
Patient
Demonstrates knowledge of pain control measures
Experiences and demonstrates periods of uninterrupted sleep
Has decreased intraocular pressure

■ **NDX:** Anxiety related to altered health status and decreased visual acuity

Assess anxiety level
Discuss previous coping methods
Encourage verbalization of anxieties
Maintain calm environment
Provide emotional support
Answer questions honestly
Explain all procedures
Reinforce physician's explanation of disease process and surgery if indicated
Visit frequently, especially at night
Explain nursing care plan
Discuss visual limitations as needed
Place all needed articles within reach and strive to keep them in same place at all times
Reassure that assistance with activities of daily living (ADLs) will be available
Assist and teach relaxation techniques; deep breathing, meditation, imagery

Expected outcome/evaluation
Patient
Demonstrates adaptive coping measures to reduce anxiety
Demonstrates understanding of disease process

■ **NDX:** Knowledge deficit related to lack of information about self-care and disease process

Teach eye drop instillation procedure to patient and significant other
Discuss possible side effects
Interactions of eye medications with those for other diseases, such as hypertension, diabetes, COPD
Maleate (Timoptic): depression, bradycardia, asthma
Miotics: blurred vision, diarrhea
Acetazolamide (Diamox): hyperkalemia, confusion, impotence
Always count drops and do not miss a dose
Keep extra bottles of drops in case of loss or breakage
Stress that drops will be needed over extended period of time
Discuss name, dose, administration times of medications

Emphasize need to wear and carry medical alert bracelet and card

Stress need to never take medication containing atropine or any over-the-counter medications without checking with physician

Discuss symptoms of IOP to report to physician

Severe pain in eye(s)

Blurred vision

Headache

Halos or rainbows

Nausea, vomiting

Refer to agencies for visually impaired*

Explain importance of follow-up care with physician

Expected outcome/evaluation

Patient

Demonstrates ability to instill eye drops

Verbalizes symptoms to report to physician

Understands medication instruction

EYE SURGERY

cataract removal with or without intraocular lens transplant Surgical removal of a lens that has become opaque because of senile degenerative changes, trauma, or systemic disease (diabetes) or a congenitally opaque lens; an intraocular lens may be implanted simultaneously as an alternative to wearing cataract glasses or contact lenses postoperatively

corneal transplant Surgical procedure to replace a damaged cornea with a healthy, clear donor cornea of equal size

scleral buckling, retinal cryopexy, photocoagulation Surgical repair of a detached retina

enucleation Surgical removal of a blind, painful eye globe while maintaining orbital integrity for insertion of a prosthesis

iridectomy, iridencleisis, trabeculectomy, sclerotomy Surgical incision to release accumulated pressure caused by glaucoma by creating a channel for the drainage of the aqueous humor

NOTE: Patients with retinal detachment may need special positioning in bed, patching of the eye, and restrictions on activity to prevent further or complete detachment

Preoperative Assessment and Teaching

Reinforce physician's explanation of surgical procedure

Encourage and allow time for verbalization of fears and anxieties

Answer all questions with honesty, empathy, and understanding

*Lions Clubs International, 300 22nd St., Oak Brook, IL 60570.

Explain postoperative nursing care plan and availability of staff

Assess present degree of sight and assist as needed

Provide a safe environment; orient patient to room floor plan, placement of call bell, personal articles, etc.

Explain surgical preparation of eye according to hospital policy and physician's order

Stress importance of wearing eye patch/shield postoperatively

Discuss with patient and teach not to bend, strain, lift heavy objects (over 5 lb) postoperatively

Discuss importance of trying not to cough, sneeze, or vomit postoperatively

Explain that all eye makeup is removed before surgery

Postoperative Assessment
Observations/findings

Nausea, vomiting

Placement of eye bandage(s)

Sudden, severe eye pain

Restlessness

Position to be maintained while in bed

Potential complications

Hemorrhage

Shock

Infection

Decreased visual acuity

Blindness

Medical Management

Analgesics

Antiemetics

Antibiotics

Stool softeners

Eye shield or patch

NPO until fully reactive, increase to presurgery diet

Ambulation and activities

Dressing changes/warm or cold sterile compresses

Prescription glasses

Nursing diagnoses/interventions/evaluation

■ **NDX:** Potential for infection related to invasive surgical procedure

Monitor dressing q2h for 4 hr, then q4h

Assess for drainage, bleeding, and/or pain; report immediately

Maintain eye shield or patch to increase protection

Caution patient not to touch, squeeze, or rub eye

Monitor vital signs q4h until stable

Expected outcome/evaluation

Patient's

Temperature remains normal

Eye remains clean, with no purulent drainage

■ **NDX:** Potential for injury; trauma related to altered visual acuity

Assess visual acuity
Keep side rails up at all times
Plan all care with patient; explain daily routines
Announce yourself on entering room to avoid startling patient
Assist with and teach deep-breathing exercises
  Stress need to avoid coughing as it increases IOP
Keep patient's articles in same place at bedside
Place call bell within easy reach
Enucleation patients have clean plastic conformer in eye socket to retain eye shape
Stress need to avoid vomiting; administer antiemetics
Increase activities and ambulation when patient demonstrates ability to remain safe
Assist with ambulation as needed; stand on affected side
Teach self-care activities and assist as needed

Expected outcome/evaluation

Patient
  Demonstrates understanding of safety precautions
  Notifies staff for assistance

■ **NDX:** Pain related to surgical procedure

Assess pain intensity using rating scale
Administer analgesics; assess pain to ensure that it is not due to increased intraocular pressure or bleeding; monitor for effectiveness
Administer back care and position changes to relieve discomfort
Teach and assist with alternate pain relief measures

Expected outcome/evaluation

Patient
  Reports a reduction of pain
  Appears calm and relaxed

■ **NDX:** Alteration in sensory perception related to impaired vision

Visit frequently to determine needs and allay anxiety, especially at night
Encourage to express feelings and thoughts
Involve significant others in care and activities
Reduce noise, traffic in area
Provide balanced rest and activity
Encourage diversional activities

Expected outcome/evaluation

Patient
  Accepts and copes appropriately with visual limitations
  Uses remaining sight or other senses adequately

■ **NDX:** Knowledge deficit related to lack of information about home care and possible complications

General

Instruct patient and/or significant other in care of the eyes
  Dressing changes using aseptic techniques
  Use of eye patch or shield at night
  Method of eye drop instillation
  Avoid rubbing, squeezing, or touching eye
  Use of eyeglasses as ordered; sunglasses to reduce glare
  Keep an extra bottle of eye drops in case of loss or breakage, and while traveling
Caution patient to avoid constipation, bending, vacuuming, straining, and lifting heavy objects (over 5 lb)
Provide list of organizations for visually impaired*
Discuss home care with patient and family/significant other
  Arrange furniture for safety and convenience
  Encourage self-care
  Avoid being overprotective
  Provide diversional activities: records, tapes, talking books; television and reading if able
  Know name of medication, dosage, time of administration, purpose, and side effects
  Avoid using over-the-counter medications, eye drops, or ointments without checking with physician
  Make and keep follow-up appointments with physicians
Discuss symptoms to report to physician
  Pain in eye
  Redness
  Drainage
  Decreased visual acuity
  Floaters
  Halos, sparks

CORNEAL TRANSPLANT

Discuss signs of graft rejection
  Pain
  Inflammation
  Drainage
Explain that sutures will remain in eye up to a year

---

*American Council of the Blind, 1010 Vermont Ave., Suite 1100, Washington, DC 20005; National Braille Press Inc., 88 Stephen St., Boston, MA 02115.

SCLERAL BUCKLING, RETINAL CRYOPEXY

Discuss symptoms of further detachment
  Sudden loss of vision
  Severe pain
  Increased floaters
Explain that reading is avoided for 1 week

ENUCLEATION

Conformer for eyeball may become dislodged; explain that this is of little consequence and it need not be reinserted
Discuss use of antibiotic drugs and need to wear eye shield until prosthesis is fitted (in about 1 month)

TRABECULECTOMY, LASER IRIDOTOMY

Discuss signs of increased intraocular pressure (IOP)
  Severe eye pain
  Headache
  Nausea
  Increased tearing
Explain importance of using glaucoma eye drops in unoperated eye

---

CATARACT REMOVAL

Without lens implant, using glasses: explain that glasses
  Usually magnify objects 25% to 30%
  Decrease peripheral vision
  Can cause visual disturbance if fit is incorrect
  Allow patient to focus; patient will be unable to focus without them
  Are temporary glasses and new ones will be prescribed in about 2 to 12 weeks
  Sometimes alter distance judgment
Without lens implant, using contact lenses: explain that contact lenses
  Will be fitted and worn after 2 to 12 weeks
  Allow patient to focus, but patient will need glasses for close vision
With intraocular lens implant: explain that lens implant
  Aids in focusing, but glasses will be fitted for close vision in 8 to 12 weeks
  Does not cause depth perception loss

Expected outcome/evaluation

Patient
  Verbalizes understanding of safety precautions, need to limit activity, and symptoms to report to physician
  Performs ADLs at optimal level for degree of impairment
  Demonstrates accurate eye management techniques

CONTACT LENS REMOVAL

Occasionally unconscious, paralyzed, disoriented, or elderly patients and patients with limited or restricted use of their arms may be wearing contact lenses; lenses must be removed to avoid eye damage

Assessment

Level of consciousness/ability to cooperate
Presence of contact lenses in unconscious patient: shine flashlight into eye from outer canthus; lenses will appear around iris or slightly beyond
Type of lenses
  Hard: covers iris, may be tinted
  Soft: covers iris, may be tinted
  Scleral: covers iris and sclera
Small suction cup apparatus for removing contact lenses is often kept in emergency room

Removal Procedure

Wash hands thoroughly before procedure
Removal of hard lenses
  Place forefinger at outer canthus of eye
  Gently push finger up and then down
  Lens will appear from under lid
  Store in distilled water, keeping right and left lenses separate and containers marked
Removal of soft lenses
  Place thumb and forefinger on lower and upper lid, respectively
  Gently open eye
  With other hand gently lift lens off iris, using thumb and forefinger
  Store in normal saline solution, keeping right and left lenses separate and containers marked
Removal of scleral lenses
  Place forefinger at edge of and parallel to lower lid
  Gently press lid downward until lower edge of lens is visible
  Continue gentle pressure, pulling lid toward ear
  Lens will slide out from under lid
  Store in distilled water, keeping right and left lenses separate and containers marked
Removal of all types of lenses using suction cup apparatus
  Depress bulb between thumb and forefinger
  Position cup over lens
  Slowly release pressure on bulb

Lens will adhere to cup

Remove lens and store in marked containers with appropriate solution

If lenses are not visible (eye rolled back) or difficulty is experienced in removal procedure, notify ophthalmologist to remove lenses

INSTILLATION OF EYE DROPS/OINTMENTS

Preinstillation Assessment

Assess patient's ability to hold eyes open and cooperate

Explain purpose of medication, procedure, and side effects

Perform medication assessment

Correct medication, patient, dosage, time, and eye

Check dropper for defects

Understand abbreviations

OD: right eye

OS: left eye

OU: both eyes

Instillation Procedure (Figure 12-2)

Eye drops are sterile, and any contamination of the dropper or squeeze bottle can cause infection

Always discard when contamination occurs

Position patient in chair with head tilted back or in dorsal recumbent position in bed

Wash hands before procedure

Draw medication into dropper (keep medication from going into bulb end) or open squeeze bottle of drops or tube of ointment

Gently pull down skin beneath lower lid with thumb and place forefinger above upper lid. Put pressure on the cheekbone, not on soft tissue of eye

Instruct patient to look upward

Allow time between drops as patient will blink after each drop

Instill drops or dab ointment into pocket formation in lower lid; do not touch conjunctiva with dropper or tube

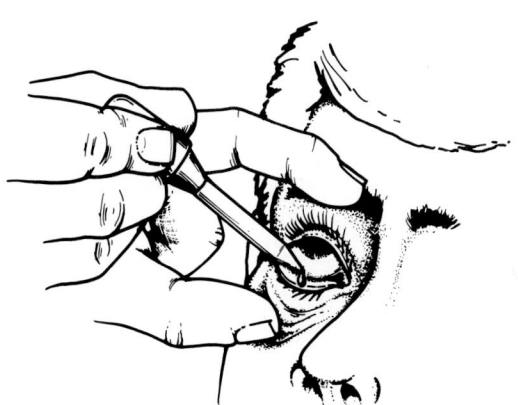

FIGURE 12-2. Instillation of eye drops.

Instruct patient to close eye gently and not to squeeze eye closed or to rub it

Wipe of excess medication with tissue

Instruct patient to open and close eye slowly for a few minutes to distribute medication evenly

AUDITORY SYSTEM ASSESSMENT

Subjective Data

Earache

Decreased, absent hearing acuity in one or both ears

Tinnitis

Feeling of fullness in ear

Own voice echoes

Popping noise when yawning or swallowing

Vertigo, dizziness

Itching in ear

Heart pulsating in ear

Ear drainage

Dark

Red

Clear

Yellow

Use of oils, cotton swabs, hairpins to clean ears

Objective Data

General appearance

Vital signs: elevated BP, T, P, and R

Ability to hear; use of hearing aid

Ability to lip-read or use sign language

Startle reflex

Tolerance of loud sounds

Type, color, and amount of ear drainage

Medication used (streptomycin, salicylates, quinine, gentamycin)

Allergies

Pertinent Background Information

CONCURRENT DISEASES OR CONDITIONS

Otitis media

Otosclerosis

Acoustic nerve tumor

Labyrinthitis

Ménierè's disease

Cerebral tumors, contusion, diseases, fractures

Diabetes mellitus

Arteriosclerosis

Hypertension

Hypotension

Mastoiditis

PREVIOUS SURGERY OR ILLNESS

Stapes mobilization

Syphilis

Otitis media

Head trauma
Mastoidectomy

SOCIAL HISTORY

Sexually transmitted diseases
Recreational hazards: swimming, diving
Exposure to loud noises
Safety precautions taken
Use of tobacco or coffee

MEDICATION HISTORY

Antineoplastics
Diuretics
Narcotics
Narcotic antagonists
Ear drops
Antibiotics
Salicylates
Quinine

Diagnostic Aids

PROCEDURES

Audiogram, audiometry
Mastoid x-ray examination
Tuning fork test (Rinne)
Otological examination
"Lateralization" tuning fork test (Weber)
Pneumatic otoscopy
Tympanometry
Caloric examination
Electronystagmography (ENG)
Electrocochleography
Tomogram
Cerebral arteriography
Computed tomography (CT) scan
Magnetic resonance imaging (MRI) scan
Schwabach test

MICROBIOLOGICAL PROCEDURES

Culture for pathogens

AUDITORY-IMPAIRED PATIENT

Assessment
Observations/findings

Assess hearing acuity and communication skills
  Lipreading or sign language
  Hearing aid
  Pad and pencil
  Flash cards
Determine status and duration of impairment
Assess acceptance of impairment and skills learned
  Well adjusted
  Fear/anxiety
  Anger, hostility

Examine ears for drainage, crusts, cerumen accumulation, and deformities

Nursing diagnoses/interventions/evaluation

■ **NDX:** Alteration in sensory perception related to hearing impairment

Assess level of hearing impairment
Reinforce physician's explanation of hearing impairment
Assess and establish means of communication
  Lipreading (speech reading)
    Speak slowly and enunciate well
    Do not exaggerate sounds
    Have only one person speak at a time
    Stand so patient can see your mouth clearly
    Speak in simple phrases first to determine expertise in the skill
    NOTE: Nurses with mustaches may be more difficult to understand
    Point to objects of conversation where appropriate
    Avoid chewing gum and shouting
    Rephrase statements if not first understood
  Sign language
    Determine if patient can communicate with pad and pencil, since most hospital personnel are not skilled in sign language
    Enlist cooperation of family/significant other in communication
  Hearing aid
    Assess patient's ability to use and care for appliance
    Make certain aid is in place and turned on before speaking
    Establish a pitch that is comfortable for patient
    Avoid shouting
  Pad and pencil
    Write messages clearly, in short, simple phrases
    Develop a checklist of phrases most often used and instruct patient to check appropriate one(s)
    Allow time for patient to understand and answer

Expected outcome/evaluation

Patient
  Accepts limitations caused by hearing impairment
  Demonstrates positive coping behaviors
  Uses learned skills for communicating

■ **NDX:** Potential for injury; trauma related to hearing impairment

Maintain safe environment
  Locate bed so door is visible, when possible
  Orient patient to surroundings; have call bell within reach
    Answer call light promptly
    Keep side rails up if appropriate

Approach patient carefully if eyes are closed; a gentle touch on patient's arm will arouse but not startle

Explain all procedures

Flag chart indicating type of impairment and ear(s) involved

Expected outcome/evaluation

Patient

Understands safety factors associated with hearing impairment

Demonstrates ability to perform activities in safe manner

Notifies staff for assistance

■ NDX: Anxiety related to hearing impairment

Maintain quiet, nonstressful environment

Assess level of anxiety

Encourage and allow time for verbalization of feelings

Explain nursing plan of care and involve patient in planning care

Display confidence and a caring, nonjudgmental manner

Use pictures when explaining procedures or treatment

Encourage communication with significant other

Avoid using electronic nurse-patient intercommunication system if patient has partial hearing since it can cause frustration

Evaluate patient's ability to use other senses (sight and touch especially) as an aid in daily living

Provide diversional activities: puzzles, cards, hobbies

Expected outcome/evaluation

Patient

Understands causes of anxiety

Demonstrates positive behaviors in coping with anxiety

Reports a reduction in anxiety level

■ NDX: Knowledge deficit related to lack of information about home and follow-up care

Reinforce physician's explanation of cause of impairment and prescribed treatment

Explain safety factors important in home environment

Discuss availability of hearing devices: amplifiers, flashing lights on telephones and door bells

Refer to local telephone company and/or hearing institute for assistance

Refer to local schools for classes on lipreading and/or sign language

Instruct patient in care of hearing aid and to have extra battery on hand at all times

Demonstrate care of ear dressings and ear drop instillation if applicable

Encourage patient to make and keep appointments with physician

Expected outcome/evaluation

Patient

Demonstrates knowledge of available outside resources

Understands and demonstrates use and care of hearing aid

Demonstrates accurate ear drop instillation

EAR SURGERIES

stapedectomy *Surgical removal of all or part of the stapes footplate and creation of a patent oval window and pathway for sound transmission using natural or artificial materials*

myringotomy with tube insertion *Surgical incision into the tympanic membrane to aspirate collected fluid and insertion of a ventilating tube to keep the pressure equal between the middle and outer ear, performed to correct serous otitis media*

tympanoplasty *Surgical repair of tympanic membrane perforated or largely destroyed by infection, trauma, otosclerosis, stenosis, or necrosis of the middle ear; type performed depends on degree of perforation and destruction as well as ossicular involvement and damage*

Preoperative Assessment/Teaching

Assess hearing acuity in both ears

Reinforce physician's explanation of procedure

Establish means of communication since hearing may be impaired

Encourage and allow time for verbalization of fears and anxieties

Explain postoperative patient care plan and availability of staff

Explain that hearing may not improve immediately

Postoperative Assessment
Observations/findings

Nausea, vomiting

Vertigo

Character and amount of ear drainage

Restlessness resulting from decreased hearing

Location and character of pain

Excessive pain

Hearing acuity

Potential complications

Infection

Hemorrhage

Decreased hearing acuity

Deafness

Medical Management

Analgesics

Antiemetics

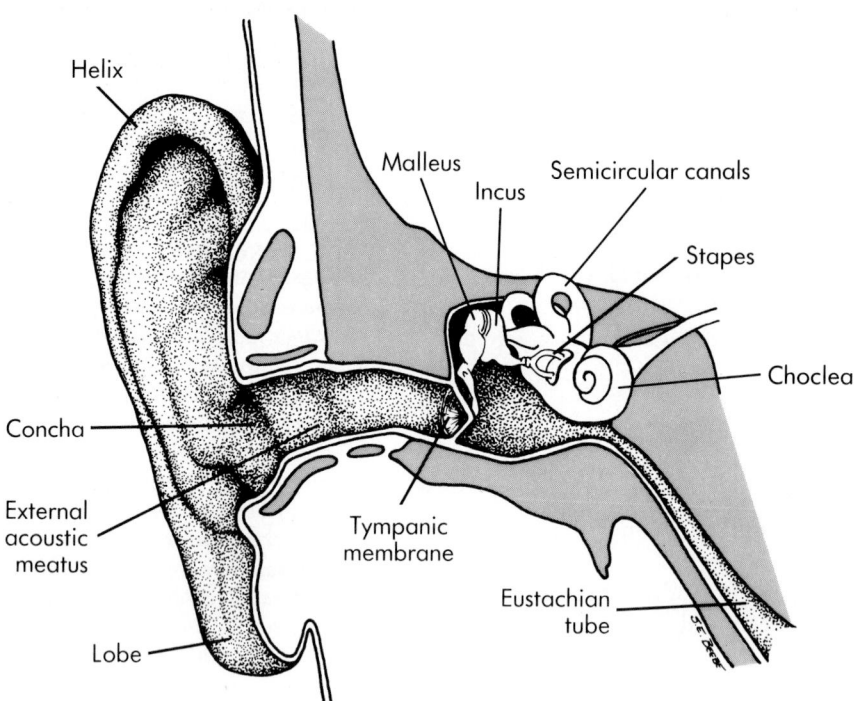

FIGURE 12-3. The ear.

Antibiotics
Dressing change schedule

Nursing diagnoses/interventions/evaluation

■ **NDX:**   Pain related to surgical procedure and position restriction

Maintain bed rest in quiet environment
   Supine position with operative side up for prescribed length of time
   Keep side rails up to promote slight position changes
   Do not turn unless ordered
   Provide back rubs prn
Assess pain intensity using a pain rating scale of 0 to 5
Administer analgesics and assess effectiveness of pain relief
Report excessive pain to physician
Have patient avoid nose blowing or sneezing since they increase pain
Have patient avoid vomiting by using antiemetics

Expected outcome/evaluation

Patient
   Expresses satisfaction with pain relief measures
   Appears calm and relaxed in position of comfort

■ **NDX:**   Potential for infection related to invasive surgical procedure

Monitor for signs of infection q4h

Increased drainage/pain
Fever
Headache
Keep outer ear plug clean and dry
Change ear plugs prn
Report excessive bleeding to physician
Monitor vital signs q4h
Maintain aseptic technique

Expected outcome/evaluation

Patient's
   Temperature remains normal
   Ear drainage is not purulent

■ **NDX:**   Alteration in sensory perception related to hearing impairment

Assess hearing acuity of affected ear
Stand at unaffected side when speaking
Explain that hearing may not improve immediately and that this is not abnormal
   Ear plugs and bleeding decrease hearing acuity
   Hearing usually improves after plugs are removed
Provide and use alternative communicating measures as needed; pen and paper, Magic Slate
Encourage verbalization of thoughts and feelings
Involve patient in self-care and assist as needed

Expected outcome/evaluation

Patient

Accepts and copes appropriately with hearing impairment

Strives to use remaining hearing or other senses adequately

■ **NDX:** Knowledge deficit related to lack of information about home and follow-up care

General

Explain importance of nutritious diet, fluid intake, rest, and activity

Discuss signs and symptoms to report to physician

Elevated temperature

Increased pain and/or ear drainage

Decrease in hearing acuity

Discuss medications: name, dosage, time of administration, purpose, and side effects

Avoid persons with URI or cold symptoms

Avoid smoking

Encourage follow-up visits with physician

Specific

STAPEDECTOMY

Instruct patient on ear care

Change only outer ear plug prn

Keep plug clean and dry

Avoid nose-blowing for 1 week

Keep ear covered while outside

Avoid sneezing; if unavoidable, open mouth wide to sneeze

Wash hair only after 2 weeks

No air travel or diving for 6 months

Plugs and packing are removed after 1 week

TYMPANOPLASTY

Discuss precautions and restrictions in ear care

Wear shower cap when bathing or place lamb's wool pledget in ear to protect ear from water

Avoid blowing nose and sneeze through mouth

Remove inner ear dressing only if prescribed by physician

May swim or fly after healing has taken place

Explain that meclizine hydrochloride (Antivert) may be needed for about 1 mo postoperatively

---

MYRINGOTOMY WITH TUBE INSERTION

Discuss special precautions and restrictions

Keep water out of ear

Place petroleum jelly–covered cotton or lamb's wool pledget in ear before showering or shampooing

Wear well-fitting ear plugs when swimming is allowed or wear a cap

Do not dive as it increases ear pressure

Explain that tube will come out naturally in 2 to 8 months and there may be bloody drainage; if tube is dislodged earlier, instruct patient or parent(s) to notify physician

Demonstrate ear drop instillation and instruct patient or parent(s) to complete prescribed course of oral or ear drop antibiotic therapy

---

Expected outcome/evaluation

Patient

Verbalizes understanding of needed restrictions and precautions

Accurately demonstrates care of ear

Expresses understanding of symptoms to report to physician

Demonstrates accurate instillation of ear drops

BIBLIOGRAPHY

Carpentino LJ: *Handbook of nursing diagnosis*, Philadelphia, 1990, JB Lippincott.

Carver JA: Cataract care made plain, *Am J Nurs* 87(5):626, 1987.

Doenges ME et al: *Nursing care plans: guidelines for planning patient care*, ed 2, Philadelphia, 1989, FA Davis.

Gulanick M et al: *Nursing care plans*, ed 2, St Louis, 1990, Mosby–Year Book.

Guzzetta CE et al: *Clinical assessment tools for use with nursing diagnoses*, St Louis, 1989, CV Mosby.

Kim MJ et al: *Pocket guide to nursing diagnoses*, ed 3, St Louis, 1989, CV Mosby.

McFarland GK, McFarlane EA: *Nursing diagnosis and intervention*, St Louis, 1989, CV Mosby.

Norris RM: Commonsense tips for working with blind patients, *Am J Nurs* 90(3):360, 1989.

Thelan LA et al: *Textbook of critical care nursing*, St Louis, 1990, Mosby–Year Book.

Thompson JM et al: *Mosby's manual of clinical practice*, ed 2, St Louis, 1989, CV Mosby.

13
CHAPTER

Immune System

IMMUNE SYSTEM ASSESSMENT

Figure 13-1
General
  Age
  Sex
  Race
  Ethnic background
  Fatigue
  Fever
  Diaphoresis, night sweats
  Rashes
  Muscular weakness
  Joint pain/swelling
  Weight loss
  Unusual masses
  Lymphadenopathy
  Poor healing
  Hepatosplenomegaly
  Vital sign changes
Central Nervous System
  General
    Headache
    Paresthesias
    Paralysis
    Neuritis
    Altered consciousness
  Cognitive
    Memory impairment
    Poor concentration
    Slowed thought processes
    Confusion
  Motor
    Unsteady gait
    Leg weakness
    Decreased hand coordination
    Tremors
    Seizures
  Behavioral
    Less animated
    Withdrawn
    Emotional lability
    Personality changes, denial, anxiety
    Psychosis
    Depression

Respiratory
  SOB
  Dyspnea
  Frequent URIs
  Cough
  Tachypnea
  Cyanosis
  Hemorrhage
  Pulmonary hypertension, fibrosis, cor pulmonale
  Wheezing
  Crackles at bases or diffuse
  Intercostal retraction
Ophthalmological
  Photophobia
  Diplopia
  Blurred vision
  Retinal cytoid bodies
  Cotton wool exudate
  Proptosis
  Papilledema
  Visual field deficits
  Blindness
  Cataracts
  Conjunctivitis
  Uveitis
Gastrointestinal
  Anorexia
  Nausea
  Dysphagia
  Abdominal pain, cramping, bloating
  Rectal itching, pain
  Weight loss, unintentional
  Vomiting
  Diarrhea
  Rectal fissures, bleeding
  Hepatosplenomegaly
Integumentary
  Sun sensitivity
  Shiny, taut skin over impaired joint
  Subcutaneous nodules over bony prominences
  Rash
  Erythema; "butterfly" cheeks and nose; nodosum
  White, gray/white patches on mucosa
  Red to purple/brown lesions

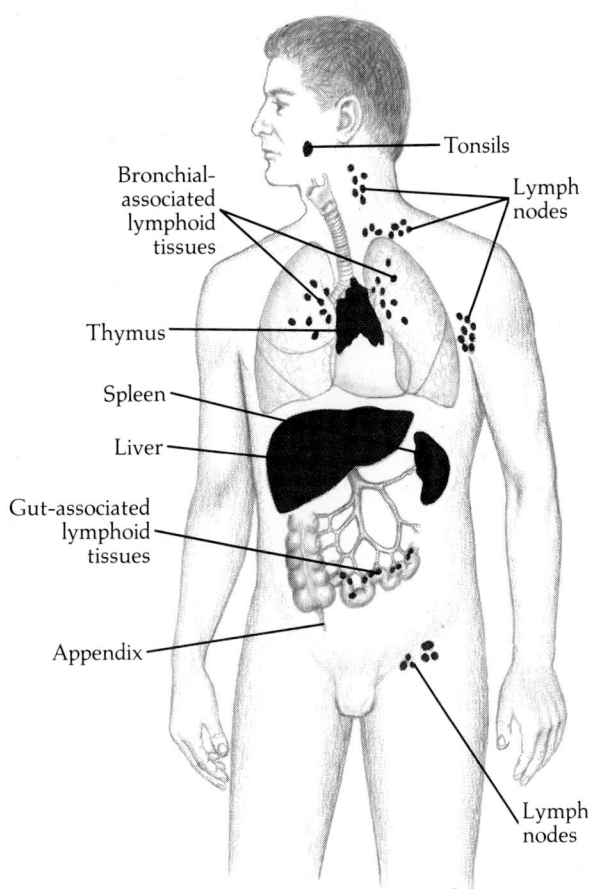

FIGURE 13-1. Organization of immune system. Cellular constituents of immune system are derived from bone marrow stem cells. On maturation, these cells are released into peripheral blood and subsequently populate organized tissues of lymphoreticular system. (From Thompson JM, McFarland GK, Hirsch JE et al: *Mosby's manual of clinical nursing,* ed 2, St Louis, 1989, Mosby–Year Book.)

Herpetic vesicles
Oral, nasal ulcerations
Bone cysts; hands, feet
Delayed wound healing
Partial alopecia
Musculoskeletal
  Joint pain and stiffness
  Muscular weakness
  Paresthesia; hands, feet
  Arthralgias
  Joint inflammation/swelling
  Impaired joint function
  Subcutaneous nodules on bony prominences
  Soft tissue edema
Genitourinary
  Hematuria
  Cellular casts

Azotemia
Flank pain
Painful urination
Cardiovascular
  Palpitations, tachycardia
  Mild to severe chest pain
  Hypertension
  Murmurs
  Cardiomegaly
  Reynaud's phenomenon
Hematological
  Petechiae
  Purpura
  Easy bruising
  Epistaxis
  Gingival bleeding
Lymphatic

Lymphadenopathy
Splenomegaly

Pertinent Background Information

CONCURRENT DISEASES OR CONDITIONS

Frequent, recurrent infections, especially viral
Opportunistic infections; fungal, protozoan, or viral
  Anemia
  Pleuritis
  Pericarditis
  Reynaud's phenomenon
  Vasculitis
  Malignancies
    Leukemia
    Immunodeficiency disease
    Kaposi's sarcoma
    Lymphoma
  IV drug use

PREVIOUS MEDICAL HISTORY

Allergies
Autoimmune disease
Infectious process
Sexually transmitted diseases
Hepatitis
Exposure to chemical agents
Irradiation

FAMILY HISTORY

Cancer
Immune disorders
Allergies

SOCIAL HISTORY

Smoking
Alcohol use
Increased stress
Sexual preference
Multiple sex partners
IV drug use, shared needles

MEDICATION HISTORY

Immunizations
Received blood or blood products before 1985
Hydralazine
Procainamide
Isoniazid
Illicit IV drug use

Diagnostic Aids

LABORATORY STUDIES

CBC
WBC, differential
Erythrocyte sedimentation rate
Coagulative profile

Lymphocytes, T_4, T_8
Serum immunoglobulin
Antigen/antibody titer
Antinuclear antibody
HAA
HAV
ASO titer
Rheumatoid factor (RF)
C-reactive protein (CRP)
Serum electrophoresis
LE cell preparation
Anti-double-standard DNA antibody
Complement (C_3, C_4)
Fluorescent treponemal antibody absorption
ELISA
Western blot assay
PCR
FBS
BUN
Bilirubin
Creatinine clearance
LDH, SGOT, SGPT
Alkaline phosphatase
Cholesterol
Iron
Electrolytes
Serology
Cultures
  Sputum, spinal fluid, oral mucous membranes, blood, and stool
Urinalysis
  Urine protein

OTHER PROCEDURES

Radiological
  Joint
  Chest
Gallium lung scan
CT scan/MRI
ECG
Nerve conduction tests
Electromyography
Pulmonary function tests
Arthroscopy
Bronchoscopy
Biopsies
  Skin, kidney, lung, bone marrow

ACQUIRED IMMUNE DEFICIENCY SYNDROME (AIDS)

AIDS includes the final stages of a wide range of health problems caused by the human immunodeficiency virus type I (HIV) (see box on p. 547). This virus attacks the cell-mediated immune system through invasion of

CENTERS FOR DISEASE CONTROL CLASSIFICATION OF HIV INFECTION

The manifestations of HIV in diagnosed patients are classified into four mutually exclusive groups

Group I   Acute infection
Mononucleosis-like syndrome in some individuals at time of exposure, associated with HIV-antibody seroconversion about 3 months after exposure

Group II   Asymptomatic HIV infection
Absence of present or previous signs and symptoms of HIV infection; seroconversion of HIV antibody or positive HIV culture

Group III   Persistent generalized lymphadenopathy
Palpable lymphadenopathy 1 cm or greater at two or more extra inguinal sites lasting for more than 3 months in the absence of concurrent illness or condition

Group IV   Other HIV disease
This group is further subdivided into subgroups independent of presence or absence of lymphadenopathy, groups C-E are classified as having AIDS

A: Constitutional disease
One or more of the following
Fever more than 1 month
Involuntary weight loss of 10% or more
Diarrhea for 1 month
Absence of concurrent illness or disease

B: Neurological disease
One or more of the following
Dementia
Myelopathy
Peripheral neuropathy
Absence of concurrent illness or disease

C: Secondary infectious diseases
Further subdivisions

C-1: Symptomatic or invasive disease of one of the following:
Pneumocystis carinii pneumonia
Chronic cryptosporidiosis
Toxoplasmosis
Extraintestinal strongyloidiasis
Isoporiasis
Candidiasis (bronchial, esophageal, or pulmonary)
Cryptococcus
Histoplasmosis
Mycobacterium avium or kansasii
Cytomegalovirus infection
Herpes simplex infection
Progressive multifocal leukoencephalopathy

C-2: Symptomatic or invasive disease of one of the following:
Oral hairy leukoplakia
Multidermal herpes zoster
Recurrent Salmonella bacteremia
Nocardiosis
Tuberculosis
Oral candidiasis

D: Secondary cancers
One or more of the following cancers indicative of a cell-mediated immunity defect:
Kaposi's sarcoma
Non-Hodgkin's lymphoma
Primary lymphoma of the brain

E: Other conditions
Presence of other clinical findings or diseases, not classified previously, that may be attributable to HIV infection or that may be indicative of a defect in cell-mediated immunity

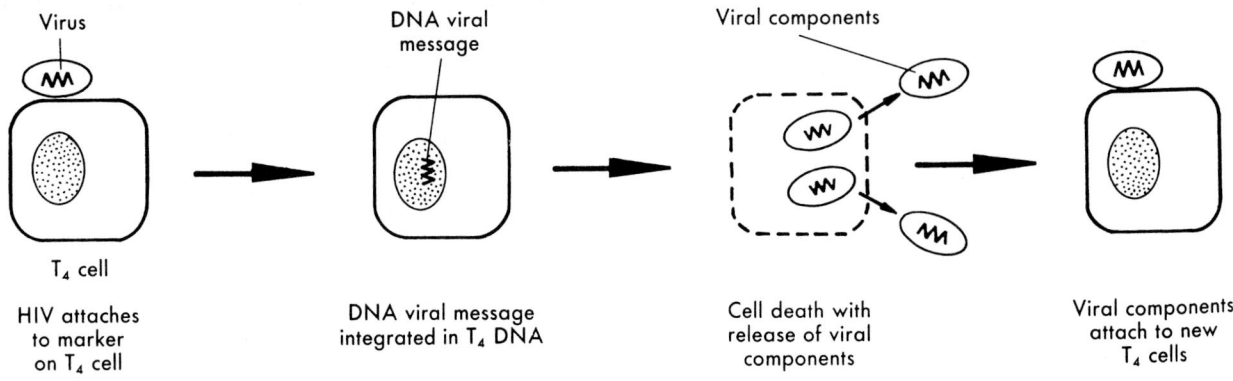

FIGURE 13-2. Mechanism of HIV action. (From Phipps WJ, Long BC, Woods NF et al: *Medical-surgical nursing: concepts and clinical practice*, ed 4, St Louis, 1991, Mosby–Year Book.)

T4 lymphocytes, causing impaired cell function and ultimately killing the individual cells, thereby depleting their number (see Figure 13-2). The infected person becomes vulnerable to opportunistic infections and cancers. HIV is transmitted from an infected person via blood/body fluids exchanged through intimate sexual contact, use of contaminated needles, use of contaminated blood or blood products, and perinatally. There have also been a few reported cases of transmission of the virus to infants via breast milk. HIV has been demonstrated in saliva, but no cases of transmission via this medium are reported. Groups most affected are homosexually or bisexually active men, IV drug users, recipients of contaminated blood or blood products, their sexual partners, and children born to HIV-infected mothers

Assessment
Observations and findings

The multiple problems associated with AIDS are included.
Pulmonary
  Cough
  SOB
  Dyspnea
  Wheezing
  Tachypnea
  Cyanosis
  Hemoptysis
  Intercostal retraction
Neurological
  AIDS dementia complex
    Cognitive
      Memory impairment
      Poor concentration
      Slowed thought processes
      Confusion
    Motor
      Unsteady gait

      Weakness, especially lower extremities
      Decreased hand coordination
      Tremors
      Seizures
    Behavioral
      Decreased animation
      Withdrawal
      Depression
      Emotional lability
      Psychosis
  Other
    Paresthesias
    Paralysis
    Headache
    Nuchal rigidity
    Altered consciousness
    Coma
Ophthalmological
  Cotton wool exudate
  Photophobia
  Blurred vision
  Papilledema
  Diplopia
  Proptosis
  Visual field deficits
  Blindness
Skin and mucous membranes
  Oral/esophageal
    White to gray/white patches
      May appear hairy if dried
    Red to purple/brown lesions
      Macular, nodular, or plaque-like
    Gingivitis
  Perioral or lips
    Corners of mouth; red fissures; crusted
    Herpatic vesicles

Skin
  Pink/purple to brown lesions
  May appear as bright red subconjunctival mass
  Vesicles
  Diaphoresis
  Rash
  Dryness
  Delayed wound healing
Lymphadenopathy: nodes not fixed or hard
Gastrointestinal
Loss of appetite
Difficulty chewing or swallowing; retrosternal pain
Nausea, vomiting
Unintentional weight loss, 10% in 1 to 2 months
Abdominal cramping/pain
Diarrhea, at least 2 stools/day for 1 month
  Intractable
Rectal: bleeding, fissures, itching, pain
Hematological
  Splenomegaly
  Petechiae
  Purpura
  Easy bruising
  Epistaxis
  Gingival bleeding
Systemic
  Night sweats
  Severe fatigue
  Elevated temperature
History
  Hepatitis
  Sexually transmitted diseases
  Frequent viral illnesses
  Amebiasis
  Exposure to contaminated needles
  IV drug use
  Recipient of blood or blood products (1978-1984)
  Multiple sex partners
  Sexual preference
  Alcohol use
  Support system
  Work/productive activities
  Fatigue
  Stress factors
  Previous losses
  Coping patterns
  Self-concept
  Conceptualization of illness

Laboratory/diagnostic studies

Antibody for HIV
  ELISA (enzyme-linked immunosorbent assay) repeatedly reactive
  Western blot assay or immunofluoresence assay positive

HIV antigen, e.g., PCR (polymerase chain reaction) positive
HIV culture confirmed positive
Decreased number of T4 (helper) cells
T8 (suppressor) cells may be increased
Inversion of T helper/T suppressor ratio
Elevated serum immunoglobulin
Leukocytopenia
Lymphocytopenia
RBC, Hct, Hgb decreased
ESR elevated
Thrombocytopenia
LDH elevated
Alkaline phosphatase elevated
Serum cholesterol decreased
Serum iron decreased
Electrolyte imbalance
Arterial blood gases
  Mild hypokalemia to respiratory alkalosis
Pulmonary function tests
  Increased flow rates
  Decreased diffusion capacity
Chest radiography
  Interstitial infiltrates
Gallium lung scan positive
Bronchoscopy with lavage/biopsy positive
Cultures
  Sputum positive for pneumocystis carinii cysts, AFB, fungi
  Sputum, spinal fluid, bone marrow positive for disseminated MAI
  Oral mucous membranes positive for candidiasis, herpes I, hairy leukoplakia
  Blood and spinal fluid positive for cryptococcal antigen test
  Spinal fluid positive for HIV, herpes I, CMV
  Stool positive for ova and parasites
CT scan/MRI
  Positive for toxoplasmosis lesions, HIV infection
Endoscopy/tissue biopsy confirm Kaposi's sarcoma
Electromyography
Nerve conduction studies

Potential complications

See Table 13-1

Medical Management

Oxygen therapy (p. 194)
Mechanical ventilatory support
Chest physiotherapy
Hemodynamic/cardiac monitoring
Central-line catheter (p. 53)
Total parenteral nutrition (p. 36)
Parenteral therapy
Chemotherapy

TABLE 13-1. Opportunistic Infections, Neoplasms, and Systems Involved in AIDS

Opportunistic infections and neoplasms	System involved
OPPORTUNISTIC INFECTIONS	
Protozoal	Pulmonary, cutaneous, ophthalmological
Pneumocystis carinii pneumonitis (PCP)	
Cryptosporidiosis	Systemic, neurological, gastrointestinal
Toxoplasmosis	Neurological, systemic, ophthalmological
Giardiasis	Gastrointestinal
Viruses	
Cytomegalovirus (CMV)	Systemic, neurological, gastrointestinal, pulmonary, ophthalmological
Herpes simplex I, II	Neurological, cutaneous
Epstein-Barr virus (EBV)	Systemic
Herpes zoster	Neurological, cutaneous
Progressive multifocal leukoencephalopathy (PML)	Neurological
Hairy leukoplakia	Cutaneous, gastrointestinal
Fungi	
Candidiasis	Neurological, cutaneous, pulmonary
Cryptococcosis	Neurological, systemic
Histoplasmosis	Pulmonary, systemic
Coccidioidomycosis	Pulmonary, cutaneous systemic
Aspergillosis	Pulmonary, ophthalmological, systemic
Bacterial	
Mycobacterium avium-intracellular (MAI)	Neurological, systemic, pulmonary, gastrointestinal
Mycobacterium tuberculosis	Neurological, pulmonary, systemic
Klebsiella pneumoniae	Pulmonary
Salmonellosis	Gastrointestinal, cutaneous, skeletal, systemic
NEOPLASMS	
Kaposi's sarcoma (KS)	Neurological, cutaneous, ophthalmological, gastrointestinal
Lymphoma (p. 632)	Neurological, systemic, gastrointestinal
OTHER	
Anemia	Hematological, systemic
Idiopathic thrombocytopenia purpura (ITP) (p. 171)	Hematological, gastrointestinal, neurological
Xerostomia	Gastrointestinal

Antiemetics
Antidiarrheals
Antivirals
Antifungals
Antineoplastics
Biological modifiers
Antibiotics
Sulfonamides
Antipyretics
Analgesics
Radiotherapy

Nursing diagnosis/interventions/evaluation

■ **NDX:**   Impaired gas exchange related to pulmonary infection (pneumocystis carinii pneumonia), lung-involved malignancy

Assess BP; apical pulse; respiratory rate, depth, pattern; level of consciousness q4h and prn; report changes to physician

Auscultate chest for breath sounds q4h and prn

Monitor cardiac rhythm and hemodynamic pressures as indicated

Monitor arterial blood gases as ordered

Report $PaCO_2$ of 50 mm Hg or above or PaO_2 of 60 mm Hg or below to physician

Administer oxygen with assisted ventilation and humidification as ordered

Suction airways as needed (p. 193)

Obtain sputum specimens for culture/sensitivity

Provide chest physiotherapy and postural drainage as ordered

Assist and teach patient to turn, cough, and deep breathe q1h to 2h

Position patient for optimal respiratory excursion and comfort, high Fowler's position or on pillow on overbed table

Teach purse-lipped or diaphragmatic breathing

Teach relaxation exercises to decrease anxiety

Avoid use of aerosol products and those with noxious odors around patient

Evaluate ADLs in relation to oxygen demands and assist if necessary

During stable period assist patient, significant other, and health team to discuss patient's goal of therapy; palliation or aggressive therapy; communicate decision to all involved in care, health team and significant others

Prepare to assist with intubation and mechanical ventilation when indicated

See Adult Respiratory Distress Syndrome (p. 225)

Expected outcome/evaluation

Vital signs are stable within patient's normal limits, breath sounds are clear; blood gases within normal limits; patient performs ADL's with or without assistance or patient is intubated and on mechanical ventilation

■ **NDX:**   Potential for infection related to profound immunological compromise and progression or onset of opportunistic infection

Institute universal precautions

Allow no infectious personnel or visitors to enter room

Be certain that all visitors and personnel entering room know and observe universal precaution procedures

Assess and record skin condition q4h to 8h

Assist with hygiene as necessary to maintain skin integrity

Use strict sterile technique for all invasive procedures

Monitor sites of invasive procedures for signs of infection

Ensure that perianal care is performed after elimination

Encourage mobility q2h

Turn and position patient q2h if on bed rest

Provide adequate uninterrupted rest and sleep periods

Assess and record condition of oral mucous membranes q4h

Remind patient to perform oral hygiene q2h; assist when necessary

Ensure required nutrient and fluid intake

Monitor intake and output; report urinary frequency, burning, or changes in character of urine

Assess and record respiratory status q4h

Report changes in breath sounds, cough, sputum, increase in respiratory rate, rhythm, use of accessory muscles, sore throat

Remind or assist patient to turn, cough, and deep breathe q2h and to use incentive spirometer q1h to 2h

Monitor and record vital signs q4h; take temperature more frequently if trend is beginning; report changes

Institute comfort and cooling measures as indicated by condition

Assess for changes in GI system

Report anorexia, nausea, vomiting, diarrhea, cramping, weight loss > 3% to 5%

Perform neurological assessment q4h

Report changes in level of consciousness, behavior, mobility; presence of headache, dizziness, confusion, speech difficulties, blurred or decreased vision

Monitor laboratory data daily; report changes

Administer medications as ordered

Antibiotics, sulfa-type medications, antipyretics, analgesics, other antiinfectives

Assess response to medications; report side or toxic effects

Expected outcome/evaluation

Current infection is controlled

No symptoms of other infections are present

■ **NDX:**   Altered thought processes related to memory deficits; impaired judgment/orientation resulting from AIDS dementia complex, HIV infection, or other opportunistic infection

Assess level of disruptions in thinking process, memory, or interpretation of stimuli and changes in attention span, routine patterns, or emotions

Assess level of consciousness and orientation q4h

Reorient to time, person, place as necessary

Identify self upon entering room

Call patient by name

Use clear, direct terms

Avoid vague comments, whispered conversations with others in room

Give one direction at a time

Avoid generalizations, "we" statements, or discussions with others in room as though patient is not present or is without hearing ability

Redirect misinterpretations of stimuli to reality-centered discussions

Assist to clarify thoughts and feelings

Verify patient's statements

Be aware that patient may be oriented at beginning of discussion but may change orientation very quickly

Assess environment and attempt to decrease stimuli that can enhance misinterpretations

Adjust lighting to prevent shadows and distortions; use night light

Keep room door closed to decrease auditory stimuli

Arrange familiar objects, pictures within patient's visual field

Keep clock and correctly dated calendar visible to patient

Provide radio, television, newspapers

Keep equipment and possessions in same place

Label bathroom, other areas with large letters

Maintain routine activities at same time; keep daily schedule posted

Encourage family, significant other to visit; assist in dealing with patient's orientation, memory loss, etc.

Enlist their aid in maintaining orientation

Protect patient from self-injury

Place furniture and equipment where clearly visible

Provide restraints as ordered if necessary to prevent unescorted wandering

Remove and check circulation, skin integrity q8h

Ensure proper placement

Encourage acceptance of responsibility for actions

Plan care with patient to enhance sense of control; make decisions

Encourage simple choices at first

Selection of menus

Choice of activity

Provide tasks that do not require new learning

Break tasks into several steps; give directions for completing one step at a time; allow patient to rest, then complete next step, etc.

Give positive reinforcement for participation in self-care activities, verbalization of independent opinions, and decisions

In collaboration with physician, refer for neuropsychiatric or psychosocial evaluation when required

Assess potential for violence directed at self or others (p. 19)

Expected outcome/evaluation

Patient uses calendar and schedule of activities to maintain orientation

Attempts ADLs by completing one step at a time

Makes limited choices (e.g., selects menu for one meal)

Discusses misinterpretations of environment

Recalls names of significant others and care givers, or condition continues to deteriorate and patient is unable to recall names of those who are familiar and remains disoriented and depressed

■ **NDX:** Pain related to neoplasm or sites of infection

Assess nature, intensity, location, duration, and precipitating and alleviating factors of pain; use pain rating scale

Assess nonverbal signs of pain

Provide nonpharmacological comfort measures

Assist patient with assuming a comfortable position

Teach relaxation techniques, music therapy, and visualization

Teach and assist with guided imagery techniques

Provide diversional activity

Provide a restful environment

Observe for desired effects and side effects of medications

Consult with physician if measures fail to provide adequate pain relief or if a dosage or interval change in pain medication is needed

Expected outcome/evaluation

Patient

Verbalizes feeling a decrease in pain

Has a relaxed facial expression and body position

■ **NDX:** Diarrhea related to GI infection, Kaposi's sarcoma, or chemotherapy

Assess usual pattern of elimination

Quantity, frequency, color, consistency of stool and use of laxatives or antidiarrheals

Assess all stools for presence of undigested food; fats; blood, overt to occult

Evaluate hydration and electrolyte status

Monitor intake and output q8h

Auscultate abdomen for bowel sounds; note distention, flatus, or cramping

Weigh daily; same time, scale, and clothing

Assess for edema; third spacing of fluids may occur because of protein deficiency and electrolyte imbalances

Assess and record status of perineal area at least each shift (q4h if frequency of stools increases)

Teach patient to perform perineal care after each stool
Wash with ABDs or soft cloth; front to back for women
Dry well by gentle patting with ABDs or soft toweling
Wash and dry hands well

Perform perineal care if patient unable to do so

Adjust diet as appropriate; avoid GI irritant and laxative foods and fluids

Provide oral electrolyte-containing fluids to 2000 ml/day unless contraindicated

Monitor replacement fluids IV or via central line when administered

Expected outcome/evaluation

Number of diarrheal stools/day is decreasing

■ **NDX:** Altered nutrition: less than body requirements related to increased metabolic demands, malabsorption, anorexia, nausea, vomiting, stomatitis, or diarrhea

Assess nutritional status; height, weight, caloric intake, electrolytes, total protein, serum albumin, Hgb, Hct, skin turgor, and muscle mass

Assess amount and types of foods and liquids tolerated and desired

Administer oral hygiene before and after intake
Use equipment appropriate to condition of mouth
Administer oral anesthetic as required

Arrange for quiet rest periods before meals

Change eating patterns to increase appetite; serve frequent, light meals; avoid food and liquids 2 hr before meals; and/or change usual place for eating

Arrange for visitors, if patient prefers, to enhance socialization

Remind patient to eat slowly and chew well

Assist with feeding when necessary

Place patient in well-ventilated room and control odors
Remove trash frequently
Empty and remove bedpans and urinals after use
Remove food trays as soon as patient has eaten

Provide high-protein drinks as a supplement

Vary textures and tastes of foods to determine those tolerated

Encourage intake of foods to increase calories
Add one cup of powdered milk to one quart whole milk
Add butter, margarine, or vegetable oil when possible
Use mayonnaise liberally
Add cream to vegetables, fruits, soups, and desserts
Use peanut butter and nuts

Eat high-calorie vegetables: avocados, carrots, beets, winter squash, legumes, sweet potatoes, canned corn or peas

Eat high-calorie fruits; bananas, grapes, prunes, raisins, dates, figs, dried apricots, canned fruits and juices

Eat high-calorie main dishes: casseroles with added powdered milk and cream, pot pies, meats, mashed potatoes with gravy or butter, macaroni and cheddar cheese, pasta with cream and butter, pizza, spaghetti

Eat high-calorie desserts; cookies with added powdered milk, dried fruits and nuts, gelatin, puddings with cream, baked custard, ice cream

Avoid foods and fluids that are poorly digested or act as irritants to GI tract
Foods high in milk fat content: patient may have lactose intolerance; use soy-based formulas
Food with high fiber content; spicy or flatus-forming foods
Foods and fluids containing caffeine

Have patient remain sitting after meal

Weigh patient daily, at same time, with same scale and clothing

Maintain calorie count daily

Notify physician when intake and output are not equivalent and/or weight decreases by 3% to 5%

Monitor electrolytes, serum albumin, and total protein; report abnormalities

Consult with nutritionist to plan diet

Administer antiemetics as ordered before meals or chemotherapy

Administer total parenteral nutrition (TPN) as ordered (p. 36)

Expected outcome/evaluation

Weight loss is controlled

Calories are maximized through use of six feedings and use of high-calorie foods or patient receives TPN

■ **NDX:** Altered oral mucous membrane related to candida infection, herpes simplex, hairy leukoplakia, Kaposi's sarcoma, or chemotherapy

Assess oral mucous membranes q8h
Note color, moisture, presence of lesions
Note color, amount, and consistency of saliva
Report presence and/or changes in lesions

Assess ability to swallow q8h; report difficulty to physician

Obtain culture of lesions as ordered; report positive results

Institute oral hygiene regimen q2h during waking hours and q6h during the night
Brush with soft-bristled toothbrush and nonabrasive toothpaste q4h
Use dilute nonalcohol mouthwash q2h
Hydrogen peroxide and normal saline: swish, gargle, and expectorate

Baking soda (1 tsp in 8 oz water): swish, gargle, and expectorate

Use toothette or cotton-tipped applicator to remove mucus and debris

Apply water-soluble lubricant to lips q2h while awake

Administer antifungal medication as ordered

Topical anesthetics may be ordered for use before meals

Administer mild analgesic as ordered

Provide time for patient to prepare for meals

Provide foods that are nonirritating, easily chewed, and high in protein

Use soft foods often: custards, yogurt, soups, soft casseroles, etc.

Avoid very sweet foods

Hot, spicy, or acidic foods are usually intolerable

Hard fruits and vegetables may be grated to make them palatable

Solid foods should be pureed or gravies and sauces added to assist with swallowing

Encourage fluids to 2000 ml/day; flavored ice pops may be appealing

Use straws or cups for liquidized foods; utensils, especially forks, may cause more discomfort

If severe stomatitis occurs increase oral hygiene to q1h to q2h

Choice of dental equipment depends on patient's comfort; toothettes or cotton-tipped swaps may be used

Moderate-to-strong analgesics may be ordered

If oral hygiene is painful, a topical anesthetic may be required 15 min before

If patient is unable to brush or rinse, irrigate mouth with rubber-tipped syringe or soft rubber catheter and irrigating container

Place patient in 60- to 90-degree position

Gently irrigate all surfaces, allowing solution to flow into emesis basin

Use saline solution

Discard unused solution

Expected outcome/evaluation

Oral lesions are healing and patient performs oral care without assistance or oral care is performed q1h to 2h; lesions are unchanged with no new lesions noted

■ **NDX:** Potential altered protection related to thrombocytopenia

Auscultate chest for heart and breath sounds q4h

Monitor cardiac status continuously

Monitor central venous pressure (CVP) q2h to 4h

Check BP, T, R, and apical pulse q4h

Assess sensorium and neurological status q4h to 8h

Check stools for bleeding

Measure intake and output; check urine for bleeding q4h to 8h

Assess skin and mucous membranes for extension or new sites of ecchymosis, hemorrhage, or hematoma q4h

If bleeding tendency or hemorrhage

Use smallest-gauge needles possible

Consolidate laboratory work; use fingersticks when appropriate

Apply pressure to site of puncture for 5 min and observe q15min for 1 hr

Do not disturb clots

Do not take rectal temperature or administer rectal medications

Have patient avoid scratching

Use soft-bristled toothbrush, towels, and nonabrasive soaps

Assist with walking when necessary to avoid bumps and falls

Keep patient warm

Encourage use of warm robes, socks

Provide extra blankets; avoid use of extra heating pads because of reduced sensation

Have patient avoid constipation

Increase fluids to 2500 ml/24 hr if permitted

Add bulk to diet

Use stool softeners or laxatives as ordered

Administer blood component transfusions as ordered

If patient is not hemorrhaging, rate of transfusion is not to exceed 1 ml/kg body weight/hr; do not extend transfusion more than 4 hr

Remember the lower the Hgb, the slower the rate of transfusion

Administer platelets as ordered

Assess for blood reactions

Maintain balance sheet

Monitor laboratory studies

Prepare for bone marrow transplantation when ordered

Expected outcome/evaluation

Vital signs remain stable; there is no evidence of bleeding; skin and mucous membranes are warm and moist with good turgor

■ **NDX:** Potential for impaired skin integrity related to malnutrition, AIDS-related infection, immobility, Kaposi's sarcoma, or chemotherapy

Assess skin condition q4h to 8h, especially sites of invasive procedure, axilla and breast folds, groin, perineal and dependent extremities; note temperature, moisture, color, texture, lesions

Report early signs of infection, skin breaks, or changes in condition of skin; note presence or changes in Kaposi's lesions

Assist with daily bath as necessary
   Use mild antibacterial soaps and soft cloths
   Rinse and dry well
   If using lotions, do not leave skin moist; avoid use of colognes and antiperspirants

Sponge patient, dry well, and change clothing when diaphoretic

Keep bed linens dry and wrinkle free; use bed cradle as necessary

Lift patient with turn sheet; avoid sliding

Prevent pressure and friction by placing pillows between pressure areas (knees, ankles)

Flotation bed may be necessary

Assist patient with turning and repositioning q2h when on bed rest, encourage small position changes q30min to 60min

Assist with and teach active or perform passive range-of-motion exercises to all extremities q4h

Increase activity as allowed; assist patient out of bed and into chair; have patient avoid sitting for more than 30 min

Teach and assist with perianal care after each elimination

Teach handwashing technique to be used after elimination and prn

Have patient avoid bumps, bruising, cuts, scratches

Explain importance of skin care to patient

Avoid IM injections and multiple venipunctures

Withdraw all blood samples for laboratory work via central line catheter using strict aseptic technique or consolidate laboratory work if no central line

See Decubitus (Pressure) Ulcer (p. 523)

Expected outcome/evaluation

Skin and tissue remain free of new areas of excoriation and breakdown

Healing of invasive sites is beginning

■ **NDX:**   Potential for body image disturbance related to Kaposi's sarcoma lesions, severe weight loss caused by malnutrition and/or diarrheal incontinence and odor, or alopecia caused by chemotherapy

Determine patient's perception of change in body image

Provide accepting and supportive atmosphere

Encourage verbalization of emotions such as anger, frustration, fear about altered functioning

Be nonjudgmental when cleaning patient after episode of incontinence or assisting with daily care

Teach methods to avoid elimination accidents and odors

Discuss potential for hair loss that occurs with specific chemotherapy; employ interventions when required (see p. 681)

Encourage discussion of physical changes in simple, direct, and factual manner

Give realistic feedback about changes

Assist significant others in adapting to change by providing resources, encouraging verbalization, and including in care of patient

Encourage patient to participate in care, especially decision-making

Give positive feedback for attempts to enhance and integrate new body image

Allow patient to progress at own rate; do not force independent functioning too soon or allow too much dependency

Assess previous adaptive and maladaptive responses to stressors and illness
   Use active listening for nonverbal cues as well as verbal statements

Assess for self-destructive behavior and intervene as appropriate

Provide assistance from other professionals to help patient to deal with changes (support groups, psychiatry)

Expected outcome/evaluation

Discusses feelings and changes in lifestyle and appearance with significant other and/or care giver

Participates in ADLs to limits of ability

Makes arrangements to meet with support group

Seeks assistance from other professionals when needed

■ **NDX:**   Potential for injury, related to visual, auditory, and tactile changes in response to CNS HIV, or opportunistic infection

Assess level of consciousness, behavior, and irritability q2h to 4h

Check pupil response, ability to fix and follow, extraocular movements, response to sound, muscle tone, q2h to 4h

Assess reflexes; test cranial nerves q2h to 4h

Assess vital signs q2h to 4h

Maintain patent airway in absence of gag reflex

Keep lights dimmed to prevent aggravation of photophobia

Approach patient and place objects within visual field

Use eye patch for diplopia; alternate patched eye

Protect eyes if corneal reflex absent; use eye medication as ordered

Talk in quiet, soothing tone

Approach patient and converse on side of greatest hearing

Establish alternate means of communication if hearing is severely diminished

Allow patient to assume position of comfort; protect from injury; keep bed in low position with rail up

Assist with meals and ADLs to prevent injury

Gradually resume activities as status improves

Assess improvements in neurological status

Assess return of vision and hearing; identify sensory losses, if any, and make appropriate referrals

Expected outcome/evaluation

Patient remains free of injury

■ **NDX:** Activity intolerance related to imbalance between oxygen supply and demand

If patient is on bed rest
  Maintain position of comfort
  Perform active or passive ROM exercises qid
  Assist with ADLs and ambulation to conserve energy
Plan undisturbed rest periods to conserve energy and permit performance of activities patient desires
Monitor pulse and respiratory rate qid and during activities
Assess adverse responses to activities: tachycardia, dysrhythmias, dyspnea, etc.
Set goals with patient to increase activities as symptoms of intolerance decrease
Explain that activity tolerance may increase with therapy

Expected outcome/evaluation

Performs ADLs without evidence of exertional dyspnea or tachycardia; activity level is progressing to pre-illness state

■ **NDX:** Sexual dysfunction related to limitations imposed by symptoms (fatigue, decreased libido, depression), fear of rejection by partner, potential for disease transmission, or impotence

Provide privacy when discussing sexuality
Determine knowledge and attitude about AIDS in relation to sexuality
Clarify any uncertainties regarding terminology, e.g., slang usage
Provide opportunities for expression of concerns, feelings of anger, anxiety, frustration
Be nonjudgmental; explain normalcy of feelings expressed
Be aware of own discomfort level and how personal attitude may affect interactions with patient
Listen actively; be aware of nonverbal cues
Provide private time and encourage patient to discuss concerns and feelings with sexual partner
  Encourage couple to focus on strengths of their relationship and to determine influence of changed sexual expression
Provide information about alternate methods for sexual expression while avoiding activities (see box above) that permit any exchange of body fluids, feces, or blood between partners
  Follow AIDS safe sex guidelines (see box above)

SAFE-SEX GUIDELINES

SAFE SEX PRACTICES

Inform previous and present partners (and those with whom you share needles) of their possible exposure; if partner is female and pregnant immediate referral for medical evaluation is advised
Inform potential partners of HIV-positive status
If female, avoid pregnancy
Limit sexual partners, preferably to one
Avoid oral-genital contact
Avoid sexual intercourse, if possible, and especially those practices that may injure tissues, e.g., anal intercourse
Modify techniques so that body fluids, blood, and feces are not exchanged, e.g., massage, hugging, dry social kissing, self-masturbation, use of sex toys (never share these)

LOW-RISK SEX PRACTICES

Vaginal or anal penetration
  Use *latex* condoms from start to finish to protect partner from contact with body fluids (natural-skin condoms allow the passage of HIV)
  Apply spermicide with nonoxol-9 inside and outside of the condom, this appears to give added protection if the condom breaks
  Use water-soluble lubricant to decrease incidence of breakage (oil-based lubricants can damage the condom)
French (wet) kissing
  This is controversial because HIV is found in saliva, but no instance of transmission via this method is reported; avoid if either partner has mouth sores
Mutual masturbation
  Use *latex* gloves to guard against possible exposure through cuts on hands

---

Expected outcome/evaluation

Patient verbalizes sexual concerns
Identifies safe sexual practices
Makes positive statements concerning altered modes of sexual expression

■ **NDX:** Social isolation related to social stigma of HIV infection, inadequate support system, fear of contracting infections from others

Determine patient's support systems: significant other, family, social groups
Encourage expression of feelings of aloneness, rejection, and isolation
Be nonjudgmental; ensure acceptance of feelings

```
┌─────────────────────────────────────────┐
│             UNSAFE SEX PRACTICES          │
│                                           │
│  Vaginal or anal intercourse without a condom │
│  Unprotected penetration of vagina or anus with │
│    hand or finger                         │
│  Blood contact of any kind                │
│  Sharing sex toys or needles              │
└─────────────────────────────────────────┘
```

Encourage visiting by significant other

Reinforce information to patient and significant other that AIDS is not transmitted through casual contact and that patient will not contract infections through socialization with healthy people

Teach significant other and visitors universal precautions to allay fears

Explain rationale for universal precautions

Assist patient in maintaining contact with others via telephone, assist with letter writing, etc.

Recognize own attitudes toward patients, lifestyle, and AIDS, and that positive or negative responses can be communicated nonverbally as well as verbally

Arrange to spend time with patient when visitors are not expected for long periods

Consider use of touch to communicate acceptance

Assist patient in assessing value of self, achievements, and environment in a positive way

Plan with significant other, family, or friends to enhance environment and provide diversional activities

Have picture albums or scrapbooks available

Provide favorite objects from home

Provide special music, videotapes, books of poetry or humor

Send unexpected gifts, e.g., balloons, special foods

Provide information about support groups; assist with arrangements for participation

Expected outcome/evaluation

Patient maintains previous relationships

Participates in support or self-help groups, forming new relationships

Verbalizes decreased sense of isolation

■ **NDX:** Dysfunctional grieving related to changes in functioning, lifestyle; life-threatening prognosis

Be sensitive to changes and restrictions in patient's and significant other's lifestyle and effect of diagnosis

Provide an atmosphere conducive to open discussion

Provide information about diagnosis, procedures, and treatment

Encourage questions; answer clearly, consistently, and clarify when necessary

Encourage patient to express feelings of anger, frustration, fear, uncertainty, etc.

Actively listen; be sensitive to nonverbal clues

Be patient and empathetic as patient experiences emotional changes and develops coping mechanisms

Set limits on maladaptive coping mechanisms if they interfere with patient's well-being

Support adaptive behaviors that suggest a progression and resolution of the grieving process

Support realistic hope, answer questions honestly, providing requested information

Provide opportunities for private time with significant other

Assist with identifying ways to adapt lifestyle as condition changes

Provide information regarding support groups that may assist patient and significant other to work through the grieving process

Provide assistance from other professional as needed and desired (social worker, clergy, psychiatrist)

Provide references for financial assistance and medical insurance assistance as needed and required

Expected outcome/evaluation

Patient begins progression through the grieving process as evidenced by expression of feelings to significant other or care giver, use of effective coping mechanisms, and compliance with treatment plans

■ **NDX:** Knowledge deficit relation to lack of information about disease process, complications/risk reduction, nutrition, activities, and continuing health care

Disease process

Explain disease process and methods to prevent transmission of HIV infection

Handwashing technique

Use of disposable latex gloves, impervious aprons or gowns for direct contact with blood or body fluids

Use of masks for care giver with URI infections or if possibility of aerosolized secretion anticipated

Protective eyewear if possibility of contact with splashes or aerosolized secretions exists

Dispose of soiled waste in separate, secured bags

Wash soiled linen separately in 1% bleach solution

Dispose of needles in impervious container

Wash dishes and utensils in hot, soapy water

Avoid sharing eating utensils, hygiene items (toothbrush, towels, etc.), sexual devices, or needles

Follow AIDS safe-sex guidelines

Never donate blood or semen

Stress importance of obtaining current, factual information about AIDS

Complications/risk reduction

Teach patient/significant other how to check for signs and symptoms of opportunistic infections and cancer complications

Teach signs and symptoms to report to care provider

Instruct in temperature-taking, recording; when to report elevation

Stress importance of maintaining clean home environment and what products to use, especially for bathroom and kitchen

Stress need to avoid cleaning cat litter box, bird cage unless wearing disposable gloves; never clean fish tanks because of toxoplasmosis

Instruct patient to wash hands after bathroom use; before eating, preparing food, and performing hygiene or procedures

Explain importance of avoiding persons who may be infectious or who may have contagious conditions, persons who have been recently vaccinated, and crowds

Explain importance of preventing injury to skin; e.g., use electric shavers, handle sharp objects with care, wear protective gloves when using strong household cleaners or handling hot cooking utensils, and avoid going barefoot

Stress importance of maintaining oral hygiene regimen, daily hygiene practices and perineal care

Discuss types of equipment to use for hygiene measures

Stress need to maintain balance between activity and rest

Explain importance of not sharing items with another person

Teach importance of stress management as well as stress reduction techniques

Stress need to avoid use of alcohol, tobacco products, and recreational drugs

Nutrition

Explain need to maintain balanced diet and liquids of choice to 2000 ml/daily

Discuss methods to use to increase intake of nutrients and liquids

Teach how to handle and store food to minimize bacterial count

Teach care of central line, heparin flush, administration of TPN (p. 36), and use of volumetric pump when in place

Activities

Explain need to perform daily self-care and to increase daily activity to tolerance

Demonstrate use of walking aids and oxygen equipment when needed

Plan exercise program
ROM and breathing exercises if on bed rest
Daily walking schedule
Use of exercise equipment as allowed

Stress importance of maintaining relationships and developing alternate diversional activities

Stress value of resuming work obligations and routine activities when possible

Stress importance of asking for and using assistance when required so that daily routine is pleasurable and satisfying

Continuing Health Care

Explain importance of on-going outpatient care
Follow-up appointments with physician or other health care provider
Routine laboratory appointments
Appointments at outpatient treatment clinics

Stress need to inform dentist, other health care providers that patient has HIV infection

Explain importance of avoiding over-the-counter medications without checking with physician and avoiding use of recreational drugs (especially IV drugs)

Teach about prescribed medications
Names, dosage, time of administration, purpose, and side or toxic effects to report

Teach medication injection and/or inhalation method when required

Stress importance of use of medical alert identification

Provide information about resources that may assist in coping with disease
Hospital, outpatient, community support, or self-help discussion groups
Psychological, psychiatric resources
Community AIDS projects and hot lines
Resources for financial assistance, medical insurance, or legal assistance
Social services available

Expected outcome/evaluation

Patient and/or significant other verbalizes understanding of home care and follow-up instructions for avoiding complications, maintenance of home environment, precautions to avoid disease transmission/reinfection, diet, activity, relationship management, and continuing health care; demonstrates temperature-taking, checking for signs of infection or cancer, oral hygiene, general hygiene and perineal measures, management of central line and TPN therapy, and medication injection/inhalation method when required

RHEUMATOID ARTHRITIS

A chronic systemic autoimmune disease of unknown etiology characterized by an inflammatory reaction in the synovial membrane leading to destruction of joint cartilage and subsequent deformities

Assessment
Observations/findings

Fatigue
Malaise
Weight loss
Joint pain and stiffness, especially on rising
Joint inflammation and swelling
Impaired joint function
Shiny, taut skin over impaired joint
Elevated temperature (low grade)
Muscular weakness, spasms, atrophy, contractions
Subcutaneous nodules over bony prominences: hands, elbows, knees
Parasthesia of hands and feet

Laboratory/diagnostic studies

Complete blood cell count (CBC), white blood cell count (WBC), erythrocyte sedimentation rate (ESR)
ASO titer, rheumatoid factor
C-reactive protein (CRP)
Serum protein electrophoresis
Antinuclear antibodies (ANA)
Arthroscopy with synovial membrane biopsy
Joint radiological study

Potential complications

Anemia
Gastrointestinal (GI) bleeding
Renal calculi
Pericarditis
Tenosynovitis
Contractures

Medical Management

Acetylsalicylic acid: buffered, enteric coated
Nonsteroid antiinflammatory agents: ibuprofen (Motrin) naproxen (Naprosyn)
Antirheumatic agents: gold, sodium thiomaleate, penicillamine
Corticosteroids
Immunosuppressive agents; azathioprine (Imuran)
Tranquilizers, antidepressants
Physical therapy: paraffin glove, whirlpool, moist heat, cold or heat
Splints, braces
Diet, activity
Surgical intervention: total arthroplasty, synovectomy, arthrodesis

Nursing diagnoses/interventions/evaluation

■ **NDX:** Pain related to joint inflammation, edema

Maintain bed rest
Use firm mattress, bedboard, and footboard as indicated

Maintain proper body alignment; assist and teach patient to
  Extend joints as tolerated
  Avoid external rotation of extremities: utilize sandbags or trochanter rolls
  Avoid use of pillow under knees
  Place pillow between knees
  Avoid flexion of neck; use thin pillow beneath head
Provide foot cradle
Apply splints, braces, or traction as indicated
Immobilize and/or support joints
Avoid jarring or quick, jerky movements
Handle affected limbs gently, giving support above and below joint
Monitor treatments for effectiveness
  Hot pack, tub baths
  Ice pack, paraffin, whirlpool
Administer skin care and gentle rubs
Use sheepskin, foam, water, or air mattress, and/or elbow and heel guards
Assess location, intensity of pain: use pain rating scale
Monitor administration of acetylsalicylic acid
  Observe for overdose: tinnitus, GI upset, or bleeding
  Assess effectiveness of pain relief measures
Discuss and promote alternate pain relief measures

Expected outcome/evaluation

Reports a tolerable level of pain
Appears relaxed, comfortable
Uses learned relaxation skills appropriately

■ **NDX:** Impaired physical mobility related to joint inflammation, swelling, and pain

Assist with and teach active and/or perform passive ROM exercises after heat treatments or apply passive ROM machine (p. 8)
Assist with and teach isometric and resistive exercises
Develop and teach planned daily exercise program
Observe patient's tolerance to exercise program and modify accordingly
Include physical therapy in program
Encourage self-care activities and independence
Promote decision-making and goal setting
Maintain planned rest periods
Maintain a safe environment
  Handrails, shower, tub, toilet
  Raised toilet seat
  Rubber-tipped walker, cane
  Raised chairs
  Wheelchair in locked position when stationary

Expected outcome/evaluation

Patient
  Functions well, within confines of disability

Participates in treatment and care

Demonstrates positive behaviors that increase level of activity

■ **NDX:** Potential for injury related to risk of side effects of pharmacological agents

Administer medications and assess for effectiveness and side effects

Monitor vital signs and observe for gastric bleeding: tarry stools, hematemesis

Monitor hemoglobin (Hgb), hematocrit (Hct), white blood cells (WBC), and platelets

Check for aspirin toxicity; headache, nausea, tinnitus, bleeding gums

Check for steroid toxicity: hypernatremia, hypokalemia, gastritis

Expected outcome/evaluation

Vital signs are within normal limits for patient

Medication side effects are minimal or absent

Laboratory results are within normal limits

■ **NDX:** Body image disturbance related to altered body function

Encourage verbalization about fears and anxiety of disease process

Assist patient in selecting adaptive coping skills

Deal with behavioral changes: denial, powerlessness, anxiety, dependence

Be supportive but firm in setting goals

Promote self-care and involve in planning care

Encourage independence and give praise for tasks accomplished

Modify environment and allow time for patient to accomplish goals

Discuss needed limitations and lifestyle changes; provide empathy and understanding

Expected outcome/evaluation

Expresses increasing confidence in coping ability

Participates in planning own care and activities

Accepts needed changes in lifestyle

■ **NDX:** Self-care deficit: feeding, bathing/hygiene, dressing/grooming, related to impaired physical ability

Assess usual level of functioning

Administer pain control before activities

Approach patient with confidence

Teach self-care activities and assist as needed

Establish and teach routine plan for ADLs

Assist with feedings prn; have patient use large-grip handles for utensils as needed

Set goals with patient; encourage short-term, easily accomplished goals

Discuss use of velcro clothing and slip-on shoes

Allow sufficient time for completing tasks

Expected outcome/evaluation

Performs self-care at optimal level within parameters of disability

Seeks needed assistance appropriately

Uses devices to increase self-care ability

■ **NDX:** Knowledge deficit related to lack of information about home care management

Stress importance of maintaining prescribed exercise, activity, and rest program

Stress importance of maintaining correct body alignment

Discuss energy-saving techniques

Reinforce physicians explanation of disease process, expectations, and limitations

Discuss diet management; stress importance of balanced diet high in vitamins, iron, and protein and no undue weight gain

Provide medication schedule, including name, dosage, purpose, side effects, and signs of aspirin and steroid toxicity

Discuss taking enteric-coated aspirin and taking medicine with meals

Explain that constipation should be avoided; use stool softeners and natural laxatives

Promote follow-up visits with physician

Provide information about support groups

Expected outcome/evaluation

Verbalizes understanding of disease process, diet, and activity regimen

Demonstrates ability to care for self within disease parameters

Expresses understanding of medication schedule/side effects

SYSTEMIC LUPUS ERYTHEMATOSUS (SLE)

A chronic, autoimmune inflammatory disease of the connective tissues that produces biochemical and structural changes in skin, joints, and muscles, usually with multiple organ involvement; the number of organs involved makes the disease an imitator of many other diagnoses

Assessment
Observations/findings

Fever

Malaise

Weakness

Anorexia

Nausea
Vomiting
Diarrhea
Abdominal pain
Weight loss
Hepatosplenomegaly
Lymphadenopathy
Drug history of hydralazine, procainamide, and/or isoniazid
Allergies
Renal system
   Hematuria
   Cellular casts*
   Proteinuria*
   Hypertension
   Edema
   Azotemia
   Hypoproteinemia
Central nervous system (CNS)
   Neuritis
   Headache
   Seizures*
Joints
   Nondeforming arthritis
   Joint warmth and swelling
Integumentary system
   Sensitivity to sun*
   Rash/erythema, "butterfly" over cheeks and bridge of nose*
   Partial alopecia*
   Oral or nasal ulcerations*
Respiratory system
   Pleuritis
   Parenchymal lung infiltrates
   Pulmonary hemorrhage
Cardiovascular system
   Pericarditis
   Murmurs
   Cardiomegaly
   Raynaud's phenomenon*
   Vasculitis: necrosis of small arteries
   Electrocardiogram (ECG) changes: dysrhythmias
Abdomen
   Peritonitis
Ocular system
   Retinal "cytoid" bodies
   Conjunctivitis
   Photophobia
   Diplopia
Behavioral changes
   Personality changes
   Depression
   Psychosis*

Hematological system
   Hemolytic anemia*

Laboratory/diagnostic studies

LE prep (positive)
Antinuclear antibodies (ANA) (positive)*
Anti-double-standard DNA antibody (positive)
Flourescent treponemal antibody absorption (FTA-ABS) (negative)
Complement (C3 and C4)
CBC, C-reactive protein, ESR, coagulation profile, rheumatoid factor, urinalysis
Thrombocytopenia
Leukopenia
False positive serology*
Creatinine clearance test
Chest radiological study
Skin and kidney biopsies

Potential complications

Infections from long-term steroid therapy
Complications from any one of the multisystems affected, such as renal failure, MI, pneumonia, CVA

Medical Management

Nonsteroid antiinflammatory agents
Corticosteroid therapy
Antiinfective agents
Antineoplastic agents
Medications related to system(s) affected; antihypertensives, analgesics, bronchodilators, topical ointments, antipyretics, antibiotics
Plasmapheresis, dialysis
Joint arthoplasty
Diet, activity, rest

Nursing diagnoses/interventions†/evaluation

■ **NDX:** Altered tissue perfusion, renal, cerebral, related to multisystem involvement

Assess renal status; observe for signs of edema, nausea, hematuria, and hypertension
   Measure urine output as needed
   Provide antihypertensive medication and monitor for effectiveness/side effects
   Provide low-salt diet
   Monitor urinalysis and kidney function studies
Assess neurological status; observe for alterations in orientation, judgment, mental acuity, speech, and muscle tone
   Provide a safe environment

---

*Four or more of these findings support the diagnosis of SLE.

*Four or more of these findings support a diagnosis of SLE.
†Patient's condition dictates amount and type of care required; modify accordingly.

Assist as needed with activity, meals, and toileting

Observe for personality changes; monitor for signs of suicide and intervene as appropriate

Encourage communication with significant other

Expected outcome/evaluation

Output balances intake; kidney function and urinalysis studies within normal range

Remains oriented: mental acuity, speech and judgment return to preacute stage

■ **NDX:** Impaired physical mobility related to joint involvement

Assess for muscle/joint involvement

Monitor ability to move, observe for pain, swelling, and limited ROM

Administer ROM exercises as ordered to unaffected joints or use passive ROM machine

Apply warm or cold compresses to area as ordered

Expected outcome/evaluation

Performs ROM with all extremities

Has no swelling nor complaints of increased pain with movement

■ **NDX:** Ineffective breathing patterns related to decreased energy/fatigue and pulmonary involvement

Assess respiratory system; observe for dyspnea, cyanosis, decreased breath sounds, tachypnea, bradypnea, rales, and rhonchi

Auscultate chest for breath sound q4h

Elevate head of bed and maintain bed rest during acute phase to conserve oxygen

Encourage patient to turn, cough, and deep breathe

Administer oxygen therapy, steroids, antiarrhythmics and bronchodilators

Assess for effectiveness/side effects

Monitor for signs of pneumonia

Culture any sputum obtained

Expected outcome/evaluation

Respirations are slow, even; and deep breaths are performed without discomfort

Participates in treatment and care with more energy and confidence

■ **NDX:** Decreased cardiac output related to alterations in mechanical/electrical factors caused by disease

Assess cardiac status

Monitor vital signs q4h; monitor apical pulse and observe for dysrhythmias, tachycardia, bradycardia

Monitor arterial pulses for bruits

Observe for peripheral edema

Administer antiarrhythmia medications as indicated

Monitor for effectiveness/side effects

Observe ECG results

Monitor jugular vein for distention

Monitor intake and output

Expected outcome/evaluation

Vital signs are normal for patient

Intake and output is balanced; skin turgor is adequate

Peripheral edema, jugular distention is absent

■ **NDX:** Impaired tissue integrity related to integumentary involvement

Assess integumentary status; observe skin and mucous membranes for color, temperature, turgor, edema, signs of infection, and rashes

Administer topical steroid and antibiotic ointments as indicated; monitor for effectiveness/side effects

Advise use of lubricants, e.g., artificial tears and vaginal water-soluble lubricants if needed

Provide nonallergenic soaps and creams

Promote sunscreen use if patient is photosensitive

Administer skin care and oral hygiene prn

Assist patient with changing position frequently and moving feet and legs to promote venous return

Encourage ambulation as soon as possible

Expected outcome/evaluation

Skin color, temperature, integrity are normal for patient

Verbalizes understanding of skin care procedure

Participates in care of skin and mucous membranes

■ **NDX:** Altered nutrition: less than body requirements, related to anorexia, fatigue, and/or electrolyte imbalance

Assess nutritional status and monitor caloric intake as indicated

Provide well-balanced, small, frequent meals; encourage patient selection; serve attractively

Assist with meals as needed

Provide calm, unhurried atmosphere

Encourage rest period after meals

Monitor electrolytes

Determine weight gain related to steroid therapy; sodium may be restricted

Weigh patient daily at same time with same clothing and scale

Provide vitamin supplement for pregnant or dieting patient

Monitor abdomen for distention, pain, and tenderness

Expected outcome/evaluation

Reports an increased appetite and finishes 90% of meals
Maintains weight normal for patient
Verbalizes an increased level of energy

■ **NDX:** Potential activity intolerance related to fatigue and arthralgia

Assess activity level and ROM of affected extremities
Provide bed rest during exacerbation
Administer analgesics to control discomfort and increase activity to tolerance
Provide a safe environment
Increase activity slowly; provide ROM exercises to unaffected joints q4h
Assist with chair sitting when allowed; support affected joint(s)
Increase ambulation as tolerated; use crutches, walker, or cane as needed

Expected outcome/evaluation

Participates in own care to tolerance
Seeks assistance as needed
Progresses toward increased activity level

■ **NDX:** Potential for infection related to altered immune system and steroid therapy

Monitor WBC and differential, ESR, C-reactive protein, urinalysis, and cultures for signs of sepsis
Culture drainage from skin rashes, breaks, injection sites, etc., and sputum, urine, etc.
Monitor temperature for febrile state
Administer antipyretics, antibiotics as indicated; monitor for effectiveness and side effects
Maintain clean environment and good personal hygiene
Institute isolation precautions as needed
Restrict infectious visitors and staff
Maintain adequate rest and sleep patterns
Provide optimal nutrition and fluid intake

Expected outcome/evaluation

Remains afebrile
Laboratory values are within normal limits
Normal skin integrity is normal for patient

■ **NDX:** Body image disturbance related to altered physical appearance

Encourage patient to express feelings and concerns; listen attentively
Reinforce physician's explanation of disease process: its chronicity, treatment, remissions, and exacerbations; clarify misconceptions

Assist with and teach stress management methods; imagery, relaxation
Provide a supportive environment, praising positive ideas and accomplishments; promote self confidence
Identify coping patterns and strengths that were successful in past experiences
Assist in and promote ways of improving body image; wig for alopecia, make-up, improved hygiene
Promote communication with significant other

Expected outcome/evaluation

Verbalizes understanding of disease process, treatment plan
Initiates suggestions for coping with altered body image
Applies learned behaviors in dealing with stressful feelings

■ **NDX:** Knowledge deficit related to lack of information about home care management

Provide and discuss written diet, activity, and rest instructions as prescribed
Stress importance of skin care; explain need to use only nonallergenic preparations on skin and hair, need to avoid exposure to sun and use sunscreen with protection factor of 15, and need to avoid hair dyes and fluorescent lights
Provide instructions on medication schedule, including name, purpose, dosage, and side effects, especially for steroids; explain that they must be taken without interruption; explain need to avoid penicillin, sulfa, phenytoin, and oral contraceptives
Stress importance of avoiding infectious individuals
Discuss signs and symptoms of exacerbation to report to physician: fever, rash, cough, joint pain
Promote and encourage patient to wear medical alert indicating dose of steroid and name and number of physician
Discuss advantages of assistance from Lupus Foundation*
Promote follow-up visits with physician

Expected outcome/evaluation

Demonstrates understanding of prescribed dietary regimen, rest and activity schedule
Verbalizes understanding of medication schedule and side effects
Expresses knowledge of symptoms to report to physician

SARCOIDOSIS

A multisystem granulomatous disorder of unknown etiology; any organ system may be involved, but pul-

---

*Lupus Foundation of America, Inc, 1717 Massachusetts NW, Suite 203, Washington, DC 20036.

monary manifestations are most common; in most cases process is benign and self-limiting without residual effects; 10% become chronic conditions; staged according to international standards, based on chest x-ray findings; fatal in 5% of cases; most common in young adults and among blacks

Assessment
Observations/findings

Weight loss
Anorexia
Fever, night sweats
Arthralgias (diffuse)
Arthritis (symmetrical, migratory)
Fatigue
Respiratory
  Clubbing of fingers
  Dyspnea
  Cough: usually unproductive but may be incapacitating and occur in paroxysms that lead to vomiting
  Hypoxemia
  Hypercapnia
  Crackles: diffuse or just at bases
Ocular
  Blurred vision
  Lacrimation
  Ocular pain
  Conjunctival infection
  Uvietis, iritis
  Blindness (rare)
Cardiovascular
  Mild-to-severe chest pain (rare)
  Palpitations
  Fatigue
  Dysrhythmias: PVCs, bundle branch or complete heart block
  Hypotension
  Jugular vein distention
  Cardiomyopathy (rare)
Cutaneous
  Skin nodules over face, neck, and extremities
  Erythema nodosum
  Bone cysts in hands and feet
  Nasal mucosal lesions
  Alopecia
Lymphatic
  Parotid and cervical lymphadenopathy
  Splenomegaly

Laboratory/diagnostic studies

Kveim skin test (intradermally injected sarcoid tissue suspension): positive in 3 to 6 weeks
Blood work
  CBC

Serum protein levels (C-reactive protein elevated); polyclonal hypergamma globulinemia (increased IgG but IgA and IgM may also be elevated)
Erythrocyte sedimentation rate (ESR): elevated
Angiotensins converting enzyme level: may be elevated
Skin and lymph node biopsy
Transbronchial biopsy via bronchoscopy
Open-lung biopsy
Bronchoalveolar lavage
Gallium-67 scan
Chest x-ray examination
  Abnormal in 90% of patients during course of illness
  Various from hilar lymphadenopathy to diffuse infiltrates and pulmonary fibrosis
  Pulmonary function tests: spirometry may be normal or show decreased vital capacity and expiratory flow rates, as well as decreased lung compliance

Potential complications

Restrictive lung disease (pulmonary fibrosis, progressive lung disability)
Complications of steroid therapy (diabetes millitus, fluid retention, electrolyte imbalances, infection)

Medical Management

No treatment if symptoms are mild
Medications
  Systemic or topical steroids
  Azathioprine (Imuran) if steroids are contraindicated
  Optic agents
  Antiarrhythmic agents
  Calcium-chelating medication if needed
Routine chest x-ray examination and pulmonary function monitoring
Low-calcium, low-salt, low-potassium diet
Vitamin D supplements
Chest physiotherapy; breathing exercises, postural drainage, and oxygen therapy
Thermal therapy and joint supports for arthritis

Nursing diagnoses/interventions/evaluation

■ **NDX:** Impaired gas-exchange related to pulmonary fibrosis or parenchymal lesions

Assess respiratory status, observing for cough, adventitious sounds, dyspnea, and abnormal rate, rhythm, or quality
Obtain sputum specimens as ordered
Instruct patient on energy conservation techniques and breathing exercises (slow, deep breaths; pursed lip breathing)
Reinforce information about proper positioning and body mechanics
Monitor pulmonary function results
Administer medications and oxygen as ordered

Expected outcome/evaluation

Maintains adequate gas exchange
Evidences normal mental status and usual skin color
Blood gases within normal range

■ **NDX:** Potential for decreased cardiac output related to dysrhythmias

Maintain bed rest
Monitor cardiac activity as indicated
Monitor vital signs q2h to 4h and prn
Monitor signs and symptoms of decreased cardiac output, including edema, dyspnea, hypotension, crackles, jugular venous distention, decreased urine output, increased heart rate, cool, clammy skin, and fatigue
Administer oxygen as ordered
Report abnormal ECG, hemodynamic, and laboratory findings
Assess heart and breath sounds q2h to 4h
Administer medications as ordered

Expected outcome/evaluation

Maintains normal cardiac output
Blood pressure within normal range
Unlabored respirations
Evidences normal mental status
Usual skin color
Normal urine output

■ **NDX:** Pain related to disease-induced arthralgias and ocular discomfort

Assess pain, location, onset, duration, and precipitating and alleviating factors
Administer analgesics as ordered
Provide comfort measures as needed
　Positioning
　Warm compresses
　Rest

Expected outcome/evaluation

Experiences decreased pain
Verbalizes pain relief
Facial expression and body positioning are relaxed
Evidences improved breathing pattern

■ **NDX:** Knowledge deficit related to lack of information about home care needs

Explain the nature of disease: even if symptoms are mild, will require ongoing evaluation and care
　Routine chest x-ray examinations
　Pulmonary function tests
　Yearly eye examination

Explain need to avoid
　Strenuous exercise
　Lengthy exposure to sun
　Smoking: recommend support group prn
　Persons who smoke
　Potential sources of infection
Explain need to restrict salt, foods high in potassium, and vitamin D supplements; to restrict calcium intake if necessary
Have patient return demonstrate pulmonary toilet activities; breathing exercises, postural drainage, and chest physical therapy to prevent pulmonary infection
Discuss symptoms to report to physician
　Shortness of breath
　Red, watery eyes
　Dizziness
　Chest pain
　Swollen joints
　Unusual fatigue
　Fever
Discuss medications: name, dosage, time of administration, purpose, and side effects of corticosteroid therapy
Take antacid with dose
Watch for signs of infection
Be aware of mood swings
Avoid taking over-the-counter medications without checking with physician

Expected outcome/evaluation

Verbalizes understanding of home care and follow-up instructions
Demonstrates pulmonary toilet activities

BONE MARROW TRANSPLANTATION (BMT)

A treatment approach that has resulted in the cure of various neoplastic and hematological diseases by replenishing depleted bone marrow cell reserves; care is divided into four phases: pretransplant (preparation), conditioning, transplant, and posttransplant (Table 3-2)
There are three sources of donor bone marrow;
Allogenic is most common; donor is often a sibling, but occasionally an unrelated person
Autologous marrow uses patient's own bone marrow; performed only for malignant disease when patient is in state of remission
Syngeneic marrow comes from an identical twin; eliminates the problem of rejection and GVHD

Indications

Several types of leukemia; usually in remission
　Acute lymphocytic leukemia (ALL)
　Acute nonlymphocytic leukemia (ANLL)
　Chronic myelocytic leukemia (CML)
Aplastic anemia
Severe combined immunodeficiency disease
Thalassemia

TABLE 13-2. Typical Bone Marrow Transplant Schedule

Day	Scheduled activity
PREPARATION PHASE	
−10 to −8	Admission
	Consents
	Bone marrow aspiration
	Lumbar puncture with intrathecal methotrexate instillation (acute leukemia)
	Administration of nonabsorbable antibiotics
	Laboratory tests
	Begin low-bacterial diet
−7	Insertion of double-lumen right atrial catheter
	Dosimetry
	Begin teaching self-care procedures and activity requirements
CONDITIONING PHASE	
−6	Insertion of three-way urinary catheter
	Leukemia: high-dose cytarabine (ARA-C) or cyclophosphamide administered
	Aplastic anemia: high-dose cyclophosphamide administered
	Lymphoma: Etoposide (Vp16)
	Neuroblastoma: cisplatin; Vp16, Melphalan
	Force fluids: 4000 to 4500 ml for adults; 3000 ml/m² for children
−5	Continue high-dose chemotherapy and increased fluid intake
−4	Three-way urinary catheter discontinued if no bleeding after completion of high-dose chemotherapy
−3	Total-body irradiation (divided dose) (ordered for leukemia; may be ordered for aplastic anemia)
−2	Total-body irradiation (divided dose)
	Begin cyclosporine
−1	Total-body irradiation (divided dose)
	Immunoglobin (given day 1 and every other week thereafter)
	Donor admitted for preoperative workup
TRANSPLANT	
0	Marrow, aspirated from donor, is infused to establish graft
	If autologous transplant, granulating colony stimulating factor (GCSF) is infused 3 hours after marrow infusion
POSTTRANSPLANT	
+1 to +30	Observe for engraftment, reactions to total-body irradiation, and complications of transplanted marrow; supportive therapy: blood products, TPN, antibiotics, pain management

Lymphoma
Some solid tumors
Neuroblastoma
Acute erythrocytic leukemia

Assessment on Admission
Observations/findings

Patient may be asymptomatic if in remission
Shortness of breath
Anemia
Bleeding tendency
Easy bruising
Petechiae
Maculopapular rash
Fever
Weakness
Chronic fatigue
Pain in joints and bones

Preparation Phase

Phase during which necessary preparation procedures are performed; these include procedures for decreasing the amount of bacteria on the body surface, as well as inside the body, and diagnostic studies

Assessment
Observations/findings

Response to diagnostic procedures or medications
    Bone marrow biopsy
    Lumbar puncture
    Right atrial catheter insertion
Ability to perform self-care procedures

Laboratory/diagnostic studies

Bone marrow studies
CBC with differential
Platelet count
Fasting blood sugar (FBS)
Serum glutamic oxaloacetic transaminase (SGOT)
Serum glutamic pyruvic transaminase (SGPT)
Bilirubin (total and direct)
Alkaline phosphatase
Blood urea nitrogen (BUN)
Creatinine
Urinalysis
Quantitative immunoglobulin
HAA
HAV
HB$_S$AG
HB$_S$AB
HB$_C$AB
Magnesium
Total protein
Toxoplasmosis titer
Herpes zoster virus

Herpes simplex virus
Cytomegalovirus
Epstein-Barr virus
HIV
VDRL
Complete red blood cell type
Chest x-ray examination
Pulmonary function test
Echocardiogram (if indicated)
Electrocardiogram (ECG)
Type/screen
Surveillance cultures on admission and weekly

Medical Management

Informed consents
Laboratory and diagnostic studies
Lumbar puncture with intrathecal methotrexate (acute
    leukemia)
Insertion of double-lumen right atrial catheter
Dosimetry
Low-bacteria diet
Nonabsorbable antibiotics
Allopurinol (except aplastic anemia patients)
Bactrim
Fluconazole (if previous fungal infection)

Nursing diagnosis/interventions/evaluation

 NDX: Knowledge deficit related to lack of information
    about transplant and informed consent, central
    line, dosimetry, self-care procedures, and diet

BMT procedure

Ensure that patient and/or significant other has read in-
    formation about BMT, outcome, and possible compli-
    cations
Encourage questions; give clear, consistent answers; be
    alert for unspoken questions
Reinforce physician's explanation
Involve other health care workers as necessary to ensure
    that patient has information required to make decisions
Explain sequence of events for each phase; discuss support
    systems available to patient and family; introduce all
    health care providers who will be involved with patient;
    orient patient to environment: room, unit, radiation
    therapy department, etc.

Expected care

Explain importance of performing self-care procedures and
    maintaining exercise and activity levels throughout hos-
    pitalization and continuing after discharge for a total
    of 100 days
Teach and have patient demonstrate performance of the
    following
    Handwashing technique
        Wash hands before self-care activities and meals, and
            after toileting

Mouth care
    Must be done at least four times each day and more
        frequently if indicated
    Never use toothbrush
    May use soft sponge cleaners to clean gums and teeth
    Rinse mouth well with entire amount of one of the
        following solutions
        Alcohol-free mouthwash, 30 ml in 150 ml of saline
            or sterile water
        Sterile normal saline: 150 to 200 ml
        Sterile water: 150 to 200 ml
    Follow with antifungal rinse and swallow as ordered;
        usually ordered on day of total-body irradiation
        (TBI)
Skin care
    Daily shower with antibacterial soap
    Rinse well
    Dry all body areas thoroughly, especially folds
        Use soft towels
        Avoid vigorous rubbing
        Apply mycostatin powder to all folds and between
            the toes
    Perineal care
        Must be performed after each voiding or bowel
            movement
        Wash hands
        Place ordered amount of povidone-iodine periwash
            solution in plastic squeeze bottle
        Add sterile water to solution; never add tap water
        Place solution on sterile pad (ABD)
        Clean perineal area, from front to back for females;
            avoid use of toilet tissue
        Discard used pad
        Wash hands
Intake and output
    Give list of measurements
    Discuss measurement tools
    Have patient record amounts on bedside record sheet
Use of incentive spirometer
Explain and demonstrate assessments that will be done
    and daily frequency (qh8 or more frequently if changes
    are noted)
    Oral status
    Skin including perianal area
    Respiratory
    Cardiac
    Gastrointestinal
    Neurological
    Hematest for stool and urine
Discuss activity level that patient will be expected to
    maintain
    Shower and bathroom activities
    Ambulation and ROM exercises
    Use of exercycle

Diversionary activities: TV watching, reading, computer/TV games, small handicrafts

Explain procedures, expected effect, and rationale

Bone marrow aspiration

Lumbar puncture

Dosimetry

Insertion of central line

Explain low-bacteria diet

Diet will be used for 100 days

Only sterile distilled water and ice cubes will be used; patient should never drink tap water

Give list of foods permitted (p. 578)

Food will not be left at bedside

Food from home must be on the approved list and cooked on the day it is brought to the hospital

Expected outcome/evaluation

Patient and/or significant other verbalizes understanding of BMT procedure, anticipated tests, procedures, medication effects, and self-care expected during hospitalization

Conditioning Phase

First phase of the clinical course; involves treatment of patient with a pretransplant "conditioning regimen"; for patients with leukemia, high-dose cytarabine (ARA-C) or cyclophosphamide and total body irradiation (TBI) have become standard treatment; for patients with aplastic anemia, high-dose cyclophosphamide is given with or without TBI; for patients with lymphomas, etoposide and TBI; and for patients with neuroblastoma, cisplatin, Etoposide, melphalan, and TBI

Assessment
Observations/findings

Side effects of medications

Nausea, vomiting

Stomatitis

Diarrhea

Pancytopenia

Hemorrhagic cystitis

Sensorineural hearing loss

Azotemia, renal tubular dysfunction

Hypomagnesia

Hypocalcemia

Hypotension related to speed of Vp16 infusion

Drug fever

Alopecia

Liver toxicity

SIADH

Side effects of TBI

Anorexia

Nausea, vomiting

Parotid gland swelling

Erythema

Decreased saliva and tears

Interstitial pneumonitis

Hepatic veno-occlusive disease (VOD)

Psychosocial

Response to treatments

Relationships and support systems

Methods of coping

Understanding of disease and treatment

Laboratory/diagnostic studies

CBC

Platelet count

RBS

Electrolytes

Blood cultures if temperature spikes

Liver function test three times a week

CMV cultures, urine and blood, twice weekly

SGOT

SGPT

Bilirubin

Alkaline phosphatase

BUN

Creatinine

Urinalysis

ECG (weekly)

Weekly PT, PTT, calcium, triglyceride

Potential complications

Pneumonia

Medical Management

High-dose cyclophosphamide

Parenteral fluids

Three-way Foley catheter with bladder irrigation

Fractionated TBI for 3 days (total: 1000 rad) or high-dose cytarabine (ARA-C) and fractionated TBI

Cardiac monitoring (during conditioning TBI and cyclophosphamide administration)

Cyclosporin

Ca-trim

Antiemetics

Antipyretics

Antibiotics

Antidiarrheals

Diuretics

Daily weights

Accurate intake and output

Isolation

TPN

Irradiated blood products

Nursing diagnoses/interventions/evaluation

■ **NDX:** Knowledge deficit related to lack of information about medications and TBI procedure

Medications

Explain effects of medications and expected care
  Premedication with antiemetics
    Insertion of three-way indwelling catheter with irrigation
    Cardiac monitor use

TBI procedure

Explain TBI procedure
  Patient will be alone in room but will be able to communicate with personnel
  Patient will be visually monitored at all times
  Nurse will remain in department and provide comfort measures as needed
  Cardiac status will be monitored throughout procedure
  Patient must remain as positioned without moving
  Patient must wear mask after completion of TBI while returning to room
  Patient will be placed in isolation at completion of procedure

Expected outcome / evaluation

Patient/significant other verbalizes understanding of medications and TBI

■ **NDX:** Altered tissue perfusion (renal) (bladder) related to local effect of cyclophosphamide

Ensure adequate hydration and diuresis 24 hr before, during, and 24 to 48 hr after medication administration (cyclophosphamide)
  Force fluids to 4000 to 5000 ml/day unless contraindicated
  Enlist patient's assistance
    Provide fluids of choice and at temperature of choice
    Offer small amounts frequently to make taking fluids less of a chore
    Serve attractively
  Administer parenteral fluids as ordered: usually dextrose in saline with electrolytes; often ordered at 200 ml/hr for 5 to 6 hr before, during, and after chemotherapy infusion
Weigh patient daily at same time with same clothing and scale
Insert indwelling catheter when ordered, using strict aseptic technique
  Connect to closed-gravity drainage system
  Perform catheter care daily
Prepare for bladder irrigation when ordered
  Administer solution as ordered for continuous irrigation
  Maintain irrigation balance sheet; report discrepancies immediately
  Test return flow for occult bleeding 2qh to 4h; report positive results and observations to physician

Administer osmotic diuretics when ordered
Check T, P, R, and BP q4h to 8h; report changes

Expected outcome / evaluation

Patient does not exhibit signs of hemorrhagic cystitis

■ **NDX:** Potential for decreased cardiac output related to effects of cyclophosphamide

Know that ECG changes are *usually* transient and not related to CHF; most ECG changes do not require treatment
Monitor heart function continuously and observe for
  Tachycardia
  Extra systoles
  ST wave changes
  Transient ECG changes
  30% decrease in limb-lead QRS voltage
Auscultate chest for heart and breath sounds qh during medication administration, then q4h
See Heart Failure (p. 101)

Expected outcome / evaluation

Heart and breath sounds remain within normal limits
ECG pattern shows transient changes (specify) but returns to patient's normal pattern

■ **NDX:** Altered nutrition: less than body requirements related to nausea and vomiting, and/or inability to ingest nutrients

Nausea and vomiting

Assess amount and types of foods and liquids tolerated and desired
Maintain calorie count
Assess predisposing factors, onset, position, frequency, and duration
Eliminate predisposing factors when possible: unpleasant odors, perfume, disturbing sights or sounds
Administer oral hygiene before and after intake
  Use equipment appropriate to condition of mouth
  Administer oral anesthetic when ordered
Change eating patterns; serve frequent, light meals; avoid food and liquids 2 to 4 hr before meals; and/or change usual place for eating
Provide foods that may be served cold or at room temperature to eliminate odors: cereal, cheese, desserts
Provide clear liquid diet to reduce nausea: juices, carbonated beverages, flavored ice pops
Provide high-protein drinks as a supplement
Vary textures and tastes of foods to determine those tolerated: bland, sour, soft, etc.
Remind patient to eat slowly and chew well
Note that sweet, highly seasoned foods are not usually well tolerated

Administer antiemetics, when ordered, as patient desires

Maintain chart of onset of symptoms, response to varying dosage of medication, and frequency of administration

Arrange for quiet rest periods before meals

Assist with preparation to conserve energy

Serve foods and liquids attractively

Arrange for visitors, if patient prefers, to enhance social aspect

Institute measures to prevent fullness, bloating, such as having patient remain in sitting position at least 30 min to 1 hr after meal; avoiding rapid position change

Use other methods to prevent onset or reduce severity of symptoms
Relaxation methods
Rhythmic breathing exercises
Imagery experiences
Self-hypnosis
Behavior modification techniques

Place patient in well-ventilated room and control odors
Remove trash frequently
Empty and remove bedpans and urinals after use
Remove food trays as soon as patient has eaten

Weight patient daily at same time with same scale and clothing

Measure intake and output qh8

Notify physician when intake and output are not equivalent and/or weight decreases by 3% to 5%

Explain low-bacteria diet

NOTE: BMT patients require 33 to 38 kcal/kg and 1.5 g protein/kg

Wash hands before food preparation

Be certain work area and utensils are clean

Keep foods at proper temperature (p. 579)

Wrap food portions individually

Use only one-serving-size canned or bottled items

Serve only foods and fluids listed on diet (p. 578)

Microwave prepared foods and fluids before serving; never reheat food

Wash thick-skinned fruits or vegetables with alcohol; peel skin off before serving

Do not leave warmed food at bedside for longer than mealtime

Cold foods may be left at bedside for 2 hr when placed in container of ice

Remove uneaten foods and liquids from room before disposal

Food from home must be on the low-bacteria food list and cooked on the day it is brought to the hospital

Refrigerate food for not more than 24 hr if not served immediately

Microwave before serving

Inability to ingest foods

Administer TPN as ordered (p. 36)

Expected outcome/evaluation

Patient maintains weight or loses less than 5% of original body weight

■ **NDX:** Potential for infection related to neutropenia secondary to TBI and/or chemotherapy

NOTE: Patient is usually isolated until absolute granulocyte level is <1000 (total WBC × percentage granulocytes)

Place patient in isolation after completion of TBI (use of isolation or laminar flow rooms is controversial)

Observe strict isolation precautions
Wash hands with povidone-iodine solution and put on cap, gown, and mask before entering room
No infectious personnel or visitors may enter room
Staff assigned to care for patient must not be assigned to care for patients who have infections
Be certain that all visitors and personnel entering room know and observe handwashing technique and other protective isolation procedures
Keep one door to isolation and anteroom closed at all times; never have both doors open at same time
Provide mask if patient must leave room
Never take flowers or plants into room
Anything taken into room must be sterilized or washed with bactericidal solution
Microwave mail or papers before taking into room (controversial)
Never use anything that has been dropped on the floor
Use tap water for bathing only
Maintain low-bacteria diet using sterile water for drinking
Be certain that visitors never use patient's equipment or bathroom
Be certain that room, all equipment, furniture, fixtures, and personal items are cleaned with bactericidal solution daily
Remove food, trash, and drainage receptacles from room immediately

Assess and record skin condition q8h with special attention to skin folds and orifices

Report any redness, swelling, drainage/discharge, pain, or tenderness

Teach signs of infection

Assist with hygiene as necessary

Maintain skin integrity
Do not give IM injections
Limit venipunctures (blood cultures only)
Observe central line site q4h
Change dressing daily if nonporous type is used, using aseptic technique
Change tubing daily

Use strict sterile technique for all procedures

Assess and record condition of oral mucous membrane q4h

Remind patient to perform oral hygiene as instructed q2h; assist when necessary; teach patient to report pain or swelling

Ensure required nutrient and fluid intake

Administer antifungal medications as ordered

Assess and record condition of perineum q4h

Ensure that perianal care is performed after elimination

Prevent constipation (p. 679) or diarrhea (p. 678); administer medications as ordered

Monitor vital signs q4h
  Take temperature more frequently if trend is beginning
  Report temperature elevations immediately

Institute comfort and cooling measures as indicated
  Change linen and clothing to keep patient dry
  Administer antipyretics as ordered
  Prevent chilling

Monitor intake and output; report urinary frequency, burning, or changes in character of urine

Use voiding measures when indicated
  If catheterization is necessary
    Use strict aseptic technique for insertion
    Perform catheter care q8h
  Obtain and monitor cultures as ordered

Assess and record respiratory status q4h

Report changes in breath sounds, cough, and sputum, increases in respiratory rate, or presence of sore throat and flu symptoms

Assist or remind patient to turn and deep breathe q2h

Administer oxygen as ordered

Encourage mobility q2h

Turn and position patient q2h if on bed rest

Provide adequate, uninterrupted rest and sleep periods

Administer antibiotics on time as ordered

Expected outcome/evaluation

Demonstrates use of preventive measures

No signs of infection are noted

■ **NDX:** Anxiety related to severity of responses to conditioning and possible poor prognosis

Assess level of anxiety and understanding of disease process when appropriate

Visit frequently or have significant other remain with patient

Use touch, reassurance, and positive body language

Provide an environment conducive to discussion and expression of worries, fears, and loss

Continue to provide information about condition and procedures

Encourage questions; answer clearly, consistently, and clarify when necessary

Reassure that patient will not be alone and that care and treatment will be given when needed

Teach methods to reduce anxiety
  Relaxation techniques

Visual imagery

Be sensitive to needs; listen to nonverbal clues

Assist with and reinforce coping strategies

Encourage continuation of relationships

Expected outcome/evaluation

Patient exhibits decreasing symptoms of anxiety

Verbalizes feelings about and understanding of condition

■ **NDX:** Body image disturbance related to sterility, alopecia, and skin and body weight changes

Assess perception of change and its effect on lifestyle and relationships

Evaluate hygiene and grooming

Provide an atmosphere for expression and discussion of changes that are occurring

Visit frequently and encourage visits by significant other

Be aware of nonverbal clues: patient and nurse

Be sensitive to needs

Provide information about process patient is experiencing

Give correct information about expected positive changes: weight regained, regrowth of hair

Assist patient with decision about temporary measures for hair loss
  Short hair style before loss
  Use of wigs, hairpieces, scarves, or caps

Plan with patient to have preferred items available before needed

Assist with gentle scalp care; use pH-balanced shampoo; expose hair and scalp to air as much as possible

Assist with and encourage routine grooming

Comment on strengths exhibited; value abilities and accomplishments of patient; assist patient with recognizing these also

Expected outcome/evaluation

Patient verbalizes feelings about losses and effects of lifestyle and relationships

Uses grooming techniques to enhance appearance

Transplant Phase

Phase in which histocompatible donor bone marrow is infused to establish a graft and to reinstate production of normal blood cellular components

Autologous transplant: Patient's marrow that was previously harvested, preserved with DMSO, and frozen is thawed and infused

Allogenic and syngeneic transplant: marrow is obtained from donor and is immediately infused

Assessment
Observations/findings

Reaction to marrow infusion

Allergic reaction to white cells in marrow

Chills, fever, hives, chest pains
Bacterial contamination of marrow
    Hypotension, fever, shaking chills
Pulmonary overload
    Tachypnea, dyspnea, rales, rhonchi, elevated BP
Pulmonary emboli
    SOB, chest pain, tachycardia
Hematuria
    Pink or red; hemostix: positive 12 to 24 hr after infusion
Increased BUN and creatinine for 24 to 48 hr after marrow infusion
Autologous transplant
    Be aware of possible side effects; the patient will immediately taste the DMSO preservative; will last 24 to 48 hr
    Pronounced odor (like garlic or oyster) from patient, related to DMSO

Nursing diagnosis/interventions/evaluation

■ **NDX:**   Potential fluid volume excess related to marrow infusion

Assess hemodynamic status before marrow infusion
Administer marrow infusion at rate ordered through central line (must be infused within 4 hr)
    Never infuse through a filter
    Never irradiate marrow
Autologous transplant
    Infuse marrow slowly initially; increase rate only after DMSO is excreted
    Use 80 micron filter
    Infuse 0.9 saline during procedure
    Maintain allergic reaction medications at bedside; epinephrine, hydrocortisone, diphenhydramine
Monitor vital signs q5min during infusion; then q15min to 30min for 2 hr
Observe for reactions q15min
    Pulmonary emboli
    Volume overload
    Allergic reaction
Never stop infusion; slow if reaction occurs and notify physician
Follow orders, continue to observe patient continuously, and monitor vital signs and ECG

Expected outcome/evaluation

Vital signs remain stable
Lungs are clear to auscultation
Reaction to infusion of marrow is minimal

Posttransplant Phase

The period after infusion of bone marrow is a critical time in which many problems can occur, the degree that the patient is affected may depend on the underlying disease and clinical status before transplant

---

GRAFT VS. HOST DISEASE (GVHD)

Condition that occurs when histocompatible differences exist between bone marrow graft and recipient

OBSERVATIONS

Skin
    Maculopapular rash
    Erythroderma
    Exfoliative dermatitis
    Bulbous formation
    Desquamation
    Hair loss
    Jaundice
GI system
    Diarrhea: 500 to 1500 ml/day
    Abdominal pain
        Ileus
    Hepatomegaly
    Splenomegaly
    Muscle wasting
    Emaciation
    Increased susceptibility to infections
    Pneumonitis
    Hemolytic anemia
    Bone marrow aplasia
    Lymphatic depletion
    Death

LABORATORY STUDIES

Bilirubin elevated from 2 mg/100 dl to >15 mg/100 dl
Lymphocytopenia
Thrombocytopenia
Electrolytes
Liver function tests
Coagulation studies

Assessment
Observations/findings

Skin and mucous membranes
    Petechiae
    Diffuse maculopapular rash; may also be first symptom of graft vs. host disease (GVHD), (see box above); onset of GVHD is usually 9 to 12 days after infusion of marrow
    Bruising
    Breaks
    Lesions
    Pruritus
    Hyperpigmentation: usually 2 to 3 weeks after TBI
Jaundice
Perianal area
    Erythema

Excoriation
Abscess
Mouth
  Irritation
  Swelling
  Erythema
  Leukoplakia
  Ulcerations
  Secretions
  Consistency
  Amount
  Color
  Taste distortion
  Herpes type 1 viral infection
Lymph nodes: cervical, axillary, groin
  Size
  Tenderness
  Pain
GI system
  Nausea, vomiting
  Anorexia
  Weight loss
  Parotitis: usually 4 to 24 hr after TBI; resolved within 24 to 72 hr
  Diarrhea
    Frequency
    Color
    Consistency
    Occult blood
    Bleeding
Renal system
  Urine
    Color
    Character
    Odor
    Amount
    Bleeding
    Occult blood
    Presence of sugar
Respiratory system
  Breath sounds
    Rales

Rhonchi
Diminished
Rate
Depth and pattern
Cough
  Type
  Frequency
Sputum
  Color
  Character
  Frequency
Cardiovascular system
  Apical rate, rhythm
  Note patient's position and activity before taking BP
  Pedal or sacral edema
Eyes
  Photophobia
  Pain
  Abnormal tear secretion
  Blurred vision
  Cataracts: late effect of TBI
Activity level: fatigue associated with activity

Laboratory/diagnostic studies

Same as for conditioning phase with increased frequency

Potential complications

Infections unresponsive to treatment
Hemorrhage
GVHD (see Tables 13-3 below, 13-4 on p. 574)

Medical Management

Supportive therapy
  TPN
  Blood products
  Pain management
  Antibiotics
  Antivirals
  Antipyretics
  Antidiarrheals
  Antiemetics
  Antifungals

TABLE 13-3. Proposed Clinical Stage of Graft vs. Host Disease According to Organ System

Stage	Skin	Liver	Intestinal tract
+	Maculopapular rash over 25% of body surface	Bilirubin 2-3 mg/dl	Greater than 500 ml diarrhea/day
+ +	Maculopapular rash over 25%-50% of body surface	Bilirubin 3-6 ml/dl	Greater than 1000 ml diarrhea/day
+ + +	Generalized erythroderma	Bilirubin 6-15 mg/dl	Greater than 1500 ml diarrhea/day
+ + + +	Generalized erythroderma with bulbous formation and desquamation	Bilirubin greater than 15 mg/dl	Severe abdominal pain with or without ileus

From Thomas ED. Reprinted by permission of *New Engl J Med* 292:896, 1975.

TABLE 13-4. Overall Clinical Grading of Severity of Graft vs. Host Disease

Grade	Degree of organ involvement
I	+ to + + skin rash; no gut involvement; no liver involvement; no decrease in clinical performance
II	+ to + + + skin rash; + gut involvement or + liver involvement (or both); mild decrease in clinical performance
III	+ + to + + + skin rash; + + to + + + gut involvement or + + to + + + + liver involvement (or both); marked decrease in clinical performance
IV	Similar to grade III with + + to + + + + organ involvement and extreme decrease in clinical performance

From Thomas ED. Reprinted by permission of *New Engl J Med* 292:896, 1975.

Antineoplastics
Fluids and electrolytes
Antibacterial diet, low bacteria diet
Daily weights
Intake and output
Isolation
Incentive spirometer
Oxygen therapy
Mechanical ventilation

Nursing diagnosis/interventions/evaluation

Note: see altered nutrition: less than body requirements; potential for infection; anxiety; and body image disturbances; under conditioning phase

■ **NDX:** Altered protection related to thrombocytopenia

Monitor platelet count daily
Inspect gums and oral cavity for bleeding q2h to 4h
Inspect skin each shift for increased bruising, petechiae, ecchymosis, and swelling
Inspect and palpate joints each shift for increased size and decreased mobility
Assess sensorium and neurological status each shift
Inspect nasal cavity at least once each shift
If epistaxis occurs
  Discourage vigorous nose-blowing
  Stay with patient at first sign of bleeding to decrease anxiety
  Apply pressure and ice at site for 10 min
  Place patient in 90-degree (sitting) position
  Instruct patient to breathe through mouth
  Reassure and encourage patient
  Record estimated blood loss
  Monitor and record vital signs q2h to 4h for 48 hr

Institute safety measures as platelet count decreases below 50,000/mm^3
  Use central line for withdrawal of blood samples and administration of parenteral medications as ordered; avoid skin punctures
  Avoid use of
    Rough towels and washcloths
    Razors
    Restraints
    Tight clothing
  Maintain clutter-free environment
  Provide night-light to prevent bumping into objects or falling
Administer careful oral hygiene
  Use sponge cleaners or gauze pads
  Avoid use of dental floss or toothpicks
  Encourage use of mouth rinse q2h to 4h
    Half saline and half water
    Half saline and half nonalcohol mouth rinse followed by saline rinse
Administer irradiated platelets as ordered; inspect IV or central line site q20min to 30min for hematoma or oozing
Administer antacids as ordered
Avoid aspirin and aspirin-containing products
Do not take rectal temperatures or administer medications rectally
Test each stool for blood
Administer stool softeners as ordered to prevent bleeding from constipation
Auscultate abdomen for bowel sounds q8h or more frequently if changes occur
Check emesis for frank or occult bleeding; record amount, color, and character; note frequency
Prepare for insertion of nasogastric lavage tube and iced saline lavage
Check and record BP, P, and T q4h
Monitor Hgb, Hct, and electrolytes as ordered
Administer platelets as ordered

Expected outcome/evaluation

Vital signs remain stable; petechiae/bruising remains minimal; no epistaxis; stools negative for blood; emesis negative for blood, or bleeding/hemorrhage from (specify) is controlled

■ **NDX:** Altered oral mucous membrane related to infection or conditioning

Assess and document mouth condition every shift
Provide/encourage mouth care q2h during waking hours and q4h during night
Choice of dental equipment will depend on state of oral cavity

Soft toothbrush if no breaks or lesions

Gauze or sponge-covered cleaners if breaks in skin or gum bleeding

Rinse mouth q2h to 4h to keep free of particles and reduce bacterial count

Commercial mouthwash may be irritating; use nonalcoholic mouthwash diluted with saline or water, or saline alone may be used

Assess denture fit

Avoid gumlike grips

Keep dentures scrupulously clean

Remove and clean before using mouth rinse

Keep mouth moist

Provide appealing, tepid liquids for sipping

Flavored ice pops may be soothing

Keep lips moist; use water-soluble gel

Provide time for patient to prepare for meals

Perform oral hygiene

Rinse mouth and gargle 15 to 20 min before meals

Use local anesthetic or mixture of antihistamine, antacid, and local anesthetic as ordered

Spray mouth with anesthetic solution in atomizer when ordered

For dry mouth, suggest saliva substitute

Administer antifungal mouthwash as ordered; diluted frozen antifungal medication may be more appealing and efficacious

If patient is unable to open mouth for oral hygiene

Prepare irrigating solution; half normal saline and half sterile water or as ordered

Place solution in irrigating container with tubing (clean, disposable tube feeding bag)

Hang 12 to 18 inches above patient's chin level

Place patient in 60- to 90-degree position

Gently irrigate all surfaces, allowing solution to flow into emesis basin

Discard unused solution each time

Provide foods that are nonirritating, easily chewed, and high in nutrition

Use soft foods often: custards, yogurt, soups, etc.

Avoid citrus and very sweet foods

Hot, spicy, or acidic foods are usually intolerable

Hard fruits and vegetables may be grated to make them palatable

Puree solid foods or add gravies and sauces to assist with swallowing

Soft casseroles or soups may be used

Use straws or cups for liquidized foods; utensils, especially forks, may cause more discomfort

Frequent, small feedings are usually more easily tolerated

Expected outcome/evaluation

Oral mucosa remains clean and moist

■ **NDX:**   Altered skin integrity related to conditioning or GVHD

Assess skin scrupulously q8h, focusing on patient's trunk, palms, soles, and ears for maculopapular erythematous rash

Assist with daily shower

Gently pat dry

If using lotions do not leave skin moist; avoid use of perfumes and antiperspirants

Use sterile gowns and sheets

Apply ointments as ordered to keep skin covered and help decrease loss of fluids

Maintain supportive fluid replacement

Keep bed linens dry and wrinkle-free; use bed cradle as necessary

Flotation bed may be ordered

Assist patient with turning and repositioning qh; encourage small position change q30min

Teach and assist with perianal care after each elimination

Teach handwashing technique to be used after elimination and prn

Avoid bumps, bruising, cuts, and scratches

Explain importance of skin care to patient

Avoid use of sharp objects: razors, cuticle scissors, etc.

Always wear slippers or shoes when out of bed

Avoid tight or constrictive clothing

Avoid use of jewelry: moisture and bacteria collect underneath, and sharp edges can cause scratches or cuts

Keep nails short

Instruct patient to avoid scratching

Use mittens for infant or small child; remove q1h to 2h; inspect skin; keep skin dry; exercise fingers and wrist

Avoid giving patient IM injections

Perform daily central line care; withdraw all blood samples for laboratory work via central line using strict aseptic technique

Expected outcome/evaluation

Patient uses appropriate skin care measures

Skin is intact and healing of disruptions is beginning

■ **NDX:**   Diarrhea related to GVHD

Check and record all stools for

Frequency

Amount

Consistency

Presence of blood, overt or occult

Teach patient to perform perineal care after each stool

Use povidone-iodine wash and water rise

Wash with ABDs or soft cloths; from front to back for women

Dry by gentle patting with ABDs or soft toweling

Wash and dry hands well

Ostomy pouch may be used for copious diarrhea

Perform perineal care if patient is unable to do so

Apply medication to perineum as ordered

Teach patient to test stool for blood after each bowel movement

Assess and record status of perineal area at least each shift (q4h if frequency of stools increases)

Weigh patient daily at same time with same clothing and scale

Monitor intake and output q4h to 8h

Monitor electrolytes daily

Encourage oral electrolyte-containing fluids to 3000 ml/day unless contraindicated (30 to 60 ml q15min to 30min)

Administer replacement fluids as ordered

Maintain food diary

Eliminate foods from diet that increase/stimulate peristalsis

Encourage foods that may decrease bowel motility, e.g., rice, bananas

Administer antidiarrheal medications as ordered; observe and report early signs of constipation

Expected outcome/evaluation

Number of stools decreases; patient uses measures to control diarrhea

■ **NDX:** Potential for injury: liver dysfunction related to GVHD

Assess skin, sclera, and mucous membranes q8h

Avoid use of artificial light when possible

Report changes in color, bleeding, and edema to physician

Bathe patient daily; provide soothing baths (i.e., use starch or oil to relieve itching)

Administer skin care as needed to decrease itching

Keep nails short to prevent scratching skin

Encourage fluids to 3000 to 4000 ml/24 hr unless contraindicated; fluids may be limited in presence of edema

Measure intake and output

Report changes in color of urine and stool

If bleeding tendency

Avoid skin puncture

Place furniture, equipment, and personal items so as to prevent injuries from falls or bumping into objects

Administer gentle oral hygiene using sponge cleaners or swabs

Avoid use of harsh soaps and rough towels and cloths

Test urine and stool for occult bleeding

Provide diet with amount of calories, carbohydrate, and protein ordered

Report changes in electrolytes, liver function, and coagulation studies

Administer immunosuppressive medications as ordered

Administer medications as ordered for itching

Expected outcome/evaluation

Skin color is within normal parameters for patient

No bleeding tendency noted—skin clear, urine light yellow, urine and stool negative for occult blood

Reports no itching

■ **NDX:** Ineffective breathing pattern related to interstitial pneumonia caused by infection (e.g., CMV, herpes, adenovirus, *p. carinii*)

Assess respiratory status q4h to 8h; rate, rhythm, excursion, breath sounds; use of accessory muscles; blood gas studies and temperature

Report cough, fever, tachypnea, dyspnea, and/or hypoxia; early sign may be increased respiratory rate at rest and/or with activity

Position patient for maximum excursion with least effort; upright supported with pillow or leaning on overbed table

Encourage deep breathing; use incentive spirometer on a regular basis

Suction airways to clear secretions; use meticulous technique

Schedule activities to prevent increased respiratory exertion and distress

Stay with patient during acute episodes to alleviate anxiety

Supportive oxygen therapy or mechanical ventilatory support may be required

Administer medications and fluids as ordered

Expected outcome/evaluation

Cough is diminishing

Respiratory rate, rhythm, and excursion are returning to patient's normal pattern

Self-care activities are performed without respiratory changes *or*

Respiratory status is maintained via mechanical ventilation

■ **NDX:** Potential fluid volume overload related to venoocclusive disease (VOD) of the liver

Assess for fluid volume overload

Weigh patient daily at same time with same clothing and scale; report abrupt weight gain

Measure abdominal girth q8h; report increasing girth

Measure intake and output q8h; report positive fluid balance

Auscultate lungs for presence of wheezes or rales

Assess respiratory rate and excursion; report increased rate and decreased excursion

Assess level of consciousness

Maintain sodium and fluid restriction as indicated

Use minimal fluid for medication administration

Monitor bilirubin and transanimase
Position patient for maximum respiratory excursion; provide oxygen when necessary

Expected outcome/evaluation

Weight is returning to normal limits
Ascites is diminishing
Breath sounds are normal
Alert and oriented

■ NDX: Pain related to oral mucositis

Assess and document pain location, onset, and duration
Determine precipitating factors
    Assess intensity by asking patient to rate pain from 0 to 5; include descriptive terms, such as dull, sharp in documentation
Maintain environment free of stress, unexpected sounds, or harsh lighting
Consider diversional, relaxation, or imagery measures
Administer pain relief medications as ordered at patient's request; assess effectiveness
Schedule analgesics to prevent severe pain; give continuous IV analgesic for continuous pain; adjust dosage to maintain pain relief without significant side effects
    Assess mental status q4h; watch for drowsiness, disorientation, agitation, and nausea

Expected outcome/evaluation

Patient verbalizes control of pain at acceptable level; posture and face appear more relaxed

■ NDX: Activity intolerance related to fatique secondary to anemia, interrupted sleep and rest patterns, or inadequate nutrition (see nursing diagnosis on altered nutrition, p. 569)

Provide adequate periods of sleep and rest
    Plan nursing activities to avoid interrupting sleep
    Provide activity-free periods throughout the day for rest
    Schedule examinations and tests carefully
Conserve patient's energy for desired activities
    Assist with meal preparation
    Keep needed items within reach
    Assist with hygiene measures
    Plan activities after rest periods
Assess response to activity; reduce or change sequence if not tolerated
Observe safety precautions
    Instruct patient to sit at side of bed before getting up; to change position slowly
Plan rest periods after meals
Maintain and increase daily activities as patient's tolerance improves
    Showering
    Mouth care

    Perineal care
    Use of incentive spirometer
    Walking in room; use of exercycle
    Active participation in all care activities
Assess response to increased activities; change daily plan as needed

Expected outcome/evaluation

Patient performs self-care activities without evidence of intolerance

Additional nursing diagnoses to consider

Ineffective coping: individual or family, related to prolonged disease; multiple life changes, or inadequate support systems
Impaired social interaction related to therapeutic isolation
Sexual dysfunction related to sterility

■ NDX: Knowledge deficit related to lack of information about self-care procedures, complications, diet, care of home environment, activities, and continuing health care

Self-care procedures

Teach care of central line, heparin flush, administration of TPN (p. 36), and use of volumetric pump
Demonstrate and explain rationale for
    Oral hygiene
    Skin care
    Perianal care
    Handwashing technique
    Use of incentive spirometer
    Measurement of intake and output
    Daily assessment of skin and mucous membranes
    Method for testing urine and stool for blood
    Method for taking and recording temperature
    Low-bacteria diet (Table 13-5)

Complications

Instruct patient and/or significant other how to assess for and report symptoms of
    Anemia
    Bleeding
    Infection
    Stomatitis
    Skin changes
    GVHD
    Nausea, vomiting
    Diarrhea
    Nephrotoxicity
Explain measures to use to avoid complications

ANEMIA

Discuss methods for conserving energy
    Planned rest periods

TABLE 13-5. Low-Bacterial Diet

Food categories	Foods allowed	Foods to avoid
Beverages	Coffee, decaffeinated coffee, tea, cereal beverages, carbonated beverages, canned or frozen fruit and vegetable juices	Fresh fruit and vegetable juices
Milk (2 or more cups)*	Skim (nonfat), low-fat, or whole milk, buttermilk, commercial milk shakes, and canned eggnog	Milk shakes made with noncommercial ice cream, yogurt, and eggnog made with raw eggs
Meat group (6 to 8 oz cooked)*	Lean meat, fish, fowl, cheese (heated), eggs (cooked), and peanut butter	Cold cuts, stir-fried foods, raw eggs, and cottage cheese
Vegetables (2 to 3 half-cup servings or more)*	All cooked fresh or frozen vegetables and canned vegetables; one serving should be a source of vitamin A (dark green leafy or deep yellow vegetables)	All raw or uncooked vegetables and salads
Fruits (2 to 3 half-cup servings or more)*	All canned or stewed fruits, fresh fruits with thick skin that can be peeled (apple, orange, banana); one serving should be a source of vitamin C (citrus fruits, cantaloupe, or guavas)	All other fresh fruits and dried fruit
Breads and other starches (5 or more servings)*	White enriched, whole wheat, and other breads, rolls, crackers, pretzels, sweet rolls, doughnuts, pancakes, waffles, French toast, all cereals, macaroni, noodles, spaghetti, rice, corn, potatoes, dried beans, and peas	Sweet rolls with custard or cream filling
Fats and oils (2 to 4 tablespoons or more)*	Liquid oil shortenings, margarine, salad dressing, nondairy creamers, nuts, and seeds	Bleu cheese and Roquefort dressing
Soups	Canned, frozen, or dehydrated soups and soups made from "allowed" ingredients	None
Seasonings and miscellaneous	Salt (iodized), spices and herbs (used in the cooking process), condiments, cocoa powder, gravies and sauces made from "allowed" ingredients	Spices, herbs, or seasonings added to food after it has been cooked
Sugars†	Jelly, jam, marmalade, honey, candy, molasses, syrups	None
Desserts†	Individually packaged commercial ice cream, ice milk, sherbet, and individually packaged cakes, cookies, canned or frozen pudding	Noncommercial ice cream, ices, sherbet; custard, gelatin, frozen yogurt

*These foods form the foundation for an adequate diet.
†These foods are not necessary for an adequate diet but add extra calories.

Adequate rest
Activities planned after rest periods
Assisting with ADLs
Keeping needed items within reach
Explain need to change position slowly; to use appliances (walker, bars, etc.) for movement if indicated
Emphasize importance of continuing to perform ADLs and other desired activities to tolerance
Explain need to maintain a diet high in iron

BLEEDING

Discuss emergency plan to follow if spontaneous hemorrhage occurs
  Have emergency numbers on hand
  Call paramedics
  Go to nearest emergency area

Explain importance of:
  Telling dentist and other medical personnel about chemotherapy, low platelet count, and BMT
  Maintaining a safe, clutter-free environment
  Avoiding over-the-counter medications, especially those containing acetylsalicylic acid (aspirin) without checking with physician
  Avoiding use of sharp objects when possible
  Use electric razor
  Use caution when handling knives or other equipment
  Avoiding harsh coughing and blowing of nose
  If cough persists, notify physician
  Take cough medication as ordered
Ensure that patient and/or significant other demonstrates method for applying pressure to bleeding site
  Apply dressing or clean material directly over site

Apply pressure for 5 min or until bleeding stops

Apply ice in covered plastic bag over site once bleeding stops

Check site for further bleeding q15min for 1 hr

INFECTION

Explain importance of:

Avoiding persons who may be infectious or who may have potentially contagious conditions, as well as persons who have been recently vaccinated and crowds

Avoiding multiple sexual partners

Reporting elevated temperature

Instruct patient to wash hands after using bathroom, before eating, or before performing any procedures

Explain importance of preventing injury to skin

Use electric razors

Handle knives and sharp objects carefully

Wear protective gloves when gardening and when using strong household cleaning solutions

Wear broad-brimmed hat and sun screen when in sun

Avoid going barefoot

Wear warm clothing and boots in cold weather

Avoid cutting cuticles, corns, or calluses

Wear padded gloves when using oven

Explain importance of:

Performing oral hygiene periodically throughout the day

Performing daily hygiene, including perineal and rectal care

Drinking up to 2500 ml of fluid each day unless contraindicated; instruct patient to avoid using common drinking fountain

STOMATITIS

Explain importance of routine oral care in the morning, after meals, and at bedtime

Discuss equipment and products to use to avoid irritation

Explain need to avoid commercial mouthwashes containing alcohol

Emphasize need to provide appetizing, high-calorie, high-protein foods in small quantities prepared to the degree of softness tolerated by patient

DIARRHEA

Explain importance of maintaining oral fluid intake at 3000 ml/day unless contraindicated

Explain need to:

Avoid diet high in fiber and roughage

Take prescribed medication during episodes of diarrhea

Discuss signs and symptoms of constipation to report

Explain need to avoid over-the-counter medications without checking with physician or nurse

Diet

Explain need to maintain low-bacteria diet (see Table 13-5)

TEMPERATURES (°F) FOR FOOD SAFENESS	
165° to 195°	This temperature kills most harmful bacteria
140° to 150°	Minimum temperature at which to cook foods to kill bacteria
45° to 140°	Danger zone for food safeness; rapid bacterial growth
34° to 45°	Cold or chill food storage; slow bacterial growth
0° to −10°	Frozen food storage

Discuss methods used during hospitalization to enhance intake of nutrients and liquids

Teach procedures for handling, storing, and cooking foods (see box above and Table 13-5)

Activities

Explain need to perform daily self-care and to increase activity daily to tolerance

Emphasize importance of planning regular rest and sleep periods

Care of home environment, equipment, and supplies

Explain that home environment must be clean and dust-free before patient's discharge

All room surfaces and furniture must be washed and/or vacuumed

All plants and flowers should be removed

Pets should be boarded elsewhere until day +100

Daily cleaning and vacuuming is necessary; use of dry dust cloths should be avoided

Equipment and supplies are to be stored in clean area

Towels and wash cloths must be changed daily

Bed linen must be changed at least twice each week

Kitchen equipment must be washed and dried immediately after use

Trash must be taken outside immediately

Continuing health care

Emphasize importance of scheduling and keeping regular appointments with physician, laboratory, and other health care workers

Explain importance of telling dentist and other health care workers about condition

Emphasize need to continue to express and discuss feelings, worries, and fears; to seek assistance as necesary

Provide patient with information concerning community resources, support groups, home care agencies, and equipment suppliers as necessary

Teach name of medication, dosage, time of administration, and side and toxic effects to report to physician

Explain need to avoid use of over-the-counter medications without checking first with physician

Expected outcome/evaluation

Patient and/or significant other verbalizes understanding of home care and follow-up instructions for avoiding complications, maintenance of home environment, diet, medications, activity management, and continuing health care; and demonstrates methods of checking for signs of complications, oral hygiene and skin/perianal care measures, management of TPN therapy, handwashing technique, use of incentive spirometer, measurement of intake, output, and calories, and procedure for taking and recording temperature

BIBLIOGRAPHY

Abernathy E: How the immune system works, Am J Nurs, April, 87(4):456, 1987.

Abernathy E: Biological response modifiers, Am J Nurs, April, 87(4):458, 1987.

American Cancer Society: Immunology and cancer reprint, CA 38:66, 1989.

Borden EC: Biologicals in cancer treatment, from National Conference on Advances in Cancer Management, American Cancer Society, Los Angeles, December, 1988.

Brochstein JA: Critical care issues in bone marrow transplantation, Crit Care Clin 4(1):147, 1988.

Centers for Disease Control: Revision of CDC surveillance case definition for acquired immunodeficiency syndrome, MMWR 36, 1987.

Centers for Disease Control: AIDS update, MMWR 38(14), 1989.

Cummings D: Caring for the HIV-infected adult, Nurse Pract 13(11):28, 1988.

Donehower MG: Malignant complication of AIDS, Oncol Nurs Forum 14(1), 1987.

Groenwald SL: Cancer nursing principles and Practice, Boston, 1987, Jones & Bartlett Publishers.

Hilton G: AIDS dementia, J Neurosci Nurs 21(1):240, 1989.

Holper J: Respiratory dysfunction: AIDS, AIDS related malignancies, AIDS dementia complex and nutrition and AIDS. In: Daeffler RJ, Petrosino BM, eds: Manual of oncology nursing practice: nursing diagnoses and care, Rockville, Md, 1990, Aspen Publishers.

Hood LE: Interferon, Am J Nurs, April, 459, 1987.

Ihde JK, Jacobsen WK, and Briggs BA: Principles of critical care, Philadelphia, 1987, WB Saunders.

Jassak PF, Spiewak P: Interleukin-2, Am J of Nurs, April, 87(4):464, 1987.

Kim MJ, McFarland GK, and McLane AM: Pocket guide to nursing diagnosis, ed 4, St Louis, 1990, Mosby–Year Book.

Lovejoy NC: The Pathophysiology of AIDS, Oncol Nurs Forum 15(5):563, 1988.

Lupus Foundation of America, Inc, Greater LA Chapter: Lupus line, Los Angeles, Aug-Sept, 1988, Oct-Nov, 1988, April-May, 1989.

McArthur J: AIDS dementia: your assessment can make all the difference, RN, March 57(3):36, 1990.

McFarland GK, McFarlane EA: Nursing diagnosis and intervention: planning for patient care, St Louis, 1989, CV Mosby.

Meisenhelder JB, LaCarite C: Fear of contagion: the public response to AIDS, Image: J Nurs Scholar, 21(1):7, 1989.

Moffatt BC et al: AIDS: A self-care manual, AIDS Project Los Angeles, Santa Monica, 1987, IBS Press.

Nass T: Helping the patient who has lupus, RN 50(10):69, 1987.

Nyamathi A, Van Servellen G: Maladaptive coping in the critically ill population with acquired immunodeficiency syndrome: nursing assessment and treatment, Heart and Lung 18(2):113, 1989.

O'Quin T, Moravec C: The critically ill bone marrow transplant patient, Semin Oncol Nurs 4(1):25, 1988.

Pagana KD, Pagana TJ: Diagnostic testing and nursing implications, ed 3, St Louis, 1990, Mosby–Year Book.

Pastan I et al: Novel cytotoxic agents created by the fusion of growth factor and toxin genes, National Conference on Advances in Management of Cancer, Los Angeles, Dec., 1988.

Perlstein LM, Ake JM: AIDS: an overview for the neuroscience nurse, J Neurosci Nurs 19(6):296, 1987.

PCR: A new test for HIV, Am J Nurs 9:1172, 1988.

Rieger PT: Monoclonal antibodies: target-specific magic bullets, Am J Nurs April, 87(4):469, 1987.

Ruggiero MR: The donor in bone marrow transplantation, Semin Oncol Nurs 4(1):9, 1988.

Sande MA, Volberding PA: The medical management of AIDS, Philadelphia, 1988, WB Saunders.

Sattler FR et al: Timethoprin-Sulfamethoxazole compared with pentamidine for treatment of pneumocystis carinii pneumonia in acquired immunodeficiency syndrome, Ann Intern Med 109:280, 1988.

Shin D, Avers JA, eds: AIDS/HIV: reference guide for medical professionals, Los Angeles, 1988, CIRD at UCLA.

Thomas ED: Bone marrow transplantation, CA 37:291, 1987.

Thompson JM et al: Mosby's manual of clinical nursing, ed 2, St Louis, 1989, CV Mosby.

Torbett MP: The immunologic system. In Armstrong ME et al, McGraw-Hill handbook of clinical nursing, New York, 1979, McGraw-Hill.

Williams AB, D'Aquila RT, and Williams AE: HIV infection in intravenous drug abusers, Image: J Nurs Scholar 19(4):179, 1987.

14
CHAPTER

Neoplasia

CANCER DETECTION AND PREVENTION

General

Obtain health history through interview
Establish rapport
Identify risk factors and symptoms of specific cancers
Determine emotional concerns about cancer
Provide information on self-examination
Teach warning signs of cancer
    Change in bowel or bladder habits
    A sore that does not heal
    Unusual bleeding or discharge
    Thickening or lump in breast or elsewhere
    Indigestion or difficulty in swallowing
    Obvious change in wart or mole
    Nagging cough or hoarseness

Skin Cancer
Determination of Risk Factors

Geographic area
Excessive exposure to sunlight (amount of absorption depends on time of day, season of year, and atmospheric conditions)
Occupational exposure to chemical irritants, such as tar, creosote, arsenic or paraffin
Familial incidence
Fair-skinned, light-colored eyes and hair
Scars from previous burns and trauma
Precancerous dermatoses and conditions
    Actinic keratoses
    Xeroderma pigmentosum
    Lupus erythematosus
    Erythroplasia
    Leukoplasia
Ionizing radiation exposure: x-rays, radium, atom bomb exposure

Signs and Symptoms

Skin lesion or rash
Firm, red or red-gray pearly lesion on face
Scaly, keratotic, slightly elevated lesion
Persistent skin growth with definite progression and/or elevation or ulceration
Any sore that does not heal
Change in a wart or mole: asymmetrical, poorly defined borders; color change; increase in diameter

Nursing diagnoses/interventions/evaluation

■ **NDX:** Knowledge deficit related to lack of information about prevention and early detection of skin cancers

Prevention

Assess knowledge level
Assess readiness and ability to learn
Ensure that patient and/or significant other is knowledgeable about
    Regular skin self-examination
    Factors that place an individual at risk
    Types of skin cancers
    Importance of reducing exposure to sunlight, especially from 10 AM to 3 PM
    Need to protect skin when exposed to sunlight
        Wear sunscreen factor specific for skin type at all times
        Cover exposed body parts
        Wear broad-brimmed hat
    Need to reduce exposure to chemical carcinogens: wear protective equipment
    Importance of reporting any skin changes to physician
    Importance of follow-up care q3 to 6 months if history of previous skin cancer

Detection

Obtain history of any recent change in skin, mole, or lesion
Obtain family history of skin cancer or dysplastic nevus syndrome
Assess skin for suspicious lesions

Head and neck area are common sites of occurrence of skin cancers

Basal cell cancers typically have pearly, shiny translucent appearance

Squamous cell cancers occur predominantly on sun-exposed skin; most appear as a solitary nodule with inflamed base and indistinct margin

Discuss procedure for and importance of monthly skin self-examination

Stress importance of medical follow-up

Expected outcome/evaluation

Patient demonstrates knowledge of definition and risk factors of skin cancer and measures for prevention and early detection of skin cancer

Cancer of Head and Neck
Determination of Risk Factors

Heavy tobacco use: cigarettes, cigars, snuff, chewing tobacco, pipe

Chronic moderate-to-heavy use of alcohol

Sun exposure

Chronic intake of extremely hot or cold liquids

History of exposure: nickel, wood dust, hydrocarbon gas, asbestos, mustard gas, radiation, uranium, syphilis, herpes simplex, Epstein-Barr virus

History of chronic inflammatory disease, chronic irritation to oral mucosa from poorly fitting dentures or defective teeth, or poor oral hygiene

Premalignant lesions
  Erythroplasia
  Leukoplasia

Sign and Symptoms

Leukoplakia

Erythroplakia

Chronic, nonhealing, often painless sores

Positive submaxillary nodes

Nasal discharge, bloody

Earache

Enlarged cervical lymph nodes

Alteration in voice tone
  Hoarseness, cough

Hemoptysis

Glossitis

Dysphagia

Sore throat lasting longer than 2 weeks

Nursing diagnoses/interventions/evaluation

■ **NDX:** Knowledge deficit related to lack of information about prevention and early detection of head and neck cancer

Prevention

Ensure that patient and/or significant other is knowledgeable about risk factors

Evaluate patient's potential for developing head and neck cancer by obtaining health history to include
  Exposure to risk factors
  Work history
  Alcohol and tobacco use
  Dental hygiene measures

Stress importance of avoiding
  Tobacco and heavy alcohol use (synergistic causation)
  Poorly fitting dentures or defective teeth
  Chemical carcinogens
  Excessive sun exposure

Stress importance of oral care with routine dental follow-up

Emphasize nutritional and fluid intake needs

Suggest programs to eliminate smoking and alcohol abuse

Refer patient to support groups for counseling and for help in coping

Detection

Obtain history of subjective symptoms: pain, visual changes (diplopia), hearing loss, taste or smell changes, changes in swallowing ability

Assess skin, eyelids, external ear and canal, and scalp and lips for lesions and visible swellings or adenopathy

Inspect external nose for loss of structure and support: test potency of nostrils by compressing one nostril at a time while patient inhales with mouth closed

Inspect oral cavity for areas of leukoplakia (white patches), erythema, or lesions that may appear infiltrating, ulcerative, or exophytic

Assess parotid, submaxillary, and sublingual glands for swelling and adenopathy; normally, thyroid gland is barely palpable

To examine thyroid, patient's neck should be slightly extended; assess for swelling; assess regional lymph nodes—observations of palpable lymph nodes include size, consistency, mobility, attachment, discoloration of overlying skin, and deep fixation to surrounding structures

Expected outcome/evaluation

Patient demonstrates knowledge of risk factors associated with head and neck cancer and measures for prevention and early detection of head and neck cancer

Lung Cancer
Determination of Risk Factors

History of tobacco use
  Number of cigarettes or cigars per day
  Number of years patient has smoked, depth of inhalation, amount of tar in cigarettes smoked

Exposure to tobacco smoke, including side-stream or passive exposure
  Hours per day
  Number of years
Exposure to ionizing radiation
Exposure to carcinogens
  Asbestos
  Aromatic hydrocarbons
  Radioactive ores
  Radon
  Bis ether
  Inorganic arsenic
  Nickel, silver, chromium, cadmium, beryllium, cobalt, selenium, steel
Exposure to atmospheric pollution
History of chronic lung disease
Low intake of vitamin A

Signs and Symptoms

Change in pulmonary habits
Respiratory infections
Chronic cough
Productive cough, usually at night
Rust-streaked sputum
Hemoptysis
Chest pain, tightness in chest
Unilateral wheeze
Dyspnea
Pneumonitis lasting longer than 2 weeks with treatment
Shoulder or arm pain; superior vena cava syndrome
Weight loss
Extrapulmonary
  Hypercalcemia
  Cushing's syndrome
  Dermatomyositis
  Clubbed fingers
  Migratory thrombophlebitis
  Nonbacterial endocarditis
  Anemia
  Disseminated intravascular coagulation (DIC)

Nursing diagnoses/interventions/evaluation

■ **NDX:** Knowledge deficit related to lack of information about prevention and detection of lung cancer

Prevention

Assess current knowledge level
Assess readiness and ability to learn
Ensure that patient and/or significant other is knowledgeable about risk factors
Obtain personal and family smoking history
Obtain patient's history of exposure to environmental carcinogens

Assess patient's history of lung disease
Ensure that patient and/or family is knowledgeable about
  Need to avoid exposure to tobacco smoke
  Correlation of smoking to lung cancer
  High-risk occupations
  Resources to help stop smoking

Detection

Obtain history of subjective symptoms: change in cough, chest pain, dyspnea, tightness in chest
Assess objective symptoms: increased sputum, hemoptysis, unilateral wheeze
Ascertain results of laboratory values: arterial blood gases, pulmonary function studies
Explain extrapulmonary signs and symptoms of lung cancer that may occur before pulmonary signs
  Superior vena cava syndrome
  Symptoms of metastatic lung tumor
    Lymph node adenopathy
    Enlarged liver, anorexia, pain in right upper quadrant
    Bone pain
    Change in mental status, seizures, headaches
  Conditions that result from ectopic hormone productions
    Inappropriate antidiuretic hormone (ADH) syndrome
    Hypercalcemia
    Cushing's syndrome
Ensure that patient and/or significant other is knowledgeable about methods of detection of lung cancer
  History and physical examination
  Chest x-ray film
  Sputum cytology
  Bronchoscopy and bronchial biopsy
  Brushings and washings
  Mediastinoscopy, lymph node biopsy
  Lung, brain, and bone scan when indicated

Expected outcome/evaluation

Patient demonstrates knowledge of risk factors associated with lung cancer, measures to reduce the risk of lung cancer, and measures for detection of lung cancer

Cancer of Esophagus and Stomach
Determination of Risk Factors

Chronic irritation from
  Heavy smoking
  Excessive use of alcohol
  Drinking and eating very hot foods
  Excessive use of hot, spicy foods and smoked meats
Exposure to foods containing nitrites and nitrates
Nutritional deficiency
Type A blood type
History of head and neck tumors, strictures, or peptic ulcer

Family history of
Pernicious anemia
Gastric polyps
Gastritis
Achlorhydria
Gastric cancer

Signs and Symptoms

Esophagus
Dysphagia
Early with swallowing hard, solid food
Constantly with swallowing saliva
Hoarseness
Coughing
Glossopharyngeal neuralgia
Foul breath
Hiccups
Esophageal obstruction
Sialism
Nocturnal aspiration
Regurgitation of saliva and food
Stomach
Vague epigastric discomfort
Vague feelings of fullness after meals
Severe steady pain
Anorexia
Weight loss

Nursing diagnoses/interventions/evaluation

 **NDX:** Knowledge deficit related to lack of information about prevention and detection of cancer of esophagus and stomach

Prevention/detection

Ensure that patient and/or significant other is knowledgeable about risk factors
Obtain patient history of
Smoking
Alcohol
Nutrition
Ensure that patient and/or significant other is knowledgeable about
Signs and symptoms to report to physician
Importance of periodic, regular physical examinations
Need to avoid foods containing nitrite and nitrate preservatives (usually smoked meats)
Need to avoid chronic irritation by tobacco, alcohol, hot and spicy foods, and tea
Importance of increasing dietary intake of vitamin C

Expected outcome/evaluation

Patient demonstrates knowledge of definition and risk factors of esophageal and stomach cancer, measures to reduce the risk of esophageal and stomach cancer, and measures for detection of esophageal and stomach cancer

Colorectal Cancer
Determination of Risk Factors

Age: over 40 years
Geographic area
High-fat, low-fiber diet
History of familial polyposis, Gardner's syndrome, adenomatous polyps, villous adenomas, or colon cancer
History of ulcerative colitis, Crohn's disease, or previous colon cancer

Signs and Symptoms

Recent changes in bowel habits
Alternating diarrhea and constipation
Note frequency, time of day, size
Symptoms depend on location of tumor
Right colon
Anemia and gastrointestinal (GI) tract bleeding
Abdominal pain
Weight loss, weakness, nausea
Sigmoid colon
Obstruction
Blood per rectum
Left colon
Mucus in stool
Constipation
Decreased-caliber stools
Blood or blood mixed with stools
Intermittent abdominal pain
Nausea, vomiting
Rectum
Rectal bleeding
Mucous diarrhea
Feeling of incomplete evacuation
Tenesmus
Abdominal and low back pain

Nursing diagnoses/interventions/evaluation

 NDX: Knowledge deficit related to lack of information about prevention and early detection of colorectal cancer

Prevention

Assess current knowledge
Assess readiness and ability to learn
Ensure that patient and/or significant other knows and understands
Risk factors
Need to schedule regular, periodic examinations that include rectal examination and Hemoccult slide test

if patient is 40 years of age or older and flexible sigmoidoscopy after age 50

Measures to promote bowel health

    Inspect stools regularly

    Include fresh vegetables, fruit, and fiber in diet; avoid excessive fat in diet

    Drink at least 8 glasses of water per day

    Exercise regularly

Detection

Ensure that patient and/or significant other is knowledgeable about

    Signs and symptoms to report to physician

    Self-detection methods

        Observation of stools (describe abnormal stools)

        Stool guaiac testing

Ensure that patient and/or significant other demonstrates hemoccult test procedure

Stress importance of reporting positive results to physician immediately

Provide written information on American Cancer Society (ACS) screening guidelines

    Annual digital rectal examination after age 40

    Guaiac stool testing annually after age 50

    Sigmoidoscopy every 2 to 5 years after two negative tests a year apart

Provide teaching and written guidelines on detection measures

    Sigmoidoscopy

    Colonoscopy

    Rectal examination

    Barium examination

    Carcinoembryonic antigen (CEA)

Expected outcome/evaluation

Patient demonstrates knowledge of risk factors associated with colorectal cancer, measures to reduce the risk of colorectal cancer, signs and symptoms that require health care follow-up, and methods to detect colorectal cancer

Renal, Pelvis, and Bladder Cancer and Cancer of Ureter and Urethra

Determination of Risk Factors

Age group: 50 to 70 years of age

Exposure to carcinogens through skin or vapor

    Aniline dye: rubber and cable industry

    Beta-naphthylamine

    4-Amino diphenyl

    Tobacco tar

    Benzedine

Exposure to pelvic irradiation

Chronic bacterial cystitis with

    Calculi

Urethral strictures

Diverticuli

Paralytic stasis

Linked with but not proved

    Coffee drinking

    High use of sodium saccharin

    Urine stasis

    Incidence high in tobacco smokers

Signs and Symptoms

Gross, painless hematuria: often intermittent

Microhematuria

Urinary

    Frequency

    Burning

    Urgency

    Pain

Dysuria

Weight loss and anemia

Back pain

Paraneoplastic syndrome associated with renal cancer

    Hypercalcemia

    Hypertension

    Polycythemia

Nursing diagnoses/interventions/evaluation

■ **NDX:** Knowledge deficit related to lack of information about prevention and detection of renal, pelvis, and bladder cancer and cancer of ureter and urethra

Prevention

Ensure that patient and/or significant other knows and understands

    Risk factors

    Importance of giving detailed occupation history

        Length of time of exposure

        Dates

        Hours per week

        Protective equipment

    Need to use safety equipment when exposed to carcinogens

    Importance of reporting signs and symptoms to physician

    Need to schedule periodic physical examinations, including rectal examination and bimanual pelvic examination for females; examinations at least q4 months for high-risk patients, including cystoscopy and cytology

Detection

Ensure that patient and/or significant other

    Recognizes signs and symptoms that require health care evaluation

Describes detection methods to determine renal, pelvis, and bladder cancer and cancer of ureter and urethra
Urinalysis (for hematuria)
Intravenous pyelography (IVP), cystoscopy
Retrograde pyelography
Nephrotomogram
Ultrasonography
Computed tomography (CT) scan
Renal arteriogram

Expected outcome/evaluation

Patient demonstrates understanding of risk factors associated with renal, pelvis, and bladder cancer and cancer of ureter and urethra; measures for prevention; signs and symptoms requiring health care evaluation; and detection measures for renal, pelvis, and bladder cancer and cancer of ureter and urethra

Testicular Cancer
Determination of Risk Factors

Between ages of 20 and 40 years
Cryptorchism (undescended testis)
Previously atrophic testes
Childhood hernia and other genitourinary anomalies
Contributing factors
Trauma
Orchitis, especially mumps
Family history of testicular cancer: father, brother
Klinefelter's syndrome
In utero exposure to diethystilbestrol (DES)

Signs and Symptoms

Feelings of discomfort in testes
Swelling
Painless
Intermittent
Scrotal heaviness
Testicular mass, palpable
Gynecomastia
Nipple pigmentation
Scrotal mass with or without pain
"Dragging" pain in lower back and abdomen
Endocrine disturbances: virilization to feminization
Metastatic presentation
Ureteral obstruction
Abdominal mass
Pulmonary lesion

Nursing diagnoses/interventions/evaluation

■ **NDX:** Knowledge deficit related to lack of information about early detection of testicular cancer

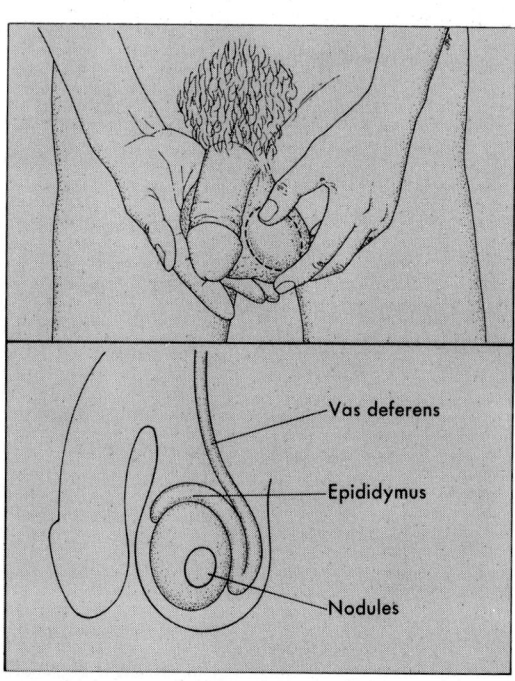

FIGURE 14-1. Testicular self-examination.

Detection

Ensure that patient and/or significant other knows and understands

Need to schedule regular, periodic physical examinations, including testicular and abdominal palpation

High-risk factors

Signs and symptoms to report to physician immediately

Importance of performing testicular self-examination every month after age 15 or earlier if history of genitourinary anomalies (Figure 14-1)

Ensure that patient and/or significant other demonstrates testicular self-examination

Perform after warm shower or bath with relaxed scrotal skin

Perform in standing position

Place middle and index fingers below one testis with thumb on top

Gently roll testis between thumb and fingers

Palpate for

Normal findings

Rubbery, spongy consistency

Smooth, without lumps

Abnormal finding: hard, painless tumor, usually on lateral or anterior surface

Hold one testicle in palm of each hand; report weight differences to physician

Expected outcome/evaluation

Patient demonstrates testicular self-examination and knowledge of signs and symptoms requiring health care evaluation

Prostate Cancer
Determination of Risk Factors

Advancing age: usually over 50 years

Black population: higher incidence

Urban environment

Family history of prostatic cancer

Linked with but not proven

First coitus at early age

Multiple sex partners

History of venereal disease

Signs and Symptoms

Early signs

Urinary hesitancy

Dysuria

Urgency

Straining to start stream

Later signs

Hematuria

Chronic urinary retention with dribbling

Bone and neuritic pain

Weight loss, lethargy

Low back pain

Nursing diagnoses/interventions/evaluation

■ **NDX:** Knowledge deficit related to lack of information about detection of prostate cancer

Detection

Ensure that patient and/or significant other knows and understands

Risk factors

Need to schedule annual physical examination that includes digital rectal examination

Yearly for men under 50 years of age

Every 6 months for men 50 years of age and older

Importance of reporting signs and symptoms to physician

Detection measures

Prostatic ultrasound

Rectal examination

Biopsy (needle or open)

Laboratory studies

Acid phosphatase

Alkaline phosphatase

Prostate-specific antigen

Expected outcome/evaluation

Patient demonstrates knowledge of signs and symptoms requiring health care evaluation and measures for detection of prostate cancer

Breast Cancer
Determination of Risk Factors

Female; 99% incidence

Increased after 40 years of age

Upper socioeconomic status; higher incidence

Nulliparous or first parity after 30 to 35 years of age

Family history of breast cancer: sister, mother

Personal history of breast disease

Adverse hormone milieu

Early menarche

Late menopause

Thyroid disorders

Diabetes

Postmenopausal hormone therapy

Lowered immunological competence

Thymic atrophy

Decreased thymus-dependent (T) lymphocytes

Exposure to excessive radiation

Use of chemotherapy

Use of immunosuppressants

Obesity

High dietary fat intake

Fibrocystic disease

Other cancers
Chronic psychologic stress

Signs and Symptoms

Palpable lump
  Usually painless
  Most often found in upper outer quadrant
Nipple discharge
Nipple retraction
Dimpling of skin
Edema (peau d'orange) erythema
Change in contour of breast
Axillary adenopathy
Symptoms associated with metastasis
  Bone pain
  Pleural effusions

Nursing diagnoses/interventions/evaluation

■ **NDX:** Knowledge deficit related to lack of information about prevention and early detection of breast cancer

Prevention

Assess level of anxiety
  Observe verbal and nonverbal behaviors
  Explore concerns regarding breast disease
Assess readiness and ability to learn
Ensure that patient and/or significant other knows and understands
  Risk factors
  Personal risks
  Importance of breast self-examination (most women discover own breast lesions)
  That most breast lumps prove to be benign on biopsy
  That prognosis for breast cancer is more favorable when discovered early
  Importance of low-fat, high-fiber diet in reducing endogenous estrogen
  Importance of weight control or reduction

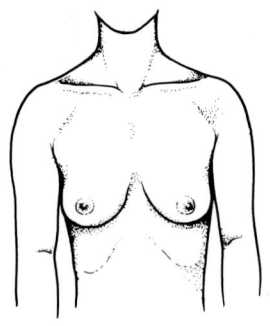
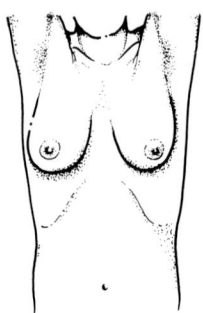
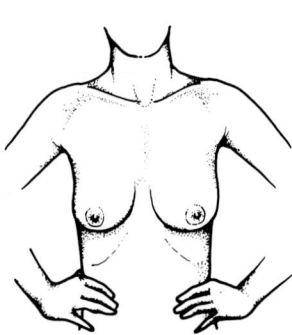
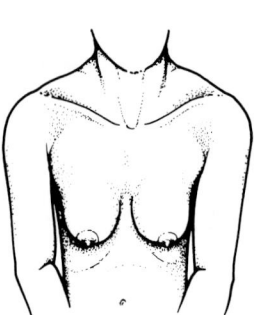

FIGURE 14-2. Breast self-examination. Visual inspection.

Detection

Ensure that patient and/or significant other knows and understands

Methods of early detection of breast cancer

Breast self-examination (monthly for all women over 20)

ACS recommendations for clinical examination by health care professional

Every 3 years for women 20 to 40 years of age

Every year for women over 40

ACS recommendations for mammography

Baseline for women 35 to 40 years of age

Every 1-2 years for women aged 40 to 49

Annual for women over age 50

Need for more frequent examinations and earlier mammograms for women with personal or family histories of breast cancer or who are at high risk

Ensure that patient and/or significant other demonstrates breast self-examination

Stand in front of mirror

Inspect breast in four positions visually; (Figure 14-2)

Standing straight with arms at side

Placing hands on waist and pressing in

Arms elevated

Leaning forward

Observe for size, differences in veins and skin, nipple irregularities, and contour

Palpate breasts

(Figure 14-3)

Place one arm over head and palpate that breast with other hand

Use flat part of fingers, beginning in upper, outer portion and continuing in circular movement to nipple

Gently milk nipple for discharge

Reverse position and palpate other breast

Lie in supine position and repeat palpation steps

Premenopausal women: perform breast self-examination 1 week after menses begin

Postmenopausal women: perform breast self-examination once a month; usually easiest to remember either first or last day of month

Expected outcome/evaluation

Patient verbalizes fears and risk factors associated with breast cancer, demonstrates breast self-examination,

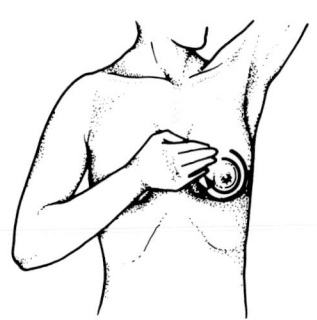
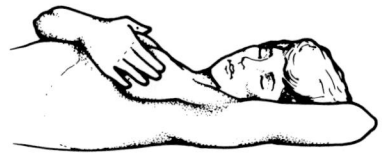
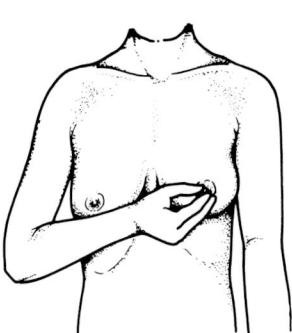

FIGURE 14-3. Breast self-examination. Palpation.

and verbalizes signs and symptoms requiring follow-up health care

Vaginal Cancer
Determination of Risk Factors

Exposure to DES in utero
Children of DES-exposed parent

Signs and Symptoms

Abnormal bleeding
Vivid red areas in vagina
Firm, indurated, cystic areas in vagina or on cervix
Vulvar pruritus

Nursing diagnoses/interventions/evaluation

■ **NDX:**   Knowledge deficit related to lack of information about prevention and early detection of vaginal cancer

Prevention/detection

Ensure that patient and/or significant other knows and understands
  Importance of maintaining accurate menstrual cycle
    history
    Frequency
    Length of menses
    Amount
    Color
  Need to maintain good gynecological hygiene
  Need to avoid frequent douching, especially during adolescent and pregnant periods
  Importance of delaying sexual function in early teen years
  Need for regular, periodic gynecological examinations
  Importance of cytological Papanicolaou (Pap) examinations
    First smear at onset of sexual activity or age 18
    Second 1 year later, then q3 years to age 35, then q5 years to age 60
    Annual smears if at high risk
  Signs and symptoms to report to physician
  Mirror method of self-examination to inspect for
    Skin excoriation
    Ulcers
    Lumps
    Leukoplakia
    Narrowing of introitus
    Atrophy

Expected outcome/evaluation

Patient demonstrates knowledge of risk factors associated with vaginal cancer, signs and symptoms requiring

health care evaluation, and detection measures for determining vaginal cancer

Ovarian Cancer
Determination of Risk Factors

Upper socioeconomic status
Hormonal factors
  Nulliparous
  Older at first parity
  Reduced fertility
  Infertility
  Exogenous therapy
Exposure to carcinogens
  Radiation
  Asbestos
History of breast cancer
Family history of breast, colon, or ovarian cancer
History of
  Pentz-Jeghers syndrome
  Mucocutaneous pigmentation
  Intestinal polyps

Signs and Symptoms

Dyspepsia
Vague abdominal discomfort
Pelvic pressure
Urinary frequency
Change in abdominal girth
Bilateral or unilateral, irregular, immobile ovarian mass
Palpable ovaries after menopause
Adnexal thickening: postmenopausal or nulliparous women
Advanced disease
  Weight loss
  Pleural/abdominal effusions
  Bowel obstruction
  Anemia
  Malnutrition

Nursing diagnoses/interventions/evaluation

■ **NDX:**   Knowledge deficit related to lack of information about detection of ovarian cancer

Prevention/detection

Ensure that patient and/or significant other knows and understands
  Risk factors
  Importance of maintaining accurate menstrual cycle
    history
    Frequency
    Length of menses
    Amount
    Color

Need to maintain good gynecological hygiene

Need for regular, periodic gynecological examinations

Importance of cytological Pap examinations

    First smear at onset of sexual activity or age 18

    Second 1 year later, then q3 years to age 35, then q5 years to age 60

    Annual smears if at high risk

Signs and symptoms to report to physician

That early detection is rare (no early symptoms)

Expected outcome/evaluation

Patient demonstrates knowledge of risk factors associated with ovarian cancer, signs and symptoms requiring health care evaluation, and detection measures for determining ovarian cancer

Cervical Cancer
Determination of Risk Factors

Low socioeconomic status: increased incidence

First coitus at early age

Multiple sex partners

Frequent genital infections; viral exposure (herpes simplex type 2, human papillomavirus)

Mismanaged parturition

Nonbarrier-type contraceptive

Chronic vaginal douching

Signs and symptoms

Early

    Unexplained vaginal bleeding or spotting

    Postcoital, postdouche bleeding

    Vaginal discharge: watery, purulent, or mucoid

Late

    Pelvic pain

    Irritation, vulvitis

    Yellow, frequently foul-smelling vaginal discharge

    Urinary symptoms, leakage of urine or feces from vagina

    Anorexia, weight loss

Nursing diagnoses/interventions/evaluation

 NDX: Knowledge deficit related to lack of information about prevention and early detection of cervical cancer

Prevention/detection

Ensure that patient and/or significant other knows and understands

    Importance of maintaining accurate menstrual cycle history

        Frequency

        Length of menses

        Amount

        Color

Risk factors and importance of realistic modifications

Need to maintain good personal and gynecological hygiene

Need to avoid frequent douching, especially during adolescence and pregnancy

Importance of delaying sexual function in early teen years

Need for regular, periodic gynecological examinations

Importance of cytological Pap examinations

    First smear at onset of sexual activity or age 18

    ACS states that women who have had normal Pap smear for 2 consecutive years can then have one every third year

    American College of Obstetrics and Gynecology (ACOG) recommends that sexually active women have a Pap smear annually

That Pap screening and physical examinations are the most effective measures of early detection and proper follow-up care to prevent cervical cancer

Signs and symptoms to report to physician

Mirror method of self-examination to inspect for

    Skin excoriation

    Ulcers

    Lumps

    Leukoplakia

    Narrowing of introitus

    Atrophy

Expected outcome/evaluation

Patient demonstrates knowledge of risk factors associated with cervical cancer, signs and symptoms requiring health care evaluation, and detection measures for determining cervical cancer

Uterine Cancer (Endometrial)
Determination of Risk Factors

Menstrual irregularities

Infertility, anovulatory

Nulliparous

Late menopause

Long-term use of estrogen drugs after menopause

History of

    Obesity

    Diabetes

    Hypertension

    Adenomatous hyperplasia

Signs and Symptoms

Any abnormal vaginal bleeding

Postmenopausal bleeding

Purulent discharge

Endometrial polyps

Enlarged, boggy uterus on examination
Lower abdominal and low back pain in late-stage disease

Nursing diagnoses/interventions/evaluation

■ **NDX:** Knowledge deficit related to lack of information about prevention and early detection of uterine (endometrial) cancer

Prevention/detection

Ensure that patient and/or significant other knows and understands
  Importance of maintaining accurate menstrual cycle history
    Frequency
    Length of menses
    Amount
    Color
  That detection by Pap smear is of low reliability
  High-risk profile
    Over 50 years of age
    No pregnancies, obesity, diabetes, hypertension with increased estrogen exposure
  Early detection helped by routine pelvic examinations
  Signs and symptoms to report to physician

Expected outcome/evaluation

Patient demonstrates knowledge of risk factors associated with uterine cancer, signs and symptoms requiring health care evaluation, and detection measures for determining uterine cancer

Leukemia
Determination of Risk Factors

Exposure to ionizing radiation
  Work environment
  Prenatal
  Treatment of preexisting cancer
Genetic factors
  Bloom's syndrome
  Trisomy 21 (Down's syndrome: 15 to 20 times the risk)
  Trisomy G (Klinefelter's syndrome)
  Fanconi's syndrome
  Philadelphia chromosome: positive
  Ataxia telangiectasis
  Family history of hematological disorder
Chemical exposure
  Benzene
  Phenylbutazone
  Arsenic
  Medications
    Chloramphenicol
    Alkylating chemotherapeutic agents
Immunodeficiency
Viral exposure

Signs and Symptoms

Anemia: pallor, fatigue, dyspnea, palpitations, headache, syncope, anorexia
Thrombocytopenia: petechiae, epistaxis, blood in excreta, bleeding gums, ecchymosis, hematoma formation, purpura
Leukopenia
  Skin infections: may appear red or dark without pus
  Fever, stomatitis, upper respiratory infection (URI) symptoms, urinary infection
Bone and joint pain
Cervical lymphadenopathy
Oropharyngeal lesions
Peridontal infections
Ocular lesions and hemorrhage
Gingival hypertrophy
GI manifestations
  Dysphagia
  Esophagitis
  Perirectal abscess
Genitourinary manifestation: uric acid nephropathy
Cardiopulmonary manifestations
  Impaired respiration
  Pneumonia
Nervous system manifestations
Lymphadenopathy
Hepatomegaly
Splenomegaly

Nursing diagnoses/interventions/evaluation

■ **NDX:** Knowledge deficit related to lack of information about prevention and detection of leukemia

Prevention

Ensure that patient and/or significant other knows and understands
  Importance of decreasing exposure time to x-ray examinations especially in young children
    Be certain diagnostic studies are essential
    Careful preparation and positioning to prevent retakes
    Shielding of gonads and other body parts during x-ray examination
    Proper shielding of health care workers when assisting with x-ray examination
  Importance of reducing exposure to toxic chemicals

Detection

Ensure that patient and/or significant other knows and understands
  Importance of regular, periodic physical examinations, including
    Palpation of lymph nodes, liver, and spleen
    Inspection of skin and mucous membranes

Palpation of sternum, bones, and joints
Importance of reporting signs and symptoms to physician
Ensure that patient/significant other is knowledgeable about detection methods
Laboratory tests
Radiologic tests
Bone marrow aspiration

Expected outcome/evaluation

Patient demonstrates knowledge of risk factors associated with leukemia, signs and symptoms requiring health care follow-up, and methods for detection of leukemia

Hodgkin's Disease
Determination of Risk Factors

Male: higher incidence
White
Young adult or over 70 years of age
High socioeconomic status
No or few siblings
History of
Infectious mononucleosis
Immunodeficiency syndrome
Use of amphetamines is questionable; not proven

Signs and Symptoms

Painless lymphadenopathy (usually supraclavicular or cervical area)
Mediastinal, axillary, and inguinal less commonly
Fever, night sweats, weight loss, lethargy, malaise, anorexia
Lymphadenopathy can cause obstruction, resulting in edema and pain
Cervical node enlargement: venous occlusion, neck edema, airway obstruction
Mediastinal adenopathy: dyspnea, cough
Inguinal involvement: dysuria, frequency, painful urination, and lumbar discomfort

Nursing diagnoses/interventions/evaluation

■ **NDX:** Knowledge deficit related to lack of information about detection of Hodgkin's disease

Detection

Ensure that patient and/or significant other knows and understands
Importance of reporting symptoms to physician
Importance of scheduling periodic physical examinations
Detection methods
Laboratory tests
Staging laparotomy

Expected outcome/evaluation

Patient demonstrates knowledge of risk factors associated with Hodgkin's disease, signs and symptoms requiring health care follow-up, and methods for detection of Hodgkin's disease

ONCOLOGY ASSESSMENT

Cancer diagnosis is based on physical and psychosocial assessment, including laboratory data, radiologic studies, biopsies, and surgical procedures. Classifications of tumor, lymph node involvement, and metastasis are used to determine the stage of the malignant condition (see the box and Tables 14-1, 14-3 on pp. 594, 595). The performance ability of the patient is evaluated and may be used to determine the type and length of treatment (see Table 14-2 on p. 594).

Current Condition

General appearance
Posture
Body movements
Hygiene
General survey of mental status
Orientation
Attention span
Speech
Behavior/mannerisms
Chief complaint
Vital signs
Weight and height
Patient's concerns
Patient's problems or needs
Patient's knowledge of
Disease process
Treatment
Outcome

Physical Assessment

Hematological system
Monitor complete blood cell count (CBC), hemoglobin, platelet count
Bleeding/hemorrhage
Petechiae
Unexplained bruises or ecchymoses
Hematomas
Bleeding from any body orifice
Prolonged oozing of blood from IM or IV sites
Change in vital signs
Change in neurological status (headache, disorientation)
Pad count high for menstruating females

TNM CLASSIFICATIONS*

PRIMARY TUMOR

T_x: Minimal requirements to assess the primary tumor cannot be met

T_0: No evidence of primary tumor

T_{IS}: Carcinoma in situ

T_1, T_2, T_3, T_4: Progressive increase in tumor size or involvement

N: Regional lymph nodes

N_0: No evidence of regional nodal involvement

N_1, N_2, N_3, N_4: Increasing degree of demonstrable abnormality of regional lymph nodes

M: Distant metastasis

M_0: Indicates absence

M_+: Indicates presence

HISTOPATHOLOGY

G_1: Well-differentiated grade

G_2: Moderately well-differentiated grade

G_3 and G_4: Poorly to very poorly differentiated grade

RESIDUAL TUMOR

R_0: No residual tumor

R_1: Microscopic residual tumor

R_2: Macroscopic residual tumor

STAGING METHOD

cTNM: Staging determined by clinical noninvasive physical examination, laboratory, and radiographic studies

sTNM: Staging information based on surgical procedures, biopsies, and histopathological analysis

pTNM: Staging determined by correlation of clinical, pathological, and residual tumor findings

*T, Primary tumor; N, regional lymph nodes; M, metastasis by vascular dissemination.

TABLE 14-1. Cancer Staging Using TNM* Classifications

Stage	T	N	M	Survival	Comments
I	1	0	0	70%-90%	Mass limited to organ of origin; nodes not involved; operable and resectable
II	2	1	0	50% ±	Local spread to surrounding tissue; nodal involvement suspected or proved; operable but without certainty of total resection
III	3	2	0	20% ±	Extensive primary tumor with fixation to deeper structures; nodes involved; operable but not resectable
IV	4	3	+	<5%	Distant metastases; inoperable

*T, Primary tumor; N, regional lymph nodes; M, metastasis by vascular dissemination.

TABLE 14-2. Host Performance Status*

Status	ECOG/Zubrod	Karnofsky (%)
H_0: Normal activity	0	90-100
H_1: Symptomatic and ambulatory; cares for self	1	70-80
H_2: Ambulatory more than 50% of time; occasionally needs assistance	2	50-60
H_3: Ambulatory less than 50% of time; requires special nursing and/or medical assistance	3	30-40
H_4: Bedridden; may need hospitalization	4	10-20

From American Joint Committee for Cancer Staging.
*The host performance status is determined at the time of classification; the condition of the patient does not enter into determination of stage but may be a factor in deciding type and time of treatment.

TABLE 14-3. Classification of Tumors

Tissue of origin	Benign	Malignant
Epithelium: surface skin and mucous membranes	Papilloma Polyp	Squamous cell or epidermoid carcinoma Basal cell carcinoma
Glands	Adenoma Cystadenoma	Adenocarcinoma
Connective tissue		
Embryonic fibrous tissue	Myxoma	Myxosarcoma
Fibrous tissue	Fibroma	Fibrosarcoma
Cartilage	Chondroma	Chondrosarcoma
Bone	Osteoma	Osteosarcoma
Fat	Lipoma	Liposarcoma
Synovial membrane	Synovioma	Synovial sarcoma
Blood vessels	Hemangioma	Hemangiosarcoma
Lymph vessels	Lymphangioma	Lymphangiosarcoma
Muscle tissue		
Smooth muscle	Leiomyoma	Leiomyosarcoma
Striated muscle	Rhabdomyoma	Rhabdomyosarcoma
Hematopoietic tissue		
Lymphoid tissue		Malignant lymphoma Non-Hodgkin's lymphoma Lymphocytic leukemia
Granulocytic tissue		Myelocytic leukemia
Erythrocytic tissue		Erythroleukemia
Plasma cells		Multiple myeloma
Nerve tissue		
Glial cells	Glioma	Glioblastoma (astrocytoma) Spongioblastoma
Meninges	Meningioma	Meningeal sarcoma
Nerve cells	Neuroma; ganglioneuroma	Neurogenic sarcoma
Neuroectoderm	Nevus	Neuroblastoma
Fibers	Neurofibroma	Neurofibrosarcoma
Retina		Retinoblastoma
Adrenal medulla	Pheochromocytoma	Pheochromocytoma
Nerve sheaths	Neurilemmoma	Neurilemmal sarcoma
Tumors of more than one tissue		
Breast	Fibroadenoma	Cystosarcoma phyllodes
Embryonic kidney		Nephroblastoma (Wilms')
Multipotent cells	Teratoma	
Uterus		Mixed mesodermal
Miscellaneous		
Melanoblasts	Pigmented nevus	Malignant melanoma Melanocarcinoma
Placenta	Hydatidiform mole	Choriocarcinoma (chorionepithelioma)
Ovary	Granulosa-theca cell tumor	Carcinoma
Testes	Interstitial cell tumor	Seminoma (spermatocytic) Carcinoma (embryonal)
Thymus	Thymoma	Thymoma

Anemia
    Palpitations, chest pain on exertion
    Dyspnea
    Dizziness, syncope
    Fatigue, weakness
    Glossitis, anorexia, indigestion
    Insomnia, hypersensitivity to cold
Infection(s), present and past
    Temperature
    White blood cell count (WBC), including differential
    Skin and mucous membrane integrity
        Skin folds (axillae, buttocks, perineum)
        Body cavities (mouth, vagina, rectum)
        Venous access sites
        Surgical wounds
    Respiratory tract
    Genitourinary system
    Eyes
        Conjunctivitis, iritis
        Infection of eyelid or lacrimal gland
Pain (p. 10)
    Type
        Acute
        Chronic
    Location, circumstances of onset
    Intensity, quality
    Activities that increase pain: eating, separation from
        significant other
    Effects on patient and family
    Relief measures
        Medication
        Distraction, meditation, relaxation, exercises
        Imagery; psychosocial and/or spiritual counseling
        Variables affecting response
            Anxiety/fear
            Ethnic/cultural background
            Past experiences with pain management
            Meaning of pain (recurrence of disease, death)
            Perceptions of pain therapy (fear of addictions)
Skin
    Color: pallor, duskiness, jaundice
    Integrity
        Breaks, lesions, ulcers
        Petechiae, bruises, erythema, ecchymosis
    Temperature
        Local and systemic
        Feeling of warmth and/or cold
    Hydration: turgor, edema, perspiration
    Hair: distribution, alopecia
    Nails: color, texture, clubbing
Eyes
    Pupil size and response
    Color
    Sclera
    Cataract formation

Nose: bleeding, drainage, crusting
Mouth, tongue, lips
    Color, moisture; presence of lesions on palate, tongue,
        buccal mucosa, inner surface of lips, and oral pharynx
    Color, amount, and consistency of saliva
    Condition of teeth
        Dental caries, rough edges
        Plaque, dental fit
    Mobility of tongue
    Ability to chew and taste
    Breath odor
Parotid gland: size, tenderness, pain
Lymph nodes
    Neck, axilla, groin
    Size, tenderness, pain
    Thyroid size
Gastrointestinal system
    Appetite
    Food and fluid intake
        Type, consistency, amount
        Frequency, preferences
    Nausea, vomiting
    Frequency, character
    Color, amount
    Factors affecting occurrence
        Anticipation
        Activities, treatments, time of day
        Other associated factors
    Relief measures used; variables affecting response
Abdomen
    Distention
    Bowel sounds
        Present: type, frequency, character
        Absent
    Rigid, flaccid, tender
Spleen and liver: size, tenderness, pain
Stool
    Normal pattern; frequency (time of last stool),
        amount, color, consistency
    Aids to normal elimination
        Dietary (food and fluid)
        Medications (laxatives)
        Enemas
    Method of elimination: toilet, commode, bedpan
    Artificial orifices
        Colostomy, ileostomy
    Method of care for excretions from artificial orifices
    Pain related to defecation
    Presence of blood (on surface or mixed throughout)
    Mucus, pus
    Level of mobility/immobility
    Stress
Diarrhea/constipation
    Frequency, amount
    Consistency, color

Bleeding, occult bleeding
Flatulence
Associated factors
Medications
Relief measures, methods of coping
Genitourinary system
  Urine, urination
    Usual pattern
    Frequency, amount
    Color, odor, specific gravity
    Presence of usual constituents
    Character, bleeding
    Any urgency felt
    Effort in starting and stopping
    Pain, burning, itching
    Nocturia
    Incontinence
    Retention
    Method of urine elimination (void, in-and-out catheter, Foley, urinary diversion)
    Care measures, methods of coping
  Fluid intake
  Medications (diuretics)
  History of urinary tract infection
Respiratory system
  Respiratory rate; depth and character of breathing
  Type of airway
  Patency of airway
  Breath sounds (normal, adventitious, increased, decreased)
  Color of skin and mucous membrane
  Chest size and shape
  Chest excursion and symmetry
  Position of trachea
  Shortness of breath on exertion
  Use of accessory muscles
  Nasal flaring, pursed-lip breathing, clubbing of extremities
  Cough: ability, frequency, depth, force, productivity
  Sputum: color, amount, odor, consistency, time of day produced
  Audible grunting, snoring, stridor
  Frequency of suctioning
  Present level and tolerance of activity
  History of
    Smoking, pulmonary infection, pulmonary diseases, exposure to air pollutants
    Chemotherapy (bleomycin), radiation therapy to thorax
  Laboratory tests: blood gas, sputum, blood cultures, WBC
  Diagnostic studies: chest x-ray examination, pulmonary function tests
Cardiovascular system
  Heart rate, blood pressure, temperature

Heart sounds
Peripheral pulses: rate, rhythm, volume
Skin color, dryness, moistness
Decreased cardiac output
  Tachycardia
  Electrocardiogram (ECG) changes
  Dyspnea on exertion, exercise intolerance
  Rales, wheezing, cough
  Edema: location, type
Neurological system
  Sensorium (awake, alert, lethargic, stuporous, comatose)
  Orientation to time, person, place, and situation
  Ability to follow commands
  Memory (recent, remote)
  Attentiveness, distractibility
  Language spoken, clarity, appropriateness
  Ability to read and write
  Motor response
    Voluntary, involuntary
    Gait, balance, paralysis, weakness
  Reflex response: pupil, gag, cough, Babinski's sign, deep tendon reflex
  Tics, trembling, seizures
  Pain
    Rate pain using pain scale
    Location, onset, duration, type
    Precipitating factors, relief measures
  Sensations: tingling, numbness, leg cramps
  Foot-drop, wrist-drop, handgrip
  Sensory
    Visual
    Auditory
    Olfactory
    Taste
    Tactile
Safety measures used

Pertinent Background Information

Sleep/rest
  Usual pattern; hours of sleep at night
  Difficulties
  Number and duration of daily naps
  Use of sleep aids: name, dosage of drug, frequency of use, length of time used
  Symptoms that may affect sleep: pain, anxiety, night sweats
  Signs and symptoms of sleep disturbance: irritability, anxiety, loss of train of thought
  Care measures
Sexuality
  Sexual history
  Current practices, reproductive history
  Impact of therapies on sexuality/sexual function; reaction of partner to illness

Expressions of affection
Methods of coping
Social
    Support system; most significant other
    Role function
    Housing/living arrangement
    Presence of dependent behaviors; presence of independent behaviors
Spirituality (p. 26): beliefs, faith, concerns
Activities of daily living (ADLs)
    Lifestyle (active, sedentary); exercise tolerance
    Degree of immobility
    Household assistance
    Employment, leisure/hobbies
    Other activities and concerns
Home environment
    Caregiver, facilities, and equipment available for meeting care needs
    Pets
    Concerns
Teaching needs
    During hospitalization
    Self-care
Previous conditions
    Acute or chronic diseases or conditions
    Surgery
    Radiation therapy
    Chemotherapy
    Biological response modifiers
    Trauma
        Physical
        Emotional

Psychosocial Assessment*
PREDIAGNOSTIC PERIOD (DETERMINATION OF FEELINGS AND PRIOR KNOWLEDGE)

Awareness of signs and symptoms; length of time known
Delay in seeking treatment
    Threats to
        Independence
        Group belongingness
        Influence on others
        Adaptive functioning
        Preexisting stability
        Decision-making ability
        Cherished values
        Desired roles
        Limitless future
        Control over destiny
Information about treatment
    Knowledge deficits
    Level of understanding

---

*Adapted from Marino LB: *Cancer nursing,* St Louis, 1981, Mosby–Year Book.

Misconceptions and myths
Ethnic/cultural beliefs
Knowledge of resources

DIAGNOSTIC PERIOD

Fears of outcome
Perceptions of threat
Significance of studies
Information about cancer and body functions
    Factual
    Deficits
    Misconceptions
        Myths
        Fantasies
Knowledge and level of understanding
    Diagnostic tests and examinations
    Schedule of tests and examinations
    Reasons for studies and preparation
    Role of patient in studies
    Physical effect of studies; expected symptoms and responses
Continuously validate patient's understanding and perceptions
Coping methods of patient, significant other, or family
    Daily activities
    Use of work and leisure activities
    Relationships
    Methods of communication
        Ability to disclose: open with family, peers, counselors, and/or medical and nursing staff
        Inability to communicate; awareness of significance
Behavioral responses
    Anxiety
        Apprehensive expectation
        Fear and worry about negative outcome
    Vigilance and scanning
        Hyperattentiveness
        Distractibility
        Concentration problems
        Impatience
        Feeling "on edge"
    Motor tension
        Jumpiness
        Restlessness
        Inability to relax
        Insomnia
        Strained facies
        Easily startled
    Autonomic hyperactivity
        Tachycardia
        Tachypnea
        Dry mouth
        Sweating
        Cold, clammy hands
        Upset stomach
        Nightmares

CONFIRMATION OF DIAGNOSIS

Knowledge of results and meaning of diagnostic studies
  X-ray examinations
  Imaging
    CT scans
    Magnetic resonance imaging (MRI)
  Isotope studies
  Ultrasound examinations
  Endoscopy
  Cytology
  Laboratory data
  Biopsy
Meaning of illness
  Perceived threat to
    Independence
    Job and economic security
    Career goals
    Relationships
    Integrity of body
    Body functions
    Recreational activities
    Sexual attractiveness and functioning
    Intimacy
  Fears of disfigurement and pain
  Secondary gains: alteration in behavior
    Acting out
    Demands for attention
    Controlling behaviors
  Methods for handling past crises
Availability of knowledgeable and supportive resources
  Family
  Significant others
  Co-workers
  Social contacts
  Religious counsel
  Community
Behavioral responses
  Shock/denial
    Rejection of reality
    Increased perspiration
    Pallor
    Faintness
    Nausea
    Anorexia
    Insomnia
    Confusion
    Difficulty in concentrating
    Difficulty in working
  Anger
    Impatience
    Bitterness
    Jealousy
    Helplessness
    Increased awareness
    Limited attention span

Uncooperative behavior
Attention-seeking behavior
Loud talking
Vulgar language
Multiple complaints
Guilt/punishment
  Underlying reasons
  Misconceptions about cancer: seen as unclean, contagious
  Diagnosis attributed to something person did or did not do
Hopelessness (p. 15)
  Quiet
  Withdrawn
  Melancholy
  Older appearance
  Poor posture
  Gait: slow, dragging
  Decreased respiration
  Feeling of fullness
  Belching
  Constipation
Bargaining
  Depression
  Exhaustion
  Attempts to avoid reality
  Self-questioning
  Shortness of breath
  Feelings of weakness
Panic attack
  Dyspnea
  Palpitations
  Chest pain
  Feelings of choking or smothering
  Dizziness
  Feelings of unreality
  Tingling of hands and/or feet
  Hot and cold flashes
  Sweating
  Faintness
  Trembling or shaking
  Fear of dying, "going crazy," or doing something uncontrollable during an attack
Be aware of importance of need to initiate appropriate interventions rapidly when the following are observed
  Agitation
  Uncharacteristic, unexplained extreme behavior
  Unrealistic perceptions and expectations
  Feelings of
    Worthlessness
    Extreme guilt
    Suicide
  Inappropriate resistance to treatment
  Use of controversial treatments (e.g., laetrile, me-

gavitamins, mechanical devices, miracle drugs, psychic surgeons, Hoxsey and Krebiozen potions)
Acceptance
    Contemplativeness
    Serenity
    Talks about condition

TREATMENT PHASE

Adequate information for informed decision making
    Options for
        Types of surgery
        Radiotherapy
        Chemotherapy
        Biological response modifiers
    Risks, benefits, and complications for each type of treatment
    Results of current research: unpredictable outcome
    Prognosis associated with each therapy
Level of understanding of chosen therapy
    Preparation
    Associated physical changes
    Complications
    Local and systemic effects
Reactions to treatment
    Follows directions
    Alterations in ADLs
Expresses needs for
    Hope associated with cure
        Future pleasurable experiences
        Ability to reach some goals
        Others being available for support
        Idea that life had meaning
    Honesty
        In answers to questions
        No protection from the truth
        In not withholding information
    Information about
        Treatment; side or toxic effects
        Special procedures or treatments
        Changes in expected outcomes
        Expected patient participation
        Availability and support of resources
        Whether patient can share what he or she has learned about care
Expresses feelings or conveys
    Anger
    Fear
    Sadness
    Helplessness
    Dependency
    Powerlessness

PREPARATION FOR DISCHARGE

Knowledge of continuing care
Methods for dealing with pain (p. 10)

Increase or decrease in functioning
Complications of treatment as disease progresses
Special procedures
Psychological needs
Daily activity allowances
Signs and symptoms of recurrence or progression
Need for follow-up care
Support groups and counselors: specific information, and contact person
Emergency care instructions

Recurrence

Expresses fears of
    Increased dependency
    Increased weakness
    Increased immobility
    Isolation
    Disintegration of relationships
Communicates need for
    Being told death is close
    Information about practical things to do before death
    Discussing pain, pain relief measures, and fear of loss of control
    Discussion of beliefs
Ability to continue treatment

Advanced or Terminal Condition

Knowledge of present diagnosis and prognosis
Symptom-control methods; patient and family participation
Responsibilities
    Relationships
    Completion of unfinished business
Ability to discuss fears of
    Inability to continue with life's activities and relationships
    Being abandoned
Hospice: alternative methods of care
Meaning of death
    Shameful
    Peaceful
Disengagement
    Life's business finished
    Goodbyes said
    Psychological withdrawal
    Few interactions

LARYNGECTOMY: RADICAL NECK DISSECTION

Removal of the larynx and surrounding neck tissue to treat a cancerous condition; a permanent stoma is formed

Preoperative Assessment
Observations/findings

Tachypnea
Dysphagia
Hemoptysis
Stridor
Hoarseness
Enlarged cervical nodes
Pain in Adam's apple; radiates to ear
Cough
Psychological problems
  Fear of surgery
  Body image change
  Loss of voice
  Panic
  Denial
  Disbelief
  Anger

Preparation

Prepare patient for surgery
  See General Preoperative Care/Teaching (p. 27)
Demonstrate
  Laryngectomy tube
  Cleaning equipment
  Suctioning equipment
Explain that nasogastric (NG) tube will be in place for feeding
Explain that IV will be in place for 24 to 48 hr
Determine level of reading, writing; identify primary language
Determine if patient can hear
Explain that patient will not be able to talk postoperatively
Prepare patient in means of communication; allow time for practice and questions
  Pad and pencil or Magic Slate
  Picture cards if patient is unable to write
Explain that patient may be in critical care for 24 to 48 hr; tour critical care area with patient and family
Instruct family to purchase a mirror with a stand
Have speech therapist visit patient preoperatively if possible
Permit opportunity for patient to meet with other individuals who have undergone similar experience

Postoperative Assessment
Observations/findings

Hemorrhage
Airway obstruction
  Restlessness
  Tachycardia
  Use of accessory muscles of respiration
  Tachypnea
  Noisy respirations
  Wheezing

Stridor
Pallor
Cyanosis
Atelectasis
Dehydration
Sensory deprivation
Fear of suffocation
Behavioral response
  Helplessness
  Fear
  Anger
Sputum
  Amount
  Character
Site of incision
  Discoloration
  Pain
  Swelling
  Drainage
  Sloughing of tissue
  Stoma
Wound drains
  Sump drains
  Hemovac
Infection
  Elevated temperature
  Purulent aspirate

Laboratory/diagnostic studies

Chest x-ray examination
Arterial blood gases
Baseline pulmonary function tests
ECG
Electrolytes
Fiberoptic endoscopy
Biopsy of suspect lesions
Skull and neck radiographic studies
Bone scan
Anti-Epstein-Barr virus antibody titers

Potential complications

Pneumonia
Respiratory failure
Metastasis
Carotid erosion
Pneumothorax
Hypovolemic shock
Tracheoesophageal fistula

Medical Management

Radiation therapy
Artificial airway and mechanical ventilation
NG tube
Oxygen therapy with humidification
Parenteal therapy
Nutritional support

Nursing diagnoses/interventions/evaluation

■ **NDX:** Ineffective airway clearance related to removal of glottis (partial/total), altering ability to cough and swallow

Assess area around laryngectomy/tracheostomy tube, noting any bleeding
Assess quality and rate of respirations
Auscultate breath sounds q2h to 4h
Monitor amount and quality of oropharyngeal secretions
Maintain patent airway
   Maintain in upright position
   Apply humidification
   Suction laryngectomy/tracheostomy tube prn: need for suction determined by auscultation of chest for breath sounds qh
   Suction if crackles or rhonchi over large airways are heard
   Use sterile technique when suctioning patient
   If on ventilatory support, hyperoxygenate and/or hyperinflate patient's lungs for four or five breaths before suctioning
   Clean inner cannula q2h to 4h and prn
   Avoid occluding airway with bed linen or when turning patient
   Have hand-held resuscitator with adaptor at bedside
   Instruct patient in suctioning and cleaning procedures
Have standby laryngectomy tube available: same size and type
Assist and teach patient to turn, cough, and deep breathe q2h

Expected outcome/evaluation

Airway is patent as evidenced by
   Clear breath sounds
   Ability to expectorate secretions
   Demonstrating skills to maintain airway clearance

■ **NDX:** Impaired skin integrity related to surgical incision, tracheostomy, and impaired wound healing secondary to preoperative radiation

Assess for signs of infection: purulent drainage around stoma, elevated temperature
Clean skin around stoma q4h and prn
   Wash with hydrogen peroxide
   Rinse with saline solution
Administer oral hygiene q2h to 4h
Elevate head of bed 45 to 60 degrees; prevent forward flexion of neck
   Remove pillows if necessary
   Place small towel under shoulders
Record drainage q8h if Hemovac or sump drains for continuous suction are in place
Pat dry

Change laryngectomy ties prn; make sure ties are loose enough not to cause pressure on neck
Place 4 × 4-inch gauze pad under laryngectomy tube
Change dressing as ordered
   Report excessive drainage to physician
   Clean area around drains with hydrogen peroxide

Expected outcome/evaluation

Maintains skin integrity as evidenced by
   Gradual reduction of redness and swelling
   Presence of granulation tissue
   No sign of elevated temperature

■ **NDX:** Impaired verbal communication related to surgical removal of larynx

Assess and review patient's understanding of methods of communication
Present calm, reassuring manner
Provide immediate means of communication
   Have call light at bedside
   Arrange signs or signals that call for immediate help
Have pad and pencil or Magic Slate available
Avoid asking questions that require "yes" or "no" answers
Wait for patient to write answer
Do not anticipate end of sentence
Read statements aloud; encourage patient to communicate feelings
Provide emotional support
   Encourage communication with significant other
   Deal with fear of suffocation, helplessness, anger
   Anticipate physical and emotional needs
   Prepare visitors for patient's appearance
   Help visitors and staff not to exclude patient from conversations or talk exclusively to one another
Assist patient with operation of artificial larynx, if available
Refer to speech therapy as indicated

Expected outcome/evaluation

Develops and uses an effective communication systems as evidenced by
   Demonstrating ability to make needs known to medical and nursing staff
   Increasing use of Magic Slate or voice box

■ **NDX:** Knowledge deficit related to lack of information about disease process and self-care management

Assess level of understanding of disease process and home care management
Assess emotional status to identify any barriers to learning
Explain importance of maintaining diet as ordered, even though food will taste dull because of loss of senses of smell and taste

Review bathing activities
  To use tub baths initially
  When showering:
    Wear shield over stoma
    Use shower hose to direct spray below neck
    Avoid getting soap into stoma
  Instruct male patients to shave with electric razor or safety razor and to avoid getting lather into stoma
Explain need to keep stoma covered at all times and to wear clothing with high necklines, natural fiber scarves, and no jewelry
Explain importance of covering stoma when coughing and reporting persistent cough to physician
Explain need to avoid
  Smoking and persons who smoke
  Persons with URIs
Explain need to wear medical alert band stating neck breather
Explain importance of
  Ongoing outpatient care
  Not using aerosol sprays around stoma
Discuss symptoms of respiratory distress to report to physician
  Difficulty breathing
  Increased temperature
Discuss medications: name, dosage, time of administration, purpose, side effects
Ensure that patient and/or significant other demonstrates
  Administration of tube feeding if ordered
  Care of incision
  Symptoms to report to physician
    Swelling
    Pain
    Drainage
Ensure that patient and/or significant other demonstrates care of laryngectomy and stoma; provide mirror
  Handwashing procedure
  Taking four or five deep breaths before suctioning
  Suctioning: clean procedure, not sterile
  Caring for inner cannula: clean procedure, not sterile
  Removing and replacing outer cannula
  Changing laryngectomy ties
  Cleansing skin around stoma bid
    Use hydrogen peroxide
    Rinse with water
    Pat dry
Refer to community support groups
  American Cancer Society
  Lost Cord/New Voice Club

Expected outcome/evaluation

Patient demonstrates knowledge of disease process and home care management, as evidenced by verbalization and return demonstration of home management principles

Additional nursing diagnoses

Body image disturbance related to cognitive-perceptual changes
Altered nutrition: less than body requirements related to changes in taste, disinterest in food, and difficulty swallowing secondary to surgery, radiation, or chemotherapy

ESOPHAGEAL CARCINOMA

Carcinoma developing in the middle or lower one third of the esophagus; usually fatal because the condition is advanced before symptoms appear

Assessment
Observations/findings

Increasing dysphagia
Painful swallowing
Substernal pain
Feeling of fullness
Pyrosis (heartburn)
Fear and anxiety
Weight loss
Generalized malaise
Dehydration
Regurgitation after eating
Increased salivation and mucus formation
Foul breath
Singultus (hiccups)
Eructation
Hoarseness and coughing
Hepatomegaly
Diaphragmatic paralysis (phrenic nerve involvement)

Laboratory/diagnostic studies

Endoscopy with biopsy and cytology
CBC and electrolytes
Chest radiologic study
Barium studies
Bronchoscopy
CT scan: liver and chest
Liver function tests

Potential complications

Malnutrition, anemia
Electrolyte imbalance
Fluid volume depletion
Aspiration pneumonia
Infection
Metastasis to other organs
Hemorrhage

Medical Management

Analgesics
Chemotherapeutic agents
Radiation therapy
Insertion of plastic tubes (Celestin tube) to maintain nutrition

Esophageal surgery (esophagogastrectomy)
Gastrostomy tube insertion

Nursing diagnoses/interventions*/evaluation

■ **NDX:** Ineffective airway clearance related to esophageal obstruction

Maintain bed rest if condition warrants
  Elevate head of bed 30 to 45 degrees
  Avoid supine position
  Do not gatch knees
Assess patient's ability to swallow and teach coughing techniques
Perform orotracheal suction as needed
Provide emesis basin and tissues for expectorating
Assist and teach patient to turn and deep breathe q2h to 4h
Administer oral hygiene q2h to 4h and prn
Monitor vital signs q4h

Expected outcome/evaluation

Patient demonstrates ability to maintain a clear airway

■ **NDX:** Altered nutrition: less than body requirements related to anorexia and dysphagia

Assess patient's ability to swallow liquids and solid foods
Provide high-calorie, high-protein diet as ordered
Encourage patient to chew foods well, to take small bites, and to eat slowly
Assist with feedings prn
Force fluids to 3000 ml/24 hr unless contraindicated
Measure intake and output
Weigh patient daily at same time with same clothing and scale
Initiate parenteral therapy with vitamins and electrolytes as ordered
Total parenteral nutrition (TPN) may be ordered (p. 36)
Assist with insertion of NG tube if ordered; connect to low, intermittent suction or closed gravity drainage as ordered
Provide gastrostomy or Celestin tube feedings if appropriate

Expected outcome/evaluation

Patient's caloric intake is maintained

■ **NDX:** Pain related to disease process

Assess pain, location, characteristics, onset, frequency, and intensity; use pain rating scale
Administer analgesics as ordered

Assess effectiveness of medication
Teach and assist with alternate pain-relieving techniques (e.g., imagery, music, relaxation)
Change position q2h to 4h
Provide planned rest periods
Assist with and teach active or perform passive range of motion (ROM) exercises q4h

Expected outcome/evaluation

Patient states that pain is minimal or absent; appears relaxed

■ **NDX:** Anxiety/fear related to poor disease prognosis

Assess patient's and/or significant other's ability to communicate feelings
Assist in dealing with emotional reactions to disease process
Recommend outside supportive groups (visiting nurses, American Cancer Society) for home care assistance
Encourage and provide time for verbalization of concerns
Involve dietitian for assistance in planning specific types of meals
Develop means of communication if patient has speaking difficulties

Expected outcome/evaluation

Patient/significant other and/or caregiver verbalizes fears and anxieties and uses effective coping mechanisms

■ **NDX:** Knowledge deficit related to lack of information about home care

Instruct patient and/or significant other on type of diet required and care of tube
  For gastrostomy tube
    Method for ascertaining correct placement and amount of residual contents
  For Celestin tube
    Elevating head at all times
    Swallowing only small amounts
    Method for clearing obstructions
Discuss and teach pain management and injection administration if ordered
Enlist support of dietitian (RD), home health agencies, etc.
Discuss schedule of radiation or chemotherapy treatments as ordered
See section on symptomatic care in chemotherapy if needed (p. 670)
Explain need to maintain physician's follow-up appointments

Expected outcome/evaluation

Patient and/or significant other demonstrates understanding of home care and follow-up instructions

---

*Patient's condition dictates type and amount of care required; modify accordingly.

GASTRIC CARCINOMA

Carcinoma most frequently occurring in the pyloric segment and along the lesser curvature of the stomach; there are no early definitive signs of the disease process

Assessment
Observations/findings

Feeling of fullness after eating
Indigestion
Eructation
Epigastric pain or discomfort after eating
Dysphagia
Anorexia
Malaise, fatigue
Generalized weakness
Weight loss
Pallor
Vertigo/syncope
Nausea, vomiting
Occult blood in stool

Laboratory/diagnostic studies

Endoscopy with biopsy and cytology
Upper GI series
CBC, hematocrit (Hct, below normal), albumin (decreased)
Gastric analysis
Tomography
Stool for occult blood (positive)
Chest radiologic examination

Potential complications

Malnutrition
Dehydration
Electrolyte imbalance
Hematemesis
Pyloric obstruction
Epigastric mass
Enlarged axillary and/or supraclavicular lymph nodes
Recurrent phlebitis
Metastasis to liver

Medical Management

Analgesics
Parenteral fluids, diet, fluid intake
Chemotherapeutic agents
Radiation therapy
Surgery (gastric resection, gastrectomy)

Nursing diagnoses/interventions*/evaluation

■ **NDX:** Altered nutrition: less than body requirements related to dysphagia and/or nausea and vomiting

*Patient's condition dictates type and amount of care required; modify accordingly.

Provide light, well-balanced, high-calorie, high-protein diet or parenteral therapy with electrolytes and vitamins as ordered
Assess and identify foods that cause discomfort
Measure intake and output
Weigh patient daily at same time with same clothing and scale
Monitor stools for occult blood
Provide adequate fluid intake, 2500 ml/24 hr, unless contraindicated

Expected outcome/evaluation

Patient's nutritional status is maintained to meet body requirements

■ **NDX:** Pain related to progressive disease process

Assess pain: location, characteristics, onset, frequency, and intensity; use pain rating scale
Administer analgesics as ordered; assess effectiveness of pain relief measures
Coordinate care to provide planned rest periods between procedures
Teach and assist with alternate pain-relieving techniques (e.g., imagery, music, relaxation)
Assist and teach patient to turn and deep breathe q4h
Change position frequently to relieve pressure
Provide diversional activities

Expected outcome/evaluation

Patient expresses minimal discomfort or absence of pain; face and body are relaxed

■ **NDX:** Ineffective individual coping related to disease process and prognosis

Provide quiet environment
Encourage and allow time for verbalization of feelings
Support positive coping behaviors and assist patient with managing stress
Encourage communication with significant other
Reinforce physician's explanation of disease process and plan of treatment
Involve patient and/or significant other in care and explain procedures and treatments

Expected outcome/evaluation

Patient expresses concerns and manages stress with positive coping behaviors

■ **NDX:** Anticipatory grieving related to poor prognosis

Assess present coping styles and interdependence in relationship with others
Provide caring and accepting environment
  Listen carefully

Encourage and allow time for communication with significant other

Encourage verbalization of feelings

Provide reassurance as needed

Offer hope realistically

Expected outcome/evaluation

Patient and significant other verbalize feelings of grief and are provided opportunities to discuss these feelings in a supportive atmosphere

■ **NDX:** Knowledge deficit related to lack of information about home care needs

Explain dietary and nutrition care plan according to patient's condition; provide written instructions as needed

Discuss performing ADLs with assistance from home health care agencies as needed

Identify appropriate support groups for assistance

Explain grieving process and ways of working through it: denial, anger, bargaining, and acceptance (p. 18)

Demonstrate methods of pain management

Encourage follow-up physician care

Expected outcome/evaluation

Patient and/or significant other demonstrates understanding of home care and follow-up instructions

INTESTINAL CARCINOMA

carcinoma of small intestine Malignancy most frequently found in the lower duodenum and lower ileum; mortality is high; early signs and symptoms are usually absent

carcinoma of large intestine Slow-growing malignancy most frequently found in the cecum, lower ascending, and sigmoid colon; prognosis is optimistic; early signs and symptoms are usually absent

Assessment

Observations/findings

SPECIFIC

Small intestine
Nausea, vomiting
Anorexia
Upper abdominal pain
Large intestine
Alteration in bowel habits and function
Rectal bleeding, tarry stool
Abdominal cramps, pain, distention

COMMON

Generalized weakness
Weight loss

Laboratory/diagnostic studies

Upper GI series
Duodenoscopy with biopsy
Radiologic abdominal series
Barium enema
Sigmoidoscopy and colonoscopy with biopsy
CBC, electrolytes

Potential complications

Electrolyte imbalance
Dehydration
Anemia
Intestinal obstruction
Bowel abscess: fistula
Metastatic involvement: lungs, kidneys, bone

Medical Management

Diet or parenteral fluids with electrolytes and vitamins
Nasogastric/intestinal aspiration
Bed rest, ambulation
Analgesics
Chemotherapeutic agents
Radiotherapy, immunotherapy
Surgical intervention (resection, ostomy, abdominoperineal resection)

Nursing diagnoses/interventions*/evaluation

■ **NDX:** Altered nutrition: less than body requirements related to vomiting and/or anorexia

Maintain NPO

Administer parenteral fluids with electrolytes and vitamins C and K as ordered

Insert NG, nasointestinal tube as ordered; connect to low, intermittent suction; observe color and amount of drainage

Measure intake and output

Monitor serum electrolytes, hemoglobin (Hgb), and Hct

Monitor vital signs

Provide high-protein, high-carbohydrate, high-calorie, low-residue diet if diet is allowed; note foods that cause irritation and anorexia

Expected outcome/evaluation

Patient's nutritional status is maintained to meet body needs

■ **NDX:** Pain related to disease process

Assess pain: location, characteristics, onset, frequency, and intensity; use pain rating scale

---

*Patient's condition dictates type and amount of care required; modify accordingly.

Maintain on bed rest in position of comfort; do not use Gatch bed on knees

Plan all care to provide rest periods

Administer analgesics as ordered: large doses are sometimes needed in terminally ill patients; assess effectiveness of pain relief measures

Teach and assess with alternate pain-relieving techniques (e.g., music therapy, relaxation, imagery)

Perform passive or assist with and teach active ROM exercises q2h to 4h

Assist and teach patient to cough and deep breathe q4h

Change position frequently; provide back rubs prn

Ambulate with assistance as ordered and tolerated

Expected outcome/evaluation

Patient expresses minimal discomfort or absence of pain

■ **NDX:** Diarrhea or constipation related to malabsorption, radiation therapy, and/or poor food and fluid intake

Assess usual elimination patterns

Auscultate abdomen for bowel sounds and measure abdominal girth q4h

Monitor stools for color, consistency, frequency, and amount

Provide low-fiber foods for diarrhea and high-fiber foods for constipation

Encourage fluid intake of 2000 ml/24 hr

Monitor for impaction as needed

Encourage activity as tolerated

Administer stool softeners/antidiarrheal agents as indicated

Expected outcome/evaluation

Patient's elimination pattern is maintained within parameters of disease process

■ **NDX:** Ineffective individual coping related to illness and prognosis

Encourage and allow time for verbalization of concerns and feelings; listen carefully

Involve significant other and encourage communication with patient

Reinforce physician's explanation of disease process and prognosis

Explain all procedures and treatments and involve patient in plan of care

Assess present coping patterns and identify strengths and provide supportive environment

Expected outcome/evaluation

Patient expresses concerns and feelings and forms adaptive behaviors in a supportive environment

■ **NDX:** Anticipatory grieving related to poor prognosis

Encourage and allow time for verbalization of feelings; assist patient in identifying steps in grieving process

Assess present patterns of coping; identify strengths

Promote family cohesiveness and communication

Provide a supportive environment in which hope is presented realistically

Provide information on outside support groups (e.g., ACS)

Expected outcome/evaluation

Patient and/or significant other expresses grief and participates in decision-making for the future

■ **NDX:** Knowledge deficit related to lack of information about home care needs and chemotherapy and/or radiotherapy

Provide patient and/or significant other with information about diet management, activity, and rest; refer to dietitian

Discuss medications: name, dosage, purpose, time of administration, and side effects

Explain side effects of chemotherapy and/or radiotherapy and ways of managing them

Refer to outside health care agencies for assistance with home care

Encourage follow-up visits with physician

Expected outcome/evaluation

Patient and/or significant other demonstrates understanding of home care and follow-up instructions

HEPATIC CARCINOMA

Malignant tumor most frequently caused by metastatic lesions in other organs; primary lesions are rare and may be asymptomatic

Assessment
Observations/findings

Slow onset of symptoms
Anorexia
Weakness, general fatigue
Progressive weight loss
Nausea, vomiting
Increased flatulence
Light-colored, bulky stools containing fat
Diarrhea
Abdominal fullness or discomfort
Abdominal pain when coughing or deep breathing
Referred pain to subscapular area
Low-grade fever
Dehydration

Melena
Anemia
Electrolyte imbalance
Abnormal liver function studies
Leukocytosis

Laboratory/diagnostic studies

Increased prothrombin time (PT), erythrocyte sedimentation rate (ESR), bleeding/clotting time
CBC, urinalysis, fasting blood sugar (FBS)
Liver function studies
Alkaline phosphatase: elevated
Decreased serum albumin
Immunoserological assay
Stools for steatorrhea
Chest radiologic study
Hepatic scintiscanning/scan, arteriography
Liver biopsy
Paracentesis cytology

Potential complications

Hypoglycemia
Hepatomegaly
Splenomegaly
Hematemesis, GI bleeding
Portal hypertension
Respiratory distress
Change in mental status
Jaundice
Ascites
Peripheral edema
Hepatic coma

Medical Management

Analgesics, antiemetics, diuretics, antacids, corticosteroids
Diet, activity
Parenteral fluids with electrolytes, vitamins, and/or salt-poor albumin
TPN
Nasogastric aspiration, urethral catheter
Percutaneous transhepatic catheter, chemotherapeutic agents
Hepatic lobectomy

Nursing diagnoses/interventions*/evaluation

■ **NDX:** Potential fluid volume deficit related to dehydration, electrolyte imbalance, NPO status, and/or nasogastric aspiration

Maintain NPO if ordered; discriminate use of ice chips may be beneficial

*Patient's condition dictates type and amount of care required; modify accordingly.

Administer parenteral fluids with electrolytes, vitamins, and salt-poor albumin as ordered
Insert NG tube and connect to low, intermittent suction apparatus as ordered; irrigate gently with measured amounts of normal saline; monitor aspirate for color and amount
Insert indwelling urethral catheter as ordered; connect to closed gravity drainage system and monitor color and amount of urine
Measure intake and output q8h
Monitor ankles for edema and measure abdominal girth q8h
Monitor vital signs q4h; provide cooling measures for temperature above 102° F (38.9° C) as ordered; take rectal temperature if NG tube is in place; observe for venous distention around rectum
Monitor electrolytes, FBS, and liver function studies
Administer medications as ordered: diuretics, antacids, corticosteroids, chemotherapeutic agents

Expected outcome/evaluation

Patient remains hydrated and electrolytes are within normal limits

■ **NDX:** Altered protection: hemorrhage and/or jaundice related to liver dysfunction and/or prolonged bleeding/clotting time

Monitor gastric aspirate and stools for bleeding; check each for occult blood with Hemastix
Observe for signs of vitamin K deficiency
  Bleeding gums, purpura
  Bleeding after injections; use small-gauge needle and apply pressure
  Monitor PT and clotting time
Monitor skin, sclera, and urine for jaundice
Administer vitamin K as ordered

Expected outcome/evaluation

Patient exhibits no signs of GI bleeding, bleeding from mucous membranes, or jaundice

■ **NDX:** Altered thought processes related to liver dysfunction and/or potential negative nitrogen balance

Monitor mental acuity frequently; observe for signs of disorientation, lethargy, personality changes, or depressed motor skills
Reorient as necessary
Provide safe environment: keep side rails in place and walking area free of obstacles; use night light; keep needed articles close
Provide clear directions; break tasks into steps; allow time for completion

Maintain continuity in schedule of care
Assist with decision making
Encourage expression of feelings
Acknowledge positive steps taken
Monitor serum albumin and blood urea nitrogen (BUN) levels

Expected outcome/evaluation

Patient is oriented to person, time and place, follows directions and begins to make decisions about care, and blood ammonia levels are within normal limits

■ **NDX:** Pain related to disease process

Assess pain: type, location, onset, frequency, and intensity; use pain rating scale
Administer analgesics as ordered; avoid morphine and sedatives; assess effectiveness of pain relief measures
Teach and assist with alernate pain-relieving techniques (e.g., relaxation; imagery, music therapy)
Maintain bed rest in quiet environment in position of comfort; no knee gatch
Assist and teach patient to turn q2h and deep breathe qh
Change position frequently and administer back rubs
Administer skin care and oronasal hygiene prn
Perform passive or assist with and teach active ROM exercises q4h
Ambulate with assistance when allowed

Expected outcome/evaluation

Patient verbalizes minimal discomfort or absence of pain; uses alternate techniques

■ **NDX:** Altered nutrition: less than body requirements related to anorexia, malnutrition, and/or fatigue

Administer TPN as ordered; monitor urine for sugar and acetone q4h
Provide diet, when allowed, with amounts of protein, fat, and carbohydrate regulated
  Avoid stress during meals
  Present meal trays attractively
  Encourage small, frequent meals
  Assist with meals as needed
  Sodium may be restricted if ankle edema or ascites is present
Weigh patient daily at same time with same clothing and scale
Monitor intake and output; institute voiding measures as needed when urethral catheter is removed

Expected outcome/evaluation

Patient's nutritional status is maintained within parameters of disease process

■ **NDX:** Ineffective family coping related to poor prognosis of disease

Reinforce physician's explanation of prognosis and clarify misconceptions
Encourage and allow time for verbalization of feelings and concerns; listen carefully
Assess present coping patterns and be supportive of those strengths that assisted in past experience
Encourage communication with significant other and assist in identifying problems
Promote feelings of self-worth and self-esteem

Expected outcome/evaluation

Patient and/or significant other verbalizes concerns and feelings and adopts positive coping behaviors in a supportive environment

■ **NDX:** Anticipatory grieving related to poor prognosis

Encourage expression of feelings about death with patient and/or significant other
Provide hope in small ways, but be realistic (short-term goals)
Provide supportive environment for patient and/or significant other to begin grieving process and assess and understand stages as they occur

Expected outcome/evaluation

Patient expresses grief and works through grieving process in supportive environment

■ **NDX:** Knowledge deficit related to lack of information about home care management

Explain chemotherapy schedule, where to come, length of procedure, and possible side effects
Provide written diet instructions regarding amounts of nutrients allowed
Demonstrate care of percutaneous transhepatic catheter if applicable
Discuss signs and symptoms to report to physician
  Decreased mental acuity
  Increased abdominal girth: weight gain
  Jaundice
  Hematemesis, tarry stools
  Mucosal bleeding
  Peripheral edema, dyspnea
Discuss medications: name, dosage, purpose, time of administration, and side effects
  Explain importance of taking only medicines prescribed by physician
  Demonstrate injection administration if applicable
Encourage follow-up visits with physician

Expected outcome/evaluation

Patient and/or significant other demonstrates understanding of home care and follow-up instructions

PANCREATIC CARCINOMA

Malignancy in the pancreas with high mortality due to lack of early symptoms, symptoms similar to those of other diseases, and rapid metastasis to other organs; 50% occur in the head of the pancreas; 50% occur in the body and tail

Assessment

Observations/findings

Midepigastric pain, varying in severity
    May radiate to lower back and subscapular area
    May be related to eating, activity, or supine position
Signs of biliary obstruction
    Jaundice
    Dark, concentrated urine
    Clay-colored stools
    Pruritus
    Increased PT
    Increased serum bilirubin and alkaline phosphatase
Rapid weight loss
Anorexia
Nausea, vomiting
Fatigue

Laboratory/diagnostic studies

Serum bilirubin, alkaline phosphatase, amylase, and lipase (elevated)
Electrolytes, FBS, liver function studies, PT
Percutaneous transhepatic cholangiography (PTC)
Endoscopic retrograde cholangiopancreatography (ERCP)
Arteriography, ultrasonography, CT scan
Percutaneous needle aspiration cytology, biopsy
Upper GI examination, abdominal radiological study
Duodenal secretion, cytology

Potential complications

Hyperglycemia
Hyperinsulinism
Steatorrhea
Hepatomegaly
Bleeding tendencies (vitamin K deficiency)
Gastric ulcer–type symptoms
Ascites
Thrombophlebitis
Diabetes mellitus

Medical Management

Analgesics, antiemetics, vitamin K, pancreatic enzymes, bile salts, insulin
Diet, parenteral nutrition with electrolytes, TPN
Nasogastric aspiration, urethral catheter

Activity, stool softeners
Chemotherapy, radiation therapy
Surgical interventions

Nursing diagnoses/interventions*/evaluation

■ **NDX:** Potential fluid volume deficit (2) related to abnormal loss of body fluids

Maintain NPO with discriminate use of ice chips
Administer parenteral fluids with electrolytes, vitamins, and insulin as ordered
Insert NG tube as ordered; connect to low, intermittent suction apparatus; irrigate gently with measured amounts of normal saline
Measure intake and output q8h
Monitor vital signs q4h; take rectal temperature
Monitor electrolytes

Expected outcome/evaluation

Patient remains hydrated, and electrolytes are within normal limits

■ **NDX:** Potential for injury related to pancreatic dysfunction

Monitor glucose, bilirubin, PT, Hgb, Hct, and serum albumin
Monitor gastric aspirate and stools for bleeding; check each for occult blood with Hemastix
Test urine for sugar and acetone q4h
Monitor skin, sclera, and urine for jaundice
Observe for signs of vitamin K deficiency
Monitor ankles for peripheral edema and calves for tenderness or pain
Perform passive or assist with active ROM exercises q4h
Auscultate abdomen for bowel sounds and measure girth q8h
Monitor mental acuity and emotional state
Administer medications as ordered: antacids, vitamin K, salt-poor albumin, diuretics
Provide skin care, and oronasal hygiene q2h

Expected outcome/evaluation

No peripheral edema observed and no tenderness or pain reported
Secretions and stool negative for bleeding
Jaundice not present

■ **NDX:** Pain related to disease process

Maintain bed rest in position of comfort and in quiet environment; no knee gatch
Assess pain: location, type, onset, frequency, and intensity; use pain rating scale

---

*Patient's condition dictates type and amount of care required; modify accordingly.

Administer analgesics as ordered; avoid opiates; methadone may be beneficial

Teach and assist with alternate pain-relieving techniques (e.g., relaxation, music therapy, imagery)

Change position frequently; sitting up and leaning forward may alleviate pain

Avoid allowing pain to become too severe

Assist and teach patient to turn q2h and deep breathe q½h

Expected outcome/evaluation

Patient verbalizes minimal discomfort or absence of pain; uses alternate techniques

■ **NDX:** Altered nutrition: less than body requirements related to anorexia, weight loss, and/or fatigue

Administer TPN as ordered

Provide high-protein, high-carbohydrate, high-calorie diet as ordered when tolerated; amounts of nutrients may depend on liver involvement

Encourage small, frequent meals and assist as needed

Monitor intake and output q8h

Administer stool softeners

Weigh patient daily at same time with same clothing and scale

Administer medications as ordered: antiemetics, antacids, pancreatic enzymes, bile salts, and insulin

Expected outcome/evaluation

Patient's nutritional status is maintained within confines of disease process

■ **NDX:** Ineffective family coping related to poor disease prognosis

Reinforce physician's explanation of prognosis; clarify misconceptions

Encourage and allow time for verbalization of fears and concerns; listen attentively

Assess present coping behaviors and support past strengths that were successful

Encourage communication with significant other and assist in identifying problems

Promote feelings of self-worth and self-esteem

Expected outcome/evaluation

Patient and/or significant other expresses concerns and feelings and moves toward adoption of positive coping behaviors

■ **NDX:** Anticipatory grieving related to poor prognosis

Encourage expression of feelings about death with patient and significant other

Provide realistic hope by setting short-term goals

Assist in identifying grieving stages; promote them as normal and assist in working through them as they occur

Expected outcome/evaluation

Patient and/or significant other expresses feelings and identifies grieving process

■ **NDX:** Knowledge deficit related to lack of information about diabetes and home care management

Explain chemotherapy and/or radiation therapy schedule: where and when to report, length of procedure, side effects, and symptom care (p. 670)

Provide written diet instructions, including amounts of rest and exercise

Demonstrate diabetes care: insulin administration, (p. 332) self-glucose monitoring and urine testing (p. 338)

Discuss medications: name, schedule, dosage, purpose, and side effects; explain importance of taking only medications prescribed by physician

Discuss signs and symptoms to report to physician
 Ascites, weight gain (abnormal)
 Jaundice, mucosal bleeding
 Increased pain
 Hematemesis, tarry stools
 Peripheral edema, dyspnea

Promote follow-up visits with physician

Expected outcome/evaluation

Patient and/or significant other demonstrates understanding of home care and follow-up instructions

OSTEOSARCOMA

Rapidly growing malignant bone tumor of unknown etiology occurring most often in the long bones of young people; secondary malignant tumors of the bone often metastasize from other primary sites

Assessment
Observations/findings

Pain over affected area of extremity, especially at night
Limited use of extremity
Anorexia
Weight loss
Fatigue
Localized swelling with or without trauma
Increased skin temperature over affected area
Elevated temperature

Laboratory/diagnostic studies

Radiologic examinations of affected bones and chest
Bone scan, CT scan, magnetic resonance imaging (MRI)
Alkaline, acid phosphatase (elevated)
Serum calcium (decreased); urine calcium (increased)

Potential complications

Cough, hemoptysis (respiratory metastasis)
Pathological fractures
Infection
Loss of limb

Medical Management

Biopsy, amputation
Antineoplastic agents
Radiation therapy
Analgesics, tranquilizers
Diet, activity, immobilization of limb

Nursing diagnoses/interventions/evaluation

■ **NDX:** Impaired physical mobility related to pain and swelling

Maintain bed rest in correct body alignment with splint, sandbags, and/or pillows
Provide foam, water, or air mattress as indicated
Assist with activity as tolerated
 Handle affected extremity gently and elevate as ordered
 Assist with and teach active or perform passive ROM exercises to unaffected extremity or use passive ROM machine
 Ambulate with assistance if tolerated; use crutches, cane, or walker as needed
Maintain planned rest periods
Encourage socialization
Promote self-care activities

Expected outcome/evaluation

Verbalizes understanding of needed position restrictions, maintains body alignment and performs ROM exercises
Alternates activity with rest periods
Demonstrates ability to use mobility devices

■ **NDX:** Altered nutrition: less than body requirements related to anorexia

Assess previous diet habits/patterns
Provide high-calorie, high-protein diet; encourage food selection
Provide small, frequent meals and snacks
Assist with feeding as needed
Provide oral hygiene before meals
Monitor intake and food tolerances
Weigh patient daily at same time with same clothing and scale
Encourage fluids to upper limits for age and weight

Expected outcome/evaluation

Selects food to enhance taste and maintain weight; weight is stable or is increasing toward ideal for height and build

■ **NDX:** Anxiety related to threatening nature of condition and treatment

Allow time for verbalization of fears/anxieties
Provide nonthreatening environment
Explain disease and correct misconceptions
Assist patient to identify prior positive coping skills
Assess present coping skills
Promote relaxation techniques, visual imagery, and physical exercise
Encourage support from significant other

Expected outcome/evaluation

Expresses understanding of disease process
Uses positive coping skills in dealing with feelings
Verbalizes a more calm and less nervous attitude

■ **NDX:** Pain related to presence of tumor

Assess pain: type, intensity, frequency, and location
 Use pain rating scale
 Observe for increasing pain and/or dysfunction
Administer analgesics; assess effectiveness of pain relief measures
Assist patient with changing position frequently; administer back rubs
Provide diversional activities
Promote a safe environment
Discuss and teach alternate pain management techniques

Expected outcome/evaluation

Verbalizes a tolerable pain level
Appears relaxed and comfortable
Initiates learned pain control methods

■ **NDX:** Knowledge deficit related to lack of information about amputation, chemotherapy, and metastasis

Reinforce physician's explanation of surgical procedure, postoperative care, and rehabilitation; clarify any misconceptions
Provide information on chemotherapy and/or radiotherapy: possible side effects, support systems available (pp. 642, 670)
Explain signs of lung metastasis: cough, hemoptysis, dyspnea
Encourage communication with significant other to discuss fears and anxieties; provide supportive environment

Expected outcome/evaluation

Verbalizes understanding of care required following surgery/chemotherapy
Expresses understanding of signs of lung involvement

ORCHIECTOMY FOR TESTICULAR TUMOR

Surgical removal of the testis; most commonly performed in the presence of testicular cancer via an inguinal incision

Assessment
Observations/findings

Scrotal mass
Testicular swelling or thickening
Backache
Weight loss
Malaise
Gynecomastia
Urine: positive reaction to any standard pregnancy test
Elevated temperature
Scrotum
    Edema
    Discoloration
Incision
    Redness
    Pain
    Swelling
    Drainage
Disturbance in self-concept

Laboratory/diagnostic studies

AFP and HCG for tumor markers
Intravenous urography (IVU)
CT scan of abdomen
Urine pregnancy test depends on type of tumor and stage
Lymphangiogram
Radionuclide imaging

Potential complications

Hemorrhage
Shock
Wound infection
Atelectasis and/or pneumonia

Medical Management

NPO until bowel sounds are audible
Parenteral IV fluids until liquids and/or diet is tolerated
BP, T, P, and R per postoperative routine
Analgesics
Antibiotics
Scrotal support
Chemotherapy
Radiation therapy
Radical lymph node dissection

Nursing diagnoses/interventions/evaluation

■ **NDX:** Pain related to surgical incision and scrotal swelling

Assess nature, intensity, location, duration, and precipitating and alleviating factors of pain; use pain rating scale
Assess nonverbal signs of pain
Provide scrotal support as ordered
Apply heat or ice to scrotum as ordered to reduce swelling; observe skin carefully to prevent injury
Assess incisional site for redness, tenderness, swelling, and drainage
Provide nonpharmacological comfort measures
    Assist patient with assuming a comfortable position
    Teach relaxation techniques
    Teach and assist with guided imagery techniques
    Provide diversional activities
    Provide a restful environment
Encourage early ambulation
Observe for desired effects and side effects of pain medications
Consult with physician if measures fail to provide adequate pain relief or if dosage or interval change for pain medication is needed

Expected outcome/evaluation

Patient verbalizes a decrease in pain and exhibits a relaxed facial expression and body position

■ **NDX:** Potential urinary retention related to postoperative scrotal swelling

Use voiding measures to facilitate bladder emptying
    Ensure privacy
    Place patient in comfortable position to urinate
    Run tap water near patient
    Flush toilet
    Place hands in warm water
    Apply heat to suprapubic areas as ordered
    Pour warm water over perineum
    Assist patient with using relaxation techniques
    Place a few drops of oil of peppermint in bedpan, on cottonball, and hold briefly in front of urinary meatus
    Pull pubic hairs slightly
    Stroke inner aspect of thigh gently
    Stroke inner aspect of thigh with ice
Catheterize patient as ordered
Measure and record urinary output qh

Expected outcome/evaluation

Patient voids normally post-operatively and shows no signs or symptoms of urinary retention

■ **NDX:** Potential body image disturbance related to fear of loss of masculinity and fertility

Provide an accepting and supportive atmosphere
Encourage expression of feelings of anxiety, fear, embarrassment, anger, frustration, and/or helplessness

Promote feelings of self-worth by stressing positive features in patient's life

Provide suggestions to help patient maintain satisfactory sexual expression

Encourage communication with significant other

Provide assistance from other professionals to help patient to deal with emotional changes (psychiatry, sexual counselor)

Emphasize positive results of surgery

Expected outcome/evaluation

Patient expresses feelings to care giver or significant other, reports feelings of increased self-esteem, and resumes ADLs

■ **NDX:** Potential for infection related to surgical incision

Monitor for and report signs and symptoms of wound infection (fever, chills, redness, swelling, tenderness, purulent and/or malodorous wound drainage)

Check surgical incision q4h for redness, swelling, tenderness, and purulent drainage

Assess temperature q4h

Monitor WBC as ordered

Obtain wound culture as ordered

Use good handwashing technique and teach and encourage patient to do the same

Instruct patient to avoid touching incision, dressings, and drainage

Maintain sterile technique when changing dressings and performing wound care

Expected outcome/evaluation

Exhibits no signs of infection

Incision is clean and dry

Temperature is within normal range

■ **NDX:** Knowledge deficit related to lack of information about postoperative routine, symptoms to report to physician, and home care and follow-up instructions

Instruct patient to
  Maintain diet as ordered
  Avoid constipation
  Exercise to tolerance, avoid fatigue, avoid heavy lifting, and plan frequent rest periods
  Report the following symptoms to physician
    Incisional redness, pain, swelling, drainage
    Pain on walking
    Thickening or any abnormality in scrotum
  Perform testicular self-examination once a month
  Care for incision
Teach medication name, dosage, schedule, purpose and side effects

Instruct patient to avoid taking over-the-counter medication without checking with physician

Prepare for chemotherapy (p. 649), radiation therapy (p. 642), or radical lymph node dissection

Teach importance of ongoing outpatient care

Expected outcome/evaluation

Patient and/or significant other verbalizes understanding of the disease process, symptoms to report to physician, and home care and follow-up instructions; and return-demonstrates care of incision and testicular self-examination

MODIFIED RADICAL MASTECTOMY

Surgical removal of the entire breast, axillary lymph nodes, and all fat, fascia, and adjacent tissues as treatment for carcinoma

Preoperative Observations

Emotional aberrations related to feelings of
  Loss of femininity
  Fear of mutilation and death

Preoperative Care

See General Preoperative Care/Teaching (p. 27)
Provide emotional support
  Encourage verbalization of fears
  Encourage communication with significant other
  Avoid false reassurances
  Help anticipate future
  Arrange for visit from Reach for Recovery, Inc.
Explain that arm will feel tight after surgery

Postoperative Assessment
Observations/findings

Hemorrhage
Edema of affected arm: lymphedema
Atelectasis
Emotional/behavioral changes related to
  Anxiety
  Depression
  Anger
  Withdrawal
  Feeling of hopelessness
  Body image change
Incision: skin donor site; nipple-grafted site
  Redness
  Pain
  Swelling
  Drainage
Wound drains
  Sump drain
  Hemovac or Jackson-Pratt

Potential complications

Hemorrhagic shock
Infection
Brachial plexus damage
    Contractures
    Shortening of muscles
Pneumonia

Immediate Postoperative Care

Place patient in position of comfort
Administer parenteral fluids as ordered; *avoid drawing blood from or administering parenteral fluids in affected arm*
Administer oral fluids as ordered
Measure intake and output; empty wound drains and measure drainage q8h and prn
Assist and teach patient to turn, cough, and deep breathe q2h
    Alternate back and unaffected side
    Support chest when coughing
Auscultate chest for breath sounds q4h
Check BP, T, P, and R q4h for 48 hr, then qid; *take BP in unaffected arm only*
Reinforce dressing prn; report excessive drainage or blood to physician
Apply pressure dressing as necessary
    Check color, sensation, and motion in fingers and hand q1h to 8h as indicated; notify physician of impaired color, sensation, or motion
    Do not release pressure dressing
If skin graft is done
    Check donor site q4h
    Reinforce dressing prn
    Notify physician if drainage is excessive
If nipple has been relocated pending future cosmetic surgery, check site q1h to 2h as ordered and perform care as explicitly as ordered by plastic surgeon
Control pain with analgesics
Perform wrist and elbow ROM exercises; gradually abduct arm and gradually raise arm over head
Ambulate prn
Monitor edema present in affected arm; measure upper arm and forearm bid

Convalescent Management

Maintain progressive diet
Encourage oral fluids to 2500 ml daily unless contraindicated
Ambulate on first postoperative day
Assist and teach arm exercises qid
    Gradually increase extent of exercises daily
    Perform hand exercises: alternately clench and extend fingers
Involve patient in care; encourage use of affected arm to wash face, brush teeth, and eat

Provide physical therapy as indicated
Notify Reach to Recovery, Inc.

Nursing diagnoses/interventions/evaluation

■ **NDX:** Potential body image disturbance related to breast removal and value of reproductive organs

Encourage patient's comments and questions about surgery, progress, and prognosis
Reinforce correct information and provide factual information to correct any misconceptions
Relate importance of communicating anything that causes anxiety
Encourage patient to verbalize and explore feelings regarding what impact missing body part might have on assuming ADLs
Encourage patient to look at and touch the changed body part
Encourage use of rehabilitation services (e.g., Reach for Recovery, wellness community)

Expected outcome/evaluation

Patient verbalizes acceptance of altered body image and confirms that she has shared her feelings with partner

■ **NDX:** Knowledge deficit related to lack of information about home care management

Explain importance of exercise to tolerance; instruct patient to stop at point of pain
Discuss types of prostheses available
Discuss types of reconstruction available
Teach care of incision
Discuss symptoms to report to physician
    Redness
    Pain
    Swelling
    Drainage
    Elevated temperature
Emphasize need to resume housekeeping duties gradually
Explain that incision and/or chest wall may feel numb
Instruct patient to shower daily
Have patient check with physician regarding use of deodorant under affected arm
Instruct patient to examine remaining breast once a month
Caution patient to avoid allowing *blood to be drawn from or IV to be started in affected arm*
Caution patient to avoid injections, vaccinations, and taking of BP in affected arm
Instruct patient to carry handbag with unaffected arm
Relate that sexual activity may be resumed when desired; position of partner should avoid any pressure on chest wall

Refer patient to Visiting Nurses Association as needed
Emphasize importance of follow-up outpatient care

Expected outcome/evaluation

Patient and/or significant other demonstrates understanding of home care and follow-up instructions

RADICAL HYSTERECTOMY

Surgical removal of the ovaries, tubes, uterus with the cervix, and parametrial tissue, along with lymph node dissection; ovarian tissue is often preserved in premenopausal patients

Preoperative Teaching and Care

Administer cleansing enema the evening before surgery if ordered by physician
Teach postoperative breathing exercises
Have practice sessions with intermittent positive-pressure breathing (IPPB) or incentive spirometer
Explain that patient will have an indwelling catheter for 24 hr and/or suprapubic catheter for 1 to 6 weeks because of denervation of bladder, causing large amounts of residual urine; reinforce that bladder function probably will resume
Explain that patient may have Jackson-Pratt or other drains present

Postoperative Assessment
Observations/findings

Hemorrhage
Vaginal drainage
    Other than serosanguineous fluid
    Foul odor of discharge
Site of incision
    Redness
    Pain
    Swelling
    Drainage
Elevated temperature
Tachycardia
Jackson-Pratt or Hemovac drains
    Leakage of urine
    Hemorrhage
Hematuria
Urinary retention
Vaginal leakage of urine
Suprapubic leakage of urine
Abdominal distention

Potential complications

Hemorrhage
Urinary tract infection
Paralytic ileus
Pneumonia
Thrombophlebitis
Constipation
Pulmonary embolus
Infection
Ureteral fistula
Ureter ligation (iatrogenic)
    Low back pain
    Decreased urine output
Lymphocyst

Immediate Postoperative Care

Check BP, T, P, and R q4h for 48 hr, then qid
Maintain NPO status until patient is passing flatus
Progress from NPO to clear-liquid diet as ordered; administer mouth care q2h while patient is NPO
Provide parenteral fluids as ordered
Connect indwelling catheter(s) to closed gravity drainage system
Measure intake and output
Assist and teach patient to turn, cough, and deep breathe q2h
Administer incentive spirometer
Auscultate chest for breath sounds q4h and prn
Empty Jackson-Pratt q1h to 2h initially and prn (decrease frequency as amount of drainage decreases to q8h)
Observe site of incision q2h to 4h
Change dressing as ordered; reinforce dressing prn
Assist patient with getting out of bed on evening of surgery as ordered
Decrease pelvic congestion
    Avoid high-Fowler's position
    Avoid pressure under knees
    Apply antiembolic stockings as ordered; reapply q6h to 8h and prn
    Perform passive leg exercises
Manage pain; provide medication as ordered
Administer perineal care with antiseptic solution q4h and prn
Auscultate abdomen for bowel sounds each shift
Give complete bed bath as necessary on first postoperative day until activity is increased

Convalescent Management

Continue with immediate postoperative care and decrease frequency of nursing functions as patient's condition improves
Progress from clear-liquid diet to high-protein or high-residue diet
Encourage fluid intake
Use voiding measures; check for residual urine
Provide abdominal support or binder as indicated
Ambulate as ordered; avoid sitting for long periods
Insert rectal tube and/or give Harris flush prn
Administer stool softeners, mild laxatives, suppositories, or small enema prn

Administer hormone therapy as ordered

Give partial bed bath progressing to self-bath or shower as indicated

Nursing diagnoses/interventions/evaluation*

■ **NDX:** Knowledge deficit related to lack of information about home care management

Ensure that patient and/or significant other demonstrates care of suprapubic catheter if patient is discharged with one in place

Teach clean, intermittent self-catheterization as indicated

Give reasons for estrogen therapy if ordered, as necessitated by surgically induced menopause

Explain that no intercourse, tampons, douching, or tub baths are allowed for 4 to 6 weeks or as indicated by physician

Caution patient to avoid sitting for long periods of time

Relate that supportive hosiery may be indicated

Caution patient to avoid constipation

Explain importance of exercise and activity to tolerance

Caution patient to avoid jarring activities, driving, and heavy lifting for 4 to 6 weeks or as indicated by physician

Explain importance of planned rest periods

Relate that abdominal support or binder may be indicated

Discuss symptoms to report to physician

Elevated temperature over 100° F (37.8° C)

Vaginal bleeding (more than slight bloody discharge)

Abdominal cramps or change in bowel habits

Difficulty in urinating

Reinforce that menstruation will no longer occur

Emphasize importance of involving family or significant other in dealing with body image changes

Caution patient to avoid activities that increase pelvic congestion (e.g., dancing, horseback riding) until allowed to do so by physician

Relate that counseling for sexually active woman and her partner is available

If a wide cuff of vagina has been removed, remaining vagina stretches with use and coitus is not affected

Sexual activity can usually be resumed 1 month after surgery

Teach name of medication, dosage, time of administration, purpose, and side effects

Emphasize importance of follow-up outpatient care for further treatment of cancer as necessary

Expected outcome/evaluation

Patient and/or significant other demonstrates understanding of home care and follow-up instructions

---

*See Total Abdominal Hysterectomy and Bilateral Salpingo-oophorectomy (TAH-BSO) (p. 518).

VULVECTOMY

vulvectomy with lymphadenectomy Excision of the vulva (labia majora, labia minora, clitoris, surrounding tissues) and the pelvic lymph nodes as a treatment for cancer

skinning vulvectomy with skin graft Excision of the upper skin layers of the vulva and placement of a skin graft from the buttock or thigh as a treatment for cancer in situ or early vulvar cancers

Preoperative Teaching and Care

Provide emotional support; encourage communication with spouse or significant other

Explain the following to patient

Bed rest may be maintained for 24 to 48 hr postoperatively

Indwelling catheter will be present

Bulky dressing may be present on surgical site; dressing may be removed 24 to 48 hr postoperatively to irrigate perineal/groin area

Alternating-pressure air mattress, convoluted foam (egg-crate) mattress, or water mattress will be used

Antiembolic stockings may be on legs

Hemovac or other drains may be present

Teach postoperative breathing exercises

Have practice sessions with IPPB or incentive spirometer

Teach leg exercises

Teach use of overhead trapeze

Explain that pain will be managed

Postoperative Assessment
Observations/findings

Perineal hemorrhage

Purulent drainage and/or foul odor from surgical site; sloughing of skin flap or graft

Elevated temperature

Body image disturbances

Psychological changes

Anger

Depression

Anxiety

Withdrawal

Hostility

Edema of lower extremities

Absence of popliteal or pedal pulses (especially with lymphadenectomy)

Skin

Excoriation

Pressure sores

Constipation or impaction

Anemia

Potential complications

Hemorrhage

Paralytic ileus

Thrombophlebitis
Infection (sepsis)
Pulmonary embolus
Pneumonia
Urinary tract infection

Immediate Postoperative Care

Provide overhead trapeze; convoluted foam (egg-crate) mattress, alternating-pressure air mattress or water mattress; and bed cradle

Maintain complete bed rest with head of bed elevated 30 to 45 degrees

Check BP, T, P, and R q2h for 6 hr, then q4h for 4 days, then q8h; do not take temperature rectally

Assist and teach patient to turn, cough, and deep breathe q2h; use pillow between legs when turning

Administer IPPB or incentive spirometer

Auscultate chest for breath sounds q8h and prn

Manage pain with analgesics

Maintain NPO status; provide mouth care q2 to 4h

Administer parenteral fluids with antibiotics as ordered

Administer low-dose heparin therapy as ordered

Connect indwelling catheter to closed gravity drainage system

Administer catheter care q24h and prn

Measure intake and output

Administer skin care to back and sides q2h to 4h and prn

Auscultate abdomen for bowel sounds each shift

Check popliteal and pedal pulses q2h to 4h and prn

Perform passive and instruct patient to do active range of motion (ROM) exercises for all extremities

Apply antiembolic stockings as ordered; reapply q6h to 8h and prn

Check circulation in extremities; report edema

Skinning vulvectomy with skin graft

Report excessive drainage

Observe dressing of graft donor site (usually buttock or thigh); report any untoward signs to physician when dressing is removed; place bed cradle over area to prevent linens from touching area

Vulvectomy with lymphadenectomy

Observe Jackson-Pratt drains and empty as indicated q2h to 4h, then each shift and prn

Observe dressing
  Reinforce if necessary q1h to 2h
  Report excessive drainage
  Do not change dressing (may remain in place 5 to 7 days)

Convalescent Management

Maintain clear-liquid diet progressing to low-residue and/or high-protein, high-carbohydrate diet

Avoid defecation with dressings in place; give diphenoxylate or paregoric as indicated

When dressings have been removed
  Irrigate surgical site (usually with half-saline solution and half-peroxide solution or plain saline solution) for vulvectomy with lymphadenectomy
  Dry with hand-held dryer on low or use heat lamp
  Use sitz baths or whirlpool as ordered bid and prn
  Check for bowel movement within 24 hr
    Avoid straining
      Administer stool softeners, laxatives, suppositories, or enemas as indicated

Elevate head of bed from 30 to 60 degrees or position patient on side with pillow between legs (upper leg bent and slightly forward)

Avoid pressure under knees; no knee gatch

Assist with active ROM exercises to all extremities tid and prn

Ambulate
  Avoid chair sitting
  Avoid crossing legs

Use voiding measures after removal of indwelling catheter

Encourage fluid intake to 2500 ml/day

Provide high-protein between-meal snacks and a variety of liquids as ordered, such as milkshakes, custards, and eggnog

Nursing diagnoses/interventions/evaluation

■ **NDX:** Potential body image disturbance related to removal of vulva and value of reproductive organs

Encourage patient's comments and questions about surgery, progress, and prognosis

Reinforce correct information and provide factual information to correct any misconceptions

Relate importance of communicating anything that causes anxiety

Encourage patient to verbalize and explore feelings regarding what impact the missing body part might have on assuming ADLs

Encourage patient to look at and touch the changed body part

Encourage use of supportive community agencies related to disease process

Expected outcome/evaluation

Patient verbalizes acceptance of altered body image and confirms that she has shared her feelings with partner

Demonstrates adaptive response related to self-concept and sexuality

■ **NDX:** Knowledge deficit related to lack of information about home care management

Involve family or significant other in all aspects of care and instruction

Emphasize importance of communicating anything that causes anxiety

Explain need for exercise and activity to tolerance

Explain need for planned rest periods

Instruct patient to take sitz baths bid and prn

Demonstrate wound irrigation and dressing change; give written instructions to patient

Discuss symptoms of wound infection to report to physician

    Unusual odor

    Fresh bleeding

    Perineal pain

    Elevated temperature above 100° F (37.8° C)

    Increased swelling of groin

    Urinary tract infection

        Frequency and urgency of urination

        Burning and pain on urination

Relate that low-dose prophylactic antibiotics may be ordered (possibly for as long as a year)

Relate that antiembolic stockings or supportive hosiery may be indicated

Instruct patient to elevate legs periodically at home

Caution patient to avoid sitting or standing for long periods or crossing legs

Caution patient to avoid constipation

Caution patient to avoid heavy lifting

Relate that counseling for sexually active woman and her partner is available

    No coitus until indicated by physician (usually 4 to 6 weeks)

    Alternate methods of achieving sexual satisfaction can be explored if clitoris has been removed; vaginal orgasm may be achieved; experiment with alternative positions

    Water-soluble lubricant may be necessary

    Fertility is not affected in woman of childbearing age

Explain need for high-protein, high-carbohydate diet

Teach name of medication, dosage, time of administration, purpose, and side effects

Relate that referrals may be indicated for Visiting Nurses Association, social service worker, or clergy

Emphasize importance of follow-up outpatient care

Expected outcome/evaluation

Patient and/or significant other demonstrates understanding of home care and follow-up instructions

PELVIC EXENTERATION

***total exenteration** Removal of all reproductive organs and adjacent tissues: radical hysterectomy, pelvic node dissection, cystectomy with formation of urinary conduit, vaginectomy, and rectal resection with colostomy*

***anterior exenteration** Excludes rectal resection with colostomy*

***posterior exenteration** Excludes cystectomy with formation of urinary conduit*

Preoperative Teaching and Care

Be aware that patient is usually admitted 1 day before surgery

Maintain clear-liquid diet until patient is NPO

Prepare bowel

    Administer cathartics as ordered 24 to 48 hr before surgery

    Give cleansing enemas as ordered 24 hr before surgery

    Give antibiotics as ordered 24 to 48 hr before surgery

Inform enterostomal therapist of patient's admission

Administer vitamin K as ordered 24 hr before surgery

Teach postoperative breathing exercises

Have practice sessions with IPPB

Teach use of overhead trapeze if appropriate

Explain the following to patient

    Bulky dressings may be present on surgical site

    Urethral catheters, colostomy, ileostomy, or urinary conduit may be present

    Patient may have Jackson-Pratt or Hemovac and other drains

    Antiembolic stockings may be on legs

    Pain will be managed

Encourage communication with enterostomal therapist, psychiatric nurse, or patient recovered from same surgery

Encourage communication with spouse or significant other

Explore sexual needs; vaginal reconstruction may be performed during exenteration or at a later time

Postoperative Assessment
Observations/findings

Site of incision

    Redness

    Pain

    Swelling

    Drainage

Colostomy, ileostomy, urinary diversion

    Necrosis

    Edema

    Stenosis

    Excoriation of skin around stoma

Oliguria progressing to anuria

Body image disturbances

Psychological changes

    Anger

    Depression

    Withdrawal

    Anxiety

    Hostility

Elevated temperature

Tachycardia
Edema of lower extremities
Absence of popliteal or pedal pulses

Potential complications

Major complications
First 48 hr: hemorrhage
Days 2 to 4: infection
Days 5 to 21: urinary or GI fistula
Shock
Electrolyte imbalance
Dehydration
Paralytic ileus
Thrombophlebitis
Pulmonary embolus
Pneumonia
Sepsis

Immediate Postoperative Care

May use overhead trapeze; convoluted foam (egg-crate) mattress, alternating-pressure air mattress, or water mattress; and bed cradle as necessary
Check BP, P, and R q4h for 48 hr, then q4h for 5 to 7 days, and as indicated by patient's condition
Check axillary or oral temperature q4h and prn; do not take temperature rectally
Measure intake and output
Assist and teach patient to turn, cough, and deep breathe q2h
Administer incentive spirometer q4h and prn
Auscultate chest for breath sounds q4h and prn
Manage pain; administer medications as ordered
Maintain NPO status; provide mouth care q2h
Connect intestinal decompression tube to intermittent, low-suction apparatus; measure carefully to calculate fluid replacement
Administer parenteral fluids with electrolytes to 3000 to 4000 ml/day; provide TPN as indicated
Give blood or blood component transfusions as needed
Check popliteal and pedal pulses q2h to 4h and prn
Apply antiembolic stockings as ordered; reapply q6h to 8h
Perform passive ROM exercises to all extremities q4h and prn
Observe surgical site, dressings, and drainage apparatus q4h for 48 hr
Reinforce dressings as necessary
Change dressings as ordered
Measure and empty drainage receptacles q8h and prn
Administer skin care to pressure areas q2h to 4h
Auscultate abdomen for bowel sounds each shift
See appropriate standard of care
Colostomy care
Urinary diversion
Do not remove pelvic packing; assist physician in its removal

Administer analgesic before removal of packing; observe closely for signs of hemorrhage
Maintain therapeutic environment
Adequate ventilation
Privacy during all nursing care activities
Room deodorants
Immediate removal of soiled dressings
Maintain planned rest periods

Convalescent Management

Continue with immediate postoperative care and decrease frequency of nursing functions as patient's condition improves
Check BP, T, P, and R q4h, decreasing to qid
Clamp nasogastric/intestinal decompression tube before clear-liquid diet as ordered
Assess nutritional status; TPN may be indicated
Slowly increase to high-protein, high-carbohydrate diet as ordered
Administer oral medication after removal of tube
Urinary antiseptics
Antibiotics
Encourage oral fluids to 3000 ml daily unless contraindicated
Provide high-protein between-meal snacks and a variety of liquids as ordered, such as milkshakes, custards, and eggnog
When dressings and packings have been removed
Irrigate perineal area with half-saline and half-peroxide solution
Pat dry
Dry with hand-held hair dryer on low or use heat lamp
Give sitz baths as ordered tid and prn
Ambulate according to patient's tolerance (at least qid)
Assist with active ROM exercises to all extremities qid and prn
Administer ostomy care*
Measure and empty colostomy appliance q8h
Measure and empty urinary conduit appliance q8h

Nursing diagnoses/interventions*/evaluation

■ **NDX:** Potential body image disturbance related to change in structure, function, and value of reproductive organs

Encourage patient's comments and questions about surgery, progress, and prognosis; reinforce correct information and provide factual information to correct any misconceptions
Relate importance of communicating anything that causes anxiety

---

*See Ostomy Management and Care and Urinary Diversion (p. 470).

Encourage patient to verbalize and explore feelings regarding what impact the missing body part might have
on assuming ADLs

Encourage patient to look at and touch the changed
body part

Encourage use of rehabilitation services (e.g., ostomy
club, wellness community)

Expected outcome/evaluation

Patient verbalizes acceptance of altered body image and
confirms that she has shared her feelings with partner

Demonstrates adaptive responses related to self-concept
and sexuality

■ **NDX:** Knowledge deficit related to lack of information
about home care management

Demonstrate colostomy care

Demonstrate urinary diversion care

Demonstrate wound irrigation procedure: give written instructions

Explain importance of sitz baths bid and prn

Discuss symptoms of wound infection to report to physician

Unusual odor and/or discharge

Fresh bleeding

Unusual pain

Elevated temperature above 100° F (37.8° C)

Upper respiratory infection (URI)

Increased swelling at groin or elsewhere

Relate that antiembolic stockings or supportive hosiery
may be indicated

Explain importance of exercise and activity to tolerance;
caution patient to avoid prolonged sitting

Explain need to plan rest periods

Explain need for high-protein, high-carbohydrate diet

Relate that estrogen therapy may be indicated

Relate that referrals may be indicated for Visiting Nurses
Association, social service worker, clergy, or ostomy
association

Relate that counseling for sexually active woman and her
partner is available

Functional vagina may be possible; check with physician

Alternate methods of achieving sexual satisfaction can
be explored

Teach name of medication, dosage, time of administration, purpose, and side effects

Emphasize importance of follow-up outpatient care

Expected outcome/evaluation

Patient and/or significant other demonstrates understanding of home care and follow-up instructions

CHORIOCARCINOMA

*Highly malignant neoplasm derived from chorionic epi-
thelium; may develop after a hydatidiform mole, a
miscarriage, or a full-term delivery*

Assessment
Observations/findings

Profuse and/or intermittent vaginal bleeding
Malodorous vaginal discharge between menses
Cough
Hemoptysis
Headache
Irritability
Nausea, vomiting
Hypertension
Tachypnea
Orthopnea
Vaginal or vulvar lesion
Anemia
Sepsis
Cachexia
Weight loss

Laboratory/diagnostic studies

Rising HCG titer
Ultrasonography

Potential complications

Metastasis (lung, vagina, oral cavity, GI tract, central
nervous system, liver)

Medical Management

Total abdominal hysterectomy and bilateral salpingo-oophorectomy (TAH-BSO)
Antineoplastic chemotherapy (methotrexate, actinomycin D, cytoxan)
Contraception

Nursing diagnoses/interventions/evaluation

See Total Abdominal Hysterectomy and Bilateral Salpingo-oophorectomy (TAH-BSO) (p. 518)
See Antineoplastic Chemotherapy (p. 649 and Table
14-6)

ACUTE LEUKEMIA

*Uncontrolled proliferation of leukocytes and their pre-
cursors in the bone marrow with infiltration of lymph
nodes, spleen, liver, and other body organs*
*acute lymphocytic (lymphoblastic) leukemia (ALL)
Lymphoblasts proliferate in bone marrow and lymph
nodes and invade other tissues; primarily a disease of
childhood*
*acute myelogenous leukemia (AML) Proliferation of
myeloblasts (immature polymorphonuclear leukocytes); occurs in all age-groups but is more common
in adults*

Assessment
Observations/findings

Central nervous system
  Elevated temperature
  Easily fatigued
  Malaise
  Irritability
  Syncope
  Headache
Skin and mucous membranes
  Pallor
  Petechiae
  Easy bruising
  Ecchymosis
  Purpura
  Gum bleeding
  Epistaxis
  Infection: may appear red or dark without pus
Gastrointestinal
  Abdominal discomfort
  Nausea, vomiting
  Dysphagia
  Esophagitis
  Anorexia
  Weight loss
  Perirectal abscess
  Hepatosplenomegaly
Cardiopulmonary
  Hypotension
  Tachycardia
  Palpitations
  Shortness of breath
  Cough
Musculoskeletal
  Bone or joint pain
  Mediastinal mass with tenderness
Enlarged lymph nodes

Laboratory/diagnostic studies

WBC
  May be low or elevated with "shift to the left"
  Excessively elevated (T cell ALL)
  Blasts
  Lymphocytes (ALL)
  Auer rods (AML)
  Phi bodies (AML)
Reticulocytopenia
  Normochromic (AML)
  Normocytic
Anemia
Thrombocytopenia
Elevated serum and urine uric acid
Elevated serum copper
Decreased zinc
Hypergammaglobulinemia (AML)
Bone marrow: proliferation of blast cells

Potential complications

Acute infection
Anemia
Hemorrhage
Organ failure

Medical Management

Antineoplastic chemotherapy
Fluid therapy
Antibiotics
Radiation therapy
Transfusions; blood components
Bone marrow transplant
Analgesics, hypnotics, narcotics

Nursing diagnoses/interventions/evaluation

■ **NDX:** Altered protection related to thrombocytopenia

Assess for bleeding q4h; more often if bleeding is suspected; report indications of bleeding to physician
  Check BP, P, R, T, and peripheral pulses
  Auscultate chest for breath and heart sounds
  Assess neurological signs
  Assess skin and mucous membranes
  Auscultate abdomen for bowel sounds
  Measure intake and output
  Hematest urine and stool
Initiate and maintain parenteral fluids as ordered
Maintain integrity of central venous line
Administer blood components as ordered
  Platelets
    Observe for changes in bleeding status during and after transfusions
    Usually ordered at fast rate of infusion to ensure therapeutic effectiveness
  Red blood cells: leukocyte poor; usually ordered
  Assess platelet count 1 hr after transfusion
Administer vasopressors and corticosteroids as ordered
  Use mechanical volume/rate controllers to maintain exact rate of infusion required
Monitor laboratory data daily; more often when ordered
  Report changes to physician immediately
  Label requests "bleeding tendency"
  Order fingersticks when possible
  Apply pressure to site for 3 to 5 min after puncture or until bleeding stops; observe for further bleeding
Intubation and mechanical ventilatory assistance may be required during periods of acute sepsis and shock
Place patient in position of comfort; use pillows or pads for support when necessary; provide care for pressure points
Use turn-and-lift sheet to move patient
Avoid restrictive clothing or bedclothes; use bed cradle or footboard

Avoid chilling; provide extra blankets, bed socks, and dry bedding when needed

Teach and assist patient to change position q1h to 2h; perform or assist with ROM exercises

Prevent trauma to decrease bleeding risk

Avoid aspirin and aspirin-containing medications

Avoid invasive procedures when possible

For IM injections use smallest-gauge needle; apply pressure until bleeding stops; recheck

Monitor invasive procedure sites for bleeding (e.g., IV, catheters)

Use soft-bristled toothbrushes or sponge cleaners

Use electric razors

Avoid vigorous nose blowing

Administer ordered antiemetics to avoid vomiting

Provide safe environment with careful arrangement of furniture and placement of personal items

Provide good lighting for ambulation

Advise use of well-fitting slippers or shoes

Prevent constipation; provide privacy; provide adequate fluids and diet; administer stool softeners or laxatives as ordered

Administer antineoplastic chemotherapeutic agents as ordered; assess for response and reactions (p. 649)

Prepare for radiation therapy (p. 642) or bone marrow transplant (p. 565) when ordered

Expected outcome/evaluation

Vital signs remain within acceptable limits; there are no further signs of bleeding, previous bleeding sites are controlled or resolving; skin and mucous membranes are warm and moist with good turgor

■ **NDX:** Potential for infection related to neutropenia or disease process

Place in noninfectious environment

Private room

Require handwashing with povidone-iodine scrub for all personnel and visitors before entering room

Remove food, trash, and drainage receptacles from room promptly

Ensure that no fresh fruits, vegetables, plants, or cut flowers are taken into room

Screen all personnel and visitors for infection

Provide support for patient to prevent feelings of isolation and alienation

Plan care with patient

Assist with daily care

Ensure that skin is dry after bathing

Assist with oral hygiene before and after meals and q2h

Handle patient carefully; prevent sheet burns and other injuries to skin

Assist with and teach perineal care after elimination and daily

Provide adequate, uninterrupted rest periods

Teach patient to turn and deep breathe q2h; avoid vigorous coughing

Assess for infection q4h in all body systems; report early signs to physician immediately

Temperature of 101° F (38.5° C)

Sore throat, "cold," "flu," coughing

Burning on urination

Small cuts or lesions that do not heal

Cooling measures may be required; avoid chilling; administer antipyretic drugs as ordered

Administer antibiotics on time when ordered

Obtain necessary cultures quickly to avoid delay in starting antibiotics

Cultures of throat, blood, urine, stool, and other lesions or areas may be ordered

Monitor results

Administer granulocyte colony–stimulating factor (G-CSF)

Monitor patient for chills and fever, pain at sites of infection, or potential infection (e.g., increased respiratory symptoms after infusion)

Expected outcome/evaluation

No signs of infection are present, previous sites of infection are healing; there is no evidence of lung congestion; urine is clear; oral temperature is within normal limits

■ **NDX:** Altered nutrition: less than body requirements related to nausea, vomiting, anorexia, abdominal discomfort, or impaired oral mucous membrane

Assess amount and types of foods and liquids tolerated and desired

Administer oral hygiene before and after intake

Use equipment appropriate to condition of mouth

Administer oral anesthetic when ordered

Assess predisposing factors, onset, position, frequency, and duration of nausea, vomiting, or discomfort

Eliminate predisposing factors when possible: unpleasant odors, perfume, disturbing sights or sounds

Change eating patterns; provide frequent, light meals; avoid foods and liquids for 2 to 4 hr before meals; and/or change usual place for eating

Serve foods cold or at room temperature to eliminate odors: sandwiches, cereal, cheese, desserts

Provide clear-liquid diet to reduce nausea: juices, carbonated beverages, flavored ice pops

Provide high-protein drinks as a supplement

Vary textures and tastes of foods to determine those tolerated: bland, sour, soft, etc.

Sweet, highly seasoned foods are not usually well tolerated

Administer antiemetics when ordered as patient desires

Arrange for quiet or rest periods before meals

Assist with preparation to conserve energy

Serve food and liquids attractively

Arrange for visitors, if patient prefers, to enhance social aspect

Weigh patient daily at same time with same clothing and scale

Measure intake and output q8h

Notify physician when intake and output are not equivalent and/or weight decreases by 3% to 5%

Administer TPN as ordered (p. 36)

Expected outcome/evaluation

Patient is taking nutritious foods and liquids or maintains TPN therapy; weight has stabilized; oral mucous membranes are intact, or healing is progressing; bowel elimination has returned to normal pattern and consistency

■ **NDX:** Pain related to bone or joint discomfort, headache, pressure of bleeding, or disease process

Maintain environment free of stress, unexpected sounds, or lighting

Assess pain: predisposing factors, intensity, frequency, duration, and effective methods of control used by patient; use pain rating scale

Place patient in position of comfort; support joints and extremities with pillows or pads

Change position qh; assist with ROM exercise if helpful

Remove restrictive clothing; use bed cradle or footboard

Provide soothing baths and back care; use warm or cold applications when helpful

Consider diversional, relaxation, or imagery measures

Administer pain relief medications as ordered at patient's request; assess effectiveness

Expected outcome/evaluation

Patient verbalizes feelings of increased comfort; uses alternate pain control methods interspersed with medication; self-care and exercise-activity tolerance are increasing

■ **NDX:** Activity intolerance related to anemia

If patient is on bed rest

   Maintain position of comfort

   Perform active or passive ROM exercises qid

   Assist with ADLs and ambulation to conserve energy

Plan undisturbed rest periods to conserve energy and permit performance of activities patient desires

Monitor pulse and respiratory rate qid and during activities

Assess adverse responses to activities (e.g., tachycardia, dysrhythmias, dyspnea)

Plan activities in small steps that patient can accomplish

Provide needed equipment to avoid expenditure of energy gathering supplies

Set goals with patient to increase activities as symptoms of intolerance decrease; encourage patient to adhere to schedule

Praise any increase in activity

Expected outcome/evaluation

Performs ADLs without evidence of exertional dyspnea or tachycardia; activity level is progressing

■ **NDX:** Fear related to poor prognosis

Assess level of anxiety and understanding of disease process when appropriate

Visit frequently or have significant other remain with patient

Use touch, reassurance, and positive body language

Provide an environment conductive to discussion and expression of worries, fears, and loss

Provide information about condition, procedures, and diagnostic studies

Encourage questions; answer clearly and consistently; clarify when necessary

Be sensitive to needs; listen to nonverbal clues

Maintain and assist with coping strategies

Encourage continuation of relationships

Provide access to others as requested: clergy, social worker, business associates, etc.

Expected outcome/evaluation

Patient expresses and discusses feelings about disease, treatment, and prognosis; sets realistic goals; seeks out resources and assistance from others when needed; and shows infrequent or no evidence of symptoms of fear or anxiety

■ **NDX:** Knowledge deficit related to lack of information about disease process, complications, activity, nutrition, anxiety/fear, and medications

Disease process

Discuss symptoms of recurrence or progression of disease to report to physician

Demonstrate how to check skin and peripheral pulses

Explain importance of regular follow-up care: physician, drug administration, laboratory studies

Complications

BLEEDING

Discuss signs and symptoms of bleeding to report to physician

Demonstrate how to check urine and stool for bleeding

Discuss accident/injury prevention

Avoid restrictive clothing

Keep home and work area free of clutter

Use assistive devices for ambulation and work when needed

Use caution when performing oral hygiene; inspect mouth for breaks or lesions; use special equipment and dentrifices as indicated

Avoid sports and hobbies that may cause injury

Handle equipment and sharp objects carefully

Prevent constipation through adequate fluids and diet and use of stool softeners or laxatives

INFECTION

Discuss signs and symptoms of infection to report: temperature elevation, sore throat, "cold," "flu," coughing, burning on urination, small cuts, hangnails, lesions that do not heal

Explain need to prevent infection

Keep environment clean

Do not handle pets and their equipment

Avoid persons with infections and large crowds

Handwashing technique for self and those assisting in the home

Daily self-care routine including perianal care after elimination

Activity

Instruct patient to balance rest and activity periods

Explain need to plan daily routine, using assistance when necessary

Instruct patient to increase activity or exercise as desired and tolerated

Nutrition

Explain need to have nutritious foods and liquids to 2500 ml/day

Emphasize need to continue planned eating pattern to enhance appetite

Give sources for delivery of prepared meals and high-protein drinks

Demonstrate how to manage TPN therapy (p. 36)

Anxiety/fear

Teach recognition of early symptoms

Explain need to continue open communication to discuss and express feelings

Discuss ways to continue problem solving and decision making

Discuss sources for assistance: psychosocial, financial, spiritual

Medications

Teach name of medication, dosage, time of administration, purpose, and side effects

Discuss side effects and complications to report to physician

Provide information about symptom care for chemotherapy (p. 670)

Demonstrate care and use of volumetric infusion device for medication administration

Explain need to avoid over-the-counter medications without checking with physician

Expected outcome/evaluation

Patient and/or significant other verbalizes home care and follow-up instructions; demonstrates methods for detecting signs of bleeding and infection, including checking urine and stool; and demonstrates oral hygiene and skin care measures, management of TPN therapy, and/or use of volumetric device for medication administration

MULTIPLE MYELOMA

Malignant disorder in which immature plasma cells proliferate in the bone marrow and form osteolytic tumors of the skeleton; initially, the pelvis, spine, and ribs are involved; other bones, the lymph nodes, spleen, liver, and kidneys are affected later; occurs primarily in males 50 to 70 years of age, diagnosis is often made in late stages, so prognosis is often poor

Assessment
Observations/findings

Medical history: increased susceptibility to infections—URI, pneumonia, urinary tract infection

Musculoskeletal

Bone pain

Predominately severe back pain on movement

Rib

Extremities

Fatigue

Weakness

Firm, nontender subcutaneous masses over area of skeletal involvement

Skeletal deformities

Pathological fractures

Shortened stature: 5 inches or more

Hematological

Anemia

Bleeding tendency

Renal: symptoms of calculi

Laboratory/diagnostic studies

Decreased Hgb

Decreased RBC

Elevated ESR, calcium level, total protein

Plasma cells: 3%

Lymphocytes: 40% to 50%
Proteinuria: Bence Jones protein
Hypercalciuria
Positive immunoelectrophoresis
Thrombocytopenia
Skeletal survey
    Diffuse osteoporosis
    Osteolytic lesions
IVP: renal involvement
Bone marrow: abnormal increase in immature plasma cells

Potential complications

Spinal cord compression (p. 413)
Nephrocalcinosis
Acute renal failure (p. 482)
Bleeding problems
Infections

Medical Management

Radiotherapy
Chemotherapy
Pain management
Laminectomy
Intake and output
Vital signs
Parenteral fluids
Treatment of complications

Nursing diagnoses/interventions/evaluation

■ **NDX:** Impaired physical mobility related to osteolytic esions and/or pathologic fractures

Explain importance of maintaining mobility to prevent further bone demineralization
Use pain relief medications before ambulation when ordered
Assist with ambulation: patient sits at side of bed, stands, gaining balance, and then walks with assistance
Avoid fast movements and stretching; encourage patient to move at own pace to avoid losing balance
Provide ambulatory aids: walkers, canes, braces, and/or crutches; provide safe environment for learning use of these aids
Assess ambulatory efforts, stance, gait, and coordination
Arrange furniture, equipment, and personal items within reach to avoid bumping, falls, or the need to reach for items
Provide night-light for safety
Assist with and teach patient the use of body mechanics and alignment
Place patient in position of comfort when on bed rest
    Maintain body alignment
    Support position with pillows or sandbags
Provide trapeze and side rails to assist with position change
Assist with turning and ROM q2h; move smoothly with care; logroll if spine is involved

Remind patient to change position qh
Assess reflexes, motor function, and sensation q8h; report changes and any sudden severe pain or inability to move a body part (may indicate new fracture or spinal cord compression)
Prepare for radiotherapy as ordered; explain rationale, expected results, and side effects
Administer chemotherapy as ordered
Prepare for laminectomy when ordered

Expected outcome/evaluation

Patient is increasing periods of ambulation using assistive aids and/or supports as necessary, is aware of surrounding environment, and avoids injury and falls
If on bed rest, patient uses trapeze, bed boards, or side rails to change position, keeping body in alignment

■ **NDX:** Pain related to severe bone pain secondary to fractures or spinal cord compression

Assess pain: predisposing factors, intensity, frequency, duration, and effective methods of control used by patient; use pain rating scale; incorporate these methods in plan
Assess neurological status q8h; report changes (may indicate vertebral compression)
Place patient in position of comfort; support joints and extremities with pillows or pads to maintain body alignment
Change position qh; assist with ROM exercise if helpful
Maintain environment free of stress, unexpected sounds, or lighting
Avoid jarring bed or chair or dropping items
Remove restrictive clothing; use bed cradle or footboard
Provide soothing baths and back care; use warm or cold applications when helpful
Encourage use of diversional, relaxation, or imagery measures
Administer pain relief medications as ordered at patient's request; assess effectiveness

Outcome/Evaluation

Patient uses alternate pain management measures interspersed with analgesics; carries out activities when pain is relieved or diminished; and verbalizes feelings of increased comfort

■ **NDX:** Potential fluid volume deficit or excess related to renal calculi, nephrocalcinosis, or renal failure

Monitor T, P, R, BP (lying and sitting), central venous pressure (CVP), and breath sounds q4h to 6h; report changes
Observe skin turgor and neck veins q4h to 6h
Measure intake and output q8h

Note frequency, amount, and color of urine; report difficulty in starting to void, pain, or presence of stones

Maintain fluids to 2000-3000 ml/day or as ordered
    Space fluids over 24 hr period
    Avoid dehydration
    Avoid fasting for laboratory work, x-ray studies, etc., without checking with physician
    Maintain urinary output ≥ 1500 ml/day

Weigh patient daily at same time with same clothing and scale; report changes of more than 3% to 5% daily

Avoid food and liquids with calcium

Ambulate or exercise q4h when possible

Expected outcome/evaluation

Vital signs are within normal limits; intake and output are in balance, with output between 1500 to 3000 ml/daily; skin turgor is good; weight is stable

■ **NDX:** Potential altered protection related to thrombocytopenia

Assess all systems for bleeding q8h; report early symptoms

Administer skin care daily and prn

Maintain skin and mucous membrane integrity
    Avoid invasive procedures when possible
    Change position qh; provide care for pressure areas
    Avoid use of harsh soaps or rough towels, cloths, and bedclothes
    Use soft-bristled toothbrush or foam swabs with evidence of gum bleeding
    Assist with and teach deep-breathing exercises; avoid vigorous coughing or nose blowing
    Avoid constipation through diet, stool softeners, or laxatives when ordered

Expected outcome/evaluation

There is no evidence of bleeding, or previous bleeding sites are resolving or controlled

■ **NDX:** Potential for infection related to increased susceptibility secondary to disturbed antibody formation

Place in noninfectious environment

Ensure that personnel and visitors observe handwashing technique

Screen all personnel and visitors for infection

Assess condition of skin and mucous membranes q8h

Maintain skin integrity; avoid invasive procedures; consolidate laboratory work

Provide mild antibacterial soaps and soft cloths and towels for skin hygiene, daily and prn

Encourage mobility q2h

Turn and position immobile patient q2h

Provide uninterrupted rest and sleep periods

Teach or assist with oral hygiene in morning, after food ingestion at bedtime, and q2h to 4h when awake

Monitor and record vital signs q4h; take temperature more frequently with elevation; report immediately

Institute comfort and cooling measures as indicated by condition
    Change linen and clothing to keep patient dry
    Avoid chilling
    Administer antipyretics as ordered

Monitor intake and output q8h; report urinary frequency, burning, or changes in character of urine

Use voiding measures when indicated to avoid catheterization

Assess and record respiratory status q4h; report changes in breath sounds, cough, and sputum, increases in respiratory rate, or presence of sore throat immediately

Assist and teach patient to turn and deep breathe q2h to 4h

Administer oxygen if ordered

Obtain cultures as ordered: blood, urine, sputum, skin, drainage, etc.

Monitor laboratory data daily; report changes

Administer IV antibiotics as ordered

Expected outcome/evaluation

No signs of infection are present; lungs are clear; skin is intact, warm and moist; urine is clear; oral temperature is within normal limits

■ **NDX:** Anxiety related to severe pain and/or poor prognosis

Assess level of anxiety and understanding of disease process when appropriate

Visit frequently or have significant other remain with patient

Use touch, reassurance, and positive body language

Provide an environment conducive to discussion and expression of worries, fears, and loss

Provide information about condition, procedures, and diagnostic studies

Encourage questions; answer clearly, consistently; clarify when necessary

Be sensitive to needs; listen to nonverbal clues

Maintain and assist with coping strategies; plan care with patient to enhance decision making and feeling of control

Encourage continuation of relationships

Provide access to others (e.g., clergy, social worker, business associates) as requested

Expected outcome/evaluation

Patient verbalizes feeling less anxious, describes feelings and makes decisions about care that are realistic

■ NDX: Knowledge deficit related to lack of information about disease process and treatment, mobility, pain management, complications, and anxiety/fear

Disease process and treatment

Discuss symptoms of recurrence or progression of disease to report to physician

Demonstrate how to monitor for spinal cord compression

Reinforce rationale, expected outcome, and side effects of radiotherapy and/or chemotherapy

Explain importance of regular follow-up with physician, radiotherapy/chemotherapy appointments, and laboratory studies

Mobility

Explain importance of ambulation and exercise on a regular basis

Discuss methods for preventing accidents and injury; use of assistive devices; arrangement of home environment

Explain use of body mechanics and need to maintain body alignment

Discuss measures to provide support and decrease musculoskeletal strain when on bed rest

Pain management

Instruct patient in alternate pain management methods

Emphasize need to have planned rest and sleep periods

Instruct patient on use of analgesics as ordered for maximal effect

Complications

RENAL DYSFUNCTION

Demonstrate method for recognizing symptoms to report

Demonstrate how to measure and record intake and output, weekly weight, and when to report

Explain importance of taking fluids, especially water, to 2500 to 3000 ml/day

Explain need to decrease calcium intake

BLEEDING

Discuss signs and symptoms to report

Demonstrate how to check urine and stool for bleeding

Explain need to avoid taking over-the-counter medications, especially aspirin or aspirin-containing products, without checking with physician

Instruct patient on how to prevent injury
  Avoid restrictive clothing
  Keep home and work area free of clutter
  Use assistive devices for ambulation and work when needed
  Use caution when performing oral hygiene; inspect mouth for breaks and lesions; use special equipment and dentrifices
  Avoid sports and hobbies that may cause injury

Handle equipment and sharp objects carefully

Prevent constipation through adequate fluids and diet and use of stool softeners or laxatives

INFECTION

Discuss signs and symptoms of infection to report to physician or nurse

Explain importance of avoiding persons who may be infectious or who may have potentially contagious conditions; explain need to avoid crowds

Explain need to avoid persons who have been recently vaccinated

Explain need to avoid multiple sexual partners

Instruct patient to wash hands after using bathroom, before eating, or before performing any procedures

Explain importance of preventing injury to skin
  Use electric razors
  Handle knives and sharp objects carefully
  Wear protective gloves when gardening and when using strong household cleaning solutions
  Wear broad-brimmed hat and sun screen when in sun
  Avoid going barefoot
  Wear warm clothing and boots in cold weather
  Avoid cutting cuticles, corns, or calluses
  Wear padded gloves when using oven

Explain need to perform oral hygiene periodically throughout the day

Explain importance of daily hygiene, including perineal care

Instruct patient to avoid using common drinking fountain

Explain need to maintain clean home environment and handle food properly

Anxiety/fear

Instruct patient on how to recognize early symptoms

Emphasize need to continue open communication to discuss and express feelings

Discuss ways to continue problem solving and decision-making

Discuss sources for assistance: psychosocial, financial, spiritual

Expected outcome/evaluation

Patient and/or significant other verbalizes understanding of home care and follow-up instructions; demonstrates methods for detecting signs of bleeding and infection, including checking urine and stool and taking oral temperature; demonstrates hygiene and skin care measures; and demonstrates use of ambulatory aids and support devices.

HODGKIN'S DISEASE

Malignant disorder characterized by painless enlargement of lymphoid tissue; usually one lymph node is affected initially, but other nodes and the spleen become involved throughout the lymphatic system

TABLE 14-4. Staging of Hodgkin's Disease

Stage*	Definition
I	Single lymph node region
II	Two or more node regions limited to one side of the diaphragm
III	Disease on both sides of the diaphragm, but limited to the lymph nodes and spleen
IV	Involvement of the bones, bone marrow, lung parenchyma, pleura, liver, skin, gastrointestinal tract, central nervous system, etc.

From Luckmann J, Sorensen KC: *Medical-surgical nursing: a psychophysiologic approach,* Philadelphia, 1987, WB Saunders.
*All stages are subclassified as A or B to describe the absence (A) or presence (B) of systemic symptoms.

(Figure 14-7 on p. 633); histiocytes called Reed-Sternberg cells proliferate and replace normal cellular structure; without treatment, other organs and structures become involved

Assessment
Observations/findings

Enlarged nodes
    Cervical and supraclavicular nodes are usually involved initially
    Firm, rubbery; become hard with sclerosing
    Vary from nontender without skin changes to tender with skin changes
Skin
    Pruritus: generalized and severe
    Temperature: alternating febrile and afebrile periods
    Night sweats
    Jaundice
    Edema: face and neck
Hematological
    Fatigue
    Malaise
Gastrointestinal
    Anorexia
    Weight loss
    Splenomegaly
    Hepatomegaly
Musculoskeletal: bone pain

Laboratory/diagnostic studies

Normocytic, normochromic anemia
WBC and differential; any combination of following
    Neutrophilia
    Monocytosis
    Eosinophilia
    Lymphocytopenia
    Abnormal ESR
    Increased alkaline phosphatase (indicates bone involvement)
    Lymph node biopsy
        Reed-Sternberg cells

Nodular fibrosis
Necrosis

Potential complications

Respiratory distress
Infection
Fractures

Medical Management

Staging procedures
    Lymph node biopsy
    Chest x-ray examination
    Bone marrow biopsy
    Liver and spleen biopsy, scans
    Peritoneoscopy
    Laparotomy
    Bone scans
    Lymphangiography (see box on p. 630)
Radiotherapy (usually Stages I, II, and III) (Table 14-4)
Antineoplastic chemotherapy (usually Stages III and IV) (Table 14-4)
Treat complications

Nursing diagnoses/interventions/evaluation

■ **NDX:** Impaired skin integrity related to pruritus, jaundice, and/or immobility

Assess condition of skin q8h
Administer daily skin care as needed
    Soothing baths: sodium bicarbonate or oatmeal
    Avoid skin dryness; apply lotions to slightly moist skin
    Cool sponge baths or tub soaks may be beneficial
    Apply powders sparingly, avoiding any buildup in tissue folds
Keep clothing light with no constrictions
Check and change q2h during night if patient is experiencing night sweats
Elevate bed clothes with bed cradle
Keep bed wrinkle free
Use linen laundered in nondetergents
Advise patient to avoid scratching; instead, apply pressure or use cool applications
Use distraction and diversion; keep needed materials within easy reach
Administer medication to relieve severe itching as ordered; assess response
Check temperature q4h to establish pattern: cool sponge baths may be helpful when temperature is elevated

Expected outcome/evaluation

Demonstrates ability to care for and protect skin
Skin is intact and turgor is adequate

■ **NDX:** Activity intolerance related to fatigue

LYMPHANGIOGRAPHY

DEFINITION

Injection of opaque dye into the lymphatic system for x-ray visualization

OBSERVATIONS

Allergic reaction to dye
  Dyspnea
  Nausea, vomiting
  Numbness of extremities
  Diaphoresis
  Tachycardia
Site of injection
  Irritation
  Redness
  Swelling
  Drainage
  Thrombus

PREPROCEDURE CARE

Explain procedure
  Local injection of dye into hands or feet
  Small surgical incision to locate lymph ducts
  Some discomfort is to be expected while lymph
    ducts are being located
  Injection of dye into lymphatic system
  Patient must lie still for long period
  Feeling of warmth is normal response to dye
  X-ray examinations of body immediately after in-
    jection, 24 hr later, and prn thereafter
  Bluish cast to skin will disappear within 1 month
Start ordered IV in extremity that is expected to be
  injected during procedure

POSTPROCEDURE CARE

Increase fluids to 2500 ml unless contraindicated
Administer back care q2h to 4h until discomfort is
  gone
Check T, P, and R q2h for four times or as ordered
Check extremities for numbness q2h for four times
Check site of incision q2h to 4h; warm compresses
  may be ordered if local tissues are infiltrated

If patient is on bed rest
  Maintain position of comfort
  Perform active or passive ROM exercises qid
  Assist with ADLs and ambulation to conserve energy
Plan undisturbed rest periods to conserve energy and per-
  mit performance of activities patient desires
Monitor Pulse and Respiratory rate qid and during activ-
  ities
Assess adverse responses to activities (e.g., tachycardia,
  dysrhythmias, dyspnea)
Plan activities in small steps that patient can accomplish

easily; provide needed equipment to avoid energy expenditure caused by frustration and gathering supplies
Set goals with patient to increase activities as symptoms
  of intolerance decrease; encourage patient to adhere to
  schedule
Praise any increase in activity

Expected outcome/evaluation

Performs ADLs without evidence of exertional dyspnea
  or tachycardia; activity level is progressing

■ **NDX:** Altered nutrition: less than body requirements
related to anorexia and/or abdominal distention secondary to splenomegaly or hepatomegaly

Assess amount and types of foods and liquids tolerated
  and desired
Provide time for oral hygiene before and after meals
Eliminate unpleasant odors, perfumes, and disturbing
  sights or sounds
Experiment with various eating patterns: small, light
  meals; liquids only; change in usual eating place and/
  or position
Vary textures and tastes of foods to determine those tol-
  erated: bland, sour, sweet, soft, dry, etc.
Add high-protein drinks as a supplement
Serve foods and liquids attractively arranged at tempera-
  ture desired by patient
Assist with preparation of tray
Arrange for visitors, if patient prefers, to enhance social
  aspect
Arrange for food-from-home treats
Provide adequate time for meal so patient does not feel
  rushed
Plan rest periods before meals to conserve energy
Weigh patient daily at same time with same clothing and
  scale
Measure intake and output q8h
Explain that sitting, rather than lying, after a meal may
  decrease full feeling
Plan periods of exercise (e.g., walking between meals)
  when possible

Expected outcome/evaluation

Patient is taking a balanced diet and liquids to 2500 ml
  daily; weight is stabilized

■ **NDX:** Pain related to bone pain or fractures

Assess pain: predisposing factors, intensity, frequency, and
  duration, and effective methods of control used by patient
Place patient in position of comfort; immobilize or support

joints and extremities with pillows or pads; maintain body alignment

Change position qh; assist with ROM exercise if helpful

Remove restrictive clothing; use bed cradle or footboard

Provide soothing baths and back care; use warm or cold applications when helpful

Encourage use of assistive devices when ambulating

Increase activity and self-care to tolerance; note responses; assist patient with being aware of body responses to attain highest level of activity without increasing frequency or intensity of pain

Consider diversional, relaxation, or imagery measures

Administer pain relief medications, as ordered, at patient's request; assess effectiveness

Expected outcome/evaluation

Patient verbalizes feelings of increased comfort and uses alternate pain control methods interspersed with medication; self-care and exercise/activity tolerance are increasing

■ **NDX:**   Anxiety related to unknown outcome of disease

Assess level of anxiety and understanding of disease process when appropriate

Visit frequently or have significant other remain with patient

Use touch, reassurance, and positive body language

Provide an environment conducive to discussion and expression of worries, fears, and potential loss

Provide information about condition, procedures, and diagnostic studies

Encourage questions; answer clearly and consistently; clarify when necessary

Reinforce physician's explanation of positive outcome

Be sensitive to needs; listen to nonverbal clues

Maintain and assist with coping strategies; plan care with patient to enhance decision making and feeling of control

Encourage continuation of relationships

Provide access to others as requested: clergy, social worker, business associates, etc.

Expected outcome/evaluation

Patient expresses and discusses feelings about disease, treatment, and prognosis; sets realistic goals; and seeks out resources and assistance from others when needed

There is infrequent or no evidence of symptoms of anxiety/fear

■ **NDX:**   Potential for ineffective airway clearance related to airway edema and/or enlarged mediastinal lymph nodes

Assess respiratory effort, breathing pattern, and breath sounds q4h to 8h (more frequently if abnormalities are noted)

Place patient in position of comfort; sitting position usually decreases respiratory effort

Assist and teach patient to turn and deep breathe q2h

Administer oxygen as ordered

Note patient's response to activities; assist as necessary to avoid respiratory distress

Keep emergency airway maintenance equipment available

Expected outcome/evaluation

Respiratory rate, excursion, and breath sounds are normal; there is no evidence of cough, stridor, or hoarseness

■ **NDX:**   Potential for infection related to increased susceptibility secondary to changes in WBC

Place in noninfectious environment

Ensure that personnel and visitors observe handwashing technique

Screen all personnel and visitors for infection

Assess condition of skin and mucous membranes q8h

Maintain skin integrity; avoid invasive procedures; consolidate laboratory work

Provide mild antibacterial soaps and soft cloths and towels for skin hygiene, daily and prn

Encourage mobility q2h

Turn and position immobile patient q2h

Provide uninterrupted rest and sleep periods

Teach or assist with oral hygiene in morning, after food ingestion, at bedtime, and q2h to 4h when awake

Monitor and record vital signs q4h; take temperature more frequently with elevation; report immediately

Institute comfort and cooling measures as indicated by condition

   Change linen and clothing to keep patient dry

   Avoid chilling

   Administer antipyretics as ordered

Monitor intake and output; report urinary frequency, burning, or changes in character of urine

Use voiding measures when indicated to avoid catheterization

Assess and record respiratory status q4h; report changes in breath sounds, cough, and sputum; increases in respiratory rate; or presence of sore throat immediately

Assist and teach patient to turn and deep breathe q2h to 4h

Administer oxygen if ordered

Obtain cultures as ordered: blood, urine, sputum, skin, drainage, etc.

Monitor laboratory data daily; report changes

Administer IV antibiotics as ordered

Expected outcome/evaluation

No signs of infection are present: skin is intact and warm, with good turgor; breathing pattern is normal; lungs are clear; respiratory excursion is normal; urine is clear; oral temperature is within normal limits

■ **NDX:** Knowledge deficit related to lack of information about disease process, treatment, complications, nutrition, activities, comfort, and anxiety/fear

Disease process and treatment

Discuss symptoms of recurrence or progression of disease to report to physician

Explain expected outcome and responses to radiation and/or chemotherapy and symptom care (p. 670)

Explain importance of regular follow-up care: physician, radiation therapy/chemotherapy, laboratory studies

Reinforce physician's explanation of need to delay pregnancy (for patients of childbearing age) until patient is in remission for a time

Complications
INFECTION

Discuss how to check for and report signs and symptoms of infection: elevated temperature, sore thoat, "cold," "flu," coughing, burning on urination, and small cuts, hangnails, and lesions that do not heal

Explain need to prevent infection

Maintain skin integrity: avoid scratching; observe careful skin care; observe for skin changes

Maintain adequate rest and sleep periods

Keep environment clean

Avoid persons with infection and crowds

Use handwashing technique for self and those assisting

RESPIRATORY DISTRESS

Discuss signs and symptoms of early respiratory distress to report: increasing cough, hoarse voice, decreased activity tolerance, any change in breathing pattern

Teach deep-breathing exercises and explain need to pace activities to avoid acute distress

Emphasize need to have emergency plan and phone numbers available for acute distress

Nutrition

Explain need to maintain balanced diet and liquids of choice to 2500 ml/day

Emphasize need to continue meal plan and eating pattern to enhance appetite

Instruct patient to weigh weekly and to report more than 5% loss

Activities and comfort

Explain importance of returning to normal lifestyle as soon as possible

Explain need to balance rest and activity periods

Instruct patient to plan daily routine and to use assistance when necessary

Instruct patient to increase activities and self-care as condition improves

Explain need to continue skin care measures to decrease pruritus

Instruct patient to continue alternate pain relief measures that are successful

Teach patient to use assistive devices when ambulating to prevent injury

Teach body alignment if patient is on bed rest, with ROM exercises and methods for preventing injury

Anxiety/fear

Instruct patient on how to recognize symptoms

Emphasize need to continue open communication to express and discuss feelings

Discuss ways to continue problem solving and decision making

Discuss sources for assistance if needed: psychosocial, spiritual, financial

Expected outcome/evaluation

Patient and/or significant other verbalizes understanding of home care and follow-up instructions, plans to increase self-care and other activities with adequate rest and sleep periods, signs and symptoms of disease or complications to report, methods for avoiding complications, diet and eating plan, plan for emergency assistance, and plan for unexpected results or side effects of radiation and/or chemotherapy; and demonstrates methods to detect complications, general hygiene care (including specific care for skin), breathing exercises, use of thermometer, and use of any needed ambulatory devices

MALIGNANT LYMPHOMA

Refers to a grouping of neoplasms originating in lymphoid tissue, which are classified by degree and differentiation of cellular content; grouping includes non-Hodgkin's lymphomas and lymphosarcoma; etiology is unknown, but a viral source is suspected; it can occur in all age-groups and is more common in males, whites, and people of Jewish ancestry

Assessment
Observations/findings

Enlarged lymph nodes (see Figure 14-4, which depicts lymphatic system)

Cervical and supraclavicular initially

Nontender, movable, rubbery

Size fluctuations

Enlarged tonsils and adenoids

Oropharyngeal and mediastinal mass

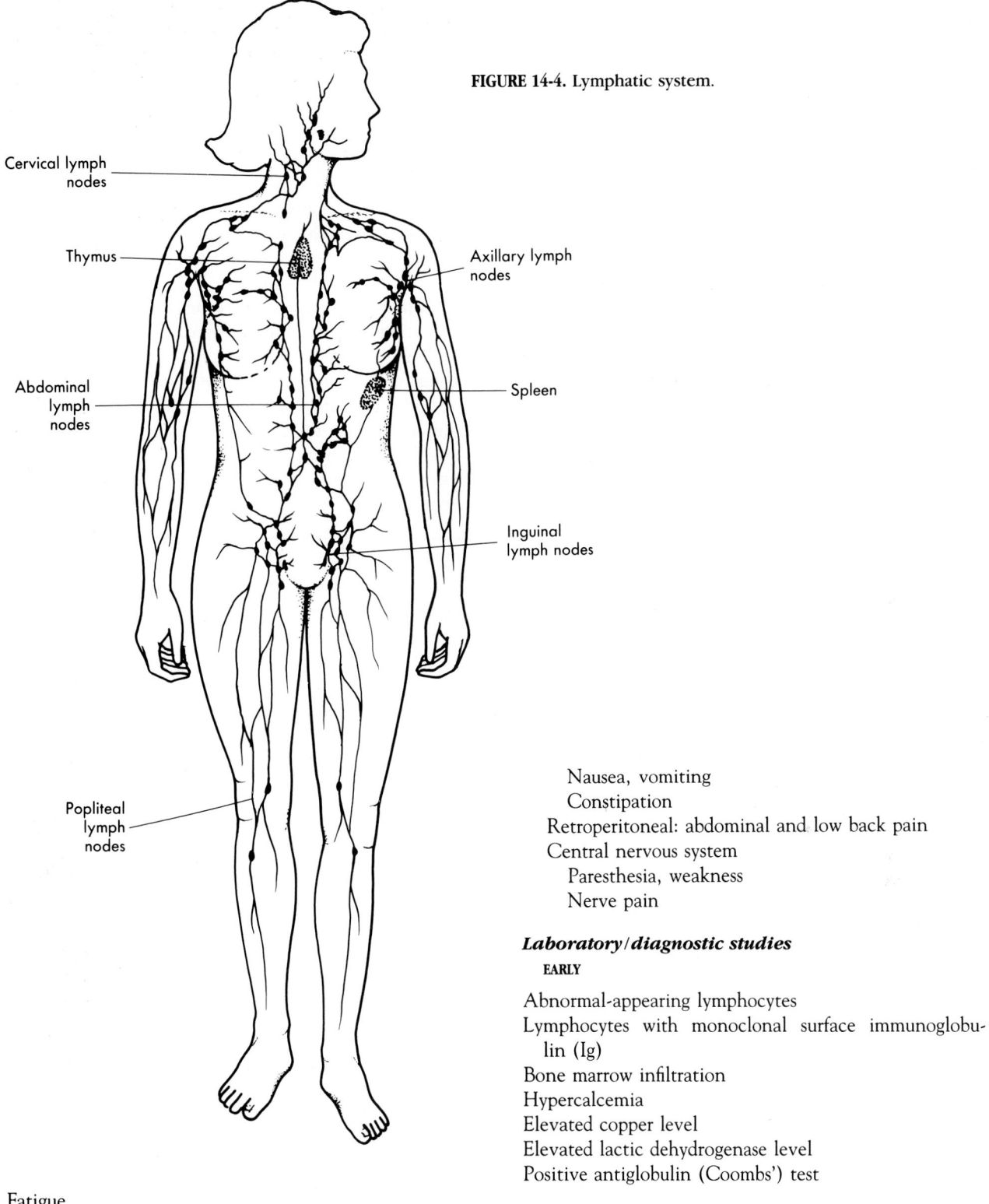

FIGURE 14-4. Lymphatic system.

Cervical lymph
nodes

Thymus

Abdominal
lymph
nodes

Axillary lymph
nodes

Spleen

Inguinal
lymph nodes

Popliteal
lymph
nodes

Nausea, vomiting
 Constipation
Retroperitoneal: abdominal and low back pain
Central nervous system
 Paresthesia, weakness
 Nerve pain

Laboratory/diagnostic studies

EARLY

Abnormal-appearing lymphocytes
Lymphocytes with monoclonal surface immunoglobu-
 lin (Ig)
Bone marrow infiltration
Hypercalcemia
Elevated copper level
Elevated lactic dehydrogenase level
Positive antiglobulin (Coombs') test

LATE

Hypoalbuminemia or hypergammaglobulinemia
Monoclonal Ig spikes

Potential complications

Pleural effusions
Bone fractures
Paralysis

Fatigue
Malaise
Weight loss
Elevated temperature
Susceptibility for infections
Pressure symptoms in areas of involvement
 GI system
 Dysphagia
 Anorexia

Medical Management

Staging procedures
    Biopsies for histological evaluation
        Lymph nodes
        Tonsils
        Liver
        Bone marrow
        Bowel
        Tissue removed during laparotomy
    Lumbar puncture
    Chest x-ray examination
    CT scans
        Spleen
        Liver
        Abdomen
        Bone
    Lymphangiography (see box on p. 630)
Radiotherapy
Chemotherapy

Nursing diagnoses/interventions/evaluation

See Hodgkin's Disease (p. 628)

Oncologic Emergencies

An oncologic emergency arises from tumor progression or metastasis and can cause irreversible morbidity or death if not promptly recognized and treated

HEMATOLOGICAL EMERGENCIES

Tumor progression may cause hemorrhage via blood vessel erosion or through coagulation abnormalities such as disseminated intravascular coagulation (DIC)

Hemorrhage
Observations

Acute hemorrhage, most commonly from
    Nose
    Bronchus
    Stomach
    Colon
    Carotid artery
    Vagina

Associated Conditions/Factors

Cancer
    Stomach
    Esophageal
    Gynecological
    Head and neck
    Colorectal

Interventions

Assess for bleeding; monitor vital signs and mental status; check mouth, nose, rectum, vagina and skin; check stools and urine for occult blood
Monitor laboratory data
Notify physician of suspected or frank bleeding
Apply direct pressure for carotid artery hemorrhage
Depending on bleeding site, prepare for
    Packing: nose, rectum, or vagina
    Occlusion balloon catheter: bronchus
    Iced saline lavage: stomach
    Iced saline enemas: colon/rectum
Monitor vital signs q15 min; decrease frequency as hemorrhage is controlled
Measure and document amount of blood loss; measure and record intake and output
Maintain calm atmosphere
Support patient and significant other psychologically
Monitor IV fluids and blood products
Prepare patient for surgery or laser surgery when ordered

Disseminated Intravascular Coagulation (DIC)
Observations

May be hemorrhagic or thrombotic
Increased bleeding from sites of invasive procedures
Ecchymotic extensions
Systemic bleeding to hemorrhage
Thromboemboli in any system
Hypotension
Tachycardia
Cool, pale, clammy skin
Shortness of breath
Loss of consciousness

Associated Conditions/Factors

Cancer
    Lung
    Prostate
Metastases
Leukemia
Sepsis
Infection
Hepatic failure

Interventions

Monitor vital signs q15 min
Assess all body systems for presence of bleeding or thromboemboli and evidence of adequate tissue perfusion
Monitor sites of bleeding
    Apply pressure
Monitor continuous heparin infusion, IV fluids, and administration of blood products and medications (e.g., vasopressors, antidysrhythmics)
Measure and record intake and output; report deficits
See p. 173 for detailed care

CARDIOVASCULAR EMERGENCIES

Superior Vena Cava Syndrome (SVCS)

Obstructed flow to the right atrium occurs from compression caused by tumor progression or enlarged mediastinal lymph nodes, from intraluminal occlusion caused by some sarcomas, or from thrombosis caused by central line devices

Observations

Prominent neck and chest veins
Telangiectasia, upper thorax
Facial plethora
Edema of face, neck, upper thorax, upper extremities
Jugular vein distention
Headache, unrelieved
Dizziness
Visual disturbances
Feeling of facial fullness
Dysphagia
Dyspnea
Cough
Hoarseness
Chest pain
Respiratory distress
Altered level of consciousness
Horner syndrome
 One-sided drooping of eye with pupil constriction and conjunctivitis with loss of sweating on same side of forehead
Enlarged heart on x-ray examination
CT scan confirmation

Associated Conditions/Factors

Lung cancer
Hodgkin's disease
Non-Hodgkin's lymphomas
Breast, thymus, testicular, and head and neck carcinomas (metastases)
Chemotherapy via indwelling central line devices
Radiation-induced fibrosis

Interventions

Assess head, neck, upper thorax, and upper extremities for signs of SVCS
Assess mental status, level of consciousness, respiratory status, vision, and voice for changes indicative of SVCS
Report findings indicative of SVCS
Position patient to reduce edema
 Semi-Fowler's to high Fowler's position
 Elevate upper extremities on pillows; overbed table may increase comfort
 Perform passive ROM q4h
Provide skin care for face, with eye care to prevent infection and breakdown
Initiate oral hygiene measures
Prevent pressure or trauma to face, thorax, and upper extremities
 Wear loose-fitting bedclothes
 Avoid use of any jewelry
 Monitor oxygen administration equipment carefully
 Avoid venous punctures for fluid or laboratory studies
 Place identification band on lower extremity
 Avoid Valsalva's maneuver, lifting, or bending
Provide easily chewed foods or full liquid diet
Assist with oral and hygiene measures and diet to decrease oxygen demand
Provide information about radiation or chemotherapy as appropriate when scheduled to reduce obstruction
Maintain calm, quiet atmosphere
Answer questions and provide information to reduce anxiety for patient and significant other
Assess effectiveness of medications administered and observe for toxic or side effects (e.g., chemotherapeutics, anticoagulants, oxygen therapy, steroids)

Cardiac Tamponade

Cardiac tamponade may be caused by pericardial effusions due to metastatic spread of malignant cells or bleeding from coagulopathies such as DIC; also may result from constrictive pericarditis caused by radiation to mediastinum

Observations

Beck's triad
 Decreased BP with narrow pulse pressure
 Increased central venous pressure (CVP)
 Muffled heart sounds
Pulsus paradoxus; 20 mm Hg or more variation
Kussmaul's sign
Tachycardia
Precordial dullness on percussion
Peripheral constriction; cold, clammy
Tachypnea
Dyspnea, cough
Chest pain
Anxiety, apprehension, feeling of doom
Low-voltage ECG
Enlarged heart on x-ray examination
Effusion on echocardiogram
Jugular vein distention
Ascites
Peripheral edema
Pulmonary congestion
Constriction of pericardial sac
 Audible knock at heart apex
 Friction rub
Shock
Cardiac arrest

Associated Conditions/Factors

Metastases from
    Lung
    Breast
    Lymphomas
    Leukemias
    Melanomas
Radiation therapy

Interventions

Assess for signs of cardiac tamponade
    Auscultate heart and breath sounds
    Assess carotid, radial, femoral, and pedal pulses
    Assess vital signs; calculate pulse pressure and presence
        of pulsus paradoxus
    Monitor respiratory status and continuous ECG
    Assess mental status and level of consciousness
Report signs of cardiac tamponade immediately
Prepare to assist with emergency pericardiocentesis or immediate transfer to ICU or OR
    Observe for dysrthythmias during and after procedure
    Auscultate breath sounds for possible pneumothorax
    Ensure venous access for fluid requirements
    Have airway intubation and suction equipment available
Support patient psychologically
    Explain need for frequent assessment and monitoring
    Provide information about emergency procedures, detailing steps as they are taken
    Remain calm; answer questions clearly
Monitor effect of oxygen therapy
Restrict activities to reduce oxygen demand; assist with positioning, toileting, etc.
Position patient to increase venous return
Provide information about further treatments, sclerosing agents, chemotherapy, radiation therapy, or pericardial windows
See p. 100 for further care

METABOLIC EMERGENCIES

Syndrome of Inappropriate Antidiuretic Hormone (SIADH)

Ectopic production of a substance similar to antidiuretic hormone (ADH) by a tumor or stimulation of the posterior pituitary gland to produce ADH by the tumor; or by specific drugs. This causes water intoxication and dilutional hyponatremia, which if unrecognized and treated, may lead to congestive heart failure

Observations

Lethargy
Weakness
Irritability
Confusion
Seizures

Nausea, vomiting
Anorexia
Sudden weight gain, usually without edema
Decreased urine output without change in intake
Congestive heart failure (CHF)
Serum sodium < 135 mEq/L
Serum osmolality < 280 mOsm/kg H_2O
Urine osmolality > 1200 mOsm/kg H_2O
Urine sodium > 20 mEq/L
Elevated BUN

Associated Conditions/Factors

Small cell lung cancer
Lymphoma
Pancreatic cancer
Prostatic cancer
Chemotherapeutic agents
    Vincristine
    Cyclophosphamide
Infections; viral/bacterial pneumonia
Increased intracranial pressure (ICP)

Interventions

Assess for fluid retention and dilutional hyponatremia
Monitor intake and output
Weigh daily: same time, scale, and clothing
Assess neurological and mental status
Evaluate laboratory values for electrolytes
Auscultate lungs for breath sounds
Report adverse signs immediately
In collaboration with physician, restrict fluids to 500 to 1000 ml/24 hr
Assess effectiveness of parenteral hypertonic saline solution and diuretics administered
    Monitor for signs of hypokalemia (pp. 38-51) and hypomagnesemia (pp. 38-51)
Provide safety measures (e.g., bed in low position with side rails up, call light within reach); assist with ambulation; assist with hygiene and diet to prevent injury
Maintain seizure precautions
Provide calm, nonstressful environment
Teach patient and significant other signs of SIADH to report

Hypercalcemia

Elevated calcium levels result from resorption of calcium from the bones. This resorption results from bone destruction by metastases to the skeleton. Prostaglandins, leukocyte cytokines, and ectopic production of a substance similar to parathyroid stimulates release of calcium from the bones; this may result in a gradual or sudden onset of renal failure

Observations

Polyuria
Nocturia
Polydipsia

Lethargy
Confusion
Disorientation
Bradycardia
Fatigue
Muscle weakness
Hypotonia
Loss of deep tendon reflexes
Dehydration
Nausea, vomiting
Anorexia
Elevated serum calcium
Serum albumin may be decreased with serum calcium within normal limits

Associated conditions/factors

Cancer
  Breast
  Lung
  Thyroid
  Kidney
  Ovarian
  Esophageal
  Parotid
  Oral
Ewing's sarcoma
Melanoma
Multiple myeloma
Leukemia
Lymphoma
Immobility
Skeletal metastases
Medications
  Thiazide diuretics
  Lithium

Interventions

Assess for signs and symptoms of hypercalcemia
  Level of consciousness and mental status
  Muscle reflexes and activity tolerance
  Nutritional status
  Intake and output
  Daily weight
  Vital signs
  Skin turgor
  Electrolyte values and albumin levels
Assess effectiveness of parenteral saline, medications administered (e.g., plicamycin, calcitonin or phosphates or diphosphonates) that inhibit calcium resorption, and diuretics (e.g., furosemide)
Encourage fluids to 2500 ml/day
Monitor diet intake of oxalates to bind dietary calcium
Teach and assist wth ROM if on bed rest; increase activity and exercise as tolerated to decrease further calcium resorption from bones
Provide safety measures when needed to prevent injury

Bed in low position with side rails up
Assist with ambulation or provide assistive devices
Call light and articles required by patient within reach; night-light available
Assist with diet and hygiene measures
Teach signs and symptoms of hypercalcemia that patient and/or significant other should report to caregiver before discharge
See p. 320 for further care

Hypoglycemia/Hyperglycemia

Abnormal blood sugar levels can occur in nondiabetic patients with cancer as a result of certain therapies, TPN, or primary tumors of pancreas

Observations

See Diabetes (p. 332)

Associated conditions/factors

Glucocorticosteroid therapy may cause hyperglycemia in patients with
  Lymphomas
  Leukemias
  Radiation therapy to reduce swelling
  Cerebral metastases to reduce edema
TPN with high glucose concentration may cause hyperglycemia
Primary beta–islet cell tumors or insulinomas cause hyperglycemia through stimulation or oversecretion of insulin
Severe malnutrition

Interventions

(See Diabetes (p. 332)

Tumor Lysis Syndrome

This emergency occurs with the rapid release of intracellular components, potassium, phosphorus, and uric acid as a result of rapid tumor cell necrosis induced by chemotherapy or radiation; the combined electrolyte disturbances may result in renal failure and cardiac arrest

Observations

Oliguria
Anuria
Flank pain
Urine crystals
Hematuria
Cardiac dysrhythmias
  Bradycardia
  Ventricular tachycardia
  Prolonged PR and QT intervals
  Depressed ST segment
  Tall peaked T waves
  Widened QRS complex
Muscular cramps; tetany

Positive Chvostek's and Trousseau's signs
Confusion
Elevated
  Serum uric acid
  BUN
  Serum creatinine
  Serume phosphate
  Serum potassium
Decreased serum calcium

Associated conditions/factors

Non-Hodgkin's lymphomas
Leukemia

Interventions

Assess cardiac status
  Apical pulse, rate, rhythm, blood pressure
  Monitor for cardiac dysrhythmias and signs of CHF
  Evaluate potassium and calcium levels
Assess neuromuscular status
  Monitor for carpopedal spasms, presence of Chvostek's
    and Trousseau's signs, seizure activity, or confusion
  Evaluate calcium and phosphate levels
Assess renal status
  Monitor intake and output, daily weight, urine pH,
    uric acid, BUN, and creatinine levels
Assess effectiveness of parenteral fluids with sodium bi-
  carbonate, calcium supplements, allopurinol, phos-
  phate binders, and diuretics when administered
Monitor dietary intake
  Restrict foods with potassium
  Encourage sodium intake if allowed
Provide safety measures, assist with ADLs, and reorient
  if confusion is present
Maintain seizure precautions; padded side rails and airway
  at bedside
Instruct patient to avoid pressure on motor nerves to de-
  crease spasms; no knee gatch or crossing of legs, etc.
See CHF (p. 101) if symptoms observed
Prepare for peritoneal or hemodialysis when necessary
  (p. 486)

NEUROLOGICAL EMERGENCY

Spinal Cord Compression

*This emergent situation occurs as a result of tumor
  growth or spread of metastases to the vertebral body
  with growth into the epidural space; usually develops
  rapidly and can cause permanent neurological deficits
  such as paraplegia*

Observations

Pain
  Neck, back, and lumbar
  Increases with motion; Valsalva's maneuver, supine po-
    sition, coughing, and sneezing; intense, localized,
    and persistent
Radicular root
  Increases with movement; related to distribution of seg-
    mental dermatome
Medullary
  Diffuse, referred, bilateral pain with shooting or burning
    in peripheral area; not increased with valsalva ma-
    neuver
Muscular weakness
  Gait and balance disturbances
  Foot-drop
  Paralysis
Increased tendon reflexes; positive Babinski's
Sensory changes, ascend from feet up
  Paresthesia
  Numbness, tingling
  Loss of sensation
  Coolness in affected area
  Sexual dysfunction
Loss of bowel and bladder control

Associated conditions/factors

Spinal cord tumors
Vertebral metastases from
  Lung
  Breast
  Lymphoma
  Multiple myeloma
  Prostate

Interventions

Assess pain: location, type, duration, radiation effects
  on movement or position change; use pain rating
  scale
Assess neuromuscular function and sensation; monitor
  tendon reflexes
Assess bowel sounds and bladder distention
Report changes immediately
Maintain on bed rest at first appearance of signs of cord
  compression
Turn and reposition using logroll method and sufficient
  personnel to prevent injury
Administer corticosteroids on time; assess effectiveness
  in reducing cord inflammation when ordered
Prepare patient for surgical decompression or radio-
  therapy (p. 642) when necessary
See Laminectomy and Paraplegia (p. 444)

PULMONARY EMERGENCIES

Pleural Effusions

*Tumor progression or metastasis causes irritation of the
  pleural membrane and results in increased production
  of fluid in the interpleural space*

Observations

Dyspnea
Cough
Tachypnea
Decreased or absent breath sounds
Pleuritic chest pain
Tachycardia
Asymmetrical bulging of intercostal space
Dullness on percussion over fluid field
Decreased fremitus
Confirmation with chest x-ray studies

Associated conditions/factors

Lymphomas
Lung cancer
Breast cancer
Leukemia
Mesothelioma
Ovarian cancer
Infection
Tuberculosis

Interventions

Auscultate chest for heart and lung sounds
Assess respiratory effort, rate, and rhythm and use of accessory muscles
Monitor vital signs; skin color, temperature, and moisture; neck vein distention; intake and output
Assess chest pain: location, character, onset, intensity
Report adverse findings to physician
Position patient for comfort and maximal respiratory excursion; usually semi-Fowler's to High Fowler's preferred
Teach and assist patient to turn, cough, and deep breathe q2h and use incentive spirometer qh
Prepare emergency equipment for respiratory depression before thoracentesis
Premedicate when ordered
Explain thoracentesis procedure and assist as necessary to increase psychological comfort
Monitor vital signs and breath sounds; check for bleeding or leakage q15 min for 1 hr then qh for 2 hr after thoracentesis
Rotate patient position to all four sides if sclerosing agent instilled
NOTE: chest tube may be clamped for defined period of time if in place; unclamp at specified time
Provide oxygen therapy and humidification when indicated
Explain and prepare for surgical procedures (pleuroperitoneal shunt, pleurectomy) if effusion unrelieved

Pulmonary Obstruction

Tumor progression causes airway obstruction; prompt intervention can prevent lung collapse beyond the obstruction

Observations

Dyspnea, severe
Progressive stridor on inhalation, exhalation, or both
Inability to speak
Use of accessory muscles
Nasal flaring
Asymmetrical chest excursion
Decreased tactile fremitus
Decreased or absent breath sounds
Rapid onset of anxiety

Associated conditions/factors

Primary lung tumors

Interventions

Assess breathing pattern, effort, respiratory rate, presence of stridor and speech, character of secretions, and breath sounds q4h; report changes indicating obstruction immediately
Maintain pharyngeal and/or endotracheal airway, tracheostomy tray, and resuscitation equipment at bedside
NOTE: tracheobronchial stents and positive-pressure devices may be used as temporary measures to prevent compression, or a tracheostomy may be required until underlying cause is treated with radioactive or laser therapy
Be prepared to administer oxygen therapy
Position patient for maximal chest excursion with least amount of effort
Provide suction for secretions patient is unable to handle
Maintain a calm atmosphere; stay with patient during times of increased anxiety and quietly coach patient in methods for breathing easier, as well as relaxation techniques
Encourage fluids to 2000 to 2500 ml/day
See Care of Patient with Tracheostomy (p. 232)

Renal Emergency

Renal Obstructions or Failure

Tumor progression can lead to obstruction of flow through ureters, bladder outlet obstruction, ureteral obstruction, or renal failure caused by a solid tumor

Observations

Urinary output <30 ml/hr
Anuria
Palpable bladder
Dysuria
Frequency
Hesitancy
Urgency

Incontinence, aware or unaware
Nocturia
Retention
Hematuria
Acute renal failure (p. 482)

Associated conditions/factors

Cancer of
Bladder
Rectum
Prostate
Cervix
Edometrium
Ovary
Lymphoma
Hodgkin's lymphoma

Interventions

Measure and record intake and output; report output of <30 ml/hr

Assess character, color, and odor of urine

Assess bladder level with decreasing output; report distention

Insert indwelling catheter and connect to closed gravity drainage as ordered

Prepare patient for surgery for obstructions
Stents may be placed for solid tumor obstructions while radiation or chemotherapy is initiated
Urinary diversion may be created for obstructions not responsive to other therapies (p. 470)

Monitor for signs of renal failure (p. 482)
Restrict fluids as ordered

Assess urinary elimination pattern, using voiding diary to determine type of incontinence or retention
See Incontinence for nursing diagnoses and interventions (p. 453)
See Urinary Retention (p. 462)

Sepsis and Septic Shock

Sepsis occurs in response to a disseminated infection, usually a gram-negative bacteria that releases endotoxins into the bloodstream; endotoxins release endogenous pyrogens, causing fever and local damage to endothelial lining of capillaries, activate clotting factor XII, and the complement system, which may result in bleeding (DIC); multiplying bacteria cause release of kinens, which enhance vasodilation; shock occurs from a generalized severe reduction in tissue perfusion caused by inadequate circulating blood volume, resulting in cellular hypoxia and decreased cardiac output

Observations

Initial
Irritability, restlessness, confusion
Fever
Chills
Warm, dry skin
Red, flushed face
Tachycardia, tachypnea
Weak peripheral pulses
Slow refill of capillary nailbed
Oliguria; <50 ml/hr
Glycosuria
Excessive thirst
Muscular weakness
Decreased BP
Mental confusion

Increasing severity
Decreased cardiac output, circulatory volume, and tissue perfusion
Dry, cool skin progressing to cold, clammy skin
Peripheral edema
Oliguria progressing to anuria
Weak, rapid heart rate
Hypotension
Hyperventilation progressing to slow, shallow respirations and respiratory failure
Greater alterations in level of consciousness

Blood culture
Chest radiograph for infiltrates
CBC for WBC changes
Arterial blood gases for metabolic acidosis
PT/PTT prolonged

Associated conditions/factors

Preexisting neutropenia
Sources of infection (Table 14-5)

Interventions

Assess vital signs, breath sounds, and cardiac status
Hypothermia may be precursor to sepsis

Monitor for skin and oral infections, URI, UTI, and vaginal discharge

Assess mental status and change in level of consciousness

Assess for changes in GI system and elimination

Obtain cultures of suspected areas of infection

Monitor laboratory values, especially absolute neutrophil count and culture reports

Report earliest signs of infection for prompt treatment

Initiate antibiotics and parenteral fluids as soon as ordered to restore volume

Measure intake and output

Institute measures to prevent infection (p. 671)

Assess for signs of bleeding; report if present; see DIC (p. 173)

Provide cooling measures for T >103.5° F; warm to tepid bath; wet towels covering body with ice applications in axilla; use cooling blanket if ineffective; administer antipyretics

Provide warmth for hypothermic patients; avoid bathing; cover with warmed blankets

TABLE 14-5. Infections in Cancer Patients

Pathogen	Sources	Common sites	Presentation
BACTERIA			
Pseudomonas	Multiple	Wounds	Purulence
		GI	Enterocolitis
		GU	UTI
		Lung	Pneumonia
Klebsiella	Multiple	Lung	Pneumonia
Escherichia coli	Multiple	GI	Enterocolitis
		GU	UTI
		Bone	Osteomyelitis
		Wounds	Purulence
		Blood	Sepsis
Staphylococcus	Multiple	Lung	Pneumonia
		Bone	Osteomyelitis
		GI	Enterocolitis
		CNS	Meningitis
		Wounds	Purulence
VIRUSES			
Herpes simplex type 1	Oral secretions	UGI	Stomatitis,
		Skin	esophagitis
		CNS	Eczema
			Encephalitis
Cytomegalovirus	Normal flora, blood products	Lung	Pneumonia
		CNS	Encephalitis
Varicella zoster	Person-to-person transmission	Skin	Shingles
FUNGI			
Candida	Normal flora	GI	Thrush, esophagitis
		Lung	Pneumonia
		GU	UTI, vaginitis
Cryptococcus	Soil, pigeon feces	Lung	Pneumonia
		CNS	Meningitis
Aspergillus	Air, building materials, pigeon feces	Lung	Bronchopneumonia
PROTOZOA			
Pneumocystis carinii	Normal flora, person-to-person transmission	Lung	Pneumonia
Toxoplasma gondii	Oocytes in cat feces, inadequately cooked meat, blood products	Disseminated	Chills, fever, diaphoresis, encephalitis, pericarditis

(Adapted from Ellerhorst-Ryan JM: Complications of the myeloproliferative system: infection and sepsis, *Semin Oncol Nurs*, November, 1(4):246, 1985.)

Observe for signs and symptoms of late shock

Monitor blood gas values

Provide oxygen therapy for decreased arterial oxygen content when ordered

Assess effectiveness of IV sodium bicarbonate when administered for metabolic acidosis

Place patient in supine or reverse Trendelenburg's position to improve cardiac output

Maintain bed rest to conserve energy and observe for signs of CHF

Turn q1h to 2h; use pillows to position edematous extremities; provide skin care

Support patient and significant other psychologically; provide information; answer questions; promote expression of feelings and fears

Be aware that patient may be transferred to ICU for invasive monitoring, mechanical ventilation, and vasopressor therapy

Cancer Therapy

SURGERY

This therapeutic modality has been the treatment of choice over the years and is performed using various methods.

Biopsy To determine a definite diagnosis and/or to establish presence of a tumor or metastasis
staging To determine the stage of the carcinoma and treatment indicated
resections
Curative: to remove tumor/organ and sufficient surrounding tissue to ensure a cure
Palliative: to relieve intractable pain, release pressure caused by tumor on other organs, control hemorrhage from eroded blood vessels, and remove infections caused by ulcerations
reconstruction To restore and regain an improved cosmetic appearance or body function

Comprehensive preoperative teaching has been found to be a critical part of this type of therapy, as well as meticulous postoperative care and teaching. The education of the patient and significant other begins on admission and continues until discharge. This ensures maximal recovery and rehabilitation.

RADIOTHERAPY

Treatment of neoplastic disease by use of gamma rays to disturb proliferation of cells by decreasing the rate of mitosis or impairing DNA synthesis, thereby reducing tumor mass; radiotherapy is administered externally (source outside of the body) or internally (source of radiation inside the body)

Assessment
Observations/findings

NOTE: Symptoms will vary depending on area(s) being irradiated; intensity of symptoms will also be affected
Skin, site of radiation
  Erythema
  Pruritus
  Edema
  Desquamation (dry or moist)
  Hyperpigmentation
  Atrophy
  Pain
Mucositis, dental caries
Altered taste
Nausea, vomiting
Anorexia, dysphagia, esophagitis
Diarrhea
Weight loss
Headache
Malaise
Fatigue
Loss of hair, itching, scaling and tanning of scalp
Tachycardia
Pericarditis
Myocarditis
Pneumonitis
Sterility
Increased susceptibility to infection

Laboratory/diagnostic studies

CBC
Decreased Hgb
Leukopenia
Thrombocytopenia
Pancytopenia
Electrolytes

Potential complications

Infection
Anemia

Medical Management

Antiemetics
Antifungals
Viscous lidocaine
Antacids
IV fluids
Antidiarrheals
Urinary anesthesia
Antibiotics
Foley catheter
Blood products

Nursing diagnoses/interventions/evaluation

■ **NDX:** Anxiety related to treatment

Pretreatment care

Patient will be seen by radiologist to determine if radiotherapy will be a useful treatment
Understand that patient is usually very anxious and fearful until treatment decision is made
Reinforce physician's explanation of procedure and benefits
Encourage discussion of fears, myths, and misconceptions surrounding treatment
Patient will be seen by radiologist once decision is made to administer radiotherapy
Understand that during this visit, area(s) to be irradiated will be marked with indelible dye
Explain procedure and what is expected of patient
  Equipment is similar to but larger than that used for x-ray examinations
  Radiologist or radiotherapist will be close by for communication during treatment
  Patient will be positioned on a table in a room by himself
  After positioning, patient must remain absolutely still
  Positioning may take 10 min or more
  Understand that treatment of one field usually lasts 1 to 3 min
  No pain results from treatment, but patient may experience discomfort from maintaining position

Expected outcome/evaluation

Patient verbalizes fears and concerns regarding treatment

■ **NDX:** Potential for impaired skin integrity related to radiation

Assess skin carefully
Teach importance of skin care
  Avoid tub bath or shower until ordered
  Do not wash skin in area being irradiated
  Do not remove skin markings between treatments
Avoid use of any product, including soap, on skin area being irradiated without checking with physician
Wear loose clothing to prevent rubbing
Avoid extremes in temperature and exposure to sunlight; do not use hot-water bottle or heating pad
Dry desquamation
  Use cornstarch sparingly
Moist desquamation
  May use water/saline to clean
  Keep clean and moist (slow healing)
Precautions to prevent infection
  Expose skin to air when possible
  Cover broken skin areas with a hydrocolloid dressing when ordered; use a stretch-type tubular dressing to hold in place
  Avoid use of tape; use nonallergenic or paper tape applied to nontreated skin areas when required
  Avoid use of cosmetics and use wigs, hairpieces, or scarves as needed
  Avoid use of deodorants if treatment is to axilla

Expected outcome/evaluation

Patient demonstrates understanding of methods to prevent or minimize skin problems

■ **NDX:** Altered nutrition: less than body requirements related to radiation

Assess nutritional status
Weigh patient daily at same time with same clothing and scale
Teach patient to maintain nutritious, high-protein diet
  Provide high-protein supplements
  Provide food when patient desires it; six small, bland feedings may be more easily tolerated
  Experiment with foods
  Serve food attractively arranged and at proper temperature
  Provide cold foods, such as ice cream and gelatins, which are more soothing to patient with stomatitis; see Stomatitis/Mucositis (p. 677)
  Avoid smoking
  Avoid spicy or hot foods
  Administer tube feedings or TPN as ordered with severe decrease in intake
  Administer vitamins as ordered
  Maintain quiet periods before and after meals

Keep room odor free and fresh
Maintain high fluid intake, to 2000 to 2500 ml/day, unless contraindicated
Administer antiemetics as ordered
Administer antacid
Record calorie count when appropriate
Assess abdomen, including bowel sounds
Assess elimination status (diarrhea or constipation)
Administer antidiarrheal/laxative as needed

Expected outcome/evaluation

Patient does not lose more than 3% to 5% of body weight

■ **NDX:** Altered oral mucous membrane related to radiation

Assess oral cavity q8h
Administer oral hygiene before and after meals, morning and night, and after vomiting
  Increase to q2h with stomatitis (p. 677)
  Use soft-bristled toothbrush
  Use foam or sponge swabs as needed
  Use diluted nonalcohol mouthwash
  Use saline rinse as needed
Administer nystatin (Mycostatin) as ordered
Note that patient may need saliva substitutes
Assess for painful or difficulty in swallowing; administer viscous lidocaine as needed

Expected outcome/evaluation

Patient prevents or minimizes discomfort

■ **NDX:** Altered patterns of urinary elimination related to radiation

Assess urinary status
Monitor for symptoms of urinary infection
Monitor intake and output
Force fluids to 3 L/day unless contraindicated
Assist with and teach care of perianal area, especially if diarrhea is present

Expected outcome/evaluation

Patient maintains balanced intake and output and exhibits no signs of urinary infection

■ **NDX:** Potential for infection related to myelosuppression

Monitor CBC (see Myelosuppression, p. 670)
Pace activities with frequent rest periods
Note that radiation therapy may have to be delayed if blood counts are very low
  Observe for signs and symptoms of infection
  Administer antibiotics and blood products as ordered

Additional nursing diagnoses

Potential fluid volume deficit related to nausea and vomiting

Fatigue related to decreased metabolic energy production

Altered tissue perfusion: cardiopulmonary related to pericarditis, myocarditis, pneumonitis

Sexual dysfunction related to sterility

Interventions for Specific Types of Sealed Sources

All types of implants

Assess psychological aspects and intervene
  Isolation: be attentive to patient's needs
  Allow verbalization and provide time for discussion of pains and anxieties
If implant, inform patient of need for personnel to observe time, distance, and shielding precautions
Personnel should wear film badges
No pregnant visitors or children

Brain implants

Assess for adverse reaction, fatigue, anorexia, possible tissue damage, neurological side effects; perform neurological assessment
Inform patient of hair loss

Gynecological cesium implants

Assess and manage adverse effects: diarrhea, cystitis, dysuria, vaginal fibrosis, and dryness
Instruct patient of mobility restrictions
  Bed rest for 48 hr
  Elevate head 30 degrees only
  No baths or pericare until unloaded; patient to have minimal care
  Encourage fluid and low-fiber diet
  May need Lomotil to stop bowel movement
  Administer pain medication as needed

Breast implants

Assess for skin erythema

Head and neck implants

Assess for side effects and manage dryness of mucous membrane of the oral cavity
  Stomatitis
  Dry desquamation
  Possible infection
  Xerostomia
Assess and maintain patent airway
Assess for and manage bleeding
Manage pain
Provide means of communicating, such as writing pad or Magic Slate
Assess for alteration in body image
  Skin markers, especially on face
  Weight loss, loss of muscle mass
  Alopecia

■ **NDX:** Knowledge deficit related to lack of information about potential complications and effects of radiation

Explain need to avoid persons with infections, especially URIs
Discuss symptoms of infection to report to physician
  "Cold," "flu," elevated temperature
  Diarrhea and frequency of or burning on urination
  Reddened, painful skin areas
  Mouth redness, swelling, ulceration, bleeding, increased salivation
Emphasize importance of maintaining nutritious diet and fluid intake to 3000 ml daily unless contraindicated
  Take six to eight small feedings
  Avoid eating immediately before or after treatment
Explain that radiation effects continue for 10 to 14 days after last treatment; tell patient signs of healing will not be seen until 18 to 21 days after last treatment
Explain need for daily oral hygiene—in the morning, after meals, and at bedtime—to keep mouth fresh and clean
Discuss the following symptoms to report to physician
  Mucositis (p. 677)
  Nausea and vomiting (p. 675)
  Inability to eat
  Increasing headache or tiredness
  Severe diarrhea (p. 678)
  Increasing redness, swelling, pain, or pruritus at site of therapy
Emphasize importance of follow-up outpatient care
Teach name of medication, dosage, time of administration, purpose, and side effects
Explain need to avoid taking over-the-counter medications without checking with physician

Expected outcome/evaluation

Patient verbalizes symptoms to report and discusses home and follow-up care

CARE OF PATIENT RECEIVING RADIUM (CESIUM) THERAPY SEALED IN A MOULD, AFTERLOADER, COLPOSTAT, OR ERNST APPLICATOR

Sealed source of radiation is inserted through the vagina and left in place for a specific length of time to treat cancer of the cervix/uterus (Figure 14-8)

Preinsertion Teaching and Care

Give low-fiber diet as ordered
Assess for potential problems with skin care and positioning
Give povidone-iodine douche as ordered
Administer enemas until clear as ordered
Insert indwelling bladder catheter if this is not to be done in the OR

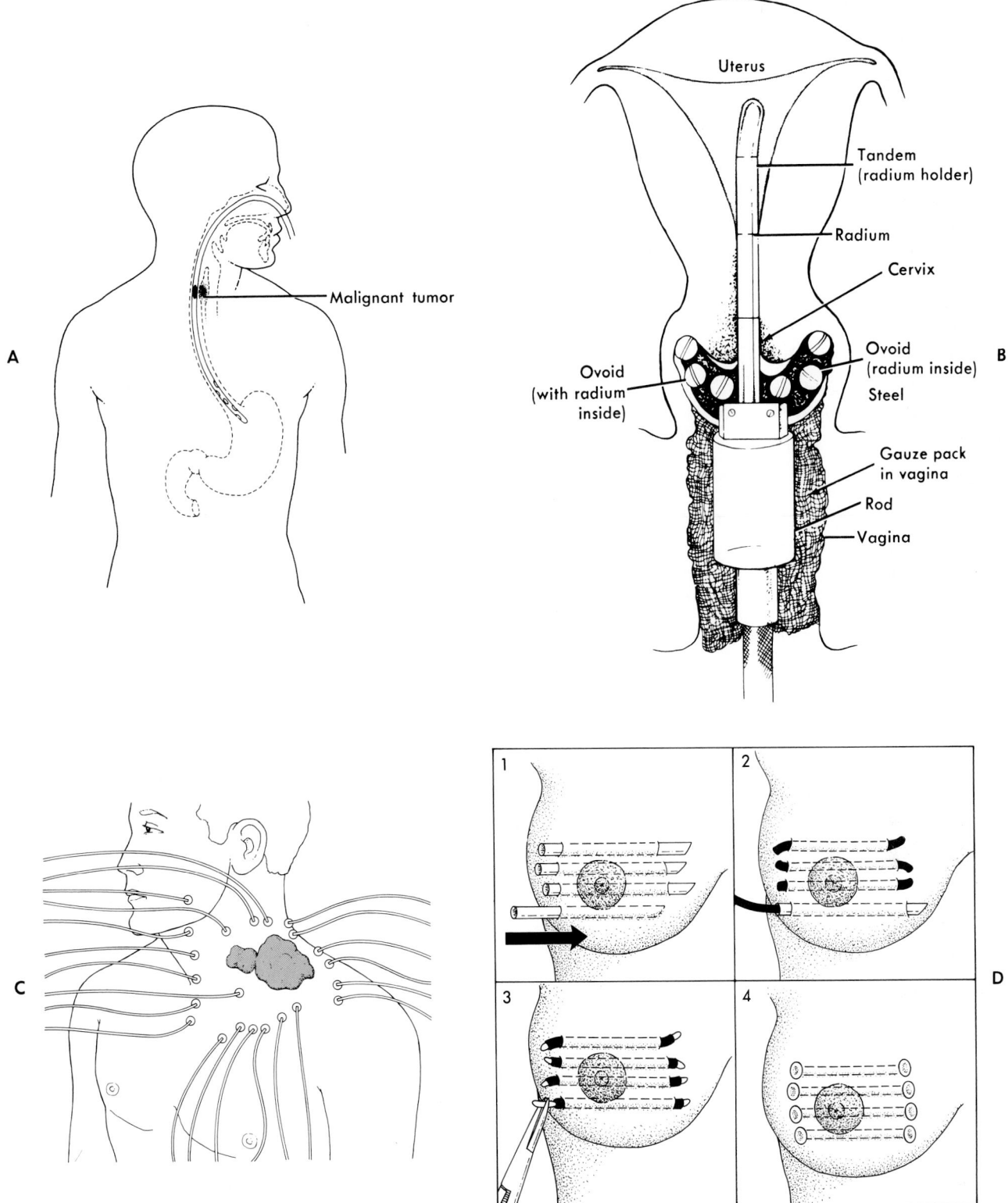

FIGURE 14-5. Examples of internal radiation therapy. **A,** Radium bougie in place for patient with cancer of the esophagus; note that radium is placed next to the tumor. **B,** Radium treatment of cancer of the cervix via application with tandem and ovoids. **C,** Iridium seeds implanted for left neck mass. **D,** Iridium seeds implanted for breast cancer. (**A** and **B** From Marino LB: *Cancer nursing,* St Louis, 1981. CV Mosby; **C** and **D** from Beare PG, Myers JL: *Principles and practice of adult health nursing,* St Louis, 1990, Mosby—Year Book.)

Explain need for bed rest; that head of bed may be elevated slightly

Explain importance of
Low-fiber diet
Bowel sedation
Reporting pain
Private room preferred and limited visitors
Minimal exposure to nursing staff

Explain that pain will be managed

Place patient in private room unless patient shares semi-private room with another patient having the same procedure done

Place needed items within patient's reach

Relate that steriliztion and cessation of menses usually occur

Postinsertion Assessment
Observations/findings

Anorexia
Nausea, vomiting
Diarrhea
Elevated temperature: over 100° F (37.8° C)
Abdominal distention
Dehydration
Tachycardia
Decreased BP
Rectal bleeding
Vaginal bleeding
Uterine contractions
Skin over pelvic area
Red
Blistered
Position of applicators
Sensory deprivation

Potential complications

Uterine perforation
Profuse bleeding
Atelectasis
Oliguria
Hematuria

Postinsertion Care

Post radiation precaution tags (Figure 14-9)
Place lead shield next to patient's pelvic area
Keep lead-lined container in room in case cesium is accidentally dislodged
Elevate head of bed 35 degrees
Maintain low-fiber diet; force fluids to 3000 ml daily unless contraindicated
Administer parenteral fluids if needed
Measure intake and output
Manage pain; give analgesics
Administer bowel and other sedation as ordered
Check BP, P, and R, and oral temperature q4h
Give partial bath daily

Wash hands, face, and upper chest
Do not bathe below waist
Do not give routine perineal or catheter care
Massage shoulders and neck instead of full back rub
Avoid routine linen change

Check position of applicator
Notify physician and radiation officer if dislodged
Use long-handled (12-inch) forceps to retrieve

Check for vaginal and rectal bleeding q2h to 4h and prn; copious discharge is common
Report bleeding to physician
Change perineal pads q4h and prn

Connect indwelling urethral catheter to closed gravity drainage system
Note character of urine
Report hematuria to physician

Use room deodorizer as needed

Removal of radium
Remove catheter as ordered; voiding measures may be necessary
Maintain adequate fluid intake to 3000 ml/day unless contraindicated
Douche as indicated
Enema as indicated
Shower
Increase activity and ambulate without assistance before discharge

Nursing diagnoses/interventions/evaluation

■ **NDX:**   Impaired physical mobility related to placement of afterloader

Assist and teach patient to deep breathe q2h during the day and evening
Auscultate chest for breath sounds q4h to 8h
Teach active ROM exercises to upper extremities q4h
Flex knees slightly and prop with pillow
Logroll patient; tilt shoulders and prop with pillow q1h to 2h
Place needed articles within patient's reach
Cautiously change perineal pad q4h

Expected outcome/evaluation

Patient maintains skin integrity and musculoskeletal function

■ **NDX:**   Anxiety related to limited social contact with others

Provide emotional support
Visit often for short periods
Encourage verbalization of fears
Provide diversional activities
Reading
Watching television

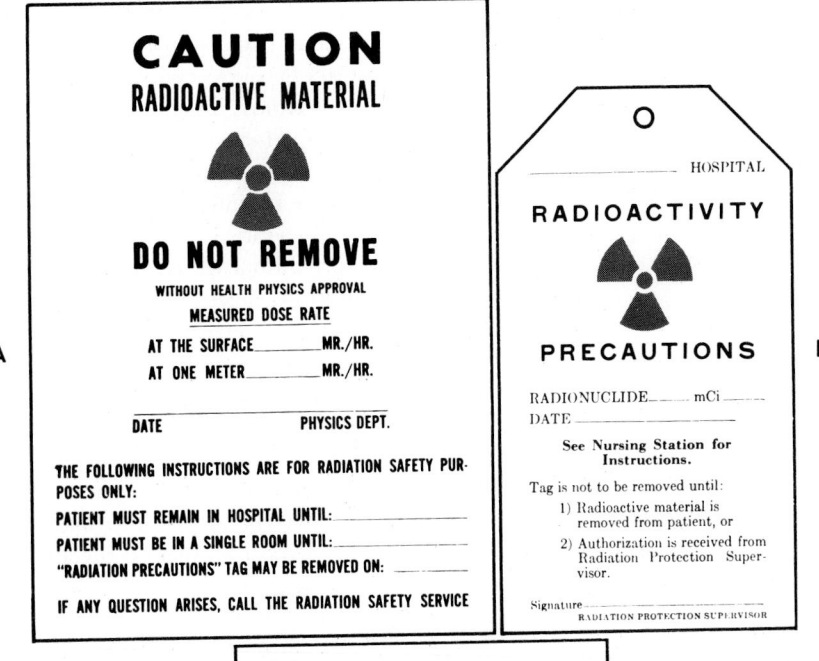

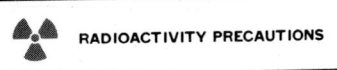

FIGURE 14-6. Radiation precaution tags. **A,** Tag placed on patient chart. **B,** Tag placed at foot of patient's bed or attached to door of patient's room. **C,** Tag placed in a wristband on patient. (From National Council on Radiation Protection and Measurement: Precautions in the management of patients who have received therapeutic amounts of radionuclides. Report No. 37, Washington, DC, 1970, The Council.)

Encourage family visits for short periods (exclude pregnant visitors and children); encourage communication with significant other via telephone

Expected outcome/evaluation

Patient demonstrates adaptive psychosocial behavior to temporary limitation of social contacts

■ **NDX:** Knowledge deficit related to lack of information about home care management

Explain need to maintain diet as ordered

Explain importance of drinking fluids to 3000 ml/day unless contraindicated

Relate that isolation will end as soon as radium is removed and that patient is not radioactive once radium is removed

Explain need to exercise to tolerance; to plan rest periods

Instruct patient to douche daily if vaginal discharge is present

Discuss symptoms to report to physician

Vaginal bleeding

Rectal bleeding

Stool or urine from vagina

Foul-smelling vaginal discharge

Abdominal distention

Abdominal pain

Nausea, vomiting, or diarrhea

Elevated temperature

Hematuria

Signs of menopause

Instruct patient to shower daily (avoid extremes in water temperature)

Caution patient to avoid exposure of pelvic area to direct sunlight; instruct patient to apply lanolin-based cream or baby oil to dry areas

Relate that sexual intercourse may be resumed when comfortable after course of treatment has ended or as indicated by physician

Demonstrate method of using vaginal dilator if ordered

Instruct patient on how to prevent urinary tract infection (UTI)

Caution patient to avoid constipation

Emphasize importance of follow-up outpatient care

Expected outcome/evaluation

Patient and/or significant other demonstrates understanding of home care and follow-up instructions

UNSEALED RADIOACTIVE THERAPY

Preparation of Room

Furniture convenient and functioning
Bed on external wall of building
 Bed freshly made
 Extra covers available
Lighting adequate
Phone and television functioning
Reading and/or hobby materials available
Flowers arranged and watered
Oral hygiene and bath equipment available
Trash baskets and linen hamper in room
Lead-lined urine containers in room
Saturated solution of potassium iodide in bathroom
Radioactive tags posted (see Figure 14-9)
 On door
 On chart cover and available for patient's use
Radioactive badges at room entrance

RADIOACTIVE IODINE

NOTE: *Pregnant staff members must not be assigned to care for patient; children should not visit*

Before Administration of Medication

Check room for needed equipment
Place items conveniently for patient's use
Order disposable dishes, utensils, and tray for diet

Ongoing Care

Wear correct badge when entering room
Limit time spent in room; plan before entering room
 Observations to be made
 Equipment needed
 Care to be done
Handle urine or stool with rubber or plastic gloves when necessary
Dispose of excreta in toilet; place one dropperful of saturated solution of potassium iodide in toilet and flush or flush toilet three times
If excreta (urine, feces, sputum, vomitus) is spilled on skin
 Run water over area for 2 min
 Wash with soap and water for 3 min
 Have area monitored by radiation therapy department
If excreta is spilled on bed or other surface in room
 Notify radiation therapy department
 Clean in usual manner after area is cleared by monitoring
Handle dressings with rubber or plastic gloves when present; discard in plastic bag and keep in room

Handle bed linens with rubber or plastic gloves if they contain excreta or perspiration; place in linen hamper in room
Do not remove linen or trash from room
Do not perform routine nursing functions for ambulatory patients
Plan care to limit exposure if patient is debilitated
 Be efficient
 Have all needed equipment on hand
 Use turn sheets; bathe soiled areas only
 Prepare and cut foods before entering room
Collect and place specimens for laboratory in lead-lined containers
After discharge or discontinuation of isolation
 Have room equipment, linen, and trash monitored by radiation therapy department
 Remove equipment, linen, and trash when permission is given by radiation therapy department; handle in usual manner

RADIOACTIVE PHOSPHORUS

Follow care as for radioactive iodine except
 No special precautions are needed for disposal of urine, feces, or sputum
 No precautions are needed for disposal of vomitus unless ^{32}P is given orally
 If chromic phosphate is given into pleural or peritoneal cavity and leakage develops, notify radiation therapy department for monitoring and instructions

Care of Patient Receiving Unsealed Radioactive Therapy
RADIOACTIVE IODINE

Administration of metabolized or absorbed radiation to treat such conditions as hyperthyroidism or thyroid cancer; usually ^{131}I or ^{32}P is administered

Assessment
Observations/findings

Response to isolation
 Depressed
 Euphoric
 Accepting
 Complaints of tender area in neck
 Progression of ophthalmopathy
 Transient productive cough
 Hypothyroidism (p. 312)
 Hyperthyroidism (p. 315)
 Hypoparathyroidism (p. 318)

Care before Administration of Medication

NOTE: *Pregnant staff members are not to care for patient; children may not visit*

Acute care

Bathe or have patient shower
Clean and arrange linen and furniture

Have personal hygiene items, reading materials, television, hobby materials, and phone accessible to patient

Remove unwanted items from room

Note food and fluid preferences and order from dietary department

Assist patient in notifying family and friends concerning visiting limitations

Allow no visiting for 24 hr after administration of medication

Allow 30 min/day visiting per person thereafter, if visitor remains 6 feet away from patient

Patient teaching

Reinforce physician's explanation of procedure and need for isolation

Involve family or significant other in care and instructions

Orient patient to plan of care

Relate that personnel will be in room for very short periods only

Assure patient that necessary care will be done

Reinforce that patient is to call for needed items or care

Daily hygienic measures are to be performed by patient if able

Hospital garments must be worn; medication is excreted via perspiration and saliva

Describe method to be used to collect 24-hr urine specimens; laboratory value of radioactivity level determines length of stay in isolation

Disposable dishes, utensils, and trays will be used for meals

Linen and waste material will remain in room

Communication with staff will be via call bell and intercommunications system

Visiting privileges will be limited

No visitors will be allowed during first 24 hr

Visitors will be allowed 2 hr/day thereafter, if visitor remains 6 feet away from patient

Routine housekeeping functions will not be performed

Care after Administration of Medication
Ongoing care

If patient vomits ^{32}P or ^{131}I immediately or within 4 hr of administration

Notify radiation safety officer and physician

All contaminated persons, materials, and surfaces must be decontaminated

Intracavity instillation

Place patient on side opposite incision after instillation

Turn patient q15 min for 2 to 3 hr

Check incision for leakage of solution q15 min for eight times, q30 min for two times, then q4h

If leakage occurs, notify radiation safety officer and physician

Visit patient briefly at least qh from doorway

Assess, anticipate, and fulfill needs and requests promptly

Deliver mail, paper, and flowers as they arrive

Provide additional diversionary activities as needed

See that additional materials and equipment are available when needed by patient for disposal of trash, excreta, and linen

Do not remove any items from room except laboratory specimens in lead-lined containers

Provide emotional support

Assess patient's reaction to therapy and isolation

Assure patient that isolation will last no longer than 8 days

Discuss concerns about radioactivity remaining after therapy is completed

Patient Teaching

Ensure that patient and/or significant other knows and understands

That patient is not continuing source of danger from radioactivity to family or others; majority of medication is excreted in 8 days

Symptoms of recurrence of hyperthyroidism to report to physician

Symptoms of hypothyroidism to report to physician

Importance of

Balanced activity and rest periods

Ongoing outpatient care

Expected outcome/evaluation

Patient identifies and manages adverse effects of radiation

ANTINEOPLASTIC CHEMOTHERAPY

chemotherapy Systemic cancer treatment using drugs that affect the cell cycle (Figure 14-10) to treat cancer; useful when there is disseminated disease or when there is a high risk of recurrence in the body; can be curative, can prolong life, or can be palliative; is often used as an adjuvant to surgery and/or radiation therapy

Assessment
Observations/findings

Physical response to specific condition

Ability and desire to learn

Barriers to learning: fatigue, denial

Knowledge of treatment plan, diagnosis, and treatment; expectations of results; patient's perception of his or her role

Attitude related to chemotherapy

Psychosocial response based on patient's coping mechanisms, support system, previous experience with chemotherapy, and amount of information received about disease process

Obtain baseline assessment before beginning chemotherapy and continue throughout treatment period (see Oncology Assessment, p. 593)

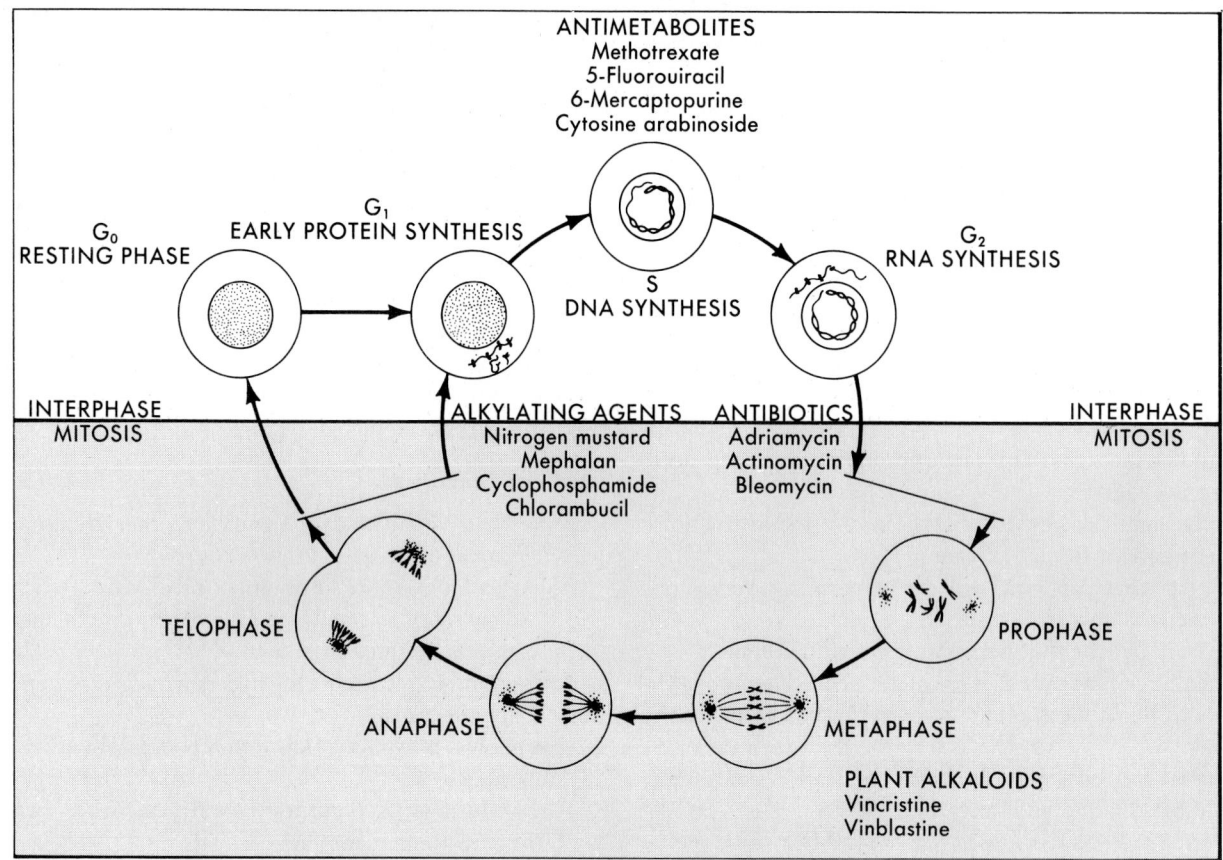

FIGURE 14-7. The cell cycle. Drugs are identified by where they exert their effect. (From Beare PG, Myers JL: *Principles and practice of adult health nursing,* St Louis, 1990, Mosby–Year Book.)

Laboratory/diagnostic studies

Specific to each medication and expected responses (see Table 14-6)

Potential complications

Side effects and toxicities specific to each medication (see Table 14-6)

Common problems
  Bone marrow suppression
  Cutaneous manifestations
  GI dysfunction
  Respiratory dysfunction
  Renal dysfunction
  Cardiac dysfunction
  Sexual and reproductive dysfunction
  Electrolyte/chemical imbalance
  Musculoskeletal dysfunction

Medical Management

Antineoplastic medications ordered according to protocol or standard regimen
Laboratory diagnostic/monitoring studies

Vital signs
Antiemetics, antacids, oral anesthetics
Parenteral fluids

Nursing diagnoses/interventions/evaluation

■ **NDX:** Fear related to disease process and/or treatment

Assess previous experience with chemotherapy
Dispel myths with factual information
Assist patient and/or significant other with recognizing and clarifying fears and with developing coping strategies for those fears
May be helpful to role play and/or coach patient by using examples of coping skills used by others

Expected outcome/evaluation

Patient verbalizes fears and begins to deal with them effectively

■ **NDX:** Pain related to disease process

Monitor and document pain characteristics, as well as associated factors such as anxiety

Assess intensity by means of asking patient to rate pain from 0 to 5; include descriptive terms such as dull, sharp

Establish a trusting relationship with patient

Schedule analgesics to prevent severe pain: regularly scheduled or continuous administration for continuous pain

Consider duration and peak effect of each analgesic

Prevent and manage side effects of analgesics, including constipation

Use supportive, noninvasive methods of pain relief (e.g., distraction, relaxation, imagery)

Provide environment conducive to rest

Evaluate patient's fears and perceptions regarding pain and pain therapy

Evaluate the meaning of the pain to patient (metastasis, punishment, recurrence, death)

Evaluate level of consciousness and note changes in sensorium

Involve significant other in care planning as much as possible

Expected outcome/evaluation

Patient expresses pain relief

■ **NDX:** Altered nutrition: less than body requirements related to nausea and vomiting, anorexia, stomatitis, disease process, and/or treatment

Assess nutritional status

Measure height and weight and compare with ideal body weight

Assess laboratory values (CBC, serum albumin) that may indicate malnutrition

Obtain history of food preferences

Perform baseline oral assessment and daily oral assessment throughout treatment period

Evaluate for presence of fatigue, depression, anxiety, and/ or pain

Describe signs and symptoms that could alter nutritional intake, such as nausea and vomiting, sore mouth, pain, difficulty swallowing, and feelings of fullness or bloating

Note any conditions that would increase energy expenditure, such as fever or infections

Describe measures to alter signs and symptoms just listed

Explain measures to maintain adequate nutritional intake (maintain ideal weight)

Frequent oral hygiene, well-fitted dentures

Avoidance of extreme temperatures of foods, and spicy foods

Encouraging significant other to make patient's favorite foods

Include basic food groups in diet

Maintain fluid intake to 2500 ml daily unless contraindicated

Provide suggestions for increasing calories and protein

in diet; offer high-calorie, high-protein in foods in small feedings

Weigh patient weekly

Describe ways to overcome alteration in taste

Experiment with different seasonings

Cold foods may be more appealing

Avoid preparation of foods with strong odors

Explain measures to prevent abdominal feeling of fullness or bloating

Limit fluid intake at meals

Avoid gas-producing foods (beans, cabbage)

Encourage small, frequent meals

Avoid greasy or spicy foods

Explain measures to control diarrhea

Reduce amount of fiber in diet

Assist patient in identifying foods, beverages, and medications that cause loose stools

Explain use of antidiarrheal medication

Evaluate hydration status and skin turgor

Monitor intake and output

Describe measures to prevent constipation

Increase liquids in diet

Eat foods with high-fiber content

Use stool softeners

Encourage activity unless contraindicated

Assess history of nausea and vomiting: cause, time of occurrence, frequency

Administer antiemetics before, during, and after chemotherapy as needed

Medicate according to pattern of nausea and vomiting

Administer chemotherapy in late afternoon or at night when possible

Encourage prophylactic oral hygiene measures before and after meals and at bedtime

Check for oral burning, pain, and changes in tolerance to foods

Teach signs and symptoms that may need health care follow-up, such as uncontrolled nausea and vomiting, diarrhea, weakness, and malaise

Expected outcome/evaluation

Patient increases weight and improves calorie intake

■ **NDX:** Impaired skin integrity related to chemotherapy

Assess skin: color, temperature, rash, tenderness, itching, turgor, peeling of palms, drainage

Inspect skin folds, especially axillary, groin, and perineum

Determine fluid and nutritional status

Teach skin care

Use mild soap and water, rinse, pat dry

Keep skin and nails meticulously clean (prevent infection)

Avoid sun exposure: wear sunscreen and protective clothing

Text continued on p. 664.

TABLE 14-6. Chemotherapeutic Drugs

Medication	Dosage	Routes of administration	Side effects and toxicities*
ALKYLATING AGENTS			

Busulfan (Myleran)	4-6 mg/day (initially); 1-3 mg/day (maintenance); given according to protocol	po	Myelosuppression
			Low doses
			  Granulocytopenia
			  Platelets, lymphoid elements spared
			Hyperpigmentation
			High doses
			  Leukopenia
			Delayed-refractory
			  Pancytopenia
			Long-term therapy
			  Pulmonary fibrosis (rare)

Chlorambucil (Leukeran)	0.1-0.2 mg/kg; given according to protocol
	2 mg/day maintenance
		po	Myelosuppression
			  Leukopenia
			Nausea and vomiting, mild
			Amenorrhea
			Depressed spermatogenesis
			Long-term therapy
			  Alveolar dysplasia
			  Pulmonary fibrosis
			  Nausea and vomiting
			  Metallic taste
			  Sinus burning

Cyclophosphamide (Cytoxan, Endoxana, CTX)	40-50 mg/kg; given according to protocol
	1-5 mg/kg/day (oral)
		po; IV	Myelosuppression
			  Leukopenia
			  Thrombocytopenia may occur
			Common with high doses
			  Stomatitis
			  Alopecia
			  Hemorrhagic cystitis
			Amenorrhea, dose-limiting
			Testicular atrophy, dose-limiting

Mechlorethamine (nitrogen mustard, HN$_2$)	0.4 mg/kg; given according to protocol	IV; intracavitary; topical; intralesional	Myelosuppression, dose-limiting
			  Lymphocytopenia, dose-limiting
			  Thrombocytopenia
			  Granulocytopenia (leukocytopenia)
			Nausea and vomiting, severe onset 1-2 hr, lasting 8 hr
			Diarrhea
			Skin rash
			Amenorrhea
			Impaired spermatogenesis
			Vesicant; pain and tissue necrosis if extravasated

Ifosfamide (Ifex)	1000-2000 mg/m^2/day for 5 days q4 weeks	IV	Myelosuppression
			  Leukopenia
			  Less thrombocytopenia
			Hematuria
			Alopecia
			CNS toxicity

*See Symptomatic Care in Chemotherapy p. 670.

Nadir	Recovery after nadir (days)	Indications	Administration and nursing implications
10-12 days	42-50	Chronic myelogenous leukemia	Oral tablets may be taken any time of the day
11-30 days 1-10 yr	24-54		
14-28 days	28-42	Chronic lymphocytic leukemia, ovarian cancer, Hodgkin's and non-Hodgkin's lymphoma	Give oral medication as ordered; no specific directions
8-14 days 24 hr to several weeks	18-25	Non-Hodgkin's lymphoma, sarcoma, breast, lung, and ovarian cancer: acute and chronic lymphocytic leukemia	Give IV push over 3-5 min through side port of patent IV Give oral doses with or immediately after meals Administer antiemetic before therapy and as indicated Force fluids to 3000 ml/day before administration and 48 hr after Check output; if falling, notify physician for parenteral therapy orders IV hydration and bladder irrigation usually ordered when high doses given Give within 15 to 30 min after reconstitution
7-15 days Within 24 hr 6-8 days	28 10-20 Several days	Hodgkin's disease, non-Hodgkin's lymphomas, lung cancer, malignant pleural effusions	Give IV push through side port of patent IV; check blood backflow before instilling each ml; flush line with 30 ml IV fluid before each blood check; flush line after administration; monitor for extravasation (p. 669); give antidote as ordered Administer antiemetic before therapy and then as indicated Tell patient a metallic taste may be experienced just after drug injection Inform patient that veins may become discolored Reposition patient q15 min for four times after intracavitary instillation
8-14 days	18-25	Testicular cancer	Give IV over a minimum of 30 min Force fluids to 3000 ml/day before administration and 48 hr after Protector such as MESNA should also be used to prevent hemorrhagic cystitis

Continued.

TABLE 14-6. Chemotherapeutic Drugs—cont'd

Medication	Dosage	Routes of administration	Side effects and toxicities*

Melphalan (Alkeran)	0.25 mg/kg/day for daily dosage; 0.1-0.15 mg/kg for interval dosage; given according to protocol	po	Myelosuppression
			  Leukopenia
			  Thrombocytopenia
			High-dose therapy
			  Nausea and vomiting
			Long-term therapy
			  Acute leukemia
			  Alopecia
			  Dermatitis
			  Stomatitis

Thio-tepa (triethylene-thio-phosphoramide)	0.2 mg/kg/day
	60 mg instillations/60 ml
	Given according to protocol; dosage reduced with hepatic or renal dysfunction
		IV intracavitary, bladder instillation	Myelosuppression
			  Leukopenia
			  Thrombocytopenia
			  Anemia
			Mild
			  Local pain
			  Nausea, vomiting
			  Dizziness
			  Headache

NITROSOUREAS			

Carmustine (BCNU)	75-100 mg/m² or up to 200 mg/m²; given according to protocol	IV
		Topical (investigational)
			Myelosuppression, dose-limiting
			  Leukopenia
			  Thrombocytopenia
			Immediate
			  Burning pain at IV site
			  Facial flushing
			  Severe nausea and vomiting onset 2 hr lasting 4-6 hr
			Long-term therapy
			  Pulmonary fibrosis

Lomustine (CCNU)	100-130 mg/m²; given according to protocol	po	Myelosuppression, dose-limiting
			  Thrombocytopenia
			  Leukopenia
			Nausea, vomiting; onset 2-4 hr
			Anorexia
			Diarrhea

Semustin (investigational) (methyl CCNU)	125-200 mg/m²; given according to protocol; dosage reduced with liver dysfunction and impaired marrow function	po	Myelosuppression, dose-limiting
			  May be cumulative
			  Thrombocytopenia
			  Leukopenia
			  Erythrocytopenia
			Nausea and vomiting; onset 4-6 hr

ANTIMETABOLITES			

Cytarabine (Ara-C, Cytosar)	1-3 mg/kg/day given according to protocol; dosage reduced with severe hepatic dysfunction	IV, intrathecal	Myelosuppression, dose-limiting
			  Leukopenia
			  Thrombocytopenia
			Nausea and vomiting especially with rapid infusion
			Stomatitis
			High dose
			  Flulike syndrome

*See Symptomatic Care in Chemotherapy p. 670.

Nadir	Recovery after nadir (days)	Indications	Administration and nursing implications
10-12 days	42-50	Breast, ovarian, and testicular cancer, myeloma, melanoma	Give oral doses 2 hr after meals
5-30 days	21-28	Papillary bladder tumors, malignant serous effusions Formerly breast and ovarian cancer and Hodgkin's lymphoma	Give IV push over 2-3 min through side port of patent IV Reposition patient q15 min for four times after intracavitary administration Bladder instillation is retained for 2 hr; reposition patient q15 min during this period
4-6 weeks 3-5 weeks	7-14	Multiple myeloma, Hodgkin's disease, non-Hodgkin's lymphoma; brain tumor, colorectal adenocarcinoma; gastric adenocarcinoma, melanoma, hepatoma	Give IV small volume for 15-45 min Apply ice pack at IV site Teach patient to report pain to staff immediately Flush vein before and after administration Administer antiemetics before administration and as ordered after
40-50 days 26-34 days 28-42 days	60 6-10 9-14 24 hr	Palliative: brain tumors, Hodgkin's disease, lung cancer, coorectal adenocarcinoma	Protect oral drug from heat and moisture Teach patient to take on an empty stomach; avoid alcohol after dose
28-63 days 21-35 days 28-42 days	82-89 6-8 hr	GI cancer, brain cancer, Hodgkin's disease, non-Hodgkin's lymphoma	Teach patient to take on an empty stomach (may lessen nausea and vomiting), observe patient preference Absorbed in 30-60 min if stomach is empty
12-14 days	22-24	Acute lymphocytic leukemia, acute granulocytic leukemia	Give IV push over 3-5 min through side port of patent IV; may be given as a continuous infusion Keep patient flat 4-6 hr after intrathecal administration

Continued.

TABLE 14-6. Chemotherapeutic Drugs—cont'd

Medication	Dosage	Routes of administration	Side effects and toxicities*

5-Fluorouracil (5-FU, fluorouracil)	12 mg/kg/day, not to exceed 800 mg/day; given according to protocol
	Maintenance dosage; 6-15 mg/kg; given according to protocol; dosage adjusted with liver or kidney dysfunction
		IV, topical, po	Myelosuppression, dose-limiting
			  Leukopenia (granulocytes)
			  Thrombocytopenia
			Nausea and vomiting
			Alopecia
			Neurotoxicity
			Diarrhea
			Stomatitis

Mercaptopurine (Purinethol, 6-mercaptopurine)	2.5-5 mg/kg/day; given po according to protocol; dosage reduced one third to one fourth with allopurinol	po	Myelosuppression
			  Thrombocytopenia, mild
			  Leukopenia, mild
			Mild nausea and vomiting
			Cumulative hyperbilirubinemia

Methotrexate (MTX, amethopterin)	2.5-5 mg po daily
	50-70 mg/m² IV (low dose)
	100-150 mg/m² IV (high dose)
	Given according to protocol
		po
		Intrathecal
		Intraarterial
		IV
			Myelosuppression
			  Leukopenia
			  Thrombocytopenia
			  Anemia
			    Hgb effect
			    Reticulocytes
			Nausea and vomiting
			Anorexia
			Mucositis
			Hepatoxicity
			Dermatitis
			Alopecia
			Increased intracranial pressure
			Nephrotoxicity

Azacytidine (t-Azacytidine) (investigational)	100-150 mg/m²/day times 5; given according to protocol	IV	Myelosuppression Leukopenia Stomatitis Nausea and vomiting; onset 1-3 hr and lasting 3-4 hr Rash Diarrhea Neurotoxicity Hepatoxicity Hypotension
Thioguanine (6-thioguanine)	2-3 mg/kg/day; given according to protocol; dosage reduced with liver or kidney dysfunction	po	Leukopenia Thrombocytopenia Anemia
VINCA ALKALOIDS			
Vinblastine sulfate (Velban)	0.1-0.4 mg/kg/wk; given according to protocol; dosage decreased with liver disease and neurologic problems	IV	Leukopenia, dose-limiting Thrombocytopenia, mild Mild nausea and vomiting Alopecia, mild Mucositis

*See Symptomatic Care in Chemotherapy p. 670.

Nadir	Recovery after nadir (days)	Indications	Administration and nursing implications
7-14 days	16-24	Breast cancer, oral lesions, gastric tumors, and colorectal cancer; topically—basal cell carcinomas	Give IV push over 3-5 min through side port of patent IV using two-syringe technique; flush line after therapy Tell patient to expect vein discoloration
7-14 days 12-21 days 11-23 days	14-21	Acute lymphocytic leukemia, chronic granulocytic leukemia	Give oral dose daily

7-14 days
4-7 days
5 days
 	
6-13 days
2-7 days
	14-21	Acute lymphoblastic and myeloblastic leukemia, trophoblastic tumors, osteogenic sarcoma, epidermoid cancer of head and neck, multiple myeloma, lung, breast, and ovarian cancer	Ensure that patient knows not to take *any* medication before checking with physician when taking methotrexate po
			Check patency of IV before administration; flush IV after administration
			High-dose (investigational)
			  Force fluids to 3000-4000 ml/day to ensure high-volume output
			  Check creatinine results with increased dosage, sodium bicarbonate may be ordered to maintain urine pH 7.0
			  Administer citrovorum (leucovorin) rescue factor on time as ordered
			  After intrathecal administration keep patient flat 4-6 hr
			  Never give with salicylates, sulfonamide, phenytoin, *p*-aminobenzoic acid (PABA), alcohol, warfarin, amphotericin B

12-14 days	—	Acute granulocytic leukemia	Give within 8 hr of preparation; usually dilute in Ringer's lactate solution; administer IV push through side port of patent IV; may be ordered as continuous infusion
14-28 days	—	Acute granulocytic and lymphocytic leukemia	Give total oral dose at one time between meals
4-10 days	7-14	Breast and testicular cancer, choriocarcinoma, Hodgkin's disease and lymphoma	Give IV push over through side port of freely running IV; check blood backflow before instilling each ml; flush line with 30 ml IV fluid before each blood check; flush line after administration

Continued.

TABLE 14-6. Chemotherapeutic Drugs—cont'd

Medication	Dosage	Routes of administration	Side effects and toxicities*
Vinblastine sulfate (Velban)—cont'd			Constipation Ileus Abdominal pain Long-term therapy Neurotoxicity
Vincristine sulfate (Oncovin)	1-2 mg/m² — adult; given according to protocol; dosage decreased with liver disease	IV	Myelosuppression, unusual Neurotoxicity, dose-limiting Peripheral neuropathy, dose-limiting Constipation Ileus Alopecia
Vindesine (Eldesine) (investigational)	2-4 mg/m²; given according to protocol; dosage decreased with impaired liver function	IV	Neutropenia, dose-limiting Thrombocytopenia Leukopenia Neurotoxicity, dose-limiting at low doses Alopecia Constipation Paralytic ileus
PODOPHYLLOTOXINS			

VM-26 (Teniposide) (investigational)	100 mg/m²/wk, 45-50 mg/m²/day; given according to protocol; dosage reduced with prior irradiation/chemotherapy	IV
		Bladder instillation (investigational)
			Myelosuppression, dose-limiting
			  Leukopenia
			  Thrombocytopenia
			Hypotension especially with rapid infusion
			Rare anaphylaxis

Etoposide	75-200 mg/m²/day × 3; given according to protocol	IV	Myelosuppression; dose-limiting
			  Leukopenia
			  Thrombocytopenia
			Mild nausea and vomiting
			Alopecia
			Severe hypotension with rapid infusion

ANTIBIOTICS			
Bleomycin sulfate (Blenoxane, "Bleo")	10-30 units/m² given according to protocol; dosage decreased with renal failure; test dose may be ordered Total cumulative lifetime dose not to exceed 400 units	IV Intracavitary Intraarterial— (investigational)	Anaphylaxis Elevated temperature with or without chills Hypotension Pulmonary toxicity Mild nausea and vomiting, dose-limiting Cutaneous reactions Alopecia
Idamycin (idarubicin HCl)	12 mg/m³/day × 3 (usually with Ara-C); 100 mg/m²/day × 7 or 25 mg/m² IV bolus, then 200 mg/m²/day × 5 continuous IV; dosage reduced with impaired renal or liver function	IV	Severe myelosuppression Nausea, vomiting, abdominal pain Severe diarrhea Mucositis Alopecia Rash: palms, soles of feet Dysrhythmias

*See Symptomatic Care in Chemotherapy p. 670.

Nadir	Recovery after nadir (days)	Indications	Administration and nursing implications*

			Monitor closely for extravasation
			  Give antidote as ordered
			  Avoid eye contact
			Experimentally given by IV infusion over 24-hr period; monitor site closely
			Administer stool softeners and laxatives as ordered

4-5 days	7	Acute lymphocytic leukemia, breast cancer, sarcomas, Hodgkin's disease, neuroblastoma, non-Hodgkin's lymphoma, small cell lung carcinoma	Ensure patent IV; give IV push over 3-5 min through side port; check blood backflow before instilling each ml; flush line with 30 ml IV fluid before each blood check;
			  Monitor for extravasation
			  Give antidote if extravasation occurs
			Administer stool softeners and laxatives as ordered

5-10 days 5-10 days	—	Acute leukemia, lung cancer, esophageal cancer, melanoma	Give IV push over 3-5 min through side port of newly inserted patent IV; flush tubing with 50-100 ml after administration Monitor for extravasation Administer stool softeners and laxatives as ordered
3-14 days	28	Hodgkin's disease, non-Hodgkin's lymphoma, malignant pleural effusions, bladder cancer; (CNS) cancer	Give IV infusion in volume five times medication volume; over at least 45 min period through patent IV Take baseline BP before therapy then 15 min into administration and at conclusion Flush line after administration
16 days	20-22	Leukemia, lung cancer, lymphoma, testicular cancer	Give through side port of patent IV over at least 30 min to avoid severe hypotension Take baseline BP before therapy then 15 min into administration and at conclusion
—	—	Squamous cell carcinoma, Hodgkin's disease, non-Hodgkin's lymphoma, mycosis fungoides, lung cancer, testicular cancer, malignant effusions	Give IV push or IV infusion as ordered after obtaining baseline Be prepared to treat anaphylaxis; have life support equipment and medications available Take T and BP q4h during infusion Assess breath sounds and respiratory function Teach patient to report signs of respiratory difficulty immediately to staff Reposition patient q15 min for four times when administering intracavitary doses
—	—	Leukemia	Give IV push over 10-15 min through side port of free-flowing IV Check blood backflow before instilling each ml; monitor continuous IV closely; flush line Monitor for extravasation; give antidote and follow policy if occurs Assess cardiac status before and during administration

*See Extravasation p. 669.

Continued.

TABLE 14-6. Chemotherapeutic Drugs—cont'd

Medication	Dosage	Routes of administration	Side effects and toxicities†

Dactinomycin (actinomycin D, Cosmegen)	0.5 mg/day for adult; 0.015-0.5 mg/kg for children; both given according to protocol	IV	Myelosuppression
			    Thrombocytopenia
			    Leukocytopenia
			    Anemia
			Nausea and vomiting, onset 1-2 hr, lasting several days
			Mucositis
			Alopecia
			Skin changes, especially irradiated areas

Daunorubicin (Daunomycin, rubidomycin)	30-60 mg/m²; given according to protocol; dosage reduced with impaired renal or liver function	IV	Myelosuppression; dose-limiting Nausea and vomiting Alopecia
Doxotrubicin (Adriamycin)	60-70 mg/m² single dose; given according to protocol; dosage decreased with hepatic dysfunction Total cumulative lifetime dose not to exceed 450-550 mg/m²	IV Intraarterial—investigational	Myelosuppression Leukopenia, dose-limiting Nausea and vomiting, onset 3-4 hr Stomatitis Marked alopecia Reactivation of irradiated skin areas Cardiotoxicity, dose-limiting

Plicamycin* (Mithracin)	0.025-0.050 mg/kg; given according to protocol	IV	Myelosuppression
			    Thrombocytopenia
			    Decreased clotting factors
			    Mild leukopenia
			Nausea and vomiting
			Diarrhea
			Stomatitis
			Neurotoxicity
			Dermatological reactions
			Nephrotoxicity
			Hepatoxicity

Mitomycin (Mutamycin, Mitomycin C)	10-20 mg/m² dose; given according to protocol	IV	Myelosuppression cumulative
			    Leukopenia
			    Thrombocytopenia
			        Erythrocytopenia
			Nausea and vomiting, onset 1-2 hr, lasting 6-8 hr
			Stomatitis
			Alopecia
			Purple bands on nails
			Mild nephrotoxicity

*Not used as an antineoplastic agent at this time.
†See Symptomatic Care in Chemotherapy p. 670.

Nadir	Recovery after nadir (days)	Indications	Administration and nursing implications*
14-21 days	22-25	Choriocarcinoma, Wilms' tumor, sarcoma, testicular cancer	Give IV push through side port of patent IV; check blood backflow before instilling each ml, flush line with 30 ml IV fluid before each blood check; flush line after administration Monitor for extravasation; give antidote if extravasation occurs Establish oral and skin hygiene care before therapy Administer antiemetic before administration and as indicated and ordered
7-14 days	—	Acute lymphocytic leukemia; acute granulocytic leukemia; neuroblastoma	Administer IV push through side port of patent IV Monitor closely for extravasation; give antidote as ordered Tell patient that urine will be colored red
10-14 days	21-24	Acute leukemia, Hodgkin's disease, non-Hodgkin's lymphoma, sarcomas, Wilms' tumor, ovarian, breast, lung, thyroid, and bladder cancer	Give IV push through side port of patent IV; check blood backflow before instilling each ml; flush line with 30 ml IV fluid before each blood check; monitor carefully to prevent extravasation that may cause severe ulceration; flush line after administration with 50-100 ml solution Teach patient to report *any sensation* during administration to staff Give antiemetics before administration and as indicated after Assess cardiac status before administration Institute oral hygiene care before administration
14 days	21-28	Hypercalcemia in malignancy	Give in small volume IV over 30-45 min through side port of patent IV; may be ordered as IV infusion given over 4-6 hr for hypercalcemia Observe for extravasation; give antidote as ordered
28-42 days	42-56	Cancer of stomach and pancreas	Give IV push over 3-5 min through side port of patent IV; check blood backflow before instilling each ml; flush line with 30 ml IV fluid before each blood check; flush line after administration Monitor closely for extravasation; give antidote if extravasation occurs Administer antiemetics before administration and then as indicated Institute oral hygiene care before therapy Observe for skin changes at IV site or distal to site for 6 weeks

*See Extravasation p. 669.

Continued.

TABLE 14-6. Chemotherapeutic Drugs—cont'd

Medication	Dosage	Routes of administration	Side effects and toxicities*
Streptozocin (Zanosar)	1.0-1.5 g/m²/wk; 500 mg-1.0 g/m²/day; given according to protocol	IV	Severe nausea and vomiting Nephrotoxicity, dose-limiting Mild hepatotoxicity Immediate burning pain at IV site; decreases after 15-20 min of infusion
MISCELLANEOUS			
Asparaginase (Elspar, L-Asparaginase)	10,000-40,000 IU/m²/day, q2-3 weeks; given according to protocol Skin test may be ordered prior to administration	IV, IM	Anaphylaxis Mild nausea and vomiting Neurotoxicity Hepatotoxicity Pancreatitis Hyperosmolar, nonketotic hyperglycemia
Cisplatin (Platinol)	80-120 mg/m²; given according to protocol Higher doses may be mixed in hypertonic saline solution to prevent nephrotoxicity	IV	Anaphylaxis Nephrotoxicity Ototoxicity Severe nausea and vomiting Hypomagnesemia
Carboplatin (Paraplatin)	360 mg/m² q4 weeks IV Should not be administered until neutraphils are >2000 and platelets >100,000	IV	Myelosuppression Leukopenia Thrombocytopenia Anemia Nausea and vomiting
Dacarbazine (DTIC)	250 mg/m²; given according to protocol	IV	Myelosuppression, dose-limiting Leukopenia Thrombocytopenia Severe nausea and vomiting, onset 1 hr, lasting to 12 hr Immediate burning pain at IV site, decreased with further dilution

*See Symptomatic Care in Chemotherapy p. 670.

Nadir	Recovery after nadir (days)	Indications	Administration and nursing implications
—	—	Pancreatic islet cell tumors, non–beta cell pancreatic tumors: stomach, carcinoid, colon	Give IV push through side port of patent IV; check blood backflow before instilling each ml; flush line with 30 ml IV fluid before each blood check; flush line after administration; monitor for extravasation (p. 669), give antidote if extravasation occurs Administer antiemetics before therapy and then as indicated Tell patient burning sensation may be experienced; slow infusion to decrease burning Force fluids to 3000 ml/day, unless contraindicated, to ensure adequate urine output Observe for hypoglycemia reactions immediately after administration Have glucose 50% available
—	—	Acute lymphocytic leukemia	Give IV push over 3-5 min through side port of patent IV Take baseline, T, P, R, and BP before administration Be prepared to treat anaphylaxis; have life support equipment readily available
—	—	Testicular and ovarian cancer; squamous cell carcinoma; lung, head and neck cancer	Assess baseline T, P, R, and BP Give by continuous IV infusion Force fluids to 3000 ml/day and give parenteral therapy as ordered 12-24 hr before drug administration Monitor intake and output Mannitol may be ordered with or after administration Ensure output of 100-150 ml/hr before giving medication Give antiemetics as ordered and indicated Be prepared to treat anaphylaxis Have life support equipment and medications available *High-dose*—investigational Parenteral hydration and bladder irrigation may be ordered
21-30	28-30	Ovarian cancer	Assess baseline TPR and BP Give by continuous IV infusion Monitor input and output Give antiemetics as ordered and indicated Be prepared to treat anaphylaxis Have life support equipment and medications available
21-28 days	36-50	Malignant melanoma, sarcoma, Hodgkin's disease	Administer small volume IV over 30-60 min through side port of patent IV Flush line after therapy Apply ice pack at IV site Give antiemetics before therapy, then as indicated

Continued.

TABLE 14-6. Chemotherapeutic Drugs—cont'd

Medication	Dosage	Routes of administration	Side effects and toxicities*

Procarbazine (Matulane)	50-200 mg/day; given according to protocol	po	Myelosuppression, dose-limiting
			    Thrombocytopenia
			    Leukopenia
			    Anemia

Amsacrine (AMSA)	75 mg/m²/day; 120 mg/m²/wk; given according to protocol; dosage reduced with hepatic dysfunctions	IV	Myelosuppression
			    Leukopenia, dose-limiting
			Neurotoxicity (cerebellar dysfunction,
			    grand mal seizures)
			Conjunctivitis
			    Nausea and vomiting, mild mucositis
			Dermatological toxicity
			Cardiac dysrhythmias
			Phlebitis

*See Symptomatic Care in Chemotherapy p. 670.

Teach patient signs and symptoms of skin changes, indicating those to report to physician

If skin tenderness or dryness is present, use water-based topical ointments

Dust on cornstarch

Wear soft cotton clothing

Expected outcome/evaluation

Patient describes measures to improve impaired skin integrity

■ **NDX:** Fluid volume deficit related to disease process and chemotherapy

Assess fluid intake and output

Inspect skin turgor and integrity

Inspect mucous membranes for moistness and integrity

Assess weight and vital signs

Evaluate laboratory values

Encourage oral fluids to 2 to 3 L/day unless contraindicated

Obtain order for parenteral fluids as needed

Identify and manage side effects that may interfere with fluid intake

Assess for factors that may contribute to fluid loss (fever, diarrhea)

Teach signs and symptoms to report to health care team

Expected outcome/evaluation

Fluid balance is maintained or restored

■ **NDX:** Potential fluid volume excess related to excess fluid intake

Regulate flow of IV at least hourly

Maintain accurate intake and output

Carefully observe for signs of fluid overload

Increased respirations

Moist rales

Auscultate chest q2h to 4h during hydration

Monitor BP and P

Weigh patient daily

Observe for signs of edema, especially in ankles and fingers

Monitor laboratory data (usually no change in Hct but may be significant drop in serum sodium)

Teach patient signs and symptoms of fluid overload to report to health care team (increased respirations, increase in weight, finger and ankle edema, puffy eyelids)

If taking diuretics, monitor administration carefully for desired results and possible side effects

Expected outcome/evaluation

Fluid balance is maintained or restored

Weight gained by fluid retention is lost

■ **NDX:** Potential or actual self-esteem disturbance related to physical and functional changes caused by chemotherapy

Assess contributing factors: disease process, treatment, patient knowledge

Evaluate how diagnosis and treatment are affecting patient's lifestyle

Evaluate support system/significant other

Determine patient's and/or significant other's coping strategies

Provide opportunity for discussion of concerns regarding physical self (physical feelings, feelings about one's body), role function (wife, mother, wage earner), and dependence/independence

Assess need for professional counseling if patient's support system is deteriorating; give information regarding necessary counseling in adaption process

Nadir	Recovery after nadir (days)	Indications	Administration and nursing implications
25-36 days	36-50	Hodgkin's disease and non-Hodgkin's lymphomas, malignant melanoma, lung and brain cancer	Avoid use of alcohol, sympathomimetic drugs, trycyclic antidepressants, CNS depressants, and heavy intake of dark beer, cheese, bananas
—	—	Acute myeloblastic leukemia, lymphoma, sarcoma, lung and breast cancer	Give within 30-60 min of preparation Dilute only in D_5W, never use saline Administer through side port of patent IV Administer corticosteroid eye medication as ordered Tell patient skin may have yellow-orange tinge

Refer patient and/or significant other to supportive group programs (e.g., I Can Cope, Reach for Recovery)

Expected outcome/evaluation

Patient recognizes changes in self-esteem

Patient demonstrates movement toward reconstruction of an altered self-concept

■ **NDX:** Self-care deficit (specify feeding, bathing/hygiene, dressing/grooming, toileting) related to weakness

Determine nature, extent, and duration of self-care deficits

Determine patient's coping techniques

Assess family/significant other's availability, willingness, and readiness to assist patient if needed

Maintain a patient, supportive attitude

Allow patient to do things that he or she is capable of doing

Provide self-help devices as needed

Praise patient for progress and emphasize achievements

Recognize dependency needs and plan care accordingly with patient/significant other input

Assist patient/significant other in planning for long-term care if needed

Arrange for nursing services as needed at home

Teach patient/significant other skills needed for home care

Expected outcome/evaluation

Patient eliminates or compensates for self-care deficits with adaptive devices or caregivers

■ **NDX:** Knowledge deficit related to lack of information about chemotherapy

Assess ability and desire to learn

Assess knowledge and level of understanding related to the disease process (factual, misconceptions)

Assess knowledge and level of understanding related to treatment (misconceptions, myths, cultural beliefs, previous experience)

Ascertain expectations of outcome of treatment

With help of audiovisual aids, explain how drugs work and expected therapeutic effects of chemotherapy treatment

Provide patient and/or significant other with written material regarding name of drug, action of drug, and potential side effects

Explain method, frequency, and duration of administration of each drug

Provide verbal and written material regarding management of side effects/toxicity

Instruct patient regarding early side effects, such as nausea and vomiting, and side effects that will be delayed, such as myelosuppression

Discuss side effects that are reversible

Instruct patient regarding side effects to report to physician

Give written information on how and where to reach health care personnel if necessary

Involve significant other in care planning as much as possible

Expected outcome/evaluation

Patient/significant other demonstrates knowledge of disease process, treatment, potential side effects and measures to manage adverse effects

ADMINISTRATION OF CHEMOTHERAPEUTIC DRUGS

Verify patient's identification

Review patient's allergy history

Assess learning needs and concerns; answer questions appropriately

Review educational materials with patient and family (films, pamphlets)

Check physician's order for drug dose, route, rate, and time of administration

Verify that informed consent has been given

Review laboratory data with knowledge of acceptable parameters

Review immediate and long-term side effects of drugs

Calculate dosage, double-check calculation, and ascertain if dosage is within normal administration range

Know amount and type of diluent to use for reconstitution (mix in biological safety hood and observe safety precautions [pp. 688-691])

Verify drug dosage with another nurse, a pharmacist, or physician

Correctly label drug with patient's name, dose, and route of administration

Administer antiemetic 30 min before administration of chemotherapy if indicated

Have emergency medications and antidote readily available for adverse reaction

Site Selection and Starting IV

Select site for venipuncture with regard to previous trauma to arm (blood drawing or lymphatic resection) and drug to be given (vesicant vs. nonvesicant); begin at distal portion of extremity

Avoid use of preexisting IV for vesicant drugs

Avoid use of lower extremities and area over joints

Wash hands

Start IV, following guidelines of facility's policy and procedures; needle gauge usually No. 23 or No. 25 scalp vein

Avoid multiple sticks; test patency of IV—blood backflows easily

Stabilize arm or hand; use pillow or board if necessary

Ensure patient's comfort

Instruct patient to notify nurse immediately of adverse effects

Interventions for Specific Types of Drugs

Nonvesicants

Can be given by IV bolus through side arm of free-flowing IV containing no additives, by continuous IV drip through a peripheral vein, or by two-syringe technique, with one syringe containing 10 ml of normal saline to test vein before drug administration and to flush vein following injection of drug

When administering through side arm of IV by bolus, check for blood backflow by pinching IV tubing and quickly releasing, before administration of drug, at halfway mark, and at end of administration; before removing needle from injection port, place 4 × 4 with alcohol swab beneath injection port to catch drop

When giving drug by continuous infusion, ensure vein patency throughout infusion period; before removing needle from injection port, place 4 × 4 and alcohol swab beneath infection port to catch drop (prevent spill)

Irritants

Can be given by infusion over 30 to 60 min depending on dosage

Check for blood backflow before administration and ensure vein patency throughout infusion period; apply ice pack prophylactically at infusion site to prevent discomfort

Vesicants

See Extravasation (p. 669)

When given peripherally, avoid sites where damage to underlying tendons or nerves are more likely to occur

Can be safely administered through side arm of newly inserted, free-flowing peripheral IV containing no additives

Check for blood backflow before instillation of each milliliter (as described for nonvesicants)

These drugs are not given as continuous infusions except through a well-established central venous access device

When administering by central venous device, obtain blood backflow before instillation of chemotherapeutic drug (see Care of Patient with Central Venous Catheter, p. 53)

Use mechanical or electrical controller for continuous chemotherapy infusion

Keep IV site and as much of limb as possible visible

Avoid obstructing view of site and vein with tape

Keep clothing well above site; remove clothing from arm when possible

General Interventions

Monitor for allergic reaction: anaphylaxis and extravasation (p. 669) on initiation, continuously during infusion, and then q4h to 8h for 24 hr

Manage pain as indicated and ordered; adjust flow rate of irritating medication to patient tolerance if possible

Know and observe for side or toxic effects and complications during administration, then for 24 to 48 hr; be aware of nadir of drugs ordered

Differentiate between effect of drug and reaction to disease when possible

Infuse parenteral fluids after drug administration to flush tubing, needle, and vein

Apply pressure over site for 3 to 4 min following removal of needle

Document medication, site, and responses or untoward effects of interventions

Specific Types of Administrations

Intrathecal or intraventricular administration

Assist with lumbar puncture or ventricular puncture

Be aware that intraventricular injection may be done through subcutaneously implanted reservoir

Observe strict aseptic technique

Be aware that a sterile isotonic diluent without preservatives is essential in minimizing neurotoxicity

Intraarterial administration

May be given in one of several arteries (e.g., hepatic artery)

See Electronic Infusion Devices (Chapter 1)

Teach patient to call staff immediately if warning symptoms are noticed

Arterial perfusion

Intraarterial administration of chemotherapeutic agent to an isolated extremity or body area

See intraarterial administration

Intraperitoneal administration: administration of chemotherapeutic agent directly into peritoneal cavity by dialysis (p. 486)

Intracavitary administration

Administration of chemotherapeutic agent into a body space to control malignant effusions

Usually excess fluid is removed from cavity before instillation of drug

Ensure free flow of medication during administration

Aspirate frequently throughout instillation for fluid return to ensure that drug is being instilled into cavity

Turn patient from side to side q15 min for four times then q2h to 4h to ensure maximal distribution throughout cavity

Drain fluids from cavity q12h to 24h after instillation and then daily or as ordered

Implantable drug delivery systems

Implantable drug infusion pumps are delivery systems intended to administer long-term chemotherapy in ambulatory patients

Device delivers a precise, continuous drug flow to selected organs or sites via a pliable, radiopaque, silicone rubber catheter

Pump is refilled by percutaneous injection and powered by a self-contained inexhaustible energy supply

SAFETY IN HANDLING CANCER CHEMOTHERAPY AGENTS

Only pharmacists, physicians, and nurses with special training should prepare chemotherapeutic agents for administration (Table 14-7)

Preparation of cytotoxic agents should be performed in a Class II biological safety cabinet (hood)

Transport parenteral drugs in plastic cover to prevent spillage and contamination

All equipment and unused drug(s) should be treated as hazardous waste and disposed of according to facility's policy and procedure: place linen in double bag marked "Caution, Chemotherapy"; instruct personnel to observe precautions in handling; wash twice

Personnel who are planning to become or who may be pregnant should not handle these medications

TABLE 14-7. Hazards Associated with Chemotherapeutic Drugs

Medication	Route	Hazard	Precaution and action
ALKYLATING AGENTS			
Cyclophosphamide (Cytoxan)	IV, po	Teratogenic and carcinogenic; skin irritation is rare	Wear protective gloves; flush spills with large amounts of water
Mechlorethamine hydrochloride (Mustargen, nitrogen mustard)	IV, intracavitary, topical, intralesional	Strong vesicant, nasal irritant, highly toxic	Wear protective gloves; protect eyes; wash skin with large amounts of water, sodium carbonate (3%), or isotonic solution of sodium thiosulfate (2.5%); wash eyes out with large amounts of water; irrigate with sodium thiosulfate in isotonic solution (contact physician)
Ifosfamide (Ifex)	IV	Teratogenic and carcinogenic; skin irritation is rare	Wear protective gloves; flush spills with large amounts of water
ANTIMETABOLITES			
Cytarabine (Ara-C, cytosar)	IV, SC, IM, intrathecal	Teratogenic; not absorbed through intact skin	Wear protective gloves; wash spills with water
5-Fluorouracil (Fluoroplex, Fluorouracil, Adrucil)	IV, po, topical	Minor inflammatory reaction if skin is broken	Flush spills with large amounts of water

Continued.

TABLE 14-7. Hazards Associated with Chemotherapeutic Drugs—cont'd

Medication	Route	Hazard	Precaution and action
Methotrexate (Mexate, Amethopterin MTX)	IV, IM, intrathecal	Teratogenic, carcinogenic skin irritant	Wear protective gloves; wash spills with water; apply nonmedicated cream for stinging; for systemic absorption of significant quantity notify physician; give folinic acid (leucovorin calcium)
ANTIBIOTICS			
Dactinomycin (Cosmegen, actinomycin D)	IV	Teratogenic; corrosive to soft tissues	Wear protective gloves; protect eyes; rinse spillage off in running water for 10 min; rinse with buffered phosphate solution
Bleomycin (Blenoxane)	IV, IM, subcutaneous, intraarterial, intratumoral, intracavitary	Cytostatic: local, toxic, or allergic reaction	Wear protective gloves; wash spills thoroughly with water
Daunomycin (Cerubidin, Daunorubicin, DNR)	IV	Skin and mucous membrane irritant	Wear protective gloves; wash spills immediately with water or isotonic saline
Doxorubicin (Adriamycin)	IV	Potential teratogenic; suspected carcinogenic skin irritant, but not absorbed into bloodstream	Wear protective gloves; wash spills immediately with large amounts of water
Plicamycin (Mithracin)	IV	Rare skin irritation	Wash spills with water
Mitomycin (Mitomycin C, Mutamycin)		Teratogenic; suspected carcinogenic skin irritant	Wear protective gloves; wash spills thoroughly and immediately with large quantities of water; irrigate contaminated eyes with large amounts of water; notify physician
PODOPHYLLOTOXINS			
Etoposide (VP-16)	IV	Suspected teratogenic and carcinogenic irritants	Wear protective gloves; wash spills with large amounts of water
Teniposide (VM-26)			
VINCA ALKALOIDS			
Vinblastine (Velban)	IV	Suspected teratogenic skin irritant	Wear protective gloves; wash spills thoroughly and immediately with large amounts of water
Vincristine (Oncovin)	IV	Suspected teratogenic skin irritant	Wear protective gloves; wash skin with large amounts of water
Vindesine	IV	Suspected teratogenic skin irritant; may produce corneal ulcers	Wear protective gloves; protect eyes; wash areas with large amounts of water
MISCELLANEOUS			
Asparaginase (L-Asparaginase)	IV, IM	Potentially teratogenic	
Azathioprine (Imuran)	IV (Investigational)	Potentially teratogenic, suspected carcinogenic skin irritant	Wear protective gloves; protect eyes; wash spills off with water immediately
Cisplatin (Platinol)	IV	Suspected teratogen and carcinogen; skin reaction in sensitive patients	Wear protective gloves; rinse spills thoroughly with water
Dacarbazine (DTIC)	IV	Teratogenic, carcinogenic irritant to skin and mucous membranes	Wear protective gloves; wash spills with soap and water immediately; irrigate eyes with water
Carboplatin (Paraplatin)	IV	Suspected teratogen and carcinogen; skin reaction in sensitive patients	Wear protective gloves; rinse spills thoroughly with water

Avoid eating, drinking, smoking, and using cosmetics while preparing and/or administering drug

Wash hands thoroughly before putting on gloves and after gloves are removed

Wear disposable cover gowns with closed front and cuffed, long sleeves and latex gloves throughout preparation, administration, and disposal period when handling medication or equipment

Wear protective garment and gloves when handling patient excreta during administration and for 48 hr following administration

Syringes and IV sets with Leur-Lok fitting should be used whenever possible to prevent spillage

When priming IV line and removing needle from injection port, place alcohol swab and 4 × 4 beneath site to collect small spills; discard in hazardous waste container

Occupational Safety and Health Adminstration (OSHA) recommends

Drug administration sets should be attached and primed within the hood before the drug is added to the fluid

Wipe up spills immediately; contain spills by gently covering them with disposable absorbent material; be careful to prevent aerosolization (wear gown, mask, double gloves); place absorbent material in double plastic bag marked "Hazardous Waste"

EXTRAVASATION

Escape of agents from a vein into the tissue; escape of certain antineoplastic agents can cause necrosis of local tissue; care must be taken when giving these agents (see Administration of Chemotherapeutic Drugs, p. 666); vesicant drugs, which can cause tissue necrosis if they infiltrate, include vincristine, vinblastine, doxorubicin (Adriamycin), dactinomycin, daunorubicin, dacarbazine, mitomycin, nitrogen mustard, mithramycin, and streptozocin

Assessment
Observations/findings

Venipuncture site
  During infusion
    Burning
    Pain
    Swelling
    Induration
    No blood return or questionable blood return (blood return is obtained, but patient questions or complains of pain—drug escape could be above injection site)
  Postinfusion
    Ulceration
    Desquamation
    Necrosis
  Phlebitis
    Pain

Increased temperature
Redness
Swelling
Predisposing factors
  Sclerotic vascular disease
  Multiple venipunctures

Medical Management

Orders to institute extravasation procedure
Sodium thiosulfate
Hydrocortisone
Hyaluronidase
Ice or warm packs

Nursing diagnoses/interventions/evaluation

■ **NDX:** Potential for impaired skin integrity related to risk of adverse effects of antineoplastic agents

Prevention of extravasation

Administer vesicant medication through a freshly inserted IV site with a good blood return

Select large veins in region with large amount of soft tissue to avoid possible involvement of tendons should IV infiltrate

Check medication dosage and dilution carefully

Administer at rate ordered; monitor closely

Monitor IV site continuously during infusion

Instruct patient to notify staff immediately if burning sensation is felt at site or IV slows or stops

After infusing medication, infuse neutral solution through IV line as ordered

Observe for possible clinical signs of extravasation: pain, burning, swelling, no blood return or questionable blood return

Observe for possible clinical signs of tissue necrosis: erythema, induration, tenderness, pain, eventual ulceration with tissue breakdown

Steps in management of extravasation once confirmed
  Discontinue IV immediately
  Apply appropriate pack (hot or cold)
  Infiltrate area with antidote using interdermal technique
  Instruct patient on follow-up

Recommended protocol

Vesicants, when extravasated, produce local necrosis; recommended treatment is
  Mechlorethamine (mustargen, nitrogen mustard)
    Discontinue IV
    Infiltrate local area with 1/6 molar (isotonic) sodium thiosulfate using intradermal technique
    Apply ice for 20 min qh for 24 hr
    Notify physician
  Dactinomycin (actinomycin D, Cosmegen); mithramycin (Mithracin, Plicamycin); mitomycin C (Mu-

tamycin); daunorubicin (Daunomycin); doxorubicin (Adriamycin); streptozocin (Zanosar), amsacrine
Discontinue IV
Infiltrate area with hydrocortisone sodium succinate 50 mg or other water-soluble corticosteroid (using intradermal technique)
Apply ice for 20 min qh for 24 hr
Notify physician
Vinblastine (Velban); vincristine (Oncovin)
Discontinue IV
Infiltrate area with hyaluronidase (150 units) using intradermal technique
Apply warm, moist packs for 24 hr
Notify physician

Ongoing care

Instruct patient on follow-up
Continue to observe site
Notify physician of skin changes

Expected outcome/evaluation

Skin is intact; there is no redness, swelling, or necrosis

SYMPTOMATIC CARE IN CHEMOTHERAPY

Hematological: Myelosuppression

Inhibition of bone marrow activity resulting in decreased production of blood cells and platelets caused by the effects of chemotherapy, the disease state, or radiation therapy; the majority of chemotherapeutic agents produce some degree of myelosuppression; since the blood count nadirs produced by most chemotherapeutic agents can be predicted, the schedule of drug delivery is designed to coincide with the recovery of the bone marrow; the nurse must be aware of the nadir (the point of lowest drop in blood count) for each chemotherapeutic drug

LEUKOPENIA

Temporary reduction in the total number of circulating white blood cells; since the life span of the leukocyte is very brief (6 to 8 hr), leukopenias occur frequently in patients receiving chemotherapy, placing them at risk for infections; a good indication of a patient's ability to fight infection is the absolute granulocyte count (AGC), which is calculated by multiplying the total WBC count by the percentage of neutrophils in the differential:

AGC = WBC × % Neutrophils (mm³)

(Bands + segs = neutrophils)

When AGC is below 1000 cells/mm³, patient is at risk of infection; opportunistic endogenous organisms can cause systemic and severe infections; severe neutropenia often defined as <500 neutrophils/mm³

Assessment
Observations/findings

Elevated temperature if not masked by corticosteroids or antiinflammatory drugs
Any sudden rise or fall of temperature of even 1° F
Elevated temperature of 100.4° F (38.3° C) lasting 24 hr or longer, not associated with blood products or drugs
Elevated temperature may be caused by other factors, such as atelectasis, tumor, or response of disease process
Sudden rise and fall in neutrophils; may be indicative of infection
In neutropenic patients, inflammatory response (redness, heat, edema, pus formation, pain) may be diminished or absent
Respiratory
  Dyspnea, especially on exertion
  Cough, sore throat, sputum production
  Changes in breath sounds (wheezes, rales, rhonchi)
  "Colds" and "flu"
Skin and mucous membrane
  Skin breaks, puncture sites
  Redness
  Swelling
  Drainage
  Ulceration
Oral cavity
  Fissures
  Redness
  Swelling
  Ulceration
Perineum
  Discomfort
  Pain
  Excoriation
Rectum
  Tenderness
  Fissures
  Abscess
Genitourinary
  Frequency, dysuria, urgency
  Neurological deficit: monitor residual urine; check urine for clarity and odor
  Vaginal discharge
  Assess vaginal hygiene and contraceptive techniques
  Prostate enlargement
Eye or ear drainage

Laboratory/diagnostic studies

WBC
Differential values
  Granulocytes
    Comprise 56% to 75% of total WBC
    Responsible for fighting bacterial and fungal infection
    Life of 6 to 7 hr
    Type: neutrophils, eosinophils, basophils

Lymphocytes
   Comprise 20% to 40% of total WBC
   Responsible for immune defenses
   B lymphocytes: humoral immunity
   T lymphocytes: cell-mediated immunity
Monocytes
   Comprise 2% to 8% of total WBC
   Defense against bacteria and fungi
Chest x-ray examination
Pulmonary function tests
Urinalysis
Cultures: blood, sputum

Potential complication

Septicemia

Medical Management

Intake and output
Cultures of blood, sputum, urine, skin, drainage, etc.
Antibiotic therapy
Antifungal medications
IV gamma globulin
Antiviral therapy
Granulocyte colony-stimulating factors (G-CSF)

Nursing diagnoses/interventions

■ **NDX:** Potential for infection related to neutropenia

Check results of WBC and differential to ensure that they are within acceptable limits; calculate ACG
Assess patient for increasing myelosuppression; nursing management will depend on severity of condition
Assess skin and mucous membranes for skin and symptoms of infection; give special attention to skin folds and body cavities
Assess respiratory and genitourinary tract for evidence of infection
Document findings and interventions
Instruct patient and/or significant other that the WBC count may decrease following most chemotherapy; WBC count usually recovers before next dose; however, recovery may be delayed, and an occasional dose of chemotherapy may be delayed
Teach patient to guard against infection by
   Maintaining meticulous total body hygiene, including perineal care
   Avoiding crowds and persons with infections
   Maintaining good nutrition and fluid intake
   Practicing good oral hygiene after meals
   Getting adequate rest and exercise
   Reporting signs and symptoms of infection to health care personnel immediately
Place patient in noninfectious environment if AGC is <1000/mm³ or as ordered; use of reverse isolation or laminar flow room are controversial based on research findings

Use physical means to reduce exposure to microbes
   Instruct and ensure that personnel and visitors follow handwashing procedure with providone-iodine before entering room
   No one with infectious condition ("cold," "flu," skin rash, etc.) may enter room
   Staff assigned to care for patient with neutropenia must not be assigned to care for patients who have infections, if possible
   Care for neutropenic patient first and take other precautions to avoid transferring any infectious agents to neutropenic patient
   Keep room clean
      Avoid any trash in room and bathroom
      Remove food and examination trays immediately after use
      Maintain furniture, fixtures, floor, and equipment free of dust and spills
   Ensure that allied health personnel (e.g., laboratory technicians) do not bring into patient's room equipment that has been in other areas of hospital
   If patient requires transportation, avoid using elevator with potentially infectious passengers present; mask for patient may be required
Maintain skin integrity
   Avoid IM injections
   Observe IV or central line site q4h
   Change dressing daily if nonporous type is used, using aseptic technique
   Change IV tubing and bottles daily
   Avoid infiltrations that necessitate restarting IV; position IV site to prevent stress and movement at site of insertion
   Consolidate laboratory work; clean skin with povidone-iodine scrub before puncture
   Assess previous puncture sites each shift
   Assess and record condition of oral cavity each shift
      Teach or assist with oral hygiene measures in morning, after food ingestion, at bedtime, and q2h to 4h when patient is awake at night
      Administer antifungal and antiviral medication as ordered
      Assess and record condition of perineum daily
      Initiate and teach perineal care to be performed after each bowel movement;
         Prevent constipation (p. 679) and diarrhea (p. 678)
         Administer medications as ordered
         Avoid use of enemas and suppositories
Monitor and record vital signs q4h; take temperature more frequently if trend is beginning; report any change in temperature immediately
Institute comfort and cooling measures as indicated by condition
   Change linen and clothing to keep patient dry
   Avoid chilling

Administer antipyretics as ordered

Mechanical cooling blanket may be ordered

Monitor intake and output; report urinary frequency, burning, or changes in character of urine

Use voiding measures when indicated to avoid catheterization

If catheterization is necessary

Use strict aseptic technique for insertion

Perform catheter care each shift

Obtain cultures as ordered: blood, urine, sputum, skin, drainage, etc.

Assess and record respiratory status q4h; report changes in breath sounds, cough, and sputum; increases in respiratory rate; or presence of sore throat immediately

Assist and teach patient to turn, cough, and deep breathe q2h

Administer oxygen if ordered

Encourage mobility each shift

Turn and position immobile patient q2h to prevent pressure sores

Provide mild antibacterial soaps and soft cloths and towels for skin hygiene, daily and prn

Administer IV antibiotics as ordered

Monitor laboratory data daily; report changes

Administer gamma globulin as ordered

Monitor for anaphylactic reaction, phlebitis, nausea, back or abdominal pain, and chills

Minimize side effects by initiating comfort measures, use of blankets, decreasing rate of infusion and premedicating with acetaminophen (Tylenol) as ordered

Administer colony-stimulating factors (CSFs) as ordered

Assess for headache; institute interventions

Instruct patient about low-bacteria diet

Instruct about need to remove flowers and plants from environment during neutropenic phase

Expected outcome/evaluation

Patient/caregiver promptly reports symptoms or signs of infection

■ **NDX:** Knowledge deficit related to lack of information about infection, activities, prevention of injury, and daily care

Discuss signs and symptoms of infection to report to physician or nurse

Emphasize importance of avoiding persons who may be infectious or who may have potentially contagious conditions

Explain need to avoid persons who have been recently vaccinated

Explain need to maintain safe sex practices

Explain need to wash hands after using bathroom, before eating, and before performing any procedures

Emphasize importance of preventing injury to skin

Use electric razors

Handle knives and sharp objects carefully

Wear protective gloves when gardening and when using strong household cleaning solutions

Wear broad-brimmed hat and sunscreen when in sun

Avoid going barefoot

Wear warm clothing and boots in cold weather

Avoid cutting cuticles, corns, or calluses

Wear padded gloves when using oven

Explain need to perform oral hygiene periodically throughout the day

Emphasize importance of daily hygiene, including perineal and rectal care

Emphasize importance of drinking up to 3000 ml of fluid each day unless contraindicated; explain need to avoid using common drinking fountain

Explain need to maintain clean home environment and handle food properly

Caution patient to avoid contact with pets or other animals during neutropenic phase

Teach name of medication, dosage, time of administration, purpose, and side effects

Explain need to tell all health care personnel, especially dentists, about need to avoid infections

Emphasize importance of follow-up outpatient care

Ensure that patient and/or significant other demonstrates

Method for taking and recording temperature

Procedure for caring for very small cuts or breaks in skin

Expected outcome/evaluation

Patient demonstrates knowledge regarding prevention of infection and remains infection free

THROMBOCYTOPENIA

Reduction in the number of circulating platelets caused by destruction of bone marrow during chemotherapy; platelets circulate for about 10 days before removal from circulation

Assessment
Observations/findings

Petechiae, easy bruising, bleeding gums or nose, purpura (especially lower extremities), hypermenorrhea, tarry stools, blood in urine and/or emesis, abdominal pain, distention, prolonged bleeding from invasive procedures, vaginal or rectal bleeding, blurred vision, headache, disorientation, decreased platelet count

Certain drugs such as mitomycin and the nitrosoureas are associated with delayed, cumulative thrombocytopenia

Laboratory/diagnostic studies

CBC and platelet count

ABO, Rh, and HLA compatability

Potential complications

Spontaneous bleeding
    <10,000 platelets: fatal central nervous system
    (CNS) hemorrhage or massive GI hemorrhage
    <20,000 platelets: hemorrhage in any system

Medical Management

Intake and output
Bleeding precautions
Stool softeners
Neurological assessment
Platelet infusion (can be random or type specific)

Nursing diagnoses/interventions/evaluation

■ **NDX:**   Potential altered protection related to thrombocytopenia

Monitor platelet count and coagulation studies
Anticipate time of nadir after chemotherapy
Identify drugs and/or other factors that may lower platelet
    count and predispose patient to bleeding
Assess and report any signs and symptoms of bleeding
Inspect gums and oral cavity for bleeding each shift
Inspect skin each shift for increased bruising, petechiae,
    ecchymosis, and swelling
Inspect and palpate joints each shift for increased size and
    decreased mobility
Assess sensorium and neurological status each shift
Inspect nasal cavity at least once each shift
If epistaxis occurs
    Have patient sit at 90-degree angle
    Apply pressure to nose
    Place ice pack at back of neck
    If nasal bleeding is not controlled in 10 to 15 min
        Notify physician
            Administer platelet transfusion immediately when
                ordered
Institute safety measures as platelet count decreases below
    50,000/mm^3
    Avoid needle sticks when possible
    Consolidate laboratory work; apply pressure to site for
        5 min and observe site q15 min for at least 1 hr
    Avoid IM injections, aspirin, and aspirin-containing
        products
    Do not take rectal temperatures or administer medi-
        cations rectally; avoid enemas
    Avoid bladder catheterization when possible
    Take BP only when necessary and pump cuff only as
        high as necessary
    Avoid use of
        Rough towels and washcloths
        Razors
        Restraints
        Tight clothing
    Maintain clutter-free environment

Provide night-light to prevent bumping into objects or
    falling
Administer careful oral hygiene
    Use toothettes or gauze pads
    Avoid use of dental floss or toothpicks
    Encourage use of mouth rinse q2h to 4h
        Half saline and half water
        Half saline and half hydrogen peroxide followed by
            saline rinse
Inspect IV or central line site q20 to 30 min for hematoma
    or oozing
    Maintain pressure at site for 5 min when IV is discon-
        tinued
    Inspect q15 min for four times
Administer antacids as ordered
Test stool for blood after each movement
Test urine for blood each time patient voids
Administer stool softeners as ordered to prevent bleeding
    from constipation
Avoid vaginal douches
Use lubricant during intercourse to avoid trauma

Expected outcome/evaluation

Patient experiences absence or control of bleeding

■ **NDX:**   Knowledge deficit related to lack of information
           about measures to prevent bleeding

Explain relationship between platelets and bleeding risk
Teach patient signs and symptoms of bleeding to be re-
    ported to physician in any of the following areas
    Skin
    Oral
    Nasal
    Rectal
    GI tract
    Vagina
    Cerebral
    Urinary tract
Discuss emergency plan to follow if spontaneous hemor-
    rhage occurs at home
    Have emergency numbers on hand
    Call paramedics
    Go to nearest emergency area
Emphasize importance of telling dentist and other medical
    personnel about chemotherapy and low platelet count
Emphasize importance of maintaining safe, clutter-free en-
    vironment
Explain need to apply pressure at blood withdrawal site
    after laboratory work is completed
Emphasize importance of avoiding over-the-counter med-
    ications, especially those containing acetylsalicylic acid
    (i.e., aspirin), without checking with physician
Caution patient to avoid use of sharp objects when possible
    Use electric razor

Use caution when handling knives or other equipment

Explain need to avoid harsh coughing, blowing of nose, straining, and strenuous exercise

    If cough persists, notify physician

    Take cough medication as ordered

Emphasize importance of follow-up outpatient care

    Routine laboratory appointments

    Return physician and nurse appointments

Ensure that patient and/or significant other demonstrates

    Method for applying pressure to bleeding site

        Apply dressing or clean material directly over site

        Apply pressure for 5 min

        Apply ice in covered plastic bag over site once bleeding stops

        Check site for further bleeding q15 min for 1 hr

    Method for testing stool and urine for occult blood

Expected outcome/evaluation

Patient

    Recognizes significance of being at risk for bleeding

    Demonstrates knowledge of measures necessary to prevent bleeding

    Has no signs of bleeding

ANEMIA

Temporary reduction in the number of circulating red blood cells and the level of hemoglobin caused by destruction of cells during chemotherapy, leading to tissue hypoxia from impaired oxygen-carrying capacity

Assessment
Observations/findings

Headache

Dizziness

Fainting

Fatigue

Irritability

Difficulty in concentrating

Dyspnea

Palpitations

Syncope

Complaints of feeling cold

Loss of color in nails and palms of hands

Laboratory/diagnostic studies

Decreased Hgb and Hct (dehydration may raise Hgb/Hct); if precipitious drop in Hgb, may be caused by hemorrhaging

CBC and platelet count

Reticulocyte count

ABO, Rh compatability

Mean cell volume (MCV)

Mean cell hemoglobin (MCH)

Mean cell hemoglobin concentration (MCHC)

Bone marrow aspirate

Total iron-binding capacity (TIBC)

Potential complications

Severe anemia can result in hypotension and myocardial infarction

Medical Management

IV fluids

Intake and output

ECG

Packed RBCs

Nursing diagnoses/interventions/evaluation

■ **NDX:** Potential activity intolerance related to anemia

Note signs and symptoms of fatigue, shortness of breath, tachycardia on exertion, and/or dizziness

Adjust ADLs to match energy level

Monitor laboratory data

    Hgb and Hct

    MCV, MCH, MCHC, reticulocyte count

Anticipate time of nadir after chemotherapy (see Table 14-6)

Provide adequate periods of rest and sleep

    Plan nursing activities to avoid interrupting sleep

    Provide activity-free periods throughout the day for rest

    Schedule examinations and tests carefully

Conserve patient's energy for desired activities

    Assist with meal preparation

    Keep needed items within reach

    Assist with hygiene measures

    Plan activities after rest periods

Gradually increase activity under supervision as problem resolves

Keep patient warm

    Encourage use of warm robes, socks, and clothing

    Provide extra blankets; cotton sheets are often more comfortable

Assess neurological status each shift

Skin: pallor, petechiae, purpura, jaundice

Nailbeds: pallor, blanching

Mucous membranes: pallor, petechiae

Bones: tenderness over ribs and sternum

Take and record vital signs each shift

Assess respiratory and cardiac status each shift; report tachycardia, irregular cardiac sounds, and presence of wheezes or rales

Place patient at 60-degree angle to facilitate breathing; position with pillows if indicated

Administer oxygen therapy as ordered

Assess extremities, abdomen, and sacrum for presence of edema; report positive findings

Observe safety precautions: instruct patient to sit at side of bed before getting up; change position slowly

Provide nutritious diet high in iron

Plan rest periods after meals

Administer blood products when ordered (p. 152); one unit of blood will usually raise Hgb 1 g/dl

Monitor for reaction to blood
  Hives
  Chills
  Elevated temperature

Expected outcome/evaluation

Patient demonstrates a progressive increase in activity tolerance while maintaining physiological response within acceptable range

■ **NDX:** Knowledge deficit regarding lack of information about anemia and home care management

Teach patient about the relationship between Hgb and availability of oxygen as required for normal tissue function

Teach signs and symptoms of anemia to report to physician

Emphasize importance of eating foods high in protein, vitamins, and minerals, which are necessary for RBC production

Explain need to include foods high in iron, vitamin, B_{12}, and folic acid

Arrange for dietitian to teach patient and significant other foods to include in diet

Discuss methods to conserve energy
  Planned rest periods
  Adequate rest
  Activities planned after rest periods
  Assisting with ADLs
  Keeping needed items within reach

Explain need to change position slowly; use appliances (walker bars, etc.) for movement if indicated

Emphasize importance of continuing to perform ADLs and other desired activities to tolerance

Emphasize importance of follow-up care

Emphasize the importance of preventing secondary problems related to tissue hypoxia: infection: tissue breakdown, and/or blood loss

Expected outcome/evaluation

Patient demonstrates knowledge of factors that contribute to anemia and measures to prevent anemia, and demonstrates adequate oxygen saturation of tissue

Gastrointestinal
NAUSEA, VOMITING, AND ANOREXIA

Caused by physiological changes resulting from cancer, the toxicities of radiation therapy or chemotherapy, and/or psychological expectation

Assessment
Observations/findings

Time of onset of nausea and vomiting before or after chemotherapy administration or radiation therapy
  Duration
  Severity

Possible cause
  Anticipation
  Foods
  Bowel obstruction
  Other medications
  Brain metastasis
Vomitus: amount, frequency, character, color
Nutritional status (p. 3): weight loss, decreased food/fluid intake
Dehydration
  Dry mucous membranes and skin
  Poor skin turgor
  Sunken, soft eyeballs
  Concentrated urine; decreased output
Antiemetics: type, frequency, and method of administration

Laboratory/diagnostic studies

Electrolytes
CBC

Potential complications

Severe dehydration
Electrolyte imbalance
Malnutrition

Medical Management

Antiemetics
Sedatives/hypnotics
IV fluids/parenteral nutrition

Nursing diagnoses/interventions/evaluation

■ **NDX:** Altered nutrition: less than body requirements related to nausea, vomiting, and/or anorexia

General

Remove food trays as soon as patient has eaten
Be aware that flowers and scents may be noxious
Instruct personnel and visitors to avoid wearing colognes and perfumes or using tobacco products if these are noxious to patient
Provide oral hygiene materials
  Keep dentifrice and mouth rinse pleasing to patient within reach
  Encourage and assist with dental and oral care before and after meals and especially after vomiting

Nausea and vomiting

Instruct patient and/or significant other about drugs that are known to cause severe emetic action, such as cisplatin and nitrogen mustard
Instruct patient and/or significant other about measures used to minimize side effects
Assess history of nausea and vomiting
Assess for known or probable preexisting disease states such as diabetes or hypercalcemia

Administer antiemetics before administration of agents and every 4 to 6 hr for 24 hr rather than as needed

Administer antihistamines or barbiturates combined with an antiemetic as ordered to decrease stimulation of the vomiting center in the brain

If metoclopramide (Reglan) is given, assess for extrapyramidal side effects; keep diphenhydramine (Benadryl) available to counteract side effects

If dexamethasone (Decadron) is given, administer slowly to prevent sensations of hot flushes and burning in perineal area

Lorazepam (Ativan) may be given as an amnesic during chemotherapy administration to help control nausea and vomiting

Provide safety measures when administering these medications

Give chemotherapy in late afternoon or at night when possible

Continually evaluate effectiveness of antiemetics to help patient find the most effective combinations of drugs

Teach patient and/or significant other methods to prevent nausea and vomiting

Small, frequent meals

Small dietary intake before treatment

Avoidance of greasy or spicy foods

Rest periods before and after meals

Quiet, restful environment

Monitor laboratory values, CBC, electrolytes

Monitor vital signs

Maintain chart of onset of symptoms, reaction to varying dosage of medication, and frequency of administration

Marijuana may be prescribed

Monitor intake and output

Administer IV replacement fluids as ordered

Weigh patient daily at same time with same clothing and scale

Experiment with several methods to reduce or alleviate nausea and/or vomiting before or after chemotherapy

Withhold food and fluids for 4 to 6 hr

Eat a light, bland meal

Eat a normal meal

Take only fluids for 4 to 6 hr

Eat dry foods only

Assist patient with belching air swallowed during feeding

Avoid motions conducive to nausea (rapid or frequent change of position)

After chemotherapy

Take liquids only

Eat dry foods only

Use methods of diversion to distract patient

Animated conversation

Absorbing projects or activities

Use other methods to prevent onset or reduce severity of symptoms

Relaxation methods

Rhythmic breathing exercises

Imagery experiences

Self-hypnosis

Behavior modification techniques

Place patient in well-ventilated room and control odors

Room should be away from food preparation area and soiled linen and waste product storage

Remove trash frequently

Empty and remove emesis basin, bedpans, and urinals after use

Anorexia

Plan appetizing meals based on patient's preference

Serve food attractively arranged and at proper temperature

Avoid liquids with meals

Provide foods high in carbohydrates to promote earlier emptying of stomach

Cool foods that are bland, soft, and odorless may be tolerated

Sweet foods are often preferred

Add calories and nutrients by adding supplements to food (e.g., high-protein supplements, dry milk products)

Encourage patient to chew food well to ensure easier digestion

Serve main meal when patient can best tolerate food

Expected outcome/evaluation

Patient maintains stable weight or increases weight and improves caloric intake and nutritional value of food ingested

■ **NDX:** Knowledge deficit related to lack of information about the control of nausea and vomiting and measures to improve nutrition

Teach method and rationale of all aspects of ongoing care to be implemented at home

Emphasize importance of maintaining adequate food and fluid intake

Emphasize importance of reporting the following to physician or nurse

Continuous vomiting for 24 hr without food or fluid intake

Signs and symptoms of dehydration

Feeling of extreme stomach fullness and/or abdominal pain relieved by vomiting

Teach name of medication, dosage, frequency of administration, purpose, and toxic or side effects; if medication causes drowsiness, caution patient to avoid driving and participating in activities that require mental alertness for safety

Emphasize importance of follow-up outpatient care

Expected outcome/evaluation

Patient demonstrates knowledge of measures to control nausea and vomiting and measures to improve nutritional status, and exhibits clinical improvement in nutritional/hydration status

STOMATITIS/MUCOSITIS

stomatitis *Temporary inflammatory response of the oral mucosa to the cytotoxic effects of chemotherapy and/or radiation; may progress to ulcerative bleeding and secondary infection*
mucositis *Temporary inflammatory response of mucous membrane*

Assessment
Observations/findings

Buccal mucosa
  General erythema
  Swelling
  Pain
  Bleeding
  Ulceration
  Infected lesions
    Candida albicans: soft whitish patches; may be localized or extensive
    Herpes simplex: painful clusters of vesicles or ulceration
    Gram positive: dry, brownish yellow, circular, raised eruptions
    Gram negative: creamy white, raised, moist, nonpurulent painful ulcer
Lips
  Red fissures at corners of mouth
  Edema
  Surface abnormalities on palpation
Changes in taste
Ability to chew and swallow
Hydration status

Laboratory/diagnostic studies

CBC, platelet count
Cultures of oral cavity

Potential complications

Infections caused by bacteria, fungi, and/or viruses
Pain associated with mucositis
Malnutrition
Dehydration
Electrolyte imbalance

Medical Management

Antibacterial agents
Antifungal agents
Antiviral agents

Diet: may require parenteral nutrition
Analgesics

Nursing diagnoses/interventions/evaluation

■ **NDX:** Potential for altered oral mucous membranes related to chemotherapy*

Establish oral hygiene regimen at initiation of chemotherapy, especially if patient is receiving 5-fluouracil (5-FU), methotrexate, or bleomycin
Assess oral cavity daily with tongue blade and light, noting color, moisture, and presence of lesions
Note color, amount, and consistency of saliva
Institute prophylactic oral hygiene regimen before, within 30 min after each meal, and q2h to 4h during waking hours
  Brush with soft-bristled toothbrush and nonabrasive toothpaste
  Use foam stick moistened with mouthwash to remove debris from mucosa if unable to tolerate brush or if platelet count is greatly decreased
  Use mouthwashes with no alcohol content
  Remove dentures and bridges, and cleanse following oral hygiene regimen
  Keep mucosa moist by frequent fluid intake and eating soft, moist food; suggest saliva substitute
Obtain order for mild analgesia if pain is present
Assess history of alcohol use, tobacco use, radiation therapy, and previous and current treatment with chemotherapy
Teach patient about oral complications of chemotherapy, how to examine mouth, and complete oral care

Expected outcome/evaluation

Oral mucosa remains clean and moist

■ **NDX:** Impaired tissue integrity related to stomatitis, pharyngitis/esophagitis, and/or rectal or vaginal mucositis secondary to chemotherapy

Stomatitis

NOTE: Stomatitis generally occurs 5 to 7 days after chemotherapy and persists for up to 10 days
If mild stomatitis occurs
  Culture oral cavity
  Assess oral cavity q8h
Encourage oral hygiene regimen q2h during waking hours and q6h during the night
  Brush with soft-bristled toothbrush and nonabrasive toothpaste q4h
  Use dilute nonalcohol mouthwash or normal saline: swish, gargle, and expectorate
  Baking soda (1 tsp in 8 oz of water): swish, gargle, and expectorate

---

*Nursing management will depend on severity of condition.

Use toothette or cotton-tipped applicator to remove mucus and debris

Apply lip lubricant q2h during waking hours

Assess need for use of antifungal or antibacterial agents

Topical anesthetics such as viscous lidocaine (Xylocaine) or Orabase may be used before meals for discomfort

Use mild analgesic q3h to 4h

Encourage bland diet high in protein

Encourage fluid to 2 L/day; avoid citrus juices

If severe stomatitis occurs:

Request order for culture for oral cavity

Assess oral cavity q8h

Practice oral hygiene q1h to 2h, including

Cleaning of teeth with soft-bristled toothbrush, toothette, or gauze soaked in mouthwash—normal saline mixture

Use of antifungal and/or antibacterial agents

Use of topical anesthetics such as equal parts diphenhydramine (Benadryl) elixir (25 mg), Maalox, and viscous lidocaine (Xylocaine)

Use of moderate to strong analgesic q3h to 4h

Encourage diet (pureed) and liquids high in protein

If patient has difficulty in eating and maintaining fluid intake, parenteral nutrition may be necessary

If oral hygiene is difficult because of pain in oral cavity, encourage patient to rinse with 1 tsp viscous lidocaine 15 min before oral hygiene

If patient is unable to brush or rinse, irrigate mouth with syringe or soft rubber catheter using saline and water q3h to 4h

Gently clean lips with saline solution

If oral candidiasis is present, instruct patient to swish and swallow an oral suspension of nystatin (Mycostatin)

Teach patient how to examine mouth and do oral care

Pharyngitis/esophagitis

Assess for difficulty in swallowing and for infection

Antacids may be helpful

Obtain physician's order for Sucralfate

Rectal or vaginal mucositis

Instruct female patients to report any pain, ulceration, or bleeding of mucous membrane lining perineum or vagina

Instruct patient to include frequent perineal washing after voiding; pat dry

Instruct patient to use sitz baths

Caution patient to avoid douches

Tell patient to avoid sexual activity while symptomatic

Instruct male patient to report signs and symptoms involving perineum

Follow above regimen

Expected outcome/evaluation

Demonstrates oral care regimen and intact oral mucosa,

states relief of oral and esophageal pain, and exhibits healing of mouth and esophagus

Demonstrates rectal and vaginal mucosa care and exhibits healing of mucositis

DIARRHEA

Passage of frequent stools of a soft or liquid consistency with or without discomfort caused by effects of chemotherapy on epithelium

Assessment
Observations/findings

Frequent stools

Watery

Bloody

Containing mucus

Tarry

Dehydration

Dry mucous membranes

Poor skin turgor

Decreased urine output

Laboratory/diagnostic studies

CBC, electrolytes

Stool cultures

Potential complications

Electrolyte imbalance

Dehydration

Malnutrition

GI bleeding

Medical Management

Antidiarrheals

Antispasmodics

IV fluids/parenteral nutrition

Nursing diagnoses/interventions/evaluation

■ **NDX:** Diarrhea related to mucosal changes secondary to chemotherapy

Assess usual pattern of elimination, including use of laxatives

Determine other probable causes of diarrhea, such as inappropriate diet, treatment side effects, infection, stress, or disease progression

Evaluate hydration and electrolyte status

Monitor intake and output, weight, and electrolytes

Assess frequency, character, and volume of stool

Assess abdomen, including bowel sounds; note distention, cramping, or flatus

Assess perineal/perianal region for skin status

Adjust diet as appropriate; include bananas and cheese; avoid hot liquids, coffee, fresh fruits, and prune juice

Include foods high in potassium if weakness is present and laboratory values indicate a low potassium level

Encourage increased fluid intake of 3 L/day if not contraindicated; suggest liquids that contain electrolytes, such as Gatorade, grape juice, and fruit drinks

Administer medications that control diarrhea, such as Kaopectate or Lomotil as ordered

Observe and report early signs of constipation

Establish protocol for care of perineal area

> Gently clean area with water and mild soap after each stool; dry thoroughly and inspect for breakdown
>
> Apply ointments as indicated
>
> Use sitz baths as indicated
>
> Use skin barrier as needed

Check and record all stools for

> Frequency
>
> Amount
>
> Consistency
>
> Presence of blood, overt or occult

Teach patient to perform perineal care after each defecation

> Use povidone-iodine wash or mild soap and water
>
> Wash with soft cloths, front to back for women
>
> Dry by gentle patting with soft toweling
>
> Wash and dry hands well

Perform perineal care if patient is unable to do

Apply medication to perineum as ordered

Teach patient to test stool for blood after each bowel movement

Assess and record status of perineal area at least each shift; q4h if frequency of stools increases

Weigh patient daily at same time with same clothing and scale

Consult with physician to determin possibility of interrupting treatment until diarrhea is controlled

Assess for edema; third spacing of fluids may occur from protein deficiency and electrolyte imbalances

Expected outcome/evaluation

Patient achieves normal bowel consistency and pattern

■ **NDX:**   Knowledge deficit related to lack of information about methods for control of diarrhea

Discuss signs and symptoms of diarrhea that must be reported to physician

Emphasize importance of maintaining oral fluid intake of 3000 ml/day unless contraindicated

Explain need to avoid diet high in fiber and roughage

Explain need to take prescribed medication during episodes of diarrhea

Explain need to avoid over-the-counter medications without checking with physician or nurse

Ensure that patient and/or significant other demonstrates

Method of performing perineal care after each bowel movement; soft cloths or tissues may be used

Handwashing technique

Method of testing stools for occult blood

Expected outcome/evaluation

Patient demonstrates knowledge of methods to correct and control diarrhea; achieves normal elimination pattern and consistency of stool

CONSTIPATION

Passage of irregular, infrequent hard feces; may be caused by disease process, chemotherapy, or other factors

Assessment
Observations/findings

Absence of stool for more than 3 days

Difficult, painful stool evacuation

Stool

> Hard, dry
>
> Red-streaked

Absence of bowel sounds

Laboratory/diagnostic studies

Depends on cause

Potential complications

Ileus

Medical Management

Stool softeners

Hydration: oral or parenteral

Laxatives or enemas if not contraindicated

Nursing diagnoses/interventions/evaluation

■ **NDX:**   Constipation related to chemotherapy

Assess usual pattern of elimination, including use of laxatives

Identify factors that could alter usual pattern of elimination, such as immobility, chemotherapeutic drugs (vincristine, vinblastine), opiate/narcotic analgesics, low-fiber diet, or inadequate fluid intake

Assess for presence of associated signs and symptoms, such as flatus, distention, or discomfort

Assess for fecal impaction

Evaluate and record time and character of bowel elimination daily

Auscultate abdomen for bowel sounds each shift

Administer enema type, amount, and solution as ordered; digital removal of feces may be necessary—follow hospital policy and procedure

If no spontaneous stool occurs within 24 hr after enema, administer stool softeners, laxative, or suppository as ordered

Monitor intake and output

Force fluids to 3000 ml/24 hr unless contraindicated

Maintain diet high in fiber and bulk

Encourage ambulation and exercise to tolerance

Perform ROM exercises q4h to 8h if patient is immobile

Provide privacy when needed

    Assist with ambulation to bathroom

    Screen patient in bed

    Do not schedule appointments or examinations at time of patient's usual evacuation

Perform perineal care after bowel movement

Assess condition of perineum daily

Apply medication to rectal area as ordered

■ **NDX:** Knowledge deficit related to lack of information about methods to prevent constipation

Emphasize importance of noting daily bowel function and consistency of stool

Discuss/demonstrate methods to enhance daily bowel movements, especially when taking vinca alkaloid medication

    Take stool softener and laxative as ordered

    Maintain fluid level at 3000 ml/24 hr unless contraindicated

    Eat diet high in fiber

    Administer enema if no bowel movement occurs in 3 days

Explain need to report to physician if these methods fail

Explain need to avoid over-the-counter medications without checking with physician

Expected outcome/evaluation

Patient demonstrates knowledge of methods to promote adequate bowel elimination; achieves regular elimination pattern and consistency of stools

Integumentary
DERMATOLOGICAL

hypersensitivity reactions *Reactions to antineoplastic agents; can be very serious and/or life threatening, particularly if an anaphylactic reaction occurs; drugs most often associated with an anaphylactoid reaction include asparaginase, cisplatin (infrequent), and bleomycin*

hyperpyrexia *Associated with bleomycin, especially in patients with lymphoma*

erythema (Adria flaré) *Associated with doxorubicin; the flare usually results when the drug is too concentrated of if the patient has very sensitive skin*

Assessment
Observations/findings
GENERAL

Urticaria
Angioedema
Bronchospasm
Abdominal cramping
Hypotension
Hyperpigmentation
Maculopapular rash
Vesicle formation
Acne
Thinning of skin and striae
Petechiae
Ecchymosis
Hives
Pruritus
Desquamation
Jaundice
Photosensitivity
Nail changes
    Horizontal or longitudinal banding
    Thickening of nailbed
Radiation "recall" phenomena
Blue discoloration of vein

HYPERPYREXIA

High fever

ERYTHEMA (ADRIA FLARÉ)

Itching
Redness (diffuse or streak above the vein)
Urticaria

Medical Management

GENERAL

Diphenhydramine (Benadryl)
Epinephrine
Parenteral corticosteroids

HYPERPYREXIA

Acetaminophen
Fluid intake

ERYTHEMA (ADRIA FLARÉ)

Ice pack to affected area

Nursing diagnoses/interventions/evaluation

■ **NDX:** Impaired skin integrity related to adverse effects of antineoplastic agents

Review patient's allergy history
Monitor vital signs and mental status

Observe patient throughout administration of drug

Ensure that appropriate drugs and equipment are immediately available for possible emergency use; in the event of an anaphylactoid reaction, have the following available

Diphenhydramine (Benadryl)

Epinephrine

Oxygen

Airway

Suction equipment

Be fully aware of facility procedure to follow in the event of such a reaction

For Adria flaré

At first signs of itching or redness, reduce the amount of drug being given (e.g., if giving 1 ml, reduce to ½ ml); flush vein well and continue administering drug; if erythema and urticaria occur, stop IV and apply ice pack; start fresh IV and administer additional drug

For hyperpyrexia

Give acetaminophen q4h as ordered

Push oral fluids

Advise patient to report adverse reactions immediately

Assess skin condition q8h, especially axillary and breast folds, groin, perirectal area, and dependent extremities

Assist with daily bath prn

Use antibacterial soaps and soft cloths

Rinse and dry well

If using lotions, do not leave skin moist

Keep linens dry and wrinkle free

Teach and assist with perianal care after each elimination

Use soft towels or cloths

Ensure that area is kept dry

Advise patient to wear cotton clothing and underwear

Teach handwashing technique to be used after elimination and prn

Caution patient to avoid bumps, bruising, cuts, and scratches

Explain importance of skin care to patient

Caution patient to avoid use of sharp objects: razors, cuticle scissors, etc.

Explain need to always wear slippers or shoes when out of bed

Caution patient to avoid tight or constricting clothing

Caution patient to avoid use of rings and watches when possible; moisture and bacteria collect underneath, and sharp edges can cause scratches or cuts

Avoid IM injections when possible

Central line may be ordered and inserted to avoid multiple IV injections—perform daily central line care if inserted

Consolidate laboratory work; use fingersticks when possible; cleanse skin with povidone-iodine before venipuncture

Avoid excessive sunlight for photosensitivity; use of sunscreens is helpful

Expected outcome/evaluation

Patient achieves and maintains skin integrity

ALOPECIA

Temporary loss of body hair as a result of chemotherapeutic agents that interact with cells that are in the anaphase of cell cycle (85% to 90% of total scalp hair cells at any one time); hair loss in area of radiotherapy; dose-dependent antineoplastics associated with alopecia include cyclophosphamide, doxorubicin, and vinblastine; antineoplastics associated with thinning rather than total hair loss include bleomycin, vincristine, 5-FU, and etoposide

Assessment
Observations/findings

Hair loss

Scalp especially affected early

Long-term therapy

Axilla

Extremities

Pubis

Alterations in body image

Medical Management

Ice cap (patient with solid tumors)

Nursing diagnoses/interventions/evaluation

■ **NDX:** Body image disturbance related to physical changes caused by chemotherapy

Establish therapeutic nurse-patient relationship

Inform patient in advance about impending hair loss; hair loss varies among individuals

Have patient obtain wigs, scarves, hats, or caps before hair loss begins

Hair loss to scalp begins about 10 days after scalp is irradiated

Understand that hair loss usually begins 1 to 2 weeks after single dose of chemotherapy; maximal loss will occur 1 to 2 months after beginning therapy

Stress temporary nature of hair loss

Complete regrowth is usual after chemotherapy is completed

Regrowth can begin during treatment

Tell patient to expect alterations in texture and color (physiology of hair follicle is changed by drugs)

Assess patient's perception of effect of hair loss

Short hairstyles may be preferred

Beginning hair loss may not be readily noticeable

Patient comfort may be increased by a short hair style when maximal amount of hair is falling out

Stress importance of periodic rather than continuous use of wigs to allow scalp to "breathe"

Assist with gentle scalp care during susceptible period

Wash hair with pH-balanced shampoo

Expose hair and scalp to air as much as possible

Application of ice bags and tourniquets around hairline may assist in minimizing hair loss (controversial)

Be aware that efficacy of these procedures has not been proved

Understand that these procedures are never used when patient has a widely metastatic tumor such as leukemia, lymphoma, or myeloma or scalp tumor implants

Be aware that these procedures, if used, could possibly create a tumor cell sanctuary in the scalp

Never use these procedures when administering drugs by IV infusion or oral route

Apply ice cap or ice bag (e.g., chipped ice in plastic bag) to scalp when ordered; usually applied 20 to 30 min before administration of IV push medication, during, and for 20 min after completion of administration

Apply tourniquet or inflatable scalp pressure cuff when ordered; usually applied during drug administration and for 5 to 10 min after completion

Manage pain as indicated and/or ordered

Headache is usually experienced with ice cap

Assess effectiveness of pain relief measure(s)

Ensure that patient and/or significant other knows and understands

Need to discuss feelings related to perceptions of hair loss

Importance of gentle hair and scalp care

To expose scalp to air as much as possible

That hair loss will be temporary throughout course of treatment

To avoid use of dyes, color rinses, permanents, and bleaches until such time as indicated by condition of scalp, hair, and physician's direction

■ **NDX:** Potential impaired skin integrity secondary to alopecia

Wash scalp with mild soap and water

Use soft-bristled hairbrush to reduce pull on hair

Use mild oil (mineral) to lubricate scalp and reduce itching

Reduce exposure to sun by using a sunscreen and/or wearing hat or cap

Expected outcome/evaluation

Verbalizes acceptance of temporary body change

Demonstrates care of scalp area

Cardiotoxicity

Cardiac damage caused by toxicity of antineoplastic medications

Assessment
Observations/findings

Tachycardia

Extrasystoles

ST-T wave changes

Transient ECG changes

Thirty percent decrease in limb-lead QRS voltage

Predisposing medications

Doxorubicin (Adriamycin)

Daunorubicin (Daunomycin)

Concurrent use of cyclophosphamide

Predisposing factors

Previous radiation therapy near heart

Aortic stenosis

Uncontrolled hypertension

Distended neck veins

Gallop heart rhythm

Ankle edema

Laboratory/diagnostic studies

ECG

Cardiac enzymes

Chest x-ray examination

Echocardiogram

Radionuclide angiography

Percutaneous endomyocardial biopsy

Potential complications

CHF

Cardiomyopathy

Medical Management

Serial ECG

Oxygen therapy

Cardiac glycosides

Nursing diagnoses/interventions/evaluation

■ **NDX:** Altered tissue perfusion: cardiopulmonary related to chemotherapy

Monitor pulse rate and rhythm

Note significant variation in vital signs, skin color, temperature, sensorium, decreased urine output, and dyspnea

Be aware that by the time cardiac toxicity is clinically detectable, it is often irreversible and debilitating

Be aware of agents that place patient at risk for cardiotoxicity, such as doxorubicin (adult total cumulative dose not to exceed 450 to 550 mg/m^2) and daunorubicin (total cumulative dose is 550 mg/m^2); see Heart Failure (p. 101)

Be aware that weekly low-dose injection of doxorubicin and continuous infusions may be associated with less cardiotoxicity

Expected outcome/evaluation

Patient demonstrates minimized cardiac dysrhythmias or decompensation

Pulmonary Toxicity

Respiratory difficulties, temporary or chronic, related to chemotherapeutic toxicities; chemotherapeutic drugs typically associated with pulmonary toxicity include bleomycin, busulfan, and carmustine

Assessment
Observations/findings

Toxicities associated with bleomycin include pneumonitis and interstitial fibrosis
Persons over 70 years of age who receive total cumulative dose of greater than 400 to 500 units are at greatest risk
Fine, crackling basilar rales
Dyspnea at rest, hypoxemia
Tachypnea, fever
Headache
Malaise
Pneumonia (noninfectious)
Pulmonary edema
Pulmonary fibrosis
Predisposing factors
   Preexisting pulmonary disease
   Radiation therapy
   Pulmonary conditions: infection, edema, emboli
   Dry, hacking cough
   Adverse pulmonary changes are also associated with cyclophosphamide (Cytoxan) in combination with bleomycin, mitomycin, melphalan, and procarbarzine
   History of smoking

Laboratory/diagnostic studies

Pulmonary function tests
Arterial blood gases
Chest x-ray examination

Potential complications

Pneumonitis
Interstitial fibrosis

Medical Management

Steroids
Antimicrobials
Bronchodilators
Oxygen

Nursing diagnoses/interventions/evaluation

■ **NDX:** Impaired gas exchange related to adverse effects of chemotherapy

Be aware that once pulmonary changes are clinically detected, the disease course is often progressive
Observe for shortness of breath
Auscultate chest for breath sounds q4h during course of chemotherapy; report abnormal breath sounds immediately
Check T, P, R, and BP q4h; report temperature of 100.4° F (38° C) or above
Monitor pulmonary function tests as ordered
Teach and assist patient to turn, cough, and deep breathe q4h
Administer oxygen cautiously when ordered; high-dose oxygen may increase reaction, especially that caused by bleomycin
Force fluids to 3000 ml/day unless contraindicated
Administer IV fluid therapy as ordered
Measure intake and output q8h
Administer medications as ordered: corticosteroids, bronchodilators, antimicrobials
See Adult Respiratory Distress Syndrome (ARDS) (p. 225)

Expected outcome/evaluation

Patient maintains optimal pulmonary function

■ **NDX:** Ineffective airway clearance related to adverse effects of chemotherapy

Encourage fluids to 2 to 3 L/day if not contraindicated
Assist with turning, coughing, and deep-breathing exercises q2h to 4h
Assess chest sounds and respiratory movement q8h
Teach necessity of raising secretions and expectorating vs. swallowing
Assit with nebulizer treatments and respiratory physiotherapy

Expected outcome/evaluation

Patient demonstrates improved ventilation and oxygenation of tissue
Secretions are removed, and airway patency is maintained

Renal
NEPHROTOXICITY

Dysfunction in any part of the renal system in the presence of chemotherapeutic agents that are excreted through the kidneys or act on the lining of the renal system; antineoplastic agents associated with renal dysfunction include cisplatin, methotrexate, mitomycin, 5-azatadine, nitrosoureas, and high-dose cyclophosphamide

Assessment
Observations/findings

Dysuria, frequency, urgency
Hematuria (mild to severe), proteinuria
Oliguria, anuria
Neuromuscular irritability
Muscle weakness
Tremors, personality change
Elevated uric acid
Hyperkalemia, hyperphosphatemia
Hypocalcemia, hypomagnesemia
Hyponatremia
Elevated BUN, serum creatinine, and creatinine clearance
Hypertension, headache, nausea, vomiting

Laboratory/diagnostic studies

Electrolytes, serum BUN, and serum creatinine
Creatinine clearance
Uric acid, calcium, magnesium
Cystoscopy

Potential complications

Renal damage

Medical Management

IV fluid (titrate according to output)
Intake and output
Medications
    Bicarbonate
    Allopurinol
    Antihypertensives
    Osmotic diuretics
    Antiemetics

Nursing diagnoses/interventions/evaluation

■ **NDX:** Altered tissue perfusion: renal related to chemotherapy

Ensure adequate hydration and diuresis 24 hr before, during, and 24 to 48 hr after medication administration
Force fluids to 3000 to 4000 ml/day unless contraindicated
Enlist patient's assistance
    Provide fluids of choice and temperature
    Dietary restrictions of protein, potassium, and sodium may be necessary
    Offering small amounts frequently makes taking fluids less of a chore
    Serve attractively
If gastric distress is present, antacids may alleviate it
Use antimetics for control of nausea
Administer IV fluids as ordered: usually dextrose in saline with electrolytes; often ordered at 200 mg/hr for 5 to 6 hr before, during, and after chemotherapy infusion
Measure intake and output; report discrepancies and output of 120 ml/hr
Test urine for occult bleeding each shift during chemotherapy infusion; slow infusion and report overt hemorrhaging to physician
Monitor vital signs
Adminsiter antihypertensive drugs as ordered
Test urine pH as ordered
Administer sodium bicarbonate as ordered to maintain urine pH of 7
Adequate renal function is maintained
Laboratory tests are within normal limits

Expected outcome/evaluation

Adequate renal function is maintained; laboratory tests are within normal limits for patient

■ **NDX:** Knowledge deficit related to lack of information about measures to enhance renal function

Explain need to measure intake and output
Emphasize importance of maintaining fluid intake to 3000 to 4000 ml/day
Discuss signs and symptoms of nephrotoxicity to report to physician
Teach name of medication, dosage, frequency, and toxic or side effects to report to physician
Emphasize importance of follow-up outpatient care
Emphasize importance of taking antihypertensive drugs when ordered

Expected outcome/evaluation

Patient and/or significant other verbalizes symptoms of toxicity to report and measures to follow to ensure adequate fluid intake

HEMORRHAGIC CYSTITIS
Dose-related chemical cystitis caused by toxic effects of cyclophosphamide's or ifosfamide's metabolite on bladder mucosa

Assessment
Observations/findings

Urinary frequency
Loss of bladder tone
Occult or gross hematuria

Laboratory/diagnostic studies

Urinalysis
CBC

Potential complications

Permanent bladder damage

Medical Management

IV fluids
Bladder irrigation
Intake and output
Antiemetics
Sedatives

Nursing diagnosis/interventions/evaluation

■ **NDX:**   Altered patterns of urinary elimination: bladder irritation related to chemotherapy

Encourage high fluid intake to 3 L/day (if not contraindicated) before and 48 hr following drug administration

Encourage frequent voiding q3h to 4h; bladder should be emptied before bedtime and when patient is awake at night

Observe and report signs and symptoms of cystitis
Test urine for hematuria (dipstick)
Monitor output closely; report decrease in urine (may be indicative of SIADH secondary to drug)

Administer cyclophosphamide early in the day to prevent urine from pooling in bladder overnight

Indwelling catheter may be ordered

Through-and-through bladder irrigation may be ordered

Administer antiemetics and sedatives as needed

Teach exercises to regain bladder tone

Expected outcome/evaluation

Urinary elimination is within normal limits

Neurotoxicity

Damage to myelin sheath, paralysis of autonomic nerves, or central nervous system (CNS) damage caused by effects of chemotherapeutic medications; antineoplastic agents typically associated with neurotoxicity are the Vinca (plant) alkaloids: vincristine, vinblastine, and vindesine

Assessment
Observations/findings

Tingling
Paresthesia
Tremors
Muscle aches/pains
Muscle weakness
Difficulty in heel walking
Inability to get out of chair
Foot-drop
Ptosis
Hyporeflexia to loss of deep tendon reflexes
Ataxia
Hemiplegia
Slurred speech
Jaw pain
Hoarseness
Irritability
Seizures
Somnolence
Personality change
Coma
Arachnoiditis (in relation to intrathecal administration)
Fever
Back pain

Dizziness
Headache
Stiff neck
Vomiting
Ototoxicity
Constipation and colicky pain
Ileus
Urinary retention

Laboratory/diagnostic studies

Neurological examination
Neuroradiologic studies

Potential complications

Paralytic ileus
Obstipation
Adynamic ileus
Raynaud's phenomenon (with combination vinblastine and bleomycin)

Medical Management

Medications
Stool softeners
Laxatives
Physical therapy

Nursing diagnoses/interventions/evaluation

■ **NDX:**   Impaired physical mobility related to toxic effects of chemotherapy

Assess for weakness/numbness of arms, hands, legs, and feet

Assess for hoarseness and jaw pain

Assess for abdominal cramping, constipation, and paralytic ileus

Perform neurological assessment before administration of medication, then q4h to 8h after infusion is completed; report changes to physician immediately

Assess ability to perform ADLs

Evaluate for discomfort or pain associated with movement

Assess pain, cardiac, respiratory, and elimination status

Provide safe, uncluttered environment to prevent falls

Instruct patient to sit on side of bed, stand, and then begin to walk; provide walkers, etc., as indicated

Instruct patient to report numbness and tingling or other signs of toxicity immediately

Assure patient and significant other that changes are usually reversible when medication is stopped; discuss specifics with physician—motor weakness may take many months to resolve

Provide environment and time conducive to discussing concerns and fears

Assess color and temperature of extremities, especially hands

Assess for CNS toxicity if methotrexate or cytarabine is given intrathecally; have patient lie flat for at least 1 hr following instillation of drug

Expected outcome/evaluation

Patient achieves and maintains mobility within usual parameters

■ **NDX:** Constipation related to chemotherapy

Auscultate abdomen for bowel sounds q4h to 8h
Check and record daily bowel elimination (constipation and colicky pain that develop within 2 days of drug administration are early manifestations of toxicity)
Administer stool softeners and laxatives prophylactically
Encourage fluid to 3 L/day unless contraindicated
Encourage diet high in fiber
Measure intake and output
Administer enemas as ordered
Encourage mobility as tolerated

Expected outcome/evaluation

Maintains mobility within normal limits
Maintains normal bowel elimination

Hepatotoxicity

Dysfunction of the liver induced by chemotherapeutic medications, other hepatotoxic drugs, or preexisting hepatic conditions; because the hepatocytes are not rapidly dividing cells, they are less affected by many drugs; antineoplastic agents associated with hepatic toxicity include nitrosoureas, methotrexate, 6-mercaptopurine (6-MP), cytosine arabinoside, mithramycin, asparaginase, and interferon

Assessment
Observations/findings

Lethargy
Weakness
Pruritus
Jaundice
Dark urine
Sweet or sour odor of urine and breath
Clay-colored stools
Bleeding tendency
 Purpura
 Epistaxis
 Melena
Abdominal tenderness
Right upper quadrant pain
Anorexia
Digestive discomfort
Ascites
Generalized edema
Palmar erythema

Spider angiomas
Irritability
Apathy
Memory defects
Asterixis
Coma
Associated factors, preexisting or concurrent
 Viral hepatitis
 Abdominal radiotherapy
 Hepatic metastasis
 Hepatotoxic drugs
 Transfusion of blood products
 Graft vs. host disease (GVHD) (p. 565)

Laboratory/diagnostic studies

Elevated
 Serum transaminase
 Bilirubin
 Alkaline phosphatase
 Cholesterol
 Fibrinogen
Decreased
 Hepatic clotting factors
 Albumin
Liver function tests
Blood clotting test, CBC
Liver biopsy
Radiologic examination

Potential complications

Cirrhosis
Ascites
Hepatomegaly

Medical Management

IV fluids
Blood products
Nasogastric tube

Nursing diagnoses/interventions/evaluation

■ **NDX:** Potential impaired skin integrity secondary to pruritus

Assess skin condition each shift
Bathe patient daily; use soothing baths (e.g., use cornstarch or oil) to relieve itching
Maintain skin hydration by application of lotion after bath and twice daily, adding bath oil to water
Protect skin from irradiation
Teach distraction, relaxation, and imagery
Administer skin care as needed to decrease itching; antihistamine drugs may be ordered
Keep nails short to prevent scratching skin
Encourage fluids to 3000 to 4000 ml/24 hr unless contraindicated; fluids may be limited in presence of edema

Expected outcome/evaluation

Skin remains intact
States itching has decreased

■ **NDX:** Potential for altered protection related to altered clotting mechanisms

Assess sensorium q2h to 4h
Report changes of increased lethargy
Avoid use of drugs such as narcotics and barbiturates that cause CNS depression
Observe for signs of bleeding: hematemesis, melena, petechiae
Assess for abdominal distention; measure abdominal girth
Assess bowel sounds
Monitor vital signs and laboratory studies; if nasogastric tube is being used, maintain patency
Provide oral care; keep nostrils clean and lubricated
Maintain proper position of tube
Place in semi-Fowler's position unless contraindicated
Report changes in color, bleeding, and edema to physician
Measure intake and output
Report changes in color of urine and stool
Manage pain as indicated or ordered
Assess response to relief measure(s)
If bleeding tendency
  Avoid IM injections
  Consolidate laboratory work
  Use fingersticks when possible
  Apply pressure at puncture or IV site for 5 min after procedure has been completed; check site q15 min for four times
  Place furniture, equipment, and personal items so as to prevent injuries from falls or bumping into objects
  Administer gentle oral hygiene using toothettes or swabs
  Avoid use of harsh soaps and rough towels and cloths
  Test urine and stool for occult bleeding
Provide diet with amount of calories, carbohydrate, and protein as ordered; avoid high-fat foods
Serve meals attractively and at correct temperature; small feedings may be more tempting
Weigh patient daily at same time with same clothing and scale
Encourage activity to tolerance; assist with and teach active ROM exercises q4h
Administer medications as ordered for itching
Continue nursing measures as indicated for primary condition

Expected outcome/evaluation

Bleeding and pruritus are controlled

Gonadal Dysfunction

Testicular or ovarian dysfunction caused by adverse effects of chemotherapeutic drugs (e.g., nitrogen mustard, cyclophosphamide, chlorambucil)

Assessment
Observations/findings

Reduction of spermatocytes
Irregular menses
Amenorrhea
Menopausal symptoms: hot flushes, insomnia, irritability, dyspareunia, vaginal dryness

Laboratory/diagnostic studies

Serum follicle-stimulating hormone (FSH)
Sperm count

Potential complication

Permanent sterility

Medical Management

Estrogen (menopausal symptoms)

Nursing diagnoses/interventions/evaluation

■ **NDX:** Sexual dysfunction related to infertility caused by chemotherapy

Obtain brief sexual history, including sexual practices, sex education and attitude, and effects of disease and treatment on sexual function
Advise male patients regarding sperm banking before chemotherapy administration if appropriate
Provide contraceptive information to patients before they initiate chemotherapy if appropriate
Initiate discussion related to infertility
Encourage ventilation of feelings
Evaluate patient's and/or partner's coping skills and response to infertility
Instruct patient that infertility may be temporary or permanent (dose related)
Inform patient that sexual drive and capability usually are not physically impaired as a result of chemotherapy
Advise that antifertility effects may be reversible in some cases after therapy is terminated
Refer patient for counseling if appropriate

Expected outcome/evaluation

Patient achieves improving or satisfying sexual role function

BIOLOGICAL RESPONSE MODIFIERS

This cancer therapy is based on the theory that if the immune system recognizes tumor cells as foreign, it will mobilize and destroy them. Through research, biological and chemical agents produced by the body, biological response modifiers (BRMs) have been discovered. A BRM is any soluble substance capable of altering (or modulating) the immune system with either a stimulatory or a suppressive effect (see Figure 14-11). BRMs can affect the host-tumor response in three ways: (1) by modulating the individual's immune response to the tumor; (2) by direct

Text continued on p. 693.

TABLE 14-8. Biological Response Modifiers *(Under Investigation)*

Agent	Route of administration	Indications under investigation	Side/toxic effects	Administration and nursing indications
Calmette-Guérin bacillus (BCG)	Scarification, intradermal by Tine technique or Heaf gun	Superficial or subcutaneous melanoma	Local, inflammatory response that increases with treatment to ulceration with eschar formation Pruritus Enlarged painful nodes, malaise, mild fever	Anesthesize area Clean skin with acetone and allow to dry Choose site that is flat and near major lymph nodes to increase absorption and that is covered by clothing that does not bind Keep areas clean and dry Use nonmedicated, hypoallergenic cream to previous sites when needed
	Intravesical (bladder) Retain for 2 hours	Bladder (FDA) approved	Bladder irritation, infection, chills, fever, cough	Prior to treatment Bladder culture, Have patient limit fluids for 12 hours Void prior to administration With first and each subsequent voiding for 6 hours add bleach equal to amount voided, close cover of toilet and flush Rehydrate patient Report fever, cough, chills to physician immediately for antibiotic therapy
	Intralesional	Cutaneous melanoma	Inflammatory reaction in 4 hr; fever, myalgia, nausea, vomiting for 2-3 days Hypersensitivity reaction can occur: fever, chills, intravascular coagulation abnormalities, hypotension, and oliguria Disseminated BCG infection: persistent fever, weight loss, malaise, nausea, and vomiting Temporary, reversible hepatic dysfunction	Have antihistamines, corticosteroids, and emergency equipment available Patients with strongly positive tuberculin reaction may need diphenhydramine (Benadryl) before and after intratumor therapy Antipyretics usually control symptoms; isoniazid may be ordered

Continued.

TABLE 14-8. Biological Response Modifiers *(Under Investigation)*—cont'd

Agent	Route of administration	Indications under investigation	Side/toxic effects	Administration and nursing indications
Interferons exhibit broad antiviral, antiproliferative and immunodulatory activity	IM, IV (bolus, short-term infusion, a continuous infusion), subcutaneous, intravesical, intrathecal, or intralesional	Hairy cell leukemia (FDA approved), non-Hodgkin's lymphoma, Kaposi's sarcoma, renal cell carcinoma, malignant melanoma, multiple myeloma untreated, chronic granulocytic leukemia, mycosis furgoides, superficial bladder (intravesical), ovarian (intraperitoneal). Clinical trials for AIDS and rhino virus.	Flulike symptoms; fever (38°-40° C) 2-4 hr after injection; malaise, chills, headache, and low-grade fever may last to 20 hr after first dose Chronic fatigue, irritability, impatience, low motivation, depression; sense of doom, and paranoia with high doses Nausea, altered taste, early satiety, anorexia, arthostatic hypertension; cardiovascular symptoms with history of problems Transient pancytopenia Proteinuria with preexisting renal disease	Reconstitute according to manufacturer's directions Premedicate with acetomenophen, then q3-4h after *Avoid* aspirin, nonsteroid antiinflammatory agents, and steroids (may hinder effectiveness) Morphine may be ordered for severe chilling (rigor) lasting over 10 min Instruct patient to plan rest periods; may need to alter work habits Provide nutritional counseling Encourage fluid intake Avoid sudden position changes Evening administration may diminish side effects
Thymosin fraction V	IM, subcutaneous	Small cell lung cancer, squamous cell carcinoma of head and neck	Allergic reaction, systemic itching	Antipruritics may be administered to relieve itching
Interleukin-2 (IL-2) Adoptive immunotherapy	IV bolus, continuous IV infusion, intrahepatic infusion, peritoneal infusion	Advanced cancer in which standard therapy is ineffective (renal cell melanoma, colon, etc.)	Symptoms are usually dose related and usually reverse in 8-21 days after IL-2 Disorientation, combativeness, psychosis, anxiety Oliguria, proteinuria, elevated creatinine and BUN Anemia, thrombocytopenia Elevated bilirubin, SGOT, SGPT, LDH Erythematous rash, pruritus, desquamation	Assess baseline status of affected systems Provide safety measure, explanations and reorient Monitor intake and output; test urine for protein; monitor laboratory values Monitor for bleeding; evaluate daily laboratory values; test stool, urine, and vomitus for blood; avoid rectal manipulation and IM injections Monitor laboratory values Benadryl may be given prophylactically; assess skin daily; use water-based lotion; avoid harsh products; pat skin dry

Continued.

TABLE 14-8. Biological Response Modifiers *(Under Investigation)*—cont'd

Agent	Route of administration	Indications under investigation	Side/toxic effects	Administration and nursing indications
			Nausea, vomiting, mucositis, decreased appetite, diarrhea	Monitor dietary intake; prophylactic antiemetic usually given; antidiarrheal given as necessary; see Mucositis (p. 677), and nausea and vomiting (p. 675)
			Hypotension	Monitor vital signs qh during infusion then q4h; albumin, dopamine, or phenylephrine may be ordered
			Weight gain, peripheral edema, ascites, dysrhythmias, dyspnea, pulmonary edema	Monitor intake and output; weigh daily; measure abdominal girth with ascites; elevate extremities with edema; monitor O_2 saturation
			Fever	Acetaminophen given prophylactically Monitor temperature qh during infusion and for 24 hr Provide cooling measures as needed
			Chills	Meperidine may be ordered for chills or rigor
			Flulike symptoms	Rest; acetaminophen q4h
IL-2 and LAK Adoptive immunotherapy	IL-2 given for 3 days; collect leukocytes through lymphopheresis (for 4 to 5 days); separated lymphocytes incubated with IL-2; prepared LAK cells are infused after test dose for 3 days; IL-2 infused also and for several days after LAK infusion	Melanoma, nodular lymphomas, renal cell cancer, colorectal cancer	Fever Headache Chills Nausea	Acetaminophen usually given Meperidine administered for chills or rigor Antiemetics manage nausea
			High dosages peripheral edema, ascites, or interstitial infiltrates	Vasopressors, diuretics and careful fluid replacement may be required
			Thrombocytopenia	May require RBC transfusion Monitor for bleeding
			Mental status changes: confusion paranoia, hallucinations, severe disorientation	Provide safety measures, reorient continuously, haloperidol may be required
Lymphotoxin effects delayed hypersensitivity; allow higher doses of chemotherapy and radiotherapy	Intralesional injection in accessible tumors	Melanoma, bladder, and prostate cancer	—	—

TABLE 14-8. Biological Response Modifiers *(Under Investigation)*—cont'd

Agent	Route of administration	Indications under investigation	Side/toxic effects	Administration and nursing indications
Monoclonal antibodies Biological tracers that react with one, specific part of the antigen's surface (an epitome) Serve as carriers of antitoxin drugs, toxins, radioisotopes or other BRMs to tumor cells	IV by infusion pump	Lymphoma, lymphocytic leukemia, T-cell leukemia, cutaneous T-cell lymphoma, gastric and colon cancer and melanoma	Fever, chills, headache, flushing, urticaria, rash Bronchospasm, dyspnea, hypotension, tachycardia, anaphylactic reaction	Diphenhydramine usually controls mild allergic response Assess patient q15 min first hr; then q30 min Infusion stopped; saline; epinephrine, hydrocortisone, and diphenhydramine may be ordered; monitor vital signs; keep resuscitation equipment nearby
Tumor cell vaccines Provide active, specific immune stimulation	Intradermal	—	Fever, chills, headache, malaise Hepatitis	Acetominophen usually relieves symptoms
Colony-Stimulating Factors (CSF): G-CSF (granulocyte CSF) and GM-CSF (granulocyte-macrophage CSF) Increase the production of granulocytes and monocytes by stimulating stem cell and precursor cell replication and maturation	IV, short or continuous infusion, Subcutaneously	Bone marrow destruction: iatrogenically induced: antiviral therapy in AIDS, cancer Chemotherapy and bone marrow transplant Intrinsic states: myelodysplasia congenital cyclic neutropenia aplastic anemia, hairy cell leukemia	Fever, myalgias, bone pain, fatigue Anorexia Pericardial Pleural effusions	Acetaminophen usually controls symptoms Monitor vital signs, intake output and assess heart and breath sounds; report negative findings
Erythropoietin Increases the production of RBC	Subcutaneously	Anemias: End-stage renal disease Associated with antineoplastic chemotherapy and A2T	Fever, fatigue rare	Follow manufacturers directions Rotate sites of injection Acetaminophen usually controls symptoms

Continued.

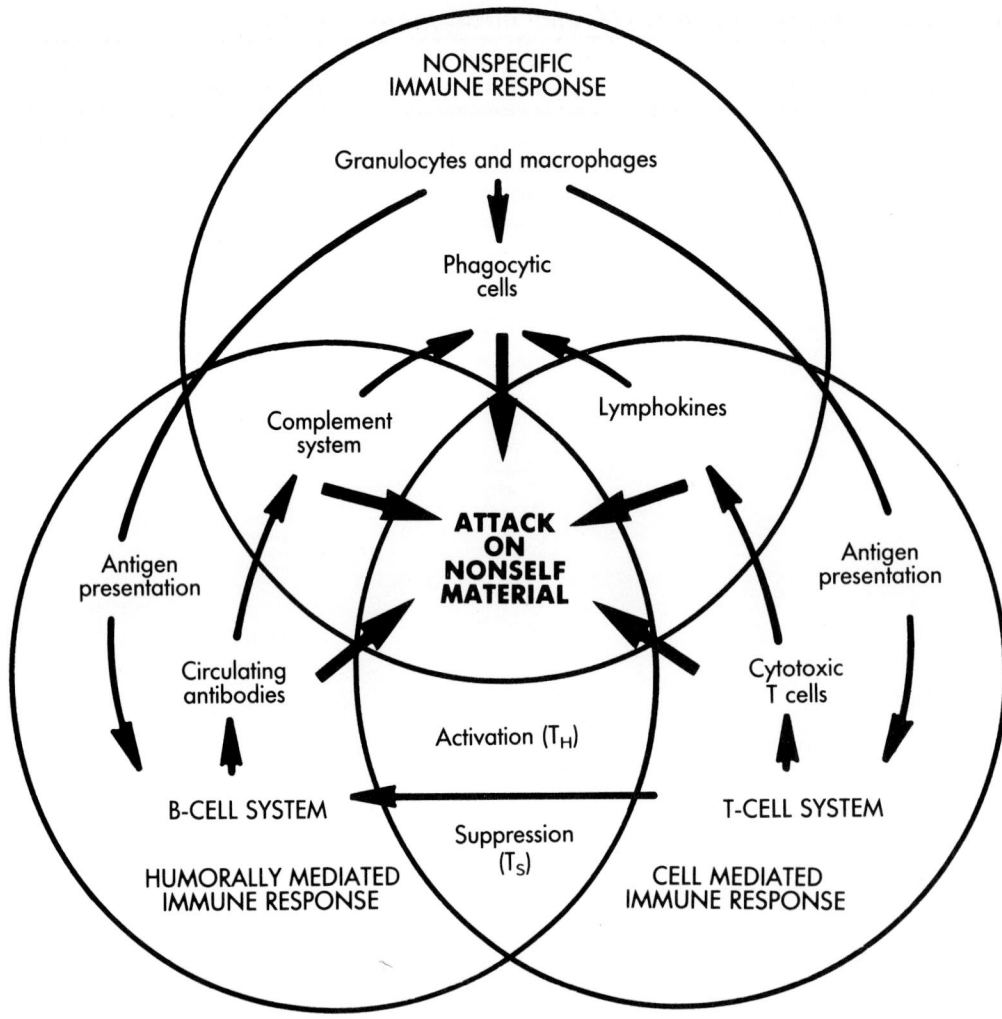

FIGURE 14-8. Interrelationship of nonspecific, humorally mediated, and cell mediated immune response systems. (From Phipps WJ, Long BC, Woods NF et al: *Medical-surgical nursing: concepts and clinical practice,* ed 4, St Louis, 1991, Mosby–Year Book.)

TABLE 14-8. Biological Response Modifiers *(Under Investigation)*—cont'd

Agent	Route of administration	Indications under investigation	Side/toxic effects	Administration and nursing indications
Tumor necrosis factor (TNF) has the capability of destroying malignant cells but not normal cells; activation of cells of the immune system has also been reported	IM, IV, bolus, short-term infusion	Metastatic melanoma, advanced renal cancer, others being studied		Agitation of the biological or rapid expulsion from a syringe may result in denaturing the molecules
			Pain, erythema at injection site	Rotate IM injection sites to reduce irritation; apply cold or warm compresses; acetaminophen may increase comfort

Continued.

TABLE 14-8. Biological Response Modifiers *(Under Investigation)*—cont'd

Agent	Route of administration	Indications under investigation	Side/toxic effects	Administration and nursing indications
			Fever, chills, fatigue, headache	Premedicate with acetaminophen, then continue q4h as needed. Encourage and monitor fluid intake during febrile episodes
			Hypotension	Monitor vital signs with BP lying and standing. Report negative findings

antitumor activity, killing or suppressing growth; (3) by altering other biological activities that indirectly affect the tumor, such as interfering with tumor cell's ability to survive or metastasize, promoting cell maturation, or interfering with transformation of normal cells into cancer cells (Table 14-8).

BIBLIOGRAPHY

Averette HE, Donato DM: Ovarian carcinoma: advances in diagnosis, staging and treatment of advanced disease, National Conference on Advances in Cancer Management, Los Angeles, Dec, 1988.

Beart RW Jr: Advances in the management of color and rectal cancer, National Conference on Advances in Cancer Management, Los Angeles, Dec, 1988.

Boronow RC: Cervical and endometrial cancers, National Conference on Advances in Cancer Management, Los Angeles, Dec, 1988.

Brady LW: Innovations in radiation oncology: experimental efforts to increase survival, National Conference on Advances in Cancer Management, Los Angeles, Dec, 1988.

Bruera E, Macdonald RN: Overwhelming fatigue in advanced cancer, *Am J Nurs*, Jan, 88(1):99, 1988.

Bruera E et al: Managing chemotherapy–induced emesis, *Am J Nurs*, March, 87(3):367, 1988.

Cady B: Advances in diagnosis, staging, and management of local-regional breast cancer, National Conference on Advances in Cancer Management, Los Angeles, Dec, 1988.

Cancer chemotherapy guidelines and recommendations for nursing education and practice, Pittsburgh, 1988, Oncology Nursing Society.

Cancer facts and figures—1988, New York, 1988, American Cancer Society.

Chemotherapy and you: a guide to self-help during treatment, NIH Pub No 86-1136, revised 1985, Bethesda, MD, National Cancer Institute

Clark J: Prevention of unsafe exposure to cytotoxic drugs, *Curr Concepts Nurs*, 2(2):3, 1988.

Cohen SM, Hollingsworth AO, and Rubin M: Another look at psychologic complications of hysterectomy, *Image* 21(1):51, 1989.

Daeffler RJ, Petrosino BM: *Manual of oncology nursing practice*, Rockville, MD, 1990, Aspen.

D'Agostino NS: Managing nutrition problems in advanced cancer, *Am J Nurs*, Jan, 89(1):50, 1989.

DeVita VT, Hellman S, and Rosenberg SA: *Cancer principles and practice of oncology*, Philadelphia, 1982, JB Lippincott.

Dillman JB: Toxicity of monoclonal antibodies in the treatment of cancer, *Semin Oncol Nurs*, May, 4(2):107, 1988.

Dodd MJ: *Suggestions for managing the side effects of chemotherapy*, East Norwalk, CT, 1987, Appleton & Lange.

Foley KM: Advances in pain management, National Conference on Advances in Management of Cancer, Los Angeles, Dec, 1988.

Foon KA: Advances in immunotherapy of cancer: monoclonal antibodies and interferon, *Semin Oncol Nurs*, May, 4(2):112, 1988.

Glaspy JA and Golde DW: The colony-stimulating factors: biology and clinical use, *Oncology*, September, 4(9):23, 1990.

Grady C: Host defense mechanisms: an overview, *Semin Oncol Nurs*, May, 4(2):86, 1988.

Groenwald SL: *Cancer nursing: principles and practice*, Boston, 1987, Jones and Bartlett.

Gulanick M et al: *Nursing care plans: nursing diagnosis and treatment*, ed 2, St Louis, 1990, Mosby–Year Book.

Hahn MB and Jassak PF: Nursing management of patients receiving interferon, *Semin Oncol Nurs*, May 4(2):95, 1988.

Hassey K: Demystifying care of patients with radioactive implants, *Am J of Nurs*, July, 85(7):788, 1985.

Hassey K: Principles of radiation safety and protection, *Semin Oncol Nurs* 4(2):23, 1987.

The Health Professional and Cancer Prevention and Detection, New York, 1988, American Cancer Society.

Irwin MM: Patients receiving biological response modifiers: overview of nursing care, *Oncol Nurse Forum*, September, 14(6):32, 1987.

Kim MJ, McFarland GK, and McLane AM: *Pocket guide to nursing diagnosis*, ed 4, St Louis, 1990, Mosby–Year Book.

Lauver D, Angerame M: Overadherence with breast self-examination recommendations, Image 22(3):148, 1990.

McFarland GK, McFarlane EA: *Nursing diagnosis and intervention: planning for patient care*, St Louis, 1989, Mosby–Year Book.

Moldawer NP and Fighin RA: Turner necrosis factor: current clinical status and implications for nursing management, *Semin Oncol Nurs*, May, 4(2):120, 1988.

Oncology Pharmacy Advisory Board: *Oncology: basic concepts for pharmacists*, Evansville, Ind, 1987, Bristol-Myers.

OSHA's new standards for hospitals' chemical hazards, *Am J Nurs*, Jan, 89(1):12, 1989.

Padavic-Shaller K: IL-Z: nursing applications in a developing science, *Semin Oncol Nurs*, May, 4(2):142, 1988.

Pagana KD, Pagana TJ: *Diagnostic testing and nursing implications*, ed 3, St Louis, 1990, Mosby–Year Book.

Portlock CS: Non-Hodgkin's lymphomas, National Conference on Advances in Management of Cancer, Los Angeles, Dec, 1988.

Psychosocial issues and cancer, *CA* 38:130, 1988.

Rogers B, Emmett EA: Handling antineoplastic agents: urine mutagenicity in nurses, *Image* 19(3):108, 1987.

Rosenberg SA: Hodgkin's disease, National Conference on Advances in Management of Cancer, Los Angeles, Dec, 1988.

Rotman M, Aziz H: Concomitant infusion chemotherapy and radiation, National Conference on Advances in Management of Cancer, Los Angeles, Dec, 1988.

Simonson GM: Caring for patients with acute myelocytic leukemia, *Am J Nurs,* March, 88(3):204, 1988.

Simpson C, Seipp CA, and Rosenburg SA: The current status and future applications of interluekin-Z and adoptive immunotherapy in cancer treatment, *Semin Oncol Nurs,* May 4(2):132, 1988.

Thelan LA, Davie JK, and Urden LD: *Textbook of critical nursing: diagnosis and management,* St Louis, 1990, Mosby–Year Book.

Thompson JM et al: *Mosby's manual of clinical nursing,* ed 2, St Louis, 1989, Mosby–Year Book.

Travaglini J, Nevidjon B: Cancer-induced oncologic emergencies, *Clin Adv Oncol Nurs* 2(1), 1990.

Walters P: Chemo: a nurse's guide to action, administration, and side effects, *RN* Feb, 53(2):52, 1990.

Woods NF, Yates BC, and Primomo J: Supporting families during chronic illness, *Image* 21(1):46, 1989.

15 CHAPTER

Perinatal/Neonatal Standards

Mother

ANTEPARTUM ASSESSMENT

Observations/findings

Age
Height
Prepregnancy weight
History of infertility
Menstrual history
   Last menstrual period (LMP)
   Interval between periods
   Expected date of confinement (EDC)
Pregnancy history
   Gravida
   Term deliveries
   Premature deliveries
   Abortions
   Stillbirths
   Date of each delivery (month and year)
      Weeks of gestation
      Duration of labor in hours
      Spontaneous or induced labor
      Type of delivery
      Children living (ages, any developmental problems)
      Multiple births
      Maternal, fetal, or neonatal complications
   BP, T, P, and R
   Fetal heart rate (FHR)
   Blood type and Rh factor
   Rubella titer
   Urine protein and glucose
   Date and results of last Papanicolaou (Pap) test
Previous major illnesses and surgeries
Current health problems
Breast changes
   Fullness
   Tingling
   Heaviness
   Darkening of areola
   Presence of colostrum
   Turgid nipples and engorged areolas with sexual stimulation
Cardiovascular changes

Increase in heart rate of 10 to 15 beats/min from baseline from 14 to 30 weeks of pregnancy
Slight decrease in BP during second trimester with increase in third trimester <15 mm Hg in either systolic or diastolic
Tendency toward dependent edema
Hematological changes during pregnancy
   Blood volume increases and peaks by 30 to 34 weeks
   Red blood cell (RBC) production accelerates
   Hgb declines because of hemodilution
   Reticulocyte count increases because of hematopoiesis
   White blood cell count (WBC) increases up to 25,000 mm³
   Total plasma proteins decrease to 3 to 3.5 g/dl (normal = 4 to 4.5 g/dl) because of fall in albumin level
   Sedimentation rate increases because of decrease in total plasma proteins
Respiratory changes
   Nasal stuffiness because of estrogen-initiated hyperemia
   Sinus stuffiness
   Prone to nose bleeds
   Increased oxygen consumption
   Decreased functional residual capacity and residual volume of air
   Increased tidal volume, minute ventilatory volume, and minute oxygen uptake
   Increased respiratory rate
Basal metabolism
   Increases by 15% to 20% at term
   Lassitude and fatigability in early pregnancy
   Heat intolerance in late pregnancy
Urinary changes
   Frequency of urination
   Increased bladder capacity
   Increased glomerular filtration rate
   Mild proteinuria
   Mild glycosuria
Gastrointestinal (GI) changes
   Tender gums
   Excessive salivation
   Transitory nausea and vomiting in first trimester
   Heartburn and acid indigestion (esophageal regurgitation and decreased emptying time)
   Unusual food preferences

Constipation
Hypercholesterolemia
Decreased gallbladder emptying time
Neurological changes
Lightheadedness or faintness in early pregnancy
Headache associated with pregnancy-induced hypertension
Sensory changes in legs with compression of pelvic nerves
Musculoskeletal changes
Decreased abdominal muscle tone
Increase in lumbosacral curve
Hypermobility of pelvic joints
Waddling gait near term
Prone to carpal tunnel syndrome
Acroesthesia (numbness and tingling of hands)
Integumentary changes
Thickened skin
Increased subdermal fat
Hyperpigmentation
Chloasma (mask of pregnancy)
Linea nigra
Increased hair and nail growth
Accelerated sebaceous and sweat gland activity
Increased fragility of cutaneous elastic tissues resulting in striae gravidarum (stretch marks)
Acne vulgaris (preexisting)
Aggravated in first trimester
Improved in third trimester
Angiomas (vascular spiders) on neck, thorax, face, and arms
Thinning and softening of fingernails and toenails
Patterns of tobacco, alcohol, and prescription/nonprescription drug use
Patterns of nutrient intake
Planned method of feeding infant
Self-esteem and perceived ability to cope with life situations
Body image resulting from physiological changes of pregnancy
Desire for participation in prepared childbirth classes
Plans for postdischarge infant care at home
Concurrent conditions
Diabetes
Cardiovascular conditions
Severe anemia
Epilepsy
Asthma or other pulmonary conditions
Drug sensitivities
Renal disorders
Sexually transmitted disease
Patterns of work or employment

Laboratory/diagnostic studies
Pregnancy test confirmation
Blood typing and Rh factor identification
Hemoglobin (Hgb) and hematocrit (Hct)
VDRL (Veneral disease research laboratories) test
Pap test (cervical cytology test)
Urinalysis
Irregular antibody screen
Rubella antibody titer
TORCH screen as indicated
SMA
Sickle cell test
GC culture at 36 weeks
Alpha fetoprotein between 10 and 16 weeks
Hepatitis BsAg
As indicated, Tb, HIV
Fasting blood sugar (FBS) screening (at 26 weeks' gestation if no high-risk factors for diabetes are present)
Glucose tolerance tests for diabetes as indicated and per facility protocol
One hour glucola at 26 weeks as indicated
Chorionic villus sampling as indicated
Amniocentesis before or at 16 weeks for genetic screening
Biophysical profile (as indicated)
Fetal breathing movements, gross body movements, fetal tone, amniotic fluid index, nonstress test

Medical Management
Uncomplicated pregnancy visit schedule
Every 4 weeks during first 28 weeks
Every 2 to 3 weeks until 36 weeks
Weekly until delivery
Nonstress testing (NST) (p. 712)
Contraction stress testing (CST) (p. 713)
Antibiotics for treatment as indicated
Prenatal vitamins and iron supplements
Counseling and other referrals as indicated for high-risk pregnancy
Genetic counseling as indicated

Nursing diagnosis/interventions/evaluation

■ **NDX:** Knowledge deficit related to lack of information about actual changes of pregnancy and potential problems (Figure 15-1)

Discuss danger signals to report to physician immediately
Any vaginal bleeding
Swelling of face or fingers
Severe or continuous headache
Dimness or blurring of vision
Muscular irritability (or convulsions)
Abdominal pain or epigastric pain
Persistent vomiting
Chills or fever
Dysuria
Diarrhea
Escape of fluid from vagina
Abrupt decrease in fetal movements during last trimester

Emphasize importance of avoiding smoking, alcohol, and illicit drugs, including opium derivatives, barbiturates, amphetamines, PCP, cocaine, marijuana, benzodiazepines

Emphasize importance of avoiding any nonprescription drugs, including aspirin and nose drops, without checking with physician and of avoiding prescription drugs that can be abused

Explain need to check with physician before traveling

Discuss methods to alleviate nausea, hemorrhoids, and/or varicose veins

Emphasize importance of ongoing outpatient care

Explain need to avoid excessive fatigue when exercising

Explain need to maintain good body mechanics when bending, lifting, or walking

Explain need to rest periodically with legs elevated

Emphasize importance of being sedentary if pregnant with two or more fetuses or if pregnancy-induced hypertension is present

Explain need to avoid use of constricting garments, especially on lower extremities

Explain need to drink adequate amounts of fluid to 3000 ml/day unless contraindicated

Emphasize importance of well-balanced diet

Explain need to wear well-fitting, supportive brassiere

Explain need to wear only low-heeled shoes if backache or unstable balance occurs with higher-heeled shoes

Emphasize importance of maintaining normal bowel habits with adequate fluid intake, reasonable exercise, and diet high in fiber

   Mild laxatives such as prune juice, milk of magnesia, bulk-producing substances, or stool softeners may be taken when necessary

   Avoid use of nonabsorbable oil preparations and any other nonprescription medications without checking with physician

Emphasize importance of avoiding intercourse when there is a threat of spontaneous abortion or premature labor

Explain need to avoid routine douching

   Never use hand bulb syringe because of danger of air embolism

   If douching is absolutely necessary, bag should not be elevated more than 2 feet above hips, and nozzle should not be inserted more than 3 inches through vulva

Discuss pros and cons of breast-feeding vs. bottle feeding

Discuss special caretaking considerations for working mothers

Expected outcome/evaluation

Patient/significant other demonstrate ability to adapt to changes of pregnancy and family verbalizes that appropriate preparations have been made for role transitions to parenthood

PREGNANCY-INDUCED HYPERTENSION (PIH; PREECLAMPSIA)

Syndrome of hypertension, edema, and proteinuria occurring during the second half of pregnancy, characteristically in primigravidas; resolves within 10 days postpartum; the etiology is unknown but could be caused by increased vasoconstrictor tone, abnormal prostaglandin action, or immunological factors

Assessment
Observations/findings
GENERAL OBSERVATIONS

Elevated BP
Proteinuria
Edema
   Face
   Fingers
   Pretibial pitting type
Irritability, emotional tension
Hyperreflexia
Nervousness

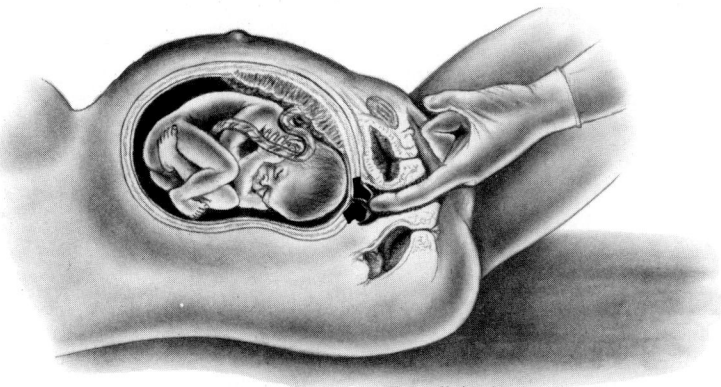
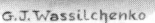
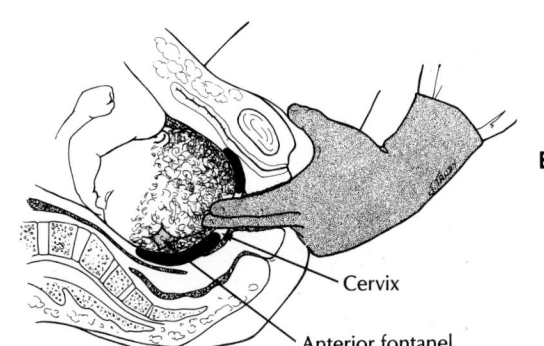

A   **B**

Cervix

Anterior fontanel

FIGURE 15-1. Vaginal examination. **A,** Undilated, unaffected cervix. Membranes intact. **B,** Palpation of sagittal suture line. Cervix effaced and partially dilated. (From Bobak IM, Jensen MD: *Essentials of maternity nursing,* ed 3, St Louis, 1991, Mosby–Year Book.)

PLACENTAL
AGING

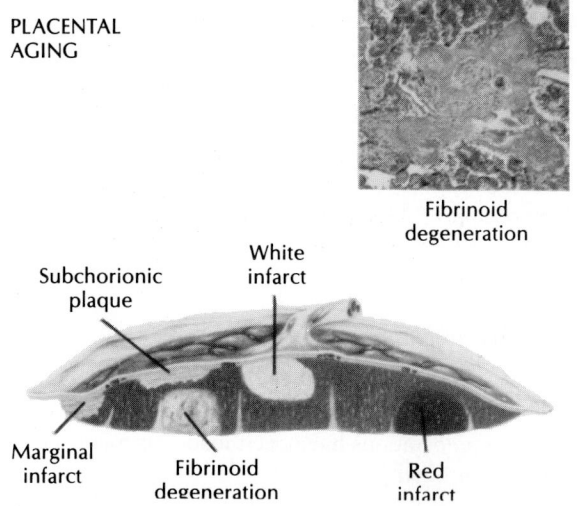

Fibrinoid
degeneration

FIGURE 15-2. Effects of severe PIH on placenta with resultant placental insufficiency. (From Bobak IM, Jensen MD, and Zalar MK: *Maternity and gynecologic care: the nurse and the family,* ed 4, St Louis, 1989, Mosby–Year Book.)

Subchorionic
plaque

White
infarct

Marginal
infarct

Fibrinoid
degeneration

Red
infarct

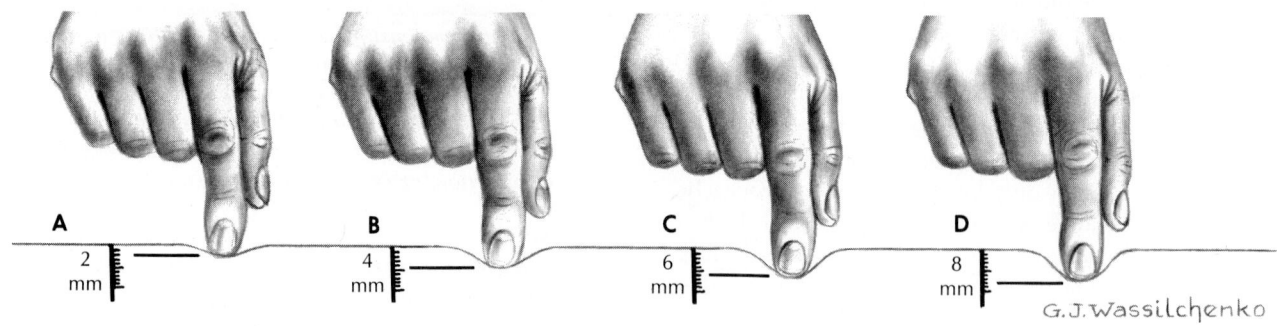

G.J.Wassilchenko

FIGURE 15-3. Assessment of pitting edema: **A,** +1; **B,** +2; **C,** +3; **D,** +4. (From Bobak IM, Jensen MD, and Zalar MK: *Maternity and gynecologic care: the nurse and the family,* ed 4, St Louis, 1989, Mosby–Year Book.)

Nausea, vomiting
Visual disturbances (scotomata, blurred vision)
Severe generalized headache
Altered level of consciousness
Epigastric pain or right upper quadrant pain
Oliguria
Pulmonary edema
Cyanosis
Onset of labor
Magnesium blood level above 7.5 mEq/L

MILD PREECLAMPSIA

BP above 140/90 mm Hg or rise in systolic pressure of 30 mm Hg above normal and in diastolic pressure of 15 mm Hg above normal on two occasions at least 6 hr apart
Proteinuria >0.3 g/L/24 hr or 1 g/L in two random specimens collected at least 6 hr apart

SEVERE PREECLAMPSIA

BP above 160/110 mm Hg or systolic pressure of 50 mm Hg above normal; diastolic pressure of 35 mm Hg above normal
Proteinuria: more than 5 g daily (or 3 + to 4 + based on semiquantitative assay)
Massive generalized edema
Cerebral or visual disturbances
Oliguria: 400 ml or less in 24 hr
Rising plasma creatinine

Laboratory/diagnostic studies

CBC, differential and platelet count
Liver enzyme (serum glutamic oxidase transaminase (SGOT), serum glutamic pyruvic transaminase (SGPT), lactate dehydrogenase (LDH), creatine phosphokinase (CPK), alkaline phosphatase
Mg^+, Ca^+ levels

Blood urea nitrogen (BUN), uric acid, creatinine
Serum electrolytes as indicated
Ultrasound profile
Urine (24 hr) for total protein and creatinine
NST and CST as indicated
Coagulation profile; fibrinogen, fibrin degradation products (fibrin split products), prothrombin time (PT), partial thromboplastin time (PPT)
Type and crossmatch
Lecithin/sphingomyelin (L/S) ratio and PG (phosphatidylglycerol) as indicated
Fetoscope/Doppler for fetal heart tones by 20 weeks' gestation
Ultrasound for size and dates as indicated
    Biparietal diameter (BPD) at 16 to 18 weeks' gestation
Amniocentesis (p. 693)
Biophysical profile

Potential complications

HELLP syndrome (H, hemolytic anemia; EL, elevated liver enzymes; LP, low platelets)
Hypertensive crisis
Vascular overload, congestive heart failure
Uteroplacental insufficiency (UPI)
Intrauterine growth retardation (IUGR)
Central nervous system (CNS) disturbances
Cerebrovascular accident (CVA)
Seizures
Fetal loss
Prematurity
Magnesium sulfate toxicity
    Respiratory arrest
    Flushing
    Thirst
    Diaphoresis
    Anxiety
    Drowsiness
    Lethargy
    Slight slurring of speech
    Ataxia
    Flaccidity
    Hypotension
    Hyporeflexia; disappearance of patellar reflex
Essential hypertension
Disseminated intravascular coagulation (DIC)
Abruptio placentae

Medical Management

Laboratory/diagnostic tests as indicated
Bed rest
Daily weights (same time, scale, and clothing)
Vital signs with blood pressure
Seizure precautions
Electronic fetal monitoring as indicated

IV fluids as indicated
Antihypertensives as indicated
    Hydralazine; if ineffective physician may progress to labetalol (Trandate), diazoxide (Hyperstat), sodium nitroprusside, nifedipine
Anticonvulsives as indicated
    Magnesium sulfate
Oxytocin infusion for delivery as indicated (p. 708)
Central venous pressure (CVP) line or Swan-Ganz catheter to manage persistent oliguria

Nursing diagnoses/interventions/evaluation

■ **NDX:**   Altered uteroplacental and renal tissue perfusion related to pregnancy-induced hypertension

Mild preeclampsia

Place patient in quiet, nonstimulating environment—subdued lighting
Maintain bed rest: lateral position is preferred; bathroom privileges may be ordered
Monitor vital signs per hospital protocol
Give complete bed bath unless otherwise ordered
Administer medication as ordered
Check urine for pH, protein, blood, glucose, and acetone q shift and more frequently as condition becomes more acute
Limit visitors as indicated by condition; permit brief but frequent visits by toddlers or other children, since they help to reduce patient's anxiety about their welfare
Maintain seizure precautions
    Padded tongue blade or oral airway at bedside
    Padded side rails; crib bumpers can be used
    Suction equipment readily available
    Oxygen ready to use
    Call light within easy reach
    Magnesium sulfate, calcium antidote, and hydralazine readily available
Collect 24 hr urine specimens as ordered
Auscultate FHR for a full minute q8h and prn or use electronic fetal monitor for 20 to 40 min q8h
Provide diversionary activities
    Television
    Painting
    Reading, books on tape
    Needlework

Severe preeclampsia

Continue with ongoing care of mild preeclampsia and *increase* frequency of nursing functions as condition progresses
Place patient in quiet, darkened room
Maintain padded side rails up at all times
Maintain complete bed rest—no visitors
Check BP and P qh and prn

Auscultate chest for breath sounds prn

Maintain seizure precautions

Connect indwelling catheter to closed gravity drainage system as ordered

Have emergency delivery pack available

Measure intake and output q4h and prn; report output <60 ml/hr

Check urine protein q4h as ordered

Monitor CVP or PAWP (pulmonary artery wedge pressure) if Swan-Ganz line is used

Administer parenteral fluids as ordered based on CVP, PAWP, or other order

Administer magnesium sulfate as ordered

    Observe patient for progressing signs of magnesium sulfate toxicity

    Check deep tendon reflexes (DTRs) q4h to 8h and before each dose of magnesium sulfate or qh if patient is receiving continuous magnesium sulfate infusion; if patellar reflex is absent, withhold next dose of magnesium sulfate until magnesium blood level is drawn, and notify physician

    Assess need for respiratory support with vital signs if magnesium sulfate is administered with a respiratory rate below 12/min

    Check respiratory rate q30min for four times and prn after administration

    Have calcium antidote at bedside

Administer hydralazine 5 mg IV bolus when diastolic blood pressure reaches 110 mm Hg as ordered

    If diastolic pressure is not lowered to 90 to 100 mm Hg in 20 min, increase the dose in 5 mg increments (10, 15, 20 mg) q20min to 30 min as ordered (maximal effect is seen in 20 to 30 min after administration)

    Take BP q5min and report to physician

    Do not leave patient unattended at any time during administration of hydralazine

Never leave patient alone when convulsion is pending

Note and report symptoms of

    Extremely high BP

    Severe headache

    Extreme irritability

    Acute anxiety

    Visual disturbances

Delivery care

See Oxytocin Infusion: Augmentation or Induction of Labor (p. 708) if labor is induced

Maintain separate IV lines for concurrent administration of oxytocin and magnesium sulfate

Ensure that cross-matched blood is immediately available from blood bank if cesarean section is performed

Prepare for neonatal stimulation and resuscitation

Notify pediatrician to be present at time of delivery

Notify admitting nursery that mother had magnesium sulfate

Postdelivery care

Continue with ongoing care of severe preeclampsia and decrease frequency of nursing functions as patient's condition improves

NOTE: Delivery is considered the "treatment" for PIH; however, symptoms may not subside for 2 to 7 days, and an eclamptic seizure is possible during that time

Expected outcome/evaluation

Patient's

    Level of consciousness does not change and patient does not have seizures

    Fetus does not show signs of distress

    Physiological metabolic needs are minimized

    Tissue perfusion is maximized

    Blood pressure readings are maintained or lowered

 NDX: Fluid volume excess related to increased fluid retention and edema associated with pregnancy-induced hypertension

Weigh patient daily at same time with same clothing and scale

Check BP and P q4h and prn; same arm in same position; report tachycardia of 120 bpm or more and tachypnea to physician

Report increased CVP or PAWP, neck vein distention, pulmonary rales, cyanosis, or pallor to physician

Measure intake and output

Check urine protein as ordered

Maintain diet as ordered

Administer medication as ordered

Maintain availability of blood products for immediate use if necessary

Administer IV fluids as ordered

Maintain separate IV lines for concurrent administration of magnesium sulfate and oxytocin

Document use of pump and infusion rates per hospital policy

Expected outcome/evaluation

Patient's

    Signs and symptoms do not indicate congestive heart failure

    Edema is minimal

    Circulating fluid volume is adequate

 NDX: Knowledge deficit related to lack of information about home care for pregnancy-induced hypertension

Undelivered patient

Discuss symptoms of recurrence or progression to report to physician

Discuss procedure for urine collection and appropriate storage based on type of laboratory test, if ordered

Emphasize importance of planned rest periods

Emphasize importance of keeping physician's appointments

Teach name of medication, dosage, time of administration, purpose, and side effects

Explain need to avoid taking over-the-counter medications without checking with physician

Explain need for bed rest as indicated

Discuss symptoms indicating maternal and fetal distress

Explain signs of labor and when to call physician/report to hospital

Delivered patient

See appropriate standard, depending on method of delivery: Cesarean Delivery (p. 718), or Postpartum Care (p. 714)

Emphasize importance of sixth postnatal week physician's appointment to rule out chronic hypertension

Discuss conception control methods to use until no longer indicated by physician

Expected outcome/evaluation

Patient verbalizes intent to comply with plan of care and assists in interventions as able and patient and fetus have good delivery outcome

ECLAMPSIA

Progression of preeclampsia characterized by tonic and clonic convulsions

Assessment
Observations/findings

Seizure
  Twitching and blinking of eyes
  Crying or screaming
  Loss of consciousness
  Tachypnea
  Description of seizure
    Tonic
      Rigid body
      Jaws fixed
      Hands clenched
      Legs inverted
      Cyanosis
      Breath-holding
    Clonic
      Twitching of facial muscles
      Frothing at mouth; may be blood tinged
      Biting of tongue
      Urinary or fecal incontinence
Postseizure
  Altered level of consciousness

Headache
Oliguria
Amnesia of events preceding seizure
Nausea and/or vomiting
Muscle soreness: backache
Aspiration: choking

Laboratory/diagnostic studies

Magnesium sulfate levels
Blood chemistries as indicated
Ultrasound/x-ray examination as indicated
Electronic fetal monitoring
Cardiac monitoring
See Pregnancy-Induced Hypertension (PIH) (p. 687)

Potential complications

Respiratory distress
  Difficulty in breathing
  Diminished breath sounds
  Cyanosis
  Tachycardia, tachypnea
Fetal distress (p. 710)
Signs of onset of labor
See Pregnancy-Induced Hypertension (PIH) (p. 687)

Medical Management

Anticonvulsives as indicated
Magnesium sulfate therapy as indicated (for 24 hr after delivery)
Neurological checks with vital signs
Sedatives as indicated
Antihypertensives
IV fluids as indicated
NPO
Delivery of infant when stabilized
Oxygen therapy

Nursing diagnosis/interventions/evaluation

■ **NDX:** Potential for injury related to physiological processes and effects of seizure

During and after seizure

Prevent injury by
  Removing surrounding furniture if on floor
  Supporting and protecting head; turn head to side if possible
  Gently restraining limbs
  Never leaving patient unattended
Insert oral airway or padded tongue blade when able; *never attempt to force jaws open*
Loosen constrictive clothing
Suction oropharynx and nasopharynx prn
Administer oxygen per nasal cannula or face mask at 10 to 12 L/min for 10 min as ordered when possible
Maintain NPO

Give mouth care when reactive and inspect for damage

Auscultate FHR q1h to 2h and prn or monitor FHR with electronic monitor

Connect indwelling urinary catheter to closed gravity drainage system

Measure urinary output qh

Report output <30 ml/hr to physician

Maintain parenteral fluids as ordered

Monitor central venous pressure (CVP) or pulmonary artery wedge pressure (PAWP) as ordered

Measure intake and output

Do neurological check immediately after seizure and prn

Pupillary size and reaction to light

Level of consciousness

Check BP and P q15min for six times and prn; leave BP cuff on arm continuously

Do not take temperature unless necessary; take axillary temperature

Do not move patient unnecessarily

Reorient patient to environment when conscious

Provide emotional support

Administer medication as ordered: anticonvulsives, sedatives, hypotensives

Protect from extraneous stimuli

Keep room darkened; light only enough to make observations and provide care

Avoid sudden noises

Avoid jarring bed

Converse only if absolutely necessary

Observe for onset of labor

Reinforce physician's explanation of what has happened and maternal and fetal prognosis to both patient and spouse or significant other

See interventions for severe preeclampsia (p. 689)

See Pregnancy-Induced Hypertension (PIH) (p. 687)

Expected outcome/evaluation

Patient is protected from injury to self and fetus

HYPEREMESIS GRAVIDARUM

Excessive or pernicious vomiting during pregnancy, potentially leading to dehydration and/or starvation

Assessment
Observations/findings

Nausea and vomiting usually in morning and/or after meals

Epigastric pain

Hiccups

Heartburn

Thirst; may be severe

Weight loss

Oliguria

Concentrated urine

Dry skin

Poor skin turgor

Emesis of food, mucus, and/or bile

Metabolic acidosis evidenced by headache, mental dullness, disorientation

Laboratory/diagnostic studies

Blood chemistries/electrolytes

Hgb/Hct

Coagulation profile

CVP monitoring as indicated

Cardiac monitoring

Potential complications

Dehydration

Jaundice

Tachycardia

Elevated temperature

Alkalosis

Starvation

Emotional disturbances regarding pregnancy and family relationships

Withdrawal

Depression

Medical Management

IV fluids as indicated

Total parenteral nutrition (TPN)/intralipids as indicated

Central venous catheter as indicated

Frequent small meals

Continuous nasogastric tube feedings as indicated

Nursing diagnoses/interventions/evaluation

■ **NDX:** Fluid volume deficit(2) related to vomiting and altered nutrition related to dehydration and hyperemesis

Acute care

Maintain complete bed rest

Maintain NPO status for 24 to 48 hr

Administer parenteral fluids with B complex vitamins and vitamin C as ordered

Administer electrolyte replacement or TPN as ordered

Dipstick urine for pH, protein, blood, glucose, acetone, and specific gravity q shift

Maintain feeding/parenteral nutrition as ordered

Maintain patent IV access

Measure intake and output q2h to 4h

Administer medications as ordered; may include antihistaminics, antiemetics, anticholinergics, and sedatives

Administer oral hygiene q2h and prn, especially after episodes of vomiting

Check BP, T, P, and R q4h and prn

Monitor CVP readings as ordered

Convalescent care

Continue with acute care and decrease frequency of nursing functions as patient's condition improves

Encourage activity as tolerated

Serve small, frequent feedings of solid foods high in carbohydrate, such as crackers, dry toast, and cereal five to six times each day

Serve small amounts of liquids such as hot tea, crushed ice, carbonated beverages, and cold fruit juices an hour after each meal

Increase amounts of solid food and fluids slowly according to tolerance

Serve food attractively and at proper temperature

Provide foods patient craves; avoid foods and fluids high in fat content

Remove meal tray from bedside as soon as patient has finished

Avoid exposing patient to odors that are nauseating
- Certain foods
- Room deodorizers
- Colognes and perfumes
- Mouthwash solutions

Expected outcome/evaluation

Patient does not lose weight and is less than 10% dehydrated

■ **NDX:** Anxiety related to change in health status and situational crisis

Provide private room if possible

Have same person care for patient each shift, if possible

Limit/control visitors for first 24 hours as indicated by patient's condition; inform family of patient's progress by telephone

Maintain calm and safe environment
- Decrease stimuli
- Talk with and reassure patient
- Explore coping mechanisms

Encourage verbalization

Request psychiatric evaluation if indicated

Talk to patient in a soothing voice

Expected outcome/evaluation

Patient
- Verbalizes feeling less anxious
- Evidences relaxed facial expression
- Responds to staff in an appropriate manner
- Asks questions about care and prognosis

■ **NDX:** Knowledge deficit related to lack of information about care for hyperemesis

Explain need for well-balanced diet with adequate fluid intake at scheduled times

Discuss symptoms of recurrence to report to physician

Emphasize importance of planned rest periods

Reinforce physician's explanation of effect of condition on fetus

Explain that symptoms nearly always disappear by fourth month of pregnancy

Teach name of medication, dosage, time of administration, purpose, and side effects

Explain need to avoid taking over-the-counter medications without checking with physician

Emphasize importance of ongoing outpatient care

Relate that referral to Visiting Nurse's Association may be indicated

Relate that termination of pregnancy may be indicated for unwanted pregnancy

Explain that therapeutic abortion may be indicated for deteriorating physical and/or mental condition, such as that caused by persistent elevated temperature despite adequate hydration, tachycardia, jaundice, retinal hemorrhage, profound depression, or delirium

Expected outcome/evaluation

Patient adjusts to special needs, demonstrates self-care, and verbalizes understanding of instructions

AMNIOCENTESIS

Withdrawal of amniotic fluid through a needle inserted through the maternal abdominal and uterine wall to assess fetal health, maturity, genetic karyotype, and/or sex

Assessment
Potential complications

Fainting

Abdominal pain

Nausea

Premature labor

Fetal hyperactivity or hypoactivity

Fetal tachycardia: above 160 beats/min

Fetal bradycardia: below 120 beats/min

Maternal hemorrhage

Amnionitis
- Tachycardia
- Elevated temperature
- Foul odor of amniotic fluid

Medical Management

Obtain consent

Laboratory tests as indicated

Ultrasound just before or during procedure

Nursing diagnosis/interventions/evaluation

■ **NDX:** Potential for injury related to invasive procedure; transabdominal access to intrauterine cavity

Auscultate FHR

Explain that procedure is usually not harmful to mother or fetus

Explain that procedure is virtually painless

Postprocedure care

Apply adhesive bandage to site of injection

Palpate fundus for fetal activity

Monitor FHR with electronic monitor if possible or auscultate FHR q15min twice

Check BP, P, and R

Position on left side if patient experiences profuse diaphoresis, fainting, or nausea

Reinforce physician's explanation of reason for procedure

    Assessment of fetal maturity and health

    Diagnosis of genetic defects

    Sex determination

Discuss symptoms to report to physician

    Any vaginal drainage, discharge, spotting, or bleeding

    Fetal hyperactivity, diminished activity, or absence of fetal movement

    Any signs of infection

        Elevated temperature

        Chills

    Abdominal pain

    Cramps

Expected outcome/evaluation

Patient does not experience injury (complications) to self or fetus

CARE OF DIABETIC MOTHER DURING LAST TRIMESTER OF PREGNANCY

Diabetic mothers are frequently hospitalized during the last trimester of pregnancy to monitor insulin needs, which are usually higher than during the previous two trimesters, and to monitor fetal well-being because of the increased fetal and neonatal morbidity and mortality associated with maternal diabetes

Assessment
Observations/findings

Large weight gain

Presence of risk factors

    Previously diagnosed glycosuria

    Insulin dependent

    Positive family history

    Obesity > 200 lb

    Previous large-for-gestational-age (LGA) baby

    Previous stillbirth

    Previous congenital anomalies

    Habitual abortion

    Maternal age ≥25 years

Laboratory/diagnostic studies

Blood glucose screening

Glucose loading test, oral glucose tolerance test (OGTT)

Urine glucose/acetone

NST/CST

Blood chemistries as ordered

Potential complications

Hypoglycemia (pp. 332, 343)

Diabetic ketoacidosis (p. 340)

PIH (p. 687)

    Hypertension

    Edema (especially of face and hands)

    Proteinuria

Anxiety

Spontaneous abortion

Hydramnios

Worsening diabetes: increasing insulin requirements

Pyelonephritis

Increased congenital anomalies in infant

    Cardiac defects

    Neural tube defects

    Caudal regression syndrome

    See Infant of Diabetic Mother (IDM) (p. 734)

Infant respiratory distress

Infant macrosomia

Infant hypocalcemia

Infant hypoglycemia

Medical Management

Glucose screening tests as indicated

Insulin as indicated on sliding scale

    Continuous insulin infusion pump may be preferred

IV fluids as indicated

American Dietetic Association (ADA) diet as indicated

Monitored weight gain

Urine testing as indicated for blood, glucose, ketones, protein, bilirubin and pH

Nursing diagnoses/interventions/evaluation

■ **NDX:**   Potential for injury to mother and fetus related to hypoglycemia/hyperglycemia

Maintain patient on NPH or other long-acting insulin as ordered; as EDC approaches, patient's insulin may be regulated by home monitoring of blood glucose and regular insulin on a sliding scale

Monitor blood glucose as ordered

Replace foods not eaten with appropriate exchange; see Diabetic Food Replacement (p. 847)

Auscultate FHR tid and prn

Weigh patient daily at same time with same clothing and scale

Measure intake and output

Assist physician with amniocentesis

Encourage verbalization about concerns for fetus and self

Reinforce physician's explanation of status of fetus and reasons for laboratory studies

Explain procedure for and implications of nonstress testing or contraction stress test

Expected outcome/evaluation

Patient
Achieves and maintains euglycemia
Has no injuries (complications to self or fetus)

■ **NDX:** Knowledge deficit related to lack of information about changes in diabetic regimen during pregnancy

Discuss need for compliance with diabetic regimen
Discuss maternal perception of fetal movement
Explain need for antepartum surveillance
Explain potential need for planning delivery if cesarean section
Discuss symptoms of hypoglycemia and appropriate treatment
Discuss symptoms of diabetic ketoacidosis and appropriate treatment (p. 340)
Discuss symptoms to report to physician
Diminished fetal activity
Signs of PIH
Signs of labor
Signs of uncontrolled diabetes
Demonstrate and have patient and/or significant other return-demonstrate
Home glucose monitoring
Use of sliding scale insulin dosing for injection
See Insulin Therapy Teaching Guide (p. 335)

Expected outcome/evaluation

Patient and significant other verbalize understanding of diabetic regimen during pregnancy and intent to comply with plan of care

Additional nursing diagnoses to consider

Anxiety
Noncompliance
Altered nutrition; less or more than body requirements
Situational low self-esteem

CARE OF DIABETIC MOTHER DURING LABOR AND DELIVERY

Insulin needs vary during labor and delivery, necessitating careful patient observation and monitoring of glucose levels

Assessment
Observations/findings

Hypoglycemia
Hunger

Perspiration
Palpitation
Tachycardia
Weakness, fatigue
Tremor
Pallor
Blurred or double vision
Dizziness
Headache
See Care of Mother in First Stage of Labor (p. 704)
See Care of Mother during Delivery (p. 708)

Laboratory/diagnostic studies

Blood glucose monitoring
Electrolytes as ordered
Electronic fetal monitoring
Real-time ultrasound

Potential complications

See Care of Diabetic Mother during Last Trimester of Pregnancy (p. 694)
Hypoglycemia of mother and infant after delivery
See Infant of Diabetic Mother (IDM) (p. 734)

Medical Management

Decreased insulin
Continuous IV infusion of insulin if blood glucose is >420 mg/dl
Capillary blood glucose monitoring q1h to 2h
IV fluids as indicated
NPO as indicated
For elective cesarean section
No insulin in morning
Early morning delivery (8 to 9 AM preferred because of glucose levels)
Monitoring of glucose after delivery
Observation for insulin reaction
Family planning counseling and implications for future pregnancies

Nursing diagnoses/interventions/evaluation

■ **NDX:** Potential for injury to mother and fetus related to hypoglycemia/hyperglycemia and possible uteroplacental insufficiency during labor

Labor and delivery care

Administer parenteral fluids; electrolyte solutions may be ordered
Monitor fetus internally if possible
Check blood glucose as ordered q1h to 3h
Be aware that regular insulin is preferred to long-lasting insulin
See Care of Mother in First Stage of Labor (p. 704)
See Care of Mother during Delivery (p. 708)
See Fetal Distress (p. 710)
See Care of Mother on Fetal Monitor (p. 712)

Postdelivery care

See Postpartum Care (p. 714)

Observe for symptoms of hypoglycemia

Be aware that insulin dosage will be adjusted to pre-pregnant state needs

Use regular insulin based on blood glucose tests for first 24 to 48 hr as ordered

Progress to NPH or other long-acting insulin after first 24 to 48 hr as ordered, when patient is maintaining stable diet

Check blood glucose levels periodically if ordered

Expected outcome/evaluation

Mother maintains euglycemia, and fetus does not experience distress

■ **NDX:** Knowledge deficit related to lack of information about changes in diabetic regimen during labor

Explain need for NPO status during labor

Explain need for changes in insulin requirements

Explain that insulin and dietary needs may vary because of lactation postpartum

Discuss changes in administration of insulin

Explain need for more frequent capillary glucose monitoring

Explain need to avoid persons with infections, especially upper respiratory infections (URIs), during puerperium

See Care of Diabetic Mother during Last Trimester of Pregnancy (p. 694)

Expected outcome/evaluation

Patient and significant other demonstrate knowledge of diabetic regimen changes and intent to comply with plan of care

PREMATURE RUPTURE OF MEMBRANES (PROM)

Rupture of the bag of waters (RBOW) 12 hours or more before the onset of labor; the etiology is unknown but it is associated with hydramnios, multiple gestation, preterm labor, cervical incompetence, trauma, and amnionitis

Assessment
Observations/findings

Fluid leaking from vagina

Positive nitrazine paper test (alkaline amniotic fluid)

Laboratory/diagnostic studies

Nitrazine paper test (positive)

False positives may occur with contact with cervical mucus, blood, semen, antiseptics, and alkaline urine

"Fern" pattern on dried microscope slide

Fluid cultures as indicated

Presence of amniotic fluid pool in vagina

Potential complications

Bleeding

Amnionitis

Foul odor of vaginal discharge

Maternal elevated temperature

Maternal tachycardia

Maternal leukocytosis

Meconium-stained amniotic fluid

Umbilical cord protruding from introitus

Compression of the umbilical cord

Fetal distress

Fetal tachycardia: above 160 beats/min

Fetal bradycardia: below 120 beats/min

Variable decelerations on electronically monitored patient

Preterm delivery of premature infant

See Care of Mother in First Stage of Labor (p. 704)

Medical Management

Oxytocin induction of labor as indicated based on gestational age

Fetal heart rate monitoring

Introital and rectal culture for group B streptococcus

Fetal maturity testing

IUPC (intrauterine pressure catheter) as indicated

CBC and differential

Nursing diagnoses/interventions/evaluation

■ **NDX:** Potential for infection related to premature rupture of membranes

Check T, P, and R q4h

Auscultate FHR or use electronic FHR monitor q1h to 4h and prn

Avoid vaginal examinations

Observe drainage of amniotic fluid for color, amount, and odor q2h to 4h and prn

Administer perineal care with antiseptic solution after each elimination, q2h to 4h and prn

Keep patient clean and dry

Change pad under buttocks q2h to 4h and prn

Palpate fundus for uterine activity q1h to 2h and prn

Report onset of contractions to physician

Administer antibiotics if ordered

Prepare oxytocin induction as ordered if labor does not begin within 24 hr of PROM and if patient is near EDC

Decrease frequency of nursing functions as patient's condition stabilizes

Carefully clean perineal region; wipe from front to back after elimination

Make note of PROM on infant's chart so that nursery will observe infant for possible respiratory distress, meconium aspiration, and pneumonia at delivery and after

Expected outcome/evaluation

Patient is treated for infection or does not have symptoms of infection and fetus/newborn does not have undesirable sequelae or infection is treated

■ **NDX:**   Knowledge deficit related to lack of information about premature rupture of membranes

Discuss with patient that because amniotic fluid is continually produced, she will not experience a "dry" labor
Report any signs of onset of labor; labor usually begins within 24 hr after rupture of membranes

Expected outcome/evaluation

Patient verbalizes understanding of signs of labor to report and that leaking will continue as amniotic fluid is continually produced

PLACENTA PREVIA

Total, partial, or low implantation of the placenta over the internal cervical os (Figure 15-4); occurs most often in multiparas; total and partial placenta previa prohibits vaginal delivery (the fetus is delivered by cesarean section); with low implantation the fetus can sometimes be delivered vaginally with the presenting part acting as a tamponade against the placenta

Assessment
Observations/findings

Painless vaginal bleeding: intermittent to constant flow
Soft, relaxed uterus

Laboratory/diagnostic studies

Ultrasound to identify position of placenta
Amniography
Speculum vaginal examination
Hgb/Hct; complete blood cell count (CBC)
Amniocentesis for fetal maturity as indicated

Clotting studies
Electronic fetal monitoring: continuous

Potential complications

Fetal bradycardia: below 120 beats/min
Monitored fetus: late decelerations
Absence of fetal heart tones
Maternal shock
Fetal hyperactivity, hypoxia
Neonatal anemia, shock (hypovolemic)
Cesarean section

Medical Management

Cesarean section for fetal distress or to control hemorrhage
Tocolytic agents as indicated if patient is preterm
IV fluids as indicated
Type and cross match 2 to 4 units of fresh whole blood and/or other blood products as available

Nursing diagnoses/interventions/evaluation

■ **NDX:**   Altered fetal tissue perfusion related to maligned placenta and hypovolemia associated with bleeding

NOTE: *Amount of bleeding and position of placenta determine care and the frequency of monitoring vital signs*
Maintain complete bed rest
Never do a manual vaginal or rectal examination
Avoid rectal stimulation; no enemas
Monitor intake and output
Initiate parenteral fluids as ordered
    Monitor IV site and flow to ensure patency
Place patient in high Fowler's or lateral position if membranes are ruptured; avoid supine position
Place patient in position of comfort if membranes are not ruptured
Check BP, P, and FHR q¼h to 2h and prn

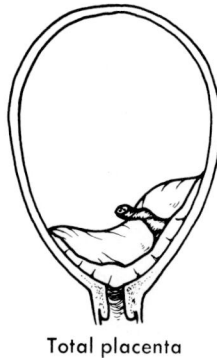
Total placenta
previa

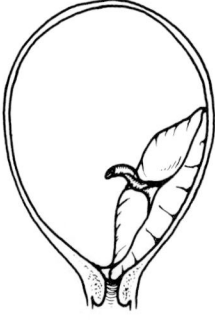
Partial placenta
previa

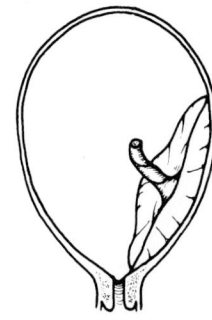
Low
implantation

FIGURE 15-4. Placenta previa (abnormal implantation).

Check random pulse oximeter oxygen saturation if respiratory complications are present or impending

Observe amount, color, and character of vaginal drainage q15min to 2h and prn depending on amount of bleeding

Administer perineal care with antiseptic solution after every elimination and/or q4h and prn

Report saturation of more than one perineal pad q30min

Weigh pads and linen to estimate blood loss as ordered

Administer transfusions and volume expanders as ordered

Report any sign of onset of labor to physician immediately

Monitor FHR electronically as indicated

Prepare for double setup and/or delivery as indicated

Administer oxygen by mask or nasal cannula as indicated

Continue with care and decrease frequency of nursing functions as patient's condition stabilizes

Explain and prepare for diagnostic tests if ordered
Ultrasonography
Amniography
Placenta scan

Prepare for delivery as ordered

See Cesarean Delivery (p. 718) or Postpartum Care (p. 714)

Expected outcome/evaluation

Patient does not hemorrhage and fetus does not show signs of distress

■ **NDX:**   Anticipatory grieving related to potential loss of fetus

Encourage patient and family to verbalize fears

Correct any misconceptions

Avoid defensive responses to patient's criticisms of health care

Provide ongoing information about status and plan of care

Facilitate discussion between patient/family

Expected outcome/evaluation

Patient expresses feelings and concerns and maintains constructive interpersonal relationships with family and health care providers

ABRUPTIO PLACENTAE

Premature separation of the placenta occurring before the third stage of labor (Figure 15-5) (may be associated with cocaine use)

Assessment
Observations/findings

Uterus
Extreme tenderness
General or localized pain
Pain: may be absent to severe
Sudden enlargement: symmetrical or asymmetrical
Progressive decrease of relaxation between contractions developing into continuous boardlike rigidity
Uterine tachysystole and hypertonus on monitored patient
Low back pain
Hyperactive fetus

Vaginal bleeding may or may not be present

Hemorrhage: usually concealed

Rising uterine fundus
Fetal heart rate
Bradycardia: below 120 beats/min
Heart tones: may be absent
Monitored fetus: may have late decelerations
Absence
Extreme anxiety
Hypovolemia

Port wine colored amniotic fluid may be present

Laboratory/diagnostic studies

CBC, coagulation profile (platelets, fibrinogen, prothrombin time [PT], partial thromboplastin time [PTT], fibrin degradation products [fibrin split products])

Continuous external fetal monitoring

Potential complications

Fetal distress (p. 710)
DIC (p. 173)

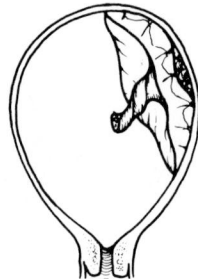 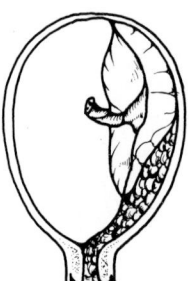 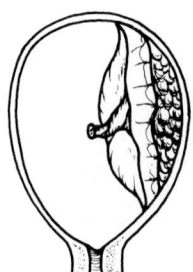

Partial separation (concealed hemorrhage)

Partial separation (apparent hemorrhage)

Complete separation (concealed hemorrhage)

FIGURE 15-5. Abruptio placentae (premature separation).

Hypofibrinogenemia
Hypoprothrombinemia
Bleeding from mucous membranes
Bruising; ecchymosis
Oliguria progressing to anuria
Maternal hypovolemic shock (p. 105)
Renal failure

Medical Management

Cesarean delivery for compromised fetus, maternal hemorrhage, or unstable maternal condition
IV fluids as indicated
NPO (if near or in shock or delivery imminent)
Volume expander or blood transfusion as indicated
Oxygen 8 to 10 L/min as indicated
Analgesics

Nursing diagnoses/interventions/evaluation

■ **NDX:** Altered placental tissue perfusion related to hypovolemia associated with hemorrhage of abrupted placenta

Immediate care

Administer oxygen as ordered
Remain with patient at all times
Maintain complete bed rest in position of comfort
Palpate fundus for presence of uterine contractions and relaxation
    Report increasing uterine intensity or sustained uterine contraction to physician
    Instruct patient to report any sudden increase in pain
Prepare for immediate delivery and neonatal resuscitation
Order type and cross match of 2 to 4 units of packed cells if ordered by physician
Assist with amniotomy if done by physician
Monitor fetus internally with spiral electrode if possible
Check BP, P, and FHR q5min to 15min
Perform tilt test prn
Administer transfusions or volume expanders as ordered

Stabilization care

Control pain carefully as ordered; small doses of analgesics are preferred
Weigh pads and linens to estimate blood loss as ordered
Allay anxiety as much as possible
Explain all actions taken
Ask patient to verbalize any changes in feeling and sensorium
Reinforce physician's explanation for cesarean section if done
Notify postpartum nurses to observe patient for
    Incisional hematoma
    Disparate intake and output
See Cesarean Delivery (p. 718) or Postpartum Care (p. 714)

Expected outcome/evaluation

Patient's condition does not develop into hypovolemic shock and fetus' hydration is maintained and fetus does not experience a negative sequelae

■ **NDX:** Fluid volume deficit related to active loss of blood from abrupted placenta before delivery

Initiate and maintain parenteral fluids as ordered
Monitor CVP as ordered
Maintain patent IV line
Measure intake and output q1h
Connect indwelling catheter (Foley) to closed gravity system as indicated

Expected outcome/evaluation

Patient's
    Hgb/Hct is restored to/maintained at previous levels
    Skin turgor is adequate

■ **NDX:** Fear related to unanticipated complication requiring immediate obstetrical care

Explain aspects of care to patient/family
Reinforce physician's explanation of plan of treatment and expected prognosis
Attempt to maintain a calm, reassuring demeanor and environment
Assist with rhythmic breathing and relaxation techniques during episodes of pain associated with uterine hypertonus

Expected outcome/evaluation

Patient and family exhibit coping behaviors and interact appropriately with staff and one another

PROLAPSED UMBILICAL CORD

Protrusion of the umbilical cord in advance of the presenting part; this should be suspected after amniotomy or spontaneous gross rupture of membranes and should be ruled out by vaginal examination (Figures 15-6 and 15-7)

Assessment
Observations/findings

Umbilical cord: may or may not be visible at introitus
Meconium-stained amniotic fluid
Fetal bradycardia: below 120 beats/min
Slowing pulsations of visible cord
Severe, variable decelerations of FHR

Laboratory/diagnostic studies

Vaginal examination for prolapse verification

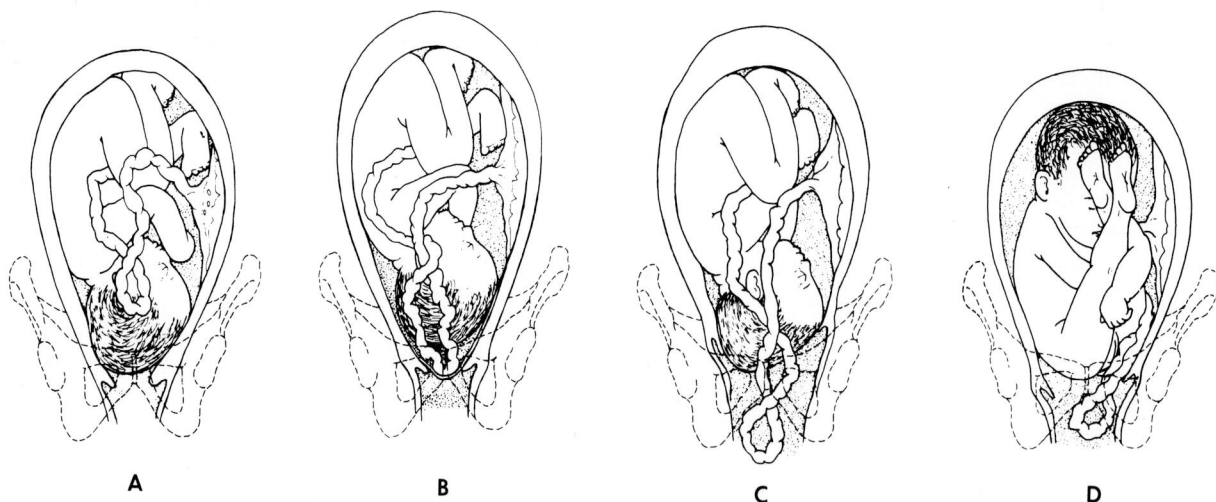

FIGURE 15-6. Prolapse of umbilical cord. Note pressure of presenting part on umbilical cord, which endangers fetal circulation. **A,** Occult (hidden) prolapse of cord. **B,** Complete prolapse of cord. Note membranes are intact. **C,** Cord presenting in front of fetal head and may be seen within vagina. **D,** Frank breech presentation with prolapsed cord. (From Bobak IM, Jensen MD: *Essentials of maternity nursing,* ed 3, St Louis, 1991, Mosby—Year Book.)

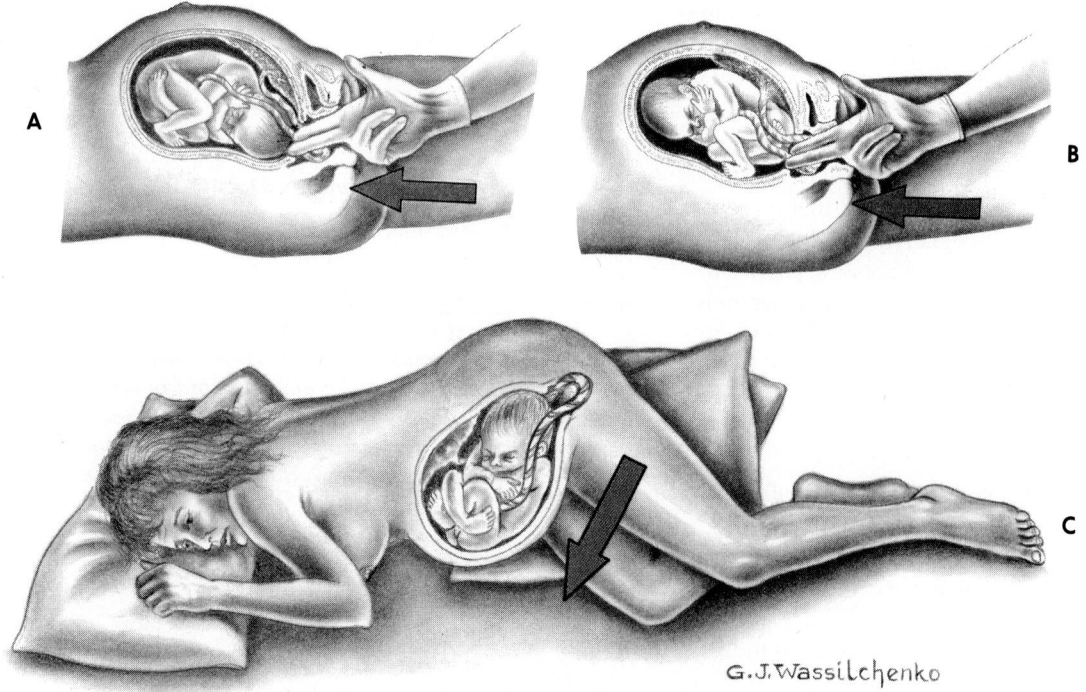

FIGURE 15-7. Arrows indicate direction of pressure against presenting part to relieve compression of prolapsed umbilical cord. Pressure exerted by examiner's fingers in **A,** vertex presentation, and **B,** in breech position. **C,** Gravity relieves pressure with woman in modified Sims' position with hips elevated as high as possible with pillows. (From Bobak IM, Jensen MD: *Essentials of maternity nursing,* ed 3, St Louis, 1991, Mosby—Year Book.)

Potential complications

Fetal distress (p. 710)
Fetal hypoxia
Fetal death, stillborn

Medical Management

Bed rest (knee-chest position for acute episode)
Cesarean section
Oxygen therapy as indicated
IV therapy as indicated

Nursing diagnoses/interventions/evaluation

■ **NDX:**   Potential for fetal injury related to potential cord compression associated with prolapse of umbilical cord

Maintain absolute bed rest
Never attempt to replace a prolapsed cord into vagina
Avoid cord compression
  Elevate presenting part sufficiently to relieve pressure on the umbilical cord until delivery
  Pressure of examiner's sterile gloved hand (cord between two spread fingers)
  Knee-chest or exaggerated Trendelenburg's position
  Do not manipulate cord
  Rapid filling of urinary bladder with 500 to 700 ml of normal saline through indwelling catheter may help to elevate the presenting part
Prepare for immediate delivery; cesarean section is usually done
Check FHR q2min to 5min, preferably with an electronic fetal monitor
Administer oxygen (10 to 12 L/min) by face mask as ordered
Gently cover exposed cord with sterile saline compresses
Stay with patient at all times
Allay anxiety as much as possible by explanation to patient about importance of maintaining special position and not bearing down or pushing with contractions
Teach patient panting and blowing techniques for use during uterine contractions
Reinforce physician's explanation of need to do immediate delivery
See Postpartum Care (p. 714) or Cesarean delivery

Expected outcome/evaluation

Circulation is maintained through umbilical cord as evidenced by absence of fetal compromise
Fetal heart rate is in the normal range and there is absence of severe variable decelerations on an electronically monitored fetus

Additional nursing diagnoses to consider

Altered fetal tissue perfusion
Maternal fear

PRETERM LABOR

Physiological process by which the fetus is expelled from the uterus before the completion of the thirty-seventh week of gestation

Assessment
Observations/findings

Uterine contractions
  Every 10 min or less (six to eight uterine contractions/hr)
  Lasting 30 sec or more
Progressive cervical dilatation: ≥50% effacement or ≥2 cm dilatation
Complaints of back pain or pressure

Laboratory/diagnostic studies

Electronic fetal monitoring (EFM)
Fetoscope/Doppler as indicated
Urinalysis
CBC
Cervical cultures, including group B streptococcus
Amniocentesis to assess fetal lung maturity and presence of infection
Maternal and fetal baseline ECG
Electrolytes
Blood glucose

Potential complications

Compromised infant at birth
  Prematurity
  Small-for-gestational-age infant
  Respiratory distress syndrome
Tocolysis (magnesium sulfate, terbutaline, or ritodrine)
Magnesium sulfate therapy
  Maternal effects
    Flushing, sense of warmth
    Headache
    Dizziness
    Respiratory depression
    Hypotension
    Hyporeflexia
    Nystagmus
    Nausea, vomiting
    Lethargy
    Pulmonary edema
  Fetal/neonatal effects
    Decreased muscle tone
    Respiratory depression
    Lethargy, drowsiness
    Lower Apgar scores with prolonged maternal treatment
Sympathobetamimetics (Ritodrine, Terbutaline)
  Maternal effects
    Tachycardia

Palpitations
Hypotension
Arrhythmias
Hypokalemia
Chest pain
Pulmonary edema
Tremors
Agitation
Headache
Elevated blood glucose
Hyperlipidemia
Fetal/neonatal effects
Fetal distress
Tachycardia
Bradycardia if severe maternal hypotension
Neonatal hypotension
Neonatal hypoglycemia
Neonatal hypocalcemia
Neonatal irritability

Medical Management

Bed rest in left lateral position
Continuous EFM and uterine contraction monitoring for a minimum of 1 hour
Home uterine monitoring as indicated by condition, uterine activity, fetal gestational age, and maternal compliance with this regimen
Laboratory tests as indicated
IV fluids as indicated
Intake and output
Ultrasound for evaluation of placenta, fetal/uterine anomalies, and gestational age confirmation
Glucocorticoids as indicated
Tocolysis as indicated (magnesium sulfate terbutaline or ritodrine hydrochloride)
Antibiotics as indicated

Nursing diagnoses/interventions/evaluation

■ **NDX:** Potential for injury to fetus related to potential for preterm delivery; potential for injury to mother related to tocolysis therapy

Maintain complete bed rest in side-lying position
Administer IV fluids as ordered
Note frequency, duration, and strength of contractions q15 min and prn; monitor uterine activity with toco-transducer (tocodynamometer) if available
Auscultate FHR q15 min to 30 min or electronically monitor with ultrasound
Measure intake and output as ordered
Assist with amniocentesis and/or ultrasound if ordered
Administer any other medications, including corticosteroids, in exact dose, time, and route as ordered
Decrease frequency of nursing functions as patient's preterm labor is arrested

Continuous labor

See Care of Mother in First Stage of Labor (p. 704)
In addition
Prepare for high-risk infant
Notify neonatologist or pediatrician
Have resuscitative equipment ready for use
Plan to have infant's blood cross matched if less than 32 weeks' gestation
Monitor FHR electronically if possible
Assist physician with fetal blood sampling as indicated
Consider plotting labor dilation and descent on square-ruled graph paper (labor is usually rapid, but a high frequency of abnormal labors occurs as well—Friedman curve)
Provide comfort measures before administering minimal doses of analgesics as ordered
Retain placenta for pathology as ordered
See Care of Premature Infant (p. 731)

Tocolytic therapy

Magnesium sulfate
Maintain patent IV access
Administer 3 to 6 g IV in a 10% solution over 15 to 30 min for initial dose as ordered
Continue and monitor IV infusion titrated according to uterine response and side effects (i.e., 2 g/hr)
Watch for symptoms of toxicity; discontinue, administer oxygen therapy, and notify physician if toxicity occurs
Respiratory depression
Hypotension
Absence of deep tendon reflexes
Keep antidote for magnesium sulfate toxicity (10% calcium gluconate) at bedside
Monitor and decrease dosage after 24 hr or when uterine contractions subside as ordered
Check vital signs and DTRs q30min to 1h
Continue to monitor uterine activity
Monitor intake and output q1h; should be at least 30 ml urine per hour
Auscultate lungs q4h to 8h for presence of fluid
Monitor fetus with EFM as ordered
Check fetal heart rate with vital signs if no EFM is done
Monitor magnesium sulfate levels
Obtain baseline electrolytes and calcium levels by venipuncture
Terbutaline
Parenteral administration
Administer loading dose of 0.25 mg slowly
For continued therapy add 15 mg terbutaline to 250 ml of 5DW or NS (this will deliver 60 μgms/ml)
Give 5 μg/min and increase dose in 5 μg increments q10 min until tocolysis is achieved or 55 μgms/min is reached
Oral therapy

Administer first dose before discontinuing parenteral
therapy
Dosage 2.5 to 5.0 mg q4h po until 36 weeks' gestation
Ritodrine hydrochloride
Obtain laboratory data as ordered (may include CBC,
electrolytes, and glucose)
Place in left lateral position during infusion
Monitor maternal electrocardiogram (ECG) as ordered
Administer ritodrine (usually 50 μg/min) via infusion
pump or controller with drug piggybacked into main
IV line, being careful not to exceed maximum dosage
of 350 μg/min
Monitor rate and dosage and increase by 50 μg/min
q10min based on maternal and fetal responses as or-
dered
Do not increase dose and/or discontinue ritodrine:
If patient demonstrates unacceptable side effects
If maternal heart rate exceeds 140 beats/min
If fetal tachycardia of 180 beats/min or greater per-
sists
If systolic blood pressure is <90 mm Hg or more than
a 20% decrease, or diastolic BP is <40 mm Hg
Check BP, P, and FHR q10min while increasing dos-
age, then q30min while patient is receiving IV rito-
drine maintenance dose
Monitor FHR and uterine contractions continuously if
possible
Measure intake and output
Report undesirable side effects, including headache and
palpitations, to physician
Continue to maintain IV infusion for 12 hr after arrest of
labor, using smallest dose possible to maintain tocolysis
Adjust dosage of tocolytic agent for patients with diurnal
patterns of uterine activity
Auscultate lungs q8h to check for fluid overload
Monitor intake and output q1h
Initiate oral therapy 30 min before discontinuing IV ther-
apy as ordered
Decrease frequency of nursing functions as preterm labor
is arrested

Expected outcome/evaluation

Preterm delivery is avoided and there are no maternal
complications of tocolysis therapy

■ **NDX:** Potential situational low self-esteem related to
perceptions and expectations of pregnancy and
delivery

Encourage patient to verbalize fears and concerns
Note and document
Minimal eye contact
Self-defeating statements and/or behaviors
Overt expressions of guilt or blame
Negativity or inadequacy in actions or verbal commu-
nications

Demonstrations of anger
Include significant other in discussions
Provide factual information about placement of blame for
initiation and continuation of uterine contractions
Provide positive feedback and encouragement to patient
for seeking early interventions

Expected outcome/evaluation

Patient verbalizes positive feelings about self

■ **NDX:** Pain related to uterine contractions

Use nonpharmacological measures when appropriate
Positioning
Muscular relaxation techniques
Breathing techniques
Distraction techniques
Eliminate or minimize other factors that could contribute
to pain
Encourage frequent voiding
Explain all procedures before executing them
Answer all questions if possible
Offer choices to allow for control as patient is able
Keep patient and significant other informed of changes
in labor and fetal status
Explain reasons why analgesic agents may not be appro-
priate
Effect on fetal heart rate
Possible masking of contractions
Combined side effects of tocolytic agents and analgesia
Provide positive reinforcement and touch as appropriate
Plan nursing care to provide rest periods to promote com-
fort, sleep, and relaxation
Assess and document factors contributing to stress or per-
ception of pain
Assess and document q30min
Frequency and duration of contractions
Location of pain
Intensity and duration of pain

Expected outcome/evaluation

Patient verbalizes decreasing or more tolerable discomfort

■ **NDX:** Knowledge deficit related to lack of information
about potential premature labor and delivery

Explain arrested labor
Emphasize importance of maintaining bed rest in sidelying
position with bathroom privileges as ordered
Emphasize importance of avoiding intercourse, douching,
or nipple stimulation, including preparation of breasts
for breastfeeding
Teach name of medication, dosage, frequency of administration, purpose, and toxic side effects
Teach or reinforce instructions if patient will be monitored

at home with periodic modem transmission of uterine activity

Emphasize importance of having supportive person to perform housekeeping, cooking, and child care tasks

Discuss signs of labor to report to physician

Emphasize importance of follow-up medical care

Discuss development and gestational stage of fetus

Expected outcome/evaluation

Patient demonstrates self-care and patient and significant other verbalize understanding of premature labor and purpose of treatment

CARE OF MOTHER IN FIRST STAGE OF LABOR

Physiological process by which the fetus is expelled from the uterus

early labor Dilation of 0 to 4 cm with mild to moderate irregular contractions

active labor Dilation of 4 cm with moderate to strong regular contractions q2min to 5 min

transitional labor Dilation of 8 cm to complete dilation with strong contractions

Assessment

Observations/findings

Behavior
    Surge of energy and activity
    Talking frequently
    Anxious
    Fear of isolation
Rupture of membranes
Uterine contractions: regular with increasing intensity and frequency
Transitional labor
    Nausea and vomiting
    Irritability
    Loss of coping mechanisms
    Hiccups and/or belching
    Trembling and/or shaking of legs
    Chilling
    Perspiration
    Rectal pressure
    Urge to push
    Hypersensitive abdomen

Laboratory/diagnostic studies

Baseline laboratory tests
    CBC with differential
    Hgb/Hct
    VDRL serology
    Chemistries
Urinalysis
Cultures as indicated by history of signs and symptoms
Ultrasound/x-ray examination as indicated
Electronic fetal monitoring
Fetal scalp pH testing

Potential complications

Nonreassuring findings
    Fetal tachycardia: above 160 beats/min
    Fetal bradycardia: below 120 beats/min
    Meconium-stained amniotic fluid
    Foul-smelling amniotic fluid
Fetal hyperactivity
Monitored labor (p. 712)
    Severe variable decelerations: <70 beats/min for more than 30 sec
    Uncorrectable, repetitive late decelerations of any magnitude
    Absence of variability
    Prolonged deceleration
    Unstable FHR; sinusoidal pattern
Supine hypotension syndrome
Inadequate uterine relaxation
    Contractions lasting longer than 90 sec
    Relaxation between contractions less than 30 sec
Arrest of labor
Amnionitis secondary to prolonged rupture of membranes
Elevated temperature
Distended bladder
Dehydration
Hemorrhage

Medical Management

Laboratory tests as indicated
IV fluids as indicated
Prenatal chart and previous medical chart ordered to labor and delivery unit
Vital sign monitoring according to facility policy
Analgesia as indicated
Preparation for selected/indicated anesthesia by anesthesiologist/nurse anesthetist
Fetal heart rate-uterine contraction (FHR-UC) monitoring

Nursing diagnoses/interventions/evaluation

■ **NDX:** Potential for injury to mother related to physiological processes of labor

Check temperature q2h after rupture of membranes

Consider plotting cervical dilation and fetal descent over time on square-ruled graph paper (Friedman curve)

Give enema in early labor if ordered

Administer clear liquids as ordered

Measure intake and output

Have patient void q2h and prn

Check urine for glucose and protein

Maintain complete bed rest in position of comfort if membranes are ruptured, especially if presenting part is not yet engaged; otherwise, patient may ambulate as tolerated

    Allow patient up to bathroom if presenting part is well applied to cervix as ordered

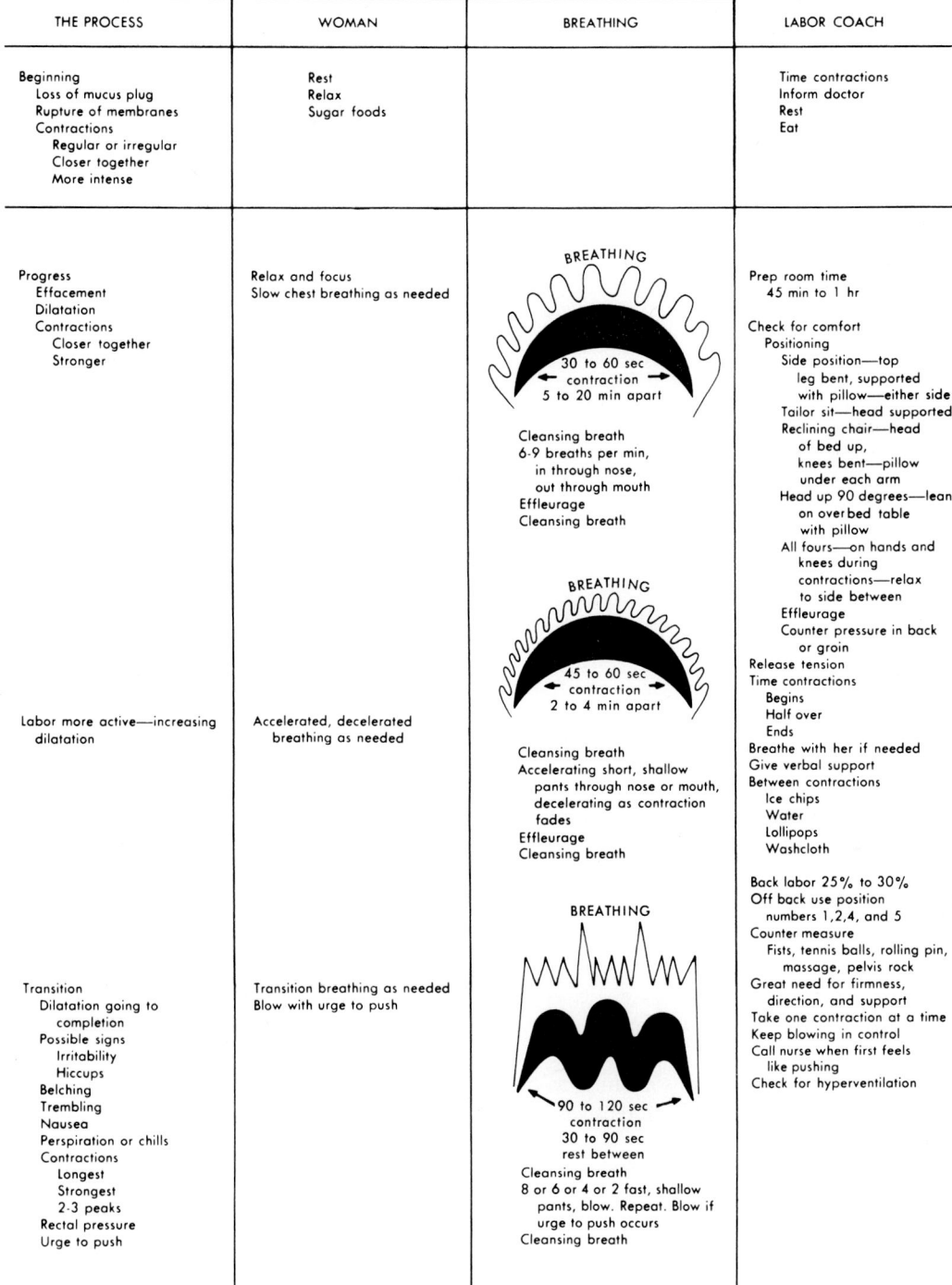

THE PROCESS	WOMAN	BREATHING	LABOR COACH
Beginning Loss of mucus plug Rupture of membranes Contractions Regular or irregular Closer together More intense	Rest Relax Sugar foods		Time contractions Inform doctor Rest Eat
Progress Effacement Dilatation Contractions Closer together Stronger	Relax and focus Slow chest breathing as needed	**BREATHING** 30 to 60 sec contraction 5 to 20 min apart Cleansing breath 6-9 breaths per min, in through nose, out through mouth Effleurage Cleansing breath	Prep room time 45 min to 1 hr Check for comfort Positioning Side position—top leg bent, supported with pillow—either side Tailor sit—head supported Reclining chair—head of bed up, knees bent—pillow under each arm Head up 90 degrees—lean on overbed table with pillow All fours—on hands and knees during contractions—relax to side between Effleurage Counter pressure in back or groin
Labor more active—increasing dilatation	Accelerated, decelerated breathing as needed	**BREATHING** 45 to 60 sec contraction 2 to 4 min apart Cleansing breath Accelerating short, shallow pants through nose or mouth, decelerating as contraction fades Effleurage Cleansing breath	Release tension Time contractions Begins Half over Ends Breathe with her if needed Give verbal support Between contractions Ice chips Water Lollipops Washcloth
Transition Dilatation going to completion Possible signs Irritability Hiccups Belching Trembling Nausea Perspiration or chills Contractions Longest Strongest 2-3 peaks Rectal pressure Urge to push	Transition breathing as needed Blow with urge to push	**BREATHING** 90 to 120 sec contraction 30 to 90 sec rest between Cleansing breath 8 or 6 or 4 or 2 fast, shallow pants, blow. Repeat. Blow if urge to push occurs Cleansing breath	Back labor 25% to 30% Off back use position numbers 1,2,4, and 5 Counter measure Fists, tennis balls, rolling pin, massage, pelvis rock Great need for firmness, direction, and support Take one contraction at a time Keep blowing in control Call nurse when first feels like pushing Check for hyperventilation

FIGURE 15-8. ASPO (Lamaze) review sheet. (Prepared by the teachers of the American Society of Psychoprophylaxis in Obstetrics of Los Angeles, Inc., with permission of the Board of Directors of ASPO of Los Angeles, Inc.)

THE PROCESS	WOMAN	BREATHING	LABOR COACH
Birth Good pushing routine may take several contractions Pushing may not feel good for 3 or 4 contractions	Push with contractions Stop pushing as directed by doctor or nurse	BREATHING CONTRACTION	**Labor room** Elevate bed as desired Remind her of technique Pushing position after 2 cleansing breaths, elbows into bed, push gently during contraction, think vagina, forceful pushing will alleviate discomfort, 2 cleansing breaths after contraction Coach dress for delivery now
First baby—push in labor room until baby's head shows Second baby—to delivery room as soon as completely dilated		2 cleansing breaths Perform gentle pushing 2 cleansing breaths Stop pushing Be sure to follow doctor's directions, stop pushing when directed—blow, then pant, pant blow.	**Delivery room** Take 2 pillows Encourage Push as before, support her head and shoulders as she pulls herself up Push as before, support her head and shoulders as she pulls herself up Be sure she follows doctor's directions Listen for doctor's command—stop pushing, etc., and repeat to her
As head comes to outlet may experience burning or stinging sensation on perineum, extreme pressure on anus—may feel as if it's "turning inside out"			
Expulsion of the placenta—placenta, membranes, umbilical cord are delivered	Enjoy baby with your husband!	Push as directed.	Enjoy baby with your wife!

CONGRATULATIONS

FIGURE 15-8, cont'd. ASPO (Lamaze) review sheet.

Initiate lactated Ringer's solution or other IV solution as ordered

Prehydrate with 500 to 1000 ml of fluid before anesthetic procedure as ordered

Maintain dosing of prelabor medications or drugs as ordered (i.e., anticonvulsants, antihypertensives, or methadone)

See ASPO (Lamaze) review sheet (Figure 15-8)

Expected outcome/evaluation

Patient
  Does not experience any injury related to labor as evidenced by adequate hydration, skin turgor, voiding pattern (absence of distended bladder)
  Has absence of fever

 NDX: Pain and anxiety related to physiological process of labor

Active labor

Give back rub qh and prn between contractions

Apply pressure to sacrum as needed prn during contractions

Apply cool compress to forehead prn

Change pad under buttocks when moist q30min to 60min and prn

Assist with breathing techniques and teach to significant other to assist patient

Change gown and linen as necessary

Turn off bright overhead lights when not needed

Clip call bell to bottom sheet within easy reach to ensure that staff is promptly notified of patient's needs

Relieve discomfort with medication as ordered

Assist physician with local or regional anesthetic; take BP and P q10 min for three times after anesthetic and until stabilized

Avoid talking to patient during contractions

Reposition patient q30min and prn; lateral position is preferred

Transitional phase of labor

Encourage deep ventilation before and after each contraction when patient is in active labor and during transition period

Avoid urge to push by panting and/or blowing in rapid sequence with contractions until completely dilated

Have emesis basin readily available

Have patient void to ensure empty bladder

Cover feet with blanket or have patient wear socks if chilling occurs

Tell patient that the transition stage usually lasts no more than 1 to 2 hr and then she will be allowed to push and deliver infant

Palpate abdomen very lightly and only as often as necessary if abdomen is hypersensitive

Avoid having persons in labor room who are not directly caring for patient

Accept aggression or other coping behaviors; avoid negative comments

Avoid unnecessary talking or expression of feelings to meet own needs

Focus on patient and support her
  Calm voice
  Touch
  Positive reinforcement after contractions

Expected outcome/evaluation

Patient
  Experiences manageable pain and minimal anxiety as evidenced by verbalization of same
  Complies with assistive directions by staff
  Has continuing interaction with significant other/family

■ **NDX:** Altered oral mucous membrane related to mouth breathing

Administer oral hygiene qh and prn between contractions
  Suck on ice chips, wet washcloths, or sour lollipops unless contraindicated
  Rinse mouth with water and/or mouthwash
  Apply petroleum jelly or antichapping lipsticks to dry lips prn

Expected outcome/evaluation

Patient does not experience disruption in tissue layers of oral cavity

■ **NDX:** Potential for injury to fetus related to uterine contractions of labor and/or uteroplacental insufficiency

Note frequency, duration, and strength of contractions q30min to 60min and prn in early labor; increase to q15min to 30min in active labor

Auscultate FHR immediately after uterine contractions, preferably for one full minute if not electronically monitored in second stage of labor (q15min to 30min and prn)

Check BP and P qh and prn

Check T, P, and R q2h to 4h and prn

Auscultate FHR immediately after membranes rupture or amniotomy is done

Turn mother to left-lateral position, increase rate of plain IV, administer 100% oxygen by face mask, and notify physician immediately if fetal distress is evident by auscultation or electronic fetal monitoring

See Care of Mother on Fetal Monitor (p. 712)

Expected outcome/evaluation

Patient delivers an infant in good condition at birth with Apgar score ≥8 at 5 min of age

■ **NDX:** Anxiety related to lack of knowledge and uncertainty about what to expect during labor

Allay anxiety as much as possible by doing the following
  Explain reasons for performing all procedures
  Encourage spouse or significant other to remain with patient to provide support during labor
  Let spouse or significant other listen to fetal heart tones with stethoscope, fetoscope, or ultrasound stethoscope
  Provide supportive care based on patient's knowledge of labor process
  Inform waiting family members and friends of patient's progress and let patient know that they are interested in her
  Reduce environmental stimuli that may contribute to anxiety and tension; provide relaxed, restful atmosphere
  At appropriate intervals reassure patient that labor is progressing and that both patient and infant are doing fine
  Instruct spouse or significant other when and where to change into scrub suit, cap, and mask to be ready to go into delivery room

Expected outcome/evaluation

Patient
  Understands process of labor and rationale for procedures
  Is supported by significant other in coping with anxiety

PROCEDURAL CARE OF MOTHER DURING DELIVERY: SECOND STAGE OF LABOR

The stage of expulsion of the fetus, placenta, and membranes from the mother at birth after complete dilatation of the cervix

Assessment
Observations/findings

Involuntary bearing down
Pushing
Grunting sounds
Extreme anxiety
Vomiting episode
Involuntary shaking of legs
Perspiration between nose and upper lip
Increase in bloody show
Patient stating, "Baby is coming"
Desire to defecate, fear of "making a mess"
Prolonged second stage
  More than 1 hr for multigravidas
  More than 2 hr for primigravidas

Laboratory/diagnostic studies

Electronic fetal monitoring
Cord blood: gases, pH, and other tests as ordered

Potential complications

High-risk delivery
Birth asphyxia
Difficult delivery
  Shoulder dystocia
  Breech presentation
  Cephalopelvic disproportion
Forceps delivery
Vacuum extraction
Cesarean section
Infant bruising, fractures
See Care of Newborn (p. 725)

Nursing Procedures
Care during delivery

Auscultate FHR q5min and/or after each push if electronic monitor is not used (if electronic monitor was used continuously during labor then it should be continued in the delivery room until the time of delivery)
Check BP and P q5min to 10min
Pad stirrups
Administer oxygen mask at 10 to 12 L/min as ordered
Understand that low- to semi-Fowler's position with lateral tilt is preferred while pushing
Assist with breathing techniques
  Deep ventilation before and after each contraction
  Breathing technique and pushing with contractions
Observe perineum while pushing
Notify physician if second stage is prolonged
Prepare perineum according to hospital procedure
Request patient not to touch sterile drapes if used
Place nurse, spouse, and/or labor coach at head of delivery table to encourage patient during delivery process
Encourage long, sustained pushing rather than frequent short pushes
Encourage complete relaxation between contractions

Reassure patient that she is doing well and is advancing infant with each push
Apply cool moist cloth to forehead as needed
Have DeLee suction catheter available and ready to use if meconium-stained amniotic fluid is present
Plan for suctioning of naso-oropharynx after delivery of fetal head and before delivery of thorax to prevent meconium aspiration
Assist physician or nurse-midwife as needed

Immediate postdelivery care

Permit mother to inspect infant as soon as possible
Place infant on maternal abdomen to provide skin-to-skin contact if delivery room is warm
See Care of Newborn (p. 725)
Defer neonatal eye therapy for 1 to 2 hr after birth to promote eye contact with mother
Check BP and P q10 min to 15 min for four times and prn
Add oxytocic drug as ordered to parenteral fluids
Palpate fundus, noting location and tonus q5min to 10min for four times
Administer perineal care before removing legs from stirrups
Place sterile perineal pad and/or pad under buttocks before transporting patient to recovery area
Place ice pack on episiotomy unless otherwise ordered
Assist with infant's warm water bath if infant's temperature is stable as indicated
Maintain mother's warmth with blankets as needed
Place radiant heat warmer over upper part of mother's bed or place dry, warmly blanketed infant next to mother so that she can visually inspect, touch, and/or breast-feed nude infant while preventing neonatal heat loss
Let mother and spouse and/or labor coach be with infant in delivery area, providing them with as much privacy as feasible unless this is contraindicated by maternal or fetal pathological condition
Encourage mother to freely express her feelings about herself and her infant
Explain that behaviors manifested in labor are normal and there is no reason to apologize if mother is apologetic for behavior while in labor
See Postpartum Care (p. 714)

OXYTOCIN INFUSION: AUGMENTATION OR INDUCTION OF LABOR

Oxytocin infusion may be used to either begin the labor process or to augment a labor that is progressing slowly because of inadequate uterine activity

Laboratory/diagnostic studies

FHR-UC monitoring
Cephalopelvic disproportion (CPD) measurements
Ultrasound as ordered

Assessment

Observations/findings

Dysfunctional labor pattern (Table 15-1)
Absence of cephalopelvic disproportion
Bishop score (Table 15-2)

Potential complications

Fetal distress
  Hyperactive fetus
  Fetal tachycardia: above 160 beats/min
  Fetal bradycardia: below 120 beats/min
  Late decelerations
    Prolonged deceleration
  Severe variable decelerations
Uterine hyperstimulation
  Contractions longer than 90 sec
  Contractions occurring more frequently than q2min
  Peak pressure of contraction above 90 mm Hg pressure
  Inadequate uterine relaxation: less than 30 sec between contractions
  Intrauterine resting tone above 15 mm Hg pressure between contractions
  Sustained tetanic uterine contraction
Meconium-stained amniotic fluid
Maternal hypertension
Water intoxication
  Rising BP
  Edema of face, fingers, and around eyes
  Shortness of breath
  Difficulty in breathing
  Urinary output <30 to 50 ml/hr
Abruptio placentae: sudden, severe uterine pain (p. 725)

Precipitate delivery
Hemorrhage
Shock
Uterine rupture

Medical Management

Baseline FHR-UC recording
Oxytocin infusion at a rate of 0.5 mU/min and increasing for desired results at 15 to 20 min intervals in increments of 1 to 2 mU/min not to exceed 20 mU/min
Continuous FHR-UC monitoring
Analgesia
Tocolytic agents for excessive uterine activity that persists after oxytocin is discontinued, after supportive treatment is provided (lateral position and oxygen by mask) and fetal distress is present
Terbutaline 0.25 mg IV push or magnesium sulfate 4 grams, 10% solution IV over 15 to 20 minutes

Nursing diagnoses/interventions/evaluation

■ **NDX:** Potential for injury related to augmentation of labor and potential uterine hyperstimulation

See Care of Mother in First Stage of Labor (p. 704)
Maintain complete bed rest
Ensure that physician is immediately available
Apply fetal monitoring; obtain baseline strip before start of IV oxytocin
Place patient in position of comfort; lateral position is preferred
Always piggyback oxytocin solution into main IV line (10 U oxytocin in 1000 ml IV fluid = 10 mU/ml)
Administer oxytocin via a controlled infusion device as ordered
Monitor dose in mU/min q15min to 30min and before each increase
Increase rate of oxytocic solution as ordered to produce contractions q2min to 3min of 30 to 60 sec duration
Monitor patency of parenteral system
Check BP, P, and FHR q15min to 30min or as ordered
Observe contractions for frequency, duration, strength, and relaxation q5min for five times, then q15min to 30min and prn
Administer analgesics as ordered
Assist in breathing and relaxation techniques (p. 706)
Measure intake and output q2h

TABLE 15-1. Dysfunctional Labor Patterns

	Nulliparas	Multiparas
Prolonged latent phase	> 21 hours	> 14 hours
Protracted active phase	< 1.2 cm hour	< 1.5 cm hour
Secondary arrest: *no change*	> 2 hours	> 2 hours
Prolonged deceleration phase	> 3 hours	> 1 hour
Protracted descent	< 1 cm hour	< 2 cm hour
Arrest of descent	> 1 hour	> ½ hour

TABLE 15-2. Bishop Scoring System

Score	0	1	2	3
Station of Presenting Part	−3	−2	−1/0	+1/+2
Dilatation in cm	0	1-2	3-4	>5
Effacement in cm	>2.5	2	1	<0.5
Consistency	Firm	Medium	Soft	—
Position of os	Posterior	Central	Anterior	—

Prepare for delivery as indicated

Reinforce physician's explanation of reason for augmentation or induction of labor

Expected outcome/evaluation

Mother and fetus are not compromised as a result of oxytocin infusion

■ **NDX:**   Knowledge deficit related to lack of information about oxytocin infusion procedure

Reinforce physician's explanations
Discuss indications for procedure
Explain methodology of administration
Discuss expected effects of oxytocin induction/augmentation of labor
Explain differences between induction/augmentation and normal, spontaneous contractions

Expected outcome/evaluation

Patient/significant other verbalize understanding of procedure, indications for it, and expected effects

FETAL DISTRESS

A symptom complex indicative of a critical response to stress; may include hypoxia and/or acidosis

Assessment
Observations/findings

Fetal tachycardia: above 160 beats/min
Fetal bradycardia: below 120 beats/min
Meconium-stained amniotic fluid
Fetal hyperactivity or hypoactivity
Monitored fetus
  Nonreassuring FHR patterns
    Progressive increase or decrease in baseline FHR
    Tachycardia: 160 beats/min or greater; progressive decrease in baseline variability
  Ominous FHR patterns
    Severe variable deceleration; FHR below 70 beats/min for longer than 30 sec with
      Rising baseline FHR
      Decreasing variability
      Slow return to baseline (may be with overshoot)
    Late decelerations of any magnitude
    Absence of variability
    Prolonged deceleration
    Severe bradycardia
    Unstable FHR; sinusoidal pattern

Laboratory/diagnostic studies

Electronic fetal monitoring
Amniocentesis
Cord blood studies
Fetal scalp sampling: pH < 7.2

Potential complications

Fetal death
Neonatal death
CNS disorders
Meconium aspiration syndrome
Intracranial hemorrhage
Hypoxia
Hypoglycemia

Medical Management

Discontinue tocolytic therapy as applicable
Administer oxygen to mother
Deliver infant as indicated
Fetal blood sampling as indicated
IV fluids as indicated
Laboratory tests as indicated
Continuous fetal evaluation until time of delivery
Neonatal resuscitation required at delivery

Nursing diagnoses/interventions/evaluation

■ **NDX:**   Potential for injury to fetus related to episode(s) of fetal distress

Intervene methodically; it is not necessary to proceed with subsequent steps if intervention corrects FHR pattern
Change maternal position to where FHR pattern is most improved
Correct maternal hypotension: elevate legs; increase rate of maintenance IV infusion
Discontinue oxytocin if infusing
Administer oxygen by face mask at rate of 10 to 12 L/min or as ordered
Fetal scalp or acoustic stimulation may be done to assess FHR variability if patient is making good progress toward vaginal delivery
Perform vaginal and/or speculum examination to check for prolapsed cord
Assist physician with fetal blood sampling as indicated
Prepare for termination of labor as indicated
Explain briefly to patient the reasons for actions taken

Expected outcome/evaluation

Fetus will have minimal compromise
Fetus/infant will be delivered in good condition

■ **NDX:**   Anxiety/fear related to uncertain infant outcome and unfamiliarity with care required to treat fetal distress

Explain all interventions to mother and significant other, such as
  Reasons for procedure
  How procedures are to be done
  Available options
  Results expected from procedure
Simplify explanations and repeat as necessary

TABLE 15-3. Biophysical Profile

A. Description: A Physical Examination of the Fetus with Realtime Ultrasound Measuring

Fetal breathing movements (FBM)
Fetal movement (FM)
Fetal tone (TON)
Amniotic fluid index (AFI)
Nonstress test (NST)

B. Interpretation

Biophysical variable	Normal (score = 2)	Abnormal (score = 0)
Fetal breathing movements (FBM)	At least one episode of FBM of at least 30 sec duration in 30-min observation	Absent FBM or no episode of ≥30 sec in 30 min
Gross body movements (FM)	At least three discrete body/limb movements in 30 min (episodes of active continuous movement considered as a single movement)	Two or fewer episodes of body/limb movements in 30 min
Fetal tone (TON)	At least one episode of active extension with return to flexion of fetal limb(s) or trunk; opening and closing of hand considered normal tone	Slow extension with return to partial flexion, or movement of limb in full extension, or absence of fetal movement
*Amniotic fluid index (AFI)	AFI ≤ 5 cm	AFI < 5 cm
Nonstress test (NST)	Reactive	Nonreactive

* Amniotic fluid index: The summation of deepest vertical pocket of amniotic fluid in each of the four quadrants of the amniotic sac. Measurements are done in centimeters and perpendicular to the floor.

C. Record Biophysical Profile

Parameter	Score
FBM	_____
FM	_____
TON	_____
AFI	_____
NST	_____
TOTAL:	_____

D. Management Based on Interpretation and Score

Score	Action
8-10	Equivalent to reactive NST; manage per protocol
4-6	If pulmonary maturity is favorable, deliver; if not, repeat test in 24 hours; if score persists, deliver if maturity is certain; otherwise, treat with steroids and deliver in 48 hours
0-2	Evaluate for delivery

Provide realistic, factual information regarding infant status
Provide information regarding availability of neonatal intensive care unit should infant require this type of care
Reassure patient that emergency equipment and experienced personnel are available for delivery
Encourage patient to express concerns
Offer choices where feasible
Provide information regarding
Known possible causes of fetal distress

Misconceptions
Postdelivery
Ensure that parents see infant before transport to nursery
Allow mother to hold and/or stroke infant if possible

Expected outcome/evaluation

Patient/significant other verbalize understanding of required care and are able to verbalize fears and concerns regarding infant

CARE OF MOTHER ON FETAL MONITOR

Refer to Care of the Mother During Labor (p. 704)

The following guidelines relate to patient teaching and functioning of the monitor

Explain that fetal status via FHR can be continuously assessed even during contractions

Explain that lower activity on strip chart shows uterine activity; upper panel shows FHR

Reassure patient and significant other that prepared childbirth techniques can be implemented without difficulty

Explain that effleurage performed during external monitoring can be done on sides of abdomen or upper thighs

Relate that breathing patterns based on timing and intensity of contractions can be enhanced by observation of uterine activity panel of strip chart for onset of contractions

Note peak of contraction; knowing that contraction will not get stronger and is half over is usually helpful

Note diminishing intensity

Coordinate with appropriate breathing and relaxation techniques

Reassure patient/significant other that use of internal mode of monitoring does not restrict patient movement

Explain that use of external mode of monitoring usually requires patient cooperation in positioning and movement

Reassure patient and significant other that use of monitor does not imply fetal jeopardy

External Monitoring
ULTRASOUND TRANSDUCER

Monitors FHR with high-frequency sound waves

Tap transducer before use to ensure sound transmission

Apply ultrasound transmission gel to maternal abdomen; clean abdomen and transducer and reapply gel q2h and prn

Massage reddened skin areas and reposition belt or adhesive device q2h and prn

Auscultate FHR with stethoscope or fetoscope if in doubt as to validity of tracing

Position and reposition transducer prn to ensure clear, interpretable FHR data

TOCOTRANSDUCER

Monitors uterine activity via a pressure-sensing device placed on the maternal abdomen

Position and reposition qh and prn on the fundus where least maternal tissue is in evidence

Maintain abdominal strap snugly

Adjust penset *between* contractions to print between 20 and 25 mm Hg on strip chart

Palpate fundus q30min to 60min to gauge strength of contraction; only frequency and duration of contractions can be assessed with tocotransducer

Do not assess patient's need for analgesic based on uterine activity displayed on strip chart

Massage reddened areas under transducer and belt qh and prn

Internal Monitoring
SPIRAL ELECTRODE

Obtains fetal ECG from presenting part and converts it into FHR

Ensure that color-coded wires are appropriately attached to push post on leg plate

Apply electrode paste to leg plate q2h and prn

Observe FHR panel of strip chart for long- and short-term variability

Turn electrode counterclockwise to remove; never pull straight out from presenting part

Administer perineal care after voiding during labor

INTRAUTERINE CATHETER

Catheter (may be fluid-filled) that internally monitors intrauterine pressure

Flush open system catheter with sterile water before insertion and prn

Ensure that black mark on catheter is visible at introitus

Maintain height of strain gauge at miduterine level

For open system catheters

Turn stopcock off to patient, then with pressure valve of strain gauge released, flush strain gauge, remove syringe, and set stylus to 0 line of chart paper; test further according to manufacturer's instructions q3h to 4h and prn

For closed system catheters set baseline rate between uterine contractions when uterus is relaxed

Check proper functioning by tapping catheter, asking patient to cough, or applying fundal pressure; observe appropriate inflection on strip chart

Maintain catheter taped to patient's leg to prevent dislodgement

NONSTRESS TEST (NST)

Basis for NST is that the healthy fetus will exhibit acceleration of FHR and average FHR variability with fetal movement or in response to vibroacoustic stimulation

Assessment
Observations/findings

Accelerations of FHR

Other periodic changes in FHR

Baseline changes in FHR

Evidence of fetal movement on strip chart

Blips

Spikes

Momentary increases in uterine pressure

Laboratory/diagnostic studies
INTERPRETATION OF RESULTS OF NONSTRESS TEST

Reactive: two or more accelerations of FHR with an amplitude of 15 beats/min lasting 15 sec or more associated with fetal movement in a 10 min period or five or more FHR accelerations in a 20 min period

Nonreactive: either less than two accelerations of FHR with an amplitude below 15 beats/min or lasting less than 15 sec, or absence of accelerations associated with fetal movement in a 10 min period, or less than five FHR accelerations in a 20 min period

Suspicious: definite accelerations of FHR associated with fetal movement; however, number of accelerations or amplitude and duration do not meet criteria of reactive or nonreactive test

Unsatisfactory: quality of FHR recording is not adequate for interpretation

Potential complications

Identification of fetal compromise
Detection of uteroplacental insufficiency

Medical Management

Begun at 32 to 34 weeks in high-risk patients
If nonreactive, proceed to VST and/or CST
If reactive, repeat 1 to 2 times per week until delivery or until nonreactive

Nursing Care

Explain general use of equipment and procedure to patient and significant other

Give full liquid meal (if not taken before test) to reduce bowel sounds if ordered

Request patient to void

Assist patient with assuming semi-Fowler's position with lateral uterine tilt

Monitor FHR and uterine activity externally until test can be interpreted

Confirm fetal movement by palpation or patient confirmation

Reinforce implications of reactive and nonreactive tests

VIBROACOUSTIC STIMULATION TEST (VST)

Monitor FHR and UA until at least 10 to 15 min of interpretable data is obtained

Apply artificial larynx firmly to the maternal abdomen over the fetal head

Depress the button on the artificial larynx from 1 to 10 seconds according to facility procedure

Observe the FHR strip:

Reactive test: increase in FHR of at least 15 bpm from baseline in response to vibroacoustic stimulation (Note this increase may last for 15 to 30 min and should be interpreted as tachycardia)

Nonreactive test: no response of FHR to vibroacoustic stimulation; consider proceeding to contraction stress test

CONTRACTION STRESS TEST (CST)

Assessment of uteroplacental reserve by means of "stressing" the fetus with contractions and observing the resultant FHR pattern

Assessment
Observations/findings

Periodic changes in FHR
    Accelerations
    Decelerations: early, late, variable
Baseline changes in FHR
    Tachycardia
    Bradycardia
    Absent or minimal variability
    Sinusoidal pattern

Laboratory/diagnostic studies
INTERPRETATION OF RESULTS

Negative: three contractions >40 sec duration in a 10 min period without late decelerations; there is usually a good baseline variability and acceleration of FHR with fetal movement

Positive: persistent and consistent late decelerations occurring with more than half the contractions

Hyperstimulation: contractions occurring more often than q2min and/or lasting longer than 90 sec
    Uterine hypertonus; rise of baseline uterine tone
    Late decelerations occurring during or after excessive uterine activity

Suspicious: late decelerations occurring with less than half the uterine contractions once an adequate contraction pattern has been established

Unsatisfactory: inadequate contraction pattern or tracing too poor to interpret; test is not interpretable and cannot be used for clinical management

Potential complications

Uterine hyperstimulation
Elevated BP
Onset of labor
Supine hypotension syndrome
Clarity of strip chart tracing
Fetal compromise
Emergency delivery

Medical Management
After nonreactive NST

If positive CST, imminent delivery
If negative CST, repeated per hospital protocol until delivery or until CST becomes positive

Preprocedural care and teaching

Explain general use of equipment and procedure to patient and significant other

Give full liquid meal (if not taken before test) to reduce bowel sounds if ordered

Request patient to void

Assist patient with assuming semi-Fowler's or lateral tilt position

Understand that contractions can be stimulated by dilute IV oxytocin or by nipple stimulation

Nipple-stimulated contractions

Monitor FHR and uterine activity externally to determine baseline until at least 10 min of interpretable data are obtained

Check BP and P q15min

Defer nipple stimulation if three unstimulated contractions of greater than 40 sec duration occur within a 10 min period

Apply warm, moist washcloth to both breasts for several minutes

Instruct patient to massage and/or roll nipple of one breast for 10 min; if uterine contractions do not occur, stimulate both breasts for 10 min

Restimulate breasts intermittently as needed to maintain uterine contractions

If nipple stimulation does not produce desired uterine activity, proceed to oxytocin-stimulated contraction stress test

Oxytocin-stimulated contractions (oxytocin challenge test; OCT)

Administer parenteral fluids with oxytocin piggybacked into main IV line; deliver with infusion pump in mU/min

Check BP and P q15min

Monitor FHR and uterine contractions externally to determine baseline uterine activity until 10 min of interpretable data are obtained before administration of oxytocin

Defer oxytocin infusion if three unstimulated contractions of greater than 40 sec duration occur within a 10 min period; interpret the results

Increase dosage of oxytocin q15min to 20min as ordered

Discontinue oxytocin when three uterine contractions of greater than 40 sec duration have occurred within a 10 min period

Postprocedure care

Continue to monitor FHR and uterine contractions until uterine activity is diminished to pretest baseline

Interpret results of test

Teach patient signs of onset of labor; labor almost never begins within 48 hr if fetus is less than 38 weeks' gestational age

Expected outcome/evaluation

Complications are absent or minimized

Patient complies with procedure instructions

POSTPARTUM CARE

Care after delivery of a fetus through the vaginal canal throughout the maternal recovery period to 6 weeks after birth

Assessment
Observations/desirable findings

Skin
  Mask of pregnancy
  Striae
Breasts
  Colostrum
  Breast milk
Abdomen
  Uterine involution
    Firm (Figure 15-9)
    Midline
    1 to 2 finger breadths below umbilicus and decreasing
  Relaxed abdominal muscles
Lochia
  Color: rubra, serosa, or alba
  Flow: heavy, moderate, light, or scant
Perineum: episiotomy clean and intact (Figure 15-10)
Appropriate psycho-emotional responses to childbirth

Laboratory/diagnostic studies

Hgb/Hct
Medication blood levels as ordered
CBC with differential if indicated
Electrolytes if indicated

Potential complications

Hemorrhage; soft, relaxed fundus
  Retained placental fragments
  Hematoma of episiotomy site
Infection
  Elevated temperature
  Diaphoresis
  Chilling
  Nausea, vomiting
  Tachycardia
  Foul odor of lochia
  After pains
  Drainage from episiotomy
  Edema, redness, or discoloration at incisions or lacerations
  Gaping sutures at incisions or lacerations
Bladder distention and/or inability to void
Painful hemorrhoids
Constipation

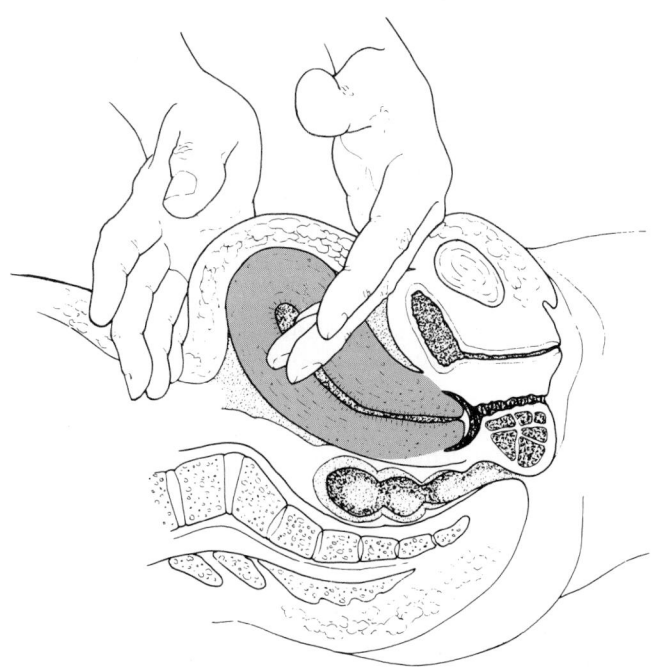

FIGURE 15-9. Palpating fundus of uterus during first hour after delivery. Note that upper hand is cupped over fundus; lower hand dips in above symphysis pubis and supports uterus while it is massaged gently. (From Bobak IM, Jensen MD: *Essentials of maternity nursing*, ed 3, St Louis, 1991, Mosby–Year Book).

Thrombophlebitis
Pulmonary embolus
Engorged breasts; sore nipples
Behavioral changes
    Depression
    Withdrawal
    Lack of contact with, or care of, newborn
    Infant abuse
    Infant neglect

Medical Management

Postpartum assessment with vital signs
Neurological checks and spinal dermatomes check with vital signs if regional anesthesia is received
IV fluids
Oxytocics as indicated
Pain medications, stool softeners, antiflatulents as indicated
Breast binder if indicated
Lactation suppression drugs
Ice bag to perineum as indicated
Topical anesthetic to episiotomy prn
Anesthetic ointment for hemorrhoids
Foley catheter if indicated
Progressive ambulation as tolerated
Laboratory tests as indicated

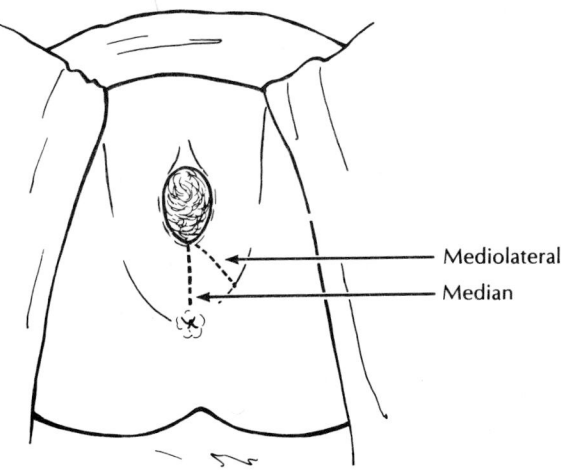

— Mediolateral
— Median

FIGURE 15-10. Types of episiotomies. (From Bobak IM, Jensen MD: *Essentials of maternity nursing*, ed 3, St Louis, 1991, Mosby–Year Book.)

Regular diet as tolerated; encourage po fluid and snacks
Intake and output
Anti-Rh globulin as indicated
Rubella vaccine as indicated

Nursing diagnoses/interventions/evaluation

■ **NDX:** Potential fluid volume deficit related to active loss associated with postpartum hemorrhage

Check the following q15min until stable then q4 to 8h per hospital policy
    Fundus location and tone
    Episiotomy condition
    Lochia amount, color, and consistency
    Level of consciousness
If fundus is soft and/or relaxed, massage until firm
Teach mother self-massage of uterine fundus
Teach mother normal parameters of lochia and instruct her to call physician if there is abnormally heavy flow
Change perineal pads q30min to 60min and/or as needed; report excessive bleeding to physician
Avoid unnecessary massage of fundus, which can cause uterine relaxation and hemorrhage
Maintain parenteral fluids with oxytocics as ordered
Encourage fluids po unless contraindicated
Measure intake and output for 24 hr or as ordered
Remain with patient during the first time out of bed in the event that hemodynamic changes and/or orthostatic hypotension result in dizziness/faintness

Expected outcome/evaluation

Patient
    Does not become hypovolemic as a result of excessive blood loss
    Has vital signs that are WNL

■ **NDX:** Pain related to episiotomy, afterbirth pains, and/or breast discomfort

Note time when sensation has returned to lower extremities after spinal anesthetic

Manage pain; administer medication as ordered

Apply ice bag to perineum as ordered

Maintain warmth with blankets; avoid drafts in patient care unit

Use sitz bath tid and prn if ordered

Administer anesthetic spray to episiotomy and hemorrhoids prn

Apply anesthetic ointment to hemorrhoids prn

Shower or bathe daily; avoiding washing nipples of breast-feeding mothers at any other time as this removes natural oils and contributes to skin irritation and discomfort

Have mother wear supportive bra at all times

Check breasts q4h to 8h and prn

If breast-feeding

Manually express breasts q4h and after nursing

Place warm moist towel packs on engorged breasts for 15 to 30 min q1h to 3h, then massage and manually express breasts or have infant nurse

If bottle-feeding

Never massage or manually express engorged breasts

Have mother wear snug-fitting breast binder over bra and use ice bags q1h to 3h for 15 min on each side if breasts are engorged

Stand with back toward water in shower to avoid stimulation of breasts

Anticipate need for pain relief

Administer pain medication as ordered and document effectiveness

Instruct mother to squeeze buttocks together when sitting down if episiotomy is painful with ambulation

Encourage mother to use relaxation techniques learned in labor for afterbirth pains during breast-feeding

Expected outcome/evaluation

Patient's

Pain is relieved or minimized

Uterine fundus is firm and pain-free

Able to demonstrate proper breast care

■ **NDX:** Potential for infection related to incision and/or lacerations

Instruct patient on perineal care per hospital policy

Change perineal pad from front to back after each elimination

Observe condition of episiotomy and document same each shift

Watch for elevated temperature or other changes in vital sign parameters

Note and report any abnormal, foul-smelling drainage or discharge

Administer antibiotics as ordered

Expected outcome/evaluation

Patient's episiotomy and/or lacerations heal without evidence of infection as evidenced by absence of edema and drainage

■ **NDX:** Potential for urinary retention related to trauma and subsequent edema associated with childbirth process

Avoid distention of bladder; encourage voiding within 6 to 8 hr after delivery or catheterize as ordered

Encourage daily fluids to 3000 ml unless contraindicated

Encourage patient to void q4 to 6h as able

Employ techniques to assist voiding as needed, including voiding in sitz bath if this is the only way the patient can comfortably void

Expected outcome/evaluation

Patient

Does not experience bladder distention

Voids q.s. following delivery

■ **NDX:** Constipation related to pain of episiotomy and hemorrhoids secondary to childbirth process

Ensure adequate fluid intake

Sitz bath may be of some help to relax perianal muscles before bowel movement

Give stool softeners or laxative as ordered

Encourage patient to ambulate as tolerated, increasing progressively

Maintain regular diet with between-meal snacks; increase amount of fruit and roughage

Anesthetic spray/ointment applied to perianal area and episiotomy site may provide pain relief and subsequently permit bowel movement

Expected outcome/evaluation

Patient has bowel movement with minimal discomfort

■ **NDX:** Potential for altered parenting related to transition to parenthood and role change

Recover mother and infant in same bed under radiant heat warmer if possible to promote visual inspection, skin to skin contact, and attachment

Assist with holding and inspecting infant as soon as possible and before 6 hr after delivery and prn until mother is able to become actively involved in infant care

Permit mother to have infant at bedside as little or as much as she desires

Meet mother's dependency needs during "taking in" phase (first 2 to 3 days)

    Encourage verbalization; mothers are usually extremely talkative, repeatedly relating experience of labor and delivery

    Understand that enthusiastic listening by nurse helps experience become more meaningful to parents

Meet mother's needs during "taking hold" phase (about 10 days)

    Reassure mother that she is performing well in all aspects of self-care and infant care

    Avoid intervening between mother and infant regardless of how awkward her skills seem

    Positively reinforce all tasks done well

    Avoid negative criticism at all times, unless solicited by parent

Assist and teach mother to perform all infant care tasks: bathing, feeding, diapering, cord care, cuddling, etc.

Teach mother and visitors proper handwashing technique

Involve spouse or significant other in infant care and teaching

Observe mother-infant interaction; report to physician

    Mother not holding infant while feeding

    Lack of eye contact between mother and infant

    Absence of verbalization of mother to infant

    Lack of physical contact with infant

Encourage verbalization about role of mothering, effect of new family member, and sibling rivalry, if applicable

Encourage visits by healthy siblings unless contraindicated

See Care of Newborn (p. 725)

Expected outcome/evaluation

Mother

    Demonstrates adequate infant caretaking skills

    Provides an optimal environment for infant growth and development

 NDX: Situational low self-esteem in response to feelings of inadequacy associated with responsibilities of parenthood related to birth experience

Encourage discussion of real and perceived problems

Help mother validate the reality of her labor and delivery experience

Give reassurance concerning her ability as a mother

Help patient accept emotional ups and downs of postpartum period and explain that these feelings and changes are common during this time

Encourage rest periods throughout the day

Provide opportunity for parent/infant interactions and involve father or significant other as possible

Support and encourage parents and/or significant other in interactions and caring for infant

Expected outcome/evaluation

Mother

    Demonstrates effective emotional adjustment and healthy self-esteem as evidenced by positive statements about self and about abilities to care for infant

■ **NDX:** Knowledge deficit related to lack of information about postpartum care

Caution patient to avoid coitus or douching for 4 to 6 weeks or as indicated by physician

Demonstrate breast care and manual expression if mother is breast-feeding

Emphasize importance of nutritious diet

Caution patient to avoid lifting anything heavier than the infant for 2 to 3 weeks

Explain need for planned rest periods

Explain need to carefully clean perineal region

    Wipe from front to back after urinating

    Administer perineal self-care

    Apply perineal pad from front to back

    Wash vulva and perineum, including sutures, before washing anal area when showering

Relate that absorbable sutures do not need to be removed

Relate that sitz bath and perineal light may be used at home prn

Instruct patient to use anesthetic spray and/or ointment to perineal area and/or hemorrhoids

Caution patient to avoid constipation; stool softeners or mild laxatives may be necessary

Discuss symptoms to report to physician

    Temperature above 100° F (37.8° C)

    Foul odor of lochia

Relate that shower or tub bath may be taken

Explain that lochia may continue for 3 to 4 weeks, changing from red to brown to white

Relate that menses will return 6 to 8 weeks after delivery, often despite breast-feeding

    Explain that some nursing mothers do not menstruate until they wean infant from breast, whereas others resume menstruation at various times while nursing

    Emphasize that pregnancy is possible 4 to 6 weeks after delivery, whether mother is breast-feeding or not; discuss availability of nonprescription methods of contraception

Explain need for mild exercise initially

    Do not start vigorous exercise until approved by physician

    Explain that Kegel exercises can be begun during early puerperium

Discuss normalcy of postpartum "blues"

Discuss need to plan for needs of other children at home and discuss possible behavioral changes as a result of new family member

Teach name of medication, dosage, time of administration, purpose, and side effects

Emphasize importance of ongoing outpatient care, including postpartum checkup

Emphasize the normalcy of feelings that may be disturbing
  Initial lack of feeling of love for infant
    Variations from prenatal expectations of what infant would look like; disappointment in sex, weight, or appearance
    Frustration caused by increased demands on time
    Feelings of being trapped
    Unsettled feelings about being a mother and parent
    Feelings of tension, nervousness, and fatigue
Discuss how to contact available community resources
  Housekeeping agencies
  Nursing care agencies
  Diaper services
  Family planning organizations
  Breast-feeding organizations: La Leche League*
  Parenting groups
  Publications on infant care
    Growth and development
    Parenting
    Health care
Discuss proper principles and practice of infant care

Expected outcome/evaluation

Patient demonstrates and verbalizes understanding of postpartum self-care and infant care

CESAREAN DELIVERY

Delivery of a fetus through a uterine incision; most common is the transverse lower segment incision, with the classic vertical cesarean incision done less frequently

Assessment
Observations/findings
INDICATIONS

CPD in current pregnancy
Fetal distress
Failure to progress in labor
Malposition of fetus
  Breech presentation
  Transverse lie
  Abnormal vertex presentation
Umbilical cord prolapse
Abruptio placentae
Placenta previa

---

*La Leche League International, 9616 Minneapolis Ave, Franklin Park, IL 60131.

Preoperative laboratory/diagnostic studies

Fetal monitoring for fetal well-being
ECG monitoring
CBC with differential
Electrolytes
Hgb/Hct
Type and cross match for blood
Urinalysis
Amniocentesis for fetal lung maturity as indicated
X-ray examination as indicated
Ultrasound as ordered

Potential complications

Hemorrhage; soft, relaxed uterine fundus
Shock
Anemia
DIC
Infection
  Elevated temperature
  Tachycardia
  Foul odor of lochia
Site of incision
  Redness
  Pain
  Swelling
  Drainage
Cystitis
Engorged breasts
Pneumonia
Paralytic ileus
Thrombophlebitis
Pulmonary embolus
Behavioral changes
  Guilt
  Depression
  Withdrawal
  Lack of contact with or care of newborn
Anesthesia reaction: malignant hyperthermia
Fetal injury during surgery
Fetal blood loss during surgery
Neonatal depression/resuscitation at birth

Medical Management

IV fluids as indicated
Anesthesia: regional or general
Agreement of significant other to attend cesarean section
Laboratory/diagnostic tests as indicated
Oxytocic administration as indicated
Vital signs per recovery room protocol
Abdominal surgery skin preparation
Consent form signed
Foley catheter insertion
See Postpartum Care (p. 714) for routine medical management

■ **NDX:** Knowledge deficit related to lack of information about procedure and precesarean delivery care

Predelivery teaching

Discuss with mother and significant other the reason for cesarean section

Explain "normal" preoperative procedures and potential variations for current situation

Witness consent form and obtain baseline vital signs

Draw blood for CBC, electrolytes, type, and screen

Obtain urine for urinalysis

Insert Foley catheter

Maintain NPO status

Perform abdominal surgery preparation per hospital policy and aseptic technique principles

Administer IV fluids as ordered

Remove contact lenses and jewelry

Discuss presence of husband/significant other in operating room as appropriate

Encourage parents to attend preparatory classes specifically for cesarean delivery if cesarean is elective

Inform father that immediately postdelivery, he may hold infant close to mother's face and arms unless contraindicated

Expected outcome/evaluation

Patient will verbalize rationale for cesarean delivery and cooperate with pre-surgical preparations

■ **NDX:** Pain related to postoperative condition

Anticipate need for pain medications and/or additional methods of pain relief

Note, document, and identify
Reports of pain at incisional site: abdomen
Facial grimace of pain
Decreasing mobility
Relief/distraction behavior

Administer pain medication as ordered and evaluate its effectiveness

Provide other comfort measures that may be helpful, such as repositioning or supporting with pillows

Expected outcome/evaluation

Pain is minimized/controlled and patient verbalizes that she is comfortable

■ **NDX:** Impaired cardiopulmonary and peripheral tissue perfusion related to interruption of flow secondary to postoperative immobility

Assess respiratory status with vital signs

Document and report increased respiratory rate, non-productive cough, audible rhonchi, rales, or upper airway congestion

Note symptoms of
Pulmonary embolus
Restlessness
Chest pain
Diaphoresis
Dyspnea
Tachycardia
Change in BP
Abnormal breath sounds

Encourage patient to cough, turn, and deep breathe q2h during first postoperative day, then prn

Demonstrate splinting to support incision

Encourage use of incentive spirometer

Encourage early ambulation

Discuss elevating feet prn and not crossing legs

Check Homan's sign with vital signs

Note symptoms of
Deep vein thrombosis formation
Localized tenderness
Calf pain
Redness
Swelling
Elevated temperature
Positive Homan's sign

Expected outcome/evaluation

Patient
Does not have respiratory congestion
Shows no signs or symptoms of pulmonary embolism or deep vein thrombosis during hospitalization

■ **NDX:** Potential for altered patterns of urinary elimination and/or constipation related to manipulation and/or trauma secondary to cesarean section

Encourage voiding q4h to 6h if possible

Employ techniques to encourage voiding as needed

Explain perineal care procedures per hospital policy

Palpate lower abdomen if patient reports bladder distention and inability to void

Encourage mother to
Ambulate as tolerated
Increase intake of fluids (2000 to 3000 ml/day)
Increase fruit and roughage in diet

Give stool softener/laxative as ordered

Administer antiflatulents as ordered

Monitor intake and output until eliminating adequately

See Postpartum Care (p. 714)

Expected outcome/evaluation

Patient
Voids spontaneously without discomfort

Has a bowel movement within 3 to 4 days after surgery

■ **NDX:** Potential for situational low self-esteem in response to feelings of inadequacy associated with unanticipated cesarean delivery and interruption of anticipated childbirth experience

Encourage mother to verbalize fears and feelings of guilt and/or blame
  Sense of failure at not delivering "normally"
  Feelings of being cheated or disappointed
  Feelings of intrusion from surgical procedure
Provide support through reassurance and open communication
Include husband/significant other in discussions
Provide positive feedback to mother and significant other

Expected outcome/evaluation

Patient
  Verbalizes feelings of self-worth
  Demonstrates appropriate coping skills

■ **NDX:** Potential for infection or injury related to surgical procedure

Monitor for elevated temperature or tachycardia as signs of infection
Observe incision for signs of infection
  Redness
  Tenderness
  Swelling at incision site
  Reports of pain
  Unusual discharge
  Elevated temperature
Change dressing prn or as ordered
Assess fundus, lochia, and bladder with vital signs as ordered
Evaluate vital signs for symptoms of infection or hemorrhage q4h and prn
Massage fundus if boggy or does not remain firm
Notify physician of deviations from normal parameters
  Boggy, displaced uterus
  Uterine tenderness at palpation
  Persistent discharge of lochia rubra
  Profuse bleeding
  Foul-smelling lochia

Expected outcome/evaluation

Patient's
  Incision is clean and dry, without any signs or symptoms of infection
  Uterine involution progresses normally

■ **NDX:** Knowledge deficit related to lack of information about postcesarean delivery care

Discuss the following with mother and significant other during the postpartum period
  Need to avoid coitus or douching for 4 to 6 weeks or as indicated by physician
  Breast care and manual expression if breast-feeding
  Need to avoid sitting for long periods of time with knees bent
  Care of incision
  Symptoms of wound infection to report to physician
  Importance of nutritious diet
  To avoid lifting anything heavier than infant for 4 to 6 weeks
  Importance of planned rest periods
  Need to avoid constipation; stool softeners or mild laxatives may be necessary
  That showers may be taken
  That lochia may continue for 3 to 4 weeks, changing from red to brown to white
  That menses will return 6 to 8 weeks after delivery unless breast-feeding
    Explain that some nursing mothers do not menstruate until weaning infant from breast
    Explain that others resume menstruation at various times while nursing
    Explain that pregnancy is possible whether mother is breast-feeding or not, 4 to 6 weeks after delivery; discuss availability of nonprescription methods of contraception
  Importance of exercise; do not start vigorous exercise until approved by physician
  Name of medication, dosage, time of administration, purpose, and side effects
  Importance of follow-up outpatient care, including postpartum check-up
  Normalcy of postpartum "blues"
  Need to plan for needs of other children at home and discuss possible behavioral changes as a result of new family member
  Normalcy of feelings that may be disturbing to mother
    Initial lack of feeling of love for infant
    Variations from prenatal expectations of what infant would look like: disappointment in sex, weight, or appearance
    Frustration resulting from increased demands on time
    Feelings of being trapped
    Unsettled feelings about being a mother and parent
    Feelings of tension, nervousness, and fatigue
How to contact available community resources
  Housekeeping agencies
  Nursing care agencies
  Diaper services
  Family planning organizations
  Breast-feeding organizations: La Leche League, lactation institutes
  Cesarean birth groups (such as C/Sec. Inc.)

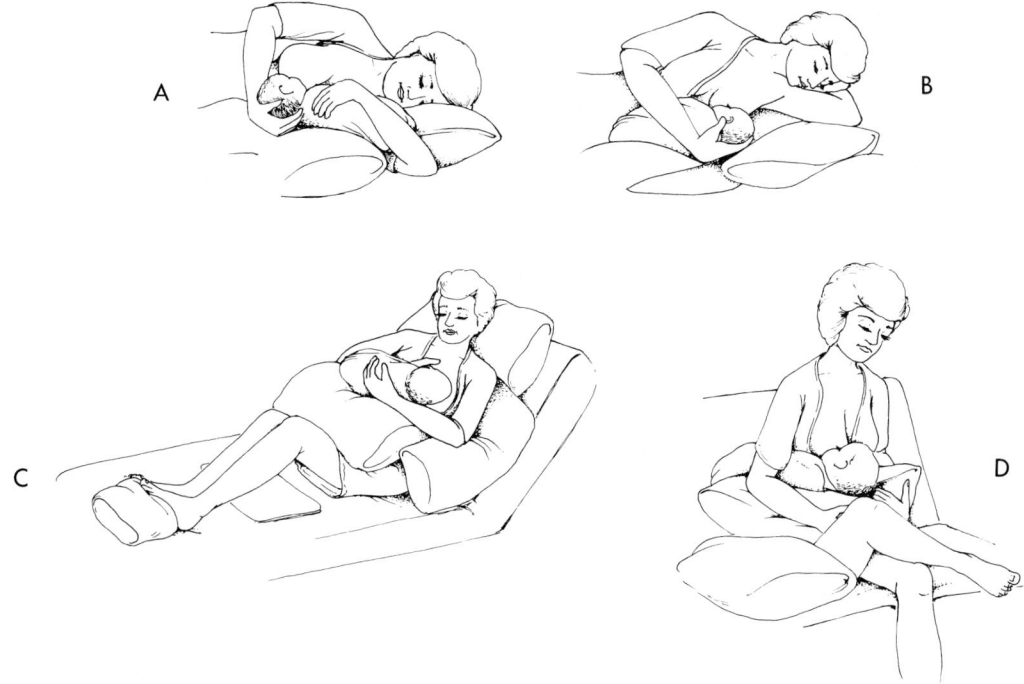

FIGURE 15-11. Comfortable breast-feeding positions after cesarean delivery. **A** and **B,** Side-lying position. **C,** Sitting in bed. **D,** "Football" hold.

Parenting groups
Publications on infant care
Growth and development
Parenting
Health care
Infant stimulation
See Care of Newborn (p. 725)

Breast-feeding

Discuss, demonstrate, and return-demonstrate breast-feeding principles related to cesarean delivery as follows
If desired, breast-feeding is possible
Feed only breast milk to baby
Do not supplement with formula or water routinely (see Breast-feeding)
Take pain medication 20 to 30 min before nursing
Proper positioning prevents and relieves discomfort
Instruct mother
When lying on either side
Put baby on his side facing you
Pull baby's buttocks toward abdomen
Use pillows to support the mother's back and protect abdomen
When sitting up in bed
Use pillows under both knees to support them
Place a pillow under each arm and another over abdomen
Put baby on his side toward the mother in "crook" of her arm, with his face and belly facing toward the mother

Instruct mother to pull baby in close
If abdomen is very sore after delivery, or baby is under 6 lb, mother can feed sitting up, using "football hold" (Figure 15-11); place baby facing up on pillow at mother's side and supported under her arm, his head toward foot of bed, feet toward head of bed

BREAST-FEEDING

Assessment
Observations/undesirable findings

Breasts
Hardness
Tenderness
Pain
Redness
Dehydration
Infant
Nursing more frequently than q2h
Voiding less than six times daily

Potential complications

Engorgement
Nipple problems
Cracked nipples
Inverted nipples
Sore nipples
Mastitis
Nipple confusion of infant

Medical Management

Antibiotics for mastitis as indicated

Referral to lactation specialist/consultant

Increase of caloric intake by 500 calories/day

Increase of fluid intake to 3000 ml daily unless contraindicated

Contraception counseling

Family planning counseling referrals as indicated

Nursing diagnoses/interventions/evaluation

■ **NDX:** Potential fluid volume deficit in infant related to inadequate breast-feeding

Instruct mother to

Feed baby when hungry

Begin feeding infant on one side for 10 to 30 min or until he begins to slow down

Break suction of baby's mouth on nipple by placing finger inside mouth between gums

Avoid pulling infant off breast without releasing suction

Burp baby in a sitting position after nursing at each breast

Place infant on opposite breast for 10 to 30 min or until he begins to slow down

Change back to other breast again until infant seems satisfied and falls asleep

Replace nursing bra after nursing is completed

Remind mother that during newborn period total feeding time can range from 20 min to 1 hr each

Remind mother that best way to tell if baby is getting enough milk is to listen for swallowing while sucking

Explain that adequate intake and nutrition is judged by six to eight wet diapers per day, baby sleeping 1 to 2 hr between feedings, and baby gaining weight by time of newborn examination with first visit to health care provider

Expected outcome/evaluation

Infant receives adequate intake for appropriate weight gain

■ **NDX:** Potential for ineffective breast-feeding related to any one of multiple factors, including previous history of breast-feeding failure, poor infant suck reflex, nonsupportive partner, interruption in breast-feeding, and lack of information about appropriate breast-feeding technique

Initiate breast-feeding as soon as mother and infant are in good condition (this may be on delivery table); manually express both breasts q4h until infant can be nursed

See Figures 15-12 and 15-13 on proper body and nipple positioning

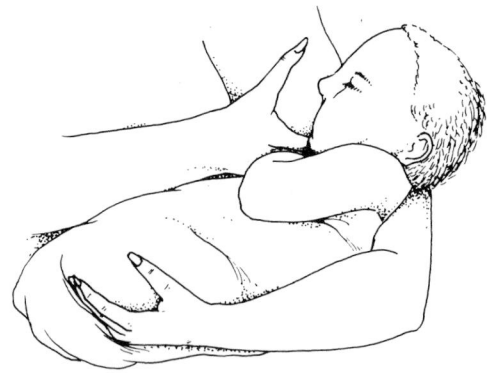

FIGURE 15-12. Correct body position for breast-feeding. Head of infant is in crook of mother's arm with front of infant facing front of mother.

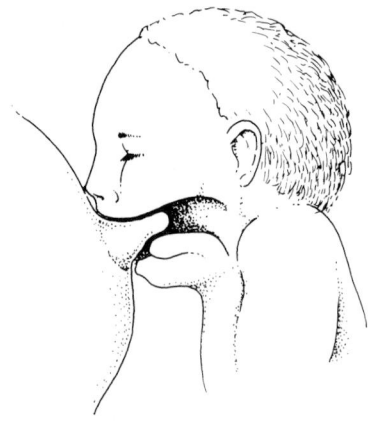

FIGURE 15-13. Correct latch-on position. Infant's mouth compresses milk-collecting sinuses in areola.

Remain with mother for at least her first two breast-feeding experiences

Have mother assume most comfortable position for her; may be sitting or lying on side

Alternate breast that is used first at each feeding: place safety pin on bra as reminder

Apply small amount of hydrous lanolin to nipples to prevent dryness and cracking if necessary as ordered; it does not need to be washed off before next feeding

Have mother shower daily for breast and general cleanliness

Do not wash breasts with any solution except water to avoid removing protective oils from breasts before each feeding

Avoid using nipple shield; if necessary, use only long enough to draw nipple out so that infant may grasp and suckle

Demonstrate hand expression of milk (Figure 15-14)

Wash hands well before starting

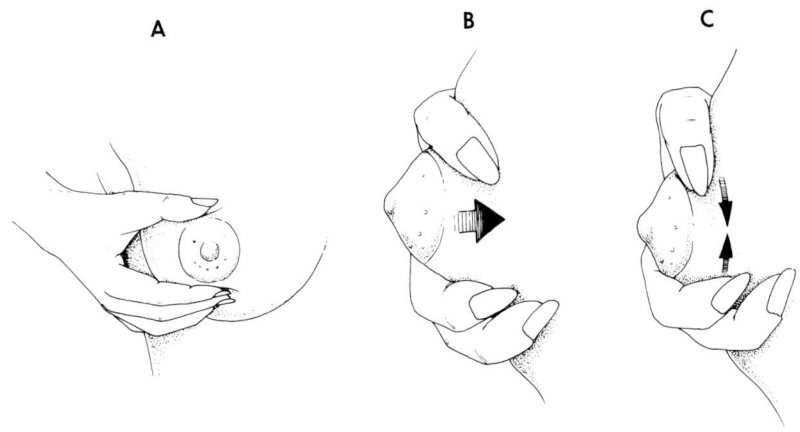

FIGURE 15-14. Hand expression of breast milk. **A,** Place thumb and fingers about 1 to 1½ inches behind nipple, forming C shape. **B,** Press in toward body. **C,** Firmly press fingers together on lacteal sinuses to express milk.

Cup breast with either hand (left hand for left breast, right hand for right breast)

Place thumb above and fingers below nipple, 1 to 1½ inches behind nipple on areola (forming the letter "C")

Press in toward back, then roll fingers down toward nipple, while gently pressing thumb and finger together

Do not let fingers slide on skin

Move fingers completely around areola to reach all milk sinuses

Alternate between breasts every few minutes

Instruct patient in appropriate techniques and relate information to promote a successful breast-feeding experience

Refer to specific instructions in next section under "knowledge deficit"

Expected outcome/evaluation

Patient

Demonstrates appropriate breast-feeding skills with a minimum of discomfort

Expresses satisfaction with the breast-feeding experience

■ **NDX:** Knowledge deficit related to lack of information about principles of breast-feeding

Discuss and assist mother with the following

Breast-feeding reflex: "let-down" reflex

Handwashing before breast-feeding

Body position (see Figure 15-6)

Nipple position (see Figure 15-7)

Inversion of nipples as indicated

Explain that supply of milk is related to demand

Giving formula only decreases milk supply

No need to supplement

Need for feeding often on demand (often up to every 1½ to 2 hr; later about every 3 hr-breast-fed babies usually eat every 3 hr)

Emphasize importance of drinking at least six to eight glasses of liquid each day (water, juice, and milk) and eating a balanced diet, including meat, milk, vegetables and fruits, grains and cereals

Advise patient to limit visitors and household duties for the first month postpartum

Suggest that patient have relatives or friends assist with household chores, shopping, and meals prn

Explain need for planned rest periods and napping when able

Relate that milk can be expressed into clean glass containers or into plastic disposable bottle liners

Explain that mother's daily fluid intake should be a minimum of 3000 ml unless contraindicated; a full 8 oz glass of fluid before each nursing session will help ensure adequate maternal hydration

Discuss adjustment of dietary intake to meet infant's needs

Eat well-balanced, high-protein diet

Avoid foods that cause infant distress (colicky, crying, wakeful); do not arbitrarily omit foods usually eaten

Explain that breast milk normally has a thin, watery appearance

Explain that milk supply will be adequate if infant nurses regularly; the more infant nurses the more milk is produced

Explain that six wet diapers daily of pale-colored urine is indicative that infant is properly hydrated

Explain that four to six bowel movements daily is normal in breast-fed infant

Explain that it may be necessary to keep infant awake

during feedings by unwrapping blanket and gently rubbing back or feet

Tell patient not to routinely give prepared formula

Explain that for several days after delivery it is normal to experience uterine cramping while nursing

Explain that milk flowing from opposite breast while nursing is normal

Caution patient to avoid plastic-coated breast shields in bra between feedings; a clean ironed handkerchief or Woolwich shield from La Leche League is preferred

Discuss treatment for engorged breasts
  Place very warm towel packs on breasts for 15 min
  Massage from outer breast to areola
  Manually express milk or nurse infant

Caution patient that a breast-feeding woman can become pregnant and should be aware of contraceptive methods other than oral contraceptives, which are usually contraindicated for at least the first 3 months

Relate that breast milk normally leaks during coitus

Discuss symptoms of complications to be reported to healthcare provider

Discuss how to contact local breast-feeding organizations for further information while at home
  La Leche League
  Lactation Institute
  Lactation specialists/consultants in private practice
  Breast-feeding clinics

Expected outcome/evaluation

Patient
  Demonstrates successful breast-feeding techniques
  Does not develop complications

POSTPARTUM HEMORRHAGE

Maternal blood loss postdelivery resulting from uterine atony, lacerations, and/or retained products of conception; predisposing factors include overdistended uterus (macrosomic baby, multiple gestation, hydramnios), unusually short, ≤4 hours, or prolonged labor, preeclampsia (PIH) treated with magnesium sulfate, chorioamnionitis

Assessment
Observations/findings

Uterine atony
  Relaxed fundus
  Dark bleeding
  Boggy, distended uterus
  Expulsion of clots
Genital lacerations
  Constant trickle of bright red blood
  Firm fundus
Retained placental tissue
  Dark bleeding
  Boggy, distended uterus

Abdominal pain
Tachycardia
Progressive hypotension

Laboratory/diagnostic studies

Vaginal examination
Clotting studies
Hgb and Hct
CVP monitoring

Potential complications

Shock
  Pallor
  Restlessness
  Weak, rapid pulse
  Decreased BP
  Chills
  Difficulty in breathing
  Air hunger
See Hypovolemic Shock (p. 105)
DIC
Postpartum infection
Anemia
Transfusion hepatitis
Hysterectomy (for placenta accreta)

Medical Management

Dilation and curettage (D & C) as indicated
Repair of lacerations
Manual removal of placental fragments
Insertion of uterine packing as indicated
IV fluids, volume expanders, or blood products
NPO
Strict intake and output
Vital signs as indicated
Antiembolic stockings as indicated
Oxygen therapy as indicated
Medications as indicated (prostaglandin, iron therapy)
Oxytocin infusion as indicated
Prostin E2 (PG E2) vaginal suppository as indicated
Vaginal packing as indicated

Nursing diagnoses/interventions/evaluations

■ **NDX:** Fluid volume deficit related to hypovolemia associated with postpartum hemorrhage

Never leave patient unattended during active bleeding
Massage relaxed, boggy fundus until firm; *do not overmassage or push hard on a relaxed fundus*
Administer oxygen at 10 to 12 L/min if ordered
Administer parenteral fluids with oxytocics as ordered
  Example: oxytocin 20 to 30 units in 1 L solution infused at rate of 200 cc/hr (DO NOT administer an undiluted IV bolus of oxytocin)
Administer volume expanders or blood as ordered
Check BP, P, and R q15min until stable, then as ordered

Palpate fundus and observe amount of vaginal bleeding q15min until stable

Measure intake and output

Weigh pads and linens to estimate blood loss

Apply antiembolic stockings to legs to enhance venous return

Maintain warmth with blankets

Allay anxiety as much as possible by remaining with patient and offering simple, brief explanations of care

Be aware that physician may order prostaglandin IM (or PG E2 vaginal suppository) to control atony

Continue with acute care and decrease frequency of nursing functions as patient's condition improves

Observe for side effects of iron therapy if ordered

Reinforce physician's explanation of the following, if done

    Vaginal examination

    Insertion of uterine packing

    D & C

Expected outcome/evaluation

Patient

    Receives adequate fluid replacement with no untoward effects

    Does not have symptoms of hemorrhagic/hypovolemic shock

■ **NDX:** Pain and discomfort related to uterine massage and uterine contraction

Explain purpose of frequent postpartum assessments

    Palpation of fundus for height, position, and tone

    Uterine massage if necessary

    Lochia flow

Encourage patient to palpate fundus and learn what good uterine tone feels like

Encourage patient to check fundus periodically and to massage as needed

Apply ice pack to perineum prn

Promote comfort by position changes

Encourage rest periods between examinations

Provide emotional support, especially if pain medication is contraindicated

Administer medications as ordered by physician and check for any reactions

Minimize other factors that could be contributing to discomfort, such as distended bladder, episiotomy pain, or "afterbirth" pain

■ **NDX:** Knowledge deficit related to lack of information about postpartum blood loss prevention/precautions

Discuss symptoms to report to physician or nurse practitioner

    Passage of large or several clots

Large amount of bleeding: more than a menstrual period

Pain

Foul odor of vaginal drainage

See Postpartum Care (p. 714)

Teach name of medication, dosage, time of administration, purpose, and side effects

Expected outcome/evaluation

Patient

    Verbalizes symptoms to report

    Demonstrates self-care as taught

Newborn

CARE OF NEWBORN

Assessment
Observations/findings
GENERAL

Apgar scores

Quality of cry and respirations

Skin color

Apical pulse and heart rate

Respiratory rate

Muscle tone

Reflexes

Thermal control

Cord condition

Feeding and sucking pattern

Stool pattern

Voiding pattern

Congenital defects

SPECIFIC

Apgar scores

Heart rate; presence of murmur

Respiratory effort

Muscle tone

Reflex irritability

Color

Abnormalities or malformations

Head circumference: normal, 33 to 35 cm

Chest circumference: normal, 30 to 33 cm

Birth-related trauma: presence of caput, cephalohematoma, and forceps marks

Amount of subcutaneous fat

Cry

    Lusty

    Feeble

    High-pitched

    Absent

    Asymmetrical facies

Umbilical cord

    Drainage

    Bleeding

Number and type of vessels
Presence or absence of Wharton's jelly
Unusually high or low temperature: normal, 97.7° F (36.5° C) axillary
Edema (except for presenting part)
Color
  Jaundice
  Pallor
  Gray, dusky
  Cyanosis
  Plethora
GI system
  Hard and soft palate intact
  Refusal to feed
  Excessive mucus
  Regurgitation; vomiting
  Abdominal distention
  Imperforate anus
  Stools
    Meconium
    Bloody
    Diarrhea
    Absent
Neurological system
  Moro's reflex: absent, asymmetrical, or hyperactive
  Sucking reflex: strong or weak
  Rooting reflex: good or poor
  Suck/swallow coordination
  Tremors
  Twitching
  Seizure activity
  Loss of motion of an extremity
State of consciousness
  Deep sleep
  Active REM sleep
  Drowsy
  Wide awake (quiet alert)
  Active awake (active alert)
  Crying
Respiratory rate: normal, 40 to 60/min
  Tachypnea
  Shallow or periodic breathing
  Nasal flaring
  Retractions
  Expiratory grunt
Cardiovascular rate: normal, 120 to 160 beats/min
  Tachycardia
  Bradycardia
  Blood pressure: normal, 60/30 to 90/50 mm Hg
Musculoskeletal system
  Muscle tone
  Muscle strength
  Limpness
  Weakness
  Rigidity

  Asymmetry
  Swelling of skull or spine
  Abnormal position or posture of extremity
Skin
  Pustules
  Abrasions
  Rash
  Petechiae
  Ecchymosis
  Condition of circumcision
Genitourinary system
  Hypospadias
  Epispadias
  Undescended testicles
  Indeterminate sex
  Failure to void

Laboratory/diagnostic studies

Cord blood samples
Phenylketonuria (PKU; newborn screening examination)
Hct

Potential complications

Altered thermoregulation
Birth injuries
Congenital defects
Need for resuscitation at delivery

Medical Management

Vitamin K IM injection
Newborn screening examination (PKU, thyroid, etc.)
Eye prophylaxis
Feeding schedule
Cord care protocol
Chemstrip as indicated
Hct
Daily weights
Rectal temperature once, then axillary temperature per protocol

Postdelivery nursing procedures

Perform stabilization procedures (Figure 15-15)
Take Apgar scores at 1, 5, and 10 min after delivery
Apply clamp to umbilical cord
Identify infant according to facility policy: bracelet, necklace, and/or footprints
Perform screening examination for congenital defects
Assist with infant's warm water bath as indicated (LeBoyer deliveries)
Show warmed infant to parents; identify sex and check identification bracelets initially and at each visit to mother and at discharge
Allow parents to hold infant as condition of infant and parents permits to promote attachment and family-centered care

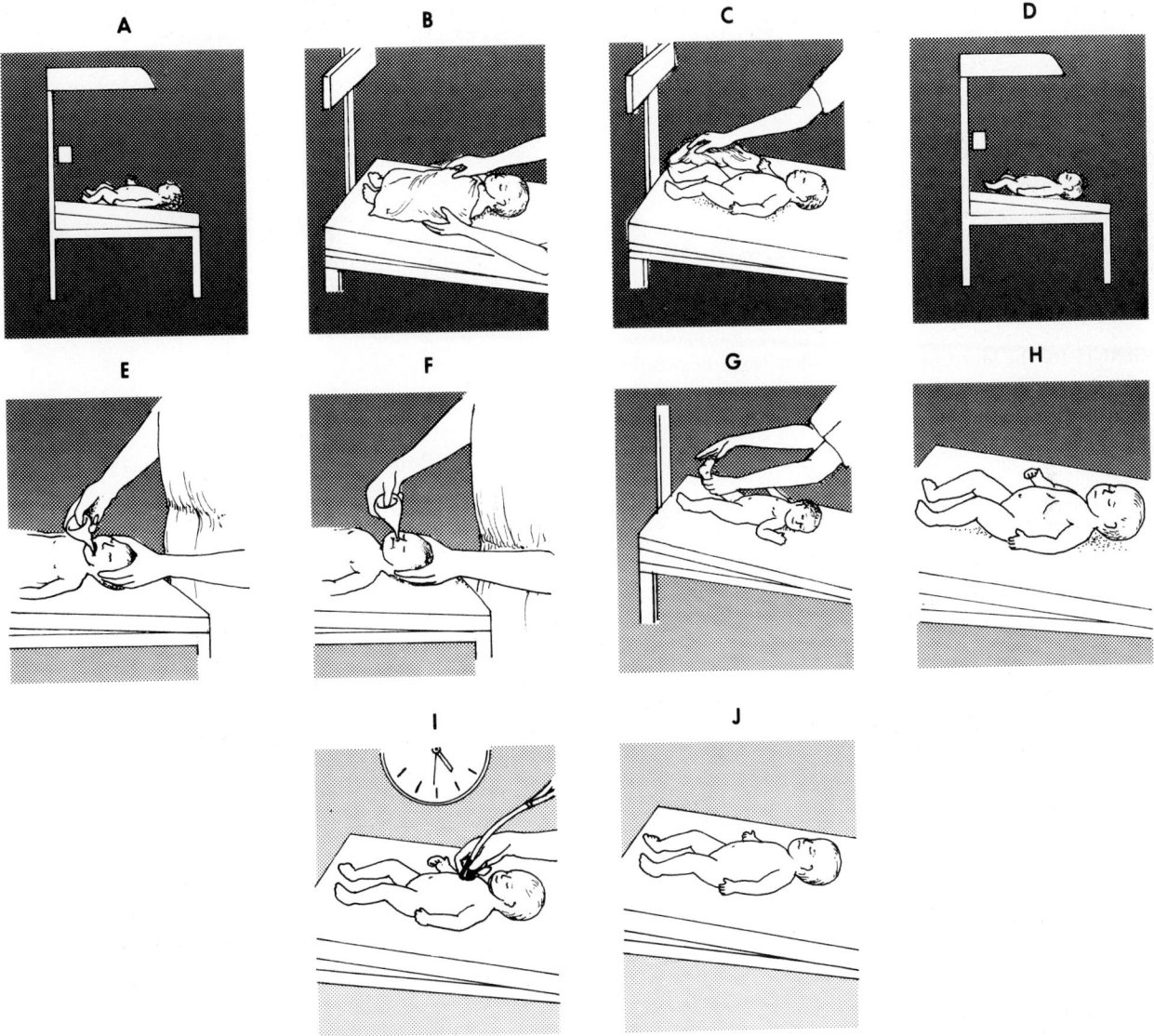

FIGURE 15-15. Immediate stabilization of newborn at delivery—sequence of interventions for assessment at delivery. **A,** Place infant under radiant heat warmer in slight Trendelenburg position. **B,** Dry immediately. **C,** Remove wet linens. **D,** Position infant with head and neck in "sniffing" position. **E and F,** Suction oropharynx, then nasopharynx with bulb syringe as needed. *Not shown:* Suction oropharynx, trachea, and stomach as necessary with 10-French catheter connected to wall suction of 80 to 100 mm Hg per gauge. **G,** Tactile stimulate by slapping twice on sole of foot. **H,** Assess respirations. **I,** Assess heart rate by apical pulse. **J,** Assess color. Resuscitate as indicated by assessment.

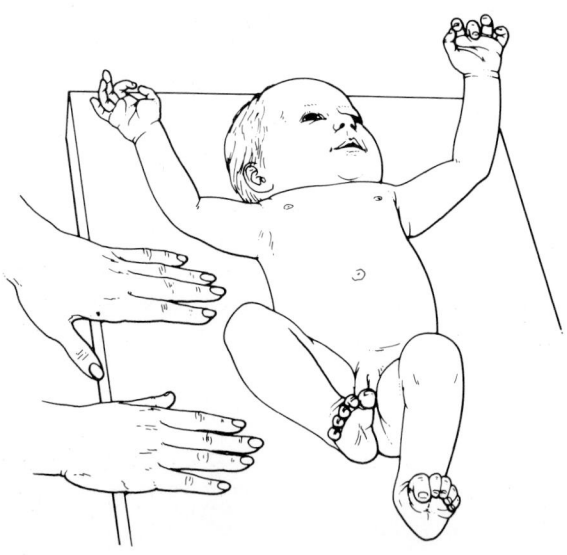

FIGURE 15-16. The Moro, or "startle," reflex. Note the position of the arms and the index finger and thumb. (From Scipien GM, Chard MA, Howe J et al: *Pediatric nursing care,* St Louis, 1990, Mosby–Year Book.)

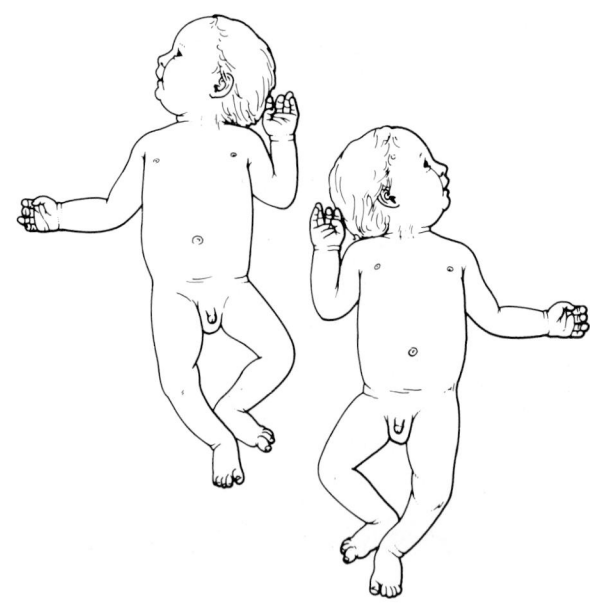

FIGURE 15-17. The tonic neck reflex demonstrating the typical asymmetrical fencer position. (From Scipien GM, Chard MA, Howe J et al: *Pediatric nursing care,* St Louis, 1990, Mosby–Year Book.)

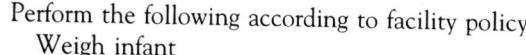

Perform the following according to facility policy
  Weigh infant
  Measure length and head circumference
  Administer medication as ordered
    Eye prophylaxis
    Vitamin K therapy
  Do resuscitation documentation
  Do newborn admitting assessment
  Perform cord care
Perform neuromuscular maturity and physical maturity assessment (Ballard rating) (Figures 15-16, 15-17, and 15-18)
Give sponge bath daily until umbilical cord falls off, then bathe daily, washing hair two to three times per week
Perform neonatal behavioral assessment and share infant responses with parents
Administer circumcision care; apply petrolatum gauze to penis
Perform newborn assessments as required by policy and/or infant condition; particularly note the following
Note time of first voiding and meconium stool
Auscultate heart rate qh twice and prn
  Report rate above 180 or below 100 beats/min to physician
  Report heart sounds heard on right side of chest
  Report murmur
Check respiratory rate q30min for four times and prn
Assess quality of respirations and report if abnormal
Perform heel puncture for blood glucose testing if infant is at risk for hypoglycemia or hypothermia

Provide for sucking needs with pacifier as indicated (be aware that homemade pacifiers are unsafe)
Check rectal temperature one time to determine patency of anus
Administer eye prophylaxis and vitamin K therapy as ordered
Administer sterile water to establish adequate sucking/swallowing if this has not been established by infant breast-feeding in the delivery room, followed a few minutes later by 5% glucose water, breast-feeding, or formula per facility policy or as ordered
Administer feedings as ordered
Apply alcohol or triple dye to cord according to facility policy; remove cord clamp when cord is dry (usually about 48 hr after birth)

Nursing diagnoses/interventions/evaluation

■ **NDX:** Potential for ineffective thermoregulation related to cold stress, hypoglycemia, hypoxemia, or immature thermoregulation mechanism

Recover mother-baby couple together under radiant heat warmer if possible; otherwise provide neutral thermal environment for infant with warmed blankets, etc.
Observe infant nude, if possible, for 1 to 2 hr postdelivery while maintaining neutral thermal environment
Maintain axillary temperature at 97.7° F (36.5° C); check every 30 min for 2 hr and until stable

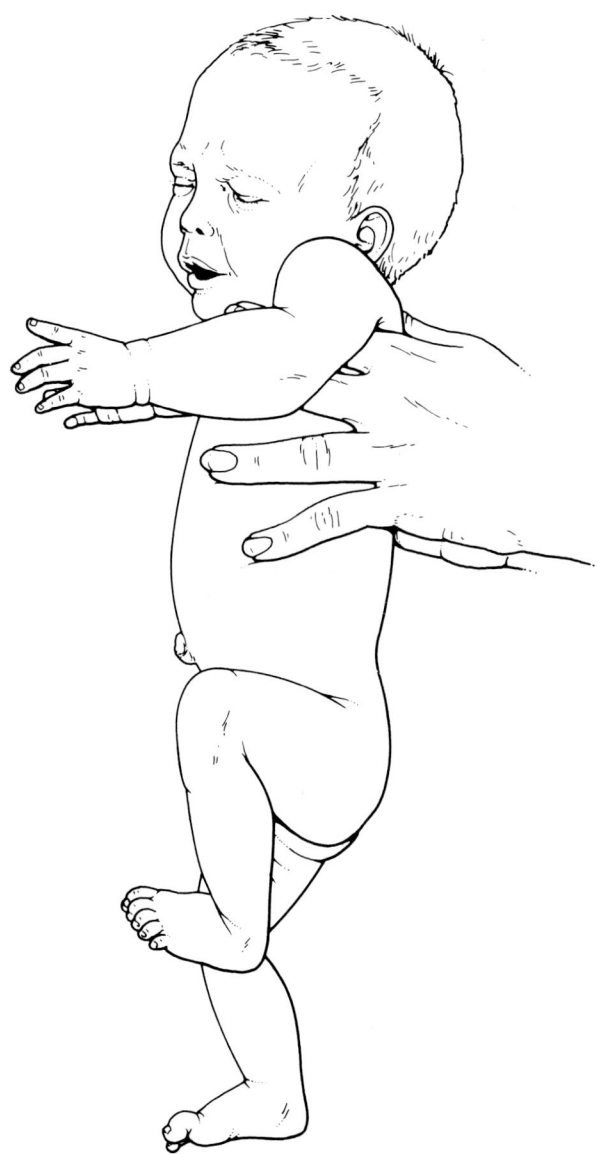

FIGURE 15-18. The stepping reflex. (From Scipien GM, Chard MA, Howe J et al: *Pediatric nursing care,* St Louis, 1990, Mosby—Year Book.)

Avoid bathing for first hour and until axillary temperature is stable at 97.7° F (36.5° C) and other vital signs are stable

Return to radiant warmer after bath until axillary temperature restabilizes to 97.7° F (36.5° C)

Expected outcome/evaluation

Infant maintains normal axillary temperature of 97.7° to 98.6° F (36.5° to 37° C)

■ **NDX:** Potential for ineffective airway clearance related to coordination of suck-swallow-gag reflexes

Keep bulb syringe in crib at all times; suction prn
Hold infant for feedings: *never prop bottles* (be aware that although demand feedings are preferred, infant may need to be awakened if longer than 4 to 5 hr intervals occur between feedings)
Reposition infant q2h and prn; place on right side or abdomen after feedings for at least 30 min
Periodically reassess respiratory rate and rhythm
Perform "football hold" and use obstructed airway maneuvers recommended by American Heart Association as needed for choking

Expected outcome/evaluation

Infant maintains patent airway as evidenced by normal respiratory rate/depth/rhythm and clear breath sounds

■ **NDX:** Knowledge deficit (parental) related to lack of information about infant care and role change

Teach principles of, demonstrate and have parents return-demonstrate, and document in patient teaching plan
    Infant care: bathing, feeding and burping, diaper change, cord care, circumcision care, temperature taking (rectal and axillary)
    Instructions for formula preparation or pumping and storage of breast milk
    Breast/formula feeding
Discuss issues related to use of disposable and recyclable cotton diapers
Review
    Importance of dressing infant according to temperature of day; avoid overheating
    Importance of natural home environment; avoid unnatural quietness and overheating of home
    How to seek assistance for infant problems and concerns of parenthood (e.g., pediatrician's phone number, support groups, etc.)
Discuss conflicts of parental roles
    Idealized versus realistic role of parenting
    Love, resentment, or indifference toward infant
    Personal needs and demands of parenting
Describe how to obtain emergency care if required
Identify abnormal signs and symptoms to report to physician
    Jaundice
    Fever lasting longer than 24 hr
    Infant pulling on ears
    Productive cough
    Vomiting
    Refusal to feed
    Diarrhea
    Lethargy

Expected outcome/evaluation

Parents and/or significant other demonstrate adequate caretaking of infant and demonstrate adjustment to parenting roles

CARE OF PREMATURE INFANT

premature infant Infant who is born before the end of the thirty-seventh week of gestation

Observations/findings

Respiratory distress syndrome (p. 745)
  Nasal flaring
  Tachypnea
  Retractions
  Expiratory grunt
Aspiration
Recurrent apnea
Irregular respiratory and cardiac rates
Hypoglycemia
  Twitching
  Diaphoresis
  Jitteriness
  Tremors
  Cyanosis
  Lethargy; limpness
  Irregular respiratory rate
  Apnea
  Weak, high-pitched crying
  Convulsions
Difficulty in feeding
Hypocalcemia
Hypothermia
Decreased muscle tone
Weak or absent sucking, swallowing, and gag reflexes
Easily fatigued
Edema

Laboratory/diagnostic studies

Blood glucose monitoring for hypoglycemia
Blood gas monitoring as needed
Blood chemistries as needed
X-ray examinations as needed
Cord blood and placenta saved at delivery for diagnostic tests

Potential complications

Skin breakdown
Jaundice
Neonatal sepsis
Physiological anemia (third to seventh week)
Iatrogenic anemia
Necrotizing enterocolitis
Congenital defects
Respiratory distress syndrome
Bronchopulmonary dysplasia (BPD)
Transient tachypnea of newborn (TTN)
Hypovolemic shock
Patent ductus arteriosus (PDA) resulting in congestive heart failure
Poor thermoregulation
Retrolental fibroplasia (retinopathy of prematurity [ROP]) with oxygen therapy
Meconium aspiration syndrome
Hypoglycemia

Medical Management

Pulmonary surfactants
Blood glucose monitoring
Blood gas monitoring as indicated
Gestational age assessment

Postdelivery Nursing Procedures

See Care of Newborn (p. 725)
Administer eye prophylaxis and vitamin K therapy as ordered
Conserve infant's energy with planned rest periods and resting after each feeding and procedure
Give sponge bath daily
Clean skin and reapply conductive gels to skin as necessary for electrodes
Use flotation pad or sheepskin
Use pressure diapers to prevent externally rotated and hyperextended hips
Perform gestational age assessment
Administer IM injections with tuberculin syringe and 25-gauge needle into mid-anterior thigh; *do not give injections into buttocks*
Perform heel puncture for Dextrostix or Chemstrip testing q30min to 60min for 3 hr and prn; if any results are below 45 mg/100 ml, perform immediate blood glucose as ordered
Measure head circumference and length of body weekly
Weigh infant at same time and on same scale daily before feeding

■ **NDX:** Potential fluid volume deficit (and electrolyte imbalance) related to water loss and inadequate nutritional replacement

Administer parenteral fluids as ordered via peripheral line or umbilical catheterization
Monitor blood gases, electrolytes, and Hct as ordered; monitor amount of blood withdrawn
Initiate oral feedings as ordered (general guidelines follow)
  Encourage mother to provide breast milk for all feedings
  Feed infants under 3 lb q2h to 3h and prn

Feed infants over 3 lb q3h to 4h and prn

Do not nipple feed if respiratory rate is above 60 breaths/min

Use soft preemie nipple

Provide oral gavage feedings or gavage feedings as ordered, alternating with nipple feedings to prevent tiring; try nipple feeding when infant sucks on gavage tube

Measure intake and output, including passage of stool

Check specific gravity of urine as ordered

Weigh daily

Expected outcome/evaluation

Infant maintains adequate fluid volume and electrolytes for growth and weight gain as evidenced by normal skin turgor, weight, intake, and urine specific gravity

■ **NDX:** Potential ineffective breathing pattern related to decreased energy, fatigue, and immaturity

Maintain respiratory and cardiac monitors until infant is stable

    Take apical pulse, counting for a full minute q2h to 4h and prn

    Check respiratory rate q2h and prn

Administer warmed and humidified oxygen by route and percentage as ordered

Chart oxygen concentration q2h and prn

Calibrate oxygen analyzer to room air q8h

Monitor arterial blood gases as ordered

Gently stimulate when apneic by rubbing chest or wiggling leg (connect loose ankle restraint to long piece of gauze and tie to tongue blade outside top hole of incubator)

Reposition q2h; avoid positioning very small infants or those with respiratory distress on abdomen

Maintain head position of incubator or radiant warmer slightly elevated

Expected outcome/evaluation

Infant achieves/maintains effective respiratory pattern as evidenced by normal color and blood gases

■ **NDX:** Potential for ineffective thermoregulation related to cold stress and immature temperature regulation mechanisms

Diaper or clothe infant as indicated by condition

Provide neutral thermal environment

Maintain axillary temperature at 97.7° F (36.5° C)

    Regulate temperature by skin sensor

    Avoid taking rectal temperatures

Organize nursing functions so that portholes do not have to be opened frequently, causing temperature fluctuations and increasing metabolic rate

Expected outcome/evaluation

Infant maintains normal temperature of 97.7° to 98.6° F (36.5° to 37° C)

■ **NDX:** Knowledge deficit (parental) related to lack of information about role of caring for premature infant

Discuss and identify

    Need to verbalize feelings of emotional unpreparedness for the parenting role

    Need to plan for infant's physical needs, such as crib, clothes, etc., since they may be unprepared because of premature delivery

    Symptoms to report to pediatrician

        Elevated temperature

        Yellow skin

        Poor feeding

        Vomiting

        Loose stools

        Lethargy

        Productive cough

    Need to dress infant according to temperature of the day

    Need to maintain constant room temperature

    Need to wake infant for every feeding and feed amount of formula ordered

    Need to avoid crowds and persons with infections, especially URIs

    Need to count from due date as birth date in anticipating growth and development patterns

    Need to keep follow-up outpatient care appointments

Teach parents how to take infant's temperature

Explain the following to parents

    Infant receives care in incubator, which simulates uterine environment in providing warmth

    Temperature, oxygen, and humidity are regulated to meet infant's needs

    Infant is not cold, even though unclothed or only diapered; this permits closer observation

    Gavage feedings are done until infant is able to suck from a nipple

    Disproportionately large head is normal for infant's stage of development

    Lanugo will disappear as infant matures

    Breast-feeding mothers can manually express breasts to maintain a supply of breast milk; see Breast-feeding (p. 721)

See Care of Newborn (p. 725) and Family-Centered Care of High-Risk Infant (p. 751)

Expected outcome/evaluation

Parents and/or significant other verbalize understanding through interactive discussion and successfully demonstrate adequate special infant caretaking skills

SMALL FOR GESTATIONAL AGE (SMALL FOR DATE, LOW BIRTH WEIGHT, INTRAUTERINE GROWTH RETARDATION, DYSMATURITY)

Infant whose weight and size at birth falls below the 10th percentile of appropriate for gestational age of infant whether delivered at term or earlier than or later than term

Assessment
Observations/findings

Physical characteristics
  Alert; appearance normal
  Cries for and has large capacity for feedings
  Reduced subcutaneous fat
  Loose and dry skin
  Diminished muscular mass, especially over buttocks and cheeks
  Sunken (scaphoid) abdomen
  Thin, yellow, and dry umbilical cord
  Irregular respiratory rate
  Apnea
  Weak, high-pitched cry
  Difficulty in feeding
  Eye rolling
  Tachypnea
  Intercostal retractions
  Expiratory grunt
  Nasal flaring
  Tachycardia
  Twitching
  Jitteriness
  Tremors
  Cyanosis
  Lethargy, limpness
  Convulsions

Laboratory/diagnostic studies

Glucose monitoring
TORCH titers as indicated
Chromosomal studies as indicated
Hct
Electrolyte monitoring
See Care of Premature Infant (p. 730)

Potential complications

Temperature instability
Hypothermia
Meconium aspiration
Respiratory distress
  High oxygen consumption
  Polycythemia
  Plethora
Hyperbilirubinemia
Hypoglycemia
Congenital infections
Chromosomal anomaly
Congenital defects

Medical Management

See Care of the Newborn (p. 725)

Nursing Care Procedures

See Care of Newborn (p. 725), Care of Premature Infant (p. 730), Family-Centered Care of High-Risk Infant (p. 751), and Large for Gestational Age
Monitor for hypoglycemia and report ≤45 mg% to physician
Monitor electrolytes as ordered
Provide neutral thermal environment; maintain axillary temperatures at 97.7° F (36.5° C)
  Check temperature q15min until stabilized, then q2h to 4h and prn
  Regulate temperature by skin sensor
  Change sensor site daily and prn
Check apical pulse and respiratory rate q30min to 60min and prn
Monitor Hgb and Hct as ordered
Initiate feedings with sterile water at 2 to 3 hr of age and follow a few minutes later with formula or glucose water as ordered; feed q3h or as ordered
Do not give formula or glucose water just before blood is drawn for testing of blood sugar level
Weigh infant daily unclothed, at same time with same scale
Measure intake and output
Continue with immediate care and decrease frequency of nursing functions as patient's condition improves

LARGE FOR GESTATIONAL AGE (DYSMATURITY, HIGH BIRTH WEIGHT)

Neonate whose size and weight at birth fall above the 90th percentile of appropriate for gestational age of infant; often born to diabetic mother, multipara, or mother with a genetic predisposition for infants with excessive birth weight

Assessment
Observations/findings

Greater than 9 lb at birth
Birth injuries

Laboratory/diagnostic studies

Blood glucose monitoring
Blood chemistries if indicated
CBC if indicated
  Hgb, Hct

Potential complications

Hypoglycemia
  Twitching

Jitteriness
Tremors
Cyanosis
Lethargy, limpness
Convulsions
Irregular respiratory rate
Apnea
Weak, high-pitched cry
Difficulty in feeding
Eye rolling
Hyperthermia
Cephalhematoma
Respiratory distress
Polycythemia
Aspiration pneumonia
Erythroblastosis fetalis
Transposition of the great vessels
Brachial paralysis
    Arm abducted
    Internally rotated arm
    Wrist flexed
    Palm limp
    Absence of Moro's reflex on affected side
Fractured clavicle
    Decreased or absent movement of arm
    Overt deformity
    Passive movement of arm produces cries of pain
Phrenic nerve paralysis
    Cyanosis
    Diminished breath sounds
    Labored respirations
    Absence of abdominal bulging on inspiration
    Tachypnea
    Weak cry
Facial paralysis—on affected side
    Asymmetrical contour and movement
    Flattened cheek
    Eye open
    Poor suck with drooling on affected side
Neurological deficit
    Convulsions
    Bulging fontanels
    Hypotonia or hypertonia
    Hyperreflexia; absence or asymmetry of reflexes
See Postterm Infant

Medical Management

Blood glucose monitoring protocol
Gestational age assessment
Feeding schedule

Nursing diagnoses/interventions/evaluation

■ **NDX:**   Potential for injury related to birth trauma associated with macrosomia

Report symptoms of birth injuries to pediatrician
Document assessment findings on nursing notes and update with changes each shift
Change position side to side q2h and prn
Implement and maintain splints, special diapering, etc., as ordered
See Care of Newborn (p. 725) and Infant of Diabetic Mother (p. 734)

Expected outcome/evaluation

Infant
    Has no unidentified/untreated injuries or neurological sequelae
    Maintains normal levels of fluids and electrolytes

POSTTERM INFANT (POSTMATURITY)

Infant born after the end of the forty-second week of gestation who has been subjected to placental insufficiency regardless of birth weight

Assessment
Observations/findings

Malnourished appearance
Reduced subcutaneous tissue
Loose, dry skin
Peeling skin, particularly creases and folds
Disproportionate head and chest circumference
Meconium-stained skin
Open-eyed and alert appearance
Absence of vernix caseosa
Deep sole creases over entire foot
Long fingernails
Thick pale skin
Absence of lanugo
Descended testes
Inability to displace cranial bones
Marked flexion of limbs
Neurological check after 24 hr reveals
    Elbow does not reach midline (scarf sign)
    Holds head when pulled up to sit
    May turn head from side to side
    Raises head above back when prone
Intrauterine history of
    Oligohydramnios
    Meconium-stained amniotic fluid, membranes, and/or umbilical cord

Laboratory/diagnostic studies

Blood glucose monitoring
Blood chemistries as indicated
Blood gases as indicated
Hct, Hgb
Placental/genetic studies

Potential complications

Hypoglycemia
  Twitching
  Jitteriness
  Tremors
  Cyanosis
  Lethargy, limpness
  Irregular respiratory rate; apnea
  Weak, high-pitched cry
  Difficulty in feeding
  Eye rolling
  Hyperthermia
Respiratory distress
Aspiration pneumonia
Meconium aspiration
Hypocalcemia: serum calcium <7 mg/100 ml
  Irritability
  Tachypnea
  Vomiting
Congenital anomalies
  Anencephaly
  Trisomy 16-18
  Seckel's dwarfism
See Large for Gestational Age (p. 732), Small for Gestational Age (p. 732), Meconium Aspiration Syndrome (p. 746), and Respiratory Distress Syndrome (p. 745)

Nursing diagnoses/interventions/evaluation

■ **NDX:**   Knowledge deficit (parental) related to lack of information about infant's condition and needs

Share information with parents and/or significant other about
  Peeling skin not harmful to infant
  Importance of keeping fingernails trimmed
  Appetite and nutritional needs despite size or appearance
  Appropriate weight gain, growth, and development
  Importance of regular feedings
See Care of Newborn (p. 725)

Expected outcome/evaluation

Parents demonstrate ability to care for infant

INFANT OF DIABETIC MOTHER (IDM)

Infant has increased risk of illness because of uteroplacental insufficiency, respiratory distress syndrome, hypoglycemia, hypocalcemia, hyperbilirubinemia, birth trauma, and congenital anomalies; generally large for gestational age if mother is class A, B, or C diabetic, although infant born to mother with cardiovascular complications and class D, E, F, or R diabetes is usually average or small for gestational age

Assessment
Observations/findings

Macrosomia
Puffy, plethoric facies (tomato face)
Large for gestational age (p. 732)
Intrauterine history of maternal diabetes and polyhydramnios
Murmur related to cardiac defect
Cyanosis related to cardiac defect

Laboratory/diagnostic studies

Blood glucose monitoring
Blood chemistries as indicated
Blood gases as indicated
Hgb, Hct
Blood typing/Coombs' tests
Total direct and indirect bilirubin tests as indicated
ECG as indicated
Chest x-ray examination as indicated
Gastric aspirate as indicated

Potential complications

Hypoglycemia
  Twitching
  Jitteriness
  Tremors
  Cyanosis
  Lethargy, limpness
  Seizure activity
  Irregular respiratory rate
  Apnea
  Weak, high-pitched cry
  Difficulty in feeding
  Eye rolling
Hypocalcemia: serum calcium <7 mg/100 ml
  Irritability
  Apnea; tachypnea
  Cyanosis
  Vomiting
Hyperbilirubinemia: jaundice
Hypermagnesemia
Hyperkalemia
Polycythemia
Respiratory distress syndrome (p. 745)
Cephalhematoma
Brachial palsy
Fractured clavicle
Phrenic nerve paralysis
Facial palsy
Prematurity (p. 731)
Congenital anomalies
  Cardiac defects
  Renal anomalies
  Neural tube defects

Medical Management

Blood glucose monitoring

Electrolyte monitoring

Blood gases as indicated for respiratory distress

Transcutaneous oxygen or pulse oximeter monitoring as indicated

Parenteral glucose administration through IV, umbilical venous catheter (UVC), or umbilical arterial catheter (UAC) as ordered

Parenteral glucose boluses as indicated by Chemstrip protocol

Hydrocortisone 5 mg/kg/day IM in two doses if parenteral glucose administration is not effective

Nursing diagnoses/interventions*/evaluation

■ **NDX:** Potential for injury related to altered blood glucose, fluids, and electrolytes

Perform heelstick blood glucose monitoring per facility protocol no less than q30min twice, then q1h three times; report values below 45 mg/100 ml and do immediate serum glucose test as ordered

Perform blood glucose monitoring before administering feedings

Observe for signs and symptoms of respiratory distress

Monitor electrolyte and Hct levels as ordered

Initiate feedings with sterile water at 2 to 3 hr of age, followed a few minutes later by formula or 5% to 10% dextrose water as ordered; follow feeding schedule as ordered

Assess changes in level of consciousness with vital signs q4h and prn

Observe for symptoms of intracranial hemorrhage and seizures

Maintain parenteral glucose administration as ordered; hydrocortisone administration may be ordered if glucose is not effective

Provide neutral thermal environment as indicated

Maintain axillary temperature at 97.7° F (36.5° C)

Administer electrolyte supplements as ordered

Expected outcome/evaluation

Patient maintains fluids and electrolytes in normal range and achieves and maintains euglycemia

■ **NDX:** Knowledge deficit (parental) related to lack of information about care of infant of diabetic mother

Discuss symptoms of hypoglycemia to report to physician

---

*See Care of Newborn (p. 725), Large for Gestational Age (p. 732), and Care of Premature Infant (p. 730).

Teach heelstick glucose monitoring if indicated

Emphasize importance of regular feedings

Emphasize importance of early and good prenatal care for future pregnancies

Teach administration of medications if indicated (include name, dosage, time of administration, purpose, and side effects)

Discuss risk of congenital defects

Expected outcome/evaluation

Parents and/or significant other are able to verbalize symptoms of hypoglycemia in an infant and are able to meet infant's special needs

CARE OF INFANT WITH HYPERBILIRUBINEMIA

Elevation of unconjugated serum bilirubin concentration demonstrated by jaundice; caused by hemolytic disorders (Rh-ABO incompatibility), infection, enzymatic deficiencies, maternal ingestion of sulfonamides or salicylates, or polycythemia

phototherapy: *A process by which blue light therapy decomposes bilirubin by photoisomerization*

Assessment
Observations/findings

Jaundice
    Head
    Trunk
    Extremities
    Palms and soles
    Sclera
    Roof of mouth
Pallor
Lethargy
Poor feeding
Dark, concentrated urine
Light stools
Thermal instability
Polycythemia
ABO incompatibility
Rh incompatibility
During phototherapy
    Loose, watery green stools (characteristic)
    Lethargy
    Skin rash
    Priapism
    Jaundice
    Green urine

Laboratory/diagnostic studies

Serum bilirubin, direct and indirect: rising bilirubin levels—above 12.5 mg/dl in a full-term newborn or above 15 mg/dl in a premature neonate

Blood typing—mother and infant—cord blood serology
Smear morphology
Direct Coombs' test on infant
Hct
CBC with differential
Reticulocyte count
Serum albumin
Liver function and thyroid tests as indicated
TORCH titers as indicated

Potential complications

Nonphysiological vs. physiological jaundice
Breast milk jaundice
Kernicterus
  Depression
    Coma
    Lethargy
    Diminished or absent Moro's reflex
    Hypotonia
    Absent sucking and rooting reflexes
  Excitation (follows depression)
    Twitching
    Generalized seizure activity
    Downward rolling of eyes
    Opisthotonos
    Hypertonia
    High-pitched cry
    Apnea
Hypoglycemia
Sepsis
Respiratory distress
During phototherapy
  Dehydration
  Hyperthermia
  Hypothermia
  Apnea
  Conjunctivitis

Medical Management

Phototherapy
Partial exchange transfusions as indicated
Parenteral and po supplemental fluids
Single- or double-light phototherapy with cool white fluorescent lamps
Bilirubin tests repeated as indicated and 4 hr after phototherapy is discontinued

Nursing diagnoses/interventions/evaluation

■ **NDX:** Potential for injury related to toxic bilirubin blood levels and complications associated with phototherapy

Note and document skin color from head, sclera, and trunk progressively for jaundice at least every shift
Provide neutral thermal environment as needed during phototherapy

Maintain axillary temperature of 97.7° F (36.5° C); avoid cold stress
Monitor vital signs q4h and more often prn for temperature instability
Reposition frequently, at least q2h
Administer feedings as ordered, being conscious of time away from phototherapy
Maintain parenteral fluid therapy as ordered
Observe for abnormal neurological findings and report to physician
Observe skin color in daylight or under white fluorescent lights
Monitor direct and indirect bilirubin blood levels as ordered
Obtain blood samples with phototherapy lights off for accurate levels
For infant undergoing phototherapy
  If holding infant is contraindicated, elevate head, talk to, and stroke infant during and after feedings
  Inspect eyes with lights off at least q8h
  Change eye pads at least twice a day
  Measure distance of lights from infant every shift and maintain at prescribed levels
  Use bilimeter to measure footcandles at head, trunk, and foot levels, figure average, and document level on nursing shift assessment; if not within prescribed limits, adjust until appropriate
  Check lamp use hours and have lamps changed if greater than 2000 hours for maximum effectiveness
  Cover closed eyelids with eye shields; avoid pressure on nose
  Check eyes for drainage and report to physician
  Maintain parenteral fluid therapy for hydration as ordered
  Hold infant during feedings, turn off phototherapy lights, and remove eye shields, keeping track of time not under lights

Expected outcome/evaluation

Infant does not develop neurological sequelae or sustain any complications of phototherapy

■ **NDX:** Potential fluid volume deficit related to insensible water loss and dehydration from phototherapy

Do not clothe or diaper infant; disposable face mask may be used as "bikini" to prevent excessive skin breakdown potential and soiling, and to minimize unexposed surface area
Maintain neutral thermal environment and axillary temperature at 97.7° F (36.5° C)
Check axillary temperature at least q2h and prn
Avoid exposure of skin temperature probe to phototherapy lights
Weigh infant daily unclothed at same time on same scale before feeding

Offer pacifier prn
Measure accurate intake and output
Check urine specific gravity every shift

Expected outcome/evaluation

Infant maintains adequate hydration and normothermia

■ **NDX:** Potential alteration in parenting related to disruption of parent-infant interaction because of phototherapy

Explain need to provide adequate fluid intake; to offer water between feedings
Discuss signs and symptoms to report to physician
    Recurrence of jaundice
    Persistence of diarrhea
    Emphasize importance of having laboratory tests done as ordered
    Emphasize importance of follow-up outpatient care
Encourage parent participation in infant care activities (feeding, changing soiled linens, etc.)
Review care of infant with hyperbilirubinemia as needed with parents
Permit siblings to visit according to hospital policy
Turn off lights and remove eye shields when parents visit according to time period ordered by physician
Reinforce explanations of phototherapy, reasons for particular interventions, and plan of care
Reinforce limited planned times out from under phototherapy
Designate duties parents can do or assist with
See Care of Newborn (p. 725)

Expected outcome/evaluation

Parent performs infant care activities as able

EXCHANGE TRANSFUSION

Replacement of 75% to 85% of circulating blood by alternating repeated withdrawal of small amounts of infant's blood and replacement with equal amounts of donor blood to remove accumulated bilirubin, replace coagulation factors in DIC, and remove antibodies (Rh, ABO) and sensitized red blood cells (RBCs) producing hemolysis of RBCs

Assessment
Observations/findings

Progressively increasing jaundice

Laboratory/diagnostic studies
BEFORE PROCEDURE

Bilirubin level
Hgb level and Hct
Blood culture
Calcium level
Random blood glucose test

Donor blood culture
Serum albumin level

AT END OF PROCEDURE (LABORATORY TESTS WITH LAST AMOUNT OF BLOOD REMOVED FROM INFANT AS ORDERED)

Bilirubin level
Calcium level
Random blood sugar test
Hgb level and Hct
Type and hold or type and cross match

Potential complications
DURING PROCEDURE

Bradycardia below 100 beats/min or sudden tachycardia
Cyanosis
Hypothermia
Vomiting
Aspiration
Apnea
Pallor of a limb
Air embolus
Abdominal distention
Sudden hypotension
Cardiac arrest

AFTER PROCEDURE

Tachycardia or bradycardia
Cardiac arrhythmias
Cardiac arrest
Tachypnea or bradypnea
Hypothermia
Lethargy or jitteriness
Increasing jaundice
Dark color of urine
Cyanosis
Edema
Convulsions
Bleeding from cord
Long-term complications
    Hemorrhage
    Heart failure
    Hypocalcemia
    Hypoglycemia
    Sepsis
    Acidosis
    Shock
    Hyperkalemia
    Hypernatremia
    Thrombus formation
    Thrombocytopenia
    Serum hepatitis
    Necrotizing enterocolitis

Medical Management

Blood amount (160 ml/kg for two-volume exchange; 25 to 80 ml/kg packed RBCs for partial exchange)

Umbilical catheterization
Permission for parents to attend (unless contraindicated)
Blood warmer (80.6° to 98.6° F [27° to 37° C])

Nursing Care Procedures
Before procedure

Prepare radiant heat warmer, cardiac and respiratory monitors, and pacifier

Maintain NPO status 3 to 4 hr before exchange transfusion or aspirate stomach contents before procedure

Have resuscitative equipment readily available: oxygen, mask, bag, suction apparatus, and drugs such as sodium bicarbonate, glucose, calcium, and epinephrine

Recheck date of blood, since it should not be more than 48 hr old

Warm blood as ordered

Restrain all four extremities; keep extremities visible to detect any color changes

Assist physician with insertion of umbilical venous line if not already in place

See Umbilical Catheterization

Check laboratory work as ordered

Administer albumin as ordered

Mix blood in amounts as ordered with fresh frozen plasma or plasmanate when fresh whole blood is not used

Place infant under phototherapy lights as ordered

Reinforce parents' and/or significant other's understanding of care to be given with primary disease process that necessitates exchange transfusion

During procedure

Note respiratory and cardiac rate q5min

Check axillary temperature q15min to 30min

Suction when necessary

Observe for abnormal behavior or symptoms

Observe all blood tubing connections for integrity periodically

Record amount of blood withdrawn and infused, noting the color

Notify physician when each 100 ml of blood is exchanged

After procedure

Handle infant gently and minimally for 2 to 4 hr

Maintain neutral thermal environment

Monitor respiratory and cardiac rates q15min for eight times, then q30min to 60min for 24 to 48 hr or as ordered

Check axillary temperature q1h to 3h for 48 hr

Measure intake and output

Observe cord for bleeding q5min to 15min for 1 to 2 hr

Perform heel puncture for Dextrostix or Chemstrip testing as ordered until infant feeds or IV therapy is established

Order laboratory tests including blood gases and electrolytes as ordered

Resume feedings 4 to 6 hr after transfusion as ordered

Ensure adequate intake by using soft nipple with large hole

Feed slowly or gavage as ordered

Turn and reposition after each feeding

Reinforce physician's explanation of reason for doing exchange transfusion

Encourage parents to see infant after procedure and involve them in as much of infant's care as possible

UMBILICAL CATHETERIZATION

Passage of a radio-opaque catheter through one of the umbilical arteries or vein to provide parenteral fluid therapy and/or obtain blood samples or through the umbilical vein for exchange transfusion or emergency administration of drugs, fluids, or volume expanders

Assessment
Observations/findings

Arterial or venous site
IV pump for continuous infusion

Laboratory/diagnostic studies

Chest/abdominal x-ray examination to confirm low or high placement
Hct as indicated
Blood sampling as indicated

Potential complications

Vasospasm
    Blanching or mottling of leg
    Absence of peripheral pulses
    Darkening of legs or toes
Infection at insertion site
    Redness
    Edema
    Drainage
Sepsis
Hemorrhage via connections or oozing from site of insertion
Thromboembolism: progressive cyanosis and blackness of toes; oliguria or anuria
Necrotizing enterocolitis (p. 742)
    Abdominal distention
    Vomiting
Dislodgment of catheter
    Ventricular fibrillation (from electrocution)

Medical Management

IV solutions and infusion rate as indicated
Flush solutions as indicated

Nursing Care Procedures

Validate position of catheter tip by x-ray examination within 1 hr of insertion
Provide neutral thermal environment

Monitor cardiac and respiratory rates qh

Check axillary temperature q2h to 3h

Deliver parenteral fluids by infusion pump

Note rate of flow qh

Never permit IV bottle to empty

Flush solutions as per facility protocol

Check all connections to umbilical line q30min to 60min

Use only grounded electrical equipment on or near infant

Observe condition of cord q2h to 3h and prn

Retape IV tubing at cord prn per facility policy

If umbilical line is displaced, apply pressure with sterile 4 × 4 inch gauze, and have another person notify physician immediately

Administer cord care as ordered

Change dressing as ordered

Apply antibiotic or antiseptic ointment to cord if ordered

Check pedal pulses q2h to 4h and prn

Reposition infant q2h and prn

Reinforce physician's explanation as to reason for umbilical line

Encourage parents to visit nursery and involve them in infant's care as much as possible

Keep running totals of blood losses until replaced by transfusion

Monitor Hct periodically with blood withdrawn qd

Measure intake and output on flow sheet

Expected outcome/evaluation

Infant

Has no complications

Has solutions administered as ordered

Has blood samples obtained as ordered

Has no catheter-related infection

NEONATAL SEPSIS

Generalized infection in the newborn, often caused by antepartal or intrapartal asymptomatic maternal infection; acquired postnatal infection is usually due to contact with personnel or contaminated equipment

Assessment
Observations/findings
EARLY SIGNS

Lethargy, especially after first 24 hr

Poor sucking

Anorexia

Regurgitation of feedings

Irritability

Pallor

Hypotonia

Hyporeflexia

Weight loss

Jaundice

Hypothermia

Jitteriness

OTHER SIGNS

Hyperthermia

Grunting

Bradypnea

Apneic spells

Tremors

Seizure activity

Vomiting

Abdominal distention

Dehydration

Cool, clammy skin

Pallor

Cyanosis

Diarrhea

Hypoglycemia

Rashes

Omphalitis

Immediate maternal history: maternal amnionitis and/or prolonged premature rupture of membranes

Low birth weight

Meconium-stained skin

Birth out of asepsis (BOA)

Laboratory/diagnostic studies

Lumbar puncture

No. 1 tube: sugar protein

No. 2 tube: culture and Gram stain

No. 3 tube: cells and differential

CBC with differential

Decreased WBC

Decreased neutrophils

Platelet count: decreased

Cultures

Urine by suprapubic tap

Blood

Nasopharynx

Tracheal aspirates

Skin lesions

Ear canal

Gastric aspirate

Maternal blood/amniotic fluid cultures as ordered

Sedimentation rate: increased

Chest x-ray examination

Potential complications

Hypoglycemia

Metabolic acidosis

Coagulopathy

Renal failure

Myocardial dysfunction

Intracranial hemorrhage

Jaundice/kernicterus

Medical Management

Septic workup (obtaining all specimens for diagnosis confirmation)

Antibiotics
Feeding schedule/IV fluids as indicated
Antipyretics as indicated

Nursing diagnoses/interventions/evaluation

■ **NDX:** Potential for injury related to neonatal sepsis

Maintain isolation: isolette care
Turn and position q2h and prn
Observe vital signs q2h, noting changes and reporting to
  physician as needed
Monitor vital signs with decreasing frequency as condition
  stabilizes and infant improves
Maintain neutral thermal environment in order to ensure
  normothermia
Check axillary temperatures q2h with vital signs
Maintain strict handwashing procedure
Teach handwashing and gowning technique to parents
  before handling infant
Administer oxygen as ordered
Use apnea monitor if indicated
Perform periodic ABGs as ordered
Plan rest periods; avoid unnecessary handling
Employ cooling measures if infant is febrile, e.g., remove
  external heat sources or blankets, provide tepid sponge
  bath
Gently stimulate when apneic by rubbing chest, tapping
  warmer or incubator, or wiggling leg (connect loose
  ankle restraint to long piece of gauze and tie to tongue
  blade outside top hole of incubator)
Maintain resuscitation equipment nearby
Observe for focal signs of convulsions
  Suction nose and mouth as necessary
  Turn head to side
  Protect from movement against side of incubator or
    falling from radiant warmer
  Give oxygen as necessary
Assist physician with septic workup as indicated
Administer antibiotics as ordered
Reinforce parents and/or significant other's understanding
  of
  Name of medication, dosage, time of administration,
    purpose, and side effects
  Importance of ongoing outpatient care
  Symptoms of recurrence to report to physician
See Family-Centered Care of High-Risk Infant (p. 751)
  and Care of Newborn (p. 725)

Expected outcome/evaluation

Infant
  Receives therapy as ordered
  Has repeat cultures after medical treatment that show
    no "growth" or other complications; normothermic

■ **NDX:** Altered nutrition: less than body requirements
      related to neonatal sepsis

Administer parenteral fluids as ordered
Keep bulb syringe at bedside for emesis/obstructed airway
  management
Measure intake and output
Urine specific gravity twice per shift
Weigh infant daily
Administer gavage feedings as ordered
Accurately chart infant's activity and feeding behavior
Insert nasogastric tube periodically as necessary to relieve
  abdominal distention if infant is unable to burp and is
  nipple feeding
Observe coordination of suck/swallow reflexes with feed-
  ings
Provide for sucking needs with pacifier as indicated

Expected outcome/evaluation

Infant
  Does not lose weight
  Demonstrates a progressive weight gain

NEONATAL DRUG WITHDRAWAL

*Withdrawal symptoms usually occur within the first 24
hr of life and are most commonly due to maternal antepartal dependence on heroin, methadone, diazepam
(Valium), PCP, cocaine, and alcohol*
*fetal alcohol syndrome Occurs in infants of chronic al-
coholics and is characterized by the following defects:
intrauterine growth retardation with microcephaly, facial anomalies (small palpebral fissures, low nasal
bridge, indistinct philtrum, thin upper lip, shortened
lower jaw), and CNS dysfunction*

Assessment
Observations/findings

Muscle tremors
Irritability
Hyperactive reflexes
  Marked flexor rigidity; resistance to extension
High-pitched, shrill cry
Increased muscle tone; twitching
Sneezing, nasal stuffiness
Frantic sucking of fists
Regurgitation, vomiting
Frequent yawning
Increased mucus production
Respiratory distress
Restlessness
Inability to sleep/shortened sleep periods
Poor feeding
Uncoordinated sucking and swallowing
Excessive sweating
Increased lacrimation
Elevated temperature
Abrasions of nose and knees
Diarrhea; dehydration
Cyanosis and/or apnea

Pallor
Seizures
Maternal history of drug/substance abuse
Previous sibling with symptoms of neonatal withdrawal
 syndrome
Increased risk of sudden infant death syndrome (SIDS)

Laboratory/diagnostic studies

Positive maternal/neonatal urine toxicology screens
Abnormal BNBAS (Brazelton examination)
Auditory screening examination as ordered
Pneumogram, EEG, CBC (as work-up for SIDS)

Potential complications

Child abuse
Child neglect
Failure-to-thrive syndrome
Delayed growth and development
Seizures
CNS damage
Respiratory distress: meconium aspiration syndrome (p.
 745)
Sudden infant death syndrome (SIDS)
Long-term consequences
 Mental retardation
 Loss of fine motor control
 Poor social/interaction skills
 Abnormal sleep-wake cycles
Difficult foster care requirements

Medical Management

Paregoric/phenobarbital therapy as needed
Neonatal Abstinence Scales for assessment of symptoms
 and drug dosing
Special discharge planning as indicated
Feeding routine
Parent-infant interaction documentation
Police hold as indicated
Social services referral as indicated

Nursing diagnoses/interventions/evaluation

■ **NDX:** Altered nutrition: less than body requirements
   related to neonatal withdrawal symptoms

Give small, frequent feedings as ordered
Swaddle in soft warm clothes and blanket for comfort
Suction infant as needed
Monitor vital signs q2h and decrease frequency as patient's
 condition improves
Weigh infant q12h unclothed, at same time with same
 scale or as ordered
Administer parenteral fluids as ordered
Administer medications as ordered: phenobarbitol or par-
 egoric
Offer pacifier prn
Position infant on side or abdomen

Monitor intake and output
Note episodes of diarrhea/loose stools
Note bowel sound hyperactivity with vital signs
Take axillary temperature with vital signs at least q4h
 and prn

Expected outcome/evaluation

Infant has normal weight gain pattern on growth curve
chart

■ **NDX:** Sensory/perceptual alteration related to involuntary withdrawal behavior

Maintain regular assessments on neonatal abstinence scale
 as available in facility
Maintain administration of anticonvulsive medications as
 ordered
Allow for routine rest periods as permitted; do not disturb
 for routine nursing care during sleep
Maintain quiet environment with minimal visual, auditory, and tactile stimulation during peak withdrawal
 time
Hold infant securely and close to one's own body when
 handling
Perform BNBAS as offered by facility

Expected outcome/evaluation

Infant's symptoms are effectively managed

■ **NDX:** Potential impairment of skin integrity related
   to excessive muscular activity and diarrhea during withdrawal

Cover hands with mitts of infant shirt
Administer judicious skin care
 Clean neck folds, ears, etc., after each regurgitation or
  vomiting, q4h, and prn
 Clean buttocks and perineum after each diarrheal stool
  and prn
Reapply paste of zinc oxide ointment q2h to 4h and prn
 to excoriated buttocks with diaper changes
Expose excoriated skin areas to air and/or heat lamp prn
Protect against abrasions of face and bony prominences,
 such as heels, head, sacrum, knees, and ankles; if flail-
 ing, swaddle infant, pad sides of crib, and/or use sheepskin under and around infant
Observe for developing skin lesions resulting from high
 incidence of gonococcal and herpes type 2 infection in
 gravid drug-addicted women

Expected outcome/evaluation

Infant has no skin excoriation or minimal skin excoriation

■ **NDX:** Potential for altered parenting related to altered
   parent-infant interaction secondary to withdrawal syndrome and lifestyle of parents

See Care of Newborn (p. 725)

Encourage mother to become involved in infant's care as soon and as much as possible

Keep mother informed of infant's condition and progress

Be honest and straightforward in answering mother's questions

Avoid getting into arguments with mother should she try to manipulate, accuse, and challenge nursing care

Do everything possible to promote maternal-infant attachment

Assist mother in exploring her own feelings about her relationship with her mother

Avoid situations that promote separation and isolation of mother and infant

Encourage visits and communication with infant's father and/or significant others

Do not force unwanted infant on a mother who cannot cope with her addiction and the responsibilities of motherhood

Involve social service worker and/or visiting nurse in predischarge planning for home care

Ensure that parents and/or significant other demonstrate positive parenting behaviors as related to attachment and the "taking hold" phase

Holds infant while feeding

Manages routine infant care

Has eye-to-eye contact with infant

Ensure that parents and/or significant other knows and understands

That infant restlessness and irritability may be present during the first few months of life

That narcotics will pass through breast milk and promote infant drug addiction but may also relieve some signs and symptoms of withdrawal

That many other drugs can pass through breast milk and may be toxic to infant

Availability of community resources to assist with parenting, foster care, and drug rehabilitation

Resource telephone numbers and name of contact individual if possible

Importance of ongoing treatment

Postpartum care (p. 714)

Expected outcome/evaluation

Mother demonstrates adequate performance of infant caretaking activities; mother and/or significant other is able to adequately care for infant

---

NECROTIZING ENTEROCOLITIS (NEC)

Ischemia of the intestinal tract and invasion of the mucosa with enteric pathogens; occurs most frequently in small and asphyxiated preterm infants, in those with Hirschsprung's disease, after exchange transfusion, or with an aggressive feeding schedule

Assessment
Observations/findings

Onset or increase in amount of feeding residuals

Abdomen

Distention; increasing circumference

Increasing bowel sounds

Skin: shiny, dry, and tender

Increase in visible vascularity

Dependent edema

Lethargy, limpness, listlessness

Apnea, bradycardia, or other respiratory distress

Decrease in bowel sounds after prolonged apnea and bradycardia

Pallor

Temperature instability

Vomiting

Increased number of stools: may progress to diarrhea

Blood in stools (hematochezia)

Laboratory/diagnostic studies

Hematest of stools and emesis: occult blood—positive stools and/or gastric contents

Hct: decreased

Platelet count: decreased

Coagulation studies: increased bleeding time

CBC with differential

Radiographic findings

Dilation of the intestine, progressing to free air in the abdomen after perforation

Blood, stool, and urine cultures as ordered

Potential complications

Sepsis

Hyperbilirubinemia

Shock

DIC

Abscess

Metabolic acidosis

Paralytic ileus

Recurrent bowel obstruction

Hyponatremia

Hyperkalemia

Medical Management

Parenteral fluids: hyperalimentation and intralipid therapy

Hematest of stools

Antibiotics

Volume expanders as indicated

NPO initially for 7 to 10 days then slowly progressive feeding schedule

Nasogastric tube to gravity drainage or intermittent low suction as indicated

Oxygen administration as indicated

No rectal temperatures or rectal probes

Abdominal girth measurements q8h and prn

Intake and output

Bowel resection if more conservative measures are unsuccessful

Nursing diagnoses/interventions/evaluation

■ **NDX:** Altered nutrition: less than body requirements related to ischemia and malabsorption of nutrients through the intestinal tract

Auscultate bowel sounds with vital signs q2h to 3h and prn

Measure accurate intake and output

Measure and record abdominal girth q4h and prn

Take vital signs as indicated by patient condition at least q2h during acute phase and then with decreasing frequency as condition improves

Continue with acute care and decrease frequency of nursing functions as patient's condition improves

Administer parenteral fluids, total parenteral nutrition (TPN), and/or fat emulsion as ordered

Maintain NPO for 7 to 14 days after absence of Hematest-positive stools and abdominal distention

Progress with oral intake as ordered: give one or two feedings of plain water followed by dilute mother's or donor breast milk

Encourage mother to continue to lactate (although infant is NPO during acute phase) and explain importance of breast milk

Avoid abdominal trauma by application of skin probes and monitor electrodes

Expected outcome/evaluation

Infant does lose weight but resumes normal oral feeding schedule after treatment

■ **NDX:** Potential for diarrhea related to bowel resection*

Perform care as described in Medical Management and as above

Maintain respiratory assistance as needed

Auscultate chest for breath sounds q2h and prn

Observe site of incision for redness, swelling, and drainage

Administer ostomy care (p. 283)

Take axillary temperatures

Avoid any rectal stimulation

Manage pain as ordered

Turn q2h and prn

Change dressings as needed

Administer formula based on infant's intolerance as ordered if breast milk is unavailable

---

*Resection of necrotic bowel is indicated after bowel perforation and in the infant whose condition rapidly deteriorates.

Look for symptoms of protein intolerance—give predigested protein formula as ordered

Look for symptoms of fat and/or sugar intolerance—give monosaccharide, triglyceride formula as ordered

Expected outcome/evaluation

Infant follows normal feeding and weight gain pattern postoperatively

■ **NDX:** Parental knowledge deficit related to lack of information about special infant care procedures

See Care of Newborn (p. 725)

Parent will discuss, verbalize, demonstrate, and return-demonstrate ostomy and incisional care

Discuss symptoms of wound infection to report to physician

Discuss other symptoms to report to physician

Diarrhea

Suspected weight loss

Diet: type, frequency, and amount

Importance of follow-up outpatient care

Expected outcome/evaluation

Parents and/or significant other perform infant care duties; infant is discharged in good condition

TORCH INFECTIONS

Refers to several infectious agents that can infect fetuses and cause similar congenital malformations or developmental abnormalities: T, toxoplasmosis; O, other; R, rubella; C, cytomegalovirus; H, herpesvirus (Table 15-4)

Assessment
Observations/findings

Maternal: history of consistent contact with cat feces, poorly cooked infected meats, exposure to rubella or other infectious agents during pregnancy; rashes, oral/genital lesions; multiple blood transfusions during pregnancy; renal transplant patient

Infant

Lethargy

Febrile episodes

Mottled skin

Poor feeding

Seizures

Vesicular lesions on skin and scalp

Neurological involvement

Temperature instability

Hepatosplenomegaly

Diarrhea

Jaundice

Cataracts

TABLE 15-4. TORCH Infections

Disease	Causative agent	Mode of transmission	Common problems in the neonate
Toxoplasmosis	*Toxoplasma gondii*	Consuming oocytes in raw or poorly cooked meat or acquiring through contact with cat feces; oocytes ultimately cross placenta	Microcephaly, hydrocephalus, intracranial calcifications, jaundice, chorioretinitis convulsions, ecchymosis, pallor, hepatosplenomegaly
Rubella	Rubella virus	After exposure to the rubella virus during pregnancy, crosses placenta and infects developing embryo/fetus (results are most severe in first trimester)	Mental retardation, congenital cataracts, retinopathy, variety of congenital heart anomalies (especially patent ductus arteriosus and pulmonary artery stenosis), deafness, thrombocytopenia; these infants continue to shed active rubella virus up to 18 mo after delivery
Cytomegalic inclusion disease (CID)	Cytomegalovirus (CMV)	Exposure to virus, which has been isolated from breast milk, saliva, urine, feces, and upper respiratory tract as well as from blood-borne infections transferred to infants who are receiving multiple transfusions	Although asymptomatic at birth, infants may display various problems several months later, including hepatosplenomegaly, microcephaly, purpura, jaundice, and cerebral calcifications as well as deafness and blindness; although spastic quadriplegia and hypotonia are common in those who are severely affected, developmental delays extend from minimal involvement to a vegetative state
Herpes simplex virus (HSV)	Herpesvirus	Direct contact with infected maternal genital secretions during delivery	Skin lesions, hypoglycemia, lethargy, irritability followed by focal or generalized seizures, disseminated intravascular coagulation

From Scipien GM, Chad MA, Howe J et al: *Pediatric nursing care,* St Louis, 1990, Mosby–Year Book.

Laboratory/diagnostic studies

Serological tests
  IgM titers: elevated
  Fluorescent antibody testing
Fluid cultures as ordered: abnormal cerebrospinal fluid (CSF) values
Urine screens/cytology as ordered
TORCH antibody screening
Viral cultures for cytomegalovirus (CMV) and herpes
Cultures of lesions as indicated
Abnormal liver function studies
Abnormal coagulation studies

Potential complications

Microcephaly
Hydrocephaly
Cerebral calcifications
Chorioretinitis
Encephalitis
Seizures
Sepsis
Respiratory distress/pneumonia
Prematurity
Hepatitis
DIC
Skin lesions
Congenital blindness
Glaucoma
Cardiac defects

Deafness
Retinopathy

Medical Management

Drug therapy as indicated by findings
Isolation as indicated
Other therapy as indicated by infant condition
See Care of Newborn (p. 725) and Care of Premature Infant (p. 731)

Nursing Care Procedures
Herpesvirus
PREDELIVERY CARE

Avoid internal fetal monitoring
Avoid frequent vaginal examinations
Prepare for cesarean delivery before rupture of membranes or within 4 to 6 hr if membranes have spontaneously ruptured before patient's hospital administration—no need to isolate infant if cesarean delivery is done before rupture of membranes

POSTDELIVERY CARE

Perform active genital herpes or positive culture cytology for herpes
Place patient in private room per facility policy
Maintain strict handwashing routine
Wear gown and gloves before having contact with contaminated area or articles
Double-bag perineal pads and other contaminated waste
Infant can be brought to mother if strict technique is followed

Supervise mother in handwashing procedure
Place clean gown on mother
Assist mother with sitting in chair
Bring infant to mother
Do not lay infant on mother's bed
See Neonatal Sepsis (p. 755)

SUSPECTED/AFFECTED INFANT

Isolate infant in nursery per hospital policy
Maintain strict handwashing
Wear gown and gloves before contacting contaminated
   area or articles
Take infant to mother under supervised conditions
Double-bag contaminated articles
Be aware that incubation period for neonatal herpes is 2
   to 12 days
Observe infant for symptoms of sepsis, convulsions, and
   other signs of neurological involvement

Inactive herpes

Provide routine maternal and neonatal care if mother has
   no active lesions but a known history of genital herpes
Do not isolate mother or infant

Nongenital herpes present

Isolate mother postdelivery per hospital policy
Isolate newborn *only* after newborn has left nursery to go
   out to mother
Expedite drying or crusting to reduce virus titer by topical
   application of ethyl ether, povidone-iodine, or tincture
   of benzoin as ordered
Follow sequence for infant visitation as described in Active Genital Herpes section
Instruct mother to wear a mask or dressing to cover lesions
   when performing infant caretaking activities

Nongenital herpes absent

Provide routine maternal and neonatal care
See Care of Newborn (p. 725) and Postpartum Care (p.
   715)

■ **NDX:** Parental knowledge deficit related to lack of
   information about infant care and isolation
   techniques

Reinforce physician's teaching and discuss with parents
   and/or significant other
   Implications for infant's future growth and development
   Incidence of complications
   Maintenance of therapy
   Importance of regular follow-up
   Isolation practices
   Infant care duties

See Care of Newborn (p. 725) and Care of Premature
   Infant (p. 731)

Expected outcome/evaluation

Parents and/or significant other verbalize understanding
   of infant care and isolation techniques through interactive discussion and actual return demonstration

RESPIRATORY DISTRESS SYNDROME (HYALINE MEMBRANE DISEASE)

*Condition of decreased pulmonary gas exchange produc-
   ing retention of carbon dioxide usually resulting from
   deficiency of surfactant in immature lungs*

Assessment
Observations/findings

Tachypnea >60 respirations/min
Nasal flaring
Expiratory grunt
Cyanosis
Pallor
Absence of and/or abnormal breath sounds
Retractions: intercostal, suprasternal, substernal
Seesaw breathing
Hypothermia
Skin pale or ashen
Pitting edema of hands or feet
Hypoactive, flaccid, or motionless
White, frothy mucus in respiratory tract
Fatigue
Bradycardia or tachycardia
Jaundice
Hypotension: mean BP, 35 to 40 mm Hg

Laboratory/diagnostic studies

Chest x-ray examination
Blood gas sampling
Oxygen saturation values by pulse oximeter
Transcutaneous oxygen/CO_2 monitor readings
CBC with differential
Coagulation studies
Hgb/Hct
Blood chemistries as ordered
Absence of phosphatidylglycerol from a tracheal aspirate
   sample
Negative shake test on gastric aspirate of swallowed am-
   niotic fluid ≤30 min of birth

Potential complications

Mechanical ventilation (alveolar rupture, e.g., pneumothorax, pneumomediastinum, pneumopericardium, or
   interstitial emphysema)
Respiratory infection/pneumonia
Hyperbilirubinemia (p. 735)

Shock
Intracranial hemorrhage
Patent ductus arteriosus
Long term
  Bronchopulmonary dysplasia (p. 748)
  Retrolental fibroplasia (Retinopathy of Prematurity [ROP])
  Neurological impairment
  Altered parent-infant relationship (bonding and attachment)

Medical Management

Supplemental oxygen therapy as indicated
Mechanical ventilation as necessary
Continuous positive airway pressure (CPAP) as required
Extra Corporeal Membrane Oxygenation (ECMO) may be indicated
Neutral thermal environment
IV fluids as indicated
Administration of human or other surfactants
Antibiotics as indicated
Sodium bicarbonate for documented metabolic acidosis
Strict intake and output

Nursing diagnoses/interventions/evaluation

■ **NDX:** Ineffective breathing pattern related to pathophysiological processes associated with respiratory distress syndrome

Provide neutral thermal environment
Maintain axillary temperature of 97.7° F (36.5° C); regulate temperature by skin sensor
Position with head slightly hyperextended
Reposition q2h
Administer warmed and humidified oxygen as ordered
Have resuscitative equipment available at all times: oxygen, suction, bagging apparatus, drugs
Maintain on respiratory and cardiac monitors; note rates and variability 60 min and prn
Maintain ventilatory support as ordered
Auscultate chest for breath sounds q1h to 2h and prn
Suction q2h and prn
Perform postural drainage and percussion as ordered
Maintain umbilical arterial and/or venous line; see Umbilical Catheterization
Administer parenteral fluids as ordered
Administer sodium bicarbonate as ordered; never give undiluted
Monitor electrolytes, Hct, and glucose as ordered
Perform blood gas determinations as ordered
Administer antibiotics as ordered
Analyze oxygen q2h and before drawing blood gases, correlate with O_2 saturation and/or transcutaneous O_2/CO_2 monitors
Check blender setting for oxygen concentration q2h and prn

Calibrate oxygen analyzer q8h
Measure intake and assess output as indicated
Omit normal hygiene at times
  Plan care to allow for rest periods
  Avoid exhausting infant
Discuss with parents and/or significant others and document
  General use of monitoring and life-support equipment and any postdischarge sequelae
  Parenting skills
  Infant caretaking skills
See Care of Newborn (p. 725), Care of Premature Infant (p. 731), and Care of Newborn on a Ventilator (p. 748)

Expected outcome/evaluation

There are no complications
Blood gas values are corrected and maintained within normal range
Respiratory distress is resolved

MECONIUM ASPIRATION SYNDROME

Fetal hypoxia frequently causes relaxation of the anal sphincter, passage of meconium, and gasping respiratory efforts, resulting in meconium aspiration in the tracheobronchial airways; suspected in a meconium-stained neonate, postmature infant, or an infant large or small for gestational age

Assessment
Observations/findings

Respiratory distress
  Tachypnea
  Tachycardia
  Nasal flaring
  Pallor
  Dusky
  Cyanosis
  Expiratory grunt
  Retractions
Meconium-stained gastric aspirate; fingernails and/or skin; umbilical cord
Rotund appearance of chest and/or abdomen
Palpable liver
Meconium in amniotic fluid
Meconium visualized below vocal cords

Laboratory/diagnostic studies

Vital signs
Chest x-ray examination shows hyperinflation (within hours of delivery)
Serum glucose levels
CBC, differential and platelet
Blood gas analysis (screen for metabolic acidosis)
Cultures as indicated
Serum calcium

Potential complications

See Respiratory Distress Syndrome (p. 745)

Medical Management

See Respiratory Distress Syndrome (p. 745)

Nursing diagnosis/interventions/evaluation

■ **NDX:** Ineffective airway clearance related to meconium obstruction of airways

At delivery, suction meconium-colored fluid from oropharynx and nasopharynx with DeLee mucous trap or wall suction after head is delivered, before delivery of shoulders

After infant is delivered and cord is clamped, take infant to radiant warmer and assist with intubation to visualize vocal cords for suction of meconium *before* initial stimulation and breaths are taken

Follow immediate stabilization of newborn at delivery procedure (Figure 15-15)

Resuscitate as indicated by assessment

Empty stomach of meconium and mucus by suctioning with DeLee mucous trap or wall suction to 80 mm Hg and 10 French catheter

Provide ventilatory support as ordered (can range from supplemental oxygen to full mechanical respirator support)

Perform postural drainage and percussion q2h to 6h as ordered; position to promote maximum drainage from affected area

Change position at least q2h and prn

Administer antibiotics as ordered

Assist with x-ray examination as ordered

See Respiratory Distress Syndrome (p. 745) for other routine care, Care of Newborn on a Ventilator (p. 748), and Care of Newborn with Endotracheal Tube

Expected outcome/evaluation

Infant has all meconium removed from airway, and respiratory distress/infection has not developed

CARE OF NEWBORN WITH ENDOTRACHEAL TUBE

Assessment

Observations for undesirable findings

Entire or partial expulsion of tube

Loose tape securing tube

Disconnected or loose adapter on endotracheal tube

Obstruction of tube

   Kink in tube or in adapter on tube

   Increased retractions

   Uneven chest excursion

   Sucking of tube

   Coughing

   Restlessness

   Cyanosis

   Mucous plug

Pressure areas on nares or side of mouth near endotracheal tube

Laboratory/diagnostic studies

Abnormal arterial or capillary blood gas values

Potential complications

Respiratory infections

Unintended extubation

Airway obstruction

Skin breakdown

Long term complications

   Tracheal stenosis

   Abnormal oral-motor development

   Inhibition of normal reflexes of sucking/feeding

Medical Management

See Respiratory Distress Syndrome (p. 745), Care of Newborn on a Ventilator (p. 748), and Meconium Aspiration Syndrome (p. 746)

Nursing Care Procedures

Observe position of tube q30min and prn

Maintain patency

   Check for kinks in tube or adapter prn

   Suction q2h and prn—¼ cm beyond end of endotracheal tube

   Check connections qh and prn

Resecure tube with tape prn

Measure length of exposed tube q2h and prn

Measure suction catheter to extend just beyond end of endotracheal tube

Provide oral care each shift and prn

When suctioning

   Hyperoxygenate with 15% more oxygen than infant is receiving for 1 min before (2 min for dusky infant) and during suctioning

   Instill 0.2 to 0.5 ml normal saline solution into endotracheal tube before suctioning

Allow two to three mechanical or manual breaths to distribute solution down tube

Insert suction catheter to carina (meets resistance), remove 0.5 cm, note demarcation line on suction catheter for future suctioning, and suction no longer than 5 sec; twirl catheter as removing if holes on catheter are not alternated

Auscultate breath sounds after suctioning for effect and potential extubation

Take extreme care not to dislodge tube when repositioning

Maintain tube in anatomically correct alignment with trachea

Maintain nasogastric tube as ordered

CARE OF NEWBORN ON A VENTILATOR

Assessment
Observations for undesirable findings

Newborn
  Restlessness
  Audible cry
  Rapid onset of cyanosis
  Excessive sucking
  Excessive mucus from mouth or nose
  Gasping respirations
  Absent or abnormal breath sounds
  Tachycardia or bradycardia
  Tachypnea or bradypnea
  Apnea
  Gastric distention
Ventilator
  Rise or fall in peak pressure on pressure gauge
  Fall in positive end expiratory pressure (PEEP)
  Low fluid level in nebulizer or humidifier
  Condensation in tubing

Laboratory/diagnostic studies

Periodic blood gas analysis to ensure adequate ventilation
Transillumination of chest wall for pneumothorax
See Respiratory Distress Syndrome (p. 745)

Potential complications

Pneumothorax
  Rapid general deterioration
  Cyanosis
  Shift of apical impulse
  Unequal percussion sounds
  Asymmetrical thorax
  Bronchiopulmonary dysplasia
  See Respiratory Distress Syndrome (p. 745)

Medical Management

Ventilator settings: FIO_2, PIP/PEEP, IMV, or CPAP
See Respiratory Distress Syndrome (p. 745)

Nursing Care Procedures

Maintain care of nasal prongs (CPAP)
  Change nasal prongs/sponge q24h
  Clean internal and external nares with applicator prn
  Clean nasal prongs prn
  Check nasal prongs q2h and prn for patency
  Suction nose gently when prongs are removed for checking
  Maintain orogastric tube at all times
  Lubricate prongs before insertion with antibiotic or steroid ointment as ordered
Maintain care of mask assembly (CPAP)

Alternate mask sizes q2h; massage reddened skin areas q30min if unable to alternate mask size
  Apply gentle massage to reddened skin areas q2h and prn
  Keep nasogastric tube inserted and open to air at all times
Maintain care of endotracheal tube
Maintain patient on cardiac monitor at all times
Auscultate chest for breath sounds q1h to 2h, before and after suctioning, and prn
Record respiratory and cardiac rates qh during acute phase, decreasing frequency as patient's condition improves
Observe pressure reading q30min
Record responses to changes in oxygen concentration and ventilator settings
Check all connections for security qh
Drain condensation in tubing prn
Maintain excess ventilator tubing within warmed environment
Administer oxygen as ordered; analyze oxygen q2h
Monitor blood gases as ordered
Calibrate oxygen analyzer q8h
Refill nebulizer or humidifier prn
Reposition infant q2h and prn
  Take extreme care not to dislodge endotracheal tube
  Maintain endotracheal tube in anatomically correct position with trachea
Protect infant's skin from contact with ventilator tubing frame
Maintain nasogastric or orogastric tube as ordered for gastric distention
Change oxygen tubing and equipment q24h to 48h to prevent gram-negative rods ("waterbugs")
Have syringe and butterfly needle with three-way stopcock in-between readily available for physician to use in event pneumothorax occurs (emergency aspiration of pneumothorax)
Have bag and mask immediately available at all times
Suction q2h and prn; see Care of Newborn with Endotracheal Tube (p. 747)
Perform postural drainage and percussion as ordered; avoid for at least 1 hr after feedings
Place infant with head raised 15 to 30 degrees during and after feedings
Restrain arms; pin soft arm restraints to diaper if necessary
Administer parenteral fluids and medications as ordered
Share information with family as appropriate

BRONCHOPULMONARY DYSPLASIA

Chronic lung condition with obstructive bronchiolitis, hyperinfiltration, and pulmonary fibrosis secondary to treatment for respiratory distress syndrome, including high oxygen concentrations delivered by positive pressure ventilation

Assessment
Observations/findings

Tachycardia
Respiratory distress
Cyanosis
Difficult weaning from oxygen and/or ventilator
Tachypnea
Retractions
Grunting, nasal flaring increasing with activity
Diminished breath sounds
Crepitant rales
Difficult maintenance of oxygenation during and after suctioning procedures
Repeated episodes of respiratory infections
Poor weight gain per growth chart

Laboratory/diagnostic studies

Confirmation by chest x-ray findings of hyperaeration, enlarged heart, and chronic lung disease changes
Blood chemistries for fluid/electrolyte imbalances
Urine specific gravities every shift
Arterial/capillary blood gases
Routine Hgb, Hct

Potential complications

Frequent upper and lower respiratory infections
Developmental lags
Failure to thrive syndrome
Congestive heart failure
Cor pulmonale
Chronic hypertension
Hypercapnea
Retrolental fibroplasia (retinopathy of prematurity [ROP])

Medical Management

Medications as indicated
    Antibiotics for respiratory infections
    Diuretics for fluid balance
    Antihypertensives
    Bronchodilators
    Vitamins
    Sedatives
    Anticonvulsants
Nasogastric or gastrostomy feedings for nutrition
Electrolyte supplements as indicated
Oxygen therapy
Mechanical ventilation as indicated (early weaning from an endotracheal tube and low peak inspiratory pressures for ventilation can be expected to decrease complications and improve outcome)

Nursing diagnoses/interventions/evaluation

■ **NDX:** Ineffective breathing pattern related to pathophysiological processes associated with chronic lung disease

Monitor vital signs including respiratory rate, rhythm, and depth
Auscultate lungs for "wet" rales with vital signs at least q4h and with decreasing frequency as condition stabilizes
Space interventions to promote maximum respiratory efficiency
Plan daily routine to promote rest periods
Avoid sensory stimuli during planned rest periods
Elevate head of bed 20 to 30 degrees
Use infant seat at 30 to 45 degrees intermittently with bed rest
Maintain oxygen therapy as ordered
Perform oral/nasal/endotracheal tube suctioning prn for secretions
Have additional endotracheal tube available
Perform chest percussion before suctioning prn
Administer bronchodilators as ordered
Monitor theophylline levels and bring nontherapeutic levels to physician's attention

Expected outcome/evaluation

Infant's
    Blood gas values remain within specific limits (specify)
    Respiratory assessment findings remain within specific limits (specify)

■ **NDX:** Alteration in nutrition: potential for more or less than body requirements related to poor intake or fluid retention

Provide orogastric, nasogastric, or gastrostomy feedings as ordered; progression from continuous to bolus feedings is desirable
Provide caloric supplements as ordered
Weigh daily or q12h as ordered
Maintain po intake to specified calories/kg/day and document on flow sheet as indicated
Observe parent-infant interactions for feeding assessment and document in nursing notes
Monitor intake and output
Observe and document emesis, stool descriptions, and other output
Measure urine specific gravity every shift—done before diuretics are given

Expected outcome/evaluation

Infant
    Maintains weight gain of 15 to 30 g/day
    Avoids weight loss
    Does not have fluid retention or overload

■ **NDX:** Potential for impaired skin integrity related to diarrhea and pharmacotherapeutics

Monitor amount of stool and note amount and description of stool on flow sheet

Monitor perineal skin condition with initial assessment at least every shift and prn with diaper changes

Give good skin cleansing with diaper changes

Apply topical ointments as ordered

Use heat lamp at 18 inches and with area open to air for 30 min q4h or more as time allows; 30 min qh is maximum for heat lamp

Report multiple episodes of diarrhea to physician

Test stool pH and blood once each shift

Monitor administration of bronchodilators and antibiotics

Expected outcome/evaluation

Infant maintains skin integrity with absence of inflammation/excoriation in perianal area

■ **NDX:** Knowledge deficit related to lack of information about prolonged hospitalization and respiratory support required for infant

Discuss long-term follow-up needs of infant

Emphasize importance of maintaining oxygen therapy if ordered by physician

Explain that infant is more susceptible to URIs and discuss when to report to physician

Teach administration of oxygen and medications

Teach suctioning of infant

Discuss special feeding needs

Teach infant stimulation

Provide infant cardiopulmonary resuscitation training

See Care of Newborn (p. 725), Care of Premature Infant (p. 731), and Care of Newborn on a Ventilator (p. 748)

Expected outcome/evaluation

Parents and/or significant other understand infant needs and become progressively involved in caretaking activities

INTERMITTENT GAVAGE FEEDING

Feeding via a tube passed into the stomach through the nose or mouth; for infant with weak sucking, uncoordinated suck and swallow, respiratory distress and/or respiratory rate above 60/min, repeated apneic spells, or fatigue in sucking on "preemie" nipple (inadequate oral intake)

Assessment
Observations for undesirable findings

Cyanosis
Choking
Gagging
Spitting
Regurgitation
Vomiting

Rate of flow: excessively slow or fast

Large amount of residual for size of neonate

Potential complications

Aspiration of formula

Insertion of gavage tube into trachea

Tissue trauma with poor ingestion technique

Nursing care procedures

Use 8 French feeding tube (5 to 6 French if infant is very small)

Place infant with head raised 15 to 30 degrees during feeding and on right side or abdomen after feeding

Hold infant during feeding by mother (or nurse) if possible

Restrain only if necessary

Measure tube length before insertion from tip of nose to earlobe to xiphoid process; mark with a small piece of tape before insertion

Check placement of tube
  Place end of tube in water; will bubble with expiration if misplaced in respiratory tract
  Aspirate; evaluate contents, return to stomach or discard, and record gastric residual as ordered
  Subtract residual amount from feeding as ordered; feeding may be skipped if residual is over amount specified by physician
  If no residual, instill air into stomach and auscultate stomach for air sounds

Hold syringe 6 to 8 inches above infant's head

Initiate flow with slight pressure on plunger; gravity flow is preferred (remove plunger)

Feed infant slowly; stroke skin during feeding

Offer pacifier during feeding to promote gravity flow, calm infant, and reinforce relationship of sucking and full stomach

Do not allow air to enter stomach when feeding is complete; immediately pinch off and withdraw tubing when feeding is complete

Burp gently by rubbing or patting back

Turn head to right side after feeding or position infant on right side

Avoid postural drainage and percussion for at least 1 hr after feeding

Indicate the following on nursing care plan
  Amount and type of feeding
  Size of catheter
  Time of feeding

See Family-Centered Care of High-Risk Infant (p. 751)

Discuss the following with parents and/or significant other
  Explanation of need for gavage feedings
  That nipple feedings may be resumed when infant shows signs of the following
    Sucking on gavage tube and/or pacifier
    Rooting actively
    Good suck and swallow coordination

Effort does not outweigh caloric intake in nipple feeding

Not tiring when nipple feeding

Gaining weight in excess of 3 lb

Respiratory rate below 60/min

See appropriate standard of care, depending on infant's condition: Care of Premature Infant (p. 731), Respiratory Distress Syndrome (p. 745), or Care of High-Risk Infant

FAMILY-CENTERED CARE OF HIGH-RISK INFANT

Philosophy and interventions promoting bonding and attachment, and a method of assessing parent-infant interaction in helping to provide individualized, need-specific parent teaching and continuity of care

Assessment
Observations/findings

Sensory deprivation of newborn and parents

Anticipatory grief and emotional separation

Laboratory/diagnostic studies

Parent-infant interaction scales

BNBAS (Brazelton) assessment scale

Potential complications

Poor parenting/infant care skills of caretakers

Lack of bonding and noninitiation of attachment process

Long-term complications

    Child abuse and/or neglect

    Poor growth and development

Medical Management

Interdisciplinary team conferences

Patient care rounds

Parent-infant interaction documentation

Social services consult

Specific discharge planning needs

Nursing diagnosis/interventions/evaluation

■ **NDX:** Potential alteration in parenting related to the birth and care of high-risk neonate

Explain to parents what infant looks like and what equipment they will see before visiting nursery

Have mother visit nursery and visually examine and touch infant before 12 hr of age

Encourage parents' questions and explain equipment usage

Involve parents in infant's care as much as possible

At mother's or parent's visit to nursery, do the following

    Welcome parent by name

    Personalize comments about infant's status

        Tell mother that she is mothering better than the nurses, since she is able to become involved in infant's care

Leave a note in infant's incubator or crib, such as "Hi Mom, I've been waiting to see you" at least daily as appropriate

Encourage mother to come back to nursery soon, that it is important for her infant to get to know her

Play radio with soft music in nursery prn

Place decals outside incubator on adjacent walls

Hang mobiles within viewing distance of infant

Encourage parents to bring in brightly colored toys or music box for their infant

Assign same nurse each shift if possible

Provide infant with experiences similar to those of normal infants, including sound, touch, and smell of primary caretaker

Talk to infant during nursing care procedures

Offer pacifier prn when infant does not tire from sucking

Respond to infant's crying

Stroke infant's head and chest; hold arm or leg during nursing procedures

Hold and cuddle infant close to body as soon as able

Promote eye contact between mother and infant by repositioning infant to face mother; for infants receiving phototherapy, turn lights off and remove eye patches when mother visits

Allow siblings to view infant through nursery window if feasible

Ascertain what parents think is going to happen to infant and reinforce physician's explanation of care plan and prognosis at parents' pace and level of understanding

Maintain records of parents' visits and telephone calls

    Report to physician fewer than two telephone calls or visits weekly

    Call parents when appropriate

For parents who have been physically and/or emotionally separated from their infant

    Provide private room close to nursery nursing staff for mother to spend 1 to 2 hr daily for 2 or 3 days with infant before discharge

    Provide mother with supplies to feed and bathe infant and assure her that she will not be disturbed unless she calls for assistance

Help parents anticipate equipment and time required and caretaker's physical ability to cope with infant's needs well in advance of discharge

Refer to Visiting Nurse's Association as indicated for predischarge and/or postdischarge home visit

See Care of Newborn (p. 725) and Care of Premature Infant (p. 731)

Expected outcome/evaluation

Parents participate in infant care and demonstrate appropriate interactions and parenting skills

BIBLIOGRAPHY
American College of Obstetricians and Gynecologists: *Ectopic pregnancy,* Technical Bulletin No 150, Dec, 1990, ACOG, Washington, DC.

American Academy of Pediatrics/American College of Obstetricians and Gynecologists (AAP/ACOG): *Guidelines for perinatal care,* Washington, DC, 1988.

Cole C: *The Harriet Lane handbook,* ed 12, Chicago, 1990, Year Book Medical Publishers, Inc.

Cropley C, Bloom R: Neonatal resuscitation, Los Angeles, 1986, Charles R Drew Postgraduate Medical School.

Danforth DN: Hypertensive disorders in pregnancy, *Obstet gynecol,* Philadelphia, 1990, Harper & Row.

Doenges M, Jeffries M, and Moorhouse M: *Nursing care plans: nursing diagnoses in planning patient care,* Philadelphia, 1989, FA Davis.

Eden R: Standards of care for the postdate pregnancy, *Contemp OB/Gyn* 34(2):39, 1989.

Fletcher M, MacDonald M, and Avery G: *Atlas of procedures in neonatology,* Philadelphia, 1983, JB Lippincott.

Frantz K: *Managing nipple problems,* reprint No 11, Oak Park, Ill, 1982, La Leche League International.

Freeman R, Garite T: *Fetal heart rate monitoring,* Baltimore, 1991, Williams & Wilkins.

Friedman M: *Family nursing,* New York, 1986, Appleton-Century-Crofts.

Furrh CB, Copley R: One precious moment, *Nursing '89* 19(9):52, 1989.

A guide to successful breastfeeding, Los Angeles, 1986, Southern California Kaiser Permanente Medical Centers.

Henrickson ML: A nursing approach to epidural anesthesia, JOGNN 17(5):316, 1988.

Jensen MD, Bobak IM: Maternity and gynecologic care, ed 3, St Louis, 1989, CV Mosby.

Lockwood CJ: Placenta previa and related disorders, *Contemp OB/Gyn* 35(1):47, 1990.

Merenstein GB, Gardner SL: *Handbook of neonatal intensive care,* St Louis, 1989, CV Mosby.

Perinatal Advisory Council of Los Angeles Communities: *Neonatal protocols,* Los Angeles, 1989, The Council.

Perinatal Advisory Council of Los Angeles Communities: *Prenatal and intrapartum protocols,* Los Angeles, 1991, The Council.

Stevens KA: Nursing diagnoses in wellness childbearing settings, JOGNN 17(5):329, 1988.

16
CHAPTER

Pediatrics

Basic Standards of Care

INFANT AGE-GROUP CARE

Usual age: 1 month to 1 year
Placement: with infants or toddlers according to diagnosis

Hygiene

Give complete bath daily
Change diaper prn with diaper area care: soap and water wash, careful drying
Use A & D ointment prn
Shampoo hair q3d and prn
Trim nails prn
Clean outer ear gently qod

Sleep

Sleep 16 to 18 hr daily
Take morning and afternoon nap

Diet and Fluids

Institute intake and output sheet
Know fluid requirement: 120 to 150 ml/kg/day
Know calorie requirement: 115 kcal/kg/day
Give appropriate diet for age
   1 to 3 months
     20 kcal/oz formula with iron or breast milk
   3 to 6 months
     20 kcal/oz formula with iron or breast milk
     Diluted juices ad lib
     Introduce foods in following order
       Cereal and fruit
       Yellow vegetables
       Green vegetables
       Meat
       Mixed puree dinners
   6 to 9 months
     Formula with iron: 20 kcal/oz three times daily and at bedtime or breast milk
     Water ad lib
     Solids: all purees by spoon three times/day
     Begin adding junior foods and cup training
     Give finger foods
   9 to 12 months (birth weight usually triples by 12 months)
     20 kcal/oz formula with iron three times/day and at bedtime or breast milk
     May drink from a cup with assistance
     Solids: all chopped table foods by spoon three times/day
     Begin adding table foods; increase cup training
Avoid overfeeding of infants; intake of formula should not exceed 32 oz in a 24-hour period
Administer liquid po medications through nipple or squirt inside cheek with oral syringe

Elimination

Record and describe all stools on intake and output sheet
   1 week to 3 months: approximately q3h to 8h
   3 months to 1 year: approximately one to three times/day
Record urinary output on intake and output sheet
   Record amount if measured
   Record "wet" if not measured
   Average urinary output
     10 to 20 ml/hr
     240 to 500 ml/day

Activity

Hold for bottle and solid feeding; leave bottle with infant when able to hold
Provide infant seat high chair for meals
Provide toys for visual, auditory, and developmental stimulation
Encourage activity appropriate for age
Infant
   Holds arms out to be picked up
   Crawls around 9 months
   Begins to use thumb and index finger in pincer grasp about 9 months of age
   Drops objects deliberately for them to be picked up

Emotional Development

Respond to infant's expressed needs for warmth, physical contact, comfort, eye contact, speech, and social playtime
Bundle for sleep and nap time
Involve parents in infant's care as much as possible
Comfort infant if distressed when mother leaves
Remember infant begins to recognize parents and fear strangers

Environmental Safety

Keep side rails up at all times and instruct parents to do the same

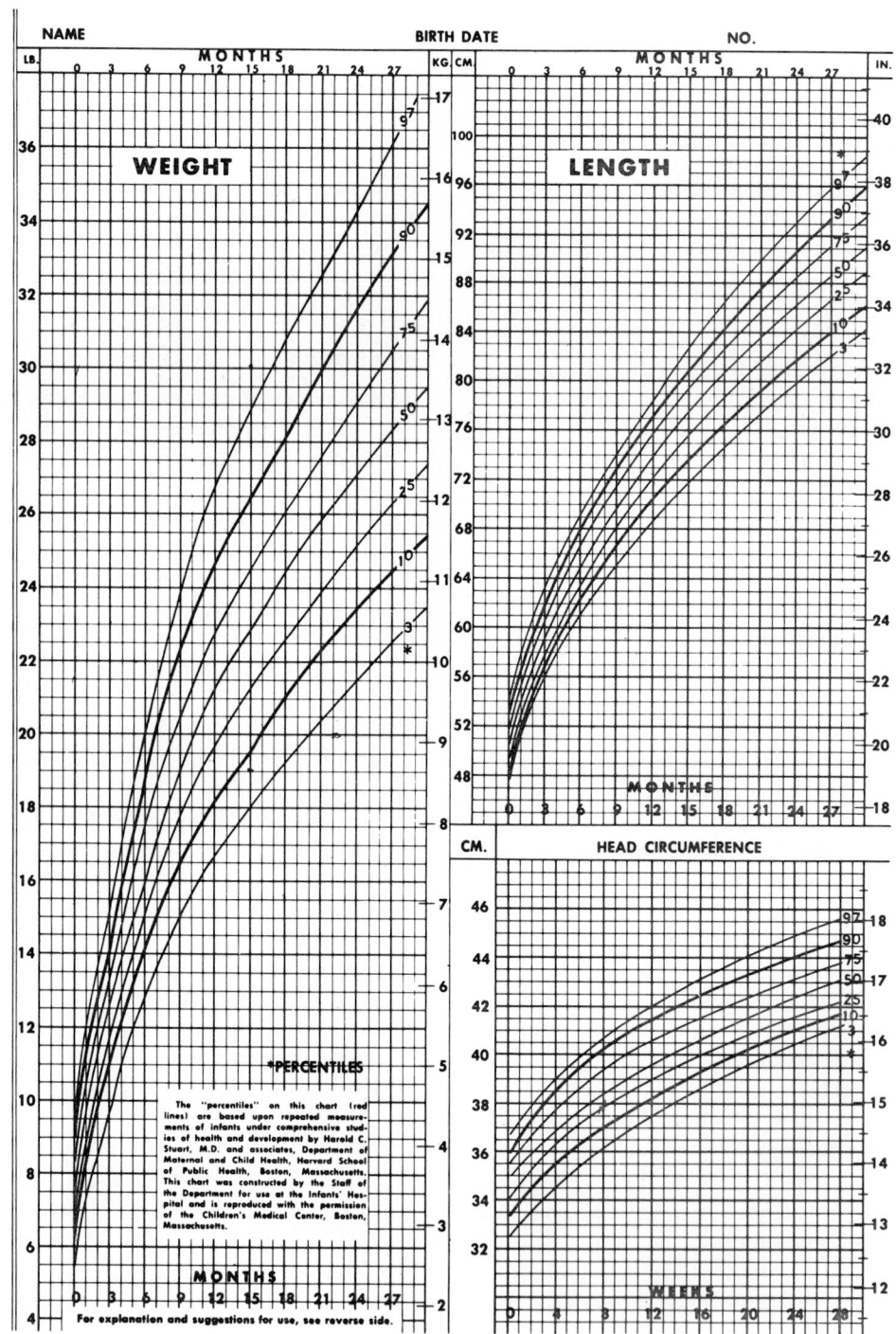

FIGURE 16-1. Percentile growth chart for infant girls. (From The Children's Hospital Medical Center, Boston, Mass. Reprinted by permission.)

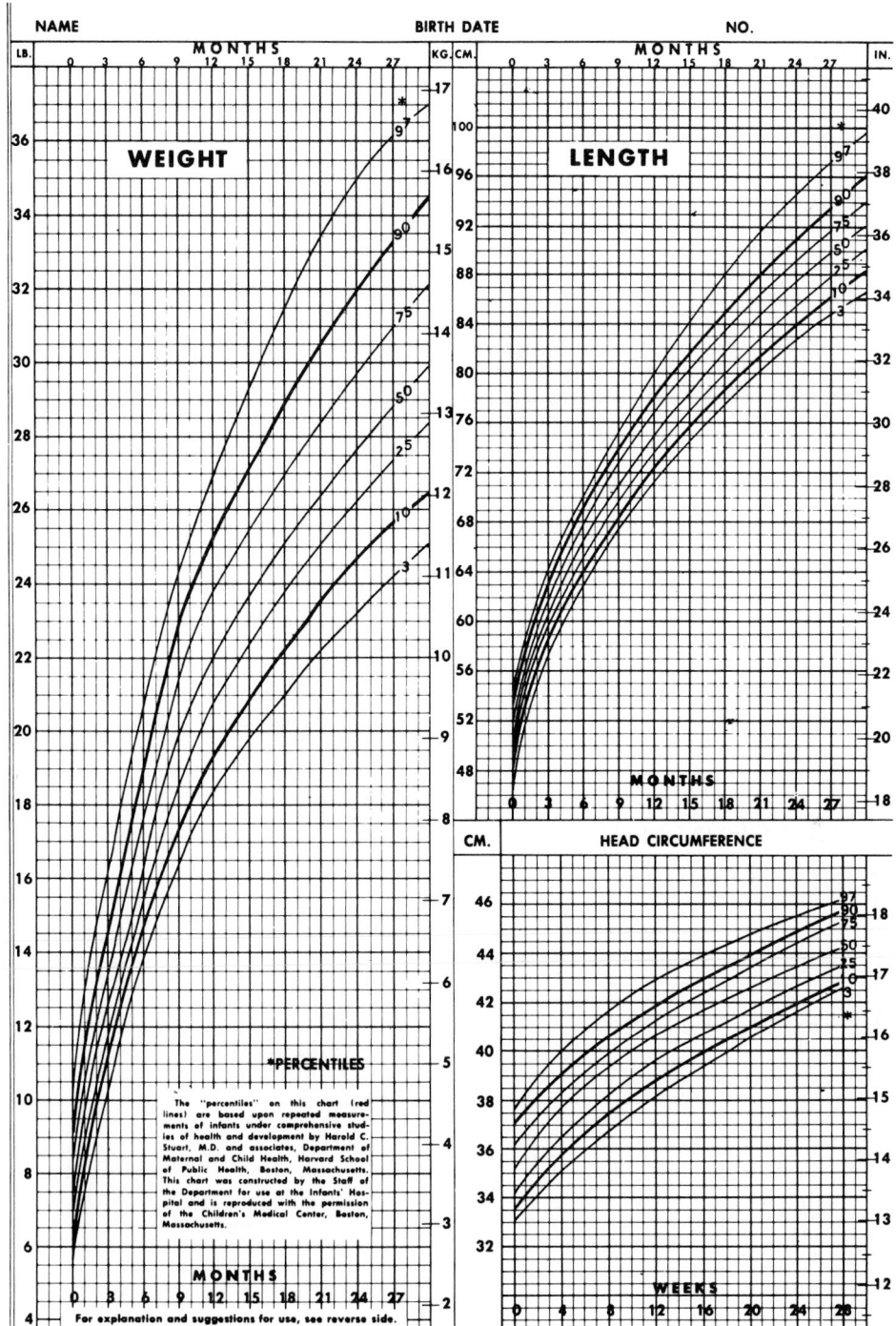

FIGURE 16-2. Percentile growth chart for infant boys. (From The Children's Hospital Medical Center, Boston, Mass. Reprinted by permission.)

Keep bed free of loose linen and absorbent pads
Allow no toys with sharp edges and points or small detachable pieces that could be detached and swallowed or aspirated
Allow no pillows

TODDLER AGE-GROUP CARE

Usual age: 1 to 3 years
Placement: with infants and toddlers according to diagnosis

Hygiene

Give complete bath daily
Initiate dental care in older toddlers
Not toilet trained
    Change diaper prn with diaper area care: soap and water wash, careful drying
    Use Desitin or A & D ointment prn
Toilet trained
    Do not use diapers
    Follow toilet training schedule as done at home
Administer hair care prn
Use pillow if desired
Cover with blanket at nap and bedtime

Sleep

Sleep 10 to 14 hr daily
Take morning and afternoon nap (1 hr each or 2 hr afternoon nap)

Diet and Fluids

Know fluid requirement: 90 to 120 ml/kg/day
Know calorie requirement: approximately 1300 kcal/day
Give appropriate diet for age
    1 year to 18 months
        Junior foods to finger foods, gradual introduction to regular diet
        Avoid carrot sticks, nuts, etc.
        Cut food into small pieces
        Milk and juices by cup
    18 months to 3 years
        Regular table food, all fluids by cup
        Avoid carrot sticks, nuts, etc.
May use spoon; do not allow fork for self-feeding

Elimination

Record and describe all stools: usual frequency, one to two times daily
Record urinary output if on intake and output
    Average urinary output
        20 to 25 ml/hr
        500 to 600 ml/day

Activity

Allow free movement in crib when possible
Understand that toddler overestimates ability to perform safely
Evaluate need to omit bumper pads in crib/play yard when child is able to use them as "stairs" to get out
Do not leave younger toddlers unsupervised in chairs, etc.
Apply appropriate restraints as necessary
Administer medication as "medicine"; do not use the word "candy"

Emotional Development

Be aware of dual stage of development: feelings of autonomy vs. dependence
Encourage child to do those things he can do safely for himself; be prepared to do for him or comfort him when he needs to be dependent
Do not reinforce normal negativism
Involve parents in care as much as possible
Comfort child when mother leaves
Protect favorite toy or blanket
Fear of separation, desertion (separation anxiety is highest in this age-group)

Environmental Safety

Keep side rails up at all times and instruct parents to do the same
Do not tie toys across crib in this age group
Prevent climbing over side rails with canopy-type crib or overbed net
Avoid balloons as playthings
Allow no toys with sharp edges and points, or those with small removable pieces that may become detached and swallowed or aspirated

---

PRESCHOOL-AGE CHILD CARE

Usual age: 3 to 6 years
Placement: with preschool age or older children, according to diagnosis

Hygiene

AM care
    Give complete bed or tub bath daily
    Administer hair care
    Shampoo weekly and prn
    Administer nail care
    Administer mouth care: including teeth brushing
HS care
    Wash face and hands
    Brush teeth
    Wash hands after using bathroom
    Place top covers on bed; pillow may be used

Sleep

Sleep 10 to 13 hr nightly

Take afternoon nap

Diet and Fluids

Know fluid requirement: 90 to 120 ml/kg/day

Know calorie requirement: approximately 1000 kcal/day

Administer medications as "medicine"; do not tell child that it is candy

Understand that need for calorie intake decreases as growth rate increases—may have periods of disinterest in food

Maintain regular diet

Cut up and prepare food; allow child to feed himself

Understand that child will eat better if portions are smaller and meal is presented one item at a time

Measure intake and output when indicated by diagnosis

Provide nourishing between-meal snacks, recognizing the long time span between meals

Elimination

Record and describe all stools: usual frequency, once daily

Record urinary output if on intake and output

  Average urinary output

    20 to 40 ml/hr

    600 to 1000 ml daily

  May still be bed-wetting; *do not chastise*

Activity

Understand that this is a period of great need for physical activity

Allow child to sit up and ambulate as much as condition allows

Involve child in care and planning as much as possible

Provide diversional activities appropriate for child's age

Emotional Development

Understand that child likes playing with other children

Understand that child needs to feel in some control of environment

Understand that child likes music and familiar stories

Understand that child needs repetitive, simple explanation for reassurance

Explain procedures honestly just before performance

Involve parents in care as much as possible

Understand that it is normal for child to have fear of bodily harm or mutilation, castration, or intrusive procedures; separation anxiety may be demonstrated less intensively than in toddler age-group

Environmental Safety

Be aware that child is more coordinated but overestimates abilities

Keep side rails up

Be aware that child is capable of putting away toys—takes pride in straightening up

Sit only in low chairs

SCHOOL-AGE CHILD CARE

Usual age: 6 to 12 years

Placement: with other school-age children according to diagnosis

Hygiene

AM care

  Give complete bed bath daily (tub or shower when feasible)—self-care advisable

  Administer hair care

  Shampoo weekly and prn

  Administer mouth care, including teeth brushing

  Administer back care, if on bed rest

HS care

  Wash face and hands

  Brush teeth

  Administer back care, if on bed rest

  Wash hands after using bathroom

  Place top covers on bed; pillow(s) may be used

Sleep

Sleep 8 to 10 hr at night

Maintain quiet rest period in afternoon—need not sleep

Diet and Fluids

Know fluid requirement: 60 to 90 ml/kg/day

Know calorie requirement: 2100 to 2500 kcal/day

Maintain regular diet

Understand that food likes and dislikes are highly developed

Provide nourishing between-meal snacks

Understand that child is self-sufficient in preparing own food

Offer food choices whenever possible and expect strong food preferences

Elimination

Record and describe all stools: usual frequency, once daily

Record urinary output if on intake and output

  Average urinary output

    30 to 50 ml/hr

    900 to 1200 ml/day

Activity

Encourage intellectual pursuits, schoolwork

Understand that child is well-coordinated and more safety conscious

May ambulate freely; bed in low position and side rails down during the day

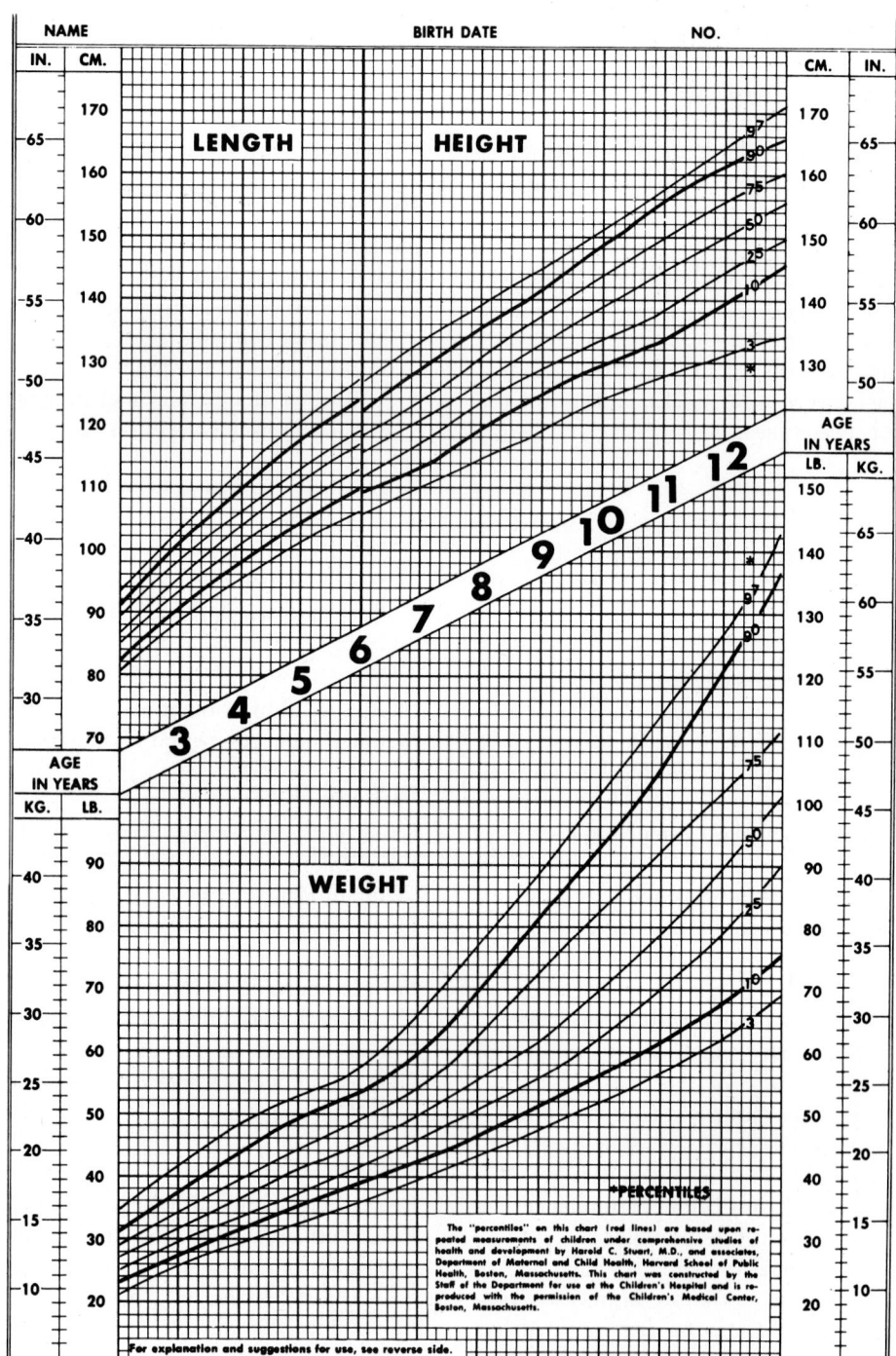

FIGURE 16-3. Percentile growth chart for girls. (From The Children's Hospital Medical Center, Boston, Mass. Reprinted by permission.)

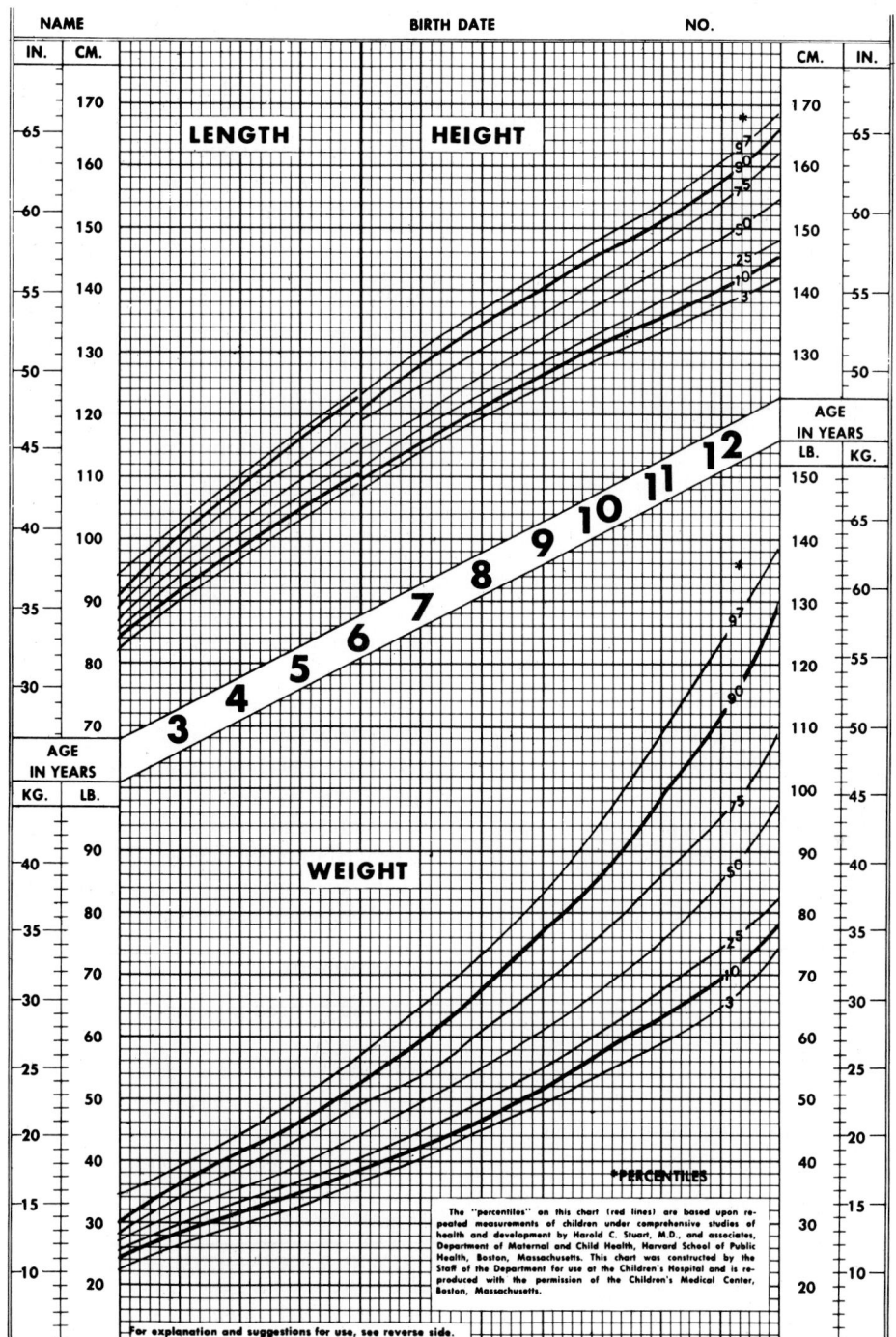

FIGURE 16-4. Percentile growth chart for boys. (From The Children's Hospital Medical Center, Boston, Mass. Reprinted by permission.)

Emotional Development

Involve child in planning care

Give child careful explanation of events with adequate time to prepare himself emotionally

Accept occasional lapses into dependence; encourage gradual return to independence

Be aware that time awareness is good

Understand that child enjoys group and competitive play

Understand that it is normal for child to fear physical nature of illness

Understand that child may exhibit concern regarding ability to hold social position in peer group because of separation

Be aware that child is modest and proud
  Do not cause embarrassment or feeling of inferiority
  Respect modesty
  Keep covered and screened when necessary

Understand that child's concept of himself is important
  Do not tease, belittle, or compare him unfavorably with other children
  Be aware that he may engage in belittling other children to build his own ego

Understand child's need to control environment

Give responsibility for child's own immediate environment and belongings

Environment

Be aware that child is more conscious of environment outside room; allow child to explore and become oriented to remainder of unit when possible

ADOLESCENT AGE-GROUP CARE

Usual age: 12 to 18 years
Placement: with other adolescents, according to diagnosis

Hygiene

AM care
  Give complete bath: bed, self-care, tub, or shower
  Administer hair care
  Shampoo as desired
  Administer mouth care, including teeth brushing
HS care
  Wash face and hands
  Brush teeth
  Offer back rub as appropriate

Sleep

Sleep 8 hr at night
Maintain quiet rest period in afternoon if desired

Diet and Fluids

Know fluid requirement: 60 to 90 ml/kg/day
Know calorie requirement: 2500 to 3000 kcal/day
Maintain regular diet

Understand that increased need for calories is related to increasing growth rate

May need double portions

Serve frequent between-meal and bedtime snacks

Offer food choices whenever possible

Elimination

Record and describe all stools; usual frequency, daily or qod

Record urinary output if on intake and output
  Average urinary output
    50 to 70 ml/hr
    1200 to 1680 ml/day

Activity

Encourage intellectual pursuits, schoolwork

Ambulate freely with bed in low position and side rail down during day

Emotional Development

Understand that adolescent considers himself adult

Understand that adolescent must have adequate explanation and involvement in planning care

Be aware that involvement with peers is of utmost importance

Understand that adolescent may exhibit concern regarding separation from peers and loss of independence, control, and identity

Understand that adolescent needs accepting attitude concerning appearance and teenage behavior

Understand that adolescent wants nurse to be an understanding adult who sets good example

Accept labile mood swings; adolescent may swing between being communicative and noncommunicative, cheerful and depressed, sensitive and cruel, etc.

Environment

Be aware of need for control of environment, especially privacy

Give responsibility for adolescent's own immediate environment and belongings

Ensure confidentiality of communication (when there is no harm to teenager or others)

Respiratory System

CROUP: LARYNGOTRACHEOBRONCHITIS

An acute viral (predominantly parainfluenza virus) infection of the larynx, trachea, and bronchi, which results in varying degrees of respiratory tract obstruction

Usual age: infant or toddler; most common in males
Seasonal occurrence: fall/winter

Assessment

Observations/findings

See Respiratory Assessment (p. 186)
Restlessness; irritability
Apprehension
Cyanosis
Nasal flaring
Retractions (suprasternal, substernal, intercostal)
Audible inspiratory stridor
Cough (brassy or barking character) with history of worsening at night
Hoarse voice
Tachypnea
Ausculated stridor, bilateral decreased breath sounds
Rhonchi, rales
Increasing tachycardia
Low-grade fever
History of cold for 1 to 2 days

Laboratory/diagnostic studies

X-ray examination (lateral neck) to rule out foreign body
White blood cell count (WBC): usually normal
Blood cultures: negative

Potential complications

Complete laryngeal obstruction
Secondary bacterial infection causing pneumonia, bronchiolitis, otitis media, or epiglottitis

Medical Management

Cool, highly humidified environment (with oxygen via mist tent as indicated)
Racemic epinephrine via nebulizer for severe respiratory distress
Cardiac monitor
Transcutaneous oxygen monitor as appropriate
Vital signs qh with acute symptoms to include pulse rate and respiratory assessment; temperature q4h and prn
NPO if in acute distress
Parenteral fluids
Corticosteroids IV (use is controversial)
Antipyretics prn for fever
Endotracheal intubation (or tracheostomy) with laryngeal obstruction

Nursing diagnoses/interventions/evaluation

■ **NDX:**   Ineffective airway clearance related to inflammation and swelling of the trachea, larynx, and bronchi

Monitor vital signs with respiratory assessment as ordered and prn
Maintain cool, moist, environment via mist tent with oxygen or compressed air
Initiate oxygen as ordered or prn for respiratory distress

Allow patient to assume position of comfort when possible
Elevate head of bed
Use nebulized mist inhaler with racemic epinephrine as ordered
Administer antiinflammatory drugs if ordered
Keep endotracheal intubation (ET) or tracheostomy equipment at bedside and assist with intubation procedure if necessary (ET size approximately that of patient's pinky finger)

Expected outcome/evaluation

Patient
   Has clear breath sounds
   Has age-appropriate respiratory rate before discharge

■ **NDX:**   Anxiety related to air hunger, hospitalization, and separation from parents

Provide nonstressful environment
   Postpone routine care while respiratory distress is severe
   Bed rest
   Allow parents to participate in child's care and encourage rooming-in
   Alleviate parental anxiety by explaining
      Need for cool, moist environment
      Need for undisturbed rest
      That their anxiety is transmitted to their child; therefore it is imperative that they remain calm
   Allow parents to play with child in mist tent when necessary
   Provide age-appropriate play activities as child's condition improves

Expected outcome/evaluation

Patient experiences a nonstressful environment that promotes normal respiratory patterns and normal child-parent relationships

■ **NDX:**   Fluid volume deficit related to insensible loss in the presence of fever, hyperventilation, and inability to tolerate fluids po

Maintain NPO status in the presence of respiratory distress and administer maintenance fluids parenterally as ordered
Record intake and output and monitor specific gravity
As respiratory status improves, urge fluids as tolerated (assess child's likes and dislikes and use of bottle vs. cup)
Give lukewarm clear liquids because they are tolerated best
Provide cooling measures prn and administer antipyretics as ordered

Expected outcome/evaluation

Patient remains hydrated and is able to tolerate age-appropriate fluid volume by mouth

Text continued on p. 776.

TABLE 16-1. Childhood Diseases

Disease	Causative agents	Transmission	Incubation	Communica-bility	Observations
Rubella (German measles)	Rubella virus	Droplet or direct contact with infected persons or articles freshly contaminated with nasopharyngeal secretions, feces, or urine	14-21 days after exposure	7 days before to 5 days after rash appears	Low-grade fever, headache, lymphadenopathy (postauricular and cervical), malaise, conjunctivitis, anorexia, sore throat, rash (maculopapular exanthema, generalized) Duration 3-5 days
Congenital rubella	Rubella virus	Transplacental during first trimester of pregnancy	Virus dangerous only to fetus	Infants may be infectious for months	Any combination possible—growth retardation, mental retardation, microcephaly, deafness, cataracts, strabismus, retinopathy, congenital heart disease, thrombocytopenic purpura, behavioral abnormalities
Rubeola (measles)	Measles virus	Direct contact with droplets	10-20 days	4 days to 5 days after rash appears	Fever, malaise, coryza, cough, conjunctivitis, Koplik's spots (small red spots with bluish white center seen on buccal mucosa opposite molars), lymphadenopathy, rash (maculopapular, erythema followed by desquamation)
Roseola infantum (exanthema subitum)	Presumably virus	Unknown; occurs between 6 mo and 2 yr	Unknown	Unknown	Fever of 104°-105° F (40°-40.5° C) for up to 3-4 days, anorexia, irritability, rash (maculopapular appearing when fever suddenly drops)
Chickenpox (varicella)	Varicella-zoster	Highly communicable via direct contact, indirect contact, droplet spread, airborne	14-21 days after exposure	Onset of fever until last vesicle is dried (5-7 days)	Malaise, fever, rash (macule to papule to vesicle)—appears first on head and mucous membranes, then concentrates on body, sparse on extremities, severe itching
Whooping cough (pertussis)	*Bordetella pertussis*	Direct contact, droplet spread, indirect contact with contaminated articles	5-21 days	7 days after exposure to 3 weeks after onset of paroxysms	See Pertussis: Whooping Cough (p. 777)

Complications	Treatment	Ongoing care	Prevention
In adolescent and adults: arthritis, encephalitis, purpura	Symptomatic: antipyretics, analgesics	Prevent exposure of nonimmune pregnant women in first trimester; provide comfort measures as necessary	12 mo or older: rubella vaccine or in combination with measles and mumps
As pertains to defect present	As pertains to defect present	Strict isolation of neonates with rubella until throat culture is free of virus; select nursing personnel who are not at risk for rubella infection; provide care as pertains to defect present	Determination of rubella titer and administration of rubella vaccine to women before pregnancy occurs
Otitis media, pneumonia, laryngitis, mastoiditis, encephalitis	Bed rest, antipyretics, vaporizer, antibiotics may be necessary	Isolate from onset of inflammation of mucous membranes through fifth day of rash; provide cooling measures for fever, especially if prone to seizures; dim lights if photophobia is present; cleanse eyelids with warm saline solution, prevent rubbing of eyes; maintain skin cleanliness with tepid baths; encourage fluids and soft, bland foods	15 mo: measles vaccine; may be in combination with mumps and rubella vaccine
Convulsions resulting from high fever	Symptomatic: antipyretics	Control high fever with cooling measures—tepid baths, antipyretics	None
Rare in normal children; encephalitis, pneumonia, bacterial skin infection possible; Reye's syndrome; severe when contracted by immunosuppressed individuals; scarring from scratching	Symptomatic: antipyretics, antihistamines for itch	Isolate until all lesions have crusted (5-7 days); prevent scratching—apply mitts, pat lesions with mixture of baking soda and warm water, keep fingernails short and clean; skin care—daily bath, change clothes and linens daily	No active immunization available; for high-risk susceptible children VZIG should be given within 72 hr of exposure; may modify varicella
Pneumonia, atelectasis, emphysema	See Pertussis: Whooping Cough (p. 777)	See Pertussis: Whooping Cough (p. 777)	DTP (diphtheria-tetanus-pertussis) at 2 mo, 4 mo, 6 mo, 18 mo, 4-6 yr

Continued.

TABLE 16-1. Childhood Diseases—cont'd

Disease	Causative agents	Transmission	Incubation	Communica-bility	Observations
Diphtheria	*Corynebacterium diphtheriae*	Direct contact with infected person, carrier, or contaminated articles	2-5 days	Variable: until bacilli are no longer present (three negative cultures)—usually 2 wk, may be up to 4 wk	Mucopurulent nasal discharge, malaise, anorexia, sore throat, tachycardia, low-grade fever, white or gray membrane in pharynx, hoarseness, apprehension, cyanosis
Mumps	Mumps virus	Direct contact with droplet or droplet spread	14-21 days	7 days before to 9 days after swelling appears	Headache, anorexia, malaise, fever, parotid gland swelling
Scarlet fever (scarlatina)	Group A β-hemolytic streptococci	Direct contact or droplet, indirect contact with contaminated articles, or ingestion of contaminated food	2-4 days	Approximately 10 days; may persist for months	High fever, tachycardia, vomiting, headache, chills, malaise, abdominal pain, enlarged tonsils, red strawberry tongue, red pinhead-sized lesions becoming generalized with flushed face followed by desquamation
Tetanus	*Clostridium tetani*	Direct or indirect contact with wound	3 days to 3 weeks	None	Stiffening of striated muscles; usually jaw, spastic rigidity
Poliomyelitis	Enterovirus	Direct contact via fecal-oral and pharyngeal routes	7-14 days	In throat—1 week after onset; in stool—4-6 weeks after onset	Headache, lethargy, anorexia, vomiting, fever, muscle pain and stiffness; CNS—loss of deep tendon reflexes, positive Kernig's and Brudzinki's signs, weakening of muscles and paralysis

Complications	Treatment	Ongoing care	Prevention
Toxemia, septic shock, airway obstruction, myocarditis, neuritis	Antitoxin, antibiotics, complete bed rest, respiratory support, tracheostomy as necessary	Strict isolation until two to three cultures are negative; maintain bed rest; observe for signs of respiratory obstruction; suction prn; provide humidified air	DTP (diphtheria-tetanus-pertussis) at 2 mo, 4 mo, 6 mo, 18 mo, 4-6 yr
Meningoencephalitis, deafness, orchitis (after puberty)	Symptomatic: analgesics, antipyretics, parenteral fluids if refuses to drink	Isolation; encourage fluids and soft, bland foods; apply warm compresses to neck; maintain bed rest; observe for neurological symptoms	15 mo: mumps vaccine, usually with measles and rubella
Glomerulonephritis, rheumatic fever	Antibiotics: usually penicillin, analgesics, bed rest	Isolate until 24 hr after initiating therapy; maintain bed rest; relieve sore throat; encourage fluids and soft diet	None available
Laryngospasms, asphyxia	Antibiotics, debridement of wound, tetanus antitoxin	Suction; minimize spasticity with medication and quiet, dark room; administer adequate fluid and nutrition—parenteral fluids, tube feeding; supply respiratory support as necessary	Tetanus vaccine (usually with diphtheria and pertussis) at 2 mo, 4 mo, 6 mo, 18 mo, 4-6 yr
Respiratory paralysis, hypertension	Supportive: analgesics, bed rest, respiratory support as necessary	Enteric isolation; maintain bed rest; administer physical therapy; administer sedation as necessary; maintain body alignment; observe for respiratory paralysis	TOPV (trivalent oral-polio vaccine) at 2 mo, 4 mo, 18 mo, 4-6 yr

■ **NDX:** Knowledge deficit related to lack of information about home care needs

Discuss diet
Explain need to encourage fluids
Discuss symptoms of recurrence to report to physician
  Increasingly labored respirations
  Poor appetite
  Restlessness
  Increasing, persistent stridor
  Fever
Explain that normal course of disease is worse at night, with improvement during waking hours
Discuss use of cool vaporizer at nap time and bedtime
Teach cooling measures
Instruct about administration of prescribed medications

Expected outcome/evaluation

Parents and/or significant other demonstrates understanding of home care and follow-up instructions and state understanding of disease, treatment, and home care needs

EPIGLOTTITIS

A severe, rapidly progressing infection of the epiglottis and surrounding areas; most commonly associated with Haemophilus influenzae *but may result from other bacteria or virus*
Usual age: 2 to 7 years; most common in males
Seasonal occurrence: none

Assessment
Observations/findings

Rapid onset and progression of respiratory difficulty within several hours
Sore throat; dysphagia

Drooling
Hoarseness or aphonia
Inspiratory stridor
Tachypnea
Retractions (suprasternal, substernal, intercostal) (Figure 16-5)
Bilateral, decreased breath sounds
Rhonchi
Pallor or cyanosis
Increasing tachycardia
Restlessness
Disorientation
Lethargy
Fever greater than 101.3° F (38.5° C) rectally

Laboratory/diagnostic studies

WBC: usually elevated
Chest and neck x-ray examination for differential diagnosis
Throat culture to isolate organism (only done *after* intubation)

Potential complications

Respiratory arrest
Septicemia

Medical Management

Laryngoscopy to visualize the epiglottis (characteristically edematous and cherry red)
Endotracheal intubation or tracheostomy
Throat culture obtained after an airway has been established
Cool, highly humidified environment
Cardiac monitor; transcutaneous O_2 monitor
Vital signs qh with acute symptoms to include pulse rate and respiratory assessment; temperature q4h and prn
NPO

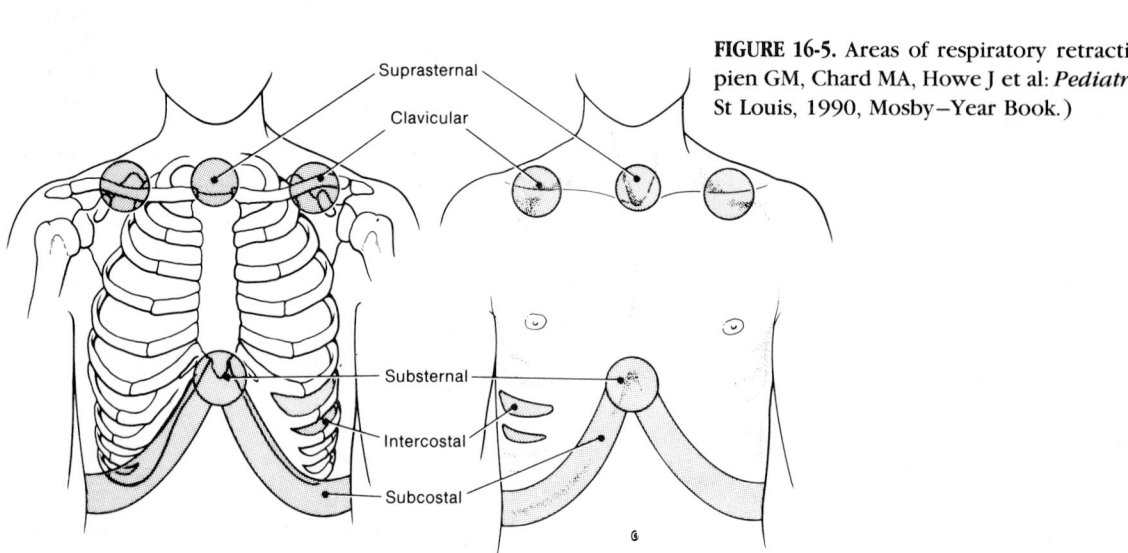

FIGURE 16-5. Areas of respiratory retractions. (From Scipien GM, Chard MA, Howe J et al: *Pediatric nursing care,* St Louis, 1990, Mosby–Year Book.)

Suprasternal
Clavicular
Substernal
Intercostal
Subcostal

Maintenance parenteral fluids
Antibiotic therapy
Corticosteroid therapy
Antipyretics prn for fever

Nursing diagnoses/interventions/evaluation

■ **NDX:** Ineffective airway clearance related to edema, copious secretions, and altered anatomic structure of airway (endotracheal tube)

Recognize signs and symptoms of epiglottitis (see observations above) and assist with establishing an artificial airway immediately (have three endotracheal tubes ready: size that approximates size of patient's pinky finger, one larger, and one smaller)
Maintain intubation (p. 230)
Maintain a patent airway with postural drainage and tracheal suctioning as ordered
Maintain cool, moist, oxygenated environment
Initiate oxygen as ordered or prn for respiratory distress
Monitor vital signs with respiratory assessment qh and prn for signs of respiratory difficulty (tachycardia, tachypnea, retractions, restlessness, cyanosis)
Postpone routine care while respiratory distress is severe
Allow child to assume position of comfort: usually high-Fowler's position
Administer antiinflammatory drugs if ordered
Administer antibiotic therapy as ordered
Implement measures to reduce anxiety
  Have parents participate in the care of their child
  Keep child and parents informed and explain all procedures

Expected outcome/evaluation

Patient has a patent airway and clear breath sounds with an age-appropriate respiratory rate before discharge
Skin color is normal

■ **NDX:** Potential fluid volume deficit related to insensible loss in the presence of fever, hyperventilation, inability to tolerate fluids po, and/or NPO status

Maintain NPO while intubated
Administer maintenance parenteral fluids as ordered
Record intake and output and specific gravity
Administer antipyretic therapy as ordered
Anticipate beginning oral fluids after extubation
Resume age-appropriate diet as tolerated

Expected outcome/evaluation

Patient remains hydrated and tolerates age-appropriate fluid volume po before discharge

■ **NDX:** Knowledge deficit related to lack of information about home care needs

Discuss diet
Explain need to encourage fluids
Teach fever management
Explain that epiglottitis rarely recurs
Teach name of medication, dosage, purpose, time of administration, and side effects

Expected outcome/evaluation

Parents/significant other verbalize understanding of disease process and child's home care needs

PERTUSSIS: WHOOPING COUGH

An acute infection of the respiratory tract caused by Bordetella pertussis *and characterized by a series of repeated spasmodic coughs ending in forced, prolonged inspiration (the "whoop") and vomiting*
Usual age: nonimmunized children under 4 years
Seasonal occurrence: spring and summer
Isolation: highly contagious and transmitted by direct contact, droplet spread, or indirectly from freshly contaminated articles

Assessment
Observations/findings

See Respiratory Assessment (p. 186)
1- to 2-week history of upper respiratory infection (URI) symptoms (catarrhal stage)
Worsening of cough to spasmodic episodes followed by vomiting (paroxysmal stage)
  Paroxysms of coughing
  Frequency usually increasing to several times an hour
  Coughing followed by vomiting of thick mucus
  Degree of respiratory distress during a spasm, particularly color change during spasm (bright red face or cyanotic)
Nutritional assessment
  Calorie intake
  Nutritional state
  Weight loss
  Dehydration (p. 841)

Laboratory/diagnostic studies

WBC: elevated
Nasopharyngeal cough plate swab or sputum sample to isolate *Bordetella*

Potential complications

Pneumonia, atelectasis, emphysema, otitis media
Respiratory arrest
Neurological complications: seizures from anoxia; intracranial hemorrhages

Nutritional deficit: weight loss, dehydration from excessive vomiting

Hernia

Prolapsed rectum

Hemorrhage (subarachnoid, subconjunctival, epistaxis)

Medical Management

Oxygen for dyspnea and cyanosis after paroxysms

Cool, humidified environment via mist tent

Parenteral fluids when vomiting is severe enough to cause nutritional deficit

Antibiotics

Bed rest while fever is present

Pertussis immune globulin (sometimes recommended in children less than 2 years of age)

Emergency intubation in the event of severely decreased oxygenation

Respiratory precautions

Nursing diagnoses/interventions/evaluation

■ **NDX:** Ineffective airway clearance related to thick pulmonary secretions

Place child in a room amenable to close observation

Be in attendance during all paroxysms to provide a calm, reassuring environment

Monitor vital signs q2h and prn

Assess respiratory status during and immediately after a coughing episode: color, respiratory rate, nasal flaring, retractions, breath sounds

Assess child's ability to clear secretions on own

Use gentle suction prn to keep airway clear (bulb suctioning is preferred, since deep nasopharyngeal suctioning can aggravate spasms)

Administer humidified oxygen prn for cyanosis

Maintain cool, humidified environment via mist tent

Elevate head of bed

Reduce child's exposure to smoke, dust, temperature changes, and excessive excitement, since they may precipitate a coughing episode

Keep child occupied with age-appropriate, quiet activities (preoccupation is associated with fewer paroxysms)

Expected outcome/evaluation

Airway remains patent and clear of mucus

Patient is supported during paroxysms to prevent complications related to anoxia

■ **NDX:** Potential fluid volume deficit related to excessive vomiting

Offer small volumes of clear liquids frequently

Offer fluids child likes via appropriate method (cup vs. bottle)

Weigh child daily

Administer parenteral fluids if ordered

Expected outcome/evaluation

Patient

Is able to tolerate age-appropriate fluid volume (p. 841)

Maintains weight

■ **NDX:** Altered nutrition: less than body requirements related to excessive vomiting

Calculate caloric requirements for age and weight

Ensure feedings of 20 kcal/oz formula or milk, despite episodes of vomiting

Offer small, frequent feedings after a coughing/vomiting episode

Offer items high in calories (items child likes)

If feeding is vomited, prevent aspiration by suctioning prn

Allow child to rest briefly, then refeed

Expected outcome/evaluation

Patient

Tolerates an age-appropriate diet reflecting appropriate caloric requirements

Maintains weight

■ **NDX:** Knowledge deficit related to lack of information about home care needs and disease process

Teach parents about stages of disease process (catarrhal stage, paroxysms stage, convalescent stage)

Explain that coughing paroxysms will continue in less severe form for several weeks after discharge

Teach parents and have them demonstrate techniques to support infant during paroxysms

Have parents demonstrate use of bulb syringe in clearing nasal and oral passages of secretions

Explain importance of refeeding if vomiting occurs

Explain need to maintain good nutritional diet

Explain need to weigh child frequently to ensure adequate hydration and nutrition

Teach name of medication, dosage, time of administration, purpose, and side effects

Emphasize need for follow-up care

Emphasize that child should avoid contact with other susceptible children

Explain to parents that the most effective treatment is prevention with the pertussis vaccine (ensure that other children are immunized)

Reassure parents that disease will not recur, because a single attack gives lifetime immunity

Expected outcome/evaluation

Parents and/or significant other state and demonstrate how to support their child during paroxysms and state that they feel comfortable caring for their child at home

PNEUMONIA

An inflammatory process of the lungs classified by the area involved and/or causative agent

Types of areas involved	Causative agents
Lobar	Bacterial
Bronchopneumonia	Viral
Interstitial	Mycoplasma
Bronchiolitis	Aspiration
Bilateral	Chemical
Right upper lobe (RUL)	Hypostatic
Right middle lobe (RML)	
Right lower lobe (RLL)	
Left upper lobe (LUL)	
Left lower lobe (LLL)	

NOTE: Nursing care is based on degree of respiratory distress and age of patient rather than on type of pneumonia

Usual age: any

Placement: respiratory isolation with suspected staphylococcal pneumonia until treated for 48 hr with antibiotics

Assessment

Observations/findings

See Respiratory Assessment (p. 186)

Signs and symptoms of respiratory distress

  Cyanosis, circumoral cyanosis
  Nasal flaring
  Retractions
  Tachypnea
  Tachycardia
  Restlessness
  Malaise
  Quality and frequency of cough
  Sputum production
  Color and character of sputum
  Chest or back pain in older children
  Apprehension, seizures, flushed cheeks, circumoral cyanosis, fretfulness, and diminished appetite in infants
  Auscultated rales, rhonchi, decreased breath sounds

Fever, chills

Anorexia

Vomiting

Abdominal pain

Abdominal distention

Nutritional assessment

Myalgia

Laboratory/diagnostic studies

WBC: very elevated with bacterial pneumonia; slightly elevated with viral pneumonia

Nasopharynx, throat, and blood culture to isolate organism

Blood gases

Sputum culture

Chest x-ray examination to localize area of infiltration, rule out pleural effusion and empyema, and locate pneumatoceles if staphylococcal pneumonia

Blood and urine for countercurrent immunoelectrophoresis (CIE) to detect specific bacterial antigens

Potential complications

Pleural effusion (with pneumococcus or Group A streptococcus)

Empyema (with *Haemophilus influenzae* or staphylococcus)

Otitis media

Meningitis

Pericarditis

Septicemia

Respiratory arrest

Medical Management

Oxygenated, cool, humidified environment

Transcutaneous O_2 monitor

Chest physiotherapy and suctioning q2h to 4h

Parenteral fluids

Antipyretic therapy prn for fever control

Antibiotic therapy

Nursing diagnoses/interventions/evaluation

■ **NDX:** Ineffective airway clearance related to thick mucous production in lungs and ineffective cough

Vital signs q2h to 4h

Initiate humidified oxygen as ordered or prn for respiratory distress via age-appropriate method (mist tent, nasal prongs, mask, or hood)

Encourage effective, sputum-raising cough

Perform postural drainage as indicated

Perform chest percussion as ordered

Auscultate lungs q2h to determine need for suctioning and/or positioning

Allow patient to assume posture of most comfort: 30-degree elevation of head or placement in infant seat is most comfortable

Change infant's position frequently, at least q2h

Administer antibiotic therapy as ordered

Expected outcome/evaluation

Patient
  Has a patent airway
  Has clear breath sounds
  Has age-appropriate respiratory rate before discharge

■ **NDX:** Activity intolerance related to fatigue from increased respiratory effort

Plan frequent rest periods for conservation of energy

Promote a nonstressful environment by
Minimizing nursing care activities during severe respiratory distress
Placing child in environment with minimal stimulation (quiet, dim lights)
Encouraging parents to participate in care of their child
Gradually increasing activity as tolerated, encouraging quiet bedside activities

Expected outcome/evaluation

Patient
Engages in age-appropriate activities in a nonstressful environment
Tolerates progressive increase in activities

 NDX: Potential fluid volume deficit related to fever, insensible water loss from tachypnea, and poor fluid intake from dyspnea

Record intake, output, and specific gravity
Assess hydration status
Encourage fluids as tolerated; give at room temperature; give cautiously to avoid aspiration
Avoid cold liquids; monitor for potential aspiration
Administer parenteral fluids as ordered
Conduct cooling measures prn
Maintain cool environment
Administer antipyretic therapy as ordered
As condition improves, gradually advance to diet appropriate for age

Expected outcome/evaluation

Patient
Is afebrile
Has age-appropriate respiratory rate
Tolerates age-appropriate fluid volume intake and diet (see standard for age under Basic Standards of Care, pp. 763-770)

 NDX: Knowledge deficit related to lack of information about disease process and home care interventions

Explain need for rest
Explain need for nourishing diet appropriate for age and extra fluids
Discuss signs and symptoms of respiratory distress
Emphasize need to avoid exposure to other persons with URIs
Demonstrate and have parents demonstrate procedure for postural drainage and percussion
Teach name of antibiotic and antipyretic, dosage, time of administration, purpose, and side effects

Expected outcome/evaluation

Patient and/or parents demonstrate understanding of follow-up instructions and verbalize plan of care for rest, fluids, diet, and follow-up care

ASTHMA

An acute inflammation and spasm of smooth muscle in the bronchi and bronchioles; with increased mucus production and plugging; most frequent cause is allergic hypersensitivity to foreign substances, but it may be triggered by infection or physical (e.g., cold air, exercise) or psychological stress; characterized by bilateral wheezing and trapped secretions

Usual age: any

Assessment
Observations/findings

See Respiratory Assessment (p. 186)
Family history of asthma
Known allergies of child
Compliance to management regimen
Posture is upright with shoulders hunched over/elevated
Nasal flaring
Cyanosis of nail beds and circumoral area
Air hunger
Retractions
Prolonged expiratory phase with pursed lips
"Tight" cough
Dyspnea
Orthopnea
Audible expiratory wheeze
Auscultated inspiratory/expiratory wheeze; note pitch (higher pitch indicates progressive obstruction)
Rales (sonorous throughout lung fields)
Rhonchi
Decreased breath sounds with increased airway resistance to airflow ("tight" chest)
Hyperresonance on percussion
Diaphoresis
Fatigue
Increasing tachycardia
Restlessness
Apprehension, anxious facial expression
Disorientation
Lips deep, dark red color
Abdominal pain
Vomiting
Anorexia
Psychobehavioral assessment
With repetitive episodes
Barrel chest
Use of accessory muscles of respiration
Facial appearance: flattened malar bones, circles beneath eyes, narrow nose, prominent upper teeth

Laboratory/diagnostic studies

Sputum examination: eosinophilia with allergic reactivity
Complete blood cell count (CBC) with differential: leukocytosis, eosinophilia, above-average hemoglobin (Hgb) and hematocrit (Hct) with chronic hypoxemia

Blood gas evaluation
  Rising P_{CO_2}: if 50 to 60, may need ventilatory assistance
  Rapidly falling pH and respiratory acidosis
Reduced O_2 saturation
Chest x-ray examination
  Overexpansion of lungs
  Rule out pneumothorax, atelectasis, pneumonia, pneumomediastinum
Pulmonary function tests
Sensitivity testing
Elimination diet as indicated

Potential complications

Atelectasis
Emphysema with chronic hyperinflation
Pneumothorax
Cor pulmonale with right-sided failure
Cardiac dysrhythmias
Emotional/behavioral problems
Respiratory failure requiring mechanical assistance
Associated URI
Side effects from corticosteroid use

Medical Management

Cool, humidified, oxygenated environment
Bronchodilators (sympathomimetics and methylxanthines) via IV line and nebulization
Monitoring for therapeutic levels of theophylline
Postural drainage, percussion, and suctioning as tolerated to clear airway (Begin *only after* airway opens and secretions become mobile)
Corticosteroids IV
IV hydration
Clear liquids or NPO depending on severity of respiratory distress
Treatment of coexisting bacterial infection with antibiotics

Nursing diagnoses/interventions/evaluation

■ **NDX:** Ineffective airway clearance, ineffective breathing pattern, and impaired gas exchange related to bronchospasm and increased pulmonary secretions

Monitor vital signs, including respiratory assessment q2h and prn
Initiate oxygen as ordered and prn for respiratory distress and/or cyanosis; transcutaneous O_2 monitoring
NOTE: Avoid use of high levels of oxygen, since it may significantly *depress* respirations
Administer bronchodilators via nebulizer as ordered and assess respiratory status before and after administration
Administer infusion of bronchodilators intravenously as ordered
Administer corticosteroids as ordered

Ensure that patient receives maximum fluids for age and weight via parenteral and/or oral route
Allow patient to assume position of most comfort
Check theophylline levels and administer bolus dosages of bronchodilators intravenously as ordered to maintain therapeutic drug levels
Monitor blood gases
Monitor for signs and symptoms of respiratory failure and prepare for emergency intubation if any of the following occur: rapid, shallow respirations; decreased breath sounds; severe retractions; cyanosis; poor capillary refill; tachycardia; decreased level of consciousness

Expected outcome/evaluation

Patient
  Has an age-appropriate respiratory rate
  States that he can breathe better
  Is able to mobilize secretions
  Has a minimal wheeze
  Is tolerant of mild activity

■ **NDX:** Anxiety related to breathlessness, air hunger, and fear

Minimize nursing routines until child's respiratory status improves
Allow child to assume position of greatest comfort
Encourage use of relaxation techniques (e.g., diversional activity, guided imagery)
Provide emotional support to child and parents by explaining all procedures to them
Allow parents to participate in care of their child *if* they can remain calm and supportive
Recognize that disorientation and panic intensify as patient becomes hypoxemic

Expected outcome/evaluation

Patient's anxiety is minimized

■ **NDX:** Potential fluid deficit related to side effects of medications and respiratory distress

Assess for anorexia, nausea, vomiting, and abdominal pain
Monitor blood levels of theophylline to avoid toxicity
Keep NPO and administer fluid requirements parenterally during severe respiratory distress
Administer small, frequent feedings of lukewarm clear fluids when tolerated
Advance to regular diet for age as tolerated
Monitor intake and output

Expected outcome/evaluation

Patient remains well hydrated

■ **NDX:** Potential activity intolerance related to precipitation of or worsening of respiratory symptoms with increased activity

Encourage bed rest with severe respiratory symptoms
Gradually increase activity while encouraging quiet bedside activities: books, games, play dough, etc.
Refer child to physical therapy or asthma camp (through local American Lung Association) for physical training
Encourage moderate exercise with at least a 15 min "warmup" session (swimming is excellent exercise and readily tolerated)
Teach proper use of physical and mental relaxation techniques to ward off an impending attack
For child with exercise-induced asthma, instruct child in proper use of inhalers before exercise

Expected outcome/evaluation

Patient is able to tolerate progressive increases in activities

■ **NDX:** Knowledge deficit related to lack of information about disease process and treatment

Teach child and/or parents to avoid known allergens
Teach parents and child early warning signs of an impending attack and encourage intervention with rest, increased fluids, and medication
Teach diaphragmatic breathing exercises
Teach parents and child how to control symptoms by proper administration of medications
Observe child's inhaler technique to ensure proper dosing of medications
Caution against overuse of bronchodilators via inhalers
Discuss possible triggers with child and/or parents and encourage them to keep records of child's activity before, during, and after attacks
Warn against exposure to known environmental irritants: smoking, URIs, cold weather, and excessive humidity
Allow parents and/or child to administer inhalation therapy at least once during hospitalization
Give parents verbal and written instructions about medications including name, action, dosage, time of administration, and side effects
Schedule medication administration just before bedtime with sufficient fluid intake; this may decrease severity of nighttime symptoms and promote needed rest
Provide guidance for parents in promoting normal growth and development; allergens should be avoided but not to the extent that child's development is inhibited or excessive family conflict is created
Tell parents that even with careful management occasional attacks may occur
Discuss desensitization when appropriate

Expected outcome/evaluation

Patient and/or parents verbalize understanding of disease and treatment and patient return-demonstrates breathing exercises and use of inhaler

BRONCHIOLITIS

A lower respiratory tract infection with obstruction at the bronchiolar level; usually of viral origin; consists of hypersecretion, edema, and inflammatory reaction of small bronchioles

Usual age: infant (rare after 2 years of age)
Seasonal occurrence: winter and early spring

Assessment
Observations/findings

Spasmodic hacking cough
Nasal flaring
Cyanosis
Dyspnea
Tachypnea
Prolonged expiratory phase
Retractions (intercostal and subcostal)
Expiratory wheeze
Rales
Rhonchi
Hyperresonance
Decreased breath sounds
Shallow respiratory excursion
Increasing tachycardia
Low-grade fever
Fatigue
Irritability
Poor feeding related to increased respiratory distress with sucking

Laboratory/diagnostic studies

Chest x-ray examination: may show segmental collapse or hyperinflation
Blood gas evaluation to monitor for respiratory acidosis
Viral studies of nasal aspirates

Potential complications

Respiratory acidosis
Respiratory arrest
Congestive heart failure (p. 835)
Atelectasis
Prolonged illness with persistent abnormal respiratory function
Asthma in childhood

Medical Management

Monitoring of blood gases and O₂ saturation
Postural drainage, percussion, and suctioning prn as tolerated to clear airway when respiratory status improves

Ribavirin via oxygen hood if RSV (respiratory syncytial virus) is suspected and criteria for use is met
(Nursing staff should exercise caution to diminish contact with aerosolized ribavirin)
Antipyretics prn
Antibiotic therapy if bacterial infection is suspected
With severe respiratory distress
NPO
Maintenance parenteral fluids or small, frequent feedings
Intubation with assisted ventilation if necessary

Nursing diagnoses/interventions/evaluation

■ **NDX:** Impaired gas exchange related to increased pulmonary secretions and inadequate ventilation

Monitor pulse, respiratory rate, and breath sounds q1h to 2h and prn
Maintain a humidified environment
Have oxygen via mask or cannula available at bedside for cyanosis
Minimize nursing care activities to conserve infant's energy
Elevate head of bed
Administer postural drainage, percussion, and suctioning prn as tolerated
Bulb suction nares prn to clear airway (infants are nose breathers)
Administer antibiotic therapy if ordered
Administer ribavirin as ordered per hospital protocol
Monitor for signs and symptoms of cardiac failure (p. 101)

Expected outcome/evaluation

Patient
Has a patent airway
Has age-appropriate respiratory rate, normal blood gases, O₂ saturation, and color indicating adequate perfusion

■ **NDX:** Potential fluid volume deficit related to decreased oral intake, increased insensible loss, and fever

Maintain NPO during severe distress
Provide maintenance fluids parenterally as ordered
NOTE: Intravenous fluids are administered cautiously; unresolved bronchiolitis can lead to cardiac failure
Monitor intake and output
Weigh infant daily
Monitor electrolytes and replace intravenously as ordered
Administer antipyretic therapy prn as ordered

Expected outcome/evaluation

Patient is well hydrated

■ **NDX:** Potential for altered nutrition: less than body requirements related to fatigue and increased respiratory distress with sucking

Begin small oral feedings of clear liquids, then dilute formula as tolerated when infant is able to suck without severe respiratory distress
Gradually increase concentration and volume of feedings to age-appropriate amount as tolerated
Clear nasal passage before feedings

Expected outcome/evaluation

Patient tolerates age/weight-appropriate fluid intake by mouth before discharge

■ **NDX:** Potential for parental anxiety related to decreased parent-infant contact with mist tent therapy, bed rest, and prolonged hospitalization

Provide emotional support and reassurance to parents
Encourage touching, holding, and cuddling by parents as tolerated by infant
Help parents feel calm so they can provide needed comfort to their child
Involve parents actively in care of their infant as soon as feasible

Expected outcome/evaluation

Parents care for infant as much as possible

■ **NDX:** Knowledge deficit related to lack of information about disease process and home care management

Teach parents to use a cool mist vaporizer at night and during daytime naps
Tell parents to avoid exposure to URIs
Explain action of medication, dosage, time of administration, and side effects
Teach parents how to manage feedings during respiratory stress
Have parents demonstrate use of nasal bulb suction

Expected outcome/evaluation

Parents and/or significant other verbalize understanding of home care instructions

CYSTIC FIBROSIS

An autosomal recessive disease involving a generalized dysfunction of exocrine glands and characterized by an increased production of thick mucus that causes a varying degree of obstruction in several organs; most commonly affected are the lungs, sweat glands, tear glands, paranasal sinuses, salivary glands, pancreas, liver, intestines, and reproductive tract (Figure 16-6)

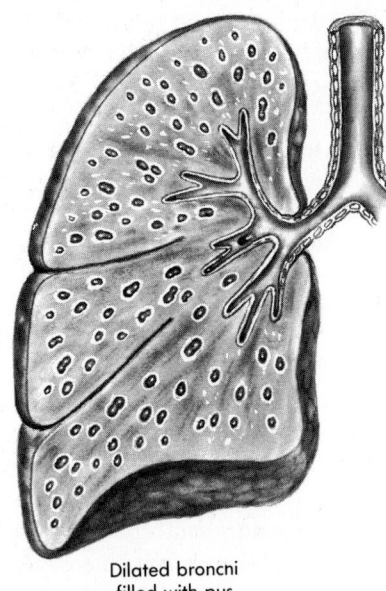

Dilated broncni
filled with pus

FIGURE 16-6. Cystic fibrosis. (From Wilson SF, Thompson JM: *Respiratory disorders, Mosby's clinical nursing series,* St Louis, 1990, Mosby—Year Book.)

Usual age: any; onset of symptoms most common in infants and toddlers

Assessment

Observations/findings

NEWBORN PERIOD

Meconium ileus: vomiting, absence of stools, abdominal distention, dehydration
"Salty" taste to skin
Poor weight gain
Failure to thrive
Listless

EXPECTED FINDINGS

Gastrointestinal (GI) system
    Poor weight gain with voracious appetite
    Tissue wasting, failure to grow
    Thin extremities with abdominal distention
    Stool
        Increased frequency
        Large, bulky, frothy
        Greasy; float in toilet
        Foul smelling
    Anorexia with infections and respiratory distress
Pulmonary system
    See Respiratory Assessment (p. 186); expect increase in respiratory distress symptoms with pulmonary infections and advanced lung damage
    History of chronic pulmonary disease
    Chronic sinusitis
    Nasal polyps

Initially dry, nonproductive chronic cough; loose productive cough with infection and advancing lung damage
Thick, tenacious mucus
Nasal flaring
Tachypnea
Prolonged expiratory phase through pursed lips
Shortness of breath with increased activity
Barrel chest
Clubbing of fingers and toes
Cyanosis
Rales
Wheeze
Decreased breath sounds
Biliary or hepatic duct obstruction
    Jaundice
    Splenomegaly
    Hepatomegaly
    Ascites
    Portal hypertension (p. 299)
    Esophageal varices with GI bleeding
Additional observations
    Sallow skin
    See Cardiovascular Assessment (p. 63): at risk for CHF (p. 835)
    Dehydration (p. 841)
    Hyponatremia (p. 38)

Laboratory/diagnostic studies

Increased sweat chloride test by pilocarpine iontophoresis (greater than 60 mEq/L is diagnostic)
Decreased or absent trypsin, lipase, and amylase from duodenal contents
Fresh stool samples studied for trypsin and fat (trypsin is minimal or absent: fat is elevated—steatorrhea)
Increased albumin content in stools: azotorrhea (greater than 20 mg%)
Chest x-ray examination
    Confirms chronic lung disease with obstructive emphysema (atelectasis, bronchopneumonia)
    Assists in identifying pulmonary complications
Pulmonary function tests
    Decreased vital capacity and tidal volume
    Increased airway resistance
    Decreased forced expiratory volume
Blood gases: reveal varying degree of respiratory acidosis

Potential complications

Lobar atelectasis
Lung abscesses
Spontaneous pneumothorax
Chronic cor pulmonale
Hemoptysis
Intestinal obstruction
Prolapsed rectum

Anemia

Diabetes mellitus

Medical Management

Inhalation therapy to liquefy mucus and prevent and treat infections

Postural drainage, percussion, and vibration two to four times a day; increased frequency with infections

Suctioning may be ordered in infants and toddlers who cannot expectorate mucus on their own

Oxygen therapy

Medications

    Bronchodilators, mucolytics, and/or expectorants via ultrasonic nebulization

    Antibiotics to treat pulmonary infections (IV, oral, or by nebulization to treat microorganism directly)

    Pancreatic enzyme replacement with meals and snacks

    Water-miscible vitamins

    Daily iron supplement

    Salt tablet supplements during hot weather

    Total parenteral nutrition (TPN) as ordered

Nursing diagnoses/interventions/evaluation

■ **NDX:**   Ineffective airway clearance related to mucopurulent secretions

Administer inhalation therapy with nebulization as ordered before postural drainage

Perform postural drainage, percussion, and vibration q2h to 4h as ordered

Schedule respiratory treatments before meals and at bedtime

Have patient cough up and spit out mucus if able

Suction prn

Note color, amount, and consistency of sputum

Administer oxygen as ordered and prn

    CAUTION: High levels of oxygen should be avoided because they may depress respirations!

Assess vital signs with respiratory assessment q2h and prn

Encourage oral fluids or increase intravenous flow rate to ensure adequate hydration for liquefication of secretions

Administer intravenous antibiotics as ordered

Administer antibiotics via nebulization if ordered *after* postural drainage routine

Protect child from contact with others who may transmit additional respiratory infections

Expected outcome/evaluation

Patient maintains a patent airway

Secretions are mobilized and removed

■ **NDX:**   Potential for altered nutrition: less than body requirements related to increased caloric and protein needs secondary to impaired intestinal absorption, and loss of fat and fat-soluble vitamins in stool

Administer pancreatic enzymes with each meal and with snacks

A low-fat, high-protein, high-calorie diet may be encouraged; however, do not enforce severe restrictions because this may impede psychological adjustment

Monitor food intake and stool frequency, character, and consistency

Alter pancreatic enzyme therapy as needed to promote normal bowel movements

Allow older child to regulate his own diet and determine need for enzyme adjustment or dietary restrictions

Record intake and output

Weigh patient daily

Administer lipid-soluble vitamins in water-miscible liquid as ordered

Encourage generous use of added salt in diet

Administer salt tablet supplements as necessary during hot weather

Expected outcome/evaluation

Patient

    Remains hydrated

    Maintains weight

    Takes a well-balanced diet

■ **NDX:**   Altered bowel elimination: diarrhea or constipation related to insufficient or excessive replacement of pancreatic enzymes

Keep accurate stool record, noting color, consistency, amount, and frequency of stools

Keep accurate record of dietary intake to identify certain foods that may contribute to altered stool patterns

Avoid known dietary irritants

Adjust pancreatic enzyme replacement as necessary in accordance with food intake and stool pattern

Encourage parents and/or child to alter diet and enzyme therapy as needed to promote growth and normal bowel movements

Expected outcome/evaluation

Patient has normal bowel elimination patterns

■ **NDX:**   Activity intolerance related to dyspnea

Encourage any aerobic activity

    Teach patient breathing exercises to help aerate lungs to maximum capacity

    In young child encourage bubble blowing or blowing out candles

    In older child teach abdominal breathing exercises

    Encourage daily exercises to promote and maintain posture

Encourage participation in swimming or hydrotherapy, since this helps strengthen muscles of respiration and promotes good breathing habits

Avoid environmental irritants such as smoke and pollutants

Perform respiratory treatments before participation in physical activity

Expected outcome/evaluation

Patient

Is able to tolerate physical activity

Participates in age-appropriate play

 NDX: Potential for ineffective individual and/or family coping related to chronicity of illness, financial burden, and/or disruption of family functioning

Encourage parents and child to communicate their feelings and concerns to you and each other

Have parents and child talk with another family who has a child with cystic fibrosis

Assess family's coping abilities and problem-solving abilities

Discuss with family the need for everyone to participate in the care of the child with cystic fibrosis

Encourage parents to foster family life by spending time with each individual member and carrying on "normal" activities

Encourage parents to promote normal growth and development in their child with cystic fibrosis

Discuss financial burden with parents

Make appropriate referral for counseling and financial assistance if necessary

Expected outcome/evaluation

Individual and family adjust to ramifications of the disease; their need for additional support is identified, and appropriate referrals are made

 NDX: Knowledge deficit related to lack of information about chronic nature of disease and home care needs

Teach child and/or parents use of nebulizer and other respiratory equipment that will be used at home: oxygen, suction, humidifier

Teach child and/or parents postural drainage, percussion, and vibration

Have child and/or parents demonstrate postural drainage routine before discharge

Set up home schedule to meet lifestyle of individual family

Have child demonstrate any newly learned breathing exercises before discharge

Involve child in ongoing exercise program, because activity increases respiratory effort and movement of mucus in airways

Tell child and/or parents to avoid persons with URIs and

known respiratory irritants such as smoke, air pollutants, and humidity

Teach need to monitor weight and stools

Encourage a high-calorie, moderate-fat diet

Teach parents to mix supplemental pancreatic enzymes with carbohydrate foods such as applesauce; protein foods will cause enzymes to break down immediately

Teach name of medications, dosage, time of administration, purpose, and side effects

Teach child and parents home IV therapy as appropriate

Yearly influenza immunizations are strongly recommended

Discuss need for salt replacement requirements during hot weather

Alert parents to symptoms that should be reported to physician

Fever

Weight loss

Poor appetite

Respiratory distress

Fatigue

Failure to raise sputum after respiratory therapy techniques

Excessive number of large, bulky, foul-smelling stools

Make appropriate referrals to community resources (Cystic Fibrosis Foundation)

Make appropriate referral for genetic counseling

Expected outcome/evaluation

Patient/parents verbalize understanding of home care and follow up instructions; child participates in ongoing exercise program; child and/or parents demonstrate and state their ability to accept and adjust to life with cystic fibrosis; parents, child, and family have ongoing community support; parents and child understand disease and its ramifications; and parents are able to care for child at home

Gastrointestinal System

CLEFT LIP REPAIR

Surgical repair of congenital interruption in the development of the upper lip; may be unilateral or bilateral

Usual age: infant

Assessment
Observations/findings
AT BIRTH

Separation of lip may range from notch in vermilion border of lip to complete extension to floor of nose

May or may not be associated with cleft palate

May or may not be associated with other congenital anomalies

PREOPERATIVE

Infant's ability to take fluids using modified feeding techniques as preferred by surgeon (Lamb's nipple, flanged nipple, Breck feeder)

Infant's tolerance of side-lying and supine position

Parents' perception of their infant

POSTOPERATIVE

Excessive bleeding, signs of infection, or separation at incision site

Security of Logan bow

Respiratory stridor, distress, or obstruction

Skin irritation under elbow restraints

Tolerance of modified feeding techniques

Fluid and caloric intake

Degree of discomfort

Parents' response to surgical repair

Laboratory/diagnostic studies

Ongoing evaluation includes
  Hearing tests
  Speech evaluation
Orthodontal and prosthodontal evaluation of teeth malposition and structural changes of maxillary arches

Potential complications

Respiratory distress postoperatively

Infection of incision

Repeated otitis media with hearing loss

Malocclusion of teeth

Speech impairment

Medical Management

Surgical correction of defect

Modified feeding technique

Type of feeding preferred (generally no milk products)

Elbow restraints

Cleaning and care of suture line

Antibiotic therapy is preferred by some surgeons

Mild sedation is preferred by some surgeons

Nursing diagnoses/interventions/evaluation

■ **NDX:** Potential for infection of suture line related to undue stress on incision, direct trauma to site, or interference with scar formation

Prevent crying by anticipating needs of infant; hold, cuddle, and use tactile, visual, and auditory stimulation to comfort infant

Use elbow restraints at all times to prevent direct trauma to area from infant's hands

Keep Logan bow in place

Position infant supine or in modified side-lying position so infant will not cause trauma to site if he turns his head

Cleanse suture line after every meal and prn

Keep suture line moist with prescribed ointment

Offer small amount of water after feedings to cleanse lip and mouth

Administer antibiotics if ordered

Administer sedative if ordered

Expected outcome/evaluation

Patient's suture line remains intact and free of infection

■ **NDX:** Potential alteration in nutrition: less than body requirements related to altered feeding techniques and inability to suck effectively

Administer parenteral fluids until oral intake is adequate

Introduce altered feeding technique preoperatively so infant can adjust to it

Do not allow nipple or pacifiers in mouth

Administer clear liquids and advance diet as tolerated and ordered

Avoid use of milk products

Feed in upright position

Burp infant after each ounce

Position in infant seat or side-lying position after feedings

Measure intake and output

Weigh infant daily

Expected outcome/evaluation

Patient
  Receives age-appropriate caloric intake (p. 841)
  Gains weight
  Remains hydrated

■ **NDX:** Impaired physical mobility related to use of elbow restraints

Remove elbow restraints, one at a time, at least q8h

Check skin under restraints for signs of irritation

Perform ROM exercises to arms

Promote age-appropriate development through auditory, visual, and tactile stimulation

Expected outcome/evaluation

Patient's
  Elbow range of motion (ROM) is maintained
  Normal growth and development are promoted

■ **NDX:** Parental role conflict related to feelings about and response to infant's physical disfigurement

Repair of lip should be performed as soon after birth as possible

Discuss with parents their perception of their infant, feelings around the time of birth, and feelings about feeding modifications

Point out positive things about their infant

Involve parents in care and feeding of their infant immediately

Have parents meet with other family whose child had cleft lip, if necessary

Expected outcome/evaluation

Parent/infant relationship is promoted and attachment occurs

■ **NDX:** Knowledge deficit related to lack of information about home care needs and follow-up care

Teach parents how to use alternative feeding technique

Have parents feed child several times before discharge

Teach lip care

Teach application of elbow restraints and need for ROM exercises

Tell parents dietary restrictions if any (usually milk products)

Discuss symptoms of incision infection to report to physician

Redness

Swelling

Drainage

Bleeding

Separation of incision

Teach name of medication, purpose, dosage, time of administration, and side effects

Ensure that parents understand need for ongoing evaluation of child's hearing, speech, and dental development

Expected outcome/evaluation

Parent(s)/significant other verbalize understanding of home care instructions and are able to care for child at home; state need for ongoing evaluation of speech, hearing, and teeth formation

CLEFT PALATE REPAIR

Surgical repair of congenital interruption of development of the oral palate; may involve the hard or soft palate, or both

Usual age: toddler

Assessment
Observations/findings
AT BIRTH

Separation of hard or soft palate, or both

Regurgitation of oral feedings through nose

Associated cleft lip, if present

Associated congenital anomalies, if present

PREOPERATIVE

Toddler's experience with Breck feeder and/or ability to drink from cup

Toddler's tolerance of prone position

Toddler's developmental status

POSTOPERATIVE

Degree of respiratory distress as a result of increased mucous secretions and swelling of incision site

Excessive bleeding

Intact sutures

Degree of discomfort

Tolerance of feeding techniques

Fluid and caloric intake

Laboratory/diagnostic studies

See Cleft Lip Repair (p. 786)

Potential complications

Airway obstruction

See Cleft Lip Repair (p. 786)

Medical Management

Surgical correction of defect

Mist tent

Diet and restrictions if any (usually milk products are avoided)

Elbow restraints

Parenteral fluids immediately postoperatively until oral intake is adequate

Antibiotics as needed

Mild sedation prn

Analgesic (usually acetaminophen) for discomfort

Nursing diagnoses/interventions*/evaluation

■ **NDX:** Potential for ineffective airway clearance related to increased oral secretions and swelling of incisional area

Administer mist tent therapy as ordered

Position child in prone, head-down position to promote drainage of oral secretions

Do not suction

Monitor respiratory status qh for first 24 to 48 hr postoperatively

Expected outcome/evaluation

Patient's airway remains patent

■ **NDX:** Potential for altered nutrition: less than body requirements related to discomfort and altered feeding techniques

---

*See Cleft Lip Repair (p. 786).

Introduce modified feeding technique before surgery to familiarize child and parent

Administer parenteral fluids as ordered until child is able to tolerate adequate oral intake

Administer liquids and purees via Breck feeder or cup

Feed in high chair

Allow parent to feed child as soon as possible

Monitor intake and output

Weigh child daily

Administer analgesics before feeding

Expected outcome/evaluation

Patient tolerates age-appropriate caloric intake and maintains weight

■ **NDX:** Potential for infection of suture site related to trauma to area and interference with healing process

Monitor temperature q4h and prn

Use elbow restraints at all times

Avoid use of straws or feeding utensils; use cup or Breck feeder *only*

Give child small amount of water after each feeding to cleanse suture line and prevent accumulation of food on incisional area

Assess child for excessive bleeding, drainage, and foul mouth odor

Administer antibiotics if ordered

Administer sedative if ordered

Expected outcome/evaluation

Patient's suture line remains clean and intact

Patient is afebrile

■ **NDX:** Knowledge deficit related to lack of information about home care needs and follow-up care

Teach feeding techniques

Tell parents dietary restrictions if any (usually milk products are avoided)

Demonstrate use of elbow restraints and ROM exercises

Discuss signs of infection

    Elevated temperature

    Drainage

    Excessive bleeding

    Foul mouth odor

Teach name of medication, purpose, dosage, time of administration and side effects

Have parents demonstrate

    Modified feeding techniques

    Application of elbow restraints

    ROM exercises

    Administration of medications

Ensure that parents understand need for ongoing evaluation of hearing, speech, and teeth formation

Expected outcome/evaluation

Parents and/or significant other demonstrate understanding of home care and follow-up instructions and return demonstrate newly learned procedures for care

TRACHEOESOPHAGEAL FISTULA

A congenital anomaly usually consisting of esophageal atresia combined with a connection of the esophagus with the trachea by way of a fistula (Figure 16-7)

Usual age: newborn; high incidence with prematurity and low birth weight

Assessment
Observations/findings

History of maternal polyhydramnios

Low weight for gestational age

Excessive salivation

Persistent drooling of salivary mucus

Bubbling from nostrils

Normal swallow with feedings followed by sudden cough and regurgitation of feeding through nose and mouth

Cyanosis, coughing, and choking with feedings

Inability to pass nasogastric tube into stomach

Abdominal distention

May have history of repeated pneumonia during first few months of life (H type)

Laboratory/diagnostic studies

X-ray studies: radio-opaque catheter is inserted into esophagus and followed by chest films; diagnosis is confirmed by failure of catheter to reach stomach or passage of catheter through abnormal channels; GI gas is also observed on x-ray examination

Potential complications

Aspiration pneumonia

Apnea/respiratory arrest

Dehydration

Inanition

Esophageal strictures (postsurgical complication)

Additional congenital anomalies (cardiac, renal, and/or gastrointestinal)

Medical Management
Postdiagnosis

NPO

Maintenance parenteral fluids and electrolyte replacement

TPN as necessary

Suctioning of nose and pharynx prn

Humidified oxygen therapy

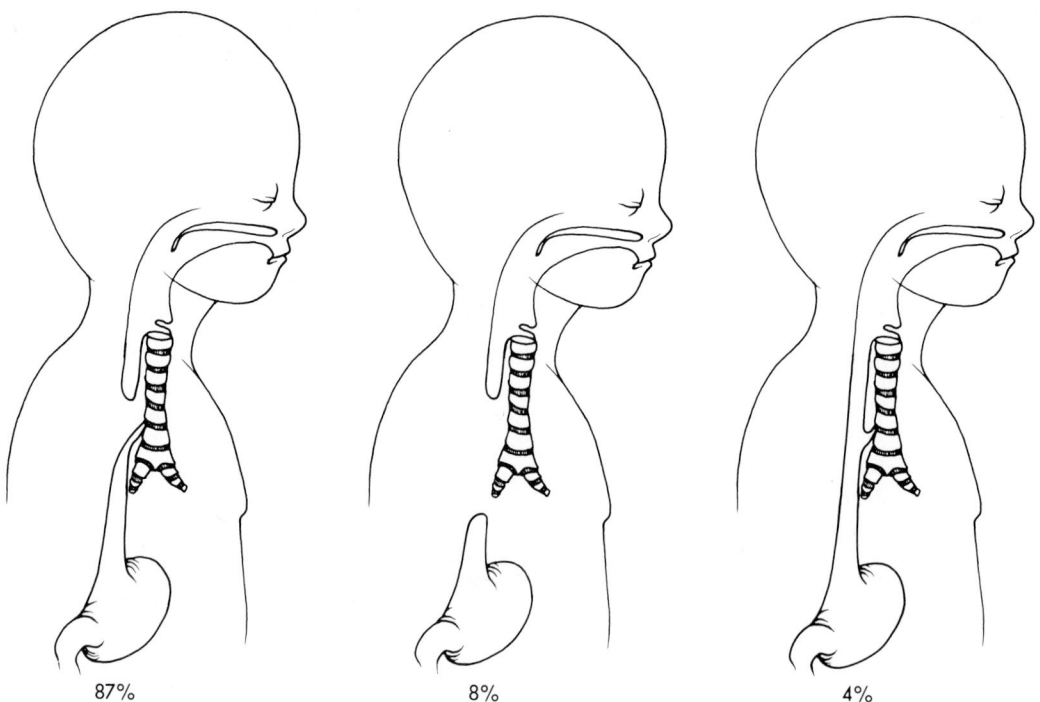

87%   8%   4%

FIGURE 16-7. Three most commonly encountered forms of esophageal atresia and tracheo-esophageal fistula, in order of frequency.

Drainage of pouch via catheter

External warming device

Endotracheal intubation and assisted ventilation with severe respiratory distress

Antibiotic therapy

Insertion of gastrostomy tube (usually done with patient under local anesthesia preoperatively to allow escape of air from stomach, thus decreasing possibility of reflux into fistula)

Surgery

Palliative surgery with ligation of fistula and insertion of gastrostomy tube *or*

Corrective surgery with ligation of fistula, anastomosis of esophagus, and gastrostomy placement; type of surgery done is determined by type of tracheoesophageal fistula and length of esophagus available for anastomosis

Postgastrostomy

Evaluation of respiratory status

Gastrostomy tube connected to gravity drainage or to low, intermittent suction

Continuation of pouch drainage

Continuation of maintenance parenteral fluids; hyperalimentation may be ordered

Replacement of gastrostomy drainage with parenteral fluids

Monitoring and replacement of fluids and electrolytes

Continuation of warm, humidified, oxygenated environment

Nursing diagnoses/interventions/evaluation (preoperative)

■ **NDX:** Ineffective airway clearance related to secretions of esophageal pouch, regurgitation of all feedings, and risk of aspiration

Maintain NPO status

Keep infant in warm, humidified, oxygenated environment

Suction frequently to clear nares and mouth of mucus

Keep pouch catheter (usually sump tube) connected to low, continuous suction as ordered

Monitor respiratory status qh and prn

Place infant in head-elevated position of at least 30 degrees

Keep infant calm and quiet by stroking, handling gently, and using pacifier; crying causes gastric regurgitation

Turn q2h

Administer antibiotics if ordered

Prepare for insertion of gastrostomy tube for gastric decompression

Postgastrostomy: maintain gastrostomy tube connected to gravity drainage or to low, intermittent suction as ordered

Expected outcome/evaluation

Patient's airway remains patent
Patient does not aspirate
Respiratory distress recognized and treated promptly

■ **NDX:** Potential fluid volume deficit related to inability to tolerate oral feedings

Monitor for signs of dehydration (p. 841)
Maintain NPO status
Administer parenteral fluids and electrolytes as ordered
Replace gastrostomy drainage with parenteral fluids as ordered
Measure intake and output and specific gravity
Weigh infant daily

Expected outcome/evaluation

Patient remains hydrated

■ **NDX:** Potential for ineffective thermoregulation related to age, an inability to raise temperature through shivering, and/or use of external warming devices

Place infant under or in an external warming device
Keep infant partially dressed; especially use cap to prevent loss of warmth through head
Keep snugly wrapped in blankets if feasible
Monitor temperature q4h and prn and regulate temperature of environment accordingly

Expected outcome/evaluation

Patient's body temperature remains between 98.6° and 100.4° F (37° and 38° C)

■ **NDX:** Knowledge deficit related to lack of information about condition and treatment

Prepare parents for necessary preoperative procedures
Explain surgical procedure to parents
Carefully explain existing problem and reason for NPO status
Provide parents with visual explanation of defect
Allow parents to continue to parent their child
Assess parent's coping ability and provide resources as necessary

Expected outcome/evaluation

Parents and/or significant other state accurate understanding of the condition and its treatment

TRACHEOESOPHAGEAL FISTULA REPAIR

Usual age: newborn

Preoperative Care

See Tracheoesophageal Fistula (p. 789)

Postoperative Care

(After surgical anastomosis of esophagus/gastrostomy placement)

Assessment
Observations/findings

Respiratory status (see Respiratory Assessment, p. 186)
Type and amount of chest tube drainage (saliva in chest tube indicates anastomotic leak)
Signs and symptoms of anastomotic leak or perforation
    Severe respiratory distress
    Assymmetrical movement of chest
    Respiratory failure (p. 223)
    Fever
    Shock (p. 105)
Tolerance to gastrostomy and oral feedings when started

Laboratory/diagnostic studies

Barium swallow under fluoroscopy may be done before oral feedings
Esophagoscopy may be performed for direct observation of anastomosis

Potential complications

Respiratory failure (p. 223)
Perforation of anastomosis
Shock (p. 105)
Hyponatremia (p. 38)
Dehydration (p. 841)
Hypothermia (p. 438)

Medical Management

Insertion of chest tube and connection to underwater seal
Determination of distance a catheter can be inserted for safe suctioning to ensure patent airway and prevent trauma to anastomosis
Warm environment
Oxygen therapy prn
NPO
Parenteral fluids and/or TPN until sufficient oral and/or gastrostomy feedings are tolerated
Gastrostomy tube connected to gravity drainage or to low, intermittent suction
Gastrostomy replacement fluids
Small, frequent feedings via gastrostomy tube begun 7 to 10 days after insertion, *without* clamping of tube after feedings; diet advanced via gastrostomy tube as tolerated
Oral feedings begun 1 to 2 weeks after anastomosis
Removal of gastrostomy tube
Prophylactic antibiotics may be ordered
Analgesics to control pain

Nursing diagnoses/interventions/evaluation

■ **NDX:** Potential for ineffective airway clearance related to anesthesia, gastric regurgitation through fistula, and/or anastomotic leak or perforation

Maintain NPO

Maintain gastrostomy tube connected to gravity drainage or to low, intermittent suction

Maintain chest tube connected to underwater seal; note amount and type of drainage qh

Monitor vital signs with respiratory assessment q1h and prn

Maintain warm environment

Administer oxygen prn as ordered

Keep infant in head-up position

Avoid hyperextension of neck to prevent pull on sutured esophagus

A suction catheter should be marked by surgeon indicating maximum length that it can be inserted when performing nasopharyngeal suctioning; before suctioning, measure suction catheter to be used against premeasured catheter

Suction *gently* and frequently to maintain airway; vigorous suctioning will traumatize tissue and increase edema already present from operation

Turn q2h

Perform postural drainage and percussion prn

Administer antibiotics if ordered

Expected outcome/evaluation

Patient's
  Respiratory rate is age appropriate
  Color is pink
  Airway is patent
  Breath sounds are clear
  Early signs of possible anastomotic leak are recognized and treated promptly

■ **NDX:** Potential fluid volume deficit related to NPO status, inability to tolerate oral feedings, and gastric suctioning

Maintain NPO status

Administer parenteral fluids as ordered

Administer gastric replacement solution parenterally as ordered

Monitor intake, output, and specific gravity

Weigh daily

Begin gastrostomy feedings as ordered

Expected outcome/evaluation

Patient remains hydrated

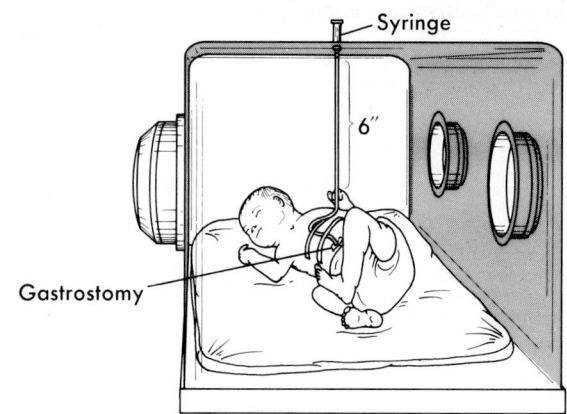

FIGURE 16-8. Feeding by gastrostomy tube.

■ **NDX:** Altered nutritional status: less than body requirements related to inability to tolerate age-appropriate caloric intake orally

Begin small, frequent clear fluid feedings via gastrostomy tube and advance amount and strength as ordered and tolerated

Check gastric residual before each feeding

Refeed gastric residual; amount of feeding to be given is determined by taking amount of formula ordered and subtracting amount of residual

Give feeding by gravity drip

Keep gastrostomy tube open to air (*do not clamp after feedings*); a 10 ml syringe barrel suspended no more than 6 inches above infant's abdomen may be used (Figure 16-8)

Give pacifier until oral feeding is begun

Begin oral feedings as ordered

Observe infant's ability to swallow without choking

Supplement oral feedings with gastrostomy feedings if necessary until infant is able to tolerate full feedings orally

Expected outcome/evaluation

Patient tolerates diet reflecting age-appropriate caloric requirements via gastrostomy tube and/or orally before discharge

■ **NDX:** Pain related to surgical incision

Assess infant for signs of pain

Provide comforting measures; allow parents to hold and cuddle infant; use quiet voices, soft music, and dim lights

Keep infant warm and dry

Administer analgesics as ordered

Expected outcome/evaluation

Patient is calm and easily consolable, without evidence of discomfort (irritability, excessive crying, disturbed sleep pattern)

■ **NDX:** Knowledge deficit related to lack of information about home care needs and follow-up care

Teach feeding techniques: if surgery was palliative, infant will go home receiving gastrostomy feedings; with corrective surgery, gastrostomy tube will be discontinued before discharge, and infant will go home receiving oral feedings

Discuss signs of respiratory difficulty
  Tachypnea
  Retractions
  Nasal flaring
Discuss signs of esophageal stricture
  Difficulty in feeding
  Vomiting
  Coughing
  Gagging
  Dysphagia
Discuss symptoms of wound infection
  Fever
  Redness
  Drainage
  Swelling
  Tenderness
Have parents demonstrate
  Feeding techniques
  Care of gastrostomy tube (if infant will be discharged with one)

Expected outcome/evaluation

Parents and/or significant other demonstrate understanding of home care and follow-up instructions and demonstrate feeding techniques and care of gastrostomy tube

PYLORIC STENOSIS

A congenital obstruction of the gastric pylorus caused by hypertrophy of the circular pyloric musculature; is most frequent in males, and symptoms usually occur in the second or third week of life

Assessment
Observations/findings

History of formula changes without resolution of symptoms
Expected findings
  Nonbilious vomiting soon after feeding, becoming progressively more severe and projectile (Projectile range may be 1 to 3 feet depending on infant's position)
  Vomitus may be blood tinged
  Eager acceptance of second feeding soon after vomiting episode
  Presence of abdominal peristaltic waves from left to right
  Distended upper abdomen
  Palpable olive-shaped pyloric mass
  Weight loss or no weight gain since birth
  Decreased stool frequency
  Hunger
  Irritability
  Dehydration

Laboratory/diagnostic studies

Hypochloremic alkalosis
  Low serum chloride
  Increased pH
  Increased bicarbonate
Elevated Hct and Hgb with hemoconcentration
NOTE: Because of hemoconcentration from extracellular fluid depletion, decreased serum levels of sodium and potassium may be masked
Upper GI series
  Delayed gastric emptying
  Elongated, threadlike pyloric channel
Palpation of "tumor" immediately after vomiting (may feel like a hard olive in epigastrum slightly to the right of the umbilicus)

Potential complications

Dehydration
Aspiration of vomitus

Medical Management
Preoperative

NPO
Rehydration with parenteral fluids
Replenishment of potassium stores and correction of alkalosis with parenteral electrolyte administration
NOTE: Replacement therapy may delay surgery 24 to 48 hr
Nasogastric tube connected to gravity drainage may be preferred by some surgeons for gastric decompression and lavage

Surgery

Surgical correction of pyloric obstruction by pyloromyotomy

Postoperative

Nasogastric tube may or may not be ordered postoperatively
Maintenance parenteral fluids until infant is able to retain age-appropriate feedings

Feedings may begin as soon as 4 to 6 hr postoperatively

Small, frequent clear liquid feedings, advancing volume and strength as tolerated

Analgesics for pain

Nursing diagnoses/evaluation/interventions

■ **NDX:** Fluid volume deficit preoperatively related to severe vomiting

Monitor improvement of symptoms of dehydration (p. 841)

Maintain NPO if ordered

Provide maintenance fluids parenterally as ordered

Maintain nasogastric tube if ordered; check drainage q2h to 4h and replace with parenteral fluids as ordered

Monitor serum electrolyte values and replace parenterally as ordered

Monitor intake and output

Expected outcome/evaluation

Patient is well hydrated with normal electrolyte values before surgery

■ **NDX:** Potential fluid volume deficit postoperatively related to inability to tolerate age-appropriate volume of feedings

Maintain NPO status as ordered

Maintain nasogastric tube connected to low, intermittent suction if ordered; empty and measure drainage q2h to 4h and replace as ordered

Administer parenteral fluids; decrease as oral intake increases

Assess infant's readiness for oral feedings: alert, bowel sounds present, flatus and/or stool, eager sucking of pacifier without being content

Monitor intake and output

Begin small, clear liquid feedings (usually electrolyte solution) q3h as ordered; increase volume and progress to formula as ordered and tolerated

Monitor for vomiting

NOTE: Some vomiting may occur for 24 to 48 hr postoperatively

Expected outcome/evaluation

Patient tolerates fluid requirements orally without vomiting

■ **NDX:** Alteration in nutrition: less than body requirements related to preoperative vomiting and inability to tolerate age-appropriate diet

Weigh infant daily

Gradually and progressively increase volume and strength of feedings as ordered and tolerated

Advance to previous formula or breast milk as soon as feasible

Keep infant prone or propped on right side after feedings

Burp infant frequently during feedings

Involve parents in care and feeding as soon as possible

Observe infant's response to feedings and feeding techniques

Expected outcome/evaluation

Patient

Tolerates feedings sufficient to meet caloric requirements (115 calories/kg) before discharge

Gains weight

■ **NDX:** Potential for infection related to surgical incision

Observe incision for signs of infection: redness, pain, swelling, drainage

Keep incision clean and dry

Monitor temperature with vital signs q4h

Expected outcome/evaluation

Patient is afebrile

Incision remains clean and intact

■ **NDX:** Knowledge deficit related to lack of information about home care and follow-up needs

Teach feeding schedule and techniques

Have parents feed infant before discharge

If infant vomits during postoperative feedings

Discuss with parents their feelings and fears about vomiting/feeding

Inform parents that some vomiting may occur 24 to 48 hr after surgery

Discuss symptoms of wound infection

Ensure that parents understand need for follow-up care

Expected outcome/evaluation

Parents and/or significant other demonstrate understanding of home care and follow-up instructions

RUPTURED (PERFORATED) APPENDIX

An obstruction of the appendiceal lumen progressively causing inflammation, distention, decreased blood supply, necrosis, and perforation of the appendix; perforation causing generalized peritonitis or a localized abscess

Usual age: any

Assessment
Observations/findings

Abdominal pain: sudden relief from pain with perforation, followed by increased diffuse pain

Rigidity

Guarding

Side-lying position with knees flexed for maximum comfort

Progressive abdominal distention

Vomiting (may occur after onset of pain)

Diarrhea or constipation

Decreased or absent bowel sounds

Fever

Tachypnea

Shallow respirations

Tachycardia

Chills

Pallor or flushing

Irritability

Restlessness

Dehydration

Laboratory/diagnostic studies

WBC count elevated, with shift of differential

Urinalysis to rule out urinary tract infection (UTI)

Abdominal x-ray examination to rule out other cause for pain (e.g., fecal impaction)

Chest x-ray examination to rule out pneumonia

Potential complications

Dehydration

Sepsis

Electrolyte imbalance

Pelvic abscess

Pneumonia

Medical Management

Preoperative

NPO

Parenteral fluids

Nasogastric tube connected to low, intermittent suction

Antibiotic therapy

Surgery

Surgical removal of appendix (appendectomy)

Postoperative

NPO

Parenteral fluids (may include TPN)

Nasogastric tube drainage replacement with parenteral fluids

Nasogastric tube connected to low, intermittent suction or sump tube to low, continuous suction

Determination of volume of nasogastric tube irrigation solution

Discontinuation of nasogastric tube

Initiation of oral feedings and advancement from clear liquids to regular diet for age

Incentive spirometer

Determination of type of incisional care

Advancement and discontinuation of Penrose drain

Antibiotics

Analgesics

Antipyretics

Nursing diagnoses/interventions/evaluation

■ **NDX:** Potential fluid volume deficit related to fever, nasogastric suctioning, and/or inability to take oral fluids

Maintain NPO status

Administer parenteral fluids as ordered

Maintain nasogastric suction as ordered

Empty and measure nasogastric tube drainage q4h to 8h and prn

Administer gastric replacement fluids parenterally as ordered

Irrigate nasogastric tube as ordered; when measuring nasogastric tube drainage, adjust volume to reflect results of irrigation

Measure intake and output, and specific gravity

Begin clear liquid diet as ordered

Conduct cooling measures prn

Expected outcome/evaluation

Patient

  Remains hydrated and afebrile

  Tolerates a sufficient amount of oral fluids to maintain hydration before discharge

■ **NDX:** Altered nutrition: less than body requirements related to increased nutritional requirements for wound healing, dietary restrictions, pain

Assess for return of peristalsis

  Flatus

  Stooling

  Decrease in quantity of gastric drainage

  Bowel sounds

  Hunger

Begin clear liquid diet and assess patient's tolerance

Advance diet gradually to regular diet for age

Encourage ambulation to promote return of peristalsis

Gradually reduce pain medication as tolerated so it will not contribute to constipation

Monitor weight

Observe for return of prehospitalization bowel pattern

Expected outcome/evaluation

Patient tolerates regular diet for age before discharge

■ **NDX:** Potential for ineffective breathing pattern related to anesthesia, postoperative immobility, pain

Monitor vital signs q4h and prn

Monitor respiratory status q2h and prn

Assist and teach patient to turn, cough, and deep breathe, and to use incentive spirometer q2h

Position patient in 45-degree head-up position

Ambulate at least 3 or 4 times qd as tolerated

Administer pain medication if necessary before ambulation and vigorous respiratory treatments

Expected outcome/evaluation

Patient's

Breath sounds remain clear

Respiratory rate is age appropriate (p. 841)

■ **NDX:** Pain related to surgical intervention

Assess for symptoms of pain (children may not verbalize pain because they fear the injection)

Facial grimacing

Crying

Poor appetite

Guarding

Refusal to increase physical activity

Administer analgesics as ordered

Change to oral preparation of analgesics as soon as patient is tolerating oral fluids

Institute other comfort and pain control measures

Relaxation

Breathing exercises

Splinting of incision with rolled blanket

Position for comfort; avoid extension of abdominal musculature

Expected outcome/evaluation

Patient is pain-free or has minimal pain before discharge

■ **NDX:** Altered skin integrity related to surgical intervention

Monitor wound for signs of infection

Fever

Redness

Swelling

Copious or foul drainage

Administer incisional care as ordered

Observe color, amount, and characteristics of drainage from Penrose drain

Administer antibiotic therapy as ordered

Encourage proper nutrition

Expected outcome/evaluation

Patient's surgical incision heals without signs of infection

■ **NDX:** Knowledge deficit related to lack of information about home care and follow-up needs

Teach wound care (packing and dressing)

Discuss symptoms of wound infection to report to physician

Redness

Pain

Edema

Drainage

Discuss diet

Explain need for exercise to tolerance with planned rest periods

Caution patient to avoid strenuous exercise for several weeks

Teach name of medication, purpose, dosage, time of administration, and side effects

Expected outcome/evaluation

Patient and/or parents demonstrate understanding of home care and follow-up instructions

HIRSCHSPRUNG'S DISEASE: AGANGLIONIC MEGACOLON

A congenital condition characterized by greatly dilated colon proximal to an area of narrowing, usually in the rectum or rectosigmoid, resulting from absence of parasympathetic ganglion cells and peristalsis (Figure 16-9)

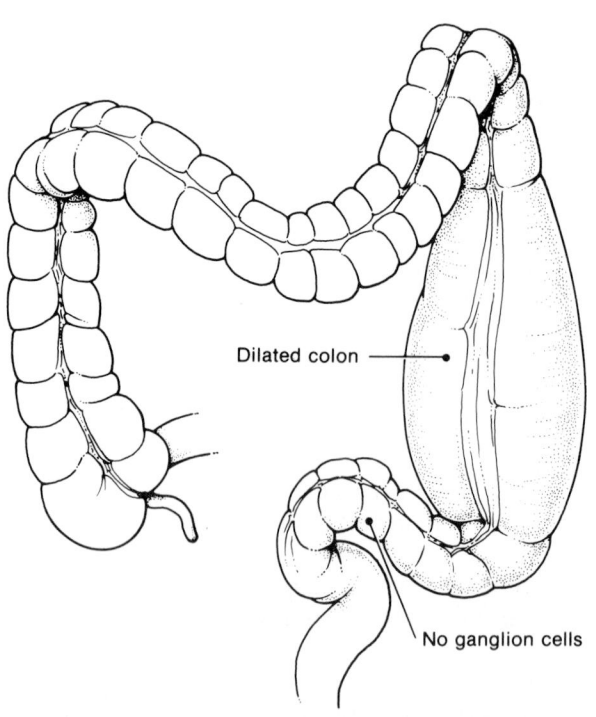

FIGURE 16-9. The affected bowel in Hirschsprung's disease. (From Scipien GM, Chard MA, Howe J et al: *Pediatric nursing care,* St Louis, 1990, Mosby–Year Book.)

Usual age: under 1 year; predominantly males

Assessment
Observations/findings
EARLY INFANCY

Failure to pass meconium within 24 to 48 hr after birth
Partial or complete intestinal obstruction
  Vomiting of bilious or fecal matter
  Abdominal distention
  Constipation
  Diarrhea: most ominous sign
Reluctance to take fluids
Weight loss

LATER INFANCY: LESS SEVERE TYPE

Gradually increasing constipation
Small pellet or ribbonlike stool
Abdominal distention
Vomiting and diarrhea episodes
Fecal mass palpable: left lower quadrant
Inadequate nutrition
  Failure to grow
  Loss of subcutaneous tissue
Anemia
Nutritional assessment

Laboratory/diagnostic studies

Rectal examination: tight internal sphincter with explosive, foul-smelling watery stool
Barium enema: retention of barium and visualization of dilated proximal colon and narrowed distal segment
Rectal biopsy: confirms lack of ganglion cells
Anorectal manometry: normal contraction of external sphincter with failure of internal sphincter to relax or contract

Potential complications

Enterocolitis (p. 800)
Septic shock (p. 105)
Dehydration (p. 841)
Hypokalemia (p. 38)
Hyponatremia (p. 38)
Hypoproteinemia
Metabolic acidosis (p. 48)

Medical Management

Surgical creation of a loop or double-barrel colostomy just above determined level of ganglionic bowel
Corrective surgery via abdominoperineal pull-through procedure (p. 798)
Parenteral fluids for hydration (may include TPN)
NPO initially; po begun after defecation through colostomy
Nasogastric tube connected to low, intermittent suction (discontinued after defecation through colostomy)
Antibiotics

Enterostomal therapist consultation as appropriate

Nursing diagnoses/interventions/evaluation

■ **NDX:** Altered nutrition: less than body requirements related to imposed dietary restriction secondary to surgery for creation of colostomy

Maintain NPO status as ordered
Maintain nasogastric tube connected to gravity drainage or to low, intermittent suction as ordered
Irrigate nasogastric tube q2h and prn to ensure patency
Note color, amount, and characteristic of nasogastric drainage
Administer parenteral fluids (and TPN) as ordered
Administer nasogastric replacement fluids as ordered
Monitor intake and output and specific gravity
Weigh patient daily
Assess abdomen for
  Distention (measure girth with vital signs)
  Return of bowel sounds
  Passage of flatus and stool through colostomy

Expected outcome/evaluation

Patient tolerates age appropriate diet (see requirements for age, p. 841) before discharge

■ **NDX:** Altered bowel elimination: constipation or diarrhea related to altered bowel evacuation via colostomy

Observe color and consistency of colostomy drainage
Measure amount of colostomy drainage; if volume is large and watery, consider increasing fluid replacement to compensate for fluid loss via colostomy
Observe rectal discharge; mucus and stool may be present, especially if loop colostomy was performed
Follow special diet if ordered (usually low-residue diet)
Observe dietary intake influence on stool pattern and avoid items that cause increase in loose stools or increased gas

Expected outcome/evaluation

Patient
  Develops normal bowel pattern
  Remains hydrated

■ **NDX:** Knowledge deficit related to lack of information about colostomy care at home and need for follow-up care

Teach and have parents demonstrate colostomy care (p. 286)
Reassure parents that they will not hurt child by touching stoma
Explain special diet as ordered
Emphasize importance of adequate fluid intake

Teach observation of colostomy drainage
Discuss need for corrective surgery
Discuss financial burden
Discuss signs and symptoms to report to physician
  Abdominal distention
  Fever
  Vomiting
  Abdominal pain
  Irritability
  Dyspnea
NOTE: If conservative dietary management is employed, patient will not have a colostomy and will be treated at home until corrective surgery is scheduled
Teach parents how to give normal saline enemas
Teach name of laxative medication, purpose, dosage, time of administration, and side effects
Discuss low-residue diet

Expected outcome/evaluation

Parents and/or significant other demonstrate understanding of colostomy care and home care needs

ABDOMINOPERINEAL PULL-THROUGH PROCEDURE

A corrective procedure for Hirschsprung's disease: Swenson, Duhamel, or Soave

Usual age: any, usually by 1 year of age or 20 lb

Postoperative Assessment for Potential Complications

Enterocolitis
  Frequent green, liquid stools
  Dehydration
  Hyponatremia
  Hypokalemia
  Magnesium deficiency
    Disorientation
    Hyperreactivity to stimuli
    Muscular twitching
    Convulsions
    Bulging anterior fontanel (if still open)
Prolonged paralytic ileus
  Abdominal distention
  Increased amount of gastric drainage
  Bilious gastric drainage
Ventilatory problems
  Tachypnea
  Tachycardia
  Decreased breath sounds
  Rales
Pelvic abscess
  Fever
  Palpable pelvic mass
  Anal discharge, purulent or bloody
  Septic shock

Medical Management
Preoperative

Clear liquid diet orally for 48 to 72 hr
Colonic irrigations with normal saline
If colostomy is present, irrigation of distal loop and rectum with normal saline
Night before operation
  Antibiotic irrigation of colostomy to cleanse bowel of bacteria; oral antibiotics may be ordered 1 day before surgery
  Parenteral fluids
  NPO

Postoperative

NPO
Parenteral fluids (may include TPN)
Nasogastric tube connected to low, intermittent suction
Irrigation of nasogastric tube q2h to 4h
Nasogastric replacement fluids
Foley catheter may be present for 1 to 2 days postoperatively
May have Penrose drain for rectal drainage
Abdominal dressing
Respiratory care: postural drainage and percussion prn
Vital signs q2h to 4h; *no rectal temperatures*
Antibiotics
Analgesics
Oral feedings begun with return or peristalsis; advancement from clear liquid diet to age-appropriate diet as tolerated

Nursing diagnoses/interventions/evaluation

■ **NDX:** Altered nutrition: less than body requirements related to imposed dietary restrictions and/or chronic poor feeding

Maintain NPO status immediately postoperatively
Administer parenteral fluids as ordered
Administer TPN solution as ordered if prolonged ileus occurs
Assess abdomen for return of peristalsis
  Presence of bowel sounds
  Nondistended abdomen (measure girth)
  Passing of flatus and/or stool
  Decrease in amount of nasogastric drainage
Discontinue nasogastric tube as ordered
Begin clear liquid diet, advancing to diet for age as ordered and tolerated (may be low-residue diet)
Observe child/parent behavior around feeding time
Do not force child to eat or make an issue out of eating
Make referral for nutritional/feeding strategy counseling as necessary

Expected outcome/evaluation

Patient tolerates age-appropriate diet before discharge

■ **NDX:** Potential fluid volume deficit related to gastric drainage, NPO status, and/or frequent loose stools

Maintain NPO immediately postoperatively

Maintain nasogastric tube to low, intermittent suction

Ensure patency of nasogastric tube by irrigating q2h as ordered

Measure nasogastric drainage q4h and prn, and replace with parenteral fluids as ordered

Measure intake and output

Monitor specific gravity as indicated

Expected outcome/evaluation

Patient remains hydrated as evidenced by good skin turgor and balanced intake and output

■ **NDX:** Altered bowel elimination: diarrhea related to poor sphincter control and/or as expected sequela of surgery

Observe frequency, consistency, color, and volume of stools

Anticipate that child may have as many as 5 to 15 loose stools per day

Assist in identifying possible dietary irritants

Ensure dietary restrictions if ordered

Anticipate and teach parents that child will be slow to toilet train

Expected outcome/evaluation

Patient eventually develops normal bowel pattern as evidenced by the establishment of a normal stooling pattern before discharge

■ **NDX:** Potential for ineffective breathing pattern related to anesthesia, postoperative immobility, and/or pain

Monitor vital signs q4h and prn

Monitor respiratory status q2h to 4h and prn

Assist patient with turning and coughing q2h initially

Administer postural drainage and percussion if necessary

Elevate head of bed; encourage parents to hold child; sit child in padded high chair; ambulate if developmentally able

Administer pain medication if necessary before vigorous respiratory treatments or ambulation

Expected outcome/evaluation

Patient's
  Breath sounds remain clear
  Respiratory rate is age appropriate

■ **NDX:** Pain related to surgical intervention

Assess for symptoms of pain
  Facial grimacing
  Crying
  Poor appetite
  Withdrawn behavior
  Refusal to increase physical activity

Administer analgesics as ordered

Institute other comfort measures
  Cuddling, sucking of pacifier, minimal auditory and visual stimulation
  Position for comfort; avoid extension of abdominal musculature

Gently cleanse anal area with soap and water; warm water squirted on area with syringe or perineal bottle is soothing

Expected outcome/evaluation

Patient is pain-free or has minimal pain before discharge

■ **NDX:** Altered skin integrity related to surgical intervention and expected frequent loose stools postoperatively

Monitor wound for signs of infection
  Fever
  Redness
  Swelling
  Copious or foul drainage

Administer incisional care as ordered

Prevent contamination of abdominal wound with urine by pinning diaper below dressing; a Foley catheter may be used immediately postoperatively for urinary diversion

Observe color, amount, and characteristic of drainage from rectal Penrose drain if present

Cleanse anal area gently with soap and water after each bowel movement

Apply protective ointments to anal and perineal area q2h and prn

Encourage proper nutrition

Expected outcome/evaluation

Patient's
  Surgical incision heals without signs of infection
  Skin of anal/perineal area remains intact

■ **NDX:** Knowledge deficit related to lack of information about home care and follow-up needs

Explain appropriate diet with restrictions if any

Teach care of anal/perineal area

Discuss symptoms of wound infection to report to physician; redness, pain, swelling, drainage

Have parents demonstrate
  Anal/perineal care
  Feeding strategies

Discuss toilet training expectations

Discuss availability of community health services for support and follow-up

Expected outcome/evaluation

Parents and/or significant other demonstrate understanding of home care and follow-up instructions

GASTROENTERITIS

A condition characterized by vomiting and diarrhea resulting from infection, allergy, intolerance of specific food substances, or ingestion of toxins

Usual age: any

Complications are most severe in infants

Child should be placed on enteric isolation precautions

Assessment

Observations/findings

Frequent loose stools
  Yellow-green, green
  May be mucoid
  May be bloody
Weight loss or failure to gain weight
Decreased appetite
Abdominal pain and/or cramping
Abdominal distention
Hyperactive bowel sounds
Vomiting
Fever
Irritability
Increasing lethargy
Excoriated buttocks
Dehydration
  Depressed anterior fontanel
  Sunken eyes
  Loss of skin turgor
  Dry mucous membranes
  No tears with crying
  High urine specific gravity
  Oliguria
Some degree of electrolyte imbalance
  Hyponatremia or hypernatremia
  Hypokalemia or hyperkalemia
  Metabolic acidosis
See Gastrointestinal Assessment
Nutritional assessment

Laboratory/diagnostic studies

WBC differential: increased bands with shigellosis
Stool specimens (culture and smear for WBC)
May have increased leukocytes or clumps of pus with enteroinvasive organisms
May be positive for occult blood
May be positive for reducing substance (sugar in stool) with disaccharide intolerance

Serum electrolytes
CBC: elevated Hct

Potential complications

Hypovolemic/septic shock (p. 105)

Medical Management

NPO until rehydrated

Parenteral fluids and electrolytes (potassium is added to parenteral solution only after renal function is ensured by passage of urine)

With chronic diarrhea, hyperalimentation may be necessary

Replacement of stool output with parenteral fluids as necessary to maintain adequate hydration

Use of oral rehydration therapy (p. 802) may be considered if child is less than 10% dehydrated, vomiting is minimal, and stool losses are less than 10 ml/kg/hr

Intake and output

Antibiotic therapy

Topical ointment for excoriated buttocks

Tests of stools for occult blood, pH, and reducing substance

Vital signs q1h to 2h

Small, frequent feedings of clear liquids begun, with gradual advancement of diet as tolerated

Examine other family members (collecting stool specimens) and treat as appropriate

Nursing diagnoses/interventions/evaluation

■ **NDX:** Fluid volume deficit related to inability to tolerate oral fluids without vomiting and diarrhea

Monitor vital signs q1h to 2h as ordered and prn

Monitor cardiac activity until fluid and electrolyte imbalances are corrected

Maintain NPO status as ordered

Administer parenteral fluids with added electrolytes as ordered

Weigh patient daily

Monitor intake and output

Determine specific gravity on each voided specimen

Describe frequency and character of stools

Describe frequency and character of vomitus (if present)

Monitor for resolving or persistent signs of dehydration

Administer stool replacement fluids if ordered

Monitor serum electrolytes

Begin small, frequent feedings of clear liquids or electrolyte solution as ordered and monitor patient's tolerance to it; advance diet gradually as tolerated

Expected outcome/evaluation

Patient
  Has tears, moist mucous membranes, normal skin tur-

gor, and adequate urinary output for age (see standard for age under Basic Standards of Care, pp. 763-770)
Gains weight

■ **NDX:** Diarrhea related to ingestion of an irritant, infectious process, or intestinal malabsorption

Maintain NPO status until stools decrease in number and volume to prevent further gastric irritation
Describe frequency, character, and color of stools
Collect stool specimen as ordered
Begin small, frequent feedings of electrolyte solution as ordered
Give liquids at room temperature; cold liquids increase bowel motility
Advance to breast milk feedings or gradually advance formula from quarter strength, half strength, and full strength as tolerated and ordered (infants)
Assess patient's tolerance to each dietary change and reduce strength of formula if stool volume increases significantly
In an older child, diet may be advanced from clear liquids to BRAT (bananas, rice, applesauce, toast) diet with elimination of all milk products (see Diet for Control of Diarrhea, below)

Expected outcome/evaluation

Patient resumes prehospitalized bowel pattern

■ **NDX:** Alteration in skin integrity related to frequent loose stools with irritation of anal area and buttocks

Keep diaper area clean and dry
Check and change diaper q1h and prn
Wash skin with mild soap and water after each stool; rinse well with water only (soap can be irritant) and dry thoroughly; apply topical ointment as ordered
Leave diaper area exposed to air as much as possible
Avoid use of heat lamp, since it can cause thermal burns and further skin irritation
Apply protective ointments after each diaper change
Ensure proper nutrition as soon as feasible to promote tissue healing
Wear gloves and wash hands before and after changing diapers

Expected outcome/evaluation

Patient
Has skin that heals without further excoriation
Has no introduction of secondary infection

■ **NDX:** Knowledge deficit related to lack of information about home care needs and procedure to follow should diarrhea recur

Explain reasons for NPO order and slow, gradual advancement of diet with restrictions
Explain need for isolation to prevent transmission of illness
Teach good handwashing techniques before and after diaper changes
Teach care of diaper area
Explain need to report recurrence of symptoms to physician
If symptoms recur, instruct parents to prevent dehydration by
Giving ad lib breast milk feedings (if breast feeding)
Avoiding lactose-containing formulas or cow's milk for 1-2 days
Giving child oral electrolyte solution (Pedialyte or Ricelyte), not to exceed 150 ml/kg/day
Giving breast milk, clear liquids, or water if child is still thirsty
Instruct patient or parents to begin BRAT diet as tolerated; as stools continue to firm, more foods should be gradually added from regular diet
Teach name of medication, purpose, dosage time of administration, and side effects

Expected outcome/evaluation

Patient and/or parents demonstrate understanding of home care and follow-up instructions and verbalize understanding of dietary instructions

DIET FOR CONTROL OF DIARRHEA

Clear liquids
Water
Tea (decaffeinated)
Carbonated beverages (served flat)
Gelatin
Flavored ice pops
Bouillon broth
Electrolyte solution (only if recommended by physician)
Apple juice (diluted to half strength—some children may not tolerate half strength; therefore, this may be eliminated from diet until stool pattern has returned)
BRAT diet
Breast milk
Bananas
Rice
Applesauce
Toast
Soup (not creamed)
Soda crackers
Pretzels
Dry sweetened cereals (no milk)
After stools begin to firm, add the following
Formula as ordered

Boiled or broiled chicken
Apples
Cottage cheese
Tapioca
Mashed potatoes
As stools continue to firm, gradually add more foods from regular diet

ORAL REHYDRATION THERAPY

The intestinal tract is used to provide adequate fluid intake for rehydration and to avoid the use of intravenous therapy; this therapy is also useful for preventing dehydration and hospitalization if initiated in the early stages of gastroenteritis

Criteria for Use

Vomiting is absent or minimal
Child is less than 10% dehydrated
Stool losses are less than 10 ml/kg/hr

Medical Management

Pedialyte or Ricelyte oral electrolyte solutions

Rehydration Therapy

If patient is 10% dehydrated or more, intravenous fluids must be used
If patient is vomiting, give 10 to 15 ml of electrolyte solution q15min for four times, then increase to 30 ml q30min twice, then
  Give 15 to 20 ml/kg/hr until rehydrated *or*
  Give entire deficit plus one third of maintenance requirements for 24 hr period plus ongoing losses over the next 8 hr (e.g., for a 10 kg child with 5% dehydration, you would give 500 ml deficit plus 333 ml maintenance plus ongoing stool losses, *all* over the next 8 hr)

Maintenance Therapy

Use same oral electrolyte solution as above and give at rate of 150 ml/kg/day; give any additional fluids ad lib as breast milk or water; lactose-free solids can be started after child is rehydrated and is not vomiting (see BRAT diet)
NOTE: Criterion for continuing oral feeding is based on how well child is doing, not necessarily how stools are; it is not recommended that child be made NPO in presence of ongoing or increasing diarrhea

INCARCERATED INGUINAL HERNIA

An obstruction of an intestinal loop, which has passed through the inguinal ring into the inguinal canal

Usual age: under 1 year

Assessment
Observations/findings

Red, firm, tender, globular, irreducible swelling in groin
Fretfulness resulting from pain
Anorexia
Nausea, vomiting
Abdominal distention
Absence of bowel movements
Dehydration
If bowel loop is ischemic or gangrenous
  Shock
  Fever
  Absence of bowel sounds
  Metabolic acidosis

Laboratory/diagnostic studies

WBC: elevated if loop is gangrenous
Serum electrolytes

Potential complications

Shock (p. 105)
Gangrenous bowel loop

Medical Management

Manual reduction of hernia if possible
Surgical reduction of hernia
Correction of hydration and electrolyte imbalances
Analgesics

*Nursing diagnosis/interventions/evaluation (preoperative)**

■ **NDX:** Pain related to intestinal obstruction

Prevent crying and straining, since this increases intestinal protrusion
Administer sedation as ordered
Position for comfort

Expected outcome/evaluation

Patient shows signs of comfort: decreased crying and increased ability to sleep without disturbance

INTUSSUSCEPTION

An intestinal obstruction resulting from one section of intestine invaginating (telescoping) into an adjacent section (Figure 16-10)

Usual age: 3 to 24 months

---

*See Ruptured (Perforated) Appendix (p. 794) for postoperative nursing diagnoses/interventions/evaluation; alter interventions appropriately for age (see standard for age under Basic Standards of Care).

Assessment
Observations/findings
FIRST 12 HR

Intermittent abdominal pain
Vomiting
Passage of one normal stool

AFTER FIRST 12 HR

Increasing vomiting
Severe pain with screaming and drawing up of knees to
   chest
Passage of red, jellylike stool (blood and mucus)
Abdominal tenderness and distention
Sausage-shaped "tumor" may be visible in right or left
   upper quadrant
Empty lower right quadrant
Developing signs of peritonitis; fever and prostration

Laboratory/diagnostic studies

Barium enema: demonstrates obstruction to flow of barium
   and is used as a nonsurgical technique to reduce telescoping of intestine (sedate as needed before procedure)

Potential complications

Shock (p. 105)
Perforation of bowel

Medical Management

Nonsurgical hydrostatic reduction by barium enema
See Ruptured (Perforated) Appendix (p. 794) for general
   abdominal surgery management

Nursing diagnoses/interventions/evaluation

See Ruptured (Perforated) Appendix (p. 794) for nursing
   concerns after abdominal surgery

Central Nervous System

HYDROCEPHALUS (Figure 16-11)

*Excessive cerebrospinal fluid (CSF) within the ventricular
and subarachnoid spaces*
noncommunicating hydrocephalus *CSF flow is blocked
somewhere within the ventricular system*
communicating hydrocephalus *CSF is not absorbed
from the subarachnoid space, but there is no interference within the ventricular system*

Usual age: first year of life but can be diagnosed at any
   age

Assessment
Observations/findings

See Neurological Assessment (p. 391)
History of meningitis, intracranial infections or hemor-
   rhage, perinatal anoxia, and/or intrauterine infection
Gradual increase in head size

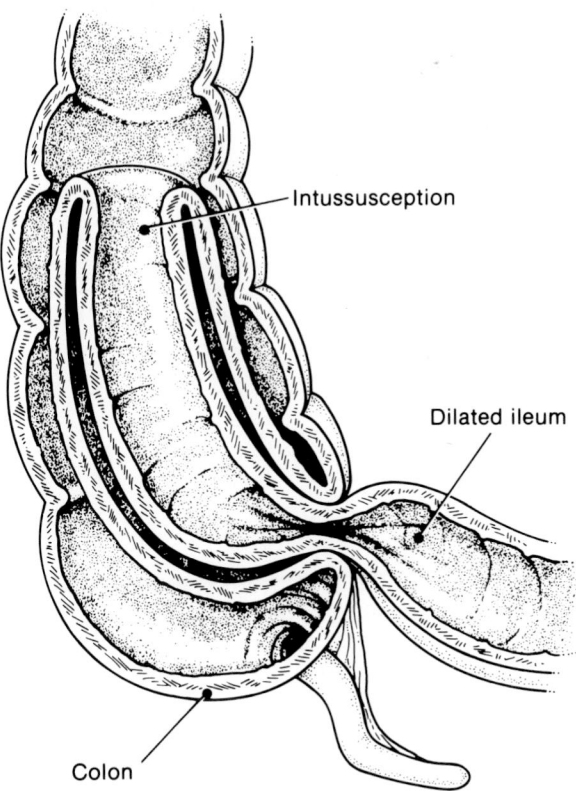

FIGURE 16-10. Telescoping bowel in the presence of intussusception. (From Scipien GM, Chard MA, Howe J et al: *Pediatric nursing care,* St Louis, 1990, Mosby–Year Book.)

Widening suture lines
Widening, bulging, nonpulsating anterior fontanel
"Bossing" of brow
Shiny scalp
Dilated scalp veins
Macewen's sign (cracked-pot sound with percussion of
   skull)
Visible sclera above iris: "sun setting"
Strabismus
Irritability
Lethargy
Poor suck or feeding difficulty
High-pitched cry
Opisthotonos
Lower extremity spasticity
Persistent primitive reflexes
Delayed development
Ataxia
Increased intracranial pressure (ICP)
   Alterations in consciousness and responsiveness
   Vomiting, especially associated with position change
   Headache on awakening
   Seizures
   Bradycardia

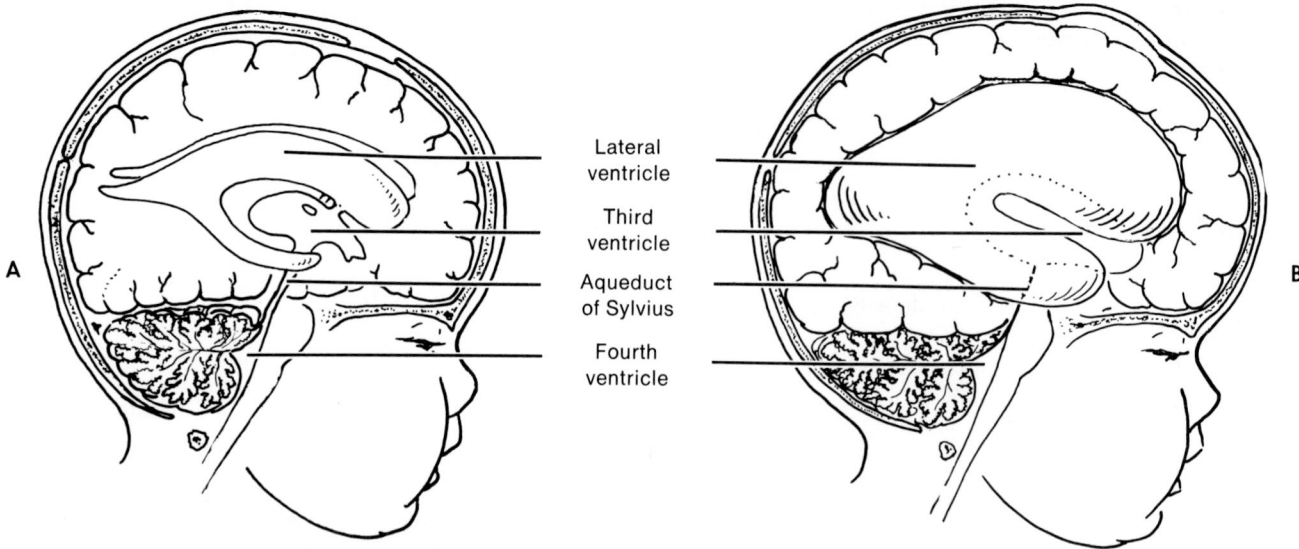

FIGURE 16-11. Hydrocephalus: a block in the flow of CSF. **A,** Patent cerebrospinal fluid circulation. **B,** Enlarged lateral and third ventricle caused by obstruction of circulation—stenosis of the aqueduct of Sylvius. (From Whaley LF, Wong DL: *Essentials of pediatric nursing,* ed 3, St Louis, 1989, Mosby–Year Book.)

Bradypnea
Hypothermia
Associated neurological defects (myelomeningocele)

Laboratory/diagnostic studies

Diagnosis made on basis of abnormal head circumference and neurological signs

Computed tomography (CT) scan: confirms presence of dilated ventricles and assists in identifying possible cause (neoplasms, cysts, congenital malformation such as Arnold-Chiari malformation or intracranial hemorrhages)

Ventricular puncture (taps) are sometimes used to measure ICP, remove CSF to reduce pressure, and obtain CSF for culture (line placed for repeated taps)

Potential complications

Associated anomalies
Mental retardation
Neurological disabilities

Medical Management

Determination of type of hydrocephalus

Insertion of shunt to carry excess CSF away from lateral ventricle to an extracranial site (usually peritoneum in infants and young children, or atrium in adolescent) where it can then be reabsorbed

Small frequent feedings to ensure adequate nutrition

Nursing diagnoses/interventions/evaluation

■ **NDX:** Potential sensory/perceptual alterations related to increased ICP secondary to CSF accumulation in ventricles

Monitor level of consciousness and responsiveness q1h to 2h
Assess vital signs q1h to 2h
Monitor blood pressure q2h to 4h
Measure head circumference q shift
Weigh patient daily
Provide therapeutic auditory and tactile stimuli

Expected outcome/evaluation

Patient is assessed for signs of increased neurological deterioration and does not experience an increasing intensity of illness

■ **NDX:** Potential for altered skin integrity of scalp related to inability of infant to turn head secondary to increased head size and weight

Change position q2h; may consider changing position of head q1h
Avoid loose linen in bed
Lay head on foam rubber pad or use water bed if available
Assess head for pressure points at least 2qh
Stimulate circulation to area with each position change
Maintain nutrition as ordered

Expected outcome/evaluation

Patient's skin integrity is maintained

■ **NDX:** Parental role conflict related to care of child with special needs

Evaluate parent's understanding of special care needs and clarify information as appropriate

Encourage parents to verbalize feelings about role confusion related to situational crisis

Expected outcome/evaluation

Parents report decreased level of stress and participate in routine caretaking tasks

■ **NDX:** Knowledge deficit related to lack of information about disorder and treatment

Explain disorder to parents
Prepare parents for surgery
Teach parents how to handle child and support child's head

Expected outcome/evaluation

Parents and/or significant other demonstrate understanding of treatment of hydrocephalus and make informed decisions about treatment

VENTRICULAR SHUNT INSERTION

Treatment for noncommunicating hydrocephalus involving surgical placement of device that bypasses cranial obstruction and carries CSF to an extracranial site where it is then reabsorbed (Figure 16-12)

Usual age: infant; reinsertion or revisions can occur at any age

Assessment
Observations/findings
PREOPERATIVE

See Hydrocephalus (p. 803)
Assessment of neurological status, especially behavior, developmental ability, and presence or absence of developmental reflexes, for postoperative comparison
Pupillary reaction
Response to auditory and visual stimulation
Head circumference
Fontanel size, protrusion, and pulsability (usually nonpulsating)
Level of consciousness
Respiratory and cardiac rate and quality
Motion present in extremities
Degree of irritability
Cry and sucking quality

POSTOPERATIVE

Reassess neurological status for improvement or deterioration
Assess for signs and symptoms of increased ICP (p. 439)
Fever
Sites of incision
  Leakage of CSF
  Swelling

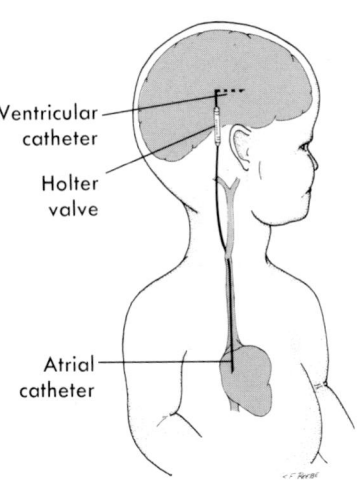

FIGURE 16-12. Ventriculoatrial shunt.

Redness
Drainage
"Tracking" along shunt

Potential complications

Shunt malfunction
Shunt infection
With ventriculoperitoneal shunt
  Peritonitis (p. 267)
  Abdominal distention
  Paralytic ileus (p. 271)
  Abdominal pain
With ventriculoatrial shunt
  Shunt block by blood clot
  Pulmonary embolus (p. 211)

Medical Management

Insertion of mechanical shunt
Monitoring of neurological status q1h to 2h after shunt insertion
Antibiotics prophylactically or for treatment of shunt infection
Gradual increase in elevation of head ordered after close assessment of neurological improvement and signs and symptoms of increased ICP
Change of surgical incision dressings and order for dressing changes
Parenteral fluids with gradual advance in diet as tolerated

Nursing diagnoses/interventions/evaluation

■ **NDX:** Potential sensory/perceptual alterations related to increased intracranial pressure associated with possible shunt malfunction or shunt infection

Measure head circumference q4h
Assess fontanel for size and bulging; level of consciousness;

pupil size, position, and reaction; extraocular movements and ability to fix and follow; muscle tone; and quality of cry qh

Assess vital signs qh and prn

Assess temperature q4h and prn

Monitor blood pressure q1h to 2h

Maintain position on nonoperative side of head; *do not position on shunt* (Figure 16-12)

Keep child flat as ordered; only advance elevation of head as ordered to prevent rapid decrease in ICP

Provide therapeutic auditory and tactile stimuli, e.g., soft cloth textures near skin, quiet/rhythmic soothing music

Expected outcome/evaluation

Patient's alteration in status is minimized by prompt recognition/resolution of shunt malfunction

Therapeutic stimuli are maintained

■ **NDX:** Potential for infection related to surgical intervention

Prevent contamination of surgical sites by keeping them covered with sterile dressings and by washing hands thoroughly before touching area

Monitor temperature q4h and prn

Assess surgical incisions q2h for redness, swelling, drainage, intactness of sutures, and "tracking" along shunt

Administer antibiotics as ordered

Expected outcome/evaluation

Patient remains afebrile with no signs of skin infection

■ **NDX:** Potential alteration in skin integrity related to decreased mobility, increased head size, and weight

See interventions and expected outcome/evaluation under Hydrocephalus (p. 803)

■ **NDX:** Knowledge deficit related to lack of information about home care and follow-up needs

Explain purpose of shunt insertion

Discuss symptoms of shunt failure or infection and increasing ICP to report to physician

Poor feeding

Vomiting

Change in behavior

Increased lethargy

Irritability

"Sun setting" eyes

Fever

Signs of skin infection around incision

Redness

Swelling

Drainage

Emphasize need for ongoing assessment and care on outpatient basis

Have parents demonstrate how to pump shunt, if ordered

Expected outcome/evaluation

Parents can state symptoms of shunt infection or malfunction and describe mechanism to contact physician to report same

MYELOMENINGOCELE

A congenital defect in the spinal vertebrae resulting in motor and sensory dysfunction of the trunk and lower extremities below the level of deformity and accompanied by nonfunctional bowel and bladder sphincters; malformed cord and roots are contained in a sac and covered by a thin vascular membrane

Usual age: diagnosed in newborn period

Assessment
Observations/findings
NEWBORN PERIOD

Meningeal sac

Location

Increasing tension

Leakage of CSF

Malodorous drainage

Rupture

Presence or absence of associated hydrocephalus

Parents' reaction to diagnosis

ANY AGE

Level of spinal defect

Degree of neurological impairment

Spastic or flaccid lower extremities

Bilateral clubfoot

Bilateral or unilateral hip dislocation

Constant dribbling of urine

Distended or flaccid bladder

Frequent small, loose stools or constipation

Progress in bowel and bladder training

Method of mobility (braces, wheelchair)

Integrity of skin

Patient and family's adjustment to diagnosis

Laboratory/diagnostic studies

Culture of CSF in presence of fever and signs of central nervous system (CNS) infection

Urinalysis and cultures in presence of urinary tract infection (UTI)

Blood urea nitrogen (BUN) and creatinine to assess renal function

Potential complications

Hydrocephalus (p. 803)
Meningitis (p. 810)
Seizure disorder (p. 399)
UTI (p. 451)
Renal failure (p. 482)
Decubitus ulcers (p. 523)
Progressive kyphoscoliosis
Death

Medical Management
Newborn period

Assessment of degree of neurological involvement
Moist, sterile normal saline dressings to sac (may also use antibacterial solution)
Dislocated hips in position of abduction
Parenteral fluids as necessary to ensure hydration and electrolyte balance
Honest information to parents about anomalies to assist them in making appropriate decisions about treatment in newborn period
Surgical closure of protruding sac
Insertion of mechanical shunt if hydrocephalus is present (see Ventricular Shunt Insertion, p. 805)

Ongoing management

Correction of orthopedic deformities; casting/bracing as necessary
Ongoing exercise regimen (physical therapy referral)
Shunt revisions as necessary
Anticonvulsants if seizure disorder is present
Assessment of renal function
Antibiotics for UTIs
Laxatives, stool softeners, and/or suppositories as necessary for bowel training
Minimal restrictions on child's activities to promote growth and development
Assessment of child and/or family's adjustment

Nursing diagnoses/interventions/evaluation

■ **NDX:**   Potential for infection related to open sac with draining, protruding spinal contents

Prevent contamination of sac from stool or urine by placing infant prone and undiapered, and securing a pad below sac
Change diapers promptly as necessary
Use aseptic technique in caring for sac
Change sterile dressing with sterile solutions as ordered
Avoid exposure to persons with known infections
Preserve intact skin around sac; avoid use of tape
Avoid pressure on sac; use protective donut as necessary
Use sterile towel while holding infant
Check temperature q4h and prn
Measure head circumference daily

Expected outcome/evaluation

Patient remains free of CNS infection related to contamination of sac

■ **NDX:**   Impaired physical mobility related to lack of nerve innervation to lower extremities (degree depends on level of involvement)

Position infant
  Keep infant prone with entire body in slightly head-up position, head turned to either side
  Place linen roll under ankles to keep foot in neutral position
  Keep legs positioned in moderate abduction
Perform passive ROM exercises as recommended by physical therapy
Turn q2h

Expected outcome/evaluation

Patient maintains physical mobility

■ **NDX:**   Parental role conflict related to intimidation by and fear of infant's care requirements

Encourage parents to express concerns and participate in infant's care
Discuss changes in parental role resulting from infant's special care needs
Encourage expression of effect on family functioning
Refer to appropriate counselor/support person

Expected outcome/evaluation

Parents verbalize intent to converse with counseling/supportive personnel and engage in infant caretaking activities, exhibiting attachment behaviors

■ **NDX:**   Potential for altered skin integrity related to decreased mobility and decreased sensation in lower extremities

Assess skin q2h and prn for pressure areas, redness, and blanching
Use water bed if available
Turn q2h and prn
Keep skin clean and dry
Ensure adequate fluid intake for hydration
Ensure adequate dietary intake of protein and carbohydrates

Expected outcome/evaluation

Patient's skin remains intact, clean, and dry

■ **NDX:**   Potential for urinary retention and bowel incontinence or constipation related to lack of nerve innervation for appropriate defecation and urination

Assess voiding and stooling pattern
Voiding
  Note color, volume, presence of constant dribbling, and presence of distended bladder after spontaneous void
  Perform Credé's maneuver on bladder q2h to 4h as necessary to promote bladder emptying
Stools
  Note frequency and consistency of stool
  Note constant dribbling of loose stool; may indicate stooling around area of constipation
  Assess abdomen for distention or palpable stool in left lower quadrant
  Administer suppositories as ordered prn

Expected outcome/evaluation

Patient establishes regular elimination pattern without constipation or urinary retention

■ **NDX:** Knowledge deficit related to lack of information about condition and treatment

Ensure that parents are given *all* the facts about myelomeningocele; *do not* allow them to receive one-sided information
Refer parents to ethics committee of physicians, social workers, nurses; and other parents of children with myelomeningocele; have the committee meet with the parents of the newborn to present factual information to them
If necessary, have parents who have a child with myelomeningocele meet with the parents of infant
Also consider having parents of infant meet with family who chose other alternatives
Allow parents sufficient time to make an informed decision
Realize that parents are grieving and decision making is difficult for them at this time

Expected outcome/evaluation

Parents have made an informed decision about infant's treatment and plan of care

Nursing diagnoses/interventions/evaluation: ongoing concerns

■ **NDX:** Potential for injury related to decreased perception of pain, touch, and temperature in lower extremities

Teach patient or parents how to assess for skin irritations
Explain need to alter position of child (shift weight) as often as q30min
Caution patient or parents to avoid use of hot baths; to check water temperature with inner aspect of forearm or with thermometer

Explain need to keep skin of feet warm, dry, and soft
Discuss age-appropriate safety precautions

Expected outcome/evaluation

Parents describe methods of protecting patient from injury so that no preventable injury occurs

■ **NDX:** Impaired physical mobility related to neurological dysfunction of lower extremities (also loss of abdominal musculature control with thoracic defects)

Perform ROM exercises; as child gets older teach him how to do this
Position patient in alignment
  Support calf with pillows
  Avoid prolonged periods in one position; change q2h
If braces are used
  Assess correct positioning of braces
  Assess for skin irritation under braces
  Have patient demonstrate application of braces
If wheelchair is used
  Use soft cushion in chair
  Support legs on pillows
  Remember to change patient's position q2h and prn
Encourage progressive mobilization
  Exercise upper extremities; push-ups, pull-ups, throwing balls, weight lifting
  Encourage self-care activities: combing hair, bathing self, dressing self
  Guide patient's legs as patient transfers self from bed to wheelchair
  Encourage independence

Expected outcome/evaluation

Patient obtains optimal mobility through use of his physical abilities and use of assistive devices

■ **NDX:** Constipation related to decreased nerve innervation, decreased abdominal muscle innervation, decreased sense of need to defecate, and decreased mobility

Meet age-appropriate fluid requirements (p. 841)
Administer well-balanced high-bulk diet: fruit, fruit juices, vegetables, bran, whole-grain breads and cereals, nuts
Involve patient in daily exercise regimen
Encourage mobilization
For individuals eligible for bowel training
  Observe stool pattern and identify normal defecation pattern
  Establish time for defecation after a meal
  Ensure privacy

Sit patient on commode or toilet (if feasible)
Administer suppositories or laxatives as ordered

Expected outcome/evaluation

Patient
    Demonstrates appropriate dietary habits
    Does not develop constipation
    Has regular bowel function

■ **NDX:** Total incontinence/retention related to decreased nerve innervation

Assess present voiding pattern
    Any sensation
    Timing in relation to fluid intake
    Constant dribbling or large volume at one time
    Amount voided
    Bladder distention after voiding
    Amount of residual urine after voiding
Maintain hydration by meeting age-appropriate fluid
Teach intermittent catheterization to patient and family
    Explain reasons for catheterization
    Demonstrate clean technique
    Explain need to empty bladder at set times because of danger of overdistention of bladder and its contribution to bladder infections
    Explain relationship between fluid intake and frequency of catheterization
Keep skin clean and dry
Administer antibiotics as ordered for UTI

Expected outcome/evaluation

Patient
    Establishes a pattern of micturition with minimal to absent dribbling
    Does not become distended

■ **NDX:** Potential for impaired skin integrity related to immobility, decreased sensation, and/or urinary/bowel incontinence

Turn patient at least q2h and prn
Assess skin frequently for redness or blanching
Use water beds if available
Position patient for comfort; eliminate wrinkles in sheets
Keep patient clean and dry
When using soap, be sure to rinse it off thoroughly
Apply lotions to keep skin soft
Also refer to nursing diagnosis of *potential for injury,* above

Expected outcome/evaluation

Patient's skin is intact, clean, and dry

■ **NDX:** Potential for altered nutrition: more than body requirements related to imbalance between intake and energy expenditure

Calculate caloric requirements (p. 841); keep in mind that actual caloric requirements for someone immobile will be less than recommended
Discuss balance between intake and energy expenditure with parents early in care of child
Assess family's eating habits
Assist family with identifying well-balanced diet
Assist family with identifying high-calorie foods and encourage them to eliminate them from family's diet
Have patient drink glass of water before meals
Increase amount of socialization and diversionary activity to distract patient from thoughts of food
Encourage patient to be involved in routine physical activity
Promote physical exercise as recommended by physical therapist
Allow patient to do as much for self as possible
Monitor weight

Expected outcome/evaluation

Patient
    Eats a diet sufficient to promote growth and development
    Does not become obese

■ **NDX:** Body image disturbance related to prolonged debilitation, inability to complete developmental tasks, and/or social isolation

Provide child with opportunities to discuss fears, concerns, grief, and anger
Ask patient to identify things patient likes about self
If patient is unable to do so, tell patient things you like about him
Encourage patient to look at self in mirror
Encourage grooming, including alternating hair styles, wearing makeup, and experimenting with different clothes, hats, jewelry, etc.
Encourage independence and reward patient for efforts to become independent
Allow patient sufficient time to accomplish a task; it may take a little longer
Encourage interaction with other children; take patient to playroom, have patient play a quiet game with roommate, etc.
Set aside time for school friends to visit child in hospital
Continue contact with school and schedule times for schoolwork so child does not fall behind
Involve child in ongoing community support group consisting of children with similar limitations

Expected outcome/evaluation

Patient verbalizes personal characteristics/attributes that patient likes about self

■ NDX: Altered family process related to chronic nature of disease and adjustment requirements for all family members

Discuss financial stress with parents

Discuss social stigma associated with disability

Discuss unresolved anger, guilt, jealousy, or grief

Assess how each family member is coping with disease

Assess ways in which child's disease has altered family functioning

Identify ways that each family member can participate in care of ill family member

Give family members insight into feelings of disabled child

Involve family in ongoing counseling

Access community resources as necessary to assist family with stress

Have family meet regularly with other families with a child with myelomeningocele

Expected outcome/evaluation

Family and/or child understand complexities of ongoing care; family members have adjusted to life with a child requiring extensive care

Family verbalizes feelings, cares for ill family member, supports each other, and uses resources appropriately

MENINGITIS

Inflammation of the meninges, usually caused by an infectious agent; bacterial viral, tubercular, or mycotic

Usual age: any; most common in infants and toddlers

Placement: patients with all types of bacterial meningitis are placed on respiratory isolation until treated for 24 hr with antibiotics

Viral (aseptic) meningitis warrants respiratory isolation for duration of hospitalization

Assessment
Observations/findings

History of preexisting infection

Irritability

Headache

Bulging anterior fontanel

Photophobia

High-pitched cry

Nuchal rigidity

Opisthotonos

Hyperactive deep tendon reflexes

Brudzinski's sign: flexing neck causes knees and hips to bend upward

Kernig's sign: leg flexed at hip cannot be straightened at knee

Disturbances in sensorium
   Delirum

Stupor

Poor feeding

Vomiting

Tachypnea

Tachycardia

Petechiae, purpuric spots with meningococcal meningitis

Laboratory/diagnostic studies

Lumbar puncture
   Bacterial
      May or may not be cloudy
      Low glucose, high protein
      High WBC: predominantly polymorphonuclear leukocytes
      Culture and sensitivities: identify specific organism and appropriate antibiotics
   Viral
      Normal glucose, normal or slightly elevated protein level
      Slightly elevated WBC: predominantly mononuclear leukocytes

Blood culture: may indicate septicemia

CBC: elevated WBC

Serum electrolytes: may be altered; serum sodium is monitored to assess for syndrome of inappropriate antidiuretic hormones (SIADH)

CT scan: may be indicated to evaluate for complications

Potential complications

Cerebral edema

Hydrocephalus

Brain abscess formation

Seizure disorder

Coma

Neurological loss: changes in behavior and motor development

Hearing loss, visual loss

SIADH

Shock (p. 105)

Disseminated Intravascular Coagulation (DIC) (p. 634)

Respiratory arrest (p. 223)

Death

Medical Management

Determination of causative organism

Respiratory or strict isolation depending on organism

Parenteral fluids given below maintenance requirements until resolution of SIADH

NPO initially, advancing diet from clear liquids to age-appropriate diet as tolerated; fluid restrictions may still prevail when diet is started; parenteral fluids are decreased as oral fluids increase

Intake and output
   High doses of intravenous antibiotics specific to isolated organism (wide spectrum coverage until organism can be isolated)

Antipyretics

Anticonvulsants if necessary

Steroids may be administered with intent of reducing sequela of deafness

Repeat lumbar puncture to assess effectiveness of therapy

Nursing diagnoses/interventions/evaluation

■ **NDX:** Sensory-perceptual alterations related to increased sensitivity to visual, auditory, and tactile stimulation

Assess child's level of consciousness, behavior, and level of irritability q1h to 2h

Check pupil response, ability to fix and follow, extraocular movements, response to sound, muscle tone, and reflexes q2h

Assess vital signs q2h and prn

Keep lights dimmed to prevent aggravation of photophobia

Talk to child in quiet, soothing tone

Allow patient to assume position of comfort with minimal handling

Encourage parents to provide comforting measures

Postpone nursing routines to decrease stimulation and allow for undisturbed sleep

Administer anticonvulsants if ordered and monitor serum levels

Gradually resume normal handling as status improves

Encourage preillness activity as muscular rigidity decreases

Have oxygen and suction available in the event that seizures occur

Expected outcome/evaluation

Patient

 Experiences reduced environmental stimulation until neurological sensitivity is decreased

 Tolerates age-appropriate stimulation before discharge

■ **NDX:** Hyperthermia related to inflammatory response to CNS infection

Assess temperature q2h to 4h and prn

Provide cooling measures prn; avoid cooling to point of shivering

Administer antibiotics as ordered

Administer parenteral fluids as ordered

Administer antipyretics as ordered

Control exposure to extremes in temperature

Keep room temperature moderately warm

Dress child in minimal clothing

Expected outcome/evaluation

Patient's temperature remains within age-appropriate temperature range

■ **NDX:** Potential fluid volume excess related to inappropriate release of antidiuretic hormone by pituitary (SIADH) unrelated to plasma osmolality

Monitor for signs and symptoms of SIADH

 Serum sodium below 130 mEq/L

 Decreased serum osmolality

 Decreased urinary output with rising specific gravities

 Elevated urine electrolytes and osmolality as compared with serum levels

 Weight gain

 Weakness and lethargy

Maintain strict measure of intake and output

Administer fluid-restrictive parenteral fluids as ordered

Gradually decrease parenteral fluid rate as oral intake increases to maintain fluid restrictions

Measure head circumference and assess fontanels for bulging q2h to 4h and prn

Expected outcome/evaluation

Patient's neurological status is not complicated by cerebral edema related to fluid retention

■ **NDX:** Knowledge deficit related to lack of information about nature of illness, home care, and follow-up needs

Explain reasons for restrictive activity, environmental stimulation, and fluids

Instruct persons to allow child to resume activity as tolerated with scheduled periods for rest

Discuss recurrence of symptoms to report to physician

 Poor feeding

 Vomiting

 Lethargy

 Irritability

 Fever

Explain need for follow-up assessment of child's visual and hearing development

Teach name of medication, purpose, dosage, time of administration, and side effects

Expected outcome/evaluation

Parents understand possible neurological sequelae and need for follow-up assessment

Patient and/or parents demonstrate understanding of treatment, and home care and follow-up instructions through actual return demonstration

Genitourinary System

ACUTE GLOMERULONEPHRITIS

An inflammatory process of the kidneys involving an antigen-antibody reaction secondary to an infection else-

where in the body; most common precipitating factor is group A beta-hemolytic streptococcus

Usual age: any; peak age is 5 years

Assessment
Observations/findings

Evidence of antecedent streptococcal infection
Hematuria: grossly bloody to smoky, brownish hue
Oliguria
Edema: facial, periorbital, slightly generalized
Weight gain
Headache
Anorexia
Vomiting
Fever
Diarrhea
Flank pain
Hypertension
Pallor
Anemia
Irritability
Lethargy
Mild to moderately elevated blood pressure

Laboratory/diagnostic studies

Urinalysis: proteinuria, elevated specific gravity, red blood cell casts, white blood cells
Blood studies
    Elevated BUN and creatinine
    Decreased serum complement activity
    Increased antistreptolysin O titer
    Mild leukocytosis
    Increased erythrocytic sedimentation rate
    C-reactive protein
    Mild anemia
Chest x-ray examination: pulmonary edema, pleural fluid, cardiac enlargement (seen with cardiac decompensation)
Throat culture
Electrocardiogram (ECG) if hyperkalemic

Potential complications

Hypertensive encephalopathy: headaches, drowsiness, restlessness, diplopia, dizziness, seizures, coma
Acute cardiac decompensation caused by hypervolemia: tachycardia, tachypnea, systolic murmur, pulmonary edema, orthopnea, abdominal distention
Acute renal failure (p. 482)
Chronic glomerulonephritis

Medical Management

Antihypertensives
Diuretics
Antibiotics with persistent streptococcal infection
Prophylactic antibiotics during convalescent period

Intake and output
Daily weight
Blood pressure q2h to 4h
Sodium-restricted diet
Potassium restriction until urine output is greater than 200 to 300 ml/day
Determination of fluid administration; may need to restrict if urine output is significantly scant; with restrictions, fluids are determined by urine output plus estimated insensible losses

Nursing diagnoses/interventions/evaluation

■ **NDX:** Fluid volume excess related to sodium and water retention secondary to decreased glomerular filtration rate

Assess vital signs with BP q2h to 4h and prn
Assess edema: color and texture of skin, areas of edema, degree of pitting
Weigh patient daily at same time with same clothing and scale
Measure intake and output
Determine specific gravity on all voided specimens
Check character and quantity of urinary output; initiate daily specimen for visual comparison
Administer fluids based on urinary output plus estimated insensible loss if ordered
Administer diuretics if ordered
Anticipate diuresis in 3 to 4 days with increased urinary output and clearing of urine color

Expected outcome/evaluation

Patient's
    Fluid balance is maintained at normal levels
    Urine output returns to normal
    Edema disappears

■ **NDX:** Altered nutrition: less than body requirements related to anorexia, fatigue, and dietary restrictions

Monitor electrolyte values to determine discontinuation of dietary restrictions
Maintain diet as ordered
    Low-protein diet with severe azotemia
    Low-potassium diet if documented hyperkalemic and during oliguric stage
    Regular diet with *no salt added*
Offer foods child likes
Have parents bring in favorite food from home if possible
Promote socialization during mealtime; have child eat with other children or with family when possible

Expected outcome/evaluation

Patient has a nutritional intake adequate to meet metabolic requirements

■ **NDX:** Activity intolerance related to lethargy, anemia, and/or fatigue

Maintain bed rest as ordered
Encourage quiet diversional play activities
Encourage educational activity appropriate for age
Encourage ambulation after diuresis occurs and blood pressure and weight have stabilized
Let child determine appropriate level of activity with guidance (usually children restrict their own activity voluntarily)
Schedule rest periods throughout the day

Expected outcome/evaluation

Patient resumes preillness activity level before discharge

■ **NDX:** Potential alteration in sensory/perceptual ability related to altered level of consciousness secondary to hypertensive encephalopathy

Assess sensorium, mental responsiveness, and vision prn
Be prepared to intervene if seizure activity occurs
Administer antihypertensive medication as ordered
Evaluate blood pressure q2h and before administering antihypertensives
Regulate fluids as ordered
Administer diuretics if ordered
Keep patient on bed rest with quiet activities as ordered

Expected outcome/evaluation

Patient's blood pressure is age appropriate
Patient is alert and oriented

■ **NDX:** Knowledge deficit related to lack of information about home care and follow-up needs

Explain need for planned rest periods and avoidance of fatigue
Caution patient and/or parents that outdoor games and sports and strenuous activity are to be avoided until there is no microscopic evidence of disease
Explain that clinical symptoms resolve in 7 to 10 days; however, laboratory findings persist for several weeks to months
Reassure patient and/or parents that recurrence is uncommon
Discuss diet: usually regular with no restrictions
Explain need to avoid individuals with known infections
Emphasize need for continued schooling
Emphasize need for continued peer contact
Teach name of medication, purpose, dosage, time of administration, and side effects
Emphasize need for ongoing outpatient care

Expected outcome/evaluation

Patient and/or parents demonstrate understanding of home care and follow-up instructions

NEPHROSIS (NEPHROTIC SYNDROME)

A syndrome resulting from degenerative changes in the kidneys without inflammation

Usual age: any, most commonly 2 to 4 years

Assessment
Observations/findings

Edema: severe, generalized, dependent
Oliguria
Dark, frothy urine
Weight gain: weight may double
Facial puffiness (around eyes, especially upon rising in the morning and dimishing later in day)
Normal blood pressure
Anorexia
Lassitude, easily fatigued
Irritability
Malnutrition
Ascites (abdominal swelling)
Diarrhea
Vomiting
Pallor, with or without anemia
Decreased activity tolerance
Respiratory difficulty

Laboratory/diagnostic studies

Urine
  Proteinuria, mainly albumin
  Casts
  Red blood cells
  Increased specific gravity
Creatinine clearance test: normal
Serum
  Hypoalbuminemia
  Hyperlipidemia
  Sodium

Potential complications

Umbilical and inguinal hernias
Rectal prolapse
Respiratory distress
Sepsis
Peritonitis
Malnutrition
Relapse
Renal failure

Medical Management

Corticosteroid therapy
For patient who is steroid resistant, cyclophosphamide in combination with steroid therapy is used

Diuretics may be used in some cases, even though the edema does not usually respond to diuretic therapy

Salt-poor albumin may be used

High-protein diet; avoidance of highly salted foods

Prophylactic broad-spectrum antibiotics to decrease risk of infection until child is on tapering dose of steroids

Eye irrigations/ophthalmic creams for eye irritation from severe edema

Nursing diagnoses/interventions/evaluation

■ **NDX:** Altered fluid volume: excess volume in interstitial spaces related to shifting of fluid from plasma to interstitial spaces, glomerular permeability to protein, and sodium and water retention; potential for fluid deficit—hypovolemia related to shifting of fluid from vascular space to interstitial spaces

Weigh patient daily

Measure intake and output

Determine specific gravity on all voided specimens

Assess degree of edema

Measure abdominal girth to monitor degree of ascites

Administer corticosteroids as ordered

Administer diuretics if ordered

Administer salt-poor albumin if ordered

Administer fluids orally as desired; *do not restrict*

Anticipate diuresis in 3 to 4 days with weight loss, increased urinary output, and decreased specific gravities

Be aware that dehydration from hypovolemia can occur in spite of excess fluid retention

Monitor for signs of hypovolemia, especially pulse quality and rate, and blood pressure

Expected outcome/evaluation

Patient

Has decreased edema and increased urinary output with decreasing specific gravities

Shows no signs of dehydration

■ **NDX:** Altered nutrition: less than body requirements related to anorexia, fatigue, and/or dietary restrictions

Plan meals and dietary approach with team consisting of nurse, dietician, parents, and child

Anticipate that high-protein diet may not be desirable to child

Make meals attractive

Give small portions more frequently

Honor food likes and dislikes

Use creative play techniques to encourage eating (games, rewards, and special treats)

Have parents feed child

Make mealtime a social time; have child eat with other children or with parents

Record food intake for calorie count evaluation

Administer diet as ordered: *no added salt*

Expected outcome/evaluation

Patient consumes adequate age/weight-appropriate caloric intake to meet metabolic demands

■ **NDX:** Altered skin integrity related to generalized edema

Assess color and texture of skin and degree of pitting (especially around eyes and dependent areas)

Elevate head on pillows to decrease periorbital edema

Keep skin warm and dry; pay particular attention to creases, fingers, and toes; use dry cloth or cotton to keep fingers and toes separated; *do not* use powders

Turn patient q2h and prn while on bed rest

Administer skin care to pressure areas q1h to 2h

Place pillows under and between legs to avoid pressure

Provide scrotal support, especially when ambulatory

Administer warm saline eye irrigations q2h to 4h

Use ophthalmic ointments as ordered

Expected outcome/evaluation

Patient's skin remains intact

■ **NDX:** Potential for infection related to increased susceptibility secondary to edema and corticosteroid therapy

Assess temperature, pulse, and respirations q4h and prn

Assess for signs of pulmonary and skin infections

Avoid persons with infections, especially URIs

Administer prophylactic antibiotics as ordered

Tell parents that child should not receive immunizations until he is no longer receiving steroids and is free of proteinuria

Expected outcome/evaluation

Patient does not demonstrate signs of infection

■ **NDX:** Activity intolerance related to fatigue

Maintain bed rest as ordered

Encourage quiet diversional play activities

Encourage educational activity appropriate for age

Encourage ambulation after diuresis occurs and blood pressure and weight have stabilized

Let child determine appropriate level of activity with guidance (usually children restrict their own activity voluntarily)

Schedule rest periods throughout the day

Expected outcome/evaluation

Patient resumes preillness activity level before discharge

■ **NDX:** Potential disturbance in body image related to rapid changes in body size and side effects of steroid therapy

Encourage patient to express feelings about self
Encourage patient to ask questions about diagnosis and treatment
Give patient encouraging information: altered body changes are temporary and reversible
Avoid reference to patient's weight or size
Promote social interaction
Promote physical activity within tolerance
Allow child access to mirror to provide visualization of self
Point out improvements in degree of edema as they occur

Expected outcome/evaluation

Patient verbalizes characteristics/attributes that patient likes about self

■ **NDX:** Knowledge deficit related to lack of information about home care and follow-up needs

Explain nature of disease
Explain need for normal activity with planned rest periods
Discuss diet: well-balanced, adequate protein; fluids as desired, no restrictions
Explain need to avoid persons with URIs
Emphasize importance of encouraging social interaction
Discuss symptoms of recurrence to report to physician
   Weight gain
   Increasing edema
   Decreasing or absent urine output
Teach name of medications, purpose, dosage, time of administration, and side effects
   Side effects of corticosteroids to anticipate: round face, increased appetite, increased hair, abdominal distention, mood swings
Have parents and/or patient demonstrate urine testing for albumin if ordered

Expected outcome/evaluation

Patient and/or parents demonstrate understanding of home care and follow-up instructions

Hematology

ACUTE LEUKEMIA

A disease characterized by uncontrolled proliferation of leukocyte precursors in blood, bone marrow, and reticuloendothelial tissues

Usual age: any; best prognosis is in child between 2 and 9 years of age

Assessment
Observations/findings
INSIDIOUS ONSET

Moderate pallor
Anorexia
Weight loss
Irritability
Abdominal pain
Malaise
Joint pains
Persistent low-grade fever
Bleeding from gums
Epistaxis
Tendency to bruise
Fatigue
Shortness of breath with exertion

ABRUPT ONSET

Fever
Tachypnea
Tachycardia
Abdominal pain
Drop in Hgb
Marked pallor
Purpura
Bone pain
Lymphadenopathy
Hemorrhagic episodes from any orifice
Buccal mucosa ulcerations
Hemorrhagic skin eruptions
Hepatomegaly
Splenomegaly
CNS leukemia infiltration
   Nausea
   Vomiting
   Headache
   Lethargy
   Irritability
   Dizziness
   Ataxia
   Convulsions
   Nuchal rigidity
Infection

Laboratory/diagnostic studies

Bone marrow aspiration/biopsy: to identify presence of blasts in marrow, to identify specific cell type involved, and to isolate null cell, T cell, and B cell markers
Chromosome analysis
Lumbar puncture: to confirm presence or absence of CNS leukemic infiltrates
Chest x-ray examination: to identify mediastinal masses
CBC with differential
   WBC: normal, depressed, or elevated
   Presence of blasts in peripheral circulation
   Thrombocytopenia

Platelet count <40,000/mm³
Identification of prognostic factors: *best prognosis*
  Age: between 2 and 9 years
  WBC <10,000/mm³
  Leukemia type: acute lymphoid leukemia (ALL)

Potential complications

Severe systemic infection
Hemorrhage
Relapse
Permanent side effects from chemotherapy/radiation: cardiomyopathy, learning disabilities
Death

Medical Management

Identification of specific type of leukemia
Determination of combination of chemotherapeutic agents to use based on type, prognostic factors, and stage of treatment (induction, consolidation, maintenance, reinduction)
Insertion of central venous catheter as appropriate
Xanthine-oxidase inhibitor (allopurinol)
Corticosteroids
Determination of CNS prevention or treatment approach: cranial irradiation, intrathecal chemotherapeutic agents, or both
Testicular biopsies in males
Testicular irradiation as necessary
Bone marrow transplantation may be considered
Treatment of complications of myelosuppression
  Protective room/bed placement during neutropenia
  Blood products as necessary: packed red blood cells (PRBCs) or platelets
  Antibiotics for ongoing infection
  Antiemetics
  Nystatin for oral *Candida albicans*
  Parenteral fluids to ensure adequate hydration when patient is receiving chemotherapeutic agents that may cause hemorrhagic cystitis
  TPN for nutritional deficit
Childhood immunizations are withheld with bone marrow depression

Nursing diagnoses/interventions/evaluation

■ **NDX:** Potential for infection related to decreased body defenses associated with neutropenia

Monitor temperature closely (*no rectal temperatures*)
Be aware that common signs of infection (redness, swelling, pus) may be missing because WBCs necessary for such responses are lacking
Administer antibiotics as ordered
Administer granulocyte transfusions as ordered

Avoid unnecessary exposure to potential sources of infection
  Scrupulous handwashing by all individuals before contact with patient
  Place in private room when patient is neutropenic
  Avoid exposure to individuals with known infections
  Use aseptic technique in caring for central venous catheter or puncture sites
Ensure adequate nutritional intake
Do *not* administer immunizations during neutropenia
If child is exposed to communicable diseases, gamma globulin may be ordered

Expected outcome/evaluation

Patient is protected from infectious organism as evidenced by absence of any sign of infection

■ **NDX:** Activity intolerance related to generalized weakness associated with anemia

Observe for signs of anemia: pallor, irritability, intolerance of normal activity, low Hgb levels
Determine patient's tolerance for activity
  Allow independence as tolerated and desired by patient
  Accept need for dependence when demonstrated
Encourage quiet bedside activities
Have planned rest periods throughout the day
Change position and provide back and pressure point care prn
Consider use of water bed or air mattress
Transfuse with PRBCs as ordered

Expected outcome/evaluation

Patient participates in age-appropriate activity in a time frame that is appropriate for the activity without complaints of tiredness/weakness

■ **NDX:** Potential for injury: bleeding related to decreased platelet counts

Postpone use of intramuscular injections and suppositories
Avoid play activity that may result in physical injury
Do not allow toys with sharp edges or points
Apply pressure for 5 to 10 min after venipuncture sticks
If nosebleed occurs, pinch nostrils against nasal septum, applying constant pressure for at least 10 min
Do *not use* aspirin or aspirin-containing products
Administer platelet transfusion as ordered
Administer maximum intravenous fluids prior to, during, and afer cyclophosphamide administration and have patient void frequently to prevent hemorrhagic cystitis

Expected outcome/evaluation

Patient does not sustain preventable trauma and has minimal/absent bleeding from nares

■ **NDX:** Altered oral mucous membrane: stomatitis-thrush related to side effects of chemotherapeutic agents

Administer oral hygiene using half-normal saline and half-hydrogen peroxide solution or diluted mouthwash prn, especially after meals

Use soft toothbrush or sponge toothettes

Administer systemic or topical anesthetics as ordered for severe pain

Allow patient to suck on ice cubes or frozen fruit-flavored ices to lessen pain from sores

Administer nystatin mouth rinse as ordered

Avoid use of lemon glycerin swabs since they are drying to mucous membranes

Expected outcome/evaluation

Patient's mucous membranes are intact and free of lesions or, if lesions are present, resultant discomfort is minimal

■ **NDX:** Altered nutrition: less than body requirements related to anorexia, malaise, nausea, and vomiting side effects of chemotherapy, and/or stomatitis

In the presence of stomatitis offer nonirritating, bland foods at moderate temperature

Monitor intake and output and dietary intake; if insufficient amounts are consumed, administer parenteral fluids or TPN as ordered

Administer antiemetics before giving chemotherapy and during administration of chemotherapy as ordered

Anticipate that child will have alternating periods of hunger and anorexia

Encourage intake of high-quality, high-calorie food of child's preference during periods of hunger

Do not force or make an issue of eating during times of anorexia; liquids may be the only thing tolerated

Allow child to participate in preparation of food if possible

Serve creative, appealing food items in small, frequent servings

Allow child choices in choosing what and when he wants to eat

Allow parents to bring favorite foods from home if feasible

Consult dietician for assistance in obtaining appealing foods and nutritional supplementation

Monitor weight daily

Expected outcome/evaluation

Patient's intake is adequate to meet metabolic demands

■ **NDX:** Pain related to physiological effects of leukemia

Organize routine nursing activities to minimize handling of patient

Maintain proper body alignment

Consider use of waterbed or air mattress

Use methods of distraction such as relaxation, breathing techniques, soft music, and guided imagery

Administer analgesics as ordered

Analgesics should be given on a round-the-clock schedule to prevent pain

When intravenous infusions of analgesics are used, the dose should be slowly titrated until maximum pain control is achieved

Alleviate any parental fears about addiction

Expected outcome/evaluation

Patient
   Reports that he is comfortable most of the time
   Denies experiencing pain for extended periods of time

■ **NDX:** Disturbance in body image related to alopecia and/or rapid changes in body appearance ranging from weight loss to weight gain secondary to treatment

Encourage patient to express feelings about self

Encourage patient to ask questions about diagnosis and treatment

Give patient encouraging information: hair will grow back, weight loss and gain fluctuations are a result of treatment and will resolve once therapy is discontinued

Promote social interaction, especially peer contact, on a regular basis

Explore possibility of wearing wigs, caps, scarves, or no head covering at all to enhance self-image (suggest purchase of wig to match hair color before hair loss occurs, if possible)

Expected outcome/evaluation

Patient verbalizes personal characteristics/attributes that patient likes about self

■ **NDX:** Potential for ineffective coping: individual and family related to diagnosis and treatment regimen

Provide consistency in care by limiting number of people caring for patient

Develop a trusting relationship with patient and family

Give them honest, accurate information

Clarify any misconceptions

Have a positive approach when possible

Determine patient and/or family's knowledge of condition and prognosis; be sensitive to their need to verbalize feelings

Recognize that parents may need to verbalize feelings of guilt, hostility, grief, or fear

Assess coping mechanisms, problem-solving abilities, and use of religious or counseling assistance

Involve parents in care of their child to the extent that *they wish* to be involved

Encourage parents to continue normal interactions with their child

Make appropriate referrals to support groups and community services

Assist patient and/or parents in explaining the disease to other family members, friends, teachers, etc.

Expected outcome/evaluation

Patient and family have adequate internal and external resources to cope effectively with diagnosis as evidenced by their verbalization of same

■ **NDX:** Knowledge deficit related to lack of information about disease process, home care, and follow-up needs

Explain nature of disease and treatment

Explain that patient and parents can anticipate at least 2 to 3 years of treatment

Explain need

For planned rest periods

To return to normal activities as tolerated

To avoid individuals with known infections

For high-quality dietary intake

For continued social contact and home teaching if activity is restricted to home environment

For good oral hygiene

For ongoing follow-up care

Discuss symptoms to report to physician

Fever

Increased fatigue

Bleeding or bruising

Pain

Teach importance of handwashing to avoid self-inoculation with infectious agents

Teach name of medication, purpose, dosage, time of administration, and side effects

Expected outcome/evaluation

Patient and/or parents feel capable of coping with diagnosis and treatment implications and are knowledgeable about home care needs

FAILURE TO THRIVE (FTT)

A general term indicating a child who fails to grow (falls more than two standard deviations below the mean height and weight for age and sex or fails to maintain a previously established growth pattern) and is developmentally delayed as part of a disease process; in its simplest sense it is a presenting symptom of an organic problem; in its most complex form it is a syndrome involving psychosocial disruption

Usual age: infant or toddler

Assessment
Observations/findings

Child admitted with this symptom is given a thorough assessment of all body systems; a possible organic cause for failure to thrive is thoroughly investigated, and nurse assists with various specimen collections and testings that are done; some 50% or more cases have a psychosocial etiology; in addition, varying degrees of psychosocial disruption occur, even with an organic cause; therefore, the nurse will assess for nonorganic indices as follows

Weight, height, head circumference below fifth percentile

Delayed physical and social development

Dull affect; apathy

Poor hygiene

Withdrawal behavior

No fear of strangers

Avoidance of eye contact: "radar gaze"

Minimal smiling or babbling

Stiffening on being held close or flaccidity and unresponsiveness

Eating disorders: self-induced vomiting, anorexia, pica, voracious appetite

Observations during mealtime

Child's reaction to food: resists and becomes irritable; spits food out; is easily distracted; is passive during meals

Mother's behavior during mealtime: tries to keep child too clean; offers too much or too little; is easily frustrated; forces child to eat

Assessment of mother-child interaction

Does child recognize mother as different from others?

Does child seek out mother?

Does mother respond? How?

Is mother sensitive to needs of her child?

Child's temperament: passive, active, fussy

Self-stimulating behaviors: head banging, thumb sucking, rocking, biting of lower lip

Is child held close, at arm's distance, turned out, or toward mother?

Does mother have realistic expectations for child?

Does mother play and talk with child?

Mother's perception of child: what does she say?

Additional assessment

Is mother-father relationship intact? Good or stressed?

Was pregnancy planned or unplanned?

How is the development of the other children?

What are their financial resources?

Who feeds child at home—consistent person or many different people?

Care giver's eating habits and knowledge of infant/toddler nutrition

Prenatal history, including reaction to pregnancy, stressors during pregnancy, and feelings toward baby

Mother's feelings about herself: be *alert* to the following

Maternal deprivation as child

Low self-concept

Stressful life with limited support system

Negative verbalizations about infant: ugly, smells, spits up, is irritable

Unrealistic expectations for infant

Poor interaction with infant: poor eye contact, little verbalization, no enthusiasm

Not responsive to needs of child: does not recognize when infant is tired, hungry, or soiled

Insists that something physical is wrong with child

Negative statements about role as mother

After admission, mother visits infrequently, misses meetings, etc.

Laboratory/diagnostic studies

CBC: often anemic

X-ray examination of long bones: determines skeletal age of bone (often delayed)

Development screening tests: identify delays in motor and social development

Several diagnostic studies are performed to identify organic cause for failure to thrive (see Failure to Thrive: Organic Workup, p. 818)

Potential complications

Child abuse

Metabolic dysfunction

Temporary placement in foster care

Medical Management

Organic cause for growth delay ruled out

Treatment of organic cause if identified

Provision of food/fluids to promote weight gain

Close community follow-up

Monitoring and evaluation of growth and development

Nursing diagnoses/interventions/evaluation

■ **NDX:** Altered nutrition: less than body requirements related to maternal deprivation

Weigh child daily: before meals, same time, same scale, naked

Keep calorie count

Keep stool record

Assign consistent care givers

Consult dietician: meet with family for nutritional teaching

Calculate caloric and fluid requirements (p. 841)

Consider the following feeding interventions

Promote a positive, nurturing environment, especially during mealtime

Keep stimulation to a minimum to avoid distraction; feed in private room if available

Always hold infant for bottle feeding

Talk softly to child and encourage eye contact

Avoid conversation with others while feeding; this is *child's* time

Set 30 min time limit for meal

Give bottle at end of meal; take bottle away after 20 min or if child is playing with it but not drinking it

If child is hungry between meals, give water only

Avoid excessive stimulation for 1 hr after meals; use soft music, vocalizations, and holding

Some children may benefit from small, frequent meals and frequent burping until able to tolerate volume of food required to meet daily metabolic requirements

Expected outcome/evaluation

Maintains age-appropriate diet reflecting adequate caloric intake

Shows progressive weight gain

■ **NDX:** Altered growth and development related to insufficient stimulation at home from primary care giver

Assist child in responding meaningfully to environment

Respond to child's cues: pick him up when he cries; verbalize to child when he babbles, etc.

Respond to child with vigor and enthusiasm

Coordinate child's daily schedule to include four to five stimulation sessions per day; each session should last only 10 to 15 min and should not be scheduled immediately before or after meals

Idenfify very specific developmental goals; each stimulation session should focus on one specific goal; for example

At 10 AM child is scheduled for gross motor stimulation

A specific goal might be: child will sit without support

For the next 15 min, stimulation is geared toward improving back and stomach muscles and balance

Consult physical therapists and/or occupational therapists as needed

Teach parents age-appropriate growth and development

Teach parents appropriate stimulation to promote growth and development

Expected outcome/evaluation

Patient shows signs of increased physical and emotional development as recorded on standardized developmental screening tests (Denver Developmental Screening Test [DDST] is frequently used)

■ **NDX:** Altered parenting related to inadequate support system, difficulty in coping with stress, and/or lack of parenting skills

Assess parent-child interactions, reinforcing any improvements in the parents' ability to identify their child's needs

Keep record of parental visiting and calling patterns

Realize that parents are under a great deal of stress at home and that this is complicated by their child's hospitalization

Establish rapport with parents; encourage sharing of feelings toward parenthood and child

Have parents discuss stressors in their life right now: financial, relationships, housing, difficulty in adjusting to new baby, recent losses, etc.

Be aware that mother, in particular, may have poor self-concept; give her positive feedback in her attempts to mother her child

Contract with parents; set up times for them to come in or call hospital (if they are unable to find transportation to hospital) to discuss care

Discuss child's progress with them

Encourage them to be involved in their child's care

Allow parents to participate in planning of child's schedule

Explain reasons for such routines

Assess parents' understanding of infant care; do not assume that they are just neglectful—they may not have learned skills

Give parents verbal and written information about infant's diet, growth and development, and age-appropriate stimulation

If parents are unable to cope with care of their child because of stressors in their home environment and no improvement is seen in their ability to relate to their child, then temporary placement in a foster home may be necessary; reinforce to parents that this is *temporary* and done as a means to assist them with their crisis; make certain that parents are referred appropriately to receive the assistance they need; make appropriate referrals to improve the support system

Visiting Nurse's Association

Early intervention/developmental programs

Social service agencies

Psychiatric services

Make certain a primary physician is identified to follow child's progress on an outpatient basis

Expected outcome/evaluation

Parents improve their coping abilities, identify and respond appropriately to their child's needs, and verbalize positive feelings regarding infant

Failure to Thrive: Organic Workup

General disease states

Infection

CBC

Red blood cell indices

Erythrocyte sedimentation rate

Purified protein derivative or tuberculin test

Serology

Nose, throat, stool, and urine cultures

Chest x-ray examination

Coccidioidomycosis and histoplasmosis skin tests

Infection

Scabies

Pediculosis

Stool ovum slides

Parasite and ameba

Pinworm slides

Nutrition: diet testing

Metabolism

Random blood sugar

BUN

Amino acid assays

Carbon dioxide level

Sodium level

Potassium level

Chloride level

Calcium level

Phosphorus level

Chronic intoxication: lead level

Malfunction of organ system

Central nervous system

Skull x-ray examination

Electroencephalogram (EEG)

CT scan

GI system

Stool fat and trypsin

Stool pH and reducing substances

Occult blood

D-Xylose tolerance tests

GI series

Barium enema

Liver function tests

Genitourinary system

Urinalysis

Urine concentration tests

Intravenous pyelogram

Cardiovascular system: ECG

Endocrine system

Protein-bound iodine level

Triiodothyronine level (T_3)

Thyroxine level (T_4)

17-Ketosteroid level

Glucose tolerance test

Growth hormone

Hematopoietic system

Sickle cell prep

Serum iron level

Bilirubin level

Respiratory system

Sweat test

Pulmonary function tests
Chromosomal or genetic disorder
  Buccal smear
  Karyotyping
  Urine for amino acids
Prenatal infection
  Rubella titer
  Cytomegalovirus culture
  Toxoplasmosis test
  Herpes

Cardiovascular System

CONGENITAL HEART DEFECTS

Noncyanotic (Acyanotic)

PATENT DUCTUS ARTERIOSUS (PDA) (Figure 16-13)

Persistence of blood flow through the fecal ductus arter-iosus, between the aorta and the main pulmonary ar-tery

Assessment
Observations/findings

INFANT

Prematurity
Respiratory distress syndrome
Congestive heart failure (CHF) (p. 835)
Tachycardia
Bounding pedal pulses
Hepatomegaly
Splenomegaly

OLDER CHILD

Exertional dyspnea
Physical underdevelopment
Widened pulse pressure

ANY AGE

Loud, continuous "machinery" heart murmur heard throughout systole and diastole: mid to upper left sternal border

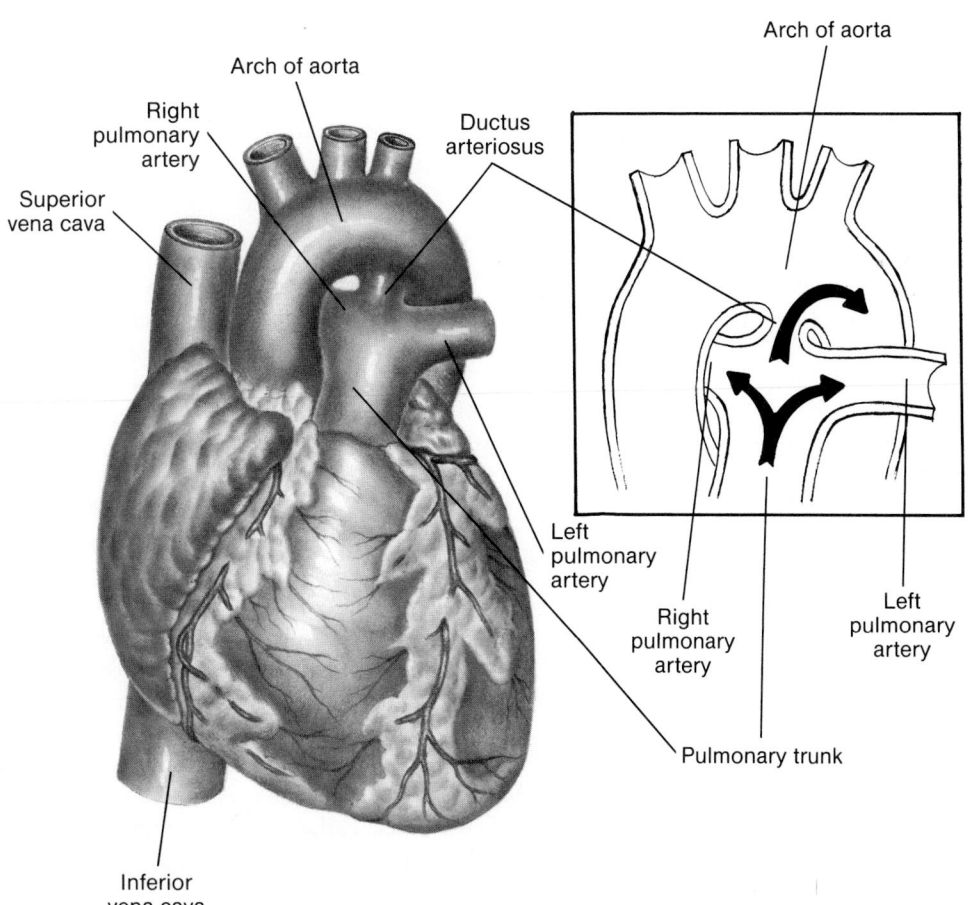

FIGURE 16-13. Patent ductus arteriosus. (From Canobbio MM: *Cardiovascular disorders, Mosby's clinical nursing series,* St Louis, 1990, Mosby–Year Book.)

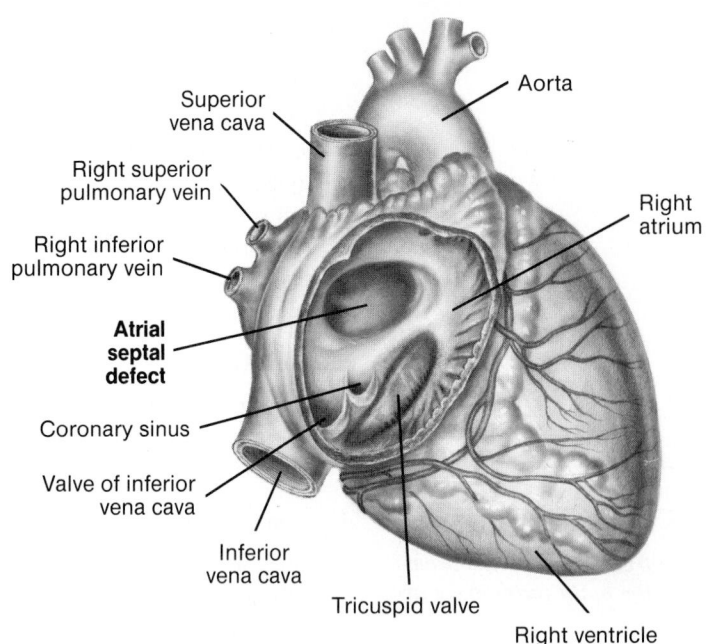

FIGURE 16-14. Atrial septal defect. (From Canobbio MM: *Cardiovascular disorders, Mosby's clinical nursing series,* St Louis, 1990, Mosby–Year Book.)

Laboratory/diagnostic studies

ECG: normal or left ventricular hypertrophy

X-ray examination: prominent pulmonary arteries, enlarged left ventricle

Echocardiogram: detects presence of PDA

Cardiac catheterization: confirms presence of defect: provides visualization of size; demonstrates increased pressures in pulmonary artery and right ventricle and presence of oxygenated blood in pulmonary artery

Potential complications

Pulmonary hypertension

After corrective surgery

Phrenic nerve injury

Subacute bacterial endocarditis (p. 91)

Medical Management

Treatment of CHF (p. 835) with fluid restriction, diuretics, and digitalization

In premature infant indomethacin is used to enhance PDA closure (this pharmacological approach does not work in older children)

Closed heart surgical intervention: ligation of PDA

PDA "plug" during cardiac catheterization may be used; this technique remains experimental

Antibiotic prophylaxis with dental work or other surgical procedures

ATRIAL SEPTAL DEFECT (ASD) (Figure 16-14)

An abnormal opening between two atria; may result from persistance of blood flow through the fetal fora-men ovale (ostium secundum) or a defect in the intraatrial septum (a low-septum is called ostium primum ASD and is often associated with a cleft mitral valve); results in some degree of left-to-right blood shunting

Assessment
Observations/findings

Symptoms vary according to size of defect

Most children are asymptomatic

Normal growth and development

Normal exercise tolerance

Soft systolic ejection murmur over second to third interspace along left sternal border is heard on examination

Ostium primum ADS with associated valve abnormalities: CHF (p. 835)

Laboratory/diagnostic studies

ECG: right ventricular hypertrophy (RVH); prolonged PR interval possible; varying degrees of heart block possible

Radiology: enlarged right atrium, right ventricle, and pulmonary artery

Echocardiogram: location of defect, size of shunt, right ventricular enlargement

Cardiac catheterization: confirms diagnosis and location of defect; oxygen content of right atrium is higher than that of superior vena cava

Potential complications

If ASD remains undetected until adulthood

CHF (p. 835)

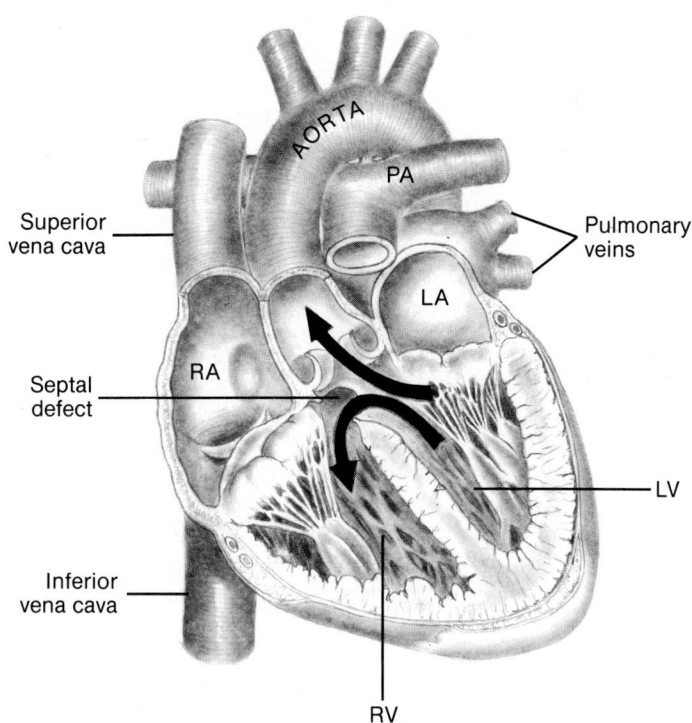

FIGURE 16-15. Ventricular septal defect. (From Canobbio MM: *Cardiovascular disorders, Mosby's clinical nursing series,* St Louis, 1990, Mosby–Year Book.)

Pulmonary vascular disease
After corrective cardiac surgery
   Transient pulmonary edema
   Heart block
   Hemorrhage
   Subacute bacterial endocarditis (p. 91)

Medical Management

CHF management (p. 835) for children with ostium primum ASD with associated valve abnormalities

Open-heart surgical intervention: closure of ASD with suture of small defect or Dacron patch on large defect

Nonoperative closure may be attempted using an ASD "umbrella," which is inserted during cardiac catheterization; this technique is presently experimental

Antibiotic prophylaxis with dental work or other surgical procedures

VENTRICULAR SEPTAL DEFECT (VSD) (Figure 16-15)

An abnormal opening between ventricles; results in left-to-right shunting of blood; often associated with other defects; can occur in either the membranous (usually moderate to large defects) or the muscular portion (usually small) of the ventricular septum

Assessment
Observations/findings

Dependent on amount of blood flow through defect
Minimal blood flow: asymptomatic
With large VSDs seen in infants

Dyspnea
Tachypnea
Tachycardia
Recurrent pulmonary infection
Feeding difficulties
Poor growth
Profuse diaphoresis
CHF (p. 835)
Rumbling or harsh pansystolic murmur is heard best at left lower sternal border and may radiate throughout precordium (not necessarily indicative of severity of defect)

Laboratory/diagnostic studies

ECG: left ventricular hypertrophy or bilateral ventricular hypertrophy
Radiology: cardiomegaly
Echocardiogram: presence of defect and quantity of shunting
Cardiac catheterization: exact size and location of defect and quantity of shunting

Potential complications

Pulmonary artery hypertension: if it progresses to degree that right ventricular pressure is greater than left ventricular pressure, blood will flow right-to-left (Eisenmenger's complex)
Pneumonia
After corrective surgery

Heart block
Residual shunt
Subacute bacterial endocarditis (p. 91)

Medical Management

CHF management (p. 835)
Palliative closed-heart surgery done with severe VSDs or those with associated complex lesions: pulmonary artery banding (PAB)—reduces diameter of pulmonary artery to decrease blood flow through pulmonary artery to lungs
Corrective open-heart surgery: closure of ventricular septal defect with either suture of small defect or Dacron patching of large defect
Antibiotic prophylaxis with dental work or other surgical procedures

COARCTATION OF AORTA (Figure 16-16)

Narrowing of the aorta, usually occurring beyond the left subclavian artery at the area of the ductus insertion; often associated with patent ductus arteriosus and aortic valve defects

Assessment
Observations/findings

NEONATE

Decreased or absent femoral pulses
Poor perfusion
Elevated blood pressure in upper extremities
Decreased blood pressure in lower extremities
Bounding pulses in upper extremities
CHF (p. 835)

OLDER CHILD (MOST COMMON PRESENTATION)

Decreased femoral pulses
Cold feet

Increased BP in upper extremities
Decreased BP in lower extremities
Epistaxis
Headache

ANY AGE

Systolic murmur possible and variable

Laboratory/diagnostic studies

ECG: usually normal
Radiology: dilated ascending aorta, cardiomegaly or normal heart size
Echocardiogram: may visualize segment of coarctation
Cardiac catheterization: confirms diagnosis, visualization of defect, and degree of narrowing

Potential complications

Damage to aorta: becomes thin and calcified as a result of persistently high pressures
Aneurysms in intercostal arteries
Cerebral hemorrhage
CHF (p. 835)
Subacute bacterial endocarditis (p. 91)
After corrective surgery
    Hypertension
    Restenosis
    Phrenic nerve injury

Medical Management

With significant hypertension in older child
    Antihypertensives
    Exercise restriction
CHF management (p. 835)
In infants who depend on patency of ductus arteriosus to provide adequate systemic blood flow, prostaglandins are used to keep ductus open until surgical correction is possible

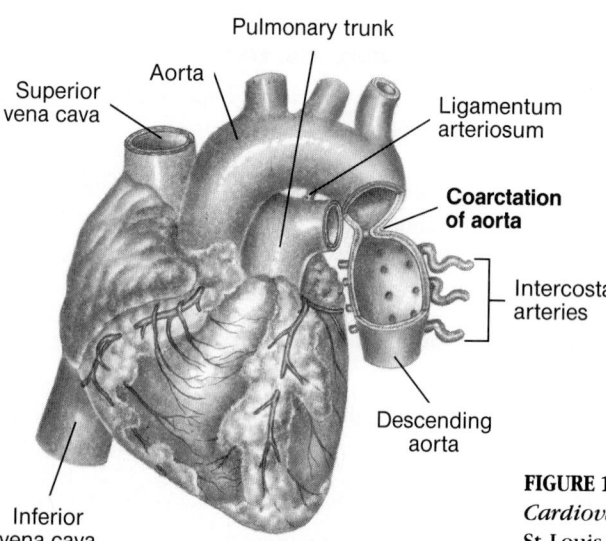

FIGURE 16-16. Coarctation of the aorta. (From Canobbio MM: *Cardiovascular disorders, Mosby's clinical nursing series,* St Louis, 1990, Mosby–Year Book.)

Closed-heart surgery
  End-to-end anastomosis *or*
  Insertion of graft replacement *or*
  Subclavian arterioplasty (infants): take down subclavian artery and use as live tissue patch for aorta
  Gore-Tex patch: patch is placed over top of aorta, allowing growth of live aortic tissue as child grows
In some children who have spontaneous recurrence of coarctation, nonoperative dilation may be done by angioplasty (balloon is inflated in narrowed area during cardiac catheterization); this procedure is still experimental
Antibiotic prophylaxis with dental work or other surgical procedures

AORTIC STENOSIS (Figure 16-17)

Narrowing or stricture of the aortic valve; stricture may be valvar, supravalvar, or subvalvar

Assessment
Observations/findings

Dependent on degree of outflow obstruction
Severe obstruction
  Symptoms occur in infancy
  Poor growth
  Poor perfusion
  Faint peripheral pulses
  Narrow pulse pressures
  CHF (p. 835)
Minimal obstruction in older child
  May be asymptomatic
  Chest pain
  Syncope

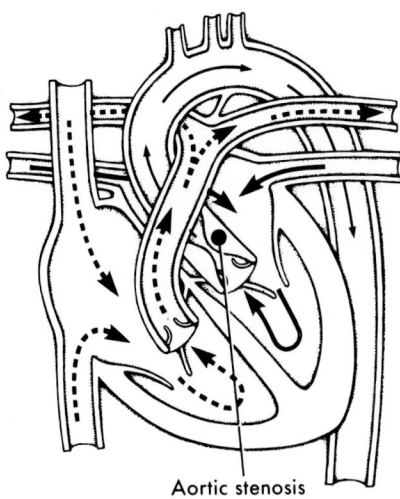

FIGURE 16-17. Aortic stenosis. (From Whaley LF, Wong DL: *Essentials of pediatric nursing*, ed 3, St Louis, 1989, Mosby–Year Book.)

Exercise intolerance
Dyspnea
Fatigue
Narrow pulse pressures
Harsh systolic ejection murmur: best heard in aortic area

Laboratory/diagnostic studies

ECG: left ventricular hypertrophy (LVH); can be normal
Radiology: LVH and enlargement of ascending aorta
Echocardiogram: thickening of aortic valve visualized; level of lesion is identified; quantitative analysis of left ventricular pressure
Cardiac catheterization: confirms diagnosis; demonstrates magnitude and site of pressure gradient from left ventricle to aorta

Potential complications

Sudden death with idiopathic hypertrophic subaortic stenosis (IHSS)
After corrective surgery
  Persistent stenosis
  Restenosis
  Aortic valve insufficiency
  Subacute bacterial endocarditis (p. 91)

Medical Management

Open-heart surgical intervention: aortic commissurotomy; valve is dilated, and commissures of valve are incised
Valve replacements may be necessary in older child in whom commissurotomy would create significant aortic insufficiency
Coumadin therapy postoperatively with valve replacement
Antibiotic prophylaxis with dental work or other surgical procedures

PULMONIC STENOSIS (Figure 16-18)

An obstructive lesion that interferes with the blood flow from the right ventricle; stricture may be valvar, supravalvar, or subvalvar

Assessment
Observations/findings

Dependent on degree of outflow obstruction
Minimal obstruction: mild exercise intolerance
Severe obstruction in older children
  Chest pain
  Dizziness
  Dyspnea or exertion
  Fatigue
Ejection or crescendo-decrescendo systolic murmur: soft in mild obstruction; loud in severe obstruction; best heard in upper left sternal border and may be transmitted back and across left chest

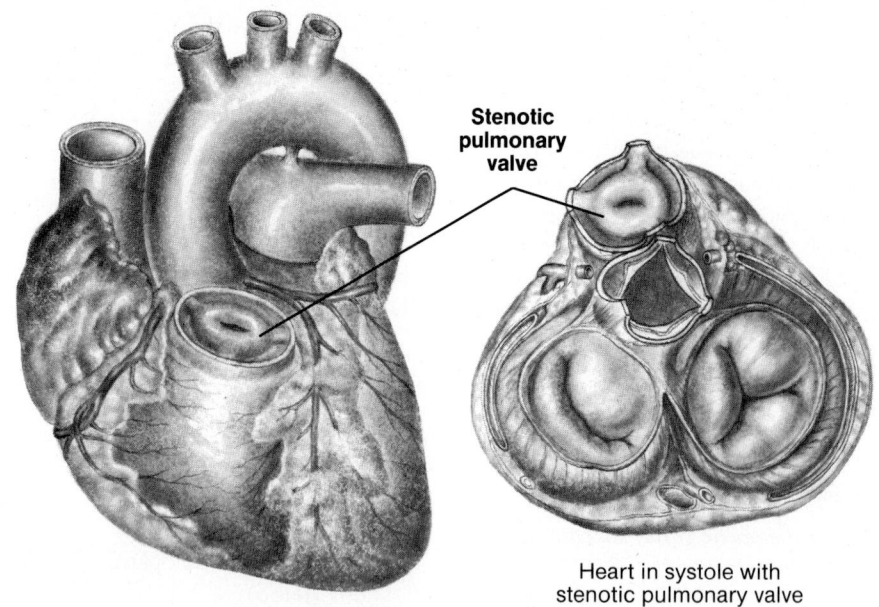

Stenotic pulmonary valve

Heart in systole with stenotic pulmonary valve

FIGURE 16-18. Pulmonic stenosis. (From Canobbio MM: *Cardiovascular disorders, Mosby's clinical nursing series,* St Louis, 1990, Mosby–Year Book.)

Laboratory/diagnostic findings

ECG: RVH

Radiology: right ventricular and main pulmonary artery enlargement

Echocardiogram: detects thickness and decreased motion of pulmonic valve

Cardiac catheterization: confirms diagnosis; identifies nature of stenotic valve and severity of stenosis; gradient measured—repair of pulmonic stenosis is recommended if pressure gradient is 60 mm Hg or more across pulmonic valve

Potential complications

Sudden death (rare)

Cyanosis and CHF (rare)

After corrective surgery
  Pulmonary regurgitation
  Transient arrythmias
  Subacute bacterial endocarditis (p. 91)

Medical Management

Monitoring of progression of stenosis as child grows

Nonoperative intervention: pulmonic valvotomy involving dilation of stenotic area during cardiac catheterization

Open-heart surgical intervention: pulmonic valvotomy—stenosis relieved by incising fused commissures as widely as possible

Antibiotic prophylaxis with dental work or other surgical procedures

Cyanotic

TETRALOGY OF FALLOT (Figure 16-19)

Includes four defects: (1) VSD, (2) right ventricular outflow obstruction (valvar and subvalvar pulmonic stenosis most common), (3) overriding aorta, and (4) RVH; results in dominant right-to-left blood flow

Assessment
Observations/findings

Cyanosis: occurs at 3 to 6 months of age (may occur only with crying/feeding in neonate because of patent ductus arteriosus)

Dyspnea

Tachypnea

Tachycardia

Delayed physical growth

Persistent right ventricular failure

Heart block

Ventricular arrhythmias

Subacute bacterial endocarditis (p. 91)

Medical Management

Adequate fluid administration to prevent dehydration

Treatment of "tet" spells

Oxygen prn

Propranolol

Knee-chest position

Morphine sulfate: relaxes right ventricular infundibulum, increases pulmonary blood flow, and decreases right-to-left shunt

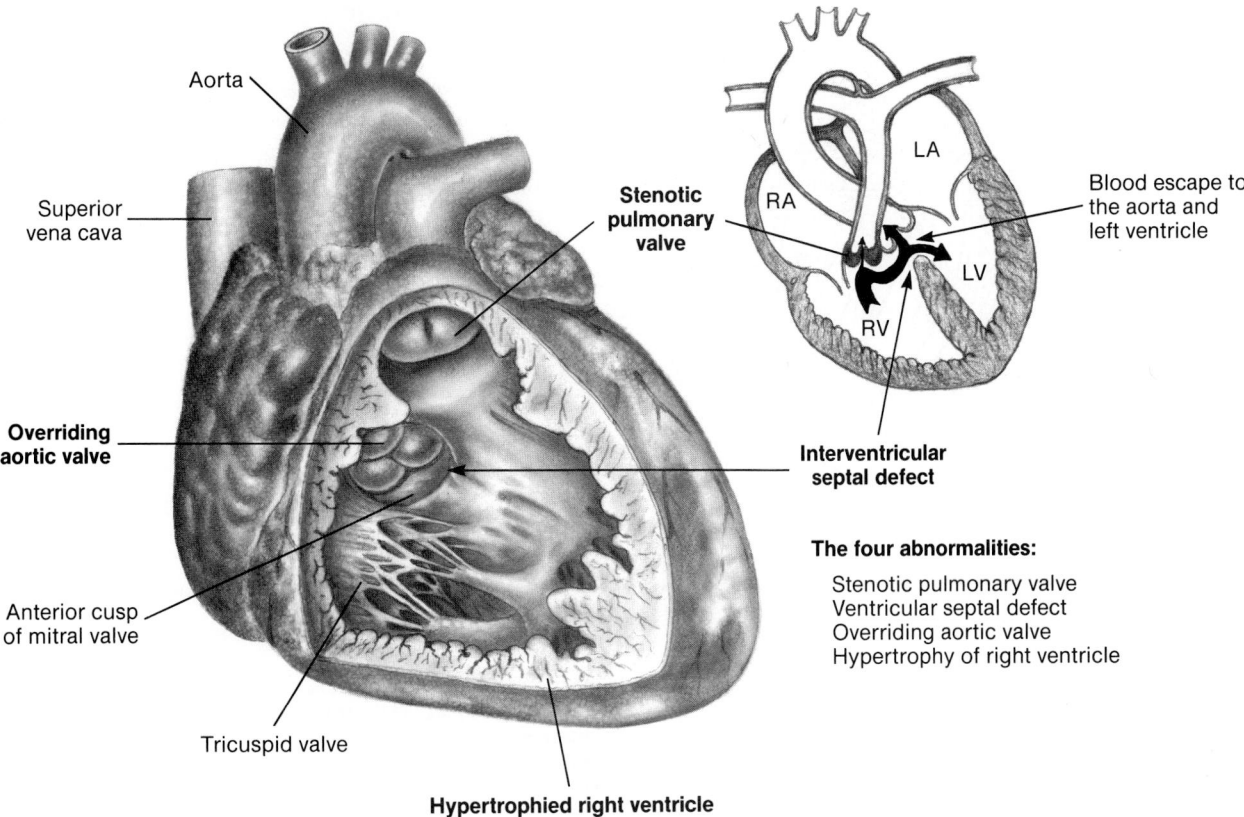

Aorta

Superior
vena cava

**Stenotic
pulmonary
valve**

LA

RA

Blood escape to
the aorta and
left ventricle

LV

RV

**Overriding
aortic valve**

**Interventricular
septal defect**

The four abnormalities:

Stenotic pulmonary valve
Ventricular septal defect
Overriding aortic valve
Hypertrophy of right ventricle

Anterior cusp
of mitral valve

Tricuspid valve

Hypertrophied right ventricle

FIGURE 16-19. Tetralogy of Fallot. (From Canobbio MM: *Cardiovascular disorders, Mosby's clinical nursing series,* St Louis, 1990, Mosby–Year Book.)

Prostaglandins are used in neonates to keep ductus arteriosus patent until surgery is possible

Palliative closed-heart surgical interventions

   Blalock-Taussig shunt: end-to-side anastomosis of right subclavian artery to right pulmonary artery or left subclavian artery to left pulmonary artery

   Modified Blalock-Taussig: Gore-Tex graft is used instead of end-to-side anastomosis

Corrective open-heart surgical intervention: complete repair of defects—closure of ventricular septal defect and correction of overriding aorta and pulmonic valvotomy

Antibiotic prophylaxis with dental work or other surgical procedures

Clubbing of fingers or toes

Paroxysmal dyspneic attacks, "blue" spells

   Severe dyspnea

   Severe cyanosis

   Hyperpnea

   Gasping

In an older child (though rare today because of early recognition and surgical intervention)

   Squatting

   Fainting

Pansystolic murmur: most intense at left sternal border

Laboratory/diagnostic studies

ECG: right axis deviation and RVH

Radiology: "boot-shaped" cardiac silhouette

Echocardiogram: demonstrates aortic override, large aorta, VSD, and thick right ventricular wall

Cardiac catheterization: actual visualization of all defects; systolic hypertension in right ventricle with sudden fall in pulmonary artery pressure

CBC: polycythemia

Blood gases: decreased PaO_2 and oxygen saturation

Potential complications

Thrombus formation

Cerebral emboli

Seizures

Brain abscess

After surgical correction

TRANSPOSITION OF GREAT VESSELS (TGV) (Figure 16-20)

Pulmonary artery leaves left ventricle, and aorta leaves right ventricle, resulting in complete separation of pulmonary and systemic circulation; life beyond birth is possible only if mixing of pulmonary and systemic

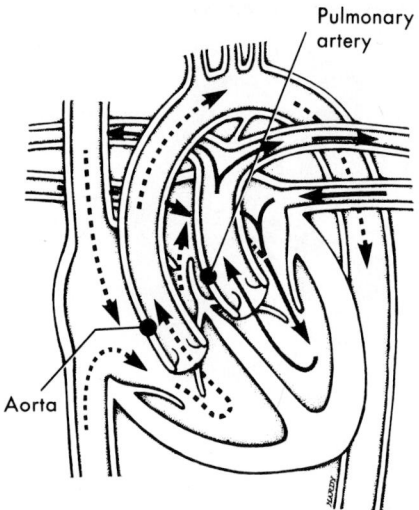

FIGURE 16-20. Transposition of great vessels (TGV). (From Whaley LF, Wong DL: *Essentials of pediatric nursing,* ed 3, St Louis, 1989, Mosby—Year Book.)

circulations occurs through patent ductus arteriosus, atrial septal defect, and/or ventricular septal defect

Assessment

Observations/findings

With minimal mixing of circulations
  Severe cyanosis
  Tachypnea
  Severe hypoxia
  Rapid onset of CHF (p. 835)
  Rapid deterioration if PDA closes
With significant mixing of circulations
  Less severe cyanosis
  Increased cyanosis with feeding/crying
  Progressive hyperpnea
  CHF
Heart murmur dependent on associated defects

Laboratory/diagnostic studies

ECG: right axis deviation, RVH
Radiology: progressive cardiomegaly
Echocardiogram: identification of aorta anterior to pulmonary artery and to the right of it
Cardiac catheterization: visualization of all defects; right ventricular hypertension; higher oxygen concentration in pulmonary artery than in aorta

Potential complications

Metabolic acidosis
After corrective surgery
  Baffle obstruction
  Baffle leaks
  Atrial dysrhythmias
  Tricuspid regurgitation
  Subacute bacterial endocarditis (p. 91)

Medical Management

In neonate
  CHF management (p. 835) with digoxin and diuretics
  Correction of metabolic acidosis: may give sodium bicarbonate
  Arterial oxygenation using palliative nonoperative interventions
  Balloon atrial septostomy during cardiac catheterization to allow mixing
  Administration of prostaglandins to maintain patency of ductus arteriosus
Corrective open-heart surgery
  Mustard procedure: atrial septum is taken down and baffle placed to redirect pulmonary and systemic circulations
  Senning procedure: similar to Mustard procedure except right atrial wall and interatrial septum are used as baffle
Antibiotic prophylaxis with dental work or other surgical procedures

CONGENITAL HEART SURGERY

Preoperative Preparation

Assessment

Obtain baseline vital signs
Ensure that child does not have infection
Ensure that laboratory studies are complete
  Chest x-ray examination
  ECG
  CBC
  Urinalysis
  Type and cross match for blood
  Electrolytes
  Coagulation studies
  Renal function tests

Nursing diagnosis/interventions/evaluation

■ **NDX:** Knowledge deficit related to lack of information about preparation for surgery

Reinforce physician's explanation of procedure
Encourage questions that will establish true understanding of surgery and alleviate fears
Gear teaching to parents and to child, depending on child's age and ability to understand
Provide diagram of heart and explain procedure
Obtain history of child's developmental status, usual daily routine, likes and dislikes, favorite toy, position in family, dietary habits, and sleep pattern in order to meet child's needs postoperatively
Explain preoperative procedures
  NPO
  Laboratory tests

Transport to operating room by way of crib or stretcher

Room where parents can wait during surgery

Reassure parents that surgeon will contact them after surgery

Describe operating room environment

    Physicians and nurses wear gowns, hats, and masks

    Allow child to try on operating room attire

Discuss anesthesia: "special sleep during which child will feel no pain"; reassure child that he will not wake up during surgery

Answer questions about operating room

    Physicians and nurses are present all the time

    Child will be helped to breathe by respirator and tube in throat

    Child will wake up soon after surgery

Describe postoperative environment

    Child will be in recovery room or intensive care unit (ICU)

    Provide visit to care unit before surgery

    Equipment

        Respiratory assistance to continue until respiration is stabilized

        Child will be unable to talk with tube in throat

        Nasogastric tube

        Monitor to chest

        Beep noises of monitor

        Chest tube(s)

        Presence of several monitoring lines

            Atrial line

            Central venous pressure (CVP) line

            Right atrial (RA) line (open heart)

            Left atrial (LA) line (open heart)

        Pacemaker wires present (open heart)

        Chest dressing or sutures

        Intravenous lines for fluid administration

        Urinary catheter

    Physicians and nurses will be present at all times

Explain that postoperative nursing care will include

    Frequent vital signs

    Coughing and deep breathing

    Pain management: explain availability of pain medication

Allow child to express self through play

    Mask, gown, cap

    Oxygen mask

    Syringe

    Doll

    Practice coughing and deep breathing

Do not overload young child with too much factual information that may be frightening; focus teaching on what child will see, hear, smell, and feel, rather than on details of surgery

Reassure child and parents concerning visitation

Allow ample time for questions and encourage feedback to ensure understanding

Expected outcome/evaluation

Patient and/or parents have expressed their concerns, fears, and anxieties about surgery and demonstrate understanding appropriate to their developmental ability

Palliative Procedures

Procedures done to either increase or decrease pulmonary blood flow as the defect demands

BALLOON SEPTOSTOMY (NONOPERATIVE)

Enlargement of foramen ovale to increase pulmonary blood flow; performed during cardiac catheterization

Assessment
Postprocedure observations

Assess for adequate mixing of blood by monitoring arterial blood gases (ABGs) and oxygen saturation

Decreased cyanosis

Increased activity tolerance

Improved feeding

Decreased oxygen requirement

Decreased respiratory effort

Potential complications (rare)

Cardiac perforation

Conduction abnormalities

BLALOCK-TAUSSIG SHUNT

Anastomosis of subclavian artery to pulmonary artery to increase pulmonary blood flow

Assessment
Postoperative observations

See Closed-Heart Surgery (below)

Decreased cyanosis

Decreased oxygen requirement

Decreased respiratory effort

Machinery-like murmur

Weak or absent BP in arm on operative side; do not draw blood or start IV in arm on operative side

Increased activity tolerance

Improved feeding

Potential complications

Thrombus formation in shunt

    Return to preoperative state of cyanosis

    Disappearance of shunt murmur

PULMONARY ARTERY BANDING (PAB)

Application of constrictive band to main pulmonary artery in order to decrease pulmonary blood flow

Assessment
Postoperative observations

See Closed-Heart Surgery (below)

With adequate restriction of blood flow

Decreasing evidence of CHF
  Improved urinary output
  Relief of edema
  Stabilization of weight
  Improved respiratory function
  Decreased need for digoxin and diuretics
  Improved feeding
With inadequate restriction of blood flow: little or no relief
  from CHF

Potential complications

Insufficient blood flow restriction

Corrective Surgery

CLOSED-HEART SURGERY
Assessment
Observations/findings

Respiratory status
  Patent airway
  Equality of chest movements and breath sounds
  Signs of respiratory distress: tachypnea, dyspnea, nasal
    flaring, cyanosis, retractions
  Presence of adventitious sounds: stridor, rales, rhonchi
  Subcutaneous emphysema (crepitus)
  Chest tube function (p. 229)
Cardiovascular status
  Peripheral perfusion: warmth, color, capillary refill,
    pulses in extremities
  Heart rate and rhythm
  Murmur status
  BP
    Coarctation repair: continued hypertension
    Patent ductus ligation: mild hypertension
    Blalock-Taussig operation: absent or faint in arm on
      operative side
Renal status
  Urinary output (minimum 1 ml/kg/hr)
  Specific gravity
Neurological status
  Level of consciousness
  Age-appropriate developmental ability
GI status: return of bowel sounds

Laboratory/diagnostic studies

ABGs
Hgb
Hct
Creatinine
Electrolytes
Chest x-ray examination: to evaluate presence of post-
  operative complications

Potential complications

See specific defect under Congenital Heart Defects
Atelectasis (p. 220)

Pneumothorax (p. 216)
Tension pneumothorax (p. 216)
CHF (p. 835)

Medical Management

Ventilatory assistance: wean from ventilatory support
Oxygen
Postural drainage, percussion, and suctioning
Order dressing changes if any
Maintenance parenteral fluids
Digitalis
Diuretics
Antibiotics
Analgesics
Antipyretics
Removal of chest tube
Removal of sutures

Nursing diagnoses/interventions/evaluation

■ **NDX:**   Decreased cardiac output related to inadequate
        myocardial contractility

Assess extremities for perfusion: warm, pink color, rapid
  capillary refill, good pulses
Maintain continuous ECG monitoring
Assess apical rate and rhythm qh
Assess level of consciousness qh
Assess breath sounds qh
Assess adequacy of urinary output (minimal 1 ml/kg/hr)
Administer digoxin if ordered
Administer diuretics if ordered

Expected outcome/evaluation

Patient has adequate cardiac output as evidenced by improved peripheral perfusion, increased urinary output,
  alertness, and clear breath sounds

■ **NDX:**   Potential for ineffective breathing pattern re-
        lated to anesthesia, incisional pain, and/or in-
        creased pulmonary secretions

Assess respiratory status qh
Initiate care of endotracheal tube if in place (p. 231)
Maintain ventilatory settings as ordered
Maintain airway patency
Administer humidified oxygen as ordered
Perform postural drainage, percussion, and suctioning q2h
  to 4h as appropriate if indicated by physician
Teach and/or assist patient to turn, cough, and deep
  breathe q2h
Use incentive spirometer in children who are old enough
  to use it
Administer analgesics before pulmonary treatments and
  as needed for pain
Initiate care of chest tube (p. 229)
Monitor blood gases

Expected outcome/evaluation

Patient has age-appropriate respiratory rate and clear breath sounds

■ **NDX:** Potential fluid volume excess related to decreased cardiac output and compensatory kidney mechanisms

Maintain parenteral fluids as ordered
Measure urinary output qh (in immediate postoperative period)
Record accurate intake and output
Observe for signs of volume excess: decreased urinary output, loose cough, pulmonary congestion, periorbital edema

Expected outcome/evaluation

Patient has minimum urinary output of 1 ml/kg/hr

■ **NDX:** Potential for infection related to surgical incision and/or invasive lines

Monitor temperature q2h and prn
Use good handwashing technique
Use strict asepsis for all dressing changes
Perform aseptic dressing change as ordered
Check incision site and puncture sites for redness, swelling, and drainage
Perform Foley catheter care as per hospital policy
Administer antibiotics as ordered
Assist in collecting specimens to determine site of infection with temperature elevation

Expected outcome/evaluation

Patient is afebrile with clean, intact surgical incision and puncture sites

■ **NDX:** Potential sensory-perceptual alterations related to anesthesia and/or cerebral hypoxia

Assess level of consciousness and motor, sensory, and developmental ability qh
Review preoperative baseline assessment
Encourage parental participation in care and stimulation

Expected outcome/evaluation

Patient returns to preoperative developmental ability

■ **NDX:** Altered nutrition: less than body requirements related to imposed NPO status postoperatively

Maintain NPO status immediately postoperatively
Assess return of bowel function
Begin clear liquid feedings and advance gradually as ordered

Monitor child's ability to consume increasing amounts of oral feedings

Expected outcome/evaluation

Patient tolerates age-appropriate diet reflecting adequate caloric intake to meet metabolic requirements

■ **NDX:** Potential for ineffective parental coping related to stress of child with chronic illness, stress of frequent hospitalizations, and separation from child

Discuss parents' feelings of fear, guilt, grief, anger, etc.
Have parents participate in care of their child as soon as possible
Encourage them to continue to do activities they normally would do with child at home: bathe, feed, dress, change diaper, hold, cuddle, play
Have parents meet with other parents with children with congenital heart disease
Involve parents in ongoing support group
Explore parents' feelings regarding overprotecting child and restricting activity of child—the "vulnerable child" feelings
Discuss ways in which parents can gradually increase child's independence
Refer to community agencies as necessary for ongoing support and follow-up

Expected outcome/evaluation

Parents demonstrate increased coping ability as evidenced by increased verbalization that they feel confident in their ability to care for their child

■ **NDX:** Knowledge deficit related to lack of information about home care and follow-up needs

Explain congenital heart defect and surgical intervention
If surgery was palliative, explain that they can expect corrective surgery in the future
Explain need for nutritious diet
   Age-appropriate type and amount
   May be salt and/or fluid restricted
Explain need for exercise to tolerance; some children will continue to be exercise restricted
Discuss symptoms to report to physician
   Fever
   Fatigue
   Increased respiratory rate
   Incisional redness, swelling, or drainage
Teach name of medication, purpose, dosage, time of administration, and side effects
Emphasize importance of follow-up care with surgeon, cardiologist, and pediatrician

Have parents demonstrate measuring and administration of medication

Expected outcome/evaluation

Parents and/or significant other demonstrate understanding of home care and follow-up instructions

OPEN-HEART SURGERY

Assessment

Observations/findings

Assessments are guided by an understanding of potential complications specifically associated with corrective surgery for specific defects (see Congenital Heart Defects, p. 821)

Review preoperative status, intraoperative course, duration of cardiopulmonary bypass, and normal growth and physiological parameters of pediatric patient

Cardiovascular status

  Peripheral perfusion

    Warmth and color of extremities

    Capillary refill

    Peripheral pulses

  Heart rate and rhythm

    Dysrhythmias are common

    Cause of rhythm disturbance must be identified: check acid-base balance, presence of hypoxia, electrolyte imbalance, and digoxin level

  Murmur status

  Presence of pacer wires

  Blood pressure

  Central venous pressure (CVP)

  Right atrial pressure (RAP)

  Left atrial pressure (LAP)

  Arterial pressure (A line)

Respiratory status

  Presence or absence of spontaneous respirations

  Equality of chest movements

  Equality of breath sounds (note any areas of decreased breath sounds)

  Presence of adventitious sounds

  Signs of respiratory distress: nasal flaring, cyanosis, retractions, restlessness, bradycardia

  Endotracheal intubation (p. 231)

  Ventilatory assistance (p. 235)

  Chest tube function and drainage (p. 229)

Renal status

  Hourly urinary output (minimum in infants is 1 ml/kg/hr)

  Specific gravity

  Presence of hemoglobinuria, pH

Neurological status

  Level of consciousness

  Neuromuscular/developmental ability

  Presence of localized or generalized neurological abnormalities

  Presence of "postoperative psychosis": disorientation, inappropriate behavior for age, restlessness, agitation

GI status

  Nasogastric drainage: monitor amount, type, pH, and for presence of blood

  Return of bowel sounds

  Abdominal girths

Temperature

  Hyperthermia

  Hypothermia: may result from surgical hypothermia

Fluid status

  Dehydration (p. 841)

  Overhydration

Laboratory/diagnostic studies

Electrolytes: monitor sodium, potassium, and calcium levels

Base deficit or excess: serum pH

ABGs: PaO_2, $PaCO_2$, pH

CBC: hematocrit, hemoglobin

Coagulation studies

BUN: elevated with renal failure

Creatinine: elevated with renal failure

Urine osmolality: elevated with renal failure

Chest x-ray examination: evaluation of lung complications

12-lead ECG: evaluation of dysrhythmia

Potential complications

Cardiac

  Dysrhythmias

  Decreased cardiac output (cardiogenic shock) (p. 105)

  Cardiac tamponade (p. 100)

Pulmonary

  Atelectasis (p. 220)

  Pulmonary edema (CHF) (p. 835)

  Pneumothorax (p. 216)

  Tension pneumothorax (p. 216)

Renal

  Acute renal failure (p. 482)

  Hemoglobinuria

Metabolic

  Acidosis

  Electrolyte disturbances

  Hypovolemia/hypervolemia

Hematological

  Coagulation abnormalities

  Hypotension

  Surgical bleeding

Neurological

  Cerebral bleeding from embolization

  Focal or diffuse CNS dysfunction

  "Postoperative psychosis"

Gastrointestinal

  Paralytic ileus

  GI bleeding

Medical Management

Validation of dysrhythmia and determination of pharmacological treatment

Cardiovascular medications

Diuretics

Initiate temporary pacing if necessary

Treatment of hypovolemia with volume expanders (PRBCs, whole blood, colloid, fresh frozen plasma [FFP], etc.)

Fluid restriction imposed until risk of hypervolemia is passed, then advancement to maintenance

Accurate intake and output

Low-dose dopamine for increased renal perfusion

Monitoring of electrolytes and replacement as necessary

Monitoring of ABGs

Order for ventilatory settings and weaning of child off ventilatory support

Postural drainage, percussion, and suctioning

Provision of caloric requirements via parenteral fluids, then orally as tolerated

Total parenteral nutrition (TPN) with prolonged complicated postoperative course

Analgesics

Antibiotics

Antacids

Antipyretics

Nursing diagnoses / interventions / evaluation

■ **NDX:**   Potential for altered cardiac output: decreased output related to inadequate contractility of heart, decreased preload, inadequate heart rate, and/or increased vascular resistance

Assess peripheral perfusion qh

Determine oxygen saturation using oximeter qh

Monitor heart rate and rhythm continuously with ECG monitor

Assess apical rate and rhythm qh

Look for underlying cause of rhythm disturbances if present: hypoxia, acid-base imbalance, electrolyte imbalance, digoxin toxicity

Monitor blood pressure qh: note decreased pulse pressure, pulsus paradoxus, or pulsus alternans

Monitor RAP, LAP, CVP, and arterial pressure qh

Assess for signs and symptoms of hypovolemia

Measure urinary output hourly; be alert for decreased urinary output

Assess for postoperative bleeding

Be alert to excessive bloody chest tube drainage

Monitor coagulation studies

Assess respiratory status qh: be alert for increased pulmonary secretions and increased respiratory distress

Be alert to changes in behavior or level of consciousness

Administer volume expanders as ordered (colloid, plasma, PRBCs)

Administer cardiovascular medications as ordered

Administer electrolytes as ordered

Administer diuretics as ordered

Maintain temporary pacing as ordered

Expected outcome / evaluation

Patient has adequate cardiac output as evidenced by age-appropriate heart rate and blood pressure, with warm, pink extremities and strong peripheral pulses

■ **NDX:**   Potential for impaired gas exchange related to altered oxygen supply secondary to ineffective breathing pattern resulting from increased pulmonary secretions, hypoventilation, and/or pain

Perform respiratory assessment (p. 186) qh

Perform postural drainage, percussion, and suctioning q2h and prn with manual administration of 100% oxygen before and after suctioning

Change position q2h

Maintain endotracheal tube if present (p. 231)

Monitor ventilatory settings as ordered (p. 235); assist in making necessary changes as ordered

Monitor ABGs and respiratory status frequently to determine effectiveness of ventilatory changes

Monitor chest tube drainage qh (p. 229)

Administer analgesics as ordered before vigorous pulmonary treatments to promote cooperation in deep breathing and coughing routines

In child who is not intubated, use incentive spirometers, and coughing and deep-breathing exercises to promote lung expansion

Expected outcome / evaluation

Patient has clear breath sounds, normal ABGs, and spontaneous effective respirations

■ **NDX:**   Potential alteration in renal tissue perfusion secondary to decreased cardiac output

Record accurate hourly intake (includes parenteral fluids, fluids used to flush lines, and oral intake) and output (urinary output, nasogastric drainage, chest tube drainage, bloods drawn for studies) measurements

Monitor urinary output; should be at least 1 ml/kg/hr

Measure specific gravity qh

Assess for presence of hemoglobinuria

Be alert to early signs of acute renal failure

   Monitor serum BUN and creatinine: increased

   Monitor electrolytes: hyperkalemia

   Monitor urine osmolality: increased

Ensure normovolemia by administering parenteral fluids as ordered

Administer electrolytes as ordered

Administer diuretics as ordered

Administer low-dose dopamine if ordered to improve renal perfusion

Expected outcome/evaluation

Patient shows evidence of adequate renal perfusion by maintaining urinary output of at least 1 ml/kg/hr

 NDX: Potential sensory-perceptual alterations related to intraoperative hypoxia, embolus, or decreased cardiac output

Assess level of consciousness, pupil response, motor and sensory function, and return of developmental abilities qh

Assess for focal (localized weakness, poor motor function, partial seizures) or diffuse neurological dysfunction (changes in behavior or level of consciousness)

Assess for presence of "postoperative psychosis": agitation, restlessness, combativeness, disorientation

Reassure child, orient to surroundings, and decrease stimulation as much as possible

Control pain

Provide frequent uninterrupted opportunities for sleep

Encourage parents to stay with child as much as possible

Have parents bring in familiar objects from home; favorite toy, tape player, books, etc.

Expected outcome/evaluation

Patient exhibits age-appropriate developmental behavior without evidence of sensory-perceptual alterations

NDX: Potential for altered nutrition: less than body requirements related to dietary restriction after surgery

Maintain gastric decompression postoperatively with nasogastric tube

Irrigate nasogastric tube q2h to 4h to ensure patency

Evaluate nasogastric drainage for volume, pH, and presence of blood

Initiate antacid therapy as ordered if drainage is positive for blood

Measure abdominal girth q2h

Assess abdomen for return of peristalsis
    Decreased nasogastric drainage
    Presence of bowel sounds
    Decreased gastric distention
    Passing of flatus or stool

Administer parenteral fluids or TPN as ordered

Begin clear oral feedings with return of bowel function

Advance diet gradually as ordered

Expected outcome/evaluation

Patient tolerates age-appropriate diet

 NDX: Potential for hypothermia related to cooling measures used during cardiopulmonary bypass procedure

Assess temperature qh

Use external warming devices to elevate child's temperature slowly

Continue use of warming devices as necessary to maintain temperature

Keep environmental temperature warm

Keep child partially dressed: hat, socks, blanket draped over extremities, etc.

Expected outcome/evaluation

Patient maintains normothermic body temperature

 NDX: Potential for infection related to surgical incision, use of cardiopulmonary bypass, and/or multiple invasive lines

Monitor temperature q2h and prn

Be aware that good handwashing is crucial

Maintain strict asepsis for all dressing changes

Perform aseptic dressing change as ordered

Check incision site and puncture sites for redness, swelling, and drainage

Perform Foley catheter care as per hospital policy

Administer antibiotics as ordered

Assist in collecting specimens to determine site of infection with temperature elevation

Monitor CBC for increased WBC count

Expected outcome/evaluation

Patient is afebrile with clean, intact surgical incision and puncture sites

NDX: Knowledge deficit related to lack of information about home care and follow-up needs

Explain congenital heart defect and surgical repair performed

Explain dietary needs: specific amount (minimal), type of formula, how often

Explain need for exercise to tolerance

Review restriction in exercise if any

Explain that child should gradually resume normal activity level and be treated as a normal child

Emphasize importance of good incisional care and hygiene if ordered

Discuss symptoms to report to physician
    Fever
    Incisional redness, swelling, drainage

Teach name of medication, purpose, dosage, time of administration, and side effects

Emphasize importance of follow-up care with cardiac surgeon, cardiologist, and pediatrician
Have patient and/or parents demonstrate
Care of child
Administration of medications

Expected outcome/evaluation

Patient and/or parents verbalize understanding of homecare and follow-up instructions

CONGESTIVE HEART FAILURE (CHF)

A state in which the cardiac output is inadequate to meet the body's metabolic needs; in infants and young children it occurs bilaterally

Assessment
Observations/findings

Signs and symptoms of decreased cardiac output
Restlessness, fussiness
Mottled, pale skin
Cool extremities
Decreased urinary output
Diaphoresis
Exercise intolerance
Poor feeding or inability to take po feedings
Increasing respiratory distress
Nasal flaring
Cyanosis
Tachypnea
Retractions
Grunting
Rales
Tachycardia
Systemic venous congestion
Rapid weight gain
Edema: periorbital
Abdominal distention
Hepatosplenomegaly

Laboratory/diagnostic studies

Chest x-ray examination: cardiac enlargement and pulmonary congestion
Arterial blood gases: acidosis
Serum glucose: hypoglycemia often occurs in infants with CHF
Serum electrolytes
Sodium: hyponatremia may occur with water retention
Potassium: hypokalemia or hyperkalemia
Serum calcium: normal levels essential for myocardial contractility
CBC
Anemia
WBC elevation may occur

Medical Management

Improvement of cardiac contractility and reduction of volume overload through use of
Digitalization (see Pediatric Digitalis Therapy p. 836)
Diuretics
Fluid restriction
Postural drainage, percussion, and suctioning in infants

Nursing diagnoses/interventions/evaluation

■ **NDX:** Altered cardiac output: decreased output related to ineffective contractility of the heart—excessive preload or afterload

Assess resting apical and respiratory rates q1h to 2h and prn
Administer digoxin accurately as ordered; do not give if heart rate is less than 100 beats/min or if rhythm is irregular
Administer diuretics as ordered
Monitor serum electrolyte levels
Restrict fluids as ordered
Monitor accurate intake and output
Weigh daily or bid at same times, unclothed, before feedings
Observe for resolution of CHF: decreased heart and respiratory rates, increased urinary output, decreased periorbital edema, decrease in and stabilization of weight, increased activity tolerance, improved feeding activity

Expected outcome/evaluation

Patient experiences improved cardiac output as evidenced by increased urinary output, decreased heart rate, decreased respiratory rate, and clear breath sounds

■ **NDX:** Activity intolerance related to dyspnea and fatigue

Reduce cardiac demands
Plan frequent rest periods
Avoid unnecessary handling of infant to prevent fatigue
Anticipate needs to prevent crying
Keep infant warm and comfortable; avoid overdressing or cold stress
Avoid overfatigue during feedings
Feed in oxgyen-enriched environment
Give small, frequent feedings
Gavage feedings in infants if sucking causes increased respiratory distress
Avoid exposure to individuals with known infections

Expected outcome/evaluation

Patient
Experiences minimal dyspnea and fatigue
Tolerates gradual increases in activity

■ **NDX:** Impaired gas exchange related to increased pulmonary secretions

Maintain warm, humidified, oxygenated environment via mist tent or oxygen hood

Monitor respiratory status q1h to 2h; especially note changes in color, respiratory rate, use of accessory muscles, and presence of rales

Monitor arterial blood gases

Monitor oxygen saturation with oximeter

Elevate head of bed: use infant seat for infants; elevate older child on pillows

Remove increased mucus via suctioning prn; suction *only* if infant needs it; avoid excessive suctioning, since it increases cardiac demands

Expected outcome/evaluation

Patient has improved gas exchange as evidenced by clear breath sounds, decreased respiratory rate, and normal blood gases

■ **NDX:** Altered nutrition: less than body requirements related to dyspnea and fatigue

Determine caloric requirements (p. 841)

Increase calories in formula to meet requirements yet remain within fluid restriction and patient's tolerance

Avoid overfatigue during feedings

Feed patient in oxygenated environment

Limit handling before feeding to prevent overexhaustion

Feed smaller amounts more frequently

Use gavage feeding in infants who cannot take adequate po feedings

Burp frequently during feedings to decrease gastric distention

Expected outcome/evaluation

Patient tolerates diet with adequate caloric intake to meet metabolic needs

■ **NDX:** Knowledge deficit related to lack of information about home care and follow-up needs

Explain need for planned rest periods

Discuss type of formula, amount, and frequency

Teach name of medications (digoxin and diuretics), purpose, dosage, time of administration, and side effects (see Pediatric Digitalis Therapy, below)

Discuss symptoms of recurrence to report to physician
  Poor feeding
  Fatigue
  Increased respiratory rate
  Loose cough
  Cyanosis
  Puffiness around eyes

Decreased urinary output

Confirm dates and times of follow-up appointments with surgeon, cardiologist, and pediatrician

Have parents demonstrate
  Proper measuring and administration of medications
  Ability to feed desired volume of formula

Expected outcome/evaluation

Parents and/or significant other demonstrate understanding of home care and follow-up instructions

PEDIATRIC DIGITALIS THERAPY

Assessment
Observations/findings
DIGITALIS EFFECT: DESIRED RESULT

Slower heart rate

Improved myocardial contractility: increased cardiac output

Slowed impulses through conduction system

DIGITALIS TOXICITY: UNDESIRABLE RESULT

Cardiac dysrhythmias: most common sign

Nausea, vomiting

Anorexia

Diarrhea

NOTE: There is an increased risk of digoxin toxicity associated with renal failure, hypoxia, acidosis, hypokalemia, and hypercalcemia

Laboratory/diagnostic studies

Serum digoxin level

Potassium and calcium levels

Nursing Responsibility

To promote safe, accurate administration of digoxin
  Ensure completeness of physician's order
    Name of preparation
    Dosage written in micrograms and milliliter equivalents
    Route of administration
    Intervals of administration
    Pulse rate under which drug is to be withheld
  Administration
    Have two people licensed to administer medications calculate dosage and volume, and double-check amount after measured
    Check resting apical pulse for rate and rhythm before each administration (count for all minute or according to hospital policy)
    If toxic symptoms are present, withhold dose, place child on cardiac monitor, and notify physician
    Monitor for dysrhythmias; check serum electrolytes if toxicity is suspected

If child vomits and you are unsure if child received dose, *do not repeat dose*

Determine best method of ensuring complete administration of oral dose: spoon, syringe, nipple, or dropper

Never dilute with anything

After administering drug in sweetened liquid form give plain water to prevent tooth decay

Objective of parent teaching is to ensure proper measuring and administration of digoxin

Teach name of medication, purpose, dosage, and time of administration; ensure that parents understand that digoxin must be given at prescribed regular intervals

Discuss signs and symptoms of toxicity

Explain need to withhold dose and notify physician if toxic symptoms occur

Explain need to give complete dose; caution parents not to mix with formula or food

Teach method of administration

Teach parents to administer drug as prescribed 1 hr before or 2 hr after meals

Caution parents not to repeat dose if unsure if child vomited it

Explain need to keep medication out of reach of children

Explain need for ongoing evaluation by cardiologist and need to refill prescription before using the last dose

Have patient and/or parents demonstrate

Measurement of dosage

Proper administration of medication

Notation of administration on calendar-type log sheet to avoid under or overdosing

Caution parents to place medication in a safe place

Give parents telephone number of nearest poison control center to be used in the event of accidental overdosage

TEMPORARY ARTIFICIAL PACEMAKER

Assessment
Observations/findings
PACEMAKER FAILURE

Bradycardia (asystole)

Possible ECG pattern changes

Absence of pacemaker artifact

No ventricular response: absence of QRS complex after pacemaker artifact

Competition: presence of pacer response complex *and* patient's own complex

Runaway pacer: pacer artifact appears at several hundred per minute

Hypotension: Stokes-Adams syndrome

Faintness

Convulsions

Coma

Pallor or cyanosis

Decreased urinary output

Fatigability

Signs of decreased cardiac output

INFECTION

Site of insertion

Redness

Pain

Swelling

Drainage

Fever

Laboratory/diagnostic studies

Continuous ECG monitoring

Potential complications

Pacemaker failure

Medical Management

Determination of pacemaker settings

Treatment of pacemaker malfunctions

Discontinuation of temporary pacemaker when feasible

Nursing diagnoses/interventions/evaluation

■ **NDX:**   Potential for altered cardiac output: decreased output related to pacemaker malfunction

Place patient on continuous ECG monitoring

Check heart rate qh

Monitor BP q4h and prn

Maintain settings on pacemaker as ordered

Protect pacemaker from falls and moisture

Prevent pull on catheter

Monitor intake and output

Position for most effective cardiac setting

Expected outcome/evaluation

Patient maintains adequate cardiac output

Any pacemaker failure is identified, and prompt treatment is given

■ **NDX:**   Potential for infection related to insertion of pacemaker wires

Observe for signs of infection at insertion site

Change insertion site dressing daily using aseptic technique and ointment if ordered

Keep wires safely taped to chest after temporary pacemaker is discontinued

Expected outcome/evaluation

Patient has clean, intact skin without evidence of infection

Pacer wires remain in place after removal of temporary pacemaker

Other Aspects of Pediatrics

CHILD ABUSE

A pattern of physical, sexual, or emotional maltreatment or neglect of children by parents, guardians, or other care givers

Assessment
Observations/findings

PHYSICAL ABUSE

Injuries are unexplained, recurrent, and/or inappropriate to history given
Bruises and welts
  In various stages of resolution
  Clustered
  Outlining shape of article used
  On different surface areas
  Circumferential on extremity
Burns
  Cigarette marks
  Scalded: socklike, glovelike, doughnut shape on buttocks and genitalia
  Having shape of instrument: iron, heater, etc.
  Infected: treatment delayed
Fractures
  Multiple
  Various stages of healing
  Frequently long bones or skull
Lacerations and abrasions
  Multiple
  Neglected
  Bite marks
  Scalp bald spots
Hemorrhage
  Intraabdominal
  Renal

Neurological injuries
  Coma
  Subdural hematoma
Optic injuries
  Hyphema
  Detached retina
  Black eyes
Genitalia
  Edematous
  Excoriated

PHYSICAL NEGLECT

See Failure to Thrive (p. 818)
Evidence of poor hygiene
No immunizations appropriate for age
Prescribed medications not given
Exposure to unsafe environment
Poor adult supervision
Abandoned
Abdominal distention
Inappropriate clothing for weather
Diaper rash
Irritable

SEXUAL ABUSE

See box below
Venereal disease
Pain or itching in genital area
Pain on urination
Poor sphincter tone
Vaginal or penile bleeding or lacerations
History of being "touched" without penile penetration

EMOTIONAL ABUSE

See Failure to Thrive (p. 818)
Disruptive behavior
Hyperactivity
Speech disorders

MOST COMMON SUBSTITUTE COMPLAINTS IN SEXUAL ABUSE CASES

Any age	Preschool age	School age	Adolescence
Abdominal pain	Excessive clinging	Decreased school performance	Same as school age plus
Anorexia	Thumbsucking	Truancy	Runaway behavior
Vomiting	Speech disorder	Lying, stealing	Suicide attempts
Constipation	Encopresis/enuresis	Tics	Sexual offenses
Sleep disorders	Excessive masturbation	Anxiety reaction	
Dysuria		Phobic and obsessional states	
Vaginal discharge		Depression	
Vaginal bleeding		Conversion reaction	
Rectal bleeding		Encopresis/enuresis	

From Zitelli BJ, Davis HW: *Atlas of pediatric physical diagnosis*, New York, 1987, Gower Medical Publishing.

BEHAVIOR

Fearful of adults
Depressed
Withdrawn
Accepting of painful procedures
Cries excessively and inconsolably
Seeks constant reassurance
Compulsive
Aggressive or compliant
Frightened of parents
Seeks parents' approval
Exhibits clinging, grabbing, or lap-hungry behavior
Chronically truant
Manipulative (p. 22)
Poor self-concept
Apprehensive when other children cry
Overanxious to please
Evasive when asked about accident
Poor peer relationships
Delinquent or runaway
Attempted suicide (p. 20)
Sleep disorders
Overly adaptive behavior
Developmental lags
Psychoneurotic reactions
Habit disorders (sucking, biting, rocking)
Sophisticated sexual knowledge
Irritable when handled

PARENT OR PRIMARY CARE GIVER

Any evidence of substance abuse (drug or alcohol)
Evidence of dysfunctional attachment process in new mother
Hostile and depressed
Unrealistic expectations for child given developmental age
Overconcerned or underconcerned about child's injury
Asks few or no questions of care givers
Behavior toward crying or injured child is aloof, not comforting or affectionate
Explains need for physical punishment because of "badness" in victim
Seductive toward child of opposite sex
Refuses to allow child to be hospitalized
Expresses feelings of loneliness, lack of friends or support systems; unhappy childhood or marriage

Laboratory/diagnostic studies

See Failure to Thrive (p. 818)
Appropriate to suspected injury
Long bone survey: to document other skeletal injury

Potential complications

Fatal traumatic injuries
Behavioral disorders

Malnutrition
Venereal disease
Pregnancy in young adolescent

Medical Management

Dependent on type and extent of injury
Thorough documentation of injuries
Report of case to appropriate authorities

Nursing diagnoses/interventions*/evaluation

■ **NDX:** Altered parenting related to stressors that contribute to abuse of a child: lack of support system, poor financial resources, abusive relationship with own parents, lack of knowledge about parenting, etc.

Do not exhibit judgmental behavior toward parents
Refer abuser to a therapist
Assess need for family therapy if the abuser is a parent or caretaker; refer to parenting class
Assess need for a support group
Assist parents in identifying their stresses
Explore more effective ways of dealing with stress
Discuss ways to use resources during times of stress to avoid injuring themselves or their child
Notify authorities of suspicion or fact of abuse or neglect as mandated by law
Make referral to social agency for purpose of
  Assessing home environment
  Providing additional support services as necessary
  Having ongoing contact with family once they return to home environment
  Having ongoiong advocate for protection of child
Cooperate with authorities in decisions made
  Understand that court order forbidding discharge of child to parents may occur
  Child may be discharged to foster home pending final decisions by legal authorities

Expected outcome/evaluation

Patient no longer experiences abuse from parents and parents obtain adequate resources to prevent further abuse of their child and seek assistance for abusive behavior

■ **NDX:** Anxiety in child related to abuse by parents and separation from parents

Perform functions slowly with sensitivity, observing child closely for emotional reactions
Have consistent care givers so child learns sense of trust
Encourage parents to visit and participate in care of their child
Observe child's reaction to parents when they visit

---

*Dependent on type and extent of injury.

If child is old enough, encourage child to talk about what happened

Reinforce that child was not injured because he was "bad"

Have child participate in play activities as soon as feasible

Encourage doll play with discussion of incident so child can express feelings and fears regarding assault

Prevent further injury if possible

Expected outcome/evaluation

Patient

Shows evidence of decreased anxiety by increased verbalization, increased interactions with other children, increased interest in play, and decreased crying

Has expressed some anxiety and fears verbally or through play

VITAL SIGNS

Temperature
When

Routinely according to hospital policy

As ordered by physician

As indicated by standard of care for disease or operation

How

Rectally: first newborn temperature

Orally: 3 years or over if no contraindication

Axillary: newborns and under 3 years as well as any child at any age since it correlates closely with core temperature

Normal Values

Rectal: approximately 97.5° to 99.5°F or 36.5° to 38°C

Oral: approximately 97° to 99°F or 36° to 37.5°C

Axillary: approximately 96.5° to 98.5°F or 35.5° to 37°C

Blood Pressure
When

Routinely according to hospital policy

As ordered by physician

As indicated by standard of care for disease or operation

How

Cuffs of several sizes should be available; cuff bladder should cover one-half to two-thirds length of upper arm; essential that size cuff being used on each child be noted in nursing care plan so that there is consistency in all pressures taken

Can use forearm or thigh if proper cuff size is not available

Can use forearm or calf of leg with electronic BP monitor

Listen at popliteal space is using high (subtract 10 mm Hg from systolic pressure)

Listen to radial artery if using forearm (add 10 mm Hg to systolic pressure)

Palpable BP can be obtained from pulse site as cuff pressure is reduced

Too large a cuff will result in lower than actual pressure

Too small a cuff will result in higher than actual pressure

Normal Values

See Table 16-2 for normal BP values by age

See Table 16-3 for classification of hypertension by age group

Heart Rate
When

Routinely according to hospital policy

As ordered by physician

As indicated by standard of care for disease or operation

TABLE 16-2. Normal BP Values for Age*

Age	Systolic diastolic
Neonate: to 1 mo	80 ± 16
	46 ± 16
Infant: 1-12 mo	96 ± 30
	65 ± 25
Preschool: 2-6 yr	60 to 110
	40 to 75
School age: 8-10 yr	105 ± 15
	60 ± 10
Adolescent: 11-16 yr	85 to 130
	45 to 85
Adults	90 to 140
	60 to 90

* Wide range of normal result in questionable value of one BP reading; greatest value of BP readings in children is in serial BP (when indicated by condition) to show upward or downward trend.

TABLE 16-3. Classification of Hypertension by Age-Group

Age group	Significant hypertension (mm Hg)	Severe hypertension (mm Hg)
Newborns (7 d)	Systolic BP ≥96	Systolic BP ≥106
(8-30 d)	Systolic BP ≥104	Systolic BP ≥110
Infants (<2 yr)	Systolic BP ≥112	Systolic BP ≥118
	Diastolic BP ≥74	Diastolic BP ≥82
Children (3-5 yr)	Systolic BP ≥116	Systolic BP ≥124
	Diastolic BP ≥76	Diastolic BP ≥84
Children (6-9 yr)	Systolic BP ≥122	Systolic BP ≥130
	Diastolic BP ≥78	Diastolic BP ≥86
Children (10-12 yr)	Systolic BP ≥126	Systolic BP ≥134
	Diastolic BP ≥82	Diastolic BP ≥90
Adolescents (13-15 yr)	Systolic BP ≥136	Systolic BP ≥144
	Diastolic BP ≥86	Diastolic BP ≥92
Adolescents (16-18 yr)	Systolic BP ≥142	Systolic BP ≥150
	Diastolic BP ≥92	Diastolic BP ≥98

Reprinted with permission from the *Report of the Second Task Force on Blood Pressure Control in Children—1987, Pediatrics* 79(1):1, 1987.

How

Apically: under 3 years of age

Radially: over 3 years of age

Apical pulse in young children will usually provide more information about quality and rhythm of heart rate than will radial pulse

Normal Values

See Table 16-4 for normal heart rate values for age

Respirations

When

Routinely according to hospital policy

As ordered by physician

As indicated by standard of care for disease or operation

How

With child quiet, at lowest activity level

Count for a full minute (or 15 seconds multiplied by 4)

Normal Values

See Table 16-5 for normal respiration values for age

NUTRITION

See Tables 16-6 and 16-7 for fluid and caloric requirements

Dehydration Checklist

Change in behavior
  Fussy
  Too quiet
Thirsty
Nauseated
Weak cry
Change in appearance
  Pale
  Ashen-gray
  Wrinkled brow
  "Worried" look
  Sunken eyeballs
  Sunken fontanelles
Tissue turgor
  Loose skin
  Skin picks up easily (tenting)
  Skin does not bounce back
Mucous membranes
  Dry mouth
  Dry tongue
  Absence of salivation
  Mucus thick, tenacious
  No tears
Weight change: severe drop from normal weight
Urinary output

TABLE 16-4. Normal Heart Rate Values for Age*

Age	Approximate beats/min
Neonate: to 1 mo	120-160
Infant	
1-6 mo	130
6-8 mo	120
8-12 mo	115
12 mo	100-140
Preschool	
2 yr	85-125
2-6 yr	90-110
6 yr	65-100
School age: 6-10 yr	85-100
Adolescent	
10-14 yr	80-90
11-16 yr	75-90
18 yr	
Males	70
Females	75
Adults	72

*Most accurate heart rates will always be those taken with child quiet, at lowest activity level, and counted for a full minute.

TABLE 16-5. Normal Respiration Values for Age

Age	Approximate rate/min
0-12 mo	30-50
1-5 yr	20-30
5-12 yr	15-25
12-18 yr	12-20

TABLE 16-6. Maintenance Fluid Requirement Calculation

Child's weight	ml/kg formula
Up to 10 kg	100 ml/kg/24 hr
11-20 kg	1000 ml + 50 ml/kg over 10 kg/24 hr
21-30 kg	1500 + 25 ml/kg over 20 kg/24 hr

TABLE 16-7. Caloric Requirement Calculation*

Age (yr)	Calories
0-1	115/kg
1-3	1300 daily
3-6	1000 daily
6-9	2100 daily
9-12	2200-2400 daily
12-15	2500-3000 daily
15-18	2300-3400 daily

*These figures are approximate; each child's needs will depend on diagnosis and current nutritional state.

TABLE 16-8. Pediatric Emergency Drugs*

Drug	Indication	Dosage
Albumin	Shock; provide serum protein	0.5-1.0 g/kg IV
Aminophylline	Bronchoconstriction	3-7 mg/kg IV; LD and MD 4-6 mg/kg/day
Atropine	Bradycardia not secondary to hypoxia	0.01 mg/kg subcutaneously
Desferoxamine mesylate (Desferal)	Iron poisoning	15 mg/kg/hr IV *or* 80 mg/kg IM q8h, 3 times
Dexamethasone (Decadron)	Cerebral edema	4 mg IM or IV stat and 0.5-1.5 mg q4h
25% dextrose	Hypoglycemia	2-5 ml/kg/dose IV push
Diazepam (Valium)	Seizures (status epilepticus)	0.1-0.3 mg/kg IV slowly q 15-30 min
Diazoxide (Hyperstat)	Hypertensive crisis	2-10 mg/kg rapid IV push
Digoxin (Lanoxin)	Congestive heart failure; paroxysmal atrial tachycardia	Digitalizing dose: divided into three doses; given at q8h intervals Infants: 0.02-0.04 mg/kg/24 hr Children: 0.04-0.06 mg/kg/24 hr
Dopamine (Intropin)	Hypotension	2-5 µg/kg/min IV drip to start; may go up to 50 µg/kg/min
Epinephrine (Adrenalin); aqueous 1:10,000	Cardiac arrest; bradycardia and/or hypotension; refractory congestive heart failure	0.01-0.02 ml/kg intracardiac 1 ml/100 5% dextrose in water at 5-10 micro-drops/min IV
Ethacrynic acid (Edecrin)	Severe congestive heart failure	1 mg/kg IV push
Furosemide (Lasix)	Pulmonary edema	1 mg/kg IV or IM
Hydralazine (Apresoline)	Hypertensive crisis (with reserpine)	1.7-3.5 mg/kg/day IV or IM divided q4h or q6h
Hydrocortisone sodium succinate (Solu-Cortef)	Asthma	3-5 mg/kg IV q6h
Isoproterenol (Isuprel)	Bradycardia and/or hypotension	0.2 mg (1 ml) in 100 ml at 3-5 microdrops/min (0.05-4.0 µg/min)
Glucagon	Hypoglycemic reactions	0.025-0.1 mg/kg IV or IM
Lidocaine (Xylocaine) (2% solution or 20 mg/ml), 1 g vial	Runs of premature ventricular contractions or ventricular tachycardia	Bolus: 1 mg/kg slow IV push, may be repeated one time only; IV drip 20-40 µg/kg/min; 1 g vial/100 ml D5W = 10 µg/ml
Mannitol (25% ampule or 20% in IV bottle)	Acute cerebral edema	1-2 g/kg in 20 min
Methylprednisolone (Solu-Medrol)	Septic shock	15-30 mg/kg IV
Naloxone (Narcan)	Narcotic toxicity	0.01 mg/kg IV; 0.4 mg/ml, 0.02 mg/ml: neonatal
Phenobarbital	Anticonvulsant	5-15 mg/kg IM or slow IV
Procainamide (Pronestyl)	Ventricular tachycardia or runs of premature ventricular contractions	2 mg/kg (maximum 100 mg) IV slowly over 5 min with ECG monitoring
Propranolol (Inderal)	Cardiac dysrhythmias; tetalogy hypercyanotic spells	0.1-0.2 mg/kg slow IV (maximum dose 3 mg)
Sodium bicarbonate	Acidosis	2-4 mEq/kg IV; 1-2 mEq/kg intracardiac; repeat q5-10 min

* Prepared by Eugene Rodriguez, RPh, Pharmacist, Kaiser Permanente Medical Center, Panorama City, Calif.

TABLE 16-9. Average Dosage of Atropine

Weight (lb)	Atropine
3 to 20	0.1 mg
20 to 30	0.15 to 0.2 mg
30 to 40	0.2 to 0.3 mg
40 to 50	0.3 to 0.4 mg
50 to 100	0.4 mg
Over 100	0.6 mg

Decreased amount and frequency
Concentrated
Increased specific gravity
Respirations
   Rapid
   Shallow
Heart rate: rapid
Body temperature: subnormal *or* fever
Neurological status
   Weak
   Depressed
   Twitching
   Convulsions

DRUGS

See Table 16-8 on pediatric emergency drugs
Atropine: see Table 16-9
Pentobarbital (Nembutal): a mg/lb of body weight
Meperidine: 60% to 75% of body weight (pounds) in milligrams
All drugs given IM (unless otherwise ordered)

BIBLIOGRAPHY

Betz CL, Poster EC: *Pediatric nursing reference,* St. Louis, 1989, CV Mosby.

Carpenito LJ: *Handbook of nursing diagnosis,* ed 2, Philadelphia, 1987, JB Lippincott Co.

Curley MAQ: *Pediatric cardiac dysrhythmias,* Bowie, Md, 1985, Brady Communications.

Engel J: *Pocket guide to pediatric assessment,* St Louis, 1988, CV Mosby.

Finberg L et al: Oral rehydration for diarrhea, *J Pediatr* 101(4):497, 1982.

Huston CJ: Epiglottis, *Nursing '88* 18(4):59, April, 1988.

Schaming D et al: When babies are born with orthopedic problems, *RN* 53(4):62, 1990.

Scipien GM, Chard MA, Howe J, et al: *Pediatric nursing care,* St Louis, 1990, Mosby–Year Book.

Waskerwitz M: Special nursing care for children receiving chemotherapy, *J Assoc Pediatr Oncol Nurses* 1(1):16, 1984.

Waskerwitz M, Ruccione K: An overview of cancer in children in the 1980's, *Nurs Clin North Am* 20(1):1985.

Whaley LF, Wong DL: *Essentials of pediatric nursing,* St Louis, 1989, CV Mosby.

Wong DL, Whaley LF: *Clinical manual of pediatric nursing,* St Louis, 1990, Mosby–Year Book.

Medical-Surgical Care

Mass Equivalents for Medications (Metric and Apothecary System)

Apothecary (grains)	Metric (mg)	Metric (g)
1/200	0.3	0.0003
1/150	0.4	0.0004
1/100	0.6	0.0006
1/60	1	0.001
1/30	2	0.002
1/20	3	0.003
1/15	4	0.004
1/10	6	0.006
1/8	8	0.008
1/6	10	0.010
1/4	15	0.015
1/3	20	0.020
1/2 *	30	0.030
3/4	50	0.050
1	60	0.060
1½	100	0.100
2	120	0.12
2½	150	0.15
3	200	0.2
4	250	0.25
5	300	0.3
7½	500	0.5
10	600	0.6
15	1000	1.0
30	2000	2.0

* From ½ to 5 grains; the following more accurate "approximate equivalents" are also acceptable.

¼ grain = 16 mg	2½ grains = 160 mg
½ grain = 32 mg	3 grains = 200 mg
1 grain = 65 mg	4 grains = 260 mg
1½ grains = 100 mg	5 grains = 325 mg
2 grains = 130 mg	

Liquid Equivalent for Medication

Apothecary and customary*	Metric (ml)
1 minim	0.06
5 minims	0.3
10 minims	0.6
15 minims	1
60 minims (1 fluid dram or ⅛ fl oz)	4
75 minims (1¼ fluid drams)	5.0
240 minims (4 fluid drams or ½ fl oz)	15
1 fl oz	30
2 fl oz	60
3 fl oz	90
4 fl oz	120
6 fl oz	180
8 fl oz	240
12 fl oz	360
16 fl oz (1 pt)	480
32 fl oz (1 qt)	960
35 fl oz	1000 (1 L)
64 fl oz	1825
128 fl oz (1 gal)	3650

* Minims, fluid drams, or fl oz.

METRIC CONVERSIONS*

LENGTH

1 inch (in)	= 2.5 centimeters (cm)
1 foot (ft)	= 30 cm
1 yard (yd)	= 0.9 meters (m)
1 mile	= 1.6 kilometers (km)

MASS (WEIGHT)

1 ounce (oz)	= 28 grams (g)
1 pound (lb)	= 0.45 kilogram (kg)
1 short ton (2000 lb)	= 0.9 tonne

VOLUME

1 teaspoon (tsp)	= 5 milliliters (ml)
1 tablespoon (tbsp)	= 15 ml
1 fluid ounce (fl oz)	= 30 ml
1 cup	= 0.24 liters (L)
1 pint (pt)	= 0.47 L
1 quart (qt)	= 0.95 L
1 gallon (gal)	= 3.8 L

* Appropriate conversions to metric measures.

24 Hr Clock System

Conventional 12 hr time	24 hr clock time
12:01 AM	0001
1:00 AM	0100
1:30 AM	0130
2:00 AM	0200
3:00 AM	0300
4:00 AM	0400
5:00 AM	0500
6:00 AM	0600
7:00 AM	0700
8:00 AM	0800
9:00 AM	0900
10:00 AM	1000
11:00 AM	1100
12 noon	1200
1:00 PM	1300
2:00 PM	1400
3:00 PM	1500
4:00 PM	1600
5:00 PM	1700
6:00 PM	1800
7:00 PM	1900
8:00 PM	2000
9:00 PM	2100
10:00 PM	2200
11:00 PM	2300
12 midnight	2400

Centigrade-Fahrenheit Equivalents*

Centigrade (C)	Fahrenheit (F)
36.0	96.8
36.5	97.7
37.0	98.6
37.5	99.5
38.0	100.4
38.5	101.3
39.0	102.2
39.5	103.2
40.0	104.0
40.5	104.9
41.0	105.8
41.5	106.7
42.0	107.6

* CONVERSION
F to C: substract 32, then multiply by $\frac{5}{9}$.
C to F: multiply by $\frac{9}{5}$, then add 32.

Linear Equivalents

Inches	Centimeters (cm)	Meters (m)
0.5	1.25	0.0125
1	2.5	0.025
2	5.1	0.051
3	7.6	0.076
4	10.2	0.10
5	12.7	0.13
6	15.2	0.15
7	17.8	0.18
8	20.8	0.20
9	23.0	0.23
10	25.4	0.25
12	30.5	0.30
18	45.7	0.46
24	61.0	0.61
30	76.2	0.76
36	91.4	0.91
42	106.7	1.07
48	121.9	1.22
54	137.2	1.37
60	152.4	1.52
66	167.6	1.63
72	182.9	1.83

Guidelines for Patient Care Planning and Nursing Care

Patient Care Standards can be used to plan individualized, goal-directed nursing care through the use of the nursing process. In planning the patient's care, the registered nurse should mutually set goals with the patient and/or family. The goals should be realistic, measurable, and based on the nursing assessment. The assessment should include considerations of biophysical, psychosocial, environmental, self-care, educational and discharge planning factors. The plan of care should be made in conjunction with the therapies of other disciplines in order to restore, promote, or maintain the patient's well-being. Needs should be reassessed when warranted by the patient's condition.

To ensure quality and appropriateness of care, it is imperative that any standard care plan be individualized to meet the patient's unique needs. Although the standards contained in this book include the nursing diagnoses, interventions, and expected outcome/evaluation one would most likely encounter in a given situation, it is expected that the nurse will individualize the plan by any number of methods, including but not limited to the following:

1. Noting the patient's name, other identification data, and the date and time of initiation of the care plan, and adding the nurse's signature.
2. Crossing through or deleting those nursing diagnoses, interventions, and evaluations that are not appropriate and initialing same.
3. Adding nursing diagnoses, interventions, and evaluations that are appropriate, as well as the date initiated and the nurse's initials.
4. Evaluating the plan on a daily basis, penciling in the current date and the nurse's initials if the interventions are still applicable. This can be done in a "review" or "evaluation" column adjacent to the nursing interventions. This provides an accountability mechanism to ensure that the plan is current each day.
5. Discontinuing the part of the plan that is no longer appropriate because of achievement of patient-centered goals. This can be done in a "discontinued/resolved" column.

It is possible that a preprinted, standard care plan will meet the needs of some individuals without any changes, especially those with a short length of stay. Therefore to demonstrate that the nurse has used the nursing process, it is important that the care plan be initiated, evaluated, and eventually discontinued by the nurse, who demonstrates accountability by dating and signing (or initialing) these items. The Nursing Care Standards of The Joint Commission on Accreditation of Healthcare Organizations requires that the patient's care is based on a plan. This can be achieved through policies and procedures describing how patient care needs will be met based on standards that serve to guide nurses in providing care to patients. A written plan of care is not required for each patient but there must be evidence that care is planned to meet the individual needs of the patient.

Documentation in the patient's record should reflect the plan of care by including nursing interventions and the patient's response to them. In addition, instructions given to the patient and/or family regarding postdischarge self-care should be documented, as well as their understanding of these instructions. A predischarge summary statement should include information about the patient's outcome, a guide for which can be found in the expected outcome/evaluation sections included with most of the standards in this text.

In summary, the nurse should use the nursing process to assess, plan, intervene, and evaluate nursing care for the patient from admission through discharge from the hospital. The plan of care should be individualized to meet each patient's needs, and documentation of care should reflect the patient's status.

A sample patient case study, accompanied by an individualized patient care plan, is provided here for your review.

CASE STUDY

Mr. Allen is a 60-year-old man admitted to the hospital with complaints of weakness, confusion, and diminishing urine output over the past week. Mr. Allen shows a history of hypertension and glomerulonephritis. On admission his vital signs are BP, 180/90; heart rate, 80 and irregular; respirations, 20; and temperature, 99.5°F (37.5°C). He is also nauseated and vomiting. Mr. Allen reports that his shoes are tight. His ankles show 2+ edema bilaterally. Mr. Allen's lungs have bilateral basal crackles. Mr. Allen's daughter states that Mr. Allen has not been taking his medications regularly and that he has not been complying with his prescribed diet. Mr. Allen has not been able to work for 2 years. He reports feeling depressed at times and has an outburst of anger in the emergency room because his toothbrush was left at home.

Laboratory findings are potassium, 5.7; blood urea nitrogen (BUN), 100; creatinine, 5.

Mr. Allen is placed on bed rest and NPO status. A Foley catheter is inserted and drains 10 ml of dark yellow, concentrated urine. An IV infusion of D5W is started at keep-open rate. Fluids are restricted to 1200 ml/24 hr. A polystyrene sulfonate (Kayexalate) enema is ordered. Furosemide (Lasix) is administered for diuresis and prazosin (Minipress) for hypertension. Blood samples for electrolyte, BUN, and creatinine studies are to be redrawn in 4 hr.

He is diagnosed as having renal failure.

DOCUMENTATION

10/1

S: "I have been urinating less and less every day"; "I've been drinking large amounts of water at home"; patient admitted to 7W from ER

O: Patient has history of diminishing urine output over past 1 week and history of glomerulonephritis; Foley catheter inserted on admission and drained 10 ml of dark yellow, concentrated urine; IV D5W started in left arm—infusing well at keep-open rate; Lasix 80 mg given IV stat with no further urine output noted; BUN, 100; creatinine 5; admission weight, 90 kg.

A: Alteration in urinary elimination (oliguria) related to decreased renal function

P: Measure urine output qh
Monitor urine specific gravity q8h
Note character of urine and report abnormalities
Measure intake and output accurately
Continue IV D5W at keep-open rate
Restrict fluids to 1200 ml/24 hr
Monitor serum BUN, creatinine, and electrolytes and report abnormalities

S: "I'm so thirsty—I've been drinking large amounts of water"; "I haven't urinated at all today"; "My shoes are really tight"; "I'm not sure what it is—I keep forgetting things"; "I'm very tired"

O: Patient awake, lethargic, oriented to person and place but requires frequent reorientation to time;

elevated BP of 180/90; bilateral neck vein distention noted; lungs show bilateral basal crackles—do not clear with cough; patient shows 2+ pitting edema in ankles bilaterally; heart tones S₃ noted; IV D5W started at keep-open rate in left arm—infusing well; patient is on NPO status; placed on 1200 ml/day fluid restriction; Lasix 80 mg given IV stat; no urine output noted; patient's weight is 90 kg on admission; potassium, 5; patient complaining of thirst

A: Fluid volume excess related to decreased ability of kidneys to extract water

P: Weigh patient daily at same time with same clothing and scale
Monitor for elevated BP
Assess level of consciousness; note changes in mental status
Assess heart sounds for presence of S₃ and S₄
Assess breath sounds for rales
Obtain chest x-ray examination as ordered
Assess for peripheral edema
Assess for distended neck veins
Restrict fluids as ordered
Administer diuretics as ordered
Maintain NPO status except for ice chips to control thirst

S: "I'm feeling nauseated"; "Sometimes I feel my heart skip a beat"; "I don't know why I can't get comfortable and rest"

O: Patient awake and restless; nauseated—vomited scant amount of green secretion; NPO at present; cardiac monitor shows frequent premature ventricular beats; apical heart rate, 80 and irregular; Kayexalate enema given—large amount of liquid brown return noted; serum potassium on admission, 5; serum potassium redrawn in 4 hr, 4.7

A: Electrolyte imbalance (hyperkalemia) related to decreasing renal ability to regulate and excrete electrolytes

P: Monitor serum electrolytes q4h as ordered
Report abnormal serum electrolyte values to physician
Dialyze as ordered
Monitor for signs and symptoms of irritability, nausea, diarrhea, intestinal colic, arrythmias, and peaked T wave on ECG
Restrict dietary potassium as ordered
Administer Kayexalate as ordered

S: "I haven't worked in 2 years because of my kidney problems"; "I can't even go to church on Sundays anymore"; "I can't stand this much longer"; "The doctor better get me well this time"; "I can't believe my daughter left my toothbrush at home—she can't do anything right"; "So, I don't take my pills all of the time—what's the difference? No one cares"

S, Subjective assessment; *O,* objective assessment; *A,* assessment (nursing diagnosis); *P,* plan.

O: Patient exhibiting anger at staff and family; daughter reports patient has been depressed at home and noncompliant with medications and treatment regimen; patient is Catholic—verbalizes desire to attend Church

A: Grieving related to loss of function of major organ system, changes in lifestyle, and life-threatening prognosis

P: Be sensitive to changes and restrictions in patient's lifestyle

Encourage patient to express feelings of frustration, anger, fear, and uncertainty

Actively listen

Observe for behavioral and emotional signs of grieving (denial, anger, crying, withdrawal, noncompliance, dependency, etc.)

Be patient and emphathetic as patient experiences emotional changes and develops coping mechanisms

Set limits on maladaptive coping mechanisms if they interfere with patient's well-being

Support adaptive behaviors that suggest a progression and resolution of grieving process

Support realistic hope; answer questions honestly, providing requested information

Arrange for visitation with clergy

Teach and reteach about disease process and management

Involve family and significant others in teaching process

Care Plan Format

Initiation date	Nursing diagnosis/problem	Expected outcome/ evaluation	Review/ evaluation date	Interventions	Resolution/ discontinue date
10/1	Altered urinary elimination (oliguria) related to decreased renal function	Patient maintains present level of urinary elimination or better (as near normal as possible) as evidenced by balanced intake and output, and normal laboratory values for BUN and creatinine within 2 weeks	10/1	Catheter care q8h: 0600, 1400, 2200 Measure urine output qh Monitor urine specific gravity q8h: 0600, 1400, 2200 Note character of urine and report abnormalities Measure intake and output accurately Administer IV D5W as ordered (keep-open rate) Restrict fluids as ordered to 1200 ml/24 hr; 500 ml, days; 400 ml, evenings; 300 ml, nights) Monitor serum BUN, creatinine, and electrolytes as ordered and report abnormalities	10/3
10/1	Fluid volume excess related to decreased ability of kidneys to extract water	Patient shows no signs of fluid volume excess within 1 week as evidenced by balanced intake and output, weight loss of 5 kg, usual mental status, clear breath sounds, and absence of pitting peripheral edema		Maintains NPO status Monitor for and report elevated BP Weigh patient on bed scale at 0600 with same scale and clothing Assess level of consciousness q4h; note and report changes in mental status at 0600, 1000, 1400, 1800, 2200, and 0200 Assess heart sounds for presence of S_3 and/or S_4 Assess breath sounds for rales q4h Assess for peripheral edema	

Continued.

Care Plan Format—cont'd

Initiation date	Nursing diagnosis/problem	Expected outcome/ evaluation	Review/ evaluation date	Interventions	Resolution/ discontinue date
				Assess for distended neck veins	
				Administer diuretic as ordered (Lasix 80 mg IV bid)	
				Provide ice chips to control thirst	
	Electrolyte imbalance (hyperkalemia) related to decreasing renal ability to regulate and excrete electrolytes	Patient maintains safe serum potassium level as evidenced by serum potassium ≤ 4.5 and absence of signs and symptoms of hyperkalemia within 2 days		Monitor serum electrolytes q4h as ordered and report abnormalities	
				Monitor and report symptoms of potassium imbalance (irritability, nausea, diarrhea, intestinal colic, arrhythmias, and peaked T-wave on ECG)	
				Restrict potassium as ordered	
				Administer Kayexalate enema as ordered	
	Grieving related to loss of function of major organ system, changes in lifestyle, and life-threatening prognosis	Patient progresses through grieving process as evidenced by expression of feelings to care giver or significant other, utilization of support systems, and effective coping mechanisms, and by compliance with treatment plan and participation in self-care activities		Be sensitive to changes and restrictions in patient's lifestyle	
				Encourage patient to express feelings of frustration, anger, fear, and uncertainty	
				Actively listen	
				Observe for behavioral and emotional signs of grieving (denial, anger, crying, withdrawal, noncompliance, dependency, etc.)	
				Be patient and empathetic as patient experiences emotional changes and develops coping mechanisms	
				Set limits on maladaptive coping mechanisms if they interfere with patient's well-being	
				Support adaptive behaviors that suggest progression and resolution of grieving process	
				Support realistic hope; answer questions honestly, providing requested information	
				Arrange for visitation by clergy	
				Teach and reteach about disease process and management	
				Involve family and significant others in teaching program	

INDEX

A

Abdominal hysterectomy and bilateral salpingo-oophorectomy, total, 518-519
Abdominoperineal pull-through procedure, 798-800
Abducens nerve, 395
Above knee amputation, 374-376
Abruptio placentae, 708-709
Abscess, brain, 432
Abuse
  child, 838-840
  substance, 434-437
Acceptance stage of dying, 32
Accessory nerve, 395
Acetazolamide for seizure disorders, 400
Acetohexamide for diabetes, 337
Achalasia, 243-244
Acid-base imbalances, 46-50
Acidosis
  metabolic, 48-51
  respiratory, 46-49
Acoustic nerve, 395
Acoustic neuromas of brain, 409
Acquired immune deficiency syndrome, 546-558
  opportunistic infections, neoplasms, and systems involved in, 550
ACTH; see Adrenocorticotropic hormone
Actinomycin D, 660-661
Active labor, 714
Activity intolerance, potential, 8
Activity/exercise functional health pattern, 8-9
Addison's disease, 322
Adenomas, pituitary, 409
ADH; see Antidiuretic hormone
Adolescents, care of, 770
Adoptive immunotherapy, 689-690
Adrenalectomy, 347-349
Adrenalin; see Epinephrine
Adrenocortical insufficiency, 322-324
Adrenocorticotropic hormone, 310
Adria flaré from chemotherapy, 680
Adriamycin; see Doxotrubicin
Adrucil; see 5-Fluorouracil
Adult respiratory distress syndrome, 225-227
Adventitious breath sound, 189
Aerolone; see Isoproterenol
Aerosol therapy, 196
Afterloader, radium therapy sealed in, care of patient receiving, 644-648
Aganglionic megacolon, 796-798
Aging, 20
Aging patient, care of, 29-30
Aging process, normal variations during, 29-30
AICD; see Automatic implantable cardioverter-defibrillator
AIDS; see Acquired immune deficiency syndrome
Airways, artificial, 230-232
Albumin
  for child, 842

Albumin—cont'd
  serum, normal, transfusion of, 182
    reactions to, 185
Albuterol as bronchodilator, 203
Alcohol intoxication, 434-437
Alcohol levels, serum, effects of, 435
Aldosterone, 310
Aldosteronism, primary, 326-328
Alkaloids, vinca, as chemotherapeutic agents, 656-659
  hazards associated with, 668
Alkalosis
  metabolic, 48-49
  respiratory, 46-47
Alkeran; see Melphalan
Alkylating agents as chemotherapeutic agents, 652-655
  hazards associated with, 667
ALL; see Lymphocytic leukemia, acute
Alopecia from chemotherapy, 681-682
ALS; see Amyotrophic lateral sclerosis
Altered consciousness, 396
  care of patient with, 396-399
Alupent; see Metaproterenol
Alzheimer's disease, 418-419
Amethopterin; see Methotrexate
Aminophylline
  as bronchodilator, 203
  for child, 842
AML; see Myelogenous leukemia, acute
Amniocentesis, 703-704
Amoxicillin for endocarditis prophylaxis, 93
Ampicillin for endocarditis prophylaxis, 93
Amputation of leg, 374-376
AMSA; see Amsacrine
Amsacrine, 664-665
Amyotrophic lateral sclerosis, 427-429
Anal reservoir, anastomosis of ileum to, 281-282
Analgesia, patient-controlled, 59
Anastomosis
  ileoanal, 279
  of ileum to anal reservoir, 281-282
Androgens, 310
Anemia
  with AIDS, 550
  aplastic, 164-169
  hemolytic, 160-162
  hypochromic microcytic, 158-160
  iron deficiency, 158-160
  macrocytic, hyperchromic, 155-158
  pernicious, 155-158
  sickle cell, 162-164
"Angel dust," abuse of, 436
Anger stage of dying, 32
Angina pectoris, 81-85
  laboratory and diagnostic findings in, 83-84
  patterns of observations in, 81
Angioplasty, transluminal, percutaneous, 140-141

851

Ankle
  arthroplasty of, 370-374
  and foot, positioning of, to prevent contractures from burns, 529
Ankylosing spondylitis, 367-368
Anorexia from chemotherapy, 675-677
Anorexia nervosa, 249-252
Antepartum assessment of mother, 695-697
Anterior pelvic exenteration, 619
Antibiotics
  as chemotherapeutic agents, 658-663
    hazards associated with, 668
  for endocarditis prophylaxis, 93
Antibodies, monoclonal, as biological response modifier, 691
Anticoagulant, 148
Anticoagulant therapy, 148-150
Antidiuretic hormone, 310
  inappropriate, syndrome of, as oncologic emergency, 636
Antihemophilic factor, cryoprecipitated, transfusion of, 181
Antimetabolites as chemotherapeutic agents, 654-657
  hazards associated with, 667
Antineoplastic chemotherapy, 649-667
Anus, construction of ileal reservoir at, 279-280
Anxiety, 13-15
Aorta, coarctation of, in child, 824-825
Aortic regurgitation, 95-96
  murmurs in, 97
Aortic stenosis
  in child, 825
  murmurs in, 97
Aortofemoral bypass graft, 77-78
APCs; *see* Premature atrial contractions
Apheresis, procedures for, 178
Apheresis therapy, 177-179
Aplastic anemia, 164-169
Apnea, posthyperventilation, 394
Apneustic respirations, 394
Appendix, ruptured (perforated), 794-796
Applicator, Ernst, radium therapy sealed in, care of patient receiving, 644-648
Apresoline; *see* Hydralazine
Ara-C; *see* Cytarabine
Aramine; *see* Metaraminol
ARDS; *see* Adult respiratory distress syndrome
Arm, burns of, placement of contracture roll for, 529
Arrest, sinus, 123
Arterial insufficiency, chronic, 73-75
Arterial system, 64
Arteriovenous fistula, internal, 491
Artery, pulmonary, banding of, 829-830
Arthritis
  gouty, 358-359
  pyogenic, acute, 355-356
  rheumatoid, 558-560
Arthroplasty
  cup, 368
  joint, total, 370-374
  Keller, 384
  Mayo, 384
Arthroscopic surgery of knee, 376-377
Artificial airways, 230-232
Artificial pacemaker, temporary, in child, 837-838
Artificial urinary sphincter, 466-469
Ascending colostomy, 264
ASD; *see* Atrial septal defect
Asparaginase, 662-663
  hazards associated with, 668

Aspergillosis with AIDS, 550
Aspergillus infection in cancer patient, 641
Aspiration of secretions, 193-194
Aspirin, effect of, on nutritional status, 4
ASPO review sheet, 715-716
Assaultive behavior, potential for, 21-22
Asthma, 202-204, 780-782
Astrocytomas, brain, 409
Asymmetric pupils, 393
Ataxic breathing, 394
Ataxic respiration, 187
Atelectasis, 220-221
Atresia, esophageal, 790
Atrial beats, premature, 123
Atrial catheter, Silastic, 55-56
Atrial contractions, premature, 123-124
Atrial fibrillation, 125
Atrial flutter, 124-125
Atrial origin, rhythms of, 123-126
Atrial septal defect in child, 822-823
Atrioventricular block, 129-132
Atrioventricular junctional biopsy, 132
Atrioventricular junctional rhythms, 132
Atropine for child, 842, 843
Auditory and optic systems, 532-543
Auditory system, assessment of, 539-540
Auditory-impaired patient, 540-541
Augmentation of labor, 718-720
AUS; *see* Artificial urinary sphincter
Automatic implantable cardioverter-defibrillator, 138-139
AV block; *see* Atrioventricular block
Axilla, burns of, placement of contracture roll for, 529
Azacytidine, 656-657
Azathioprine, hazards associated with, 668

B

Bacillus, Calmette-Guérin, as biological response modifier, 688
Bacterial infections involved in AIDS, 550
Bacterial meningitis, 432
Bacterial pneumonia, findings in, 207
Balanced suspension with Thomas' splint and Pearson's attachment, 388
Balloon septostomy in child, 829
Balloon-tipped pulmonary catheter, triple-lumen, 145
Banding, pulmonary artery, 829-830
Barbiturates, effect of, on nutritional status, 4
Bargaining stage of dying, 32
BCNU; *see* Carmustine
Beats, atrial, premature, 123
Bed, circle, care of patient on, 442
Behavior
  assaultive, potential for, 21-22
  demanding, 23
  dependent, 24
  manipulative, 22
  withdrawn, 23-24
Below knee amputation, 374-376
Beta-2; *see* Isoetharine
Bicarbonate, base
  deficit of, 46-47, 48-51
  excess of, 46-49
Bilateral salpingo-oophorectomy, total abdominal hysterectomy and, 518-519
Biliary cirrhosis, 293-295
Biliary decompression catheter, transhepatic, 292-293
Biliary lithotripsy, 290-291

Biliary obstruction, 287-288
Biliary surgery, 288-290
Biological response modifiers, 687-693
Biophysical profile of fetus, 721
Biopsy
    junctional, atrioventricular, 132
    liver, 302
Biot's respirations, 187, 394
Biphasic insulin, 336
Bishop scoring system of labor, 719
Bladder, cancer of, 585-586
Blalock-Taussig shunt, 829
Bleeding, gastric, 253-254
Bleeding esophageal varices, 244-246
Blenoxane; see Bleomycin sulfate
Bleo; see Bleomycin sulfate
Bleomycin sulfate, 658-659
    hazards associated with, 668
Blindness, 533-535
Block, atrioventricular, 129-132
Blood
    and blood components, 180-182
    loss of, signs and symptoms of, 174
    whole
        for transfusion, 181
        transfusion of, reactions to, 183-184, 185
Blood cells, human, 154
    formation and maturation of, 155
    red, transfusion of, reactions to, 183, 184
Blood pressure
    of child, 840
    high, stepped care approach for treatment of, 80
Blood transfusions, 179-185
    reactions to, 183-185
Body
    correct alignment of, body positions to maintain, 406
    positions of, to maintain correct alignment, 406
    temperature of, altered, potential, 6
Body cast, 388-389
Body image disturbance, 16-17
Bone marrow study, 165
Bone marrow transplantation, 565-580
    schedule for, 566
Bowel; see Intestine
Bowel training, 441
Bradycardia, sinus, 120, 122
Brain
    abscess of, 432
    tumors of, 408-411
BRAT diet, 801
Breast(s)
    cancer of, 587-590
        internal radiation therapy for, 645
    self-examination of, 588, 589
Breast milk, hand expression of, 733
Breast-feeding, 731-734
    correct body position for, 732
    positions for, after cesarean delivery, 731
Breath sounds, 189-190
Breathing
    ataxic, 394
    cluster, 394
    intermittent positive pressure, 237-238
    retraining techniques for, 199
Breech presentation, frank, with prolapsed cord, 710
Brethine; see Terbutaline

Bricanyl; see Terbutaline
Bricker procedure for ileal conduit, 470, 471
Bronchial breath sound, 189
Bronchiolitis, 782-783
Bronchodilators, 203
Bronchophony, 190
Bronchopulmonary dysplasia, 758-760
Bronchoscopy, therapeutic, 191-192
Bronchovesicular breath sound, 189
Bronkaid Mist; see Epinephrine
Bronkephrine; see Ethylnorepinephrine
Bronkodyl; see Theophylline
Bronkometer; see Isoetharine
Bronkosol; see Isoetharine
Brooke formula for fluid replacement for burns, 531
Bryant's traction, 387, 388
Buckling, scleral, 536, 538
Bulimia nervosa, 249-252
Bunionectomy, 384-385
Burn(s)
    classification of, 525-531
    estimation of, 526
    fluid replacement for, 531
    management of, 525-531
Busulfan, 652-653
Bypass
    gastric, 257
    jejunoileal, 257, 258
Bypass graft
    aortofemoral, 77-78
    femoropopliteal, 74

C
Calcitonin, 311
Calcium
    deficit of, 42-43
    excess, 40-41
    urinary, 479-482
Calmette-Guérin bacillus as biological response modifier, 688
Caloric requirement for child, calculation of, 841
Cancer
    bladder, 585-586
    breast, 587-590
        internal radiation therapy for, 645
    cervical, 591
        internal radiation therapy for, 645
    colorectal, 584-585
    detection and prevention of, 581-593
    endometrial, 591-592
    esophageal, 583-584
        internal radiation therapy for, 645
    head and neck, 582
    infections in patients with, 641
    lung, 582-583
    ovarian, 590-591
    pelvic, 585-586
    prostate, 587
    radiotherapy for, 642-644
    renal, 585-586
    skin, 581-582
    staging of, using TNM classifications of, 594
    stomach, 583-584
    surgery for, 641-642
    testicular, 586-587
    therapy for, 641-693

Cancer—cont'd
  ureteral, 585-586
  urethral, 585-586
  uterine, 591-592
  vaginal, 590
Candida infection in cancer patient, 641
Candidiasis with AIDS, 550
Cannabis, commonly abused, 434
Cantor tube, 282-283
CAPD; *see* Continuous ambulatory peritoneal dialysis
Captopril, 88, 91
Carbamazepine for seizure disorders, 400
Carbon dioxide tension
  decreased, 46-47
  elevated, 46-49
Carboplatin, 662-663
  hazards associated with, 668
Carcinoma
  esophageal, 603-604
  intestinal, 606-607
  liver, 607-610
  pancreatic, 610-611
  stomach, 605-606
Cardiac catheterization, 139
Cardiac cycle, 121
Cardiac rehabilitation, 116-120
Cardiac tamponade, 100-101
  as oncologic emergency, 635-636
Cardiac transplantation, 115-116
Cardiogenic shock, 105
  causes/etiologies of, 104
Cardiotomy, syndrome following, 116
Cardiotoxicity from chemotherapy, 682-683
Cardiovascular assessment, 63-68
Cardiovascular oncologic emergencies, 635-636
Cardiovascular risk factor profile, 79
Cardiovascular system, 63-151
  disorders of, in children, 821-838
Cardioverter-defibrillator, automatic implantable, 138-139
Care plan format, 849-850
Carmustine, 654-655
Carotid endarterectomy, 75-76
Cast management, 385, 388-389
Cataract removal, 536
Catheter(s)
  atrial, Silastic, 55-56
  central, peripherally inserted, 57-58
  epidural, permanent, 59-60
  intrauterine, care of mother with, 722
  peritoneal, indwelling, 487
  pulmonary, triple-lumen balloon-tipped, 145
  subclavian, multilumen, 54-55
  Swan-Ganz, 144
  transhepatic biliary decompression, 292-293
  urethral, indwelling, management of, 469-470
Catheterization
  cardiac, 139
  umbilical, 748-749
Catract removal, 538
Cauda equina lesion, 414
CCNU; *see* Lomustine
CCPD; *see* Continuous cycling peritoneal dialysis
Cell(s), blood, 154
  cycle of, 650
  formation and maturation of, 155
  red, transfusion of, reactions to, 183, 184

Cellulitis, 525
Celontin; *see* Methsuximide
Centigrade-Fahrenheit equivalents, 846
Central catheter, peripherally inserted, 57-58
Central diabetes insipidus, 330-332
Central lines, 53-58
Central nervous system
  disorders of, in children, 803-811
  surgical intervention of, 416-418
Central neurogenic hyperventilation, 394
Central spinal cord lesion, 414
Central venous nutrition, 37
Cerebellum, tumors of, 409
Cerebrovascular accident, 404-408
Cerebrovascular disruptions, 402-404
Cerubidin; *see* Daunomycin
Cervical cast, 388-389
Cervical cord injuries, 413, 414
Cervical spine, fracture or dislocation of, 365-367
Cervical traction, 387, 388
Cervix, cancer of, 591
  internal radiation therapy for, 645
Cesarean delivery, 728-731
  breast-feeding positions after, 731
Cesium therapy sealed in mould, afterloader, colpostat, or Ernst applicator, care of patient receiving, 644-648
Chambers, heart, oxygen saturation in, 143
Chemical substance abuse, 435-437
Chemotherapeutic drugs, 652-665
  safety in handling, 667-669
Chemotherapy, 649
  antineoplastic, 649-667
  hematological problems with, 670-675
  symptomatic care in, 670-687
Chest
  burns of, placement of contracture roll for, 529
  flail, 222-223
Chest tubes, 229-230
  removal of, 229-230
Chest wall, landmarks on, 66
Cheyne-Stokes respirations, 187, 394
Chickenpox, 772-773
Child(ren)
  abuse of, 838-840
  caloric requirement for, calculation of, 841
  cardiovascular system disorders in, 821-838
  central nervous system disorders in, 803-811
  digitalis therapy for, 836-837
  emergency drugs for, 842
  fluid requirement for, calculation of, 841
  gastrointestinal system disorders in, 786-803
  genitourinary system disorders in, 811-815
  growth charts for, 768, 769
  hematologic disorders in, 815-821
  preschool-age, care of, 766-767
  respiratory system disorders of, 770-786
  school-age, care of, 767-770
Childhood diseases, 772-775
Chlorambucil, 652-653
Chlorpropamide for diabetes, 337
Cholecystectomy, 288
  endoscopic laparoscopic laser, 291-292
Choledochojejunostomy, 288
Choledocholithotomy, 288
Choledyl; *see* Oxtriphylline
Cholinergic crisis, 426-427

Chronic obstructive pulmonary disease, 196-202
  diseases contributing to, 197
Circle bed, care of patient on, 442
Circulatory system of heart, 64
Cirrhosis, 293-295
Cisplatin, 662-663
  hazards associated with, 668
Cleft lip, repair of, 786-788
Cleft palate, repair of, 788-789
Clindamycin for endocarditis prophylaxis, 93
Clonazepam for seizure disorders, 400
Clonopin; *see* Clonazepam
Closed fracture, 359
Closed-heart surgery in child, 830-832
Closure, ileostomy, 281-282
Cluster breathing, 394
Coagulation, intravascular, disseminated, 173-175
  as oncologic emergency, 634
Coarctation of aorta, in child, 824-825
Coarse crackles, 189
Coccidioidomycosis with AIDS, 550
Cognitive/perceptual functional health pattern, 10-13
"Cold" shock, 105
COLD; *see* Chronic obstructive lung disease
Colectomy, temporary ileostomy, and construction of ileal reservoir at
    anus, 279-280
Colitis, ulcerative, 265-267
Colon, diverticular disease of, 272-273
Colony-stimulating factors as biological response modifier, 691-692
Colorectal cancer, 584-585
Colostomy, 283-285
  ascending, 264
  irrigation of, 285-286
  sigmoid, 264
  transverse, 264
Colpostat, radium therapy sealed in, care of patient receiving, 644-
    648
Coma
  hyperosmolar hyperglycemic nonketotic, 343
    comparison of, with diabetic ketoacidosis and hypoglycemia, 341
  myxedema, 312
Coma Scale, Glasgow, 391
Comminuted fracture, 411
Communicating hydrocephalus, 803
Communication deficit after stroke, 408
Compartment syndrome, 382, 384
Complete AV block, 131-132
Complete fracture, 359
Complete prolapse of umbilical cord, 710
Complete separation of placenta, 708
Compound fracture, 359, 411
Compression, spinal cord, as oncologic emergency, 638
Concussion, 411
Conduit
  ileal, 470, 471
  jejunal, 470
Conflict, decisional, 12-13
Congenital heart defects, 821-828
Congenital heart surgery, 828-835
Congenital rubella, 772-773
Congestive heart failure in child, 835-836
Connective tissue, tumors of, 595
Consciousness, altered, 396
  care of patient with, 396-399
Constipation, 6-7
  from chemotherapy, 679-680

Contact lens removal, 538-539
Continent ileostomy, 275-279
Continent urinary diversion, 470
Continuous ambulatory peritoneal dialysis, 486
Continuous cycling peritoneal dialysis, 487
Continuous drip narcotics, intravenous, 58-59
Continuous mechanical ventilation, 235-237
Continuous passive motion device, 389
Contraceptives, oral, effect of, on nutritional status, 4
Contraction stress test, 723-724
Contractions
  atrial, premature, 123-124
  ventricular, premature, 126-127
Contracture roll, 529
Contractures from burns, positioning to prevent, 529
Controlled cough technique, 199
Contusion, brain, 411
Convulsions, 399-402
COPD; *see* Chronic obstructive pulmonary disease
COPD disability scale, 205
Coping, ineffective, 25-26
Coping/stress intolerance functional health pattern, 25-26
Cord
  spinal; *see* Spinal cord
  umbilical; *see* Umbilical cord
Corneal transplant, 536, 537
Corticosteroids, effect of, on nutritional status, 4
Cortisol; *see* Glucocorticoids
Cosmegen; *see* Dactinomycin
Cough
  controlled, 199
  whooping, 772-773, 777-778
Coup-contracoup phenomenon, 411
Crackles, 189
Cranial nerves, functions of, 395
Craniectomy, 416
Craniocerebral trauma, 411-413
Craniotomy, 416
Crisis
  cholinergic, 426-427
  hypertensive, 78-81
  myasthenia gravis, 426-427
  sickle cell, 162-164
  thyroid, 315-318
  thyrotoxic, 315-318
Crohn's disease, 265-267
Croup, 770-771, 776
Cryopexy, retinal, 536, 538
Cryoprecipitated antihemophilic factor, transfusion of, 181
Cryptococcosis with AIDS, 550
Cryptococcus infection in cancer patient, 641
Cryptosporidiosis with AIDS, 550
CST; *see* Contraction stress test
CTX; *see* Cyclophosphamide
Cup arthroplasty, 368
Curettage, dilation and, 515-516
Cushing's disease, 324-326
Cushing's syndrome, 324-326
Cutaneous ureterostomy, 470, 471
CVA; *see* Cerebrovascular accident
Cyanotic congenital heart defects, 826-828
Cyclophosphamide, 652-653
  hazards associated with, 667
Cystic fibrosis, 783-786
Cystitis, 451
  hemorrhagic, from chemotherapy, 684-685

Cystolithotomy, 481
Cytarabine, 654-655
    hazards associated with, 667
Cytomegalic inclusion disease, 754
Cytomegalovirus with AIDS, 550
Cytomegalovirus infection in cancer patient, 641
Cytosar; *see* Cytarabine
Cytoxan; *see* Cyclophosphamide

D

D & C; *see* Dilation and curettage
Dacarbazine, 662-663
    hazards associated with, 668
Dactinomycin, 660-661
    hazards associated with, 668
Daunomycin, 660-661
    hazards associated with, 668
Daunorubicin, 660-661
    hazards associated with, 668
Deaf patient, 540-541
Death, 30
Decadron; *see* Dexamethasone
Decisional conflict, 12-13
Deep tendon reflexes, 394
Deficiency syndrome, immune, acquired, 546-558
Delivery
    care of mother during, 717-718
    cesarean, 728-731
        breast-feeding positions after, 731
    labor and, care of diabetic mother during, 705-706
    palpating fundus of uterus after, 725
    stabilization of newborn at, 737
Demanding behavior, 23
Denial and shock stage of dying, 31
Depakene; *see* Valproic acid
Dependent behavior, 24
Depressant drugs
    abuse of, 435
    commonly abused, 434
Depressed fracture, 411
Depression stage of dying, 32
Dermatological problems with chemotherapy, 680-681
Desferal; *see* Desferoxamine mesylate
Desferoxamine mesylate for child, 842
Dexamethasone for child, 842
Dextrose 50% for child, 842
Diabetes insipidus, central, 330-332
Diabetes mellitus, 332-340
    classifications of, 333
    mother with
        care of
            during labor and delivery, 705-706
            during last trimester of pregnancy, 704-705
        infant of, 744-745
    snacks before exercise with, 335
Diabetic ketoacidosis, 340-342
    comparison of, with hyperosmolar hyperglycemic nonketotic coma
        and hypoglycemia, 341
Diagnoses, nursing; *see* Nursing diagnoses
Diagnostic neurological procedures, 396
Dialysis, peritoneal, 486-490
Diamox; *see* Acetazolamide
Diarrhea, 7
    from chemotherapy, 678-679
    diet for control of, 801-802
Diazepam for child, 842

Diazoxide for child, 842
DIC; *see* Disseminated intravascular coagulation
Diet
    for control of diarrhea, 801-802
    low-bacteria, 578
Digestive system, 240-307
    anatomy of, 241
Digital replantation, 379-382
Digitalis therapy, pediatric, 836-837
Digoxin for child, 842
Dilantin; *see* Phenytoin
Dilated pupils, 393
Dilation and curettage, 515-516
Dilor; *see* Dyphylline
Diphtheria, 774-775
Discectomy, 362
Disease(s)
    Addison's, 322
    Alzheimer's, 418-419
    bowel, inflammatory, 265-267
    childhood, 772-775
    Crohn's, 265-267
    Cushing's, 324-326
    cytomegalic inclusion, 754
    diverticular, of colon, 272-273
    graft vs. host, 572
        clinical grading of severity of, 574
        proposed clinical stage of, according to organ system, 573
    Graves', 315
    heart, valvular, 95-98
        murmurs in, 97
    Hirschsprung's, 796-798
    Hodgkin's, 593, 628-632
        staging of, 629
    hyaline membrane, 755-756
    inflammatory, pelvic, 513-514
    kidney, polycystic, 475-477
    "Lou Gehrig's," 427
    Parkinson's, 419-422
    peptic ulcer, 252-253
    pulmonary, obstructive, chronic, 196-202
        diseases contributing to, 197
Dislocation of cervical spine, 365-367
Disorientation, 11-12
Dissection, neck, radical, 600-603
Disseminated intravascular coagulation, 173-175
    as oncologic emergency, 634
Disseminated sclerosis, 422-424
Dissolution, urinary stone, percutaneous, 480
Distress
    fetal, 720-721
    spiritual, 26-27
Diversion
    ureteroenterocutaneous, 470
    urinary, 470-475
        continent, 470
Diverticular disease of colon, 272-273
Diverticulitis, acute, 272-273
Diverticulosis, 243-244
DKA; *see* Diabetic ketoacidosis
DNR; *see* Daunomycin
Dopamine for child, 842
Dorsal root rhizotomy, microsurgical, 362
Doxotrubicin, 660-661
Dressler's syndrome, 116
Drip rates, IV, regulation of, 53

Drop rate-calibrated infusion controllers, 58
Drop rate-calibrated infusion pumps, 58
Drops, eye, instillation of, 539
Drugs; see Medications
DTIC; see Dacarbazine
Ductus arteriosus, patent, 821-822
Duhamel procedure, 798
Dumping syndromes, 256-257
Duodenostomy-jejunostomy, 263-264
Duodenum
    endoscopy of, 247-248
    peptic ulcer disease of, 252-253
    ulcer of, 252
Dyflex; see Dyphylline
Dying, stages of, care during, 31-32
Dying patient, care of, 30-32
Dyphylline as bronchodilator, 203
Dysfunctional grieving, 18-19
Dysfunctional labor patterns, 719
Dysmaturity, 742-743
Dysplasia, bronchopulmonary, 758-760
Dysrhythmia, sinus, 122-123

E
Ear
    anatomy of, 542
    surgery on, 541-543
Early labor, 714
ECG changes, miscellaneous, 134
ECG complex, normal, 120, 121
ECG intervals, meaning and significance of, 121
ECG rhythms, 120-134
Eclampsia, 701-702
Edecrin; see Ethacrynic acid
Edema
    pitting, assessment of, 698
    pulmonary, 209-211
Effusion, pleural, 221-222
    as oncologic emergency, 638-639
Egophony, 190
Elbow
    arthroplasty of, 370-374
    range of motion of, after stroke, 406
Eldesine; see Vindesine
Electrical nerve stimulation, transcutaneous, 60-61
Electrode, spiral, care of mother with, 722
Electrolyte imbalances, 38-46
Electronic infusion devices, 58
Elimination, urinary, altered patterns of, 7-8
Elimination functional health pattern, 6-8
Elixophyllin; see Theophylline
Elspar; see Asparaginase
Embolism, pulmonary, 211-212
Emergencies, oncologic, 634-641; see also Oncologic emergencies
Emergency drugs, pediatric, 842
Empyema, thoracic, 219-220
Encephalitis, 432
Endarterectomy, carotid, 75-76
Endocarditis, infective, 91-95
Endocrine assessment, 308-312
Endocrine glands, 310-311
Endocrine system, 308-351
    organs of, 309
    surgical interventions on, 345-351
Endometrial cancer, 591-592

Endoscopic laser cholecystectomy, laparoscopic, 291-292
Endoscopic removal of urinary stone, 480
Endoscopy, 247-248
Endotracheal tube, 231-232
    newborn with, care of, 757
Endoxana; see Cyclophosphamide
Enteral nutrition, 32-36
Enteritis, regional, 265-267
Enterocolitis, necrotizing, 752-753
Enucleation, 536, 538
Ephedrine as bronchodilator, 203
Epidural catheter, permanent, 59-60
Epidural hematoma, 411
Epidural method of intracranial pressure monitoring, 440
Epiglottitis, 776-777
Epilepsy, 399-402
Epinephrine, 310
    as bronchodilator, 203
    for child, 842
Episiotomies, types of, 725
Epithelium, tumors of, 595
Epstein-Barr virus with AIDS, 550
Equipment, special, care of patients with, 53-61
Ernst applicator, radium therapy sealed in, care of patient receiving, 644-648
Erythema from chemotherapy, 680
Erythrocytapheresis, 178
Erythromycin for endocarditis prophylaxis, 93
Erythropoietin as biological response modifier, 691
Escape rhythms, junctional, 132
Escherichia coli infection in cancer patient, 641
Esophagitis, 243-244
    from chemotherapy, 678
Esophagostomy, 263-264
Esophagus, 243-249
    atresia of, 790
    bleeding varices of, 244-246
    cancer of, 583-584
        internal radiation therapy for, 645
    carcinoma of, 603-604
    endoscopy of, 247-248
    stricture of, 243-244
    surgery on, 246-247
Estrogen, 311
ESWL; see Extracorporeal shock wave lithotripsy
Ethacrynic acid for child, 842
Ethosuximide for seizure disorders, 400
Ethylnorepinephrine as bronchodilator, 203
Etoposide, 658-659
    hazards associated with, 668
Eupnea, 394
Exanthema subitum, 772-773
Exchange transfusion, 747-748
Exenteration, pelvic, 619-621
Expression of breast milk, hand, 733
External fixation for complicated fractures, 377-379
External fixator, Ilizarov, 378
External monitoring during labor, 722
External pacemaker, temporary, 135
Extracellular fluid volume
    deficit of, 50-51
    excess of, 50-51
Extracorporeal shock wave lithotripsy, 290
    for urinary calculi, 480
Extraction, stone, surgical, 481
Extravasation as complication of chemotherapy, 669-670

Eye
  anatomy of, 533
  surgery on, 536-538
Eye drops/ointments, instillation of, 539

F

Facet joint rhizotomy, 362
Facial nerve, 395
Fahrenheit-centigrade equivalents, 846
Failure to thrive, 818-821
Fallot, tetralogy, in child, 826-827
Family-centered care of high-risk infant, 761
Feeding
  by gastrostomy tube, 792
  gavage, intermittent, 760-761
Female
  external genitalia of, 511
  genitourinary and reproductive system of, 449
  reproductive system of, 510-520
    anatomy of, 510
    assessment of, 510-513
  urinary incontinence in, surgery for, 464-466
Femoropopliteal bypass graft, 74
Fetal alcohol syndrome, 750
Fetal distress, 720-721
Fetal monitor, mother with, care of, 722
Fetus, biophysical profile of, 721
Fever, scarlet, 774-775
Fibrillation
  atrial, 125
  ventricular, 128-129
Fibroids, uterine, 518
Fibrosis, cystic, 783-786
Fine crackles, 189
Finger
  arthroplasty of, 370-374
  puncture sites in, for glucose monitoring, 338
  replacement of, 379-382
First-degree AV block, 129-130
Fistula
  arteriovenous, internal, 491
  tracheoesophageal, 789-791
    repair of, 791-793
Fixation
  external, for complicated fractures, 377-379
  internal
    Harrington rod, for scoliosis, 363
    of hip, 368
    maxillomandibular, 361-362
Fixator, external, Ilizarov, 378
Flail chest, 222-223
Flare, Adria, from chemotherapy, 680
Fluid, extracellular, volume of, imbalances in, 50-51
Fluid imbalances, 50-51
  and electrolyte imbalances, 38-51
Fluid replacement for burns, 531
Fluid requirement for child, calculation of, 841
Fluoroplex; see 5-Fluorouracil
5-Fluorouracil, 656-657
  hazards associated with, 667
Flutter, atrial, 124-125
Follicle-stimulating hormone, 310
Food
  medications to be taken with, 4
  safeness of, temperatures for, 579

Foot and ankle, positioning of, to prevent contractures from burns, 529
Formula, Brooke, for fluid replacement for burns, 531
Fractures, 359-361
  of cervical spine, 365-367
  comminuted, 411
  complicated, external fixation for, 377-379
  compound, 411
  depressed, 411
  linear, 411
Frame, Stryker, 442
Frank breech presentation with prolapsed cord, 710
Friction rub, pleural, 189
Frontal lobe brain tumors, 409
FSH; see Follicle-stimulating hormone
5-FU; see 5-Fluorouracil
Full-thickness burns, 525, 526
Functional incontinence, 453-455
Fundus of uterus, palpating, after delivery, 725
Fungi involved in AIDS, 550
Furosemide for child, 842
Fusion, spinal, 362

G

Gallbladder, 287-293
  infection of, 287-288
  removal of, 288, 292
Gallstones, 287-288
Gastric bypass, 257
Gastroenteritis, 800-801
Gastrointestinal assessment, 240-243
Gastrointestinal problems with chemotherapy, 675-680
Gastrointestinal system, disorders of, in children, 786-803
Gastroplasty, 257
Gastrostomy, 263-264
Gastrostomy tube, feeding by, 792
Gavage feeding, intermittent, 760-761
General care and nursing diagnoses, 1-62
General preoperative care/teaching, 27-28
General rehabilitative care of neurological patient, 442-444
Generalized seizures, 399
Genitalia, female, external, 511
Genitourinary assessment, 447-451
Genitourinary system, 447-509
  disorders of, in children, 811-815
  female, 449
  male, 449
  organs of, 448
Gentamicin for endocarditis prophylaxis, 93
German measles, 772-773
Gestational age
  large for, 742-743
  small for, 742
Giardiasis with AIDS, 550
Gland(s)
  endocrine, 310-311
  pituitary, 310
  thyroid, 311
  tumors of, 595
Glasgow Coma Scale, 391
Glaucoma, acute, of adult onset, 535-536
Gliomas, brain, 409
Glipizide for diabetes, 337
Glomerulonephritis, 477-479
  acute, in children, 811-813
Glossopharyngeal nerve, 395

Glucagon, 310
  for child, 842
Glucocorticoids, 310
Glyburide for diabetes, 337
Gonadal dysfunction from chemotherapy, 687
Gonads, 311
Gouty arthritis, 358-359
Graft vs. host disease, 572
  clinical grading of severity of, 574
  proposed clinical stage of, according to organ system, 573
Graft
  bypass
    aortofemoral, 77-78
    femoropopliteal, 74
  skin, skinning vulvectomy with, 617
Granulocyte colony-stimulating factor as biological response modifier, 691
Granulocyte-macrophage colony-stimulating factor as biological response modifier, 691
Graves' disease, 315
Great vessels
  oxygen saturation in, 143
  transposition of, in child, 827-828
Grieving, dysfunctional, 18-19
Growth, intrauterine, retardation of, 742
Growth chart(s)
  for boys, 769
  for girls, 768
  for infant boys, 765
  for infant girls, 764
Growth hormone, 310
Guillain-Barrè syndrome, 429-432

H
Hairy leukoplakia with AIDS, 550
Half spinal cord lesion, 414
Hallucinogens
  abuse of, 436
  commonly abused, 434
Halo traction, 387
  skull tongs and, 441-442
Hand
  positioning of, to prevent contractures from burns, 529
  range of motion of, after stroke, 407
Hand expression of breast milk, 733
Harrington rod internal fixation for scoliosis, 363
Head and neck
  cancer of, 582
  positioning of, to prevent contractures from burns, 529
Health perception/management, 1-2
Heart
  catheterization of, 139
  chambers of, oxygen saturation in, 143
  circulatory system of, 64
  congenital defects of, 821-828
  rehabilitation for, 116-120
  surgery on, 108-114
    for congenital disorder, 828-835
  tamponade of, 100-101
  transplantation of, 115-116
  valves of, location of, 66
Heart disease, valvular, 95-98
  murmurs in, 97
Heart failure, 101-105
  congestive, in child, 835-836
  vasodilator drugs used for, potential complications of, 88

Heart rate of child, 840-841
Height and weight tables, 3
Hematologic assessment, 152-154
Hematologic disorders
  in children, 815-821
  clues to, 156
Hematologic system, 152-185
Hematological oncologic emergencies, 634
Hematological problems with chemotherapy, 670-675
Hematoma
  epidural, 411
  subdural, 411
Hematopoietic tissue, tumors of, 595
Hemodialysis, care of patient after, 490-493
Hemodynamic monitoring, 143, 146-147
Hemolytic anemia, 160-162
Hemorrhage
  intracerebral, 402
  as oncologic emergency, 634
  postpartum, 734-735
  subarachnoid, 402
Hemorrhagic cystitis from chemotherapy, 684-685
Hemothorax, 217
  assessment/finding in, 216
Heparin, subcutaneous injection of, 149-150
Hepatitis, viral, 295-298
Hepatitis A, 295
Hepatitis B, 295
Hepatoxicity from chemotherapy, 686-687
Hernia, inguinal, incarcerated, 802
Herpes simplex infection in cancer patient, 641
Herpes simplex virus, 754-755
  with AIDS, 550
Herpes zoster virus with AIDS, 550
Hespan, transfusion of, 182
Hetastarch, transfusion of, 182
HHNC; *see* Hyperosmolar hyperglycemic nonketotic coma
High birth weight infant, 742-743
High blood pressure, stepped care approach for treatment of, 80
High-risk infant, family-centered care of, 761
Hip
  arthroplasty of, 370-374
  internal fixation of, 368
  surgery on, 368-370
Hip spica cast, 388-389
Hirschsprung's disease, 796-798
Histoplasmosis with AIDS, 550
HIV; *see* Human immunodeficiency virus
HN$_2$, 652-653
Hodgkin's disease, 593, 628-632
  staging of, 629
Hopelessness, 15-16
Hormone
  adrenocorticotropic, 310
  antidiuretic, 310
    inappropriate, syndrome of, as oncologic emergency, 636
  follicle-stimulating, 310
  growth, 310
  interstitial cell-stimulating, 310
  luteinizing, 310
  luteotrophic, 310
  parathyroid, 311
  thyroid-stimulating, 310
Host performance status, 594
Hostility, excessive, potential for, 21-22
Human blood cells, 154

860 Index

Human immunodeficiency virus
  infection with, Centers for Disease Control classification of, 547
  mechanism of action of, 548
Humerus, traction of, 388
Humidifiers, 196
Humidity and aerosol therapy, 196
Hyaline membrane disease, 755-756
Hydatidiform mole, 515
Hydralazine, 88, 90
  for child, 842
  effect of, on nutritional status, 4
Hydrocephalus, 803-805
Hydrocortisone sodium succinate for child, 842
Hyperbilirubinemia, infant with, care of, 745-747
Hypercalcemia, 40-41
  as oncologic emergency, 636-637
Hyperchromic macrocytic anemia, 155-158
Hyperemesis gravidarum, 702-703
Hyperglycemia as oncologic emergency, 637
Hyperglycemic nonketotic coma, hyperosmolar, 343
  comparison of, with diabetic ketoacidosis and hypoglycemia, 341
Hyperkalemia, 38-39
Hypermagnesemia, 44-45
Hypernatremia, 42-43
Hyperosmolar hyperglycemic nonketotic coma, 343
  comparison of, with diabetic ketoacidosis and hypoglycemia, 341
Hyperparathyroidism, 320-321
Hyperpyrexia from chemotherapy, 680
Hypersensitivity reactions from chemotherapy, 680
Hyperstat; see Diazoxide
Hypertension
  in child, 840
  portal, portacaval-splenorenal shunts for, 299-302
  pregnancy-induced, 697-701
  pulmonary, 212-214
  stepped care approach for treatment of, 80
Hypertensive crisis, 78-81
Hyperthyroidism, 315-318
Hypertrophy, prostatic, 501-502
Hyperventilation, neurogenic, central, 394
Hypervolemia, 50-51
Hypocalcemia, 42-43
Hypochromic microcytic anemia, 158-160
Hypoglossal nerve, 395
Hypoglycemia, 343-345
  comparison of, with diabetic ketoacidosis and hyperosmolar hyperglycemic nonketotic coma, 341
  as oncologic emergency, 637
Hypoglycemics, oral, 337
Hypokalemia, 38-41
Hypomagnesemia, 44-47
Hyponatremia, 44-45
Hypoparathyroidism, 318-320
Hypophysectomy, 349-351
Hypopituitarism, 329-330
Hypothermia, 438-439
Hypothyroidism, 312-315
Hypovolemia, 50-51
Hypovolemic shock, 105
  causes/etiologies of, 104
Hysterectomy
  abdominal, total, and bilateral salpingo-oophorectomy, 518-519
  radical, 616-617
H_2CO_3
  deficit of, 46-47
  excess of, 46-49

I

ICP; see Increased intracranial pressure
ICSH; see Interstitial cell-stimulating hormone
Idamycin, 658-659
Idarubicin HCl, 658-659
Identity, personality, disturbance of, 18
Idiopathic thrombocytopenic purpura with AIDS, 550
IDM; see Infant of diabetic mother
Ifex; see Ifosfamide
Ifosfamide, 652-653
  hazards associated with, 667
IL-2; see Interleukin-2
Ileal conduit, 470, 471
Ileal reservoir, 470, 471
  capacity of, method for increasing, 278
  construction of, at anus, 279-280
Ileoanal anastomosis, 279
Ileoanal reservoir, 279-282
Ileocecal reservoir, 470, 471
Ileostomy, 264, 283-285
  closure of, 281-282
  continent, 275-279
  temporary, 279-280
Ileum, anastomosis of, to anal reservoir, 281-282
Ileus, paralytic, 271-272
Ilizarov external fixator, 378
Image, body, disturbance in, 16-17
Imbalances
  acid-base, 46-50
  electrolyte, 38-46
  fluid, 50-51
Immune deficiency syndrome, acquired, 546-558
Immune system, 544-580
  assessment of, 544-546
  organization of, 545
Immunotherapy, adoptive, 689-690
Implant, penile, 506-508
Implantable cardioverter-defibrillator, automatic, 138-139
Implantable drug delivery system, Port-A-Cath, 56
  locations for placement of, 57
Implantation of placenta, low, 707
Implanted port, 56-57
Imuran; see Azathioprine
Inappropriate antidiuretic hormone, syndrome of, as oncologic emergency, 636
Incarcerated inguinal hernia, 802
Incentive spirometer, 238
Inclusion disease, cytomegalic, 754
Incomplete fracture, 359
Incontinence
  functional, 453-455
  reflex, 453, 457-459
  stress, 453, 455-457
  total, 453, 460-462
  urge, 453, 459-460
  urinary, 453-462
    female, surgery for, 464-466
Increased intracranial pressure, 439-440
Inderal; see Propranolol
Induction of labor, 718-720
Indwelling peritoneal catheter, 487
Indwelling urethral catheter management, 469-470
Infant
  care of, 763-766
  of diabetic mother, 744-745
  growth charts for, 764, 765

Infant—cont'd
    high-risk, family-centered care of, 761
    with hyperbilirubinemia, care of, 745-747
    large for gestational age, 742-743
    postmature, 743-744
    postterm, 743-744
    premature, 740
        care of, 740-741
    small for gestational age, 742
Infarction, myocardial
    acute, 85-88
    laboratory and diagnostic findings in, 83-84
    rehabilitation program after, 117-118
    syndrome following, 116
Infection
    in cancer patients, 641
    gallbladder, 287-288
    HIV, Centers for Disease Control classification of, 547
    neurological, 432-434
    opportunistic, involved in AIDS, 550
    potential for, 1-2
    TORCH, 753-755
    urinary tract, 451-453
Infectious hepatitis, 295
Infectious polyneuritis, acute, 429-432
Infective endocarditis, 91-95
Inflammatory disease
    of bowel, 265-267
    pelvic, 513-514
Inflatable penile prosthesis, 506, 507
Infusion, oxytocin, 718-720
Infusion devices, electronic, 58
Infusion pumps, 58
Infusion technique of tissue pressure monitoring, 384
Inguinal hernia, incarcerated, 802
Injection
    heparin, subcutaneous, 149-150
    insulin, sites for, 337
Injury
    burn, estimation of, 526
    potential for, 2
Insertion
    pacemaker, 134-138
    ventricular shunt, 805-806
Instillation of eye drops/ointments, 539
Insufficiency
    adrenocortical, 322-324
    arterial, chronic, 73-75
    placental, 698
Insulin, 310
    action of, 336
    injection sites for, 337
Insulin-dependent diabetes mellitus, 332, 333
Integumentary problems with chemotherapy, 680-682
Integumentary system, 521-531
    assessment of, 521-523
Interaction, social, impaired, 22-24
Interferons as biological response modifier, 689
Interleukin-2 as biological response modifier, 689-690
Intermittent gavage feeding, 760-761
Intermittent peritoneal dialysis, 486
Intermittent positive pressure breathing, 237-238
Intermittent positive pressure ventilator, 237
Internal arteriovenous fistula, 491
Internal fixation
    Harrington rod, for scoliosis, 363

Internal fixation—cont'd
    of hip, 368
Internal monitoring during labor, 722
Internal radiation therapy, 644-648
Interstitial cell-stimulating hormone, 310
Intestinal tube, naso-oral, care of, 282-283
Intestine, 265-287
    carcinoma of, 606-607
    inflammatory disease of, 265-267
    obstruction of, 269-271
    surgery on, 273-275
Intolerance, activity, potential, 8
Intoxication, alcohol, 434-437
Intracerebral hemorrhage, 402
Intracranial pressure
    increased, 439-440
    monitoring of, 440-441
Intraocular lens transplant, cataract removal with or without, 536
Intrauterine catheter, care of mother with, 722
Intrauterine growth retardation, 742
Intravascular coagulation, disseminated, 173-175
    as oncologic emergency, 634
Intravenous continuous drip narcotics, 58-59
Intraventricular method of intracranial pressure monitoring, 440
Intropin; see Dopamine
Intussusception, 802-803
Iodine, radioactive, 648, 649
IPD; see Intermittent peritoneal dialysis
IPPB; see Intermittent positive pressure breathing
Iridectomy, 536
Iridencleisis, 536
Iridotomy, laser, 538
Iron deficiency anemia, 158-160
Iron therapy, precautions with, 158
Irrigation, colostomy, 285-286
Ischemic cerebrovascular disruption, 402
Islets of Langerhans, 310
Isoetharine as bronchodilator, 203
Isoproterenol
    as bronchodilator, 203
    for child, 842
Isosorbide dinitrate, 89
Isuprel; see Isoproterenol
IV drip rates, regulation of, 53

J

Jejunal conduit, 470
Jejunoileal bypass, 257, 258
Jet nebulizers, 196
Joint, facet, rhizotomy of, 362
Joint arthroplasty, total, 370-374
Junctional biopsy, atrioventricular, 132
Junctional escape rhythms, 132
Junctional rhythms, atrioventricular, 132

K

Kaposi's sarcoma with AIDS, 550
Keller arthroplasty, 384
Ketoacidosis, diabetic, 340-342
    comparison of, with hyperosmolar hyperglycemic nonketotic coma
        and hypoglycemia, 341
Kidney
    cancer of, 585-586
    obstruction or failure of, as oncologic emergency, 639-640
    oncologic emergencies involving, 639-641
    polycystic disease of, 475-477

Kidney—cont'd
    problems with, from chemotherapy, 683-685
    transplant of, care of recipient of, 497-501
    transplanted, rejection of, classification of, 497
Kidney failure, 482-486
Klebsiella infection in cancer patient, 641
Klebsiella pneumoniae with AIDS, 550
Knee
    amputation above, 374-376
    amputation below, 374-376
    arthroplasty of, 370-374
    arthroscopic surgery of, 376-377
Knowledge deficit, 10-11
Kock continent ileal reservoir, 471
Kock's pouch, 275-279

L

Labor
    active, 714
    augmentation or induction of, 718-720
    Bishop scoring system for, 719
    care of diabetic mother during, 705-706
    dysfunctional patterns of, 719
    early, 714
    first stage of, care of mother in, 714-717
    monitoring during, 722
    preterm, 711-714
    second stage of, care of mother in, 717-718
    transitional, 714
Lamaze review sheet, 715-716
Laminectomy, 362
Langerhans, islets of, 310
Lanoxin; *see* Digoxin
Laparoscopic endoscopic laser cholecystectomy, 291-292
Large for gestational age, 742-743
Large intestine, carcinoma of, 606-607
Laryngectomy, 600-603
Laryngotracheobronchitis, 770-771, 776
Laser cholecystectomy, endoscopic laparoscopic, 291-292
Laser iridotomy, 538
Laser lithotripsy for urinary calculi, 480
Lasix; *see* Furosemide
Latch-on position, correct, 732
Lateral sclerosis, amyotrophic, 427-429
Leech therapy, 381
Leg, amputation of, 374-376
Lens
    contact, removal of, 538-539
    intraocular, transplant of, cataract removal with or without, 536
Lente insulin, 336
Lesions, motor neuron, upper and lower, clinical manifestations of, 413
Leukapheresis, 178
Leukemia, 592-593
    acute, 621-625
        in children, 815-818
    lymphocytic, acute, 621
    myelogenous, acute, 621
Leukeran; *see* Chlorambucil
Leukocyte concentrate, transfusion of, 181
    reactions to, 184
Leukoencephalopathy, multifocal, progressive, with AIDS, 550
Leukopenia from chemotherapy, 670-672
Leukoplakia, hairy, with AIDS, 550
Levine tube, 262
LH; *see* Luteinizing hormone

Lidocaine for child, 842
Ligation and stripping, vein, 72-73
Linear equivalents, 846
Linear fracture, 411
Linton tube, 248-249
Lip, cleft, repair of, 786-788
Liquid equivalent for medication, 845
Lithotripsy
    biliary, 290-291
    extracorporeal shock wave, 290
        for urinary calculi, 480
    laser, for urinary calculi, 480
    ultrasonic, percutaneous, for urinary calculi, 481
Liver, 293-302
    biopsy of, 302
    carcinoma of, 607-610
    surgery on, 298-299
Lobectomy, 227-229
Lomustine, 654-655
"Lou Gehrig's disease," 427
Low birth weight infant, 742
Low implantation of placenta, 707
Low-bacteria diet, 578
Lower motor neuron lesions, clinical manifestations of, 413
Lower urinary tract infections, 451
LSD, abuse of, 436
Lufyllin; *see* Dyphylline
Lumbar cord injuries, 413, 414
Lumbar puncture, 437-438
Luminal; *see* Phenobarbital
Lund and Browder chart for estimation of burn injury, 526
Lung
    cancer of, 582-583
    chronic obstructive disease of, 196-202
        diseases contributing to, 197
    edema of, 209-211
    embolism in, 211-212
    oncologic emergencies involving, 638-639
    rehabilitation, 204-205
    tuberculosis of, 214-216
Lupus erythematosus, systemic, 560-563
Luteinizing hormone, 310
Luteotrophic hormone, 310
Lymphadenectomy, vulvectomy with, 617
Lymphangiography, 630
Lymphatic system, 633
Lymphocytic leukemia, acute, 621
Lymphoma
    with AIDS, 550
    malignant, 632-634
Lymphotoxin as biological response modifier, 690
Lysergic acid diethylamide, abuse of, 436
Lysis syndrome, tumor, as oncologic emergency, 637-638

M

Macrocytic anemia, hyperchromic, 155-158
Magnesium
    deficit of, 44-47
    excess, 44-45
Male, genitourinary and reproductive system of, 449
Malignant lymphoma, 632-634
Manipulative behavior, 22
Mannitol for child, 842
Marrow, bone, transplantation of, 565-580
    schedule for, 566

Marshall-Marchetti-Krantz operation, 464
Mass equivalents for medications, 845
Mastectomy, radical, modified, 614-616
Matulane; see Procarbazine
Maxillomandibular fixation, 361-362
Mayo arthroplasty, 384
Measles, 772-773
  German, 772-773
Mechanical ventilation, continuous, 235-237
Mechlorethamine, 652-653
  hazards associated with, 667
Meconium aspiration syndrome, 756-757
Medications
  abuse of, 434-437
  chemotherapeutic, 652-665
    safety in handling, 667-669
  effect of, on nutritional status, 4
  emergency, pediatric, 842
  liquid equivalent for, 845
  mass equivalents for, 845
  for seizure disorders, 400
  to be taken with food, 4
  vasodilator, 88-91
    potential complications of, 88
  withdrawal from, by neonate, 750-752
Medium crackles, 189
Megacolon, aganglionic, 796-798
Melphalan, 654-655
Membrane(s)
  mucous, oral, altered, 4-5
  premature rupture of, 706-707
Meningiomas, brain, 409
Meningitis, 432
  in children, 810-811
Mephenytoin for seizure disorders, 400
Mercaptopurine, 656-657
Mesantoin; see Mephenytoin
Mescaline, abuse of, 436
Metabolic acidosis, 48-51
Metabolic alkalosis, 48-49
Metabolic oncologic emergencies, 636-638
Metaprel; see Metaproterenol
Metaproterenol as bronchodilator, 203
Metaramine; see Metaraminol
Metaraminol for child, 842
Methosuximide for seizure disorders, 400
Methotrexate, 656-657
  effect of, on nutritional status, 4
  hazards associated with, 668
Methyl CCNU; see Semustin
Methylprednisolone for child, 842
Metric conversions, 845
Mexate; see Methotrexate
Microsurgical dorsal root rhizotomy, 362
Mild anxiety, 13-14
Mild preeclampsia, 698, 699
Milk, breast, hand expression of, 733
Miller-Abbott tube, 282-283
Mineral oil, effect of, on nutritional status, 4
Mineralocorticoids, 310
Mithracin; see Plicamycin
Mitomycin C; see Mitomycin
Mitomycin, 660-661
  hazards associated with, 668
Mitral regurgitation, 95-96
  murmurs in, 97

Mitral stenosis, 95-96
  murmurs in, 97
Mobility, physical, impaired, 8-9
Mobitz type I, 130-131
Mobitz type II, 131
Moderate anxiety, 14
Modified radical mastectomy, 614-616
Mole, hydatidiform, 515
Monitor, fetal, mother with, care of, 722
Monitoring
  hemodynamic, 143, 146-147
  intracranial pressure, 440-441
  pressure, tissue, 383, 384
Monoclonal antibodies as biological response modifier, 691
Moro reflex, 738
Mother
  antepartum assessment of, 695-697
  in first stage of labor, care of, 714-717
  in second stage of labor, care of, 717-718
  diabetic
    during labor and delivery, care of, 705-706
    during last trimester of pregnancy, care of, 704-705
    infant of, 744-745
  with fetal monitor, care of, 722
Motor neuron lesions, upper and lower, clinical manifestations of, 413
Mould, radium therapy sealed in, care of patient receiving, 644-648
MTX; see Methotrexate
Mucositis from chemotherapy, 677-678
Mucous membrane, oral, altered, 4-5
Multifocal leukoencephalopathy, progressive, with AIDS, 550
Multifocal premature ventricular contractions, 127
Multilumen subclavian catheters, 54-55
Multiple myeloma, 625-628
Multiple sclerosis, 422-424
Mumps, 774-775
Murmurs, valvular heart disease, 97
Muscle tissue, tumors of, 595
Musculoskeletal assessment, 353-355
Musculoskeletal system, 353-390
  anatomy of, 354
Mustargen; see Mechlorethamine
Mutamycin; see Mitomycin
Myasthenia gravis, 424-426
Myasthenia gravis crisis, 426-427
Mycobacterium avium-intracellulare with AIDS, 550
Mycobacterium tuberculosis with AIDS, 550
Myelogenous leukemia, acute, 621
Myeloma, multiple, 625-628
Myelomeningocele, 806-810
Myelosuppression, 670-675
Myleran; see Busulfan
Myocardial infarction
  acute, 85-88
  laboratory and diagnostic findings in, 83-84
  rehabilitation program after, 117-118
  syndrome following, 116
Myomas of uterus, 518
Myringotomy with tube insertion, 541, 543
Mysoline; see Primidone
Myxedema, 312-315
Myxedema coma, 312

N

Naloxone for child, 842
Narcan; see Naloxone

Narcotics
  abuse of, 435
  commonly abused, 434
  intravenous continuous drip, 58-59
Nasal airway, 230-231
Nasogastric tubes, 262-263
Naso-oral intestinal tube, care of, 282-283
Nasopharyngeal airway, 230
Nausea from chemotherapy, 675-677
Nebulizers
  jet, 196
  ultrasonic, 196
NEC; see Necrotizing enterocolitis
Neck
  and head
    cancer of, 582
    positioning of, to prevent contractures from burns, 529
  radical dissection of, 600-603
Necrotizing enterocolitis, 752-753
Neglect, physical, in child, 838
Neomycin, effect of, on nutritional status, 4
Neonatal drug withdrawal, 750-752
Neonatal sepsis, 749-750
Neoplasia, 581-694
Neoplasms involved in AIDS, 550
Nephrectomy, 481, 493-497
Nephrolithotomy, 481
Nephrolithotripsy, 480
Nephrosis in children, 813-815
Nephrostomy, percutaneous, 480
Nephrotic syndrome in children, 813-815
Nephrotoxicity from chemotherapy, 683-684
Nerve stimulation, electrical, transcutaneous, 60-61
Nerve tissue, tumors of, 595
Nerves, cranial, functions of, 395
Nervous system
  anatomy of, 392
  central, surgical intervention of, 416-418
Neurogenic hyperventilation, central, 394
Neurological assessment, 391-396
Neurological dysfunction, patterns of respiration in, 394
Neurological infections, 432-434
Neurological patient, general rehabilitative care of, 442-444
Neurological procedures, diagnostic, 396
Neurological system, 391-446
Neuromas, acoustic, of brain, 409
Neurotoxicity from chemotherapy, 685-686
Newborn
  care of, 735-740
  with endotracheal tube, care of, 757
  stabilization of, at delivery, 737
  on ventilator, care of, 758
Nifedipine, 88, 91
Nipride; see Sodium nitroprusside
Nitrates, 88, 89-90
Nitrogen mustard, 652-653
  hazards associated with, 667
Nitroglycerin, 88, 89-90
Nitroprusside, 88-89
Nitrosoureas as chemotherapeutic agents, 654-655
Non-A, non-B hepatitis, 295
Noncommunicating hydrocephalus, 803
Noncyanotic congenital heart defects, 821-826
Non-insulin-dependent diabetes mellitus, 332, 333
Nonstress test, 722-723
Nonvolumetric infusion devices, 58

Norepinephrine, 310
Norisodrine; see Isoproterenol
NPH insulin, 336
NST; see Nonstress test
Nursing care, patient care planning and, guidelines for, 847-850
Nursing diagnoses
  general care and, 1-62
  standards of care related to, 1
Nutrition
  altered
    less than body requirements, 3-4
    potential for more than body requirements, 3
  for child, 841, 843
  enteral, 32-36
  parenteral, total, 36-37, 52-53
  venous, 37
Nutritional status, effect of drugs on, 4
Nutritional/metabolic functional health patterns, 3-6

O

Obesity, surgical intervention for, 257-262
Obstruction
  biliary, 287-288
  intestinal, 269-271
  kidney, as oncologic emergency, 639-640
Obstructive pulmonary disease, chronic, 196-202
  diseases contributing to, 197
Occipital lobe brain tumors, 409
Occult prolapse of umbilical cord, 710
Oculomotor nerve, 395
Ointment, eye, instillation of, 539
Olfactory nerve, 395
Oncologic emergencies, 634-641
  cardiovascular, 635-636
  hematological, 634
  metabolic, 636-638
  pulmonary, 638-639
  renal, 639-641
Oncology assessment, 593-600
Oncovin; see Vincristine sulfate
Open fracture, 359
Open-heart surgery, 108-114
  in child, 832-835
Operation, Marshall-Marchetti-Krantz, 464
Opiates, abuse of, 435
Opportunistic infections involved in AIDS, 550
Optic and auditory systems, 532-543
Optic nerve, 395
Optic system, assessment of, 532-533
Oral airway, 230
Oral contraceptives, effect of, on nutritional status, 4
Oral hypoglycemics, 337
Oral mucous membrane, altered, 4-5
Oral rehydration therapy, 802
Orchiectomy for testicular tumor, 613-614
Organic solvents, commonly abused, 434
Organs of endocrine system, 309
Oropharyngeal airway, 230
Orthopedic sepsis, 355-356
Osteomyelitis, acute, 355-356
Osteosarcoma, 611-612
Ostomy, 283
Ovarian cancer, 590-591
Oxtriphylline as bronchodilator, 203
Oxygen saturation in heart chambers and great vessels, 143
Oxygen therapy, 194-196

Oxytocin, 310
  infusion of, 718-720

P

Pacemaker, 134
  artificial, temporary, in child, 837-838
  external, temporary, 135
  insertion of, 134-138
  permanent, 136
    management of, 137
  temporary, management of, 137
  ventricular, 135
PACs; *see* Premature atrial contractions
Pain, 10
Painful respiration, 187
Palate, cleft, repair of, 788-789
Palpation of fundus of uterus after delivery, 725
Pancreas, 302-306
  carcinoma of, 610-611
  surgery on, 304-306
Pancreatectomy, 304
Pancreatitis, acute and chronic, 302-304
Pancreatoduodenectomy, 304
Panic, 15
PAP; *see* Pulmonary artery pressure
Paradione; *see* Paramethadione
Paraldehyde for child, 842
Paralytic ileus, 271-272
Paramethadione for seizure disorders, 400
Paraplatin; *see* Carboplatin
Paraplegia, 444-445
Parathyroid hormone, 311
Parathyroidectomy, 347
Parenteral nutrition, total, 36-37, 52-53
Parietal lobe brain tumors, 409
Parkinson's disease, 419-422
Partial nephrectomy, 493-497
Partial placenta previa, 707
Partial seizures, 399
Partial separation of placenta, 708
Partial-thickness burns, 525
Partitioning, stomach, 257
Passive motion device, continuous, 389
Patent ductus arteriosus, 821-822
Patient(s)
  aging, care of, 29-30
  auditory-impaired, 540-541
  dying, care of, 30-32
  position of, degrees of, 67
  with special equipment, care of, 53-61
  with special needs, care of, 27-53
  visually impaired, 533-535
Patient care planning and nursing care, guidelines for, 847-850
Patient-controlled analgesia, 59
PCA; *see* Patient-controlled analgesia
Pco$_2$
  decreased, 46-47
  elevated, 46-49
PCWP; *see* Pulmonary capillary wedge pressure
Pearson's attachment, Thomas' splint and, balanced suspension with, 388
Pectoriloquy, whispered, 190
Pediatrics, 763-843
Pelvic exenteration, 619-621
Pelvic inflammatory disease, 513-514
Pelvic traction, 387

Pelvis, cancer of, 585-586
Penicillin, effect of, on nutritional status, 4
Penile implant, 506-508
Penile prosthesis, inflatable, 506, 507
Peptic ulcer disease, 252-253
Percutaneous nephrostomy/nephrolithotripsy, 480
Percutaneous transluminal angioplasty, 140-141
Percutaneous ultrasonic lithotripsy for urinary calculi, 481
Percutaneous urinary stone dissolution, 480
Pereya procedure, 464
Perforated appendix, 794-796
Pericardiocentesis, 100
Pericarditis, 98-99
Perinatal/neonatal standards, 695-762
Perineal prostatectomy, 502
Peripheral vascular assessment, 68-70
Peripheral venous nutrition, 37
Peripherally inserted central catheter, 57-58
Peritoneal catheter, indwelling, 487
Peritoneal dialysis, 486-490
Peritonitis, 267-268
Permanent epidural catheter, 59-60
Permanent pacemaker, 136
  management of, 137
Permanent pacemaker mode, 136
Pernicious anemia, 155-158
Personality identity disturbance, 18
Pertussis, 772-773, 777-778
Pharyngitis from chemotherapy, 678
Phencyclidine, abuse of, 436
Phenobarbital
  for child, 842
  for seizure disorders, 400
Phenomenon
  coup-contracoup, 411
  Wenckebach, 130-131
Phenytoin for seizure disorders, 400
Pheochromocytoma, 328-329
Phlebitis, 70
Phlebothrombosis, 70
Phosphorus, radioactive, 648
Photocoagulation, retinal, 536
Phototherapy, 745
Physical mobility, impaired, 8-9
Physical neglect in child, 838
PID; *see* Pelvic inflammatory disease
PIH; *see* Pregnancy-induced hypertension
Pinpoint pupils, 393
Pitting edema, assessment of, 698
Pituitary adenomas, 409
Pituitary gland, 310
Placenta
  abnormal implantation of, 707
  effects of pregnancy-induced hypertension on, 698
  premature separation of, 708
Placenta previa, 707-708
Placental insufficiency, 698
Plasma, transfusion of, 181
  reactions to, 185
Plasmapheresis, 178
Platelet concentrate, transfusion of, 182
Plateletpheresis, 178
Platelets, transfusion of, reactions to, 185
Platinol; *see* Cisplatin
Pleural effusion, 221-222
  as oncologic emergency, 638-639

Pleural friction rub, 189
Plicamycin, 660-661
    hazards associated with, 668
Pneumocystis carinii infection in cancer patient, 641
Pneumocystis carinii pneumonitis with AIDS, 550
Pneumonectomy, 227-229
Pneumonia, 205-209, 779-780
    bacterial
        causes of, 206
        findings in, 207
    nonbacterial, causes of, 206
    Pneumocystis carinii, with AIDS, 550
    viral, findings in, 207
Pneumonitis, 205-209
    bacterial and nonbacterial causes of, 206
Pneumothorax, 216-219
    assessment/finding in, 216
    spontaneous, 217
    tension, 216, 217
    traumatic, 217
Podophyllotoxins as chemotherapeutic agents, 658-659
    hazards associated with, 668
Poliomyelitis, 774-775
Polycystic kidney disease, 475-477
Polycythemia, 169-171
    relative, 169
    secondary, 169
Polycythemia vera, 169
Polymorphous ventricular tachycardia, 129
Polyneuritis, infectious, acute, 429-432
Polyradiculitis, 429-432
Port, implanted, 56-57
Port-A-Cath implanatable drug delivery system, 56
    locations for placement of, 57
Portacaval shunt, 299
Portacaval-splenorenal shunts for portal hypertension, 299-302
Portal cirrhosis, 293-295
Portal hypertension, portacaval-splenorenal shunts for, 299-302
Position(s)
    body, to maintain correct alignment, 406
    for breast-feeding after cesarean delivery, 731
    latch-on, correct, 732
    patient, degrees of, 67
    to prevent contractures from burns, 529
Positive pressure breathing, intermittent, 237-238
Positive-pressure ventilator
    intermittent, 237
    pressure-limited, 236
    volume-cycled, 236-237
Post-cardiac injury syndrome, 116
Postcardiotomy syndrome, 116
Posterior pelvic exenteration, 619
Posthyperventilation apnea, 394
Postmature infant, 743-744
Postmyocardial infarction syndrome, 116
Postnecrotic cirrhosis, 293-295
Postpartum care, 724-728
Postpartum hemorrhage, 734-735
Postterm infant, 743-744
Potassium
    deficit of, 38-41
    excess, 38-39
Pouch, Kock's, 275-279
PR interval, 121
Prazosin, 88, 90
Preeclampsia, 697-701

Preexcitation, ventricular, 132-133
Pregnancy
    care of diabetic mother during last trimester of, 704-705
    tubal, 516
        ruptured, 517
        and salpingectomy, 516-518
Pregnancy-induced hypertension, 697-701
Premature atrial beats, 123
Premature atrial contractions, 123-124
    nonconducted, 124
Premature infant, 740
    care of, 740-741
Premature rupture of membranes, 706-707
Premature separation of placenta, 708
Premature ventricular contractions, 126-127
    multifocal, 127
Preoperative care/teaching, general, 27-28
Preschool-age child, care of, 766-767
Pressure monitoring, tissue, 383, 384
Pressure ulcer, 523-525
Pressure wave forms, 145
    problems associated with, 146
Pressure
    blood
        of child, 840
        high, stepped care approach for treatment of, 80
    intracranial
        increased, 439-440
        monitoring of, 440-441
    pulmonary artery, 143
    pulmonary capillary wedge, 143
Pressure-limited positive-pressure ventilator, 236
Preterm labor, 711-714
Primary adrenocortical insufficiency, 322
Primary aldosteronism, 326-328
Primatene; *see* Epinephrine
Primidone for seizure disorders, 400
Prinzmetal's angina, 81
    laboratory and diagnostic findings in, 83-84
Procainamide for child, 842
Procarbazine, 664-665
Progesterone, 311
Progressive multifocal leukoencephalopathy with AIDS, 550
Progressive systemic sclerosis, 356-358
Prolactin, 310
Prolapsed umbilical cord, 709-711
PROM; *see* Premature rupture of membranes
Prone position, 406
Pronestyl; *see* Procainamide
Propranolol for child, 842
Prostate
    cancer of, 587
    transurethral resection of, 502
Prostatectomy, 502-506
    perineal, 502
    retropubic, 502
        radical, 502, 503
    suprapubic, 502
Prostatic hypertrophy, 501-502
Prostatitis, 451
Prosthesis, penile, inflatable, 506, 507
Protamine zinc insulin, 336
Protozoal infections involved in AIDS, 550
Proventil; *see* Albuterol
Pseudomonas infection in cancer patient, 641
PTCA; *see* Percutaneous transluminal angioplasty

PTH; *see* Parathyroid hormone
Ptosis, 393
Pull-through procedure, abdominoperineal, 798-800
Pulmonary artery banding, 829-830
Pulmonary artery pressure, 143
Pulmonary capillary wedge pressure, 143
Pulmonary catheter, triple-lumen balloon-tipped, 145
Pulmonary edema, 209-211
Pulmonary embolism, 211-212
Pulmonary hypertension, 212-214
Pulmonary rehabilitation, 204-205
Pulmonary toxicity of chemotherapy, 683
Pulmonary tuberculosis, 214-216
Pulmonic stenosis in child, 825-826
Pumps, infusion, 58
Puncture
    finger, sites for, for glucose monitoring, 338
    lumbar, 437-438
Pupils, response of, variations in, 393
Purinethol; *see* Mercaptopurine
Purpura, thrombocytopenic, idiopathic, with AIDS, 550
PVCs; *see* Premature ventricular contractions
Pyelolithotomy, 481
Pyelonephritis, 451
Pyloric stenosis, 793-794
Pyogenic arthritis, acute, 355-356
Pyridoxine for child, 842

Q
QRS interval, 121
QT interval, 121
Quadriplegia, 445-446

R
Radiation precaution tags, 647
Radical hysterectomy, 616-617
Radical mastectomy, modified, 614-616
Radical neck dissection, 600-603
Radical retropubic prostatectomy, 502, 503
Radioactive iodine, 648, 649
Radioactive phosphorus, 648
Radioactive therapy, unsealed, 648-649
Radiotherapy for cancer, 642-644
Radium therapy sealed in mould, afterloader, colpostat, or Ernst applicator, care of patient receiving, 644-648
Rales, 189
Range of motion
    of affected shoulder and elbow after stroke, 406
    of affected wrist and hand after stroke, 407
Reactions, hypersensitivity, from chemotherapy, 680
Recovery room care, 28-29
Rectal mucositis from chemotherapy, 678
Rectal surgery, 286-287
Red blood cells, transfusion of, reactions to, 183, 184
Reflex(es), 394
    Moro, 738
    "startle," 738
    stepping, 739
    tonic neck, 738
Reflex incontinence, 453, 457-459
Regional enteritis, 265-267
Regular insulin, 336
Regurgitation
    aortic, 95-96
        murmurs in, 97

Regurgitation—cont'd
    mitral, 95-96
        murmurs in, 97
Rehabilitation
    cardiac, 116-120
    pulmonary, 204-205
Rehabilitative care, general, of neurological patient, 442-444
Rehydration therapy, oral, 802
Rejection of transplanted kidney, classification of, 497
Relative polycythemia, 169
Renal failure, 482-486
Repair
    cleft lip, 786-788
    cleft palate, 788-789
Replantation, digital, 379-382
Reproductive system
    female, 449, 510-520
        anatomy of, 510
        assessment of, 510-513
    male, 449
Resection of prostate, transurethral, 502
Reserpine for child, 842
Reservoir
    ileal, 470, 471
    ileocecal, 470, 471
Respiration
    apneustic, 394
    ataxic, 187
    Biot's, 187, 394
    Cheyne-Stokes, 187, 394
    in child, 841
    normal, 187
    painful, 187
    patterns of, 187
        in neurological dysfunction, 394
    sighing, 187
Respiratory acidosis, 46-49
Respiratory alkalosis, 46-47
Respiratory assessment, 186-191
Respiratory distress syndrome, 755-756
    adult, 225-227
Respiratory failure, 223-225
Respiratory findings, normal, 188
Respiratory system, 186-239
    disorders of, in children, 770-786
Response, pupil, variations in, 393
Retardation, intrauterine growth, 742
Retention, urinary, acute, 462-464
Retina, photocoagulation of, 536
Retinal cryopexy, 536, 538
Retraining, breathing, techniques for, 199
Retropubic prostatectomy, 502
    radical, 502, 503
Rheumatoid arthritis, 558-560
Rhizotomy
    dorsal root, microsurgical, 362
    facet joint, 362
Rhonchi, 189
Rhythm(s)
    of atrial origin, 123-126
    ECG, 120-124, 133-134
    escape, junctional, 132
    junctional, atrioventricular, 132
    of sinus origin, 120-123
    of ventricular origin, 126-129
Role performance, altered, 19

Role/relationship functional health pattern, 18-24
Roll, contracture, 529
Roseola infantum, 772-773
Rub, friction, pleural, 189
Rubella, 754, 772-773
  congenital, 772-773
Rubeola, 772-773
Rubidomycin; *see* Daunorubicin
Rule of nines, 526
Rupture, premature, of membranes, 706-707
Ruptured appendix, 794-796

S

Safe-sex guidelines, 556
Safety in handling cancer chemotherapy agents, 667-669
Salem sump tube, 262
Salmonellosis with AIDS, 550
Salpingectomy, tubal pregnancy and, 516-518
Salpingo-oophorectomy, bilateral, total abdominal hysterectomy and,
     518-519
Sarcoidosis, 563-565
Sarcoma, Kaposi's, with AIDS, 550
Saturation, oxygen, in heart chambers and great vessels, 143
Scarlatina, 774-775
Scarlet fever, 774-775
School-age child, care of, 767-770
Scleral buckling, 536, 538
Scleroderma, 356-358
Sclerosis
  disseminated, 422-424
  lateral, amyotrophic, 427-429
  multiple, 422-424
  systemic, progressive, 356-358
Sclerotomy, 536
Scoliosis, Harrington rod internal fixation for, 363
Secondary adrenocortical insufficiency, 322
Secondary polycythemia, 169
Second-degree AV block, 130
Secretions, aspiration of, 193-194
Seizure disorders, 399-402
  classification of, generally recognized, 399
  drugs used for, 400
  generalized, 399
  partial, 399
Self-esteem disturbance, 17-18
Self-examination, breast, 588, 589
Self-perception/self-concept functional health pattern, 13-18
Semilente insulin, 336
Semustin, 654-655
Sengstaken-Blakemore tube, 248-249
Sensory abnormality, common patterns of, 414
Sepsis
  neonatal, 749-750
  as oncologic emergency, 640-641
  orthopedic, 355-356
Septal defect
  atrial, in child, 822-823
  ventricular, in child, 823-824
Septic shock as oncologic emergency, 640-641
Septostomy, balloon, in child, 829
Serpasil; *see* Reserpine
Serum albumin, normal, transfusion of, 182
  reactions to, 185
Serum alcohol levels, effects of, 435
Serum hepatitis, 295
Severe anxiety, 14-15

Severe preeclampsia, 698, 699-700
Sexual abuse of child, 838
Sexual practices
  safe, 556
  unsafe, 557
Shock, 105-108
  cardiogenic, 105
    causes/etiologies of, 104
  "cold," 105
  hypovolemic, 105
    causes/etiologies of, 104
  septic, as oncologic emergency, 640-641
  vasogenic, 105
    causes/etiologies of, 104
  "warm," 105
Shock and denial stage of dying, 31
Shock syndrome
  causes/etiologies of, 104
  signs of, 105
  toxic, 514-515
Shock wave lithotripsy, extracorporeal, 290
  for urinary calculi, 480
Short bowel syndrome, 268-269
Shoulder
  arthroplasty of, 370-374
  range of motion of, after stroke, 406
Shunt
  Blalock-Taussig, 829
  portacaval, 299
  portacaval-splenorenal, for portal hypertension, 299-302
  splenorenal, 299
  ventricular, insertion of, 805-806
  ventriculoatrial, 805
SIADH; *see* Syndrome of inappropriate antidiuretic hormone
Sibilant wheeze, 189
Sickle cell anemia, 162-164
Sickle cell crisis, 162-164
Side arm traction, 387
Side-lying position, 406
Sighing respiration, 187
Sigmoid colostomy, 264
Silastic atrial catheter, 55-56
Simple fracture, 359
Sinus arrest, 123
Sinus bradycardia, 120, 122
Sinus dysrhythmia, 122-123
Sinus rhythms, 120-123
  normal, 120, 121
Sinus tachycardia, 122
Skeletal traction, 386
Skin
  cancer of, 581-582
  integrity of, impaired, potential, 5
  structures of, 522
Skin graft, skinning vulvectomy with, 617
Skin traction, 386
Skinning vulvectomy with skin graft, 617
Skull tongs and halo traction, 441-442
SLE; *see* Systemic lupus erythematosus
Sleep pattern disturbance, 9-10
Sleep/rest functional health pattern, 9-10
Small for date infant, 742
Small for gestational age, 742
Small intestine, carcinoma of, 606-607
Soave procedure, 798
Social interaction, impaired, 22-24

Sodium
  deficit of, 44-45
  excess, 42-43
Sodium bicarbonate for child, 842
Sodium diphenylhydantoin for seizure disorders, 400
Sodium nitroprusside, 88-89
Solu-Cortef; *see* Hydrocortisone sodium succinate
Solu-Medrol; *see* Methylprednisolone
Solvents, organic, commonly abused, 434
Somatotropin, 310
Sonorous wheeze, 189
Sounds, breath and voice, 189-190
Sphincter, urinary, artificial, 466-469
Spinal column, anatomy of, 393
Spinal cord
  compression of, as oncologic emergency, 638
  injuries of, 413-416
  lesions of, sites of, and corresponding sensory loss, 414
Spinal fusion, 362
Spinal tap, 437-438
Spine
  cervical, fracture or dislocation of, 365-367
  surgery on, 362-365
Spiral electrode, care of mother with, 722
Spiritual distress, 26-27
Spirometer, incentive, 238
Splenectomy, 175-177
Splenorenal shunt, 299
Splint, Thomas', and Pearson's attachment, balanced suspension
      with, 388
Spondylitis, ankylosing, 367-368
Spontaneous pneumothorax, 217
ST-T segment changes, 85, 86
Stable angina pectoris, 81
  laboratory and diagnostic findings in, 83-84
Standards of care related to nursing diagnoses, 1
Stapedectomy, 541, 543
Staphylococcus infection in cancer patient, 641
"Startle" reflex, 738
Stenosis
  aortic
    in child, 825
    murmurs in, 97
  mitral, 95-96
    murmurs in, 97
  pulmonic, in child, 825-826
  pyloric, 793-794
Stepping reflex, 739
Stimulant drugs
  abuse of, 436
  commonly abused, 434
Stimulation, nerve, electrical, transcutaneous, 60-61
Stomach, 249-264
  bleeding of, 253-254
  cancer of, 583-584
  carcinoma of, 605-606
  endoscopy of, 247-248
  partitioning of, 257
  peptic ulcer disease of, 252-253
  surgery on, 254-256
  ulcer of, 252
Stomatitis from chemotherapy, 677-678
Stone basket and ureteroscopy with ultrasonic fragmentation for uri-
      nary calculi, 480
Streptozocin, 662-663
Stress incontinence, 453, 455-457

Stress test, contraction, 723-724
Stricture, esophageal, 243-244
Stripping, vein ligation and, 72-73
Stroke, 404-408
Stryker frame, 442
Subarachnoid hemorrhage, 402
Subarachnoid method of intracranial pressure monitoring, 440
Subarachnoid precautions, 403
Subclavian catheters, multilumen, 54-55
Subcutaneous heparin injection, 149-150
Subdural hematoma, 411
Substance abuse, 434-437
Subtotal pancreatectomy, 304
Subtotal thyroidectomy, 345
Suicide, potential for, 20-21
Sump tube, Salem, 262
Superficial burns, 525
Superficial reflexes, 394
Superior vena cava syndrome as oncologic emergency, 635
Supine position, 406
Suprapubic prostatectomy, 502
Supraventricular tachycardia, 125-126
Surgery
  biliary, 288-290
  cancer, 641-642
  cardiac, 108-114
  closed-heart, in child, 830-832
  ear, 541-543
  esophageal, 246-247
  eye, 536-538
  for female urinary incontinence, 464-466
  gastric, 254-256
  heart, congenital, 828-835
  hepatic, 298-299
  hip, 368-370
  intestinal, 273-275
  of knee, arthroscopic, 376-377
  for obesity, 257-262
  open-heart, 108-114
    in child, 832-835
  pancreatic, 304-306
  rectal, 286-287
  spinal, 362-365
  for urinary calculi, 480-482
Surgical intervention of central nervous system, 416-418
Surgical stone extraction, 481
Suspension, balanced, with Thomas' splint and Pearson's attachment,
      388
SVCS; *see* Superior vena cava syndrome
SVT; *see* Supraventricular tachycardia
Swan-Ganz catheter, 144
Swenson procedure, 798
Symptomatic care in chemotherapy, 670-687
Syndrome
  acquired immune deficiency, 546-558
  adult respiratory distress, 225-227
  compartment, 382, 384
  Cushing's, 324-326
  Dressler's, 116
  dumping, 256-257
  fetal alcohol, 750
  Guillain-Barrè, 429-432
  of inappropriate antidiuretic hormone as oncologic emergency, 636
  meconium aspiration, 756-757
  nephrotic, in children, 813-815
  post-cardiac injury, 116

Syndrome—cont'd
 postcardiotomy infarction, 116
 postmyocardial infarction, 116
 respiratory distress, 755-756
 shock
  causes/etiologies of, 104
  signs of, 105
 short bowel, 268-269
 toxic shock, 514-515
 tumor lysis, as oncologic emergency, 637-638
 vena cava, superior, as oncologic emergency, 635
 Wolff-Parkinson-White, 132-133
Systemic lupus erythematosus, 560-563
Systemic sclerosis, progressive, 356-358

T

T tube, 292
 management of, 292
T₃, 311
T₄, 311
Tachycardia
 sinus, 122
 supraventricular, 125-126
 ventricular, 127-128
  polymorphous, 129
Tamponade, cardiac, 100-101
 as oncologic emergency, 635-636
Tap, spinal, 437-438
Teaching, preoperative, general, 27-28
Tegretol; see Carbamazepine
Temperature, body
 altered, potential, 6
 of child, 840
Temporal lobe brain tumors, 409
Temporary artificial pacemaker in child, 837-838
Temporary external pacemaker, 135
Temporary ileostomy, 279-280
Temporary pacemaker, management of, 137
Teniposide; see VM-26
TENS; see Transcutaneous electrical nerve stimulation
Tension, carbon dioxide
 decreased, 46-47
 elevated, 46-49
Tension pneumothorax, 216, 217
 assessment/finding in, 216
Terbutaline as bronchodilator, 203
Test
 nonstress, 722-723
 stress, contraction, 723-724
Testicular cancer, 586-587
 orchiectomy for, 613-614
Testosterone, 311
Tetanus, 774-775
Tetracycline, effect of, on nutritional status, 4
Tetralogy of Fallot in child, 826-827
Theolair; see Theophylline
Theophylline as bronchodilator, 203
Therapeutic bronchoscopy, 191-192
Therapy
 anticoagulant, 148-150
 apheresis, 177-179
 cancer, 641-693
 digitalis, pediatric, 836-837
 humidity and aerosol, 196
 iron, precautions with, 158

Therapy—cont'd
 leech, 381
 oxygen, 194-196
 radioactive, unsealed, 648-649
 radium, sealed in mould, afterloader, colpostat, or Ernst applicator, care of patient receiving, 644-648
 rehydration, oral, 802
 thrombolytic, 142-143
Thiazides, effect of, on nutritional status, 4
Thioguanine, 656-657
Thio-tepa, 654-655
Third-degree AV block, 131-132
Thomas' splint and Pearson's attachment, balanced suspension with, 388
Thoracentesis, 192-193
Thoracic cord injuries, 413, 414
Thoracic empyema, 219-220
Thoracotomy, 227-229
Thought processes, altered, 11-12
Thrive, failure to, 818-821
Thrombocytopenia, 171-173
 from chemotherapy, 672-675
Thrombocytopenic purpura, idiopathic, with AIDS, 550
Thromboembolism, 70
Thrombolytic therapy, 142-143
Thrombophlebitis, 70
Thrombosis, venous, 70-72
Thumb, replacement of, 379-382
Thymosin fraction V as biological response modifier, 689
Thyroid crisis, 315-318
Thyroid gland, 311
Thyroid storm, 315-318
Thyroidectomy, 345-347
Thyroid-stimulating hormone, 310
Thyrotoxic crisis, 315-318
Thyroxine, 311
Tissue pressure monitoring, 383, 384
TNM classification, 594
Tocotransducer, care of mother with, 722
Toddlers, care of, 766
Tolazamide for diabetes, 337
Tolbutamide for diabetes, 337
Tongs, skull, and halo traction, 441-442
Tonic neck reflex, 738
TORCH infections, 753-755
Torsades de pointes, 129
Total abdominal hysterectomy and bilateral salpingo-oophorectomy, 518-519
Total ankle arthroplasty, 371
Total hip arthroplasty, 371
Total incontinence, 453, 460-462
Total joint arthroplasty, 370-374
Total knee arthroplasty, 371
Total nephrectomy, 493-497
Total pancreatectomy, 304
Total parenteral nutrition, 36-37, 52-53
Total pelvic exenteration, 619
Total placenta previa, 707
Total spinal cord lesion, 414
Total wrist arthroplasty, 371
Toxic shock syndrome, 514-515
Toxoplasma gondii infection in cancer patient, 641
Toxoplasmosis, 754
 with AIDS, 550
TPN; see Total parenteral nutrition
Trabeculectomy, 536, 538

Tracheoesophageal fistula, 789-791
  repair of, 791-793
Tracheostomy, 232-234
Traction
  Bryant's, 387, 388
  cervical, 387, 388
  halo, 387
    skull tongs and, 441-442
  of humerus, 388
  management of, 385, 386-387
  pelvic, 387
  side arm, 387
  skeletal, 386
  skin, 386
Training, bowel, 441
Transcutaneous electrical nerve stimulation, 60-61
Transducer, ultrasound, care of mother with, 722
Transfusion of blood, 179-185
  and blood components, reactions to, 183-185
  exchange, 747-748
Transhepatic biliary decompression catheter management, 292-293
Transitional labor, 714
Transluminal angioplasty, percutaneous, 140-141
Transplant
  corneal, 536, 537
  intraocular lens, cataract removal with or without, 536
  renal, care of recipient of, 497-501
Transplantation
  bone marrow, 565-580
    schedule for, 566
  cardiac, 115-116
Transplanted kidney, rejection of, classification of, 497
Transposition of great vessels in child, 827-828
Transurethral resection of prostate, 502
Transverse colostomy, 264
Trauma, craniocerebral, 411-413
Traumatic pneumothorax, 217
Tridione; *see* Trimethadione
Triethylene-thiophosphoramide, 654-655
Trigeminal nerve, 395
Triiodothyronine, 311
Trimethadione for seizure disorders, 400
Triple-lumen balloon-tipped pulmonary catheter, 145
Trochlear nerve, 395
TSH; *see* Thyroid-stimulating hormone
TSS; *see* Toxic shock syndrome
Tubal pregnancy, 516
  ruptured, 517
  and salpingectomy, 516-518
Tube(s)
  Cantor, 282-283
  chest, 229-230
    removal of, 229-230
  endotracheal, 231-232
    newborn with, care of, 757
  gastrostomy, feeding by, 792
  insertion of, myringotomy with, 541, 543
  intestinal, naso-oral, care of, 282-283
  Levine, 262
  Linton, 248-249
  Miller-Abbott, 282-283
  nasogastric, 262-263
  Salem sump, 262
  Sengstaken-Blakemore, 248-249
  T, 292
    management of, 292

Tuberculosis, pulmonary, 214-216
Tumor(s)
  classification of, 595
  testicular, orchiectomy for, 613-614
Tumor cell vaccines as biological response modifier, 691
Tumor lysis syndrome as oncologic emergency, 637-638
Tumor necrosis factor as biological response modifier, 692-693
TURP; *see* Transurethral resection of prostate
24 hour clock system, 846
Tympanoplasty, 541, 543

U
Ulcer
  duodenal, 252
  peptic, 252-253
  pressure, 523-525
  stomach, 252
Ulcerative colitis, 265-267
Ultralente insulin, 336
Ultrasonic fragmentation, stone basket and ureteroscopy with, for urinary calculi, 480
Ultrasonic lithotripsy, percutaneous, for urinary calculi, 481
Ultrasonic nebulizers, 196
Ultrasound transducer, care of mother with, 722
Umbilical catheterization, 748-749
Umbilical cord, prolapsed, 709-711
Unsealed radioactive therapy, 648-649
Unstable angina pectoris, 81
  laboratory and diagnostic findings in, 83-84
Upper motor neuron lesions, clinical manifestations of, 413
Upper urinary tract infection, 451
Urea for child, 842
Ureter, cancer of, 585-586
Ureteroenterocutaneous diversion, 470
Ureterolithotomy, 481
Ureteroscopy, stone basket and, with ultrasonic fragmentation for urinary calculi, 480
Ureterostomy, cutaneous, 470, 471
Urethra, cancer of, 585-586
Urethral catheter, indwelling, management of, 469-470
Urethritis, 451
Urge incontinence, 453, 459-460
Urinary calculi, 479-482
Urinary diversion, 470-475
  continent, 470
Urinary elimination, altered patterns of, 7-8
Urinary incontinence, 453-462
  female, surgery for, 464-466
Urinary retention, acute, 462-464
Urinary sphincter, artificial, 466-469
Urinary stone, surgical extraction of, 481
Urinary tract infection, 451-453
Urolithiasis, 479-482
Uterus
  cancer, 591-592
  fundus of, palpating, after delivery, 725
  myomas of, 518
UTI; *see* Urinary tract infection

V
Vaccines, tumor cell, as biological response modifier, 691
Vaginal cancer, 590
Vaginal mucositis from chemotherapy, 678
Vagus nerve, 395
Valium; *see* Diazepam
Valproic acid for seizure disorders, 400

Value/belief functional health pattern, 26-27
Valves, cardiac, location of, 66
Valvular disorders, common, 95
Valvular heart disease, 95-98
  murmurs in, 97
Vancomycin for endocarditis prophylaxis, 93
Vaponefrin; see Epinephrine
Variable pressure limit volumetric infusion pumps, 58
Variant angina, 81
  laboratory and diagnostic findings in, 83-84
Varicella, 772-773
Varicella zoster infection in cancer patient, 641
Varices, esophageal, bleeding, 244-246
Vascular assessment, peripheral, 68-70
Vasodilator drugs, 88-91
  potential complications of, 88
Vasogenic shock, 105
  causes/etiologies of, 104
Vein ligation and stripping, 72-73
Velban; see Vinblastine sulfate
Vena cava syndrome, superior, as oncologic emergency, 635
Venous nutrition, 37
Venous system, 64
Venous thrombosis, 70-72
Ventilation, mechanical, continuous, 235-237
Ventilator
  intermittent positive pressure, 237
  newborn on, care of, 758
  pressure-limited positive-pressure, 236
  volume-cycled positive-pressure, 236-237
Ventolin; see Albuterol
Ventricular contractions, premature, 126-127
  multifocal, 127
Ventricular fibrillation, 128-129
Ventricular origin, rhythms of, 126-129
Ventricular pacemaker, 135
Ventricular preexcitation, 132-133
Ventricular septal defect in child, 823-824
Ventricular shunt insertion, 805-806
Ventricular tachycardia, 127-128
  polymorphous, 129
Ventriculoatrial shunt, 805
Ventriculostomy, 440
Vesicular breath sound, 189
Vessels, great
  oxygen saturation in, 143
  transposition of, in child, 827-828
Vinblastine sulfate, 656-659
  hazards associated with, 668
Vinca alkaloids as chemotherapeutic agents, 656-659
  hazards associated with, 668
Vincristine sulfate, 658-659
  hazards associated with, 668
Vindesine, 658-659
  hazards associated with, 668

Violence, potential for, 19-22
  directed at others, 21-22
  self-directed, 20-21
Viral encephalitis, 432
Viral hepatitis, 295-298
Viral pneumonia, findings in, 207
Virus
  herpes simplex, 754-755
  HIV, mechanism of action of, 548
  involved in AIDS, 550
Visually impaired patient, 533-535
Vital signs in child, 840-841
VM-26, 658-659
  hazards associated with, 668
Voice sounds, 189-190
Volume-cycled positive-pressure ventilator, 236-237
Volumetric infusion controllers, 58
Volumetric infusion devices, 58
Volumetric infusion pumps, 58
Vomiting from chemotherapy, 675-677
VP-16; see Etoposide
VSD; see Ventricular septal defect
Vulvectomy, 617-619

W

Warfarin, 148-149
Warm shock, 105
Wave forms, pressure, 145
  problems associated with, 146
Weight and height tables, 3
Wenckebach phenomenon, 130-131
Wheezes, 189
Whipple procedure, 304
Whispered pectoriloquy, 190
Whiteside technique of tissue pressure monitoring, 383, 384
Whole blood
  for transfusion, 181
  transfusion of, reactions to, 183-184, 185
Whooping cough, 772-773, 777-778
Withdrawal, drug, neonatal, 750-752
Withdrawn behavior, 23-24
Wolff-Parkinson-White syndrome, 132-133
Wrist
  arthroplasty of, 370-374
  range of motion of, after stroke, 407

X

Xanthine derivatives as bronchodilator, 203
Xerostomia with AIDS, 550
Xylocaine; see Lidocaine

Z

Zanosar; see Streptozocin
Zarontin; see Methosuximide

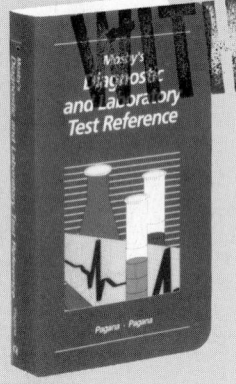
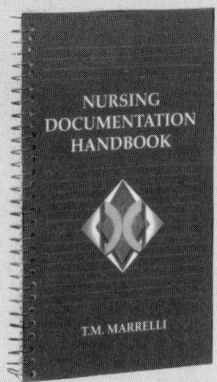
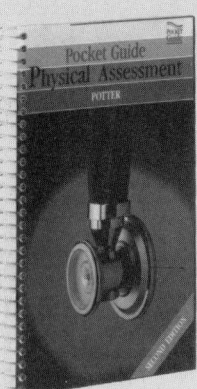
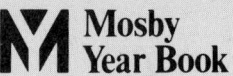